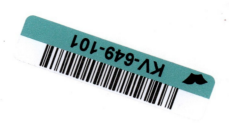

Synopsis of
GYNECOLOGIC ONCOLOGY

Synopsis of GYNECOLOGIC ONCOLOGY

Fifth Edition

C. PAUL MORROW, MD
Professor and Director, Division of Gynecologic Oncology
Department of Obstetrics and Gynecology
University of Southern California School of Medicine
Los Angeles, California

JOHN P. CURTIN, MD
Associate Attending Surgeon, Gynecology Service
Department of Surgery
Memorial Sloan-Kettering Cancer Center
Associate Professor
Department of Obstetrics and Gynecology
Cornell University Medical College
New York, New York

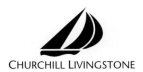

CHURCHILL LIVINGSTONE

New York, Edinburgh, London, Madrid, Melbourne, San Francisco, Tokyo

CHURCHILL LIVINGSTONE
A Division of Harcourt Brace & Company

The Curtis Center
Independence Square West
Philadelphia, Pennsylvania 19106

Library of Congress Cataloging-in-Publication Data

Morrow, C. Paul
    Synopsis of gynecologic oncology / C. Paul Morrow, John P. Curtin;
with contributions by John A. Blessing . . . [et al.]. — 5th ed.
        p.   cm.
    Includes bibliographical references and index.
    ISBN 0-443-07509-3
    1. Generative organs, Female–Cancer.   I. Curtin, John P.
II. Title.
    [DNLM: 1. Genital Neoplasms, Female.   WP 145 M883s   1998]
RC280.G5M67   1998
616.99'265–dc21
DNLM/DLC   98–21396

SYNOPSIS OF GYNECOLOGIC ONCOLOGY   ISBN   0-443-07509-3

Printed in the United States of America.

Last digit is the print number: 9   8   7   6   5   4   3   2   1

To all women who have suffered from cancer

Contributors

John A. Blessing, PhD

Assistant Research Professor, State University of New York at Buffalo; Director of Statistics, Gynecologic Oncology Group, Roswell Park Cancer Institute, Buffalo, New York

Principles of Statistics

Jeff Boyd, PhD

Director, Gynecology and Breast Research Laboratory, Department of Surgery, Memorial Sloan-Kettering Cancer Center; Associate Attending Biologist, Departments of Surgery and Human Genetics, Memorial Sloan-Kettering Cancer Center, New York, New York

Molecular Genetics of Gynecologic Cancers

John E. Byfield, MD, PhD

Medical Director, Radiation Therapy Associates Medical Group, Bakersfield, California; Formerly, Professor and Chief, Division of Radiation Oncology, Department of Radiology, University of California, San Diego, School of Medicine, La Jolla, California

Principles of Radiation Therapy

Augustin A. Garcia, MD

Assistant Professor of Medicine, University of Southern California/Norris Cancer Center, Division of Medical Oncology, Los Angeles, California

Principles of Chemotherapy

Cheryl C. Gurin, MD

Gynecology Service, Department of Surgery, Memorial Sloan-Kettering Cancer Center, New York, New York

Principles of Immunology and Immunotherapy

William H. Hindle, MD

Professor, Clinical Obstetrics and Gynecology, University of Southern California School of Medicine; Director, Breast Diagnostic Center, Women's and Children's Hospital, LAC/USC Medical Center, Los Angeles, California

Breast Disease

Conley G. Lacey, MD

Clinical Professor of Gynecology, Division of Gynecologic Oncology, Department of Obstetrics and Gynecology, University of Southern California School of Medicine; Director of Gynecologic Oncology, Ida M. Green Cancer Center, Scripps Clinic and Research Foundation, La Jolla, California

Principles of Radiation Therapy

Malcolm S. Mitchell, MD

Professor of Medicine, University of California, San Diego; Head, Biological Therapy and Melanoma Research Group, University of California, San Diego, California

Principles of Immunology and Immunotherapy

J. Tate Thigpen, MD

Professor of Medicine, Director, Division of Oncology, Department of Medicine, University of Mississippi Medical Center, Jackson, Mississippi

Principles of Chemotherapy

Duane E. Townsend, MD

Clinical Professor, Department of Obstetrics and Gynecology, University of Utah School of Medicine, Salt Lake City, Utah

Premalignant and Related Disorders of the Lower Genital Tract

Preface

Synopsis of Gynecologic Oncology is intended to be a guide to the practice of gynecologic oncology for the physician in training, the general gynecologist, and the cancer specialist. The contents integrate the essential clinical characteristics of the numerous gynecologic tumors with detailed, explicit information concerning their diagnosis, treatment, and outcome. While specific recommendations are made for managing the various premalignant and malignant gynecologic conditions, the reader is provided with sufficient background information to understand the reasons for the recommendations and to form a basis for individualized management. The "cookbook" approach has been purposely avoided.

In this, the fifth edition, nearly every chapter has been extensively revised to include all the important information which has appeared in the literature since the last edition of the book relevant to changes in clinical practice. Thus, this fifth edition, like its predecessors, has undergone major changes to present the reader with the most up-to-date information, to broaden the scope of the database, and to eliminate whatever has become obsolete. The breadth and depth of the book's contents, we believe, make this volume uniquely qualified to serve as a basic textbook as well as a reference work for clinical practice.

As we noted in the last edition, the volume and quality of new information in the field of gynecologic oncology continue to increase at a formidable pace. It is clearly beyond the capacity of a single individual to master. All of us, then, must rely upon the work, advice, and experience of others. In addition to the specialty experts who contributed to the last edition (John A. Blessing, John E. Byfield, Conley G. Lacey, Malcolm S. Mitchell, J. Tate Thigpen, and William H. Hindle), in this edition Jeff Boyd, PhD, has contributed a new chapter on the genetic basis of carcinogenesis, and Cheryl Gurin, MD, has revised Dr. Mitchell's chapter on immunology. We are grateful to all of these contributors.

We wish to acknowledge the secretarial assistance of Sylvia P. Rivera in putting the manuscript together, as well as the editorial assistance of Denise Haller and Guillermo Metz. We also wish to acknowledge the forbearance of our wives and families for the time lost with them in accomplishing this project.

C. Paul Morrow, MD
John P. Curtin, MD

Contents

1

Etiology and Detection of Gynecologic Cancer

EPIDEMIOLOGY

Gynecologic malignancies account for approximately 15 percent of all cancers in women. Based on U.S. population estimates, 81,800 women will be diagnosed with gynecologic cancer in 1997. In the same year, an estimated 26,500 women will die as a result of these cancers (Table 1–1; Parker et al, 1997). Gynecologic cancers are also very common worldwide, particularly squamous cancer of the cervix. In some Central and South American countries, cervical cancer is the most common cancer among women.

Carcinoma of the Vulva, Vagina, and Anus

Squamous carcinomas of the lower genital tract, including the vagina, vulva, and anus, share common risk factors with squamous cancer of the cervix (Peters et al, 1984). The risk of vulvar squamous cancer is related to the number of lifetime sexual partners, smoking, and a history of genital warts (Brinton et al. 1990). On average, 10 percent of women with invasive vaginal carcinoma have a history of invasive cervical carcinoma. Anal carcinoma has also been shown to be associated with sexual activity and a history of condyloma. As is true for cervical cancer, incidence rates for these anogenital cancers are highest in women of low socioeconomic status.

The average age of women who develop squamous carcinoma of the vagina is 62 years. This cancer does occur, however, as early in life as the fourth decade. In the past, 5 to 10 percent of the reported cases were associated with the use of pessary, which was thought to be of etiologic significance. This finding is rare today. Another factor considered to be a contributing cause of vaginal squamous carcinoma is radiation therapy. Pride et al (1979) noted that 20 percent of their patients had prior irradiation, usually for cervical carcinoma. This evidence is confounded, however, by the difficulty in differentiating a recurrence from a new vaginal carcinoma. The well-known propensity of the lower genital tract to develop asynchronous squamous neoplasms of the cervix, vagina, and vulva must also be taken into account. For example, Kolstad and Klem (1976) reported that 2.1 percent of their patients with in situ cervical carcinoma subsequently developed invasive vaginal cancer. It appears that cervical and vaginal squamous cancers are etiologically and epidemiologically similar, occurring almost exclusively in women who have been sexually active and arising from an in situ form.

Vulvar squamous cancer is very uncommon. Typically the disease is diagnosed in women age 70 to 80, although studies suggest that there is an increased incidence among young women. The risk factors and etiology may also be different depending on the age of the patient. Human papillomavirus (HPV) is found in only one third of patients with vulver cancer, a significantly lower rate than in cervical cancer (Iwasawa et al, 1997). Older women with vulvar cancer tend to have a history of vulvar dystrophy, especially lichen sclerosus, whereas smoking and previous cervical neoplasia are less commonly associated factors (Crum, 1992).

Cervical Cancer

Squamous Carcinoma

Most epidemiologic data regarding cervical carcinoma pertain to squamous cancers,

TABLE 1–1

Annual Female Cancer Cases and Deaths in the
United States, 1997*

Site	New Cases	Site	Deaths
Breast	181,600	Lung	66,000
Lung	79,800	Breast	43,900
Colorectal	64,800	Colorectal	27,900
Endometrium	34,900	Pancreas	14,600
Lymphoma	26,900	Ovary	14,200
Ovary	26,800	Lymphoma	12,000
Bladder	15,000	Leukemia	9,540
Cervix	14,500	Endometrium	6,000
Pancreas	14,200	Stomach	5,700
Leukemia	12,400	Multiple myeloma	5,400

*Data from Parker SL, Tong T, Bolden S, Wingo PA: Cancer statistics,
1997. CA Cancer J Clin 47:5, 1997, with permission.

TABLE 1–2

Cervical Carcinoma: Relative Risk of
Selected Factors*

Factor	Relative Risk
Age at coitarche (years)	
<16	16
16–19	3
>19	1
Years from menarche to coitarche	
<1	26
1–5	7
6–10	3
>10	1
Total number of sexual partners	
1 vs. >4	3.6
Number of sexual partners before age 20 years	
0 vs. >1	7
Genital warts	
Never vs. ever	3.2
Smoked >5 cigarettes/day	
<1 year vs. >20 years	4.0

*Data from Peters et al (1986).

which account for 80 to 90 percent of all
cases (Schiffman and Brinton, 1995). In the
United States, cervical cancer ranks as the
seventh most frequent cancer in women.
Among gynecologic cancers, it is surpassed in
frequency by both endometrial and ovarian
cancers.

As Figure 1–1 shows, there has been a dramatic, progressive drop in the incidence rate
of cervical cancer from 1947 to 1970, even
antedating the introduction of population
screening by cervical/vaginal cytology. Similar observations have been reported from
Canada, the United Kingdom, and Scandinavia. Mortality rates have also declined. In
1960, an estimated 8,000 women died of cervical cancer compared with 5,200 deaths in
1977 (DeVesa, 1984). Incidence rates for cervical cancer are highest in lower socioeco-

nomic groups, which probably accounts for
differences in the racial incidence of this cancer in the United States (DeVesa, 1984; Baquet et al, 1991). The probability at birth that
a white women will eventually develop invasive cervical cancer is approximately 0.7 to
1.0 percent, while the risk for a black, His-
panic, or American Indian woman is 1.6
percent.

In addition to race and socioeconomic
status, numerous other risk factors for cervical
cancer have been recognized, many of which
relate to sexual behavior (Table 1–2). Among

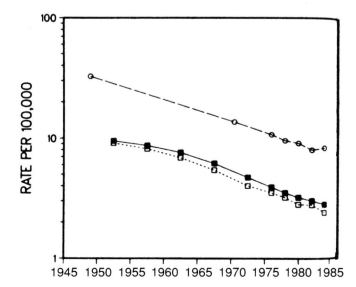

FIGURE 1–1. Age-adjusted incidence
and mortality trends of cervical carcinoma in white women. 1947–1984.
5GA, five geographic areas, SEER program. ○, Incidence—5GA; □, Mortality
—5GA; ■, Mortality—United States.
(From DeVesa SS, Silverman DT, Young
JL, et al: Cancer incidence and mortality
trends among whites in the United
States, 1947–84. J Natl Cancer Inst 79:
701, 1987, with permission.)

the most consistent and significant is age at first intercourse, especially when sexual activity is initiated within 1 year of menarche (Peters et al, 1996). The number of sexual partners and the number of children are also associated with an increased risk for cervical cancer (Bornstein et al, 1995).

The characteristics of a woman's sexual partner (the so-called high-risk male) may put her at increased risk as well. Women whose husbands have had penile cancer or who have been previously married to a woman with cervical cancer have a higher than predicted incidence of cervical cancer (Graham et al, 1979). In addition, the husbands of women with cervical cancer have been reported to be more likely to have had sexually transmitted diseases and many sexual partners (Zunzunegui et al. 1986). A history of cigarette smoking, herpes simplex infection, or venereal warts has also been associated with an increased risk of cervical cancer (DeVesa, 1984; Peters et al, 1986; Brinton, 1991; Winkelstein, 1991). In agreement with these observations are the reports that prostitutes, prisoners, and sexually transmitted disease clinic populations have a high risk of cervical cancer, whereas nuns, the Amish, Mormons, Seventh Day Adventists, Jews, and Muslims have a lower risk.

The use of barrier methods of contraception may provide protection, but circumcision of male sexual partners is no longer believed to lower the risk of cervical cancer. Oral contraceptives are probably associated with an increase in the incidence of invasive cervical cancer as well as an increase in cervical intraepithelial neoplasia (CIN) (Beral et al, 1988).

Invasive and preinvasive cervical neoplasias are more prevalent in chronically immunocompromised women. This increased risk was initially reported in renal transplant patients who were on immunosuppressive agents (Alloub et al, 1989). More recently, women infected with the human immunodeficiency virus (HIV) have been shown to be at risk for preinvasive and invasive cervical cancer. As of 1993, 217 of 16,692 women (1.3 percent) with acquired immunodeficiency syndrome (AIDS) were reported to have an invasive cervical cancer (Klevens et al, 1996).

Adenocarcinoma

The incidence of adenocarcinoma of the cervix appears to be increasing. In a population-based study of cervical adenocarcinoma in women under age 35 years, Peters et al (1986) calculated an average annual increase of 8 percent from 1972 to 1982 in Los Angeles County. An association with prolonged oral contraceptive use has been reported in which the increase in the incidence of cervical adenocarcinoma parallels the use of oral contraceptives. Contrary to this theory, however, histopathologic review of patients with adenocarcinoma failed to link oral contraceptives with adenocarcinoma of the cervix (Jones and Silverberg, 1989).

Adenocarcinoma is commonly associated with preinvasive squamous neoplasia of the cervix. Women with Peutz-Jeghers syndrome are reported to have a 5 percent incidence of minimal deviation or "adenoma malignum," a rare subtype of adenocarcinoma of the cervix (see Chapter 5).

Endometrial Carcinoma

General Factors

Endometrial carcinoma (EC) is the most common invasive neoplasm of the female genital tract in the United States. A total of 34,900 new cases are estimated to be diagnosed in 1997, which is approximately equal to the total number of ovarian and cervical cancers combined. The incidence of EC has remained stable over the past 10 to 12 years. This stability follows a doubling in the incidence of endometrial cancers in the early 1970s, presumably related to the widespread use of unopposed estrogen replacement therapy (Fig. 1–2), although part of the increase may have been related to decreased childbearing (Tretli and Haldorsen, 1990).

EC is predominantly a disorder of postmenopausal women. The average age at diagnosis is 58 years. Only 2 to 5 percent of all cases are diagnosed in women less than age 40 years, and the disease is rare before age 25 years. Nearly all women with a diagnosis of EC prior to age 40 have either chronic anovulation disorder or a hereditary predisposition (e.g., Lynch II syndrome). There is a racial difference in the incidence rates of EC: a white woman has a lifetime risk of 2.4 percent compared with the 1.3 percent risk for a black woman.

A number of constitutional factors have been identified in women who develop EC (Table 1–3). In addition to race and postmenopausal status, some other associated factors are reported to be tallness; a history

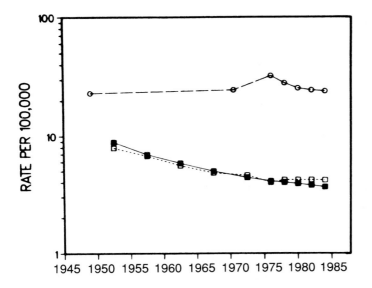

FIGURE 1–2. Age-adjusted incidence and mortality trends of endometrial cancer in white women, 1947–1984. 5GA, five geographic areas, SEER program. ○, Incidence—5GA; □, Mortality—5GA; ■, Mortality—United States. (From DeVesa SS, Silverman DT, Young JL Jr, et al: Cancer incidence and mortality trends among whites in the United States. 1947–84. J Natl Cancer Inst 79:701, 1987, with permission.)

of ovarian, colon, or breast cancer; and a family history of EC, polycystic ovarian disease, hormonally active ovarian stromal tumors (e.g., granulosa cell), and hypothyroidism. A history of pelvic radiation therapy is a risk factor for both endometrial adenocarcinoma and carcinosarcoma (Meredith et al, 1986). In these patients EC tends to be less well differentiated and have a poorer outcome than EC in patients without prior pelvic rediation (Gallion et al, 1987). Protective factors include the use of combination oral contraceptives (Beral et al, 1988) and smoking (Lesko et al, 1985). Worldwide, the variable incidence of EC is most strongly associated with socioeconomic status and total dietary fat consumption (Thomas and Chu, 1986).

TABLE 1–3

Risk Ratio Estimates for Certain Factors Correlated With Endometrial Cancer*

Factor	Relative Risk
Overweight (lb)	1.9–11
20–50	3[†]
>50	9[†]
Parous vs. nulliparous	0.1–0.9
Late menopause (age ≥52 years)	1.7–2.4
Diabetes	1.3–2.7
Radiation therapy	8.0
Exogenous estrogen use	1.6–12.0
Oral contraceptive use	
Sequential	0.9–7.3
Combined	0.1–1.0
Hypertension	1.2–2.1

*Data from Parazzini et al (1991b).
†Data from Wynder et al (1966).

Estrogen Carcinogenesis

As mentioned previously, an increase in the use of estrogens for menopausal symptoms was followed by a surge in the incidence of EC during the early 1970s. Physicians had suspected for many years that postmenopausal estrogens played a role in endometrial carcinogenesis (Fremont-Smith, 1946). Smith et al (1975) were the first of many to study the problem as recognized in the 1970s. Using a case-control study method, they compared 317 patients with EC to the same number of women with other gynecologic malignancies. The calculated increased risk of EC in estrogen users was 4.5 times the risk in the control group. Since the publication of that study in 1975, many additional studies have confirmed the increased rate of EC in women who take estrogen replacement. This risk is related to the dose of estrogen, the duration of therapy, and possibly the schedule of administration, that is, continuous versus cyclic.

Women with presumed estrogen-induced endometrial cancers typically have well-differentiated, superficially invasive tumors, although the increased risk is not limited to these favorable cases (Rubin et al, 1990). Nevertheless, the overall survival rate exceeds that of all women with EC. Women who stop estrogen replacement continue to have an increased risk of endometrial neoplasia for several years. There is considerable evidence that progestins, combined with estrogen, reduce the risk of EC (Kelsey and Whittemore, 1994). However, since this protection is not absolute, some women who take both estrogen and progestin will still develop EC.

Tamoxifen is an estrogen-like competitive agonist that acts primarily by blocking the binding of estrogen receptors. Tamoxifen is most commonly prescribed as adjuvant therapy for postmenopausal women following initial therapy for breast cancer. It has a weak stimulatory effect on the endometrium, and women who take tamoxifen may be at increased risk of developing EC. In a report on a cohort of breast cancer patients randomized to adjuvant tamoxifen therapy versus placebo, the estimated risk of developing EC was approximately 6 cases per 1,000 women (Fisher et al, 1994) among the tamoxifen-treated women (see Chapter 6).

Metabolic Abnormalities

The longstanding recognition that women with EC tend to have clinical features suggestive of an endocrine disorder (i.e., obesity, diabetes, infertility, late menopause) has led to intensive studies of their metabolic status, especially in relation to the sex steroids and their precursors. Many of these findings are discordant or inconclusive. The extraovarian conversion of adrenal androstenedione to estrone increases with advancing age and weight in obese women, but it is unclear whether there is a different rate of conversion in women with and without EC (MacDonald et al, 1978; Gambone et al, 1982). Jasonni and co-workers (1984), in a study of obese and nonobese postmenopausal women with and without EC, reported a statistically significant increase in plasma estrone sulfate, but not estrone, in nonobese cancer patients versus controls. In a more recent study, Nagamani et al (1992) found that the ovarian stroma of postmenopausal women with EC secretes significantly greater amounts of androgens than the stroma of postmenopausal women without EC, and that luteinizing hormone and insulin may contribute to the increase in ovarian steroidogenesis. It is still possible, however, that many, if not all, of the differences observed in patients with EC are due to changes associated with age and obesity.

Uterine Sarcomas

According to data from the National Cancer Institute's Surveillance, Epidemiology, and End-Result (SEER) program, which are derived from nine population-based cancer registries in the United States, uterine sarcomas account for 4.3 percent of all uterine corpus cancers (Harlow et al, 1986). Histologically, 48 percent are carcinosarcomas, 38 percent leiomyosarcomas (LMS), and 10 percent endometrial stromal sarcomas (ESS) (low and high grade combined). Carcinosarcoma is nearly three times as common, and LMS 1.5 times as common, among black women as white women. The incidence of uterine LMS is highest in women ages 30 to 50 years and declines thereafter, whereas the incidence of carcinosarcoma is low prior to age 50 years but rises sharply after that. LMS risk is associated with early age at menarche, late menopause, and history of induced abortion (Schwartz et al, 1991). Breast-feeding appears to protect against the development of LMS. Carcinosarcoma and LMS are both more common among women who have never married. No association with the use of oral contraceptives has been reported for any of the uterine sarcomas. The risk for carcinosarcoma is increased by low-dose irradiation (Meredith et al, 1986). Among patients with prior pelvic radiation, sarcomas account for 17 percent of uterine corpus cancers compared with less than 5 percent of corpus cancers diagnosed in women with no history of pelvic radiation.

Ovarian Cancer

Epithelial Ovarian Cancer

From the viewpoint of morbidity and mortality, ovarian malignancies are the most important group of neoplasms in the field of gynecologic oncology. In the United States, only 35 percent of all women diagnosed as having ovarian cancer survive 5 years. The number of deaths per year increased by 250 percent from 1930 to 1970, although the mortality rate has been stable over the past 20 years (Fig. 1–3). The U.S. estimates for 1997 (Table 1–1) anticipate approximately 26,800 new cases and 14,200 deaths due to this malignancy. The number of deaths from ovarian cancer surpasses the combined number of deaths from endometrial cancer (6,000/year) and cervical cancer (4,800/year).

Ovarian cancer is predominantly a disease of peri- and postmenopausal women, with an average age of 54 years at diagnosis (Fig. 1–4). The histologic type of neoplasm and the overall frequency of occurrence vary with age. In children and young women of less than 20 years of age, 60 percent of ovarian neoplasms are of germ cell origin. However, over 80 percent of ovarian tumors that occur

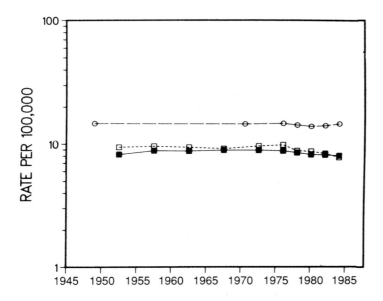

FIGURE 1–3. Age-adjusted incidence and mortality trends of ovarian cancer in white women, 1947–1984, 5GA, five geographic areas, SEER program. ○, Incidence—5GA; □, Mortality—5GA; ■, Mortality—United States. (From DeVesa SS, Silverman DT, Young JL Jr, et al: Cancer incidence and mortality trends among whites in the United States, 1947–84. J Natl Cancer Inst 79:701, 1987, with permission.)

in postmenopausal women are epithelial adenocarcinomas. Borderline ovarian tumors occur most often in younger women and are more commonly confined to the ovary than are invasive ovarian tumors (Harlow et al, 1987).

The worldwide incidence rate varies from 2.5 per 100,000 women in Japan to 15 per 100,000 women in Scandinavian countries (Parazzini et al, 1991a). In the United States, the annual incidence for white women is 13 per 100,000 women, which is one of the high-est rates in the world. The rate for black women is 10 per 100,000 women.

Many epidemiologic studies have related reproductive events to the risk of epithelial ovarian cancer (Table 1–4). Women who are nulliparous, have not used oral contraceptives (Fig. 1–5), or are infertile have a higher rate of ovarian cancer (Bristow and Karlan, 1996). The theory of incessant ovulation (Fathalla, 1972) has been addressed in several case-control studies. The greater the duration of ovulation (i.e., no pregnancies, no ovula-

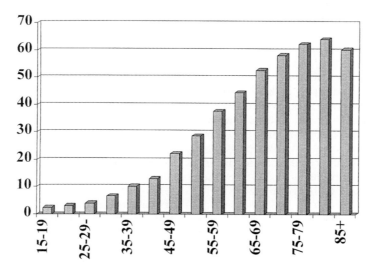

FIGURE 1–4. Ovarian cancer age adjusted and age specific incidence rates (per 100,000 population) in the United States, 1990–1994. SEER Program data. (Data from the American Cancer Society, 1996, with permission.)

TABLE 1–4

Risk Factors and Ovarian Carcinoma*

Risk Factor	Relative Risk
Positive family history	
One first-degree relative	1.9–3.6
Hereditary	17–50
Breast cancer	1.0–1.6
Nulliparous vs. parous	4.0–5.0
Oral contraceptive use (>3–5 years)	0.5
White vs. black race	1.5
High-fat diet	1.5–4.0
Talc use	3.0

*Data from Casagrande et al (1979), Cramer et al (1982a,b), Mori et al (1984), Lynch et al (1985), Schildkraut and Thompson (1988), and Beral et al (1988).

tion suppression, and late versus early menopause), the greater the risk of developing ovarian cancer (Casagrande et al, 1979; Beral et al, 1988). Other risk factors, such as high socioeconomic status and ethnic background, merely reflect the associated low parity and/or high-fat diet in this subset of the general population (Heintz et al, 1985; Rose et al, 1986). There is an increased risk of ovarian cancer in women with a prior history of malignancy, particularly breast and colon cancers (Rosen et al, 1989). EC is also associated with ovarian cancer, usually synchronously.

Familial and Hereditary Ovarian Cancer

Among women with ovarian cancer, approximately 5 to 7 percent will report a family history of ovarian and/or breast cancer. Broadly speaking, there are three categories of patients: (1) those with no significant family history of cancer; (2) those who have a positive family history (i.e., one or more first-degree relatives with ovarian and/or breast cancer) and who therefore may have an increased risk of an ovarian malignancy; and (3) those with a hereditary or genetic predisposition to develop epithelial ovarian cancer. A careful family history and, if possible, review of pertinent pathology allows the clinician to make a preliminary determination as to whether the patient is at increased risk of developing ovarian cancer. Schildkraut and Thompson (1988) estimated that the increase in relative risk for women with a history of ovarian cancer in first-degree relatives was 3.6, and for second-degree relatives was 2.9, compared with women who reported a negative family history.

When a hereditary syndrome is suggested by the family history, referral to a clinical genetics service is recommended. Ovarian cancer risk is increased in three syndromes: ovarian-specific cancer syndrome, breast/ovarian cancer syndrome, and hereditary nonpolyposis colorectal cancer or Lynch II syndrome. These can be presumptively identified by pedigree analysis or by testing for the responsible gene (Lynch et al, 1991, 1996; Claus et al, 1996). Among all women with ovarian cancer, approximately 2 to 5 percent develop their cancer as a result of a genetic susceptibility (Whittemore et al, 1997). Previously, these women were identified when there was evidence of two or more first-degree female relatives with ovarian cancer plus or minus breast cancer. The most common form of hereditary ovarian cancer is a component of the breast/ovarian cancer syndrome; mutations of a gene designated BRCA-1, located on the long arm of chromosome 17, are thought to account for the majority of hereditary ovarian cancers (Miki et al, 1994). Another gene, BRCA-2, which is located on the long arm of chromosome 13, has also been linked to hereditary ovarian cancer. Both the BRCA-1 and BRCA-2 genes have been cloned, and it is now possible to test an individual for germline mutations of either of these genes. Among women with BRCA-1 mutations, the estimated lifetime risk of developing ovarian cancer ranges from 10 to 70 percent (Claus et al, 1996). Given the far-reaching implications of testing positive for a gene mutation associated with a hereditary predisposition to cancer, the testing should be carried out in a setting that can provide comprehensive counseling, as well as long-term followup of the patient and her extended family.

Nonepithelial Ovarian Cancer

Because of the relative rarity of nonepithelial ovarian neoplasms, epidemiologic data regarding their incidence and risk factors are not as extensive as those available from studies of epithelial ovarian cancers. Familial occurrences have been reported for dysgerminoma, Sertoli–Leydig cell tumors (sometimes associated with thyroid nodules), and benign cystic teratomas.

Certain genetic syndromes are known to be commonly associated with ovarian neoplasms. Women who have an XY karyotype or a Y fragment (i.e., gonadal dysgenesis) are predisposed to develop gonadoblastomas,

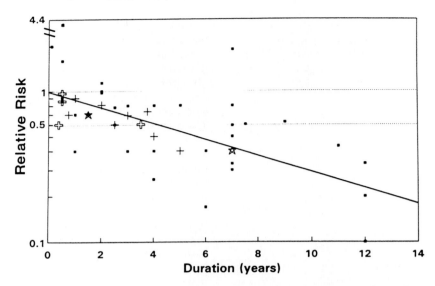

FIGURE 1–5. Effect of oral contraceptive use on incidence of ovarian cancer: the estimated risk reduction related to duration of use. (From Hankinson SE, Colditz GA, Hunter DJ, Rosner B: A quantitative assessment of oral contraceptive use and risk of ovarian cancer. Obstet Gynecol 80:708, 1992, with permission.)

which often give rise to dysgerminomas and occasionally other germ cell malignancies. Case-control studies of patients with ovarian germ cell tumors have suggested that in utero exposure to high levels of estrogen (exogenous or endogenous) may be a risk factor for development of these rare tumors (Walker et al, 1988). Patients who have a history of surgical resection of a benign cytic teratoma are reported to be at increased risk of developing a malignant germ cell tumor of the ovary (Anteby et al, 1994). The Peutz-Jeghers syndrome of buccal pigmentation and intestinal polyposis is associated with a 5 percent incidence of gonadal stromal tumors. Women with Gorlin's syndrome (multiple nervoid basal carcinomas) may develop ovarian fibromas.

SCREENING AND PREVENTION OF GYNECOLOGIC MALIGNANCY

Cancer of the Vulva, Vagina, and Anus

Screening methods and results for noncervical squamous neoplasms of the lower genital tract are poorly described, partly because of the relatively uncommon nature of these cancers. One group that has been identified is patients with a history of invasive or preinvasive lesions of the cervix. On the average,

10 percent of patients with either a vulvar or a vaginal cancer will have a history of cervical cancer. Routine cytologic screening of this population should be done annually (Pearce et al, 1996).

Cervical Cancer

When exfoliative cytology was introduced for cervical cancer screening 45 years ago, it offered the hope of eliminating deaths from this malignancy in an adequately screened population because it was capable of detecting occult cancer and, even more importantly, precancerous conditions. Successful programs have been reported from many countries (Boyes and Worth, 1981; Yajima et al, 1982; Christopherson, 1983; Day, 1984; Duguid et al, 1985). In general terms, the incidence and mortality rates for cervical cancer, which had been declining before the introduction of mass screening, have been reduced by 40 to 80 percent, with a concomitant increase in the incidence of preinvasive lesions and early-stage cancers.

Screening for cervical cancer depends on three important assumptions: (1) that cervical cancer is preceded by a long preinvasive phase for which treatment is highly effective, (2) that cervical cytology is an accurate screening test, and (3) that all patients at risk will present for their screening examinations. Two disturbing aspects of cervical cancer screening are the frequency with which invasive carcinoma is diagnosed in women who have had normal Pap smears, and the inadequate screening among high-risk segments of the population. There are several possible explanations for the apparent shortened interval from a "normal" test to an invasive lesion (Boyce et al, 1990):

1. There is a false-negative rate for Pap tests of approximately 20 percent.
2. Retrospective reviews of negative smears often demonstrate misdiagnosis (Dunn and Schweitzer, 1981; Carmichael et al, 1984).
3. A higher incidence of nonsquamous cancers, which are less likely to be detected by cervical cytology, is noted in patients who report a normal Pap test within 3 years of diagnosis of cervical cancer (Benoit et al, 1984).
4. There is growing evidence that some squamous carcinomas evolve from cytologically normal epithelium during a 2- to 5-year period (Morell et al, 1982; Bain and Crocker, 1983; Dunn et al, 1984; Peters et al, 1988).

Because of the lack of coverage of routine screening, including cervical cytology, by many health insurance plans, the indigent and those in the middle age groups are least likely to obtain one or serial Pap smears (Brown, 1996). In contrast, the lower risk groups tend to be overscreened.

One-half or more of the false-negative Pap test results are due to sampling techniques (Beilby et al, 1982). This rate can be minimized by observing a few essential points (Richart, 1979; American College of Obstetricians and Gynecologists, 1984):

1. Take a cervical specimen by scraping the squamocolumnar junction and exocervix with a wooden or plastic spatula.
2. Take an endocervical specimen by using an endocervical brush or a moist, cotton-tipped applicator.
3. Spread the specimen(s) on a glass slide and fix them immediately.
4. Avoid using a lubricating jelly, Lugol's solution, acetic acid, or any other substance on the cervix before obtaining the cytology specimen.

Although the annual Pap smear test was widely accepted by many gynecologists as the standard of care, reports have challenged this concept on both an epidemiologic and a cost-effectiveness basis. The Walton report, based on a study commissioned by the Canadian Health Service, was the first to suggest that annual Pap smears were unnecessary for most women, and were not cost-effective for women over the age of 65 years. The Walton report suggested that, after two negative smears, a women should have a Pap test done every 3 years until age 65. A more recent analysis that considered the incidence and risk factors, as well as the cost-effectiveness and potential benefits in terms of increased survival, supported a 3-year interval for screening to age 65 years (Eddy, 1990). Screening every 1 to 2 years rather than every 3 years was calculated to improve the effectiveness of the screening Pap test by less than 5 percent.

These calculations by epidemiologists and medical economists stand in contrast to the observational studies previously mentioned, which have documented the reduction in the incidence and mortality rates of cervical cancer. The majority of these population-based studies used annual screening of women; women not screened have an increased risk of developing cervical cancer and are more likely to have a more advanced stage than are women who have been screened in the past. Shy et al (1989) found that the risk of squamous cervical cancer was increased 3.9 times for women who have Pap smears at 3-year intervals than for women with annual screening. The American College of Obstetricians and Gynecologists (ACOG) recommendations for Pap smear screening are summarized in Table 1–5.

Cervical Cytology — Current Status

In the late 1980s, following concerns raised about quality control in cervical cytology screening laboratories, several initiatives were begun to improve the accuracy and utility of the Pap smear. The Bethesda System for reporting the results of cervical cytology was first published in 1988 and revised in 1992 (see Appendix III). The majority of Pap smears are now reported using the Bethesda descriptions. Quality control within the laboratories was standardized by the 1989 federal Clinical Laboratories Improvement Act (CLIA); the main provisions in regard to Pap smears include a limit on the number of Pap smears read by individual cytotechnologists per day and the mandate that 10 percent of all smears be rescreened.

TABLE 1–5

Recommended frequency of Pap Smears: ACOG Recommendations*

1. *Initial screening:* Smears should be obtained from all women by age 18 years and from sexually active women regardless of age.[†]
2. *Frequency*
   a. High-risk patients[‡]: Should be screened annually.
   b. Low-risk patients: After three or more consecutive, satisfactory annual examinations, the interval of screening is arbitrary and should be based on the informed decision of the patient and physician. The risk of an abnormality occurring within 3 to 5 years is minimal.
3. *Diethylstilbestrol (DES)-exposed patients:* Screening should begin at menarche, at age 14 years, or at the onset of symptoms. Subsequent Pap smears should be done at 6- to 12-month intervals.
4. *Following hysterectomy:* Vaginal cytology is recommended at minimum intervals of 3 to 5 years.[§]
5. *Following therapy for preinvasive disease of the cervix:* Screen at approximately 2-year intervals.
6. *Following therapy for invasive cervical malignancy:* Screening is customarily performed at 3-month intervals for 2 years and every 6 months thereafter.

*Adapted from ACOG: Recommendations on Frequency of Pap Test Screening. Committee Opinion No. 152. Washington, DC, The American College of Obstetricians and Gynecologists, 1995.

[†]*Author's comment:* It is, of course, entirely unnecessary to do cervical cancer screening on asymptomatic, non-DES-exposed virgins. They do not get cervical squamous neoplasms, and the occasional glandular carcinomas are not readily detected by exfoliative cytology.

[‡]*Author's comment:* High-risk patients are defined as those with a history of early sexual intercourse or multiple sexual partners, immunosuppressed patients, and smokers.

[§]*Author's comment:* Patients with epidemiologic high-risk features should be followed the same as those in category 5.

In addition to improved quality control and a standardized reporting system, new methods have been introduced to aid in the interpretation of cervical cytology specimens. Automated devices are currently approved for the rescreening of Pap smears. These automated devices use computerized image analysis to identify abnormal cells. Another potential improvement is in the preparation of the cervical specimen, by which the cells are collected in a medium and then processed and placed on a slide in the cytology lab. This method has the advantage of avoiding air-drying artifacts in cell morphology as well as producing a uniform monolayer cell preparation. Preliminary studies suggest that the monolayer technique results in a higher detection rate for cervical dysplasia (Wilbur et al, 1994).

Techniques other than cytology have also been proposed to improve screening for cervical cancer, including HPV screening to define a high-risk population, routine colposcopic examination of the cervix, and colpophotography. While each of these may improve the overall sensitivity and specificity of cervical cancer screening, of concern is the added cost, especially in light of the fact that the population at risk can ill afford to pay for conventional cervical cytology.

Endometrial Cancer

No satisfactory technique is available for the routine screening of large populations of women for EC and its precursors. Since the majority of endometrial cancers are stage I at diagnosis and the outcome of these patients is relatively favorable, it may be argued that mass screening is unlikely to be cost-effective or to increase survival rates. Annual endometrial biopsy cannot be recommended for all women. For patients who are symptomatic, prompt biopsy is indicated. In addition, annual endometrial biopsy is appropriate for postmenopausal women who are taking estrogen without progestin and whenever unscheduled bleeding occurs (ACOG, 1992). There is considerable debate regarding screening of tamoxifen-treated women. Some clinicians have advocated periodic endometrial sampling and/or sonographic measurement of endometrial thickness. This approach may be appropriate for clinical studies; however, routine application of these procedures is not recommended. Endometrial biopsy is indicated when tamoxifen-treated patients have symptoms.

There are numerous devices for obtaining endometrial specimens in the outpatient setting, and biopsy, as opposed to cytology, has proven to be the more accurate procedure for detecting EC and hyperplasia. Complications are unusual, but the failure rate, which averages 10 to 15 percent, increases with the age of the patient.

Ultrasonic measurement of the thickness of the endometrium may be an adjunct to endometrial biopsy in the evaluation of a patient with symptoms. When the endometrial "stripe" is less than 3 to 5 mm in thickness, the incidence of endometrial neoplasia in postmenopausal women is very low (Granberg et al, 1991). Conversely, when the endometrium is thicker than 10 mm, 10 to 20 percent of patients will have hyperplasia or carcinoma. Any patient who is noted to have a thickened endometrium on ultrasound should have an endometrial biopsy.

Routine cervical cytology occasionally leads to the diagnosis of EC. Findings suspicious for endometrial pathology are (1) numerous histiocytes in the postmenopausal smear, (2) normal-appearing endometrial cells obtained during the second half of the menstrual cycle or anytime after the menopause, and (3) atypical or malignant glandular cells in any age group. These findings are indications for endocervical and endometrial sampling. If these studies are normal and the Pap smears contains atypical or malignant cells, laparoscopy, and possibly even hysterectomy with removal of the tubes and ovaries, may be warranted, because tubal or ovarian origin of malignant cells cannot be excluded (Zucker et al, 1985; Pretorius et al, 1996) (see Chapter 6).

Ovarian Cancer

Screening for ovarian cancer, the most deadly of all gynecologic cancers, is an unrealized goal. Despite therapeutic advances in the treatment of advanced ovarian cancer, it is unlikely that these methods will provide a means of regularly eradicating disease that has spread beyond the ovary at diagnosis. A more reasonable prospect for improving the prognosis of ovarian cancer is early diagnosis. Routine pelvic examination is ill suited to mass screening for ovarian cancer. MacFarlane et al (1955) discovered six ovarian carcinomas during 18,753 pelvic examinations of 1,319 women ages 30 to 90 years in a 15-year study. Five of the six died of ovarian cancer.

Atypical or malignant cells found in a Pap smear when the lower genital tract is normal should lead to prompt evaluation of the tubes and ovaries. Culdocentesis, which provides convenient access to the peritoneal cavity, has been used to obtain fluid for cytologic studies in hopes of detecting early asymptomatic ovarian cancer. Although initial reports of this technique were encouraging, the overall results have been disappointing in terms of unsatisfactory specimens and the yield of asymptomatic, early ovarian cancer. The most significant drawback is patient discomfort, which limits the usefulness of this technique in terms of compliance.

The greatest hope for early diagnosis of ovarian cancer lies in the development of sufficiently sensitive and reliable tests that are suitable to repetitive screening of the population at risk. The evolution of diagnostic pelvic ultrasonography, as well as the development of sensitive laboratory tests for serum antigens associated with ovarian cancers, have shown mixed results for early detection of ovarian neoplasms.

The first clinically useful serum tumor marker for epithelial ovarian cancer was reported by Bast et al (1983). With a monoclonal antibody, the CA-125 ovarian cancer–associated antigen is detectable in more than 80 percent of nonmucinous ovarian carcinomas. One limitation of serum CA-125 as a screening tool is that often the patients with early disease confined to the ovary have a normal (<35 U/ml) level of CA-125. Another limitation is that many benign gynecologic conditions of reproductive-age women may cause an elevated serum CA-125 level. Zurawski et al (1990) reported the preliminary results from a trial of serial serum samples tested for CA-125. Limiting the definition of a positive test to those patients with an initial elevated level, followed by a subsequent doubling of the initial level, they report that the specificity was 99.9 percent. The one patient in the initial population of 1,000 screened had a stage III ovarian cancer at surgery. As previously discussed, a screening test must be sensitive enough to detect cancers confined to the ovary if overall survival is to be improved. Jacobs and colleagues (1993) suggest that serum CA-125 can be used to screen the general population, and, for those women who are found to have an elevated level, sonography can be used for follow-up.

Screening of women for ovarian cancer by transabdominal and/or transvaginal sonography has focused primarily on identification of abnormal morphology or, in some studies, on volumetric measurement of the postmenopausal ovaries (Campbell et al, 1989; van Nagell et al, 1993). The encouraging results of the initial reports of ultrasonic screening for ovarian cancer have been updated and reviewed by Karlan (1995). While it is true that most cases of ovarian cancer diagnosed by ultrasound screening are confined to the ovary, many of the stage I cases are either low-malignant-potential (LMP) tumors or stromal cell cancers that are known to be predominantly stage I at diagnosis. When the cases of invasive epithelial cancers are considered alone, nearly one half of those discovered in screening studies have advanced-stage disease. Thus ultrasound screening requires further investigation, particularly in regard to interval between screenings and the use of serum tumor markers.

The NIH Consensus Development Conference on Ovarian Cancer (Ovarian Cancer,

TABLE 1–6

Recommendations for Ovarian Cancer Screening*

Number of First-Degree Relatives Affected	Lifetime Risk of Ovarian Cancer	Recommendations for Screening
None	1.4%	Annual pelvic examination
One	3–5%	Participation in clinical trials: counseling by a gynecologic oncologist
Two or more, Positive test (BRCA-1, BRCA-2)	10–70%	Counseling by a gynecologic oncologist, genetic counseling, annual pelvic examination, serum CA-125, and transvaginal sonogram beginning at age 25–30

*From Ovarian cancer: screening, treatment, and follow-up. NIH Consensus Statement 1994. JAMA 273:491, 1995.

1995) recommended that women who are at high risk for ovarian cancer should be screened by annual rectovaginal examinations, serum CA-125 measurement, and transvaginal ultrasound (Table 1–6). The best age to begin screening is uncertain; age 25 to 30 may be appropriate unless the pedigree analysis demonstrates very-early-onset ovarian cancer. If the patient is at risk because of Lynch II syndrome, emdometrial biopsy should be performed on an annual basis in addition to ovarian cancer screening. Mammography and colonoscopy may be indicated depending upon the risk analysis provided by the genetics consult. There are limited data as to whether oral contraceptives and/or pregnancy provide the same protection against ovarian cancer to women with a hereditary ovarian cancer syndrome as that demonstrated in the general population.

Elective oophorectomy has been recommended for those patients who are at risk of developing ovarian cancer as a result of a genetic predisposition. In most cases, this will first require a genetics consult and possibly genetic testing to confirm the presence of a genetic marker. Testing positive for the BRCA-1 gene is strong evidence that the patient is at increased risk of developing ovarian cancer (Berchuck et al, 1996). However, if the patient has a family pedigree strongly suggestive of an autosomal dominant inheritance pattern and tests are negative for the known gene alterations associated with hereditary ovarian cancer, the patient may still be at significant risk and ultrasonic screening or prophylactic oophorectomy should be considered. If the patient with hereditary breast/ovarian or ovarian cancer syndrome has completed planned reproduction and she is age 35 years or older, a prophylactic bilateral salpingo-oophorectomy should be offered to her. If the patient is thought to have Lynch II syndrome, a prophylactic hysterectomy and bilateral salpingo-oophorectomy should be

recommended since endometrial cancer is the most common form of noncolonic cancer in these women. A laparoscopic procedure is the preferred method of prophylactic surgery. Thorough histologic examination of the ovaries is essential (Salazar et al, 1996). The patient should be informed that the prophylactic removal of the ovaries is not 100 percent effective in preventing "ovarian" cancer. The reported incidence of a peritoneal papillary adenocarcinoma, which mimics ovarian cancer, ranges from 2 to 10 percent following a prophylactic oophorectomy (Tobachman et al, 1982; Piver et al, 1993).

In addition to the familial epithelial ovarian carcinoma, there are other indications for oophorectomy to prevent malignancy (Table 1–7). These include XY gonadal dysgenesis, because of the risk for germ cell malignancy see Chapter 11), and incidental oophorectomy in women near or beyond menopause who are undergoing pelvic surgery, usually hysterectomy. The latter could reduce the overall incidence of ovarian carcinoma by 5 percent, since that is approximately the portion of women who develop ovarian carcinoma after having undergone hysterectomy without oophorectomy. Of course the majority of these women underwent vaginal hys-

TABLE 1–7

Prophylactic Oophorectomy

As primary indication for surgery
   XY gonadal dysgenesis
   Familial ovarian carcinoma
Incidental to hysterectomy
   Prior benign or malignant epithelial ovarian neoplasm
   Ovarian failure
   Age beyond 45 years*
   Epidemiologic high-risk patient below age 45 years*
   Cancer phobia

*Arbitrary and needs to be discussed with patient. Ovaries continue to function until age 55 or later.

terectomy. Perhaps laparoscopic surgery will allow more high-risk women to have prophylactic oophorectomy at the time of hysterectomy.

Because women at increased risk for ovarian carcinoma also may be at increased risk for breast and colon cancer, periodic mammography, breast self-examination, testing of the stool for occult blood, and colonoscopy are recommended.

REFERENCES

Alloub MI, Barr BBB, McLaren KM, et al: Human papillomavirus infection and cervical intraepithelial neoplasia in women with renal allografts. Br J Med 298:153, 1989.

American College of Obstetricians and Gynecologists: Cervical Cytology: Evaluation and Management of Abnormalities. Technical Bulletin No. 81. Washington, DC, American College of Obstetricians and Gynecologists, 1984.

American College of Obstetricians and Gynecologists: Hormone Replacement Therapy. Technical Bulletin No. 166. Washington, DC, American College of Obstetricians and Gynecologists, 1992.

American College of Obstetricians and Gynecologists: Recommendations on Frequency of Pap Test Screening. Committee Opinion No. 152. Washington, DC, American College of Obstetricians and Gynecologists, 1995.

Anteby EY, Ron M, Revel A, et al: Germ cell tumors of the ovary arising after dermoid cyst resection: a long-term follow-up study. Obstet Gynecol 83:605, 1994.

Bain RW, Crocker DW: Rapid onset of cervical cancer in an upper socioeconomic group. Am J Obstet Gynecol 146:366, 1983.

Baquet CR, Horm FW, Gibbs T, Greenwald P: Socioeconomic factors and cancer incidence among blacks and whites. J Natl Cancer Inst 83:551, 1991.

Bast RC Jr, Klug T, St John E, et al: A radioimmunoassay using a monoclonal antibody to monitor the course of epithelial ovarian cancer. N Engl J Med 309:883, 1983.

Beilby JOW, Bourne R, Guillebaud J, Steele ST: Paired cervical smears: a method of reducing the false-negative rate in population screening. Obstet Gynecol 60:46, 1982.

Benoit AG, Krepart GV, Lotocki RJ: Results of prior cytologic screening in patients with a diagnosis of stage I carcinoma of the cervix. Am J Obstet Gynecol 148:690, 1984.

Beral V, Hannaford P, Kay C: Oral contraceptive use and malignancies of the genital tract: results from the Royal College of General Practitioners' oral contraception study. Lancet 2:1331, 1988.

Berchuck A, Cirisano F, Lancaster JM, et al: Role of BRCA1 mutation screening in the management of familial ovarian cancer. Am J Obstet Gynecol 175:738, 1996.

Bornstein J, Rahat MA, Abramovici H: Etiology of cervical cancer: current concepts. Obstet Gynecol Surv 50:146, 1995.

Boyce JG, Fruchter RG, Romanzi L, et al: The fallacy of the screening interval for cervical smears. Obstet Gynecol 76:627, 1990.

Boyes DA, Worth AJ: Treatment of early cervical neoplasia: definition and management of preclinical invasive carcinoma. Gynecol Oncol 12:S317, 1981.

Brinton LA: Editorial commentary: smoking and cervical cancer—current status. Am J Epidemiol 131:958, 1991.

Brinton LA, Nasca PC, Mallin K, et al: Case-control study of cancer of the vulva. Obstet Gynecol 175:859, 1990.

Bristow RE, Karlan BY: Ovulation induction, infertility, and ovarian cancer risk. Fertil Steril 66:499, 1996.

Brown CL: Screening patterns for cervical cancer: how best to reach the unscreened population. Monogr J Nat Cancer Inst 21:7, 1996.

Campbell S, Bhan V, Royston P, et al: Transabdominal ultrasound screening for early ovarian cancer. Br Med J 299:1363, 1989.

Carmichael JA, Jeffrey JF, Steele HD, Ohile ID: The cytologic history of 245 patients developing invasive cervical carcinoma. Am J Obstet Gynecol 148:685, 1984.

Casagrande JT, Louie EW, Pike MC, et al: "Incessant ovulation" and ovarian cancer. Lancet 2:170, 1979.

Christopherson WM: Cytologic detection and diagnosis of cancer: its contributions and limitations. Cancer 51:1201, 1983.

Claus EB, Schildkraut JM, Thompson WD, Risch NJ: The genetic attributable risk of breast and ovarian cancer. Cancer 77:2318, 1996.

Cramer DW, Hutchison GB, Welch WR, et al: Factors affecting the association of oral contraceptives and ovarian cancer. N Engl J Med 307:1047, 1982a.

Cramer DW, Welch WR, Scully RE, Wojciechowski CA: Ovarian cancer and talc: a case-control study. Cancer 50:372, 1982b.

Crum C: Carcinoma of the vulva: epidemiology and pathogenesis. Obstet Gynecol 79:448, 1992.

Day NE: Effect of cervical cancer screening in Scandinavia. Obstet Gynecol 63:714, 1984.

DeVesa SS: Descriptive epidemiology of cancer of the uterine cervix. Obstet Gynecol 63:605, 1984.

DeVesa SS, Silverman DT, Young JL Jr, et al: Cancer incidence and mortality trends among whites in the United States, 1947–84. J Natl Cancer Inst 79:701, 1987.

Duguid HLD, Duncan ID, Currie J: Screening for cervical intraepithelial neoplasia in Dundee and Angus 1962–1981 and its relation with invasive cervical cancer. Lancet 2:1053, 1985.

Dunn JE Jr, Crocker DW, Rube IF, et al: Cervical cancer occurrence in Memphis and Shelby County, Tennessee, during 25 years of its cervical cytology screening program. Am J Obstet Gynecol 150:861, 1984.

Dunn JE Jr, Schweitzer V: The relationship of cervical cytology to the incidence of invasive cervical cancer and mortality in Alameda County, California, 1960 to 1974. Am J Obstet Gynecol 139:868, 1981.

Eddy DM: Screening for cervical cancer. Ann Intern Med 113:214, 1990.

Fathalla MF: Factors in the causation and incidence of ovarian cancer. Obstet Gynecol Surv 27:751, 1972.

Fisher B, Constantino JP, Redmond CK, et al: Endometrial cancer in tamoxifen-treated breast cancer patients: findings from the National Surgical Adjuvant Breast and Bowel Project (NSABP) B-14. J Natl Cancer Inst 86:527, 1994.

Fremont-Smith M, Meigs JV, Graham RM: Cancer of the endometrium and prolonged estrogen therapy. JAMA 131:805, 1946.

Gallion HH, van Nagell JR Jr, Donaldson ES, Powell DE: Endometrial cancer following radiation therapy for cervical cancer. Gynecol Oncol 27:76, 1987.

Gambone JC, Partridge WM, Lagasse LD, Judd HL: In vivo availability of circulating estradiol in postmenopausal women with and without endometrial cancer. Obstet Gynecol 59:416, 1982.

Graham S, Priore R, Graham M, et al: Genital cancer in wives of penile cancer patients. Cancer 44:1870, 1979.

Granberg S, Wikland M, Karlsson B, et al: Endometrial thickness as measured by endovaginal ultrasonography for identifying endometrial abnormality. Am J Obstet Gynecol 164:47, 1991.

Hankinson SE, Colditz GA, Hunter DJ, Rosner B: A quantitative assessment of oral contraceptive use and risk of ovarian cancer. Obstet Gynecol 80:708, 1992.

Harlow BL, Weiss NS, Lofton S: The epidemiology of sarcomas of the uterus. J Natl Cancer Inst 76:399, 1986.

Harlow BL, Weiss NS, Lofton S: Epidemiology of borderline ovarian tumors. J Natl Cancer Inst 78:71, 1987.

Heintz APM, Hacker NF, Lagasse LD: Epidemiology and etiology of ovarian cancer: a review. Obstet Gynecol 66:127, 1985.

Iwasawa A, Nieminen P, Lehtinen M, Paavonen J: Human papillomavirus in squamous cell carcinoma of the vulva by polymerase chain reaction. Obstet Gynecol 89:81, 1997.

Jacobs I, Davies AP, Bridges J, et al: Prevalence screening for ovarian cancer in postmenopausal women by CA 125 measurement and ultrasonography. BMJ 306:1030, 1993.

Jasonni VM, Bulleti C, Franceschetti F, et al: Estrone sulphate plasma levels in postmenopausal women with and without endometrial cancer. Cancer 53:2698, 1984.

Jones MW, Silverberg SG: Cervical adenocarcinoma in young women: possible relationship to microglandular hyperplasia and use of oral contraceptives. Obstet Gynecol 73:984, 1989.

Karlan BY, Platt LD: Ovarian cancer screening: the role of ultrasound in early detection. Cancer 76:2011, 1995.

Kelsey JL, Whittemore AS: Epidemiology and primary prevention of cancers of the breast, endometrium, and ovary: a brief overview. Ann Epidemiol 4:89, 1994.

Klevens RM, Fleming PL, Mays MA, Frey R: Characteristics of women with AIDS and invasive cervical cancer. Obstet Gynecol 88:269, 1996.

Kolstad P, Klem V: Long-term followup of 1,121 cases of carcinoma in situ of the cervix. Obstet Gynecol 48:125, 1976.

Lesko SM, Rosenberg L, Kaufman DW, et al: Cigarette smoking and the risk of endometrial cancer. N Engl J Med 313: 593, 1985.

Lynch HT, Scheulke GS, Weels IC, et al: Hereditary ovarian carcinoma: biomarker studies. Cancer 55:410, 1985.

Lynch HT, Smyrk T, Lynch JF: Overview of natural history, pathology, molecular genetics and management of HNPCC (Lynch syndrome). Int J Cancer 69:38, 1996.

Lynch HT, Watson P, Bewtra C, et al: Hereditary ovarian cancer: heterogeneity in age at diagnosis. Cancer 67:1460, 1991.

MacDonald PC, Edman CD, Hemsell DL, et al: Effect of obesity on conversion of plasma androstenedione to estrone in postmenopausal women with and without endometrial cancer. Am J Obstet Gynecol 130:448, 1978.

MacFarlane C, Sturgis MC, Fetterman FS: Results of an experiment in the control of cancer of the female pelvic organs and report of a fifteen-year research. Am J Obstet Gynecol 69:294, 1955.

Meredith RF, Eisert DR, Kaka Z, et al: An excess of uterine sarcomas after pelvic irradiation. Cancer 58:2003, 1986.

Miki Y, Swenson J, Shattuck-Eidens D, et al: A strong candidate for breast and ovarian cancer susceptibility gene BRCA1. Science 266:66, 1994.

Morell ND, Taylor JR, Snyder RN, et al: False-negative cytology rates in patients in whom invasive cervical cancer subsequently developed. Obstet Gynecol 60:41, 1982.

Mori M, Kiyosawa H, Miyake H: Case-control study of ovarian cancer in Japan. Cancer 53:2746, 1984.

Nagamani M, Stuart CA, Doherty MG: Increased steroid production by the ovarian stromal tissue of postmenopausal women with endometrial cancer. J Clin Endocrinol Metab 74:172, 1992.

Ovarian cancer: screening, treatment, and follow-up. NIH Consensus Statement 1994. JAMA 273:491, 1995.

Parazzini F, Franceschi S, La Vecchia C, Fasoli M: The epidemiology of ovarian cancer. Gynecol Oncol 43:9, 1991a.

Parazzini F, La Vecchia C, Bocciolone L, Franceschi S: The epidemiology of endometrial cancer. Gynecol Oncol 41: 1, 1991b.

Parker SL, Tong T, Bolden S, Wingo PA: Cancer statistics, 1997. CA Cancer J Clin 47:5, 1997.

Pearce KF, Haefner HK, Sarwar SF, Nolan TE: Cytopathological findings on vaginal Papanicolaou smears after hysterectomy for benign gynecologic disease. N Engl J Med 335:1559, 1996.

Peters RK, Mack TM, Bernstein L: Parallels in the epidemiology of selected anogenital carcinomas. J Natl Cancer Inst 72:609, 1984.

Peters RK, Thomas D, Hagan DC, et al: Risk factors for invasive cervical cancer among Latinas and non-Latinas in Los Angeles County. J Natl Cancer Inst 77:1063, 1986.

Peters RK, Thomas D, Skultin G, Henderson BE: Invasive squamous cell carcinoma of the cervix after recent negative cytologic test results—a distinct subgroup? Am J Obstet Gynecol 158:926, 1988.

Piver MS, Jishi MF, Tsukada Y, Nava G: Primary peritoneal carcinoma after prophylactic oophorectomy in women with a family history of ovarian cancer. Cancer 71:2751, 1993.

Pretorius R, Binstock M, Sadeghi M, Hodges W: Cervical and vaginal smears suggestive of adenocarcinoma. J Reprod Med 41:478, 1996.

Pride GL, Schultz AE, Chuprevich TW, Buchler DA: Primary invasive squamous carcinoma of the vagina. Obstet Gynecol 53:218, 1979.

Richart RM: Screening techniques for cervical neoplasia. Clin Obstet Gynecol 22:701, 1979.

Rose DP, Boyar AP, Wynder EL: International comparisons of mortality rates for cancer of the breast, ovary, prostate and colon, and per capita food consumption. Cancer 58: 2363, 1986.

Rosen PP, Groshen S, Kinne DW, Hellman S: Nonmammary malignant neoplasms in patients with stage I ($T_1N_0M_0$) and stage II ($T_1N_1M_0$) breast carcinoma: a long-term follow-up study. Am J Clin Oncol 12:369, 1989.

Rubin GL, Peterson HB, Lee NC, et al: Estrogen replacement therapy and the risk of endometrial cancer: remaining controversies. Am J Obstet Gynecol 162:148, 1990.

Salazar H, Godwin AK, Daly MB, et al: Microscopic benign and invasive malignant neoplasms and a cancer-prone phenotype in prophylactic oophorectomies. J Natl Cancer Inst 88:1810, 1996.

Schiffman MH, Brinton LA: The epidemiology of cervical carcinogenesis. Cancer 76:1888, 1995.

Schildkraut JM, Thompson WD: Familial ovarian cancer: a population-based case-control study. Am J Epidemiol 128: 456, 1988.

Schwartz SM, Weiss NS, Daling JR, et al: Incidence of histologic types of uterine sarcoma in relation to menstrual and reproductive history. Int J Cancer 49:362, 1991.

Shy K, Chu J, Mandelson M, et al: Papanicolaou smear screening interval and risk of cervical cancer. Obstet Gynecol 74:838, 1989.

Silverberg E: Statistical and Epidemiological Information on Gynecological Cancer. New York, American Cancer Society, 1986.

Smith DC, Prentice R, Thompson DJ, Herrmann WL: Association of exogenous estrogen and endometrial carcinoma. N Engl J Med 293:1164, 1975.

Thomas DB, Chu J: Nutritional and endocrine factors in reproductive organ cancers: opportunities for primary prevention. J Chronic Dis 39:1031, 1986.

Tobachman JK, Tucker MA, Kane R: Intraabdominal carcinomatosis after prophylactic oophorectomy in ovarian cancer-prone families. Lancet 2:795, 1982.

Tretli S, Haldorsen T: A cohort analysis of breast cancer, uterine corpus cancer, and childbearing pattern in Norwegian women. J Epidemiol Community Health 44:215, 1990.

van Nagell Jr JR, DePriest PD, Gallion HH, et al: Ovarian cancer screening. Cancer 71:1523, 1993.

Walker AH, Ross RWC, Henderson BE: Hormonal factors and risk of ovarian germ cell cancer in young women. Br J Cancer 57:418, 1988.

Whittemore AS, Gong G, Itnyre J: Prevalence and contribution of BRCA1 mutations in breast cancer and ovarian cancer: results from three U.S. population-based case-control studies of ovarian cancer. Am J Hum Genet 60: 496, 1997.

Wilbur DC, Cibas ES, Merritt S, et al: Thin-Prep processed clinical trials demonstrate an increase detection rate of abnormal cervical cytology specimens. Am J Clin Pathol 101:209, 1994.

Winkelstein W: Smoking and cervical cancer, current status: a review. Am J Epidemiol 131:945, 1991.

Wynder EL, Escher GC, Mantel N: An epidemiologic investigation of cancer of the endometrium. Cancer 19:489, 1966.

Yajima A, Mori T, Sato S, et al: Mass screening for cancer of the uterine cervix in Miyagi prefecture. Obstet Gynecol 59:565, 1982.

Zucker PK, Kasdon EJ, Feldstein ML: The validity of Pap smear parameters as predictors of endometrial pathology in menopausal women. Cancer 56:2256, 1985.

Zunzunegui MW, King M-C, Coria CF, Charlet J: Male influences on cervical cancer risk. Am J Epidemiol 123:302, 1986.

Zurawski VR, Sjovall K, Schoenfeld DA, et al: Prospective evaluation of serum CA-125 levels in a normal population, phase I: the specificities of single and serial determinations in testing for ovarian cancer. Gynecol Oncol 36:299, 1990.

2

Premalignant and Related Disorders of the Lower Genital Tract

Duane E. Townsend
Revised by C. Paul Morrow

HUMAN PAPILLOMAVIRUS (HPV) INFECTION

General Considerations

Condylomata acuminata, also known as anogenital or venereal warts, are caused by a family of highly infectious, primarily sexually transmitted variants of the human papillomavirus (HPV). Three benign epithelial lesions of the female genital tract attributed to HPV have been described: (1) the typical verrucous or papillary (filiform or acuminate) wart, (2) the flat or intraepithelial condyloma (grade 1, squamous intraepithelial neoplasia), and (3) the giant condyloma (the so-called cauliflower wart). Multiple sites of involvement are common. The presence of extensive warts suggests an immune-suppressed state such as pregnancy, organ transplantation, diatetes, or an immune deficiency disease (e.g., acquired immunodeficiency syndrome [AIDS]).

During the past two decades, the prevalence of anogenital warts has reached epidemic proportions. The accumulating evidence that certain HPV subtypes can be oncogenic in humans has intensified the general concern regarding the prevalence of HPV infections. HPV types 16, 18, and 33 are usually associated with invasive cervical carcinoma as well as the more severe, aneuploid dysplasias. The Bowenoid dysplasias of the vulva and anus are typically associated with HPV type 16. Types 6, 11, 42, 43, and 44, which do not integrate into the DNA of the infected cells, occur primarily in the lesser dysplasias and benign condylomas, which

have a polyploid DNA distribution. Since aneuploidy confers a substantial risk of progression, and since polyploidy is associated with regression, the oncogenic risk of HPV infection is, among other things, dependent upon the infecting viral strain (Ferenczy, 1995; Kiviat, 1996; Stoler, 1996).

There are numerous approaches to the treatment of anogenital warts, none of which is entirely satisfactory because of the high failure rate attributable to latent virus infection of the surrounding epithelium (Table 2–1). Topical chemical therapies are trichloroacetic acid (TCA), which coagulates the condylomatous tissue, and podophyllin, which is an antimitotic agent. A solution of podofilox (podophyllotoxin), the active ingredient in podophyllin, is available (Condylox). This preparation, unlike podophyllin, can be applied by the patient. TCA is not absorbed and can therefore be employed in pregnancy, whereas podophyllotoxin is absorbed systemically and cannot be used in pregnancy. Furthermore, podophyllotoxin cannot be applied to a large surface area because systemic neuro- and bone marrow toxicity may result. Topical 5-fluorouracil (5-FU; Efudex) has also been used successfully to treat anogenital warts, but systemic absorption occurs and ulceration of the vagina and vulva can be a serious problem. Courses of 5-FU are repeated only after complete healing occurs. In general, local treatments are repeated until the condyomas are gone or resistance develops. None of the topical chemicals is appropriate for treatment of heavily keratinized lesions. Condylomas can also be treated by surgical means such as laser abla-

TABLE **2–1**

Nonsurgical Treatment Methods for Anogenital Warts*

Therapeutic Modality	Regimen or Dose	Site of Treatment	Precautions
Trichloroacetic acid (TCA)	50–75% solution applied to lesions weekly in office	Vulva, vagina, cervix	Do not apply to large area of vagina
0.5% Podofilox (Condylox)	Patient applies b.i.d. × 3 days; repeat after 4 days rest up to 4 cycles	Vulva	Not in pregnancy Not perianal Not large areas (<10 cm²)
5% 5-FU (efudex)†	1–2 times/day × 7; repeat in 7–10 days; 1/4 applicator full nightly × 3	Vulva Vagina	Not in pregnancy
Interferon alfa-2b (Intron A)	1 million IU/wart (max. 5) 3 times/week for 3 weeks Intralesional	Vulva	Resistant warts "Flu" syndrome Not in pregnancy
Interferon alfa-n3 (Alferon N)	250,000 IU/wart, (max. 10) 2 times/week for up to 8 weeks Intralesional	Vulva	See Intron A
Aldara 5% (Imiquimod)	Cream applied to lesions 3 times/week h.s. maximum 16 weeks	Vulva, anus	Wash with mild soap and water after 6–10 hours

*Data from: Baker et al (1990), Gall (1995), Hatch (1995), Schering Corporation, Purdue Frederick Company, Oclassen Pharmaceuticals, Inc.
†Off-label use of drug.

tion, liquid nitrogen, electrodessication, loop electrosurgical excision procedure (LEEP), or scalpel excision. Warts resistant or not amenable to these therapies can sometimes be treated successfully with intralesional or intramuscular interferon. There are two alpha-interferons produced commercially and approved for treatment of condylomata acuminata: interferon alfa-2b (Intron A) and interferon alfa-n3 (Alferon N Injection). Interferon therapy is commonly attended by a "flu-like" syndrome of variable severity, depending upon the dose, but seldom necessitates cessation of treatment. Imiquimod is an immune response modifier that induces cytokine activity including interferon-α.

Vulvar Condylomas

The spiculated or filiform perineal warts are usually managed initially with podofilox or bitrichloroacetic acid applications (Baker et al, 1990; Hatch, 1995). If the warts fail to regress with chemical therapy, biopsy should be performed a month or so after the last treatment (podophyllin preparations may cause a transient, dysplasia-like change in the wart). Since the incubation period of HPV infection is 3 to 12 weeks or longer, new lesions may develop under treatment, and these should not be considered as treatment failures. The management of a typical case also requires treatment for associated infections such as trichomonas and monilia. Twice-daily direct application of Efudex (5%

5-FU) to vulvar warts for 1 week, repeated on a 2 to 3 week cycle, has been reported to be highly effective (Pride, 1990).

Refractory lesions that have been proven on biopsy not to be malignant can be managed by destructive therapy such as laser or electrocautery. Intramuscular and intralesional interferon therapy has been reported to be effective in clearing 30 to 50 percent of resistant genital warts (Gall, 1995). Long-standing giant condylomas and squamous papillomas (Fig. 2–1) do not respond to chemical therapy. Excision with a knife, laser, or wire loop cautery is recommended after adequate tissue sampling has excluded the presence of carcinoma.

Flat condylomas of the vulva may be similar in clinical appearance to the dysplastic lesions of Bowenoid papulosis, and consequently biopsy diagnosis is recommended. Treatment of flat condylomas is primarily by laser vaporization or excision with loop cautery. This may be accomplished in the office under local anesthesia when there are few lesions, but extensive disease requires regional or general anesthesia. The treatment depth should be about 1 mm since the lesions are intraepithelial. For the first month after therapy, intercourse is interdicted.

Vaginal Condylomas

Condylomata acuminata of the vagina may be isolated, but most are associated with cervical and/or vulvar condylomas, with which they

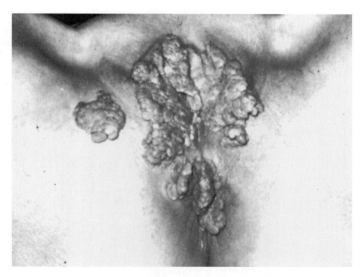

FIGURE 2–1. Giant condylomas. These cauliflower-like growths have been present for over 30 years. When removed from the patient, who was 65 years of age, foci of severe squamous dysplasia were present. This form of condyloma does not respond to medical therapy.

share many common features. Their occurrence in conjunction with high-grade dysplasia is frequent. Vaginal condylomas of the spiculated variety generally present with vaginal discharge and pruritus, whereas flat (intraepithelial) condylomas are often detected only by routine cytology.

Evaluation begins with a careful gross examination of the vulva and anus. Next the vagina is thoroughly palpated. Some condylomas will feel like grains of sand. Colposcopy with acetic acid solution and Lugol staining is then performed, with directed biopsies of the vagina and cervix if any atypical areas are noted. TCA treatment of fresh filiform condylomas can be successful if only a few lesions are present. Extensive papillary lesions and the "flat" wart are best managed by intravaginal 5-FU. One-fourth applicator full (1.5 gm) of Efudex is inserted into the vagina on three consecutive nights. The patient applies petrolatum around the introitus and on the perineum for protection against leakage of the Efudex, which may cause painful perineal ulcerations. Careful monitoring of the patient for vaginal ulceration is recommended to avoid vaginal damage and stricture. In some series laser vaporization has been relatively ineffective. Vaporizing extensive areas of the vaginal epithelium may produce stenosis.

Cervical Condylomas

The cervix is involved less frequently with the typical spiculated venereal wart. Consequently, the high frequency of cervical HPV

lesions was not appreciated until the 1970s, when Meisels and associates first described the flat condyloma (Meisels and Fortin, 1976; Meisels and Morin, 1981). The inconspicuous epithelial hyperplasia and cytologic abnormalities characteristic of flat condylomas closely resemble mild squamous dysplasia clinically, colposcopically, cytologically, and histologically. Thus it is not surprising that the true nature of CIN I remained unknown until the technology to identify the HPV virus was developed.

Diagnosis

Flat condylomas develop within as well as outside the transformation zone. They are not usually visible until acetic acid is applied, after which they turn white. The typical colposcopic features include a micropapillary contour, inconspicuous vascular patterns, feathered margins, satellite lesions, and a shiny snow-white color (Reid and Scalzi, 1985). Biopsy is required to document the nature of the lesion. An intimate admixture of flat condylomas and higher grade dysplasia is common. Histologically, the distinctive feature of the intraepithelial condyloma is koilocytosis accompanied by atypism, multinucleation, acanthosis, and parakeratosis (Fig. 2–2).

Management

Although many flat condylomas (CIN I) regress spontaneously, it is advisable to treat those that persist longer than 6 months, es-

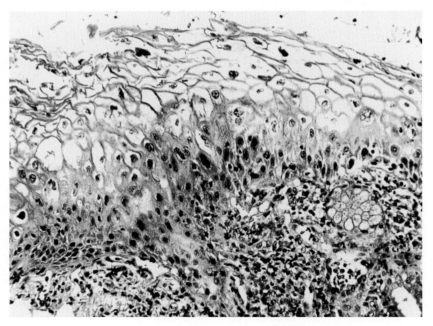

FIGURE 2–2. Cervical intraepithelial (flat) condyloma. Characteristic vacuolization and ballooning of the upper cell layer is termed *koilocytosis*. In the parabasal cells there is nuclear enlargement without abnormal mitoses. This lesion is now included in the term CIN I.

pecially when follow-up may be unreliable, because there is no satisfactory way to determine which are potentially malignant. Tests that identify the various types of HPV are relatively expensive, and it has not been demonstrated that typing has a clinically useful role in determining management of patients with suspected or documented HPV-related disease.

The treatment for cervical condylomas, whether flat or papillary, is by destruction or excision. Laser vaporization, cryosurgery, and LEEP have all been shown to be effective. The last has the advantage of a specimen for pathologic examination. It is no longer recommended that the patient's sexual partner be examined routinely. The reinfection/failure rate is not influenced by treatment of the sexual partner. Should a monogamous woman have several relapses, however, it might be prudent to examine her partner. The success rate of treating flat condylomas of the cervix is somewhat better than that of high-grade cervical dysplasia. The patient should be examined 2 to 3 months after treatment, allowing for resolution of the reparative process, which might be misinterpreted as persistent disease on the Pap smear (see section on "Cervical Intraepithelial Neoplasia").

VULVAR DYSTROPHIES

Classification and Definition

The 1987 International Society for the Study of Vulvar Diseases (ISSVD) classification of vulvar dystophies divides these disorders into non-neoplastic and neoplastic categories. The former includes lichen sclerosus, squamous cell hyperplasia, and other dermatoses. All vulvar intraepithelial malignancies, including Paget's disease and in situ melanoma (atypical melanocytic hyperplasia), are placed under the heading of neoplastic disorders (Table 2–2). The squamous dysplasias are subdivided into vulvar intraepithelial neoplasia (VIN) I, II, and III (i.e., mild, moderate, and severe dysplasia). Although the ISSVD recommends against using the term *Bowenoid papulosis*, as discussed later, we believe the term is appropriate since it describes a discrete clinical entity.

The non-neoplastic vulvar dermatoses have now been sorted out on a histopathologic basis, providing the clinician with a far simpler, more useful working classification than that based on the gross morphology of these lesions. Instead of the red/white, keratinized/nonkeratinized grouping, the more specific

TABLE 2–2

ISSVD Classification of Vulvar Dystrophies

Non-neoplastic disorders
  Lichen sclerosus
  Squamous cell hyperplasia
  Other dermatoses
Neoplastic disorder (in situ)*
  Squamous
    VIN I: mild dysplasia
    VIN II: moderate dysplasia
    VIN III: severe dysplasia and CIS
  Nonsquamous
    Paget's disease
    Melanoma in situ (level 1)

*VIN = vulvar intraepithelial neoplasia; CIS = carcinoma in situ.

diagnostic categories of lichen sclerosus (LS) (formerly lichen sclerosus et atrophicus [LSA]), squamous cell hyperplasia (formerly hyperplastic dystrophy), and mixed forms, all with or without dysplasia, are determined by tissue biopsy. The treatment is based on the specific histologic diagnosis and the presence or absence of dysplasia. In general, when VIN II or III is present, ablation or resection is indicated, whereas medical therapy predominates in the absence of significant dysplasia. The goals of treatment are to relieve symptoms, to prevent the development of carcinoma, and to restore tissue normalcy. In most instances, these goals can be achieved only in part.

Lichen Sclerosus

Etiology

Lavery and Pinkerton (1983) have proposed that the hyperplastic, atrophic, and mixed dystrophies are phases of a single disease process most likely of autoimmune origin. The association of LS with autoimmune phenomena is well documented. Various authors have reported an increased incidence of achlorhydria, vitiligo, diabetes, thyroiditis, pernicious anemia, and antibodies to gastric parietal cells and intrinsic factor in patients with LS (Harrington and Dunsmore, 1981). Meyrick-Thomas et al (1982) found that 75 percent of their LS study group had at least one autoantibody and 20 percent had evidence of an autoimmune disease. Fifteen instances of familial LS have been documented, with evidence suggesting a human leukocyte antigen (HLA) linkage (Friedrich and Mac-Laren, 1984).

Lavery and Pinkerton suggest that the association of LS with achlorhydria may result from abnormal levels of gastrointestinal hormones, especially urogastrone. This peptide in excess inhibits the production of hydrochloric acid while stimulating the production of epidermal growth factor. The latter, it is postulated, causes hypertrophy of the vulvar skin accompanied by increased levels of somatostatin, a neurotransmitter, which in turn causes pruritus. The high somatostatin levels then induce atrophic changes in the skin. In this scenario, there tends to be an alternation between the atrophic and hypertrophic states, with a mixture of the two at times. Lavery and Pinkerton report that such reversals do occur. Furthermore, they have found high levels of somatostatin in vulvar skin that had progressed from the hypertrophic to the atrophic state.

Because skin, especially genital and axillary skin, is stimulated by testosterone, it has been considered that LS, an atrophic condition, might represent target tissue failure. The response of skin to testosterone has been shown to be dependent upon its capacity for converting testosterone to dihydrotestosterone (DHT) by the enzyme 5-alpha-reductase. Friedrich and Kalra (1984) measured serum hormone levels in 10 patients with LS. Significantly lower levels of DHT, androstenedione, and free testosterone were detected. Women with complete testicular feminization have absent 5-alpha-reductase activity in their vulvar skin. While their skin does show features similar to those of LS histologically, these women do not seem to be at greater risk for developing the full-blown clinical picture of LS. Thus the etiology of LS is more complicated than end-organ insensivity to androgen.

Clinical Features

LS occurs predominantly in postmenopausal women, although it is occasionally encountered in the reproductive age group and rarely in children. The predominant symptoms are pruritus, which may be severe, and dyspareunia. There is a progressive loss of tissue elasticity with narrowing of the introitus, causing cracking or fissuring, especially with intercourse. The typical distribution is in a figure-of-eight or hourglass configuration over the glabrous vulvar skin, perineal body, and perianal region. Extragenital involvement is quite unusual. The labia minora become effaced or obliterated, while progressive phi-

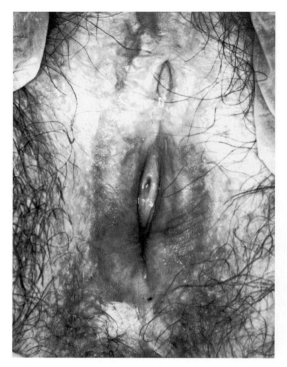

FIGURE 2–3. Lichen sclerosus. Typical features are the symmetrical involvement of the glabrous vulvar skin, effacement of the labia minora, phimosis, introital stenosis, and a shiny, parchment-like skin. Perianal involvement is common.

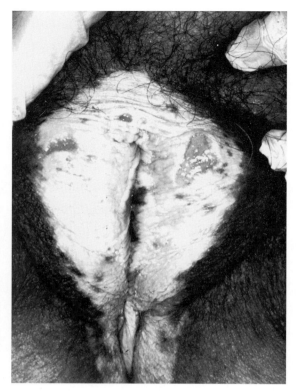

FIGURE 2–4. Lichen sclerosus. Hyperkeratosis and ulceration in this case are due to scratching. The most frequent symptom of this disorder is pruritus, which is often severe.

mosis tends to bury the clitoris under the atrophic, shiny mucosa (Fig. 2–3). Visible changes secondary to scratching, such as ulceration, ecchymoses, edema, and hyperkeratosis, can be extensive (Fig. 2–4). Approximately 5 percent of cases have an associated vulvar carcinoma at presentation (DiPaola, 1980). As Wallace (1971) reported, based on his experience with 290 cases, there is a long-term risk of vulvar cancer of a similar magnitude.

Management

The diagnosis is established by adequate biopsy, typically requiring tissue from several areas, to exclude the presence of an associated dysplasia or carcinoma. Medical therapy is the treatment of choice for LS (Table 2–3). Both surgery and laser therapy have a high failure rate. For many years topical testosterone propionate has been the first line of therapy, but studies indicate that, at least for the more advanced cases, treatment with the superpotent corticosteroid clobetasol propionate cream (Temovate) is superior. In a ran-

domized trial involving 79 patients with longstanding LS, Bracco et al (1993) compared the efficacy of clobetasol, testosterone, progesterone, and a nonmedicated cream. In the clobetasol group 75 percent of the women achieved remission of symptoms, compared to 20 percent in the testosterone-treated group. Clobetasol was the only therapy in the study producing a statistically significant improvement in the gross lesions of the vulva.

The variability in the reported success of these agents probably reflects differences in the severity of the study populations. Using a graded scoring system for symptoms and visible changes due to LS, Cattaneo et al (1991) observed in a study group of 138 patients that 80 percent or more with a score of 1 or 2 had improvement or remission with 2% testosterone propionate. In contrast, only half the patients with a score of 3 had symptomatic relief with this therapy and less than 20 percent had regression of the vulvar lesions. The severe cases accounted for approximately 20 percent of the total group.

T A B L E 2–3

Management of Lichen Sclerosus of the Vulva*

Severe lichen sclerosus
  0.05% clobetasol propionate cream (Temovate; 45-gm tube)
  Maximum 2 gm/day
  b.i.d. applications for 1–2 months; *then*
  Twice weekly applications for 2 months; *then*
  Clobetasol or a less potent steriod p.r.n
  Reinstitute clobetasol therapy for significant excerbation of symptoms
Mild to moderate lichen sclerosus
  2% testosterone propionate in petrolatum can be used instead of clobetasol therapy
  b.i.d. or t.i.d. applications for 6–12 weeks until optimal symptom relief is achieved; then reduce gradually to 1–2 times weekly

*Data from Bracco et al (1993) and Cattaneo et al (1991).

When the patient presents with severe vulvar pruritus, pain, burning, traumatic excoriations, and ecchymoses (purpura), in the absence of an obvious cancer, biopsy can be deferred until the local conditions are more favorable. Treatment is begun with 0.05% clobetasol propionate cream (45-gm tube) as described in Table 2–3. Because the pruritus is typically most severe during the night, an application at bedtime is recommended. During the first few days more frequent application of the cream may be necessary to break the scratch-itch cycle. This is very important since the scratching results in more intense itching. With the pruritus under control, the vulvar edema will subside, the ulcerations heal, and the hyperkeratosis abate. This may take 10 to 14 days, after which the vulva can be re-examined and the biopsies taken. In the absence of dysplasia and carcinoma, the steroid therapy is continued until maximum benefit is obtained. Breakthrough pruritus over the long term is managed with 0.5 to 2% hydrocortisone cream or a more potent agent, depending upon the severity of the symptoms. Moderate- to low-potency steroid preparations are preferable because chronic use does not damage the skin. If significant dysplasia is present on biopsy, treatment should be the same as for VIN. Monitoring for the appearance of carcinoma is advised (Rodke et al, 1988).

Topical testosterone propionate 0.5 to 3% in petrolatum has been the standard treatment of LS for many years but, as alluded to earlier, it is only effective for the mild to moderate cases. In the severe cases it not only does not work well, but often the patients cannot tolerate it except in attenuated doses. The medication is applied two to three times daily for 6 to 12 weeks. Once optimal symptom control is achieved the frequency of application is gradually reduced until a maintenance regimen of once or twice weekly is reached. Discontinuation of therapy may be followed by a recrudescence of symptoms. When used diligently, testosterone is reported to be highly effective for symptomatic relief. DiPaola (1980) observed a 95 percent success rate with respect to pruritus control among 121 patients, and 75 percent had remission of dyspareunia. In a literature review, Friedrich (1985) noted that 65 percent of 85 patients got complete relief of their symptoms and a similar percentage had complete clearance of the vulvar changes.

Testosterone has a number of side effects that are related to the frequency and duration of use. Among these are increased pubic and facial hair, enlargement of the clitoris, enhanced libido, acne, hoarseness, burning, and ulceration. For some patients, one or more of these side effects are intolerable or unacceptable.

An alternative to topical testosterone propionate is topical progesterone in oil (Jasionowsky and Jasionowsky, 1979). This agent appears to be similar in its overall effectiveness but slower in its action. Consequently, when pruritus is a problem, alternating progesterone with a corticosteroid may be desirable. Progesterone is particularly suitable in treating the child with symptomatic LS, since the side effects of testosterone are especially undesirable in children. The formulation is 200 mg of progesterone in 2 oz of hydrophilic ointment. In the event of corticosteroid and testosterone failure, progesterone and other medications may be tried, but they are unlikely to be successful.

Vulvar dystrophies characterized by prominent keratin production ("leukoplakia") have been treated with some success by the topical application of 13-*cis*-retinoic acid (tretinoin; Retin A) an agent marketed for the treatment of acne vulgaris. Its action appears to decrease the cohesiveness of the epithelial cells, producing a "peel." Severe local irritation (erythema, edema, blistering) may occur if it is applied to eczematous skin. Clinical studies indicate that one or two daily applications of the 0.05% cream formulation for 1 to 3 months can produce a partial or complete clearance of the skin lesions in 50 percent of cases (Markowska and Wiese, 1992; Kwasniewski et al, 1993).

A proven method to relieve the itching of LS, usually for 1 or more years, is the injection, under general or regional anesthesia, of 0.1 to 0.3 ml of absolute ethyl alcohol at the intersections of a 1-cm grid drawn on the vulva. If it is not done properly, however, tissue necrosis may result (Ward and Sutherst, 1976; Woodruff and Babaknia, 1979). Another alternative is the Mering (1956) procedure, which involves "extremely wide undercutting of the vulvar skin" to sever the nerves and "increase the vascularity" of the region. Complete relief of symptoms for 1 or more years, often with restoration of the vulvar tissues toward normal, was reported in 33 of 38 cases. It is generally agreed that this should be a procedure of last resort.

Squamous Cell Hyperplasia

Squamous cell hyperplasia (SCH), a term replacing "hyperplastic dystrophy," includes those dermatoses formerly called neurodermatitis, hyperplastic vulvitis, and lichen simplex chronicus. Friedrich (1971) and DiPaola (1980) believe that SCH results from external irritants such as nylon underwear, soaps, detergents, hygienic sprays, douches, tight clothes, and/or perspiration. From 25 to 50 percent of vulvar dystrophies are of the SCH variety. These patients tend to be younger than those with LS. The disease is unifocal and always exhibits evidence of hyperkeratosis. SCH and mixed dystrophies are more often associated with dysplasia or carcinoma than is pure LS. For this reason, their malignant potential is considered to be greater than that of LS.

Recommendations for treatment include excision (DiPaola, 1980), corticosteroids (Kaufman et al, 1974; Friedrich, 1977; Lavery and Pinkerton, 1983), or testosterone with or without corticosteroids (Birch, 1984). Lavery and Pinkerton found testosterone to cause a marked aggravation of the pruritus in all patients with SCH. Our recommended therapy for SCH, after dysplasia and carcinoma was excluded, is clobetasol, employing the same regimen as for severe LS. The response is usually rapid, with clearing of the lesions within 6 weeks. Recurrence is unusual. If more than mild dysplasia is present on biopsy, treatment should be the same as for VIN. A mixture of SCH and LS may be seen. This most likely represents LS with hyperplastic changes secondary to scratching.

VULVAR INTRAEPITHELIAL NEOPLASIA (VIN)

Clinical Features

VIN occurs in women from the teenage years to the ninth decade in life. The mean age at diagnosis is 43 years, but it has declined by 10 or more years during the past two decades. One half of the cases have multiple lesions (multifocal) and one fourth or more also involve the cervix or vagina (multicentric). Multicentric squamous neoplasia of the lower genital tract may be either synchronous or metachronous. The etiology of VIN is unknown, but clinically the patients can be subdivided into two groups: (1) premenopausal women (average age 35 years) with extensive, multifocal, warty or basaloid, HPV-positive lesions (Bowenoid papulosis) (Figs. 2–5 and 2–6); and (2) predominantly postmenopausal women with unifocal, HPV-negative keratinizing lesions. Nearly all lesions of Bowenoid papulosis are HPV positive, usually type 16, and a history of or concomitant condylomata acuminata is common. The HPV-associated cases occur predominantly in cigarette smokers (Friedrich et al, 1980; Jones et al, 1990; Andersen et al, 1991; Park et al, 1991; Rusk et al, 1991; Crum, 1992; Kurman et al, 1993; Kaufman, 1995).

The most common presenting symptom is pruritus, which is reported in up to 60 percent of patients, while 25 to 50 percent of cases are diagnosed during routine gynecologic examination. There is an increased incidence of VIN among women with HIV, chronic lymphocytic leukemia, and other conditions associated with long-term immune suppression, such as corticosteroid and organ transplant therapy.

Malignant Potential

Untreated VIN clearly has the potential for conversion to invasive carcinoma. For women over age 40, the risk is undisputed and may approach 100 percent with sufficient follow-up (Jones et al, 1990). However, among younger women several cases of spontaneous remission have been reported. Furthermore, numerous cases have been observed for a period of years without progression. This has led to the speculation that VIN, especially multifocal VIN in young women, is a benign, self-limited manifestation of a viral

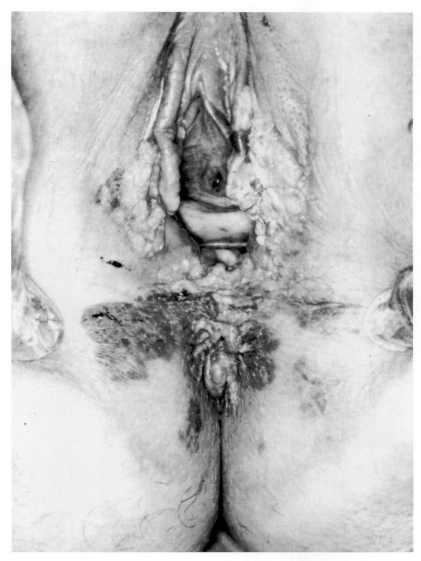

FIGURE 2–5. Vulvar dysplasia. Lesions tend to be symmetrical and are frequently multifocal. Involvement of the perianal skin and anal mucosa is common. In this patient the lesions of the labia minora are keratinized; those around the anus are pigmented.

(HPV) infection. However, the reported cases of spontaneous remission have invariably been associated with pregnancy and/or condylomata acuminata in women under 30 years of age. Further evidence of the malignant potential of Bowenoid papulosis is the fact that about 10 percent of reported cases have foci of microinvasion upon histologic examination (Fig. 2–7), and some cases present with one or more areas of frankly invasive carcinoma (Forney et al, 1977; Friedrich et al, 1980; Wilkinson et al, 1981; Benedet and Murphy, 1982; Ulbright et al, 1982; Bernstein et al, 1983; Crum et al, 1984; Hørding et

al, 1995). A similar condition has been described in young males (Patterson et al, 1986). It is multifocal and pigmented and occurs on the shaft of the penis.

Findings and Evaluation

Single lesions are predominantly located in the navicular fossa, the adjacent mucosa of the vestibule, and the labia minora. Occasionally unifocal VIN occurs on the posterior perineum or in the periclitoral region. It is distinctly unusual for single lesions to be confined to the hair-bearing skin of the vulva

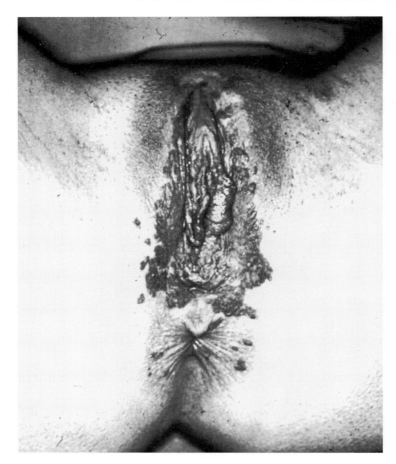

FIGURE 2–6. Pigmented vulvar squamous dysplasia. The color varies in different patients from light brown to violaceous to mahogany. Even the small perianal lesions were severely dysplastic on histologic evaluation. Typically, VIN lesions are sharply demarcated from the surrounding normal skin. Appearance is consistent with "Bowenoid papulosis."

or glans clitoridis. Multifocal VIN typically involves the clitoral prepuce, labia minora, navicular fossa, and perineal body. The labia majora and/or the posterior perineum are involved in one half to one third of these cases. When the posterior perineum is involved, the disease almost invariably extends beyond the anus to the intergluteal cleft. In addition, the mucosa of the anal canal is often involved, in which case the dysplasia may extend up the anal canal to the squamocolumnar junction (Kaplan et al, 1981; Schlaerth et al, 1984). Involvement of the glans clitoridis or urethra is rare.

The lesions of Bowenoid papulosis may be multiple and discrete, or confluent. Typically they are raised, often papular in configuration, with distinct borders and a granular surface. The color is gray, white, or pigmented, depending upon the race or complexion of the patient, and the lesions may have a shiny, smooth surface. Heavy keratinization is unusual. Bowenoid papulosis can be misinterpreted clinically as condylomata acuminata (Fig. 2–7), although the lesions never have the configuration typical of the filiform or acuminate wart. Individual lesions of pigmented Bowenoid papulosis and pigmented unifocal VIN can mimic the nevocellular nevus and seborrheic keratosis. VIN in the absence of keratinization and pigmentation may have the same color as the background mucosa or skin, making it remarkably inapparent to causal observation.

Single lesions of VIN generally have clinical features similar to those of Bowenoid papulosis, but are less often pigmented and more often keratinized. Rarely, when the vestibule is involved, the VIN may be red and velvety in character, the so-called erythroplasia of Queyrat.

Localization of the lesions of VIN in almost all cases can be satisfactorily accomplished with the alert, trained naked eye. However, magnification with a hand lens or the colposcope can be of value in identifying very small lesions (Fig. 2–8). This is facilitated by the application of 3 to 5% acetic acid (vine-

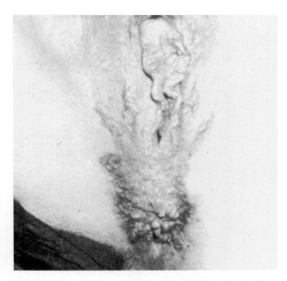

FIGURE 2–7. Extensive perineal dysplasia in a 43-year-old woman. She had been treated intermittently over a 7-year period for "warts." The labia minora and majora were also involved, but not the clitoris. Histologically all of the lesions showed dysplasia. Focal invasion (<1 mm) was present in the perianal region. Treatment consisted of excision of the involved skin and mucous membranes followed by split-thickness skin grafting. The donor site was the right buttock.

gar). The acetic acid may cause burning that can be quite painful in the presence of inflammation or excoriation. The acetic acid produces an increased whiteness of certain epithelial lesions, including condylomata acuminata and VIN. The former often have the typical double-loop capillary pattern, but the lesions of VIN seldom have the classic punctation and mosaic vascular patterns of cervical intraepithelial neoplasia (CIN) (Wright and Chapman, 1993).

Toluidine blue staining has been recommended for identifying and localizing the lesions of VIN. The test, however, has largely fallen into disuse because of a high false-negative rate (up to 40 percent) and a 5 to 20 percent false-positive rate, depending upon whether apparently normal or abnormal vulvar epithelium is being stained (Broen and Ostergard, 1971; Friedrich et al, 1980; Mashberg 1980). Keratin will prevent VIN from staining and any ulceration will retain the dye, since it is simply an in vivo nuclear stain. Lugol's solution can be of minor assistance in localizing the extent of VIN because the mucosa of a well-estrogenized vestibule will take the stain, whereas VIN will not.

The diagnosis of VIN is based upon adequate tissue biopsy and the clinical findings. The most satisfactory method of tissue biopsy is with a 3-mm Keye's or Baker's circular punch. The lesions are characteristically homogeneous in appearance. Sites of keratinization, induration, ulceration, and colposcopically abnormal vascular pattern should be preferentially biopsied. A sufficient number of biopsies of sufficient size must be obtained to exclude the presence of carcinoma. If there is a single lesion less than 1 cm in diameter, then office excision biopsy under local anesthesia is recommended.

Because of the propensity of lower genital tract squamous neoplasia for multicentric involvement, when VIN has been diagnosed, concurrent evaluation as well as long-term follow-up of all patients for CIN, vaginal intraepithelial neoplasia (VAIN), and dysplasia of the posterior perineum is necessary in addition to surveillance for local recurrence.

Treatment

The treatment of significant VIN has undergone major changes in the past two decades. The most important difference is the general recognition that total, simple vulvectomy is seldom warranted and usually contraindicated. In addition, the documentation that spontaneous regression can occur requires that this behavior be recognized in the treatment plan. Thus, the premenopausal woman who has newly diagnosed nonkeratinized, multifocal, or extensive VIN should be observed for a period of at least 6 months after her most recent pregnancy (or systemic steroid therapy) for evidence of regression, unless biopsy indicates that the lesion is aneuploid or invasion is suspected. The more severe the dysplasia, however, the greater is the risk of cancer being already present or developing subsequently (Jones and McLean, 1986; Hørding et al, 1995). Prolonged observation of patients with a VIN III lesion is proportionately less acceptable than for patients with a VIN I lesion.

Unifocal lesions are characteristically confined to the labia minora and intervening mucosa of the introitus. They are preferably treated by laser ablation, although this requires the most expertise in pretreatment evaluation. At the same time, laser therapy is the least destructive and least mutilating. Surgical and LEEP excision are also applicable. Laser ablation is especially suited to treating

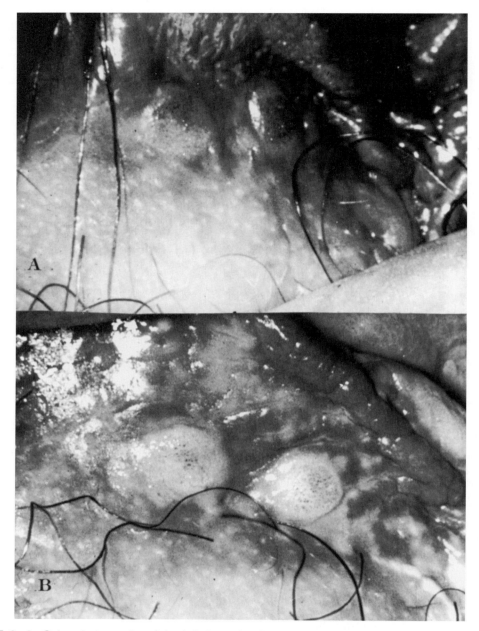

FIGURE 2–8. Colpophotographs of the inferior pole of the right labium majus in a 26-year-old woman with VIN III. *A,* The lesions are barely visible. *B,* The same lesions have been treated with acetic acid. The acetic acid has accentuated the lesions, which are now white and have vascular punctation.

VIN on the labia minora and clitoris. Healing after laser ablation occurs within 2 to 4 weeks, with minimal scarring.

Therapy for extensive VIN has been more controversial. Prior to the 1980s the most widely employed means of treating extensive VIN, while preserving the structure and function of the vulva in a reasonably normal state,

was the skinning vulvectomy with the split-thickness skin graft of Rutledge and Sinclair (1968). During the past decade, several reports have appeared documenting the superiority of laser therapy for very extensive VIN (Bagish and Dorsey, 1981; Townsend et al, 1982b; Leuchter et al, 1984; Reid, 1985). Failure rates appear to be similar to those of surgical therapy. The advantage of laser therapy is successful treatment of extensive disease without the cost and morbidity of skin grafting, and without the scarring that would result from healing by secondary intention after surgical excision. The major disadvantage is the possibility of inadvertently vaporizing early invasive carcinoma. This is of particular concern when dealing with lesions of the posterior perineum, in which as many of 10 percent of patients may have foci of microinvasion (Buscema and Woodruff, 1980; Schlaerth et al, 1984). Nevertheless, with adequate evaluation and proper patient selection, laser therapy is now considered the treatment of choice for extensive VIN.

When the anus is involved, which is frequent in these cases, clinical assessment of the upper limits of the dysplasia is unreliable. Margin checks have often been positive up to and including the squamocolumnar junction at the dentate line (Forney et al, 1977; Kaplan et al, 1981; Schlaerth et al, 1984). In this situation, routine treatment of the entire anal mucosa is recommended. The split-thickness skin graft has produced very good cosmetic and functional results (Fig. 2–9). Laser therapy produces equally effective, if not better, results.

CO_2 laser therapy can be done in the office under local anesthesia in over half of the cases. For extensive disease, regional or general anesthesia is recommended. It is necessary to treat to a depth of 1 to 2 mm for the

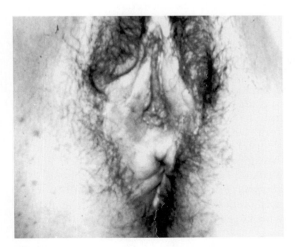

FIGURE 2–9. Skinning vulvectomy. This 24-year-old woman had extensive, severe dysplasia of the vulva and anus. A split-thickness skin graft from the buttock was used to cover the defect, including the anal canal. This picture was taken 1 year after surgery.

non-hair-bearing areas and 2 to 3 mm in the hair-bearing areas, because VIN can involve the skin appendages, especially the hair follicles and associated sebaceous glands. Recurrences are most frequent in untreated areas of the vulva.

Patients often experience much pain following laser vaporization. In addition to oral analgesics, sitz baths with artificial sea salt and 5% tannic acid (two or three tea bags in a quart of lukewarm water) or Epsom salts three to four times a day are helpful. The topical application of povidone-iodine or an antibiotic ointment reduces the chance of infection. Topical and oral analgesics are required for patients who have extensive treatment. Scarring is minimal even when large areas are vaporized (unless the treatment is too deep), and patient acceptance is excellent.

The Cavitron ultrasonic aspirator (CUSA) utilizes ultrasound to precisely and selectively fragment tissue with a high water content. A few investigators have applied the CUSA to the management of vulvar lesions, especially VIN and condylomata acuminata. Wu et al (1992), for example, reported on a series of 24 patients with VIN or vulvar condylomas and noted that the specimen was suitable for limited pathologic evaluation. No follow-up data regarding efficacy were given.

For elderly women, simple vulvectomy with primary closure may be a reasonable choice, especially since the vulva is often shrunken and occult invasion more likely to be present. Most women with extensive VIN are under 40 years of age, however, and more conservative therapy is required. Topical 5-FU has been used. It is frequently unsuccessful, is slow to heal, and in some women causes severe pain. It is not recommended (Lifshitz and Roberts, 1980).

Results

The longer patients with VIN are followed post-treatment, the higher the recurrence rate (Shafi et al, 1989). The interpretation of recurrence rates for specific therapies is difficult because more radical therapies are usually applied to patients with more extensive disease. Roy (1988) reviewed the literature on VIN and reported the following "failure" rates for the various treatments: vulvectomy, 28.8 percent; excision, 26.5 percent; superficial vulvectomy, 46.0 percent; and laser vaporization, 10.9 percent. The recurrence rate for cases with positive margins is substantially higher (70 percent) than that for cases with negative margins (6.5 percent). Patients most likely to have recurrence or new disease at the same or other lower genital tract sites are those with multifocal and extensive unifocal VIN. Such high "recurrence" rates exaggerate the apparent shortcomings of the various treatments for VIN. In the majority of cases recurrent disease consists of one or two focal lesions that are easily dispatched with the laser or local excision in the office. Recurrence has been reported in the graft following vulvar skinectomy (Cox et al, 1986).

VAGINAL INTRAEPITHELIAL NEOPLASIA (VAIN)

Etiology

Preinvasive lesions of the vaginal squamous epithelium occur in only 1 to 3 percent of patients with cervical neoplasia. The majority of women with this lesion, however, have had CIN. In a series of over 50 cases of VAIN reviewed at our institution, 40 percent of the patients had prior and 15 percent coexisting cervical or vulvar neoplasia (Bernstein et al, 1983). As discussed earlier in this chapter, HPV is thought to be a major factor in the etiology of VAIN, as well as in CIN and VIN. Other predisposing causes of VAIN are radiation and immunosuppressive therapy.

In a review of patients developing VAIN after hysterectomy, Ireland and Monaghan (1988) reported the average age to be 50 years. Two thirds of the hysterectomies were done for CIN or invasive carcinoma of the cervix. Among those women developing VAIN following hysterectomy for benign indications, the average time to diagnosis of VAIN was 11 years, whereas VAIN was diagnosed in 40 percent of the cervical neoplasia group within 1 year of hysterectomy. However, VAIN appeared as long as 15 years after surgical treatment for cervical neoplasia. Most cases of VAIN are diagnosed in women who have had a hysterectomy for CIN in the recent or distant past. Occult invasive cancer appears to be more common in this group than in women with VAIN and an intact cervix (Ireland and Monaghan, 1988). One explanation of this phenomenon is that the transformation zone (or undiagnosed VAIN) extends onto the vagina. After hysterectomy, dysplasia develops in this abnormal epithelium buried in the cuff closure or lining the inaccessible angles of the vagina.

Detection and Evaluation

The Pap smear is the single most important means of bringing the preinvasive vaginal lesion to the attention of the physician. A saline-moistened, cotton-tipped applicator or moistened cytology brush is used for cytologic sampling as the speculum is withdrawn and rotated. Vaginal cytology is suggested yearly for those patients who have had a hysterectomy for CIN and every 3 to 5 years if the hysterectomy was done for benign conditions in patients not epidemiologically at high risk for genital tract squamous dysplasia.

One means of evaluating the patient for VAIN is with the colposcope. The vaginal tube is thoroughly moistened with vinegar. To provide an end-on view of the tissues, the speculum is withdrawn and rotated, causing the vaginal mucosa to fold over the end of the speculum blades. The lesions of VAIN are typically white, sharply bordered, and finely granular, often with areas of punctation (Fig. 2–10). Mosaic structure is rarely seen. Evaluation by Lugol's stain is simpler than the colposcopy method. Aqueous Lugol's solution is applied to the vaginal mucosa with a Q-tip or cotton ball. Excess iodine is removed to prevent burning. Lugol's iodine dehydrates the epithelium, so it may be necessary to add a thin film of lubricating jelly in order to reinsert the speculum. The most significant lesions usually stain a light yellow and have sharp borders, in contrast to the mahogany color of the normal mucosa (Fig. 2–11). Less significant lesions have a variegated iodine uptake with indistinct borders.

After the number and distribution of the lesions are determined, biopsies are taken of representative areas. This is seldom painful. If pain is a problem, a vaginal tampon soaked in a topical anesthetic is placed in the vagina for 3 to 5 minutes before proceeding. The patient with postmenopausal or postradiation atrophy of the vaginal mucosa should use intravaginal estrogen cream daily for 2 to 4 weeks before evaluation, because the atrophic epithelium is often difficult to interpret colposcopically and does not stain well with Lugol's solution. Moreover, if the abnormal cytology is due to atrophic cells, the topical estrogen cream will convert the cytology to normal.

The most common location of VAIN is the upper third of the vagina; the middle and lower thirds are involved less than 10 percent of the time. The lesions are often multifocal

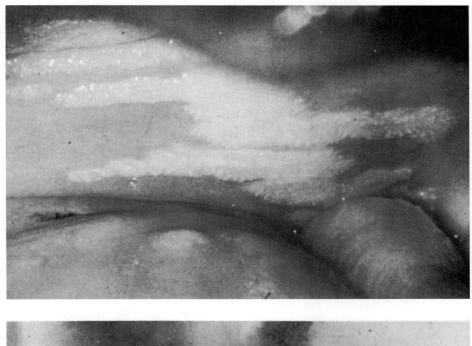

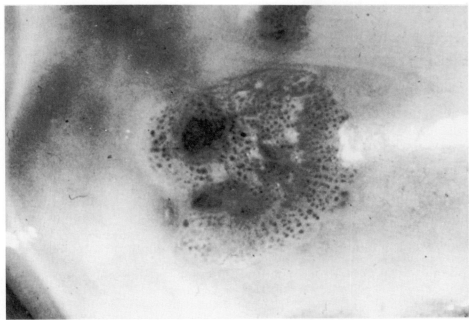

FIGURE 2–10. *A*, Colpophotograph of the right vaginal wall displaying white epithelium. Biopsy results revealed VAIN II (moderate dysplasia). The patient had an abnormal Pap smear, and the cervical examination was negative. The cause of the abnormal Pap smear was in the vagina. Treatment was by CO_2 laser. *B*, Colpophotograph of the apex of the vagina in a 35-year-old woman depicting VAIN III. Note that the lesion is raised, with vascular punctation.

and may be found within the vaginal folds. The posthysterectomy recesses at the 3 and 9 o'clock "corners" are especially common sites for VAIN. In this situation, the fold can be everted with an iris hook or exposed with an endocervical speculum to obtain a satisfactory view. Bimanual rectal–vaginal palpation of the vagina is essential because the patient may have an occult invasive carcinoma, especially at the vaginal cuff.

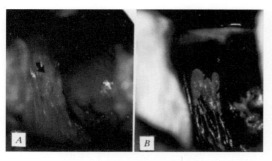

FIGURE 2–11. Multifocal vaginal dysplasia in a patient with an intact uterus. *A,* The most dominant lesion is visible at the arrow. *B,* Note the dramatic contrast provided by iodine staining. The cervix is in the right half of each frame.

Treatment

In the past, irradiation or surgical excision by partial or total vaginectomy have been the standard treatments for VAIN. Although it is effective, there is rarely an indication today for radiation treatment in the management of VAIN. Many of these women are young, and vault radiation may induce ovarian failure. Furthermore, irradiation of the vault can cause vaginal shortening and dyspareunia. For limited VAIN, surgical (Lenehan et al, 1986) or LEEP excision is an effective means of treatment. Shortening of the vagina can result if the excision is very large and the defect is closed. In this case it is better to secure hemostasis and pack the upper vagina, removing the pack the following day. The vaginal epithelium will regenerate, covering the denuded area, although a dilator will probably be necessary to prevent synechiae from forming until healing occurs. For most cases of vaginal dysplasia, however, CO_2 laser vaporization or excision provides a simple and effective means of treatment (Capen et al, 1982; Townsend et al, 1982a; Jobson and Homesley, 1983). It is imperative of course, that invasion be excluded prior to destructive therapy. When doubt exists, VAIN should be excised. Because postmenopausal women are at greater risk for having occult invasion or developing vaginal carcinoma subsequent to therapy for VAIN, these patients in particular require careful evaluation and follow-up. It is also advisable to treat VAIN by excision in this patient population.

The posthysterectomy patient may present a difficult management problem if the VAIN lesions involve the corners of the vaginal cuff. When this situation exists, surgical excision is the treatment of choice, although the laser can be used successfully in favorable situations. Excision of lesions in this location must take into account the close proximity of the ureter. In some cases the abdominal approach is advisable for complete excision and patient safety. Failure to eradicate the entire VAIN lesion carries the risk of invasive cancer developing in addition to recurrent VAIN.

Perhaps the most challenging clinical problem among women with VAIN is multifocal disease involving many levels of the vagina. Total vaginectomy and skin grafting have been used with success, as has radiation therapy. Topical 5% 5-FU (Efudex) has gained popularity because it offers a relatively simple and effective method of eradicating the dysplastic lesions on an outpatient basis without compromise of vaginal function (Petrilli et al, 1980; Stokes et al, 1980; Peters et al, 1985; Krebs, 1989). Approximately 80 percent of patients can expect to have all clinical and cytologic evidence of vaginal dysplasia remit after one or two courses of Efudex therapy. A treatment course consists of one third to one half of an applicator of Efudex inserted to the top of the vagina at bedtime once weekly for 10 weeks. The perineum is protected by applying a coat of zinc oxide paste or petrolatum before each treatment and douching the next morning. The vagina should be well estrogenized during treatment. Because of its simplicity, we recommend topical 5-FU as the treatment of choice for this group of patients.

Follow-up

The major considerations on follow-up are the recurrence of VAIN and the appearance of invasive carcinoma. An initial gynecologic examination and vaginal cytology should be obtained at 3 months post-treatment and thereafter at 6-month intervals. During the early weeks and months after treatment, more frequent visits may be necessary to monitor healing, detect the development of synechiae, and evaluate the vaginal capacity.

CERVICAL INTRAEPITHELIAL NEOPLASIA (CIN)

Classification

Cervical dysplasia is an intraepithelial neoplasm with a variable potential for progression to invasive cancer. The term encom-

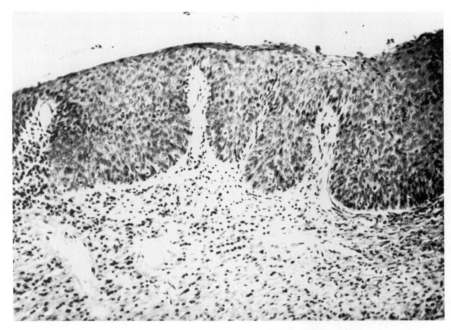

FIGURE 2–12. Photomicrograph of CIN III. Note the complete loss of cellular polarity; all layers are pleomorphic.

passes a continuum of morphologic and molecular changes, from the earliest identifiable abnormalities arising in the deep layers of the stratified squamous epithelium to the appearance of overt malignant features that persist through the full thickness of the epithelium. The progression is arbitrarily subdivided into three phases termed mild, moderate, and severe intraepithelial neoplasia (dysplasia) or CIN I, II, and III (Fig. 2–12). Historically, the term *carcinoma in situ* was reserved for the most severe degree of intraepithelial abnormality, but this term is no longer in favor because of the confusion it causes with respect to the diagnosis of cancer.

Clinical Features

The patients with a diagnosis of CIN are predominantly in the reproductive age group. Typically CIN produces no symptoms, although many patients report vaginal spotting or discharge. Cervical dysplasia has no features visible to the naked eye, with the exception of the occasional keratinizing lesion, which has the appearance of a white plaque. Consequently nearly all cases of cervical dysplasia are detected by screening cervical cytology.

Etiology

There is a great body of experimental and epidemiologic evidence that CIN and cervical carcinoma are caused by various subtypes of HPV in concert with a co-carcinogen such as might be derived from cigarette smoking. HPV, which is thought to be transmitted primarily by sexual contact, is highly infectious, producing initially an intraepithelial or acuminate condyloma of the cervix (vagina or vulva). The histologic and cytologic changes found in these lesions are similar to, if not the same as, those of mild dysplasia. HPV DNA can be detected in virtually all cases of CIN I, II, and III. Predisposing factors are essentially the same as those for invasive carcinoma of the cervix: early age at first intercourse, multiple sexual partners, cigarette smoking, genital HPV or herpes simplex virus infection, oral contraceptive use, and intercourse with a promiscuous male.

Progression to Cancer

It is now believed that CIN I lesions frequently regress spontaneously, and perhaps revert again to dysplasia. This is also true for CIN II, but once the lesion progresses to CIN III it may be irreversible. CIN III carries with it a high risk for progression to invasive carcinoma, which, given a long enough observation period, may approximate 100 percent (Mitchell et al, 1994). The generally accepted idea is that the dysplasia progresses systematically through the mild, moderate, and severe forms before invasion occurs, although there are exceptions, such as the keratinizing lesions. Nasiell and co-workers (1983, 1986) reported that 62 percent of mild and 54 percent of moderate cervical dysplasias regressed to normal with an average follow-up of 39 and 78 months, respectively. Only 16 percent of the mild dysplasias and 30 percent of the moderate dysplasias progressed to severe dysplasia during this time period, and only 0.3 percent of each group progressed to cancer. Syrjänen et al (1992), in a similar study, noted that almost two thirds of mild dysplasias regressed and only 8.5 percent progressed during a median observation period of 70 months. The corresponding figures for CIN III were 38 and 39 percent. The reported transit time from CIN III to invasive carcinoma ranges up to 20 years and longer, and the rate of progression to invasive cancer varies from 20 to 75 percent or more. For example, McIndoe et al (1984) reported that 22 percent of 137 patients with cytologic evidence of dysplasia persistent after cone or punch biopsy developed invasive carcinoma over a median follow-up of 6 years. The rate of progression and regression is strongly associated with HPV type. Thus the majority of high-grade lesions are positive for HPV 16, 18, and 33, whereas types 6 and 11, among others, account for most of the low-grade lesions.

Detection

Cervical cytology is the pre-eminent means for detecting premalignant and malignant changes in the cervix, but there are numerous sources of error (Drake, 1985). The false-negative rate for a single Pap smear is 10 to 20 percent. Thus serial or repetitive screening is necessary for optimal results. Sampling error accounts for about 50 percent of the misses. The most effective method of obtaining a specimen for cervical cytology is to sample the cervical canal with a cytology brush and to sample the ectocervix by scraping it with a spatula. The moistened cotton-tipped applicator, a common instrument for taking a specimen from the endocervical canal, has a false-negative rate substantially higher than that of the cytology brush. Another source of error in cervical cytology is the failure to fix the slide properly. Once the cervical mucus and exfoliated cells have been placed onto the glass slide, the specimen should be cytofixed within a few seconds. Air drying can lead to misinterpretation of subtle details (unless the laboratory requests air-dried smears). Laboratory error accounts for a minority of cytology misses. Consequently, the taking of the Pap smear and fixation are critical steps in assuring optimal results.

The Bethesda Reporting System

The Bethesda classification of cervical cytology (Bethesda System, 1990), reproduced in Appendix III, was developed in order to standardize reporting results, which are considered to be a pathology consultation. Representative frequencies of the major subgroups are given in Table 2–4. Low-grade squamous intraepithelial lesion (SIL) includes cases with cytologic evidence of HPV infection only, evidence of HPV infection with mild dysplasia, and mild dysplasia without specific cytologic evidence of HPV infection. High-grade SIL includes cases suspicious for moderate and severe dysplasia. Squamous cell abnormalities that are more abnormal than those typical of a reparative or inflammatory process, but not severe enough to qualify for dysplasia, are termed "atypical squamous cells of undetermined significance" (ASCUS). Similarly glandular cells with abnormalities exceeding the changes of a reparative or inflammatory process but not consistent with malignancy are classified as AGCUS or AGUS (Isacson and Kurman, 1995; Korn, 1996). The recommendations in the following paragraphs are consistent with the Interim Guidelines developed in 1992 by a National Cancer Institute (NCI) workshop (Kurman et al, 1994).

ASCUS. The percentage of Pap smears in this category varies widely but should not account for more than two to three times the number of cases allotted to low-grade SIL or 5 percent of all Pap smears. This type of smear is rarely associated with invasive carcinoma. After clinical evaluation, the most common diagnoses associated with ASCUS smears are squamous metaplasia and HPV lesions. However, a significant dysplasia may be found in 5 to 20 percent of cases. Kaufman (1996) found that only 9 percent had CIN II/III while 8 percent had CIN I. Our recommended management is follow-up Pap smear in 3 to 6 months for the patient who

TABLE 2–4

Frequency of Various Abnormal Pap Smears Reported by the
Bethesda System*

Cytologic Abnormality[†]	N	Percent of Total
Atypical squamous cells of undetermined significance (ASCUS)	408	3.4
Low-grade SIL (HPV, HPV with mild dysplasia, or mild dysplasia alone)	651	5.5
High-grade SIL (moderate or severe dysplasia/CIS)	288	2.2
Squamous carcinoma	18	0.1
Atypical glandular cells of undetermined significance (AGUS)	94	0.7
Adenocarcinoma	39	0.3

*Based upon 12,789 total smears. From Bottles K, Reiter RC, Steiner AL, et al: Problems encountered with the Bethesda System: the University of Iowa experience. Obstet Gynecol 78: 410, 1991, with permission.
[†]SIL = squamous intraepithelial lesion; HPV = human papillomavirus; CIS = carcinoma in situ.

had a normal Pap smear history, a normal-appearing cervix, and no symptoms, and whose ASCUS designation is not qualified by terms such as "favor dysplasia or carcinoma." Prior to repeat cytology, the patient should be treated for vaginitis or estrogen deficiency as indicated. All other patients and the patient with persistent ASCUS smears should undergo colposcopy.

Low-Grade SIL. Five to 40 percent or more of Pap smears with low-grade SIL are associated with a significant dysplasia (CIN II or III), but rarely is there an underlying invasive carcinoma. Furthermore, there is a high rate of spontaneous regression of low-grade SIL, although the reported rates vary widely (25 to 75 percent; Nasiell et al, 1986; Montz et al, 1992; Flannelly et al, 1994). For these reasons the management of patients with low-grade SIL on the Pap smear is controversial. One option is to rescreen these patients in 3 months, in the absence of any suspicious finding on gynecologic examination, if the patient has a known normal Pap smear history and is reliable for follow-up. If the repeat smear is abnormal, then colposcopy is warranted. Gross lesions are best evaluated by biopsy, or colposcopy plus biopsy, not a Pap smear. A second option is to perform colposcopy on all patients with a low-grade SIL on Pap smear. Flannelly et al (1994), in a randomized study in Britain, concluded that this option is more cost-effective than follow-up Pap smears because 70 percent of these women eventually underwent colposcopy and 40 percent proved to have CIN III. However, their results are not typical of screening studies in the United States.

High-Grade SIL. All patients with even a single Pap smear consistent with high-grade SIL should undergo colposcopic evaluation with directed biopsies and endocervical curettage (ECC).

AGUS. This category includes atypical endometrial-like cells, atypical endocervical-like cells, and atypical glandular cells that cannot be placed in either of these two groups. The cells may originate from cervical, endometrial, tubal, or ovarian epithelium or neoplasms. The spectrum of cellular abnormalities that are incorporated into this category runs the gamut from atypical inflammatory changes to in situ adenocarcinoma. Therefore, it is not surprising that a substantial percentage of patients with AGUS have endometrial or cervical carcinoma (Goff et al, 1992; Isacson and Kurman, 1995; Kennedy et al, 1996). Kennedy et al reported AGUS in 0.2 percent of Pap smears. Work-up disclosed the following abnormalities: cervical adenocarcinoma, 4 percent; cervical adenocarcinoma in situ, 6 percent; CIN II/III, 5 percent; endometrial carcinoma, 1 percent; and pancreatic carcinoma, 1 percent. The mean patient age was 43.7 years. In the absence of an obvious malignancy on clinical examination, the patient with AGUS needs evaluation by colposcopy, directed biopsy, and ECC. If the cells are of endometrial or indeterminate type, pelvic ultrasound and endometrial biopsy are recommended.

Evaluation

Colposcopy is a diagnostic prerequisite for any woman with an abnormal Pap smear suggesting high-grade intraepithelial neoplasia or carcinoma. Colposcopy should also be performed as part of the office evaluation of women with an abnormal-looking cervix or persistent low-level Pap smear abnormalities, and for all potentially premalignant lesions of the vulva, vagina, and anus. Colposcopy permits the physician to determine easily the precise nature of most squamous lesions of the lower genital tract, and, in expert hands, it can eliminate the need for diagnostic conization of the cervix in most cases.

Evaluation of the patient with a cytologic diagnosis of SIL begins with a visual examination of the perineum, vagina, and cervix, keeping in mind the propensity of squamous neoplasia to be multifocal and multicentric. The cervix is treated with a 3 to 5% acetic acid solution (white vinegar), and then examined with colposcopic magnification, typically ×10 to ×20. The vinegar not only removes mucus from the cervix but enhances areas of squamous metaplasia, condyloma, dysplasia, and carcinoma, making them take on a thickened, white appearance relative to the normal squamous and columnar epithelium. These lesions are nearly always located within the transformation zone with one edge at the active squamocolumnar junction (SCJ). Repeated application of the vinegar is normally required to optimize the colposcopic detection of the lesions. Representative colposcopic-directed biopsy of any acetowhite lesion is undertaken, favoring those lesions that are the thickest or have coarse or atypical vessels. Except in the pregnant patient and the patient with acetowhite epithelium extending into the endocervical canal beyond visualization with the colposcope, an ECC is also performed. The ECC specimen is easily retrieved with an endocervical cytology brush. Slight bleeding may occur. The rectovaginal bimanual pelvic examination completes the evaluation. After receiving the pathologic diagnoses on these specimens, the treatment plan can be formulated based upon four tests: the Pap smear, the colposcopic findings, the cervical biopsies, and the ECC.

Management

Principles

The fundamental objectives of managing cervical dysplasia are to (1) find the lesion, (2) rule out concurrent invasive cancer, (3) prevent the evolution of dysplasia to invasive cancer, (4) preserve fertility and reproductive integrity, and (5) employ the most cost-effective, least morbid diagnostic and treatment techniques. To achieve these ends, patients are separated into three groups based upon the results of the initial evaluation. In one group it can be concluded that no invasive cancer is present; for the second group it can be said that no invasion was detected during the work-up but invasion has not been excluded with certainty; and the third group has invasive cancer on biopsy but the extent of the invasion is not sufficiently clear to determine the optimal therapy. A diagnostic and management algorithm for these groups is outlined in Fig. 2–13.

Management guidelines for CIN can be summarized as follows: (1) a cervical lesion (e.g., an "erosion") is never ablated without evaluation by Pap smear, colposcopy, and biopsy; (2) cervical dysplasia per se is never treated in pregnancy (vide infra); (3) cervical dysplasia is never ablated without excluding the presence of invasive carcinoma; (4) exclusion of invasive cancer requires that the Pap smear, colposcopic findings, ECC, and cervical biopsies are concordant, and that the entire SCJ is visible; (5) when treating cervical dysplasia, the entire transformation zone should be excised or ablated; and (6) a keratinizing dysplasia must always be excised, never ablated, because it cannot be satisfactorily evaluated by colposcopy.

The evaluation and management of cervical squamous dysplasia is predicated upon several observations with respect to its natural behavior. First, squamous dysplasia almost invariably arises in the transformation zone with one edge of the lesion at the active SCJ. Second, there are no skip lesions in the endocervical canal. While the glandular epithelium on the ectocervix may have multiple islands of squamous metaplasia and squamous dysplasia, the more proximal glandular epithelium is not exposed to the acid vaginal milieu. It becomes involved with dysplasia only by contiguous spread from the SCJ. Third, the endocervical canal is typically about 30 mm long and 7 mm wide, and fourth, the endocervical glands do not extend deeper than 5 mm from the surface. Consequently, excision or ablation of CIN does not need to be deeper than 5 mm. In one study the maximum depth of crypt involvement by dysplasia was calculated to be 3.6 mm, and the maximum linear extent of the dysplasia was 14.8 mm (Boonstra et al, 1990).

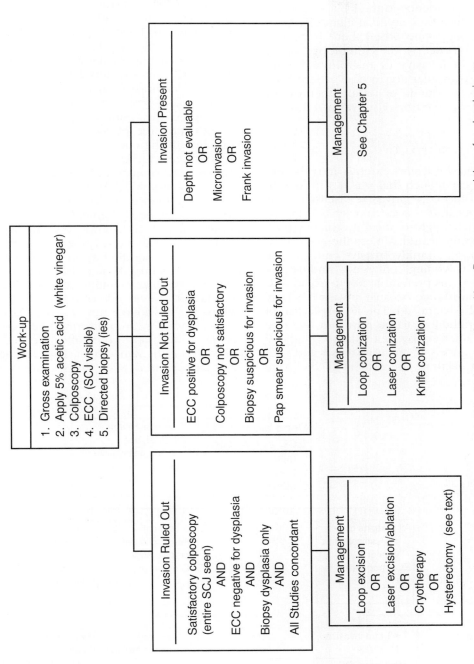

FIGURE 2–13. Outpatient management of the patient with a Pap smear suspicious for dysplasia or carcinoma. SCS = squamocolumnar junction; ECC = endocervical curettage.

INVASION RULED OUT

When the colposcopic examination is satis-factory—that is, when the entire limits of the lesion and the SCJ are visible, and the ECC is negative (no evidence in the EC specimen of squamous dysplasia, atypical glandular cells, or malignancy)—and when there is no evi-dence on colposcopy, directed biopsy, or the Pap smear of invasive or microinvasive car-cinoma or glandular atypia, the patient is el-igible for outpatient or office therapy by means of loop excision, laser vaporization, or cryosurgery.

INVASION NOT RULED OUT

If the dysplastic lesion extends into the en-docervical canal such that it is not fully eval-uable by colposcopy, invasive disease cannot be ruled out and a cone biopsy is required (Fig. 2–14). Therefore, local destructive ther-apy is contraindicated. Unless there is a clin-ical suspicion of frankly invasive endocervical carcinoma (bleeding; enlarged, nodular, or hard cervix), it is preferable not to do an ECC in this circumstance because invasion is only occasionally diagnosed. The ECC will disrupt the very epithelium to be removed by cone biopsy for microscopy, potentially complicat-ing the diagnosis of microinvasion and pre-venting an accurate assessment of the cone

tip margin. When there is no ectocervical le-sion, ECC is always necessary. In about 20 percent of patients who have an abnormal Pap smear, the ECC is positive for squamous dysplasia, but the positive rate is 50 percent for cases with unsatisfactory colposcopy. Older patients have a higher positive ECC rate, because the SCJ migrates into the canal with advancing age. Patients with evidence of CIN on ECC (no invasion demonstrated) must undergo diagnostic conization.

If only CIN is present and the cone biopsy has cleared the lesion (i.e., all margins and the ECC are free of dysplasia), treatment is complete. If the cone biopsy has not cleared the lesion and the ECC is positive, repeat con-ization is recommended because there is a substantial risk of undiagnosed invasive car-cinoma (Roman et al, 1997). Simple vaginal hysterectomy or abdominal hysterectomy is appropriate when the endocervical cone mar-gin (tip) is positive for dysplasia and the ECC is negative, depending upon the patient's re-productive status. When the patient elects conservative management, repeat conization is indicated if evidence of persistent CIN de-velops on the follow-up. A repeat ECC and cervical cytology are performed 12 weeks af-ter the cone biopsy; thereafter the patient is followed with semiannual Pap smears. In over 80 percent of such cases, there is no re-

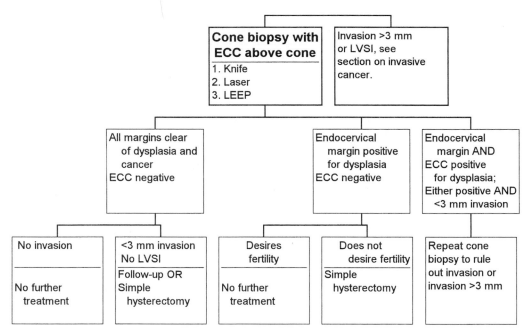

FIGURE 2–14. Management of patient based on cone biopsy results. LVSI = lymphovascular space invasion.

sidual dysplasia. For these cases, observation is the treatment of choice during the reproductive years.

DEPTH OF INVASION UNCERTAIN

Not uncommonly a cervical biopsy or ECC specimen will show areas suspicious for invasive carcinoma, or unambiguous evidence for invasive carcinoma, but the depth of invasion cannot be determined. In these cases, if the cervix appears to be involved by a frankly invasive carcinoma, LEEP biopsy should be done rather than a conization. However, in the absence of an overt carcinoma, conization is indicated to delineate the extent of invasion so the appropriate therapy may be applied (i.e., cone only, simple hysterectomy, modified or radical hysterectomy; see Chapter 5).

FALSE-POSITIVE ENDOCERVICAL CURETTAGE

The ECC is positive up to 15 percent of the time when the colposcopist finds that the entire limits of the lesion are easily visible. A careful review of these curettings will often reveal a single fragment of dysplastic epithelium, which is usually a contaminant or floater inadvertently dislodged from the visible ectocervical component of the dysplasia. According to Spirtos et al (1987), if the ECC is done before the directed biopsies, the false-positive rate is less than 5 percent. Dysplasia in a "floater" requires that the ECC be repeated in 3 to 4 weeks (to permit healing). If the repeat ECC is positive, however, cone biopsy is clearly indicated.

Specific Treatments

During the past 30 years the preferred treatment of cervical dysplasia has changed several times. The movement from the traditional knife cone biopsy to cryotherapy was made possible by the colposcopic identification of a target lesion. However, cryosurgery did not produce a specimen for pathologic evaluation, and some patients suffered from having an occult invasive cancer frozen, leading to delay in diagnosis and progression of disease (Townsend et al, 1981; Schmidt et al, 1992; Anderson, 1993). Cryosurgery was replaced by the laser, despite the laser's much greater cost, because the laser caused less tissue damage, was more precise, and could be used to excise as well as ablate tissue. The laser, however, was quickly replaced by the

LEEP procedure, which can be performed in the office, is cheaper than the laser, and yields a pathology specimen. Electrocoagulation diathermy, which has never become popular in the United States, may be, along with cryosurgery, the most cost-effective means of treating cervical dysplasia (Chanen and Rome, 1983; Deigan et al, 1986). Generally speaking, LEEP is the quickest and least expensive way to do a cone biopsy, and it is attended by less blood loss and less discomfort. However, in one small study the LEEP (and laser) cone volume was only half that obtained by the knife cone technique (Mathevet et al, 1994). This fact, plus the often multiple tissue fragments, means that more LEEP cones will have positive margins. Regardless of the technique employed to obtain the cone specimen, the management of the patient following cone biopsy is the same (Fig. 2–14).

SURGICAL CONIZATION

Conization of the cervix has two indications —diagnostic and therapeutic. In many cases, a diagnostic conization becomes therapeutic, particularly in the young patient. The indications for cone biopsy are listed in Table 2–5. The technique of conization, as well as the amount of disease excised, varies with the indications for the procedure and the extent of the disease. For example, if a patient is to have a diagnostic conization followed by a hysterectomy, the amount of tissue excised

---

TABLE 2–5

Indications for Excision/Cone Biopsy and Ablative Management of Cervical Dysplasia

Cone biopsy (knife, laser, LEEP)
  Cervical punch biopsy diagnosis of dysplasia with colposcopically inevaluable canal disease
  Cervical punch biopsy diagnosis of microinvasion or colposcopic suspicion of invasion
  Dysplasia on ECC and unsatisfactory colposcopy
  Leukoplakia resulting from keratinizing dysplasia
  Atypical glandular epithelium on biopsy or ECC
  Persistent Pap smears indicative of dysplasia or carcinoma with a negative evaluation
Ablative therapy (cryotherapy, laser, cautery)
  Excluding invasion is an absolute prerequisite:
    Colposcopic evaluation, biopsies, ECC, Pap smears, and gross appearance of cervix must be concordant
    SCJ entirely visualized and ECC negative
  Cryotherapy is most suited to treating small CIN I and II lesions without gland duct or canal involvement
  Laser therapy is preferred for large CIN I and II lesions; extension into the canal but colposcopically evaluable is acceptable

will depend upon whether or not the colposcopy and biopsy have excluded invasive ectocervical disease, and the extent of disease within the endocervical canal. Once invasive cancer on the ectocervix has been excluded, only the canal and surrounding glands need to be excised for proper diagnosis (Fig. 2–15A). When hysterectomy is carried out, however, it is important that all remaining abnormal epithelium on the ectocervix be excised. Removal of a vaginal cuff is necessary only when the dysplasia extends onto the vagina. Even in this situation it is probably better to treat the vaginal component by laser ablation/excision prior to hysterectomy.

If conization is to be used as a therapeutic technique, all abnormal epithelium must be treated. When the disease is confined to the ectocervix, only the ectocervical disease need be removed. The canal may be ignored (Fig. 2–15B). Conversely, if there is disease on the ectocervix and in the canal, then all ectocervical disease and all canal disease must be removed (Fig. 2–15C). In some instances, usually in older patients, only the canal harbors disease. In these cases, the shape of the cone is more cylindrical (Fig. 2–15D). Another technique that we have found particularly applicable to the woman who desires to maintain her fertility is combining the shallow cone for colposcopically evaluable ectocervical disease with the cylindrical cone. This double conization can be performed with a scalpel and/or the CO_2 laser, or the wire loop.

Although the technique of knife conization appears simple, it is one of the more troublesome procedures in gynecology. None of the numerous methods and stratagems devised to reduce the complication rate of cone biopsy has proved to be clearly superior. The procedure is most commonly done under general anesthesia in a hospital or surgical center, although local/regional anesthesia is often satisfactory. After the pelvic examination is done, the vagina is carefully prepped. Colposcopy is repeated to delineate the extent of ectocervical and endocervical disease. The cervical canal and uterine cavity are sounded, but cervical dilatation is postponed until after the cone biopsy has been done.

Lugol's stain is applied and the results correlated with the colposcopic and visual findings. In some cases, excision can be performed under colposcopic guidance. The cervix is brought into position with a tenaculum or lateral traction sutures, carefully avoiding trauma to the cervical epithelium.

Operative bleeding can be minimized by injecting the tissues with a dilute vasoconstrictor such as vasopressin 1:30. Usually a No. 15 or No. 11 scalpel blade is utilized. All Lugol's-negative or colposcopically abnormal ectocervical tissue is removed with the endocervix unless hysterectomy is planned and ectocervical invasion has been ruled out by colposcopy and biopsy. The initial incision is made around the abnormal ectocervical epithelium. Then the incision is carried deeper into the cervix, tapering toward the canal. The average cone will remove 2.0 to 2.5 cm of canal.

After the cone specimen is removed, it is marked for orientation. Next, the cervix is dilated and the residual endocervix is curetted. The presence or absence of dysplasia in this specimen assists in making decisions about further treatment. Unless otherwise indicated, endometrial curettage is performed routinely only in the postmenopausal patient. Hemostasis is secured with figure-of-eight PGA sutures.

The observed frequency of complications from knife cone biopsy varies widely, but the types of reported complications are typically similar: intraoperative, early postoperative, and delayed postoperative blood loss; infection; cervical stenosis (with dysmenorrhea, hematometra, amenorrhea); and cervical perforation. Intraoperative blood loss of more than 200 ml is seldom reported, but postoperative bleeding requiring evaluation, hospital admission, packing, suturing, and even transfusion is reported in 3 to 15 percent of cases. The bleeding is often delayed for 1 to 2 weeks after the cone biopsy. The risk of clinical infection after cone biopsy may be as high as 5 percent if prophylactic antibiotics are not used. Symptoms of cervical stenosis are reported in 1 to 5 percent of cases or more. In these patients cervical dilatation is indicated.

CRYOSURGERY

Before performing cryosurgery, a careful gynecologic history is taken. Emphasis is placed on intermenstrual bleeding, menorrhagia, the quality and character of any discharge, salpingitis, and the date of the last menstrual period. Cryosurgery, like conization, is best performed during the week immediately after the menstrual period to avoid treating a patient with an early pregnancy. This timing also permits the most active phase of regen-

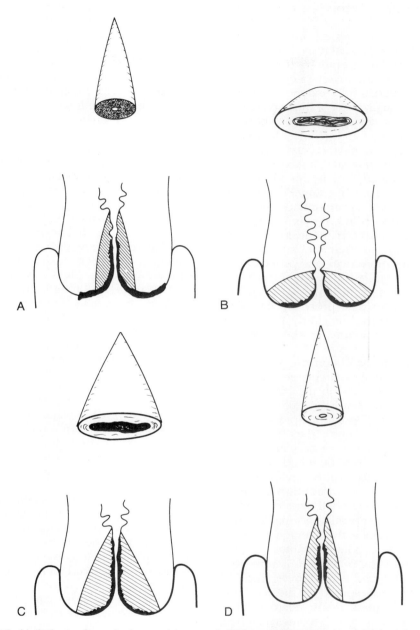

FIGURE 2–15. Variations of cervical cone biopsy. *A*, Patient with ectocervical and endocervical lesion. When invasion has been excluded on the ectocervix by colposcopy and office biopsy and the patient will undergo hysterectomy after the cone biopsy, the ectocervical lesion does not need to be removed at the time of conization. In this instance, the cone design is more cylindrical, removing most of the endocervical canal to rule out invasion. ECC is always performed proximal to the cone biopsy. *B*, Patient with ectocervical disease only. This is the ideal situation for office LEEP management because diagnosis and therapy can be completed in one step. *C*, When the lesion involves the ectocervix and the endocervix and the patient wishes to retain her uterus, diagnosis and therapy are performed by cone biopsy, which removes the ectocervical lesion, the transformation zone, and most of the endocervical canal. This can be performed by the LEEP procedure, but if the disease extends deeply into the canal, it may be easier to get clear margins by knife cone biopsy. *D*, When there is endocervical disease only, typically in the postmenopausal woman, diagnostic knife cone biopsy is the preferred procedure, especially with an atrophic cervix.

eration to take place before the onset of the next menses.

Cryosurgery is performed in the office without anesthesia or analgesia. Nitrous oxide is the preferred refrigerant for treating CIN of any degree. An adequate speculum is inserted and the blades fully extended to provide optimum visualization of the cervix. This also reduces the chance of freezing the vaginal wall. All mucous and cellular debris are removed from the vagina and cervix with cotton balls soaked in vinegar. The extent of the disease to be treated is determined colposcopically and by applying Lugol's solution. The probe that best approximates the anatomic configuration of the cervix is attached to the cryosurgical unit. If the lesion is more than 1.5 times greater than the surface area of the probe tip, more than one probe application will be required. The cervix is thoroughly moistened with saline to ensure proper heat transfer. The probe tip, at room temperature, is firmly but gently positioned so that the greater extent of the lesion is covered.

When the probe has been properly positioned, the refrigerant is circulated. Ice crystallization initially occurs on the back of the probe tip and then spreads laterally from the edge of the probe. The lateral spread of the ice ball should begin within 10 to 15 seconds after the refrigerant has been circulated. If the duration of the freeze is to be timed, the clock is started when the ice ball begins its lateral spread. However, it is more important to make certain that the ice ball extends at least 5 mm onto colposcopically normal epithelium. In our experience, the average duration of a single freeze is about 3 minutes.

During the freezing process, it is unnecessary to know the probe tip temperature. If there is rapid lateral spread of the ice ball, there will be adequate tissue necrosis. If a small portion of the vagina becomes attached to the probe during the freezing process, no serious sequelae will occur. If a large area of the vagina becomes attached to the probe, the tip should be defrosted and reapplied. After completing the freeze, the probe is defrosted and removed. Then the cervix is carefully inspected to make certain that the ice ball has extended the necessary 5 mm onto normal epithelium. Any area that does not appear to be adequately frozen should be immediately retreated. If multiple freeze applications are required, it is important that the ice balls overlap. Only a single freeze-thaw cycle is needed when nitrous oxide is the refrigerant. Some authors, however, prefer the freeze-thaw-freeze cycle.

Postcryotherapy side effects and complications related to treatment of CIN are rarely serious. Included are uterine cramps during the freeze, facial flushing immediately after the freeze, and a heavy watery, sometimes malodorous discharge that begins with a few hours and lasts for 2 to 3 weeks. Tampon use, intercourse, and douching are prohibited until the discharge stops. Postcryotherapy bleeding is very unusual. Infection and cervical stenosis are reported in fewer than 3 percent of cases.

Nearly all treatment failures are, with adequate follow-up, diagnosed during the first year. The risk of new disease developing subsequently is similar to that of the high-risk population at large. It is advisable to review the pathology of "failure" diagnosed as mild dysplasia, since actively regenerating epithelium may be confused with CIN I. The most common causes of cryotherapy failure are an inadequate freeze (low refrigerant pressure, poor probe application, insufficient freeze time), gland duct involvement, a greater than 3-cm lesion, extension of disease into the endocervical canal, and a high lesional grade (Hatch et al, 1981; Savage et al, 1982; Townsend and Richart, 1983; Creasman et al, 1984; Ferenczy, 1985; Benedet et al, 1992). The generally reported success rate for cryosurgery with satisfactory colposcopy is 90 percent (Tables 2–6 and 2–7). Selective retreatment can improve the overall success rate to more than 95 percent. Patients with dysplasia persisting after a second freeze should be subjected to cone biopsy. Cryosurgery, as well as any other ablative technique for CIN, should be performed by, or in consultation with, an experienced colposcopist because the risk of masking invasive cancer, thereby delaying its diagnosis and proper treatment.

LASER THERAPY

Laser is an acronym for *l*ight *a*mplification by *s*timulated *e*mission of *r*adiation. The CO_2 produces electromagnetic radiation of high intensity by the controlled discharge of a carbon dioxide, nitrogen, and helium gas mixture. This energy, in the form of infrared light, is emitted at a wavelength of 10.6 Å with a power range of 10 to 10,000 W. At this wavelength, vaporization of biologic tissue is achieved with little difficulty. Tissue destruction results from raising the temperature of

TABLE 2–6
Treatment Results for Cervical Dysplasia

Modality	CIN I		CIN II		CIN III	
	N	(%) NED[§]	N	(%) NED[§]	N	(%) NED[§]
Knife cone*	—	—	208	(99)[‖]	87	(100)
Cryotherapy[†]	156	(93)	275	(88)	475	(87)
Laser[†]	312	(96)	472	(91)	773	(91)
LEEP[‡]	158	(90)	103	(89)	243	(90)

*Data from Abdul-Karim and Nunez (1985).
[†]Data from Benedet et al (1992).
[‡]Data from Wright et al (1992a) and Luesley et al (1990).
[§]NED = no evidence of disease.
[‖]CIN I and CIN II combined.

the cell until the intracellular water turns into steam, vaporizing the cell. Heat from the laser can also coagulate vessels up to 1 mm in diameter. As a consequence, blood loss is less than that encountered utilizing the knife.

Perhaps the most important advantage of laser therapy is its ability to destroy tissue with a very narrow zone of injury around the treated tissue (50 to 100 μm). This is possible because there is no lateral scatter of the beam below the tissue surface. Significant lateral tissue injury will result, however, when the laser beam is delivered with insufficient power density to convert the tissue water rapidly to steam. In this situation there is time for the heat to dissipate into, and raise the temperature of, the surrounding tissues. If the temperature rises above 55°C, thermal necrosis results (Fisher, 1983).

The power density is a function of the laser spot size and the beam power:

$$\text{Power density} = \frac{\text{Beam power in watts}}{\text{Beam diameter in cm}^2}$$

For most purposes in gynecology, the CO_2 laser is operated with a power density of 750 to 1,500 W/cm². A lower power density (350 to 450 W/cm²) is used for hemostasis. The latter is most readily achieved by defocusing the spot, which increases its effective size and thereby decreases the power density. Laser units are generally equipped to permit the release of energy in four modes: single pulse, repeat pulse, continuous wave, and superpulse. The latter releases laser energy in very rapid bursts (250 to 750 per second) which reduces the heat buildup in the surrounding tissues.

There are several *safety procedures* that must be followed when employing the laser. First, the eyes of all personnel in the laser room, including the patient, must be protected by wearing goggles of glass or plastic; nonreflecting instruments also should be used. Second, precautions must be taken to avoid explosions and fires. Thus, flammable anesthetics and flammable prep solutions should not be used, and the drapes must be wet or fireproof. Third, since cervical neopla-

TABLE 2–7
Results of Comparative Treatment Studies of CIN

Laser			Cryotherapy			LEEP		
Grade	N	(%) NED[‡]	Grade	N	(%) NED[‡]	Grade	N	(%) NED[‡]
*CIN I	87	(97)	CIN I	89	(98)	—	—	—
II	154	(91)	II	153	(93)	—	—	—
III	109	(91)	III	106	(84)	—	—	—
[†]CIN I	54	(83)	—	—	—	CIN I	43	(67)
II	96	(78)	—	—	—	II	96	(95)
III	74	(86)	—	—	—	III	77	(77)

*Data from Berget et al (1987), Townsend and Richart (1983) and Ferenczy (1985).
[†]Data from Gunasekera et al (1990) and Oyesanya et al (1993).
[‡]NED = no evidence of disease.

sia may contain virus particles, and since the viral DNA may be present in the laser plume, special precautions need to be taken to evacuate the plume. The tip of the fume evacuator should be placed within 1 cm of the tissue being treated. The filtration system in the evacuator apparatus also disposes of the carbon particles so they cannot be inhaled (Lipow 1986; American College of Obstetricians and Gynecologists, 1990; Ferenczy et al, 1990). An additional safety procedure is to test the laser prior to anesthetizing the patient. The laser spot size and power density are set and then checked with a few pulses applied to a tongue blade. The alignment of the helium–neon aiming beam with the laser beam is also checked.

The selection of patients for laser ablation of cervical dysplasia follows the same rules as for the use of cryotherapy. The laser is more effective than cryotherapy for larger lesions, high-grade lesions, and those lesions that extend into the endocervical glands or the cervical canal (Ferenczy, 1985; Kirwan et al, 1985). When treating CIN, the entire transformation zone on the cervix is destroyed to a depth of 5 to 7 mm. This causes sufficient discomfort that local anesthesia is often necessary. Mixing the anesthetic agent with vasopressin (30:1) will enhance the hemostatic effect of the laser beam.

For 1 to 2 weeks following laser therapy for cervical dysplasia, spotting and vaginal discharge may occur. The patient is advised not to exercise vigorously or to have sexual intercourse for 3 weeks, the time required for healing. Either of these activities can cause excessive bleeding. Despite these precautions, about 1 percent of patients will have sufficient bleeding to require examination. Cure rates reported for laser therapy for essentially the same as those for cryosurgery (Tables 2–6 and 2–7), but laser therapy is less likely to result in cervical stenosis or a recessed SCJ (Baggish, 1980; Baggish and Dorsey, 1985; Anderson, 1982; Townsend and Richart, 1983; Wright et al, 1983).

Laser conization has been recommended by some authors as similarly effective as, but safer than the knife cone biopsy (Larsson et al, 1983; Wright et al, 1984; Baggish and Dorsey, 1985). This requires a small spot size (0.25 to 0.8 mm) and a power density greater than 5,000 W/cm^2, which allow rapid cutting but make the beam harder to control. Lower power density and/or a larger spot size produces too much thermal tissue damage to obtain a satisfactory cone specimen. The endocervical mucosa is undermined for 2 to 3 mm to promote eversion and prevent canal stenosis.

LOOP ELECTROSURGICAL EXCISION PROCEDURE

Also known as large loop excision of transformation zone (LLETZ, LETZ), this is the latest of the many techniques employed to diagnose and treat cervical neoplasia. LEEP has the advantages of simplicity, low cost, and full pathologic evaluation of the neoplastic tissue. Its current popularity is undoubtedly attributable to the many cases of invasive cervical cancer that were diagnosed following cryotherapy, electrocoagulation, and laser ablation. With these destructive methods, because no specimen is available for histopathology, invasive cancer must be absolutely excluded prior to treatment. Unfortunately, the means of excluding cancer are not absolutely reliable.

The modern era of loop excision for cervical dysplasia began when Cartier (1984) utilized a small, fine wire loop to excise part or all of the abnormal transformation zone. His technique did not receive much attention because of the popularity of cryosurgery and the CO_2 laser. The clinical potential of loop excision was fully developed by Prendiville et al (1989), who enlarged the loop to permit the removal of the entire transformation zone with a single pass. Electricity cuts tissue by an arcing phenomenon. The arc extends out from and around the thin wire, causing steam to be released from the water-filled cells. A small steam envelope is created around the wire loop, and, as the loop is passed through the tissue, the steam envelope cuts the tissue. If the wire loop itself touches the tissue, stalling occurs. Anything that interferes with this arcing increases the thermal artifact. To maintain arcing, a shiny tungsten-quality wire of approximately 0.007 inches in thickness is required.

Reports of clinical studies soon appeared in the literature pointing out the utility of LEEP in women with abnormal Pap smears (Gunasekera et al, 1990; Mor-Yosef et al, 1990; Murdoch et al, 1991; Wright et al, 1992a). The advantages, moreover, became most apparent in those clinics where women with abnormal Pap smears were seen and treated at the initial visit. This "see and treat" philosophy has been used to greatest advantage by physicians in England, reducing the backlog of patients awaiting evaluation and treatment for an abnormal Pap smear.

When first beginning to utilize this technique, it is recommended that physicians follow the traditional protocol in evaluating the woman with an abnormal Pap smear (i.e., repeat cytology, colposcopy, biopsies, ECC, etc.). Patients then return to the physician's office for LEEP at a second visit. Once the physician becomes comfortable with this method, then the single-visit approach can be utilized more effectively. The major drawback to the one-visit approach is overinterpretation of colposcopically benign white epithelium (e.g., squamous metaplasia) by the colposcopist. In some reports the specimens from almost one third of patients did not contain any significant pathology (i.e., dysplasia) or HPV-related lesions (Murdoch et al, 1991).

Method. In general, patients who are candidates for LEEP will have a Pap smear suspect for high-grade SIL (CIN II or III). Those individuals who have persistent low-grade SIL should also be treated, but not necessarily by loop excision. If there is no lesion seen colposcopically, then the patient must have the traditional evaluation of repeat cytology, ECC, and evaluation for VAIN. The LEEP technique will not only biopsy the area but also remove it in its entirety in most instances. In other words, both diagnosis and treatment are performed simultaneously. LEEP should not be performed in the presence of severe cervicitis, pelvic infection, or early pregnancy.

During the examination, a liberal application of vinegar is used. The physician should locate the transformation zone and when possible the SCJ. Instead of taking a directed biopsy, the entire lesion, including the transformation zone and the SCJ, is excised with the electrosurgical loop. If the physician notes disease within the endocervical canal, a smaller loop is utilized to remove the canal disease. To ensure that no dysplasia remains in the canal, an ECC, a cytology brush sample, or a small margin check excision is performed.

The loop excision is performed under local anesthesia using 2% xylocaine, a vasoconstrictor such as 1:100,000 epinephrine or 1:30 vasopressin, and a 27-gauge needle. Four to eight sites are injected with 0.2 to 0.3 ml at the junction between normal and abnormal tissue (total 3 ml). After the lesion is localized colposcopically, Lugol's solution is applied to the cervix. The iodine stain lasts much longer than the vinegar effect, making it easier to locate the lesion. The anesthetic needs to be injected no deeper than 1 to 2 mm into the tissue. If it appears that a conization (i.e., removal of canal tissue) will be necessary, the injection of additional anesthetic around the cervical canal to a depth of 5 to 10 mm is recommended. It is important that the mouth of the speculum is opened wide and that the speculum is insulated to prevent conduction of electricity. A low-powered vacuum is necessary to remove the plume, about 10 percent of that created by the laser. It is also important to select a loop of proper width and depth. Many loops excise too much tissue, which, in a nulliparous patient, can approximate a cervical amputation. Loops have been designed for shallow biopsy as well as conization. Loop R2007 (Fig. 2–16) is used to excise the ectocervix and loops R1010 and S1010 are used to remove the canal tissue. It bears repeating that removal of excessive tissue is not only unnecessary but may be deleterious.

After attaching the appropriate loop to a hand piece the electrosurgical generator is activated. The unit is placed on Blend I, and the wattage is set according to the loop being used (Fig. 2–17). The area to be excised is confirmed grossly by Lugol's iodine staining. After the cervix is moistened with saline, the loop is positioned 3 mm beyond the lesion and the current is activated. The loop is then brought into contact with the tissue and passed horizontally or vertically through the tissue at a slow, even pace. The specimen should be dish shaped and no more than 5 to 10 mm deep. The cervix is reinspected and additional passes are made excising all of the nonstaining tissue. The canal is inspected colposcopically using a vinegar-soaked cotton-tipped applicator. If there is canal disease as noted by a "white rim," then a canal loop is used to remove the canal disease. Once all disease has been removed, a final canal check is performed. The raw bed is cauterized with a ball electrode and thick ferric subsulfate (Monsel's solution) is applied.

Loop excision may require several passes, and it is not uncommon in large lesions, or disease that involves the canal, to have "positive" margins since the loop is cutting through the field of dysplasia. However, the status of the ectocervical margins should be known to the operator since the excision margins are outlined with Lugol's solution. The endocervical canal margin status should also be known to the operator based upon the colposcopic assessment. To avoid the

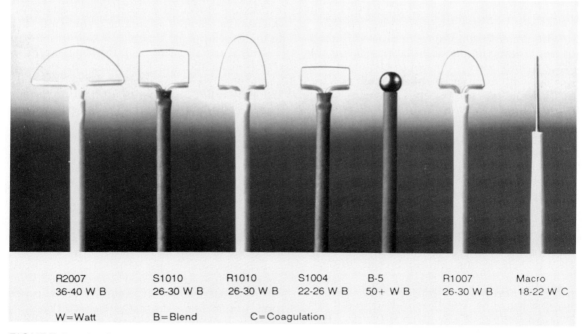

R2007	S1010	R1010	S1004	B-5	R1007	Macro
36-40 W B	26-30 W B	26-30 W B	22-26 W B	50+ W B	26-30 W B	18-22 W C

W=Watt   B=Blend   C=Coagulation

FIGURE 2–16. Variety of loops designed for LEEP with matched power output for electrosurgical generator shown in Figure 2–17. The electrode or probe is made of fine tungsten wire attached to an insulated T-bar and shaft. It inserts into a standard electrosurgical hand unit.

problem of a histologically positive canal margin, a separate small portion of the remaining colposcopically normal canal can be removed. The surgical margins can be inked by the operator as the specimens are removed to assist the pathologist's interpretation.

Patients may have a cramping pain during the performance of the loop excision. Delayed bleeding is reported in about 3 percent and cervical stenosis in about 1 percent of patients, and infection is rare (Luesley et al, 1990; Wright et al, 1992a). Following LEEP, a watery discharge may be present for 1 to 2 weeks. Patients are advised not to have sexual intercourse or to exercise for 3 weeks. The reported treatment outcome is similar to that for cryosurgery and laser therapy (Tables 2–6 and 2–7).

HYSTERECTOMY

The clearest indication for simple hysterectomy in the treatment of CIN is the presence of dysplasia at the cone tip in a postreproductive woman. In most other situations, the advantage of hysterectomy over cone biopsy must be weighed against other patient benefits such as sterilization, since both cone biopsy and hysterectomy have a similar high degree of effectiveness in eradicating cervical dysplasia. Combining two large series (Boyes et al, 1970; Kolstad and Klem, 1976), the observed rate of recurrent CIN III was 3.0 percent for 1,603 women treated by cone biopsy and 0.9 percent for 3,087 women treated by hysterectomy. The corresponding rates for invasive carcinoma were 0.6 percent and 0.2 percent. The data of Bjerre et al (1976) emphasize the importance of a negative cone margin. In a study of 1,336 cone biopsies for CIN III, the recurrence rates were 2.9, 14.0, and 29.6 percent, respectively, for patients with a negative, equivocal, and positive cone margin. Thus, while the failure rate after cone biopsy is three times that after hysterectomy, conization is 97 percent effective when the margins are negative. The routine use of hysterectomy after cone biopsy for CIN does not seem to be justified in the absence of other patient benefits.

Treatment Failure

The success rates of the various methods for the treatment of cervical neoplasia are similar, as shown in Table 2–6. Risk factors for CIN treatment failure include poor technique, gland duct involvement, severity of CIN, size

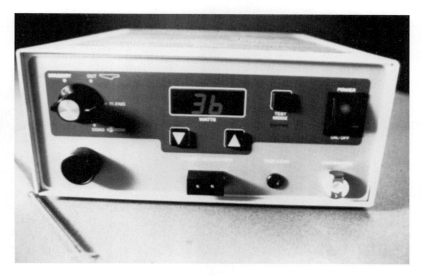

FIGURE 2-17. Photograph of electrosurgical generator matched to electrodes in Figure 2-16.

of lesion, margin status, and the presence of canal disease (Townsend and Richart, 1983; Ferenczy, 1985; Demopoulos et al, 1991; Shafi et al, 1993). A number of controlled and randomized studies have compared the cure rates of CIN treated by LEEP, laser, and cryosurgery (Table 2-7). The patient selection and endpoint definitions have not been uniform in these reports, but, taking into consideration the results of single-arm studies, there is nothing in the controlled studies to indicate a distinct superiority of treatment efficacy for any of these methods.

Technical Factors

The most important difference in the various techniques available for the treatment of CIN relates to whether the cervical tissue is destroyed or excised for pathologic evaluation. Thus there are two basic methodologies: the excision techniques of knife cone biopsy, laser excision, LEEP, and hysterectomy; and the ablative techniques of cryosurgery, laser vaporization, cold coagulation, and electrofulguration. The importance of excision in terms of a definitive pathologic diagnosis is illustrated by the report of Burger and Hollema (1993), who found that the colposcopically directed biopsy underestimated the diagnosis in 22 percent of 121 patients with squamous dysplasia and satisfactory colposcopy. Five invasive carcinomas were missed (four microinvasive, one invasive to 6 mm). Similarly, Chappatte et al (1991) reported that 16 of 100 patients with cervical dysplasia suitable for ablative therapy had a worse lesion on excision biopsy (LEEP), including three cases of

microinvasion. It is understandable, then, that ablative therapy occasionally obscures the presence of an invasive carcinoma, leading to delay in diagnosis and progression of disease (Townsend et al, 1981; Schmidt et al, 1992; Anderson, 1993). Errors underlying the failure to diagnose invasive cancer include deviations from the prescribed pretreatment protocol and misinterpretation of cervical biopsies or ECC. Morbidity, expense, degree of difficulty, and quality of the specimen are significant but less important differences in the treatment modalities.

Thermal Artifact

A critical issue with respect to the excision techniques of LEEP and laser is the pathologic evaluability of the specimen, especially the margins of resection (Fig. 2-18). This issue arises because both techniques are capable of causing significant thermal damage to the specimen, and the reported magnitude of the problem ranges widely. Krebs et al (1993), in a review of a community hospital experience, found that 48 percent of the LEEP cones had moderate to severe thermal artifact that interfered with the histologic interpretation of the specimens. Naumann et al (1994) observed that the thermal artifact correlated with the number of slices in the specimen. In 75 percent of their cases the artifact was minimal, in 23.5 percent the artifact interfered with interpretation of the margin, and in 1.8 percent the damage was so extensive that it interfered with the histologic diagnosis. In contrast, Oyesanya et al (1993) reported that only 3 percent of 150 LEEP specimens had sufficient

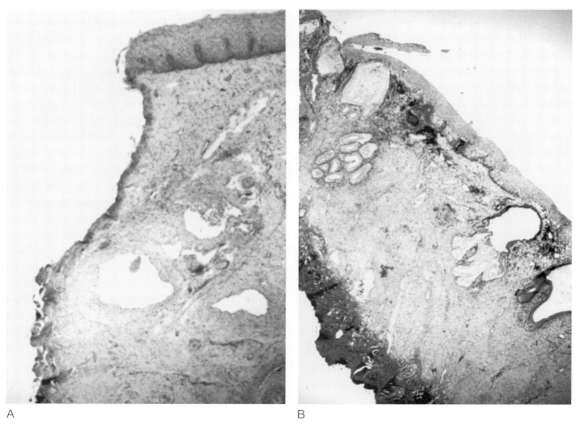

A   B

FIGURE 2–18. Photomicrographs of thermal artifact from cervical loop specimen. *A*, Depth of artifact is 100 μm. *B*, Depth of artifact is 300 μm.

artifact to impair the assessment of the margins, and Felix et al (1994) had no problem in the interpretation of all 57 of their specimens obtained by obstetrics/gynecology residents. The reports of serious thermal damage attending laser cone biopsy range from 0 to 50 percent (Howell et al, 1991; Fowler et al, 1992; Krebs et al, 1993; Oyesanya et al, 1993; Mathevet et al, 1994). Two investigators used micrometers to measure the extent of coagulation and charring of LEEP and laser cone specimens. Wright et al (1992b) found the mean thickness of the injured zone in the laser and LEEP groups to be 411μ and 396μ, respectively, but all specimens were evaluable. Baggish et al (1992) reported the mean depth of thermal injury to be 187μ and 164μ for the LEEP and laser specimens, respectively, and in neither group did the artifact interfere with the histologic evaluation of the specimens. One can only conclude that the thermal artifact is heavily operator, and perhaps equipment, dependent. Failure to use a proper generator and electrodes can result in

excessive thermal artifact. The best systems have a digital readout, a cut blend mode (Blend 1), and a coagulation mode. Even more important is that the electrodes used in performing this procedure be matched to the system. That is, there should be a predetermined power setting already established for each electrode to ensure maximum ease of excision and minimal thermal artifact. The reuse of loops increases the thermal artifact.

Follow-up Regimen

Regardless of the method of treatment for cervical dysplasia, the patient is re-examined in 4 to 6 weeks for healing of the cervix and patency of the external os. In the meantime, vaginal rest is recommended to reduce the possibility of bleeding and infection. The patient is then asked to return in another 6 weeks for repeat Pap smear (ectocervical scrape and endocervical brush specimen). Neither an ECC nor colposcopy is necessary on a routine basis. If the first follow-up Pap smear is normal, it is repeated in 3 months and then 6 months. If these smears are also normal, the patient is put on a 6-month follow-up schedule thereafter. Colposcopy is indicated whenever the Pap smear is abnormal, the cervix appears abnormal, or the patient has relevant symptoms.

COLPOSCOPY

The colposcope is basically a stereoscopic dissecting microscope with increased illumination. Various levels of magnification are available, the most practical being between ×8 and ×18. A blue–green filter is inserted between the light source and the tissue to accentuate the color tone differences between normal and abnormal patterns, as well as to enhance the vascular patterns. The examination of the visible portion of the female genital tract by colposcopy usually takes no more than a few minutes in the uncomplicated case. In patients with an abnormal Pap smear, a complete evaluation usually takes 15 to 20 minutes.

Cervical Disease

Normal Transformation Zone

One of the major concepts on which contemporary colposcopy is based is the transformation zone, defined as the area of the cervix and vagina initially covered by columnar epithelium that, through a process called metaplasia, has been replaced in whole or in part by squamous epithelium.

At one time, it was believed that the cervix was normally covered by squamous epithelium and that the presence of endocervical columnar epithelium on the ectocervix was an abnormal location for this tissue. However, studies in Australia and the United States have established that columnar tissue normally exists on the ectocervix at puberty in at least 70 percent of girls and extends onto the vagina in an additional 5 percent. Moreover, the location of columnar epithelium on the ectocervix is determined early in embryologic development.

The replacement of columnar by squamous epithelium by the process of squamous metaplasia probably occurs throughout an individual's lifetime; however, this normal physiologic transition is most active during fetal life, adolescence, and the first pregnancy. The process is enhanced by an acid environment

and is no doubt influenced by sex steroids such as estrogen and progesterone.

Embryologically the fallopian tubes, uterus, cervix and vagina are derived from the paired müllerian ducts. Initially the vagina is lined with simple columnar epithelium, but early in fetal life, a stratified cuboidal epithelium, which eventually differentiates into squamous epithelium, begins to displace this müllerian-derived columnar tissue. Virtually all of the columnar epithelium in the vagina and a variable portion of the ectocervical columnar tissue are replaced during normal fetal development. The location of columnar tissue on the ectocervix and, in a few cases, in the vagina is therefore not the result of outward growth from the cervix, as was once believed. The replacement of the columnar tissue apparently stops around the fifth gestational month. After the initial replacement of müllerian columnar epithelium by the urogenital sinus cuboidal epithelium is completed, and any further replacement of the columnar tissue by squamous tissue is accomplished by metaplasia. This begins in the fetus during the latter half of pregnancy, probably as a result of the influence of maternal sex steroids. After delivery, the metaplastic process slows because of the loss of maternal steroids and the resultant normalization of the neutral vaginal pH. With the onset of puberty and menstruation, the vaginal fluid again becomes acidic as a result of colonization by the adult bacterial population. When the columnar ectocervical tissue is exposed to this acid environment, the transformation process is once again activated.

The metaplastic squamous epithelium originates both as a peripheral ingrowth from the squamous epithelium laid down early in fetal life and from multipotential cells (reserve cells) that are usually found subjacent to the columnar epithelium. The multipotential cells differentiate into immature squamous epithelium when exposed to an acid environment. The squamous cells then displace the overlying columnar epithelium, producing multiple foci or islands that broaden, coalesce, and eventually join the squamous epithelium growing in from the periphery. Gland openings develop that permit the egress of mucus from the deeper secreting columnar cells. In some instances the gland openings become occluded and the nabothian cysts form. The complete transformation of columnar to squamous epithelium probably requires many years. Patients who take oral contraceptives seem to have a slower transformation rate, probably because of the buffering effect caused by increased production of mucus.

In the reproductive years, the transformation zone is characterized by areas of columnar epithelium interspersed with areas of metaplastic squamous epithelium, gland openings, and nabothian cysts. With advancing age, the transformation zone matures, nabothian cysts and gland openings disappear, and the constantly changing SCJ gradually migrates into the endocervical canal. The upward migration is relatively slow because of the anatomic location of the canal and the neutral pH of the environment. Also with advancing age, the transformation zone becomes less apparent and only a very fine vascular structure reveals its location. Occasionally, the metaplastic squamous epithelium appears slightly whiter than the original squamous epithelium. This is due to an increased number of relatively large nuclei in the intermediate and parabasal cell layers. The immature metaplastic epithelium lacks glycogen and only partially stains with iodine. In most women a normal transformation zone develops, and cytology is normal. However, in a few instances, perhaps in some cases because of HPV, a DNA change occurs in the immature metaplastic squamous epithelium and potentially malignant cells develop. As a consequence, an abnormal transformation zone evolves. It is the abnormal transformation zone where patterns characteristic of the earliest forms of cervical neoplasia are found (Table 2–8).

Abnormal Transformation Zone

A transformation zone is classified as abnormal when one or more of the following patterns are viewed: white (acetopositive) epithelium, mosaic structure, punctation, leukoplakia, or abnormal blood vessels. Although each pattern may exist as a separate and distinct entity, a mixture of patterns is not unusual. The basic component of all patterns is white epithelium resulting from an increased number of nuclei that have an increased DNA content. Light from the colposcope illuminating an area with increased nuclear density is reflected through the lens of the instrument, giving the area an enhanced white appearance. The optical density and, therefore, the degree of whiteness vary directly with the nuclear concentration. Normal epithelium is pinkish white, whereas CIN, with its greater

TABLE 2–8

Colposcopic Terminology*

Normal colposcopic findings
　Original squamous epithelium
　Columnar epithelium
　Transformation zone (TZ)
Abnormal colposcopic findings
　Within the transformation zone
　　Acetowhite epithelium
　　Punctation
　　Mosaic
　　Iodine-negative epithelium
　　Leukoplakia
　　Atypical blood vessels
　Outside the transformation zone
　（same as within TZ）
Suspect frank invasive cancer
Unsatisfactory colposcopy
　Squamocolumnar junction not visible
　Severe inflammation or severe atrophy
　Cervix not visible
Miscellaneous findings
　Non-acetowhite micropapillary surface
　Exophytic condyloma
　Inflammation
　Atrophy
　Ulcer
　Other

*From Stafl A, Wilbanks GD: An international terminology of colposcopy: report of the Nomenclature Committee of the International Federation of Cervical Pathology and Colposcopy. Obstet Gynecol 77: 313, 1991. From the American College of Obstetricians and Gynecologists, with permission.

nuclear density, is significantly whiter. In some instances the white epithelium exhibits vascular patterns referred to as mosaic and punctation. These are due to the retention and/or crowding out of the individual villus capillaries of the columnar epithelium. Leukoplakia is a raised, white plaque of keratin that is visible with the naked eye before the application of acetic acid (vinegar), an agent that assists in the removal of mucus. Acetic acid also has a dehydrating effect, causing a relative increase in the nuclear/cytoplasmic ratio and, therefore, in the optical density, which further accentuates the differences between normal and abnormal squamous epithelium.

Invariably, the peripheral border of the white epithelium abuts the native squamous epithelium, while the inner limit is defined by the active or physiologic SCJ. Leukoplakia seldom abuts the physiologic SCJ; however, it is almost always found within the transformation zone. Atypical vessels form highly irregular patterns termed "commas," "spaghetti," "corkscrews," or "earthworms." They are to be differentiated from the regular branching of normal vessels frequently seen over large nabothian cysts. Atypical vessels are more important than other features of the atypical transformation zone, since they are indicative of early invasive carcinoma. Examples of the various colposcopic abnormalities of the transformation zone are seen in Figures 2–19 through 2–25. The intraepithelial condylomas or flat warts are properly included in the atypical transformation zone because, in some cases, they are associated with dysplasia or have a premalignant poten-

tial. This is discussed in detail at the beginning of this chapter.

With experience it is possible to grade the colposcopic abnormalities and to make an accurate prediction of the histologic diagnosis. Factors considered in grading include the vascular structures (regular or irregular), surface contour (flat, depressed, raised, and/or irregular), color and opacity (degree of whiteness), and the line of demarcation from normal epithelium. The green filter enhances the

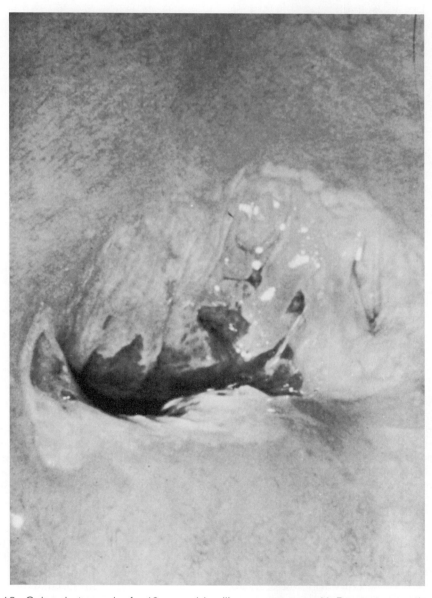

FIGURE 2–19. Colpophotograph of a 19-year-old nulliparous woman with Pap test sugestive of moderate dysplasia. An abnormal transformation zone characterized by white epithelium is present. Directed biopsy showed moderate dysplasia. The entire limits of the physiologic SCJ are seen; therefore, diagnostic conization is unnecessary.

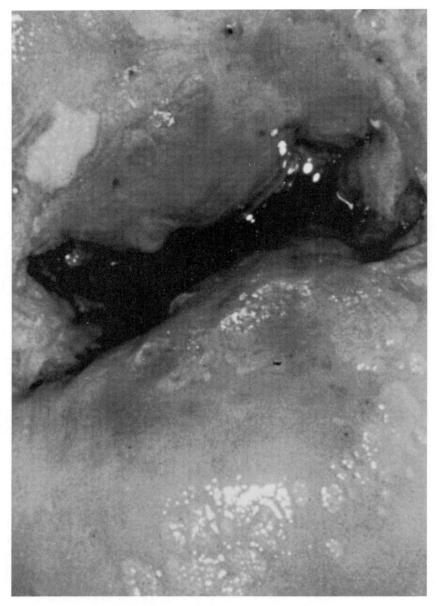

FIGURE 2–20. Colpophotograph of a 27-year-old gravida 2, para 2 woman whose Pap smear was consistent with mild to moderate dysplasia (CIN I to II). Leukoplakia is present at the 11 o'clock position in the transformation zone but not at the SCJ. The patient had white epithelium extending into the canal, and the upper limits of the lesion could not be seen. ECC revealed moderate dysplasia, and diagnostic conization was necessary for complete evaluation of the endocervical canal. The small area of leukoplakia was visible to the naked eye before the application of acetic acid.

color tone differences and the vascular changes. The latter are best viewed before acetic acid application, but acetic acid is essential to enhance the color tone differences. In addition to dysplasia, immature metaplastic squamous epithelium also appears white because the immature squamous cells are relatively small, with a resultant increased nuclear/cytoplasmic ratio. It is possible to differentiate squamous metaplasia from mildly dysplastic epithelium, however, because the border between metaplastic and normal epithelium is highly irregular, whereas the border between normal and dysplastic tissue is usually sharp.

Most dysplastic lesions are unifocal, although multifocality does occur, and they are invariably confined to the transformation

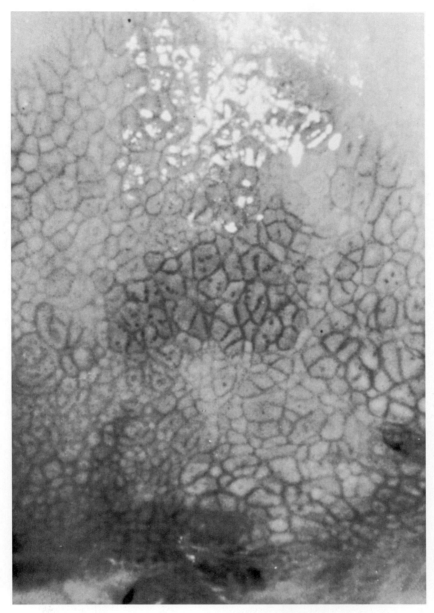

FIGURE 2–21. Atypical transformation zone characterized by mosaic structure, with an occasional area of punctation. The mosaic structure is regular, and the punctation has a moderate increase in intercapillary distance. Directed biopsy showed CIN III. The entire limits of this lesion could be seen; therefore, diagnostic conization was unnecessary.

zone. We have not seen a single patient with CIN in the canal and on the ectocervix without an intervening bridge of dysplastic epithelium.

The flat condyloma is now a well-recognized colposcopic abnormality (Fig. 2–24). Unfortunately, the white lesion of squamous metaplasia is often interpreted by the colposcopist as a flat condyloma. Distinguishing between the flat condyloma, squamous meta-

plasia, and the low-grade SIL/CIN lesion by colposcopy is virtually impossible. Even the histologic interpretation can be difficult. Therefore, it is not surprising that colposcopy suffers from the inability to reliably distinguish benign from so-called premalignant lesions. Consequently, tissue biopsy must be performed to clarify the diagnosis. Even then differences of opinion may exist among pathologists and consultation may be required.

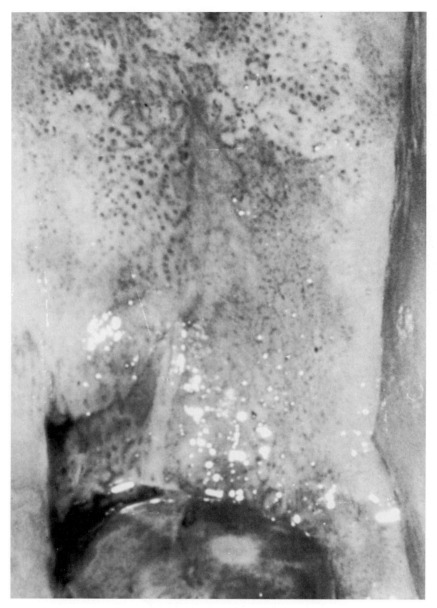

FIGURE 2–22. Atypical transformation zone characterized by punctation. A large polyp occluding the external os is present at the bottom of the colpophotograph. Directed biopsy revealed CIN III, but the entire limits of the lesion could not be viewed. ECC showed strips of neoplastic squamous epithelium consistent with CIN III. Conization was negative for invasion.

Colposcopically Overt Carcinoma

There are instances in which the naked eye can detect no evidence of invasive carcinoma, but colposcopic examination reveals features consistent with invasive cancer: raised, irregular surface contour; thick epithelium; and a markedly atypical vascular pattern. In these cases the colposcope is particularly valuable in pinpointing the exact area to biopsy for early diagnosis and prompt initiation of therapy.

Satisfactory or Unsatisfactory Examination

Critical to every colposcopic evaluation of the cervix is the ability to view the entire limits of the active or physiologic SCJ. If the entire

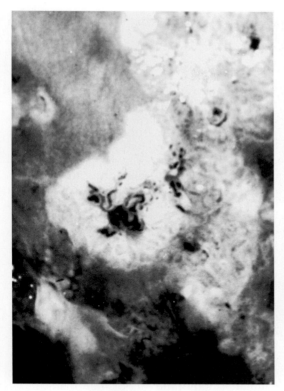

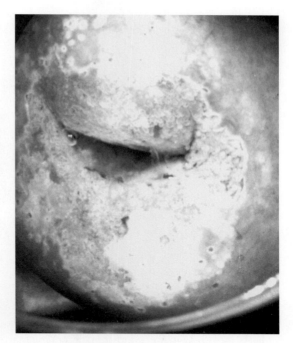

FIGURE 2–24. Colpophotograph of flat condyloma in a 19-year-old patient with a Pap smear consistent with HPV/low-grade SIL.

FIGURE 2–23. Atypical transformation zone characterized by heavy white epithelium, with a focus of atypical vascular structure in the center of this epithelium. Directed biopsy of the atypical vascular pattern revealed microinvasive carcinoma. Conization was necessary to assess the lesion completely, since microinvasive cancer was present and the lesion extended well into the canal. An ECC revealed severely dysplastic epithelium.

limits of this most important landmark cannot be seen, the examination must be judged unsatisfactory, and the possibility of invasive cancer in a patient with an abnormal Pap test cannot be excluded by colposcopy. However, if invasive cancer has been recognized and confirmed by a biopsy on the visible portion of the cervix, the patient has had an appropriate evaluation. In cases where CIN is present but the entire SCJ cannot be seen, the examination is considered unsatisfactory and a diagnostic cone biopsy is required if invasive cancer is not found by the office biopsies.

Other Colposcopic Findings

The single largest subdivision of colposcopic abnormalities consists of those lesions that are of relatively minor significance. Most fre-

quently encountered are condylomata acuminata, cervical polyps, true erosions (usually the result of speculum insertion), vaginocervicitis, and atrophic epithelium. The most important of these are the condylomas. The benign, spiculated condylomas, more frequently seen during pregnancy, are usually recognized because of their striking surface contour (Fig. 2–25) and vascular structure. Most are associated with vulvar and vaginal components and are almost invariably multifocal.

Benign Cervical Changes

Physicians are often faced with a patient who has a red, granular, angry-appearing cervix. In these cases, colposcopic examination often permits an accurate evaluation of the abnormality, thereby assuring both the physician and the patient that a more serious problem is not present. The appearance of the cervix in these patients is invariably due to the single-celled columnar epithelium overlying the highly vascular stroma, an appearance that is sometimes exaggerated by oral contraceptives. It is normal for columnar epithelium to be located on the ectocervix, and therapy is not necessary. Endocervical polyps can

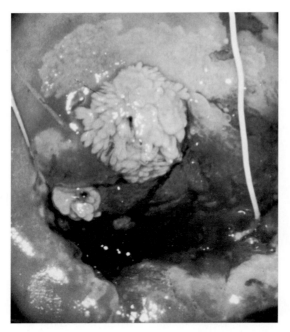

FIGURE 2–25. Typical condylomata acuminata present at the 12 o'clock position. The patient had a Pap test suggestive of mild to moderate dysplasia. White epithelium present on the anterior lip with a very irregular border is consistent with squamous metaplasia or intraepithelial condyloma. The entire limits of the lesion could be seen. Directed biopsy of the lesion at the 12 o'clock position revealed condyloma, and directed biopsy of the white epithelium revealed active metaplasia. An intrauterine device string is present, passing out of the os at the 4 o'clock position.

also be assessed by colposcopy. In most cases the base of the polyp can be viewed to assist in removal.

Vulvar Disease

VIN is amenable to colposcopic evaluation, although the patterns are not as striking as those of the cervix. VIN is frequently multifocal, and with the colposcope it is easier to identify the true extent of the disease. Keratinized lesions, however, are not evaluable by colposcopy and must be totally excised. The most frequent colposcopic pattern encountered on the vulva is white epithelium, which may have a keratinized surface. Mosaic structure and punctation are infrequent because the lack of columnar epithelium precludes the formation of these patterns. Condylomas are quite assessable by colposcopic examination, which can exclude the presence of a

more serious problem, avoiding biopsy in most cases.

Vaginal Disease

Some benign and malignant vaginal lesions can be evaluated by colposcopy. Posthysterectomy granulation tissue that is abnormally persistent, however, should be assessed by biopsy if the patient had surgery for malignant disease. Colposcopic evaluation of granulation tissue is not reliable because this tissue normally has atypical vascular features. VAIN has a tendency to be multifocal. It is well suited to colposcopic evaluation, with the help of Lugol's solution to assist in the location of tiny foci that may be hidden in the vaginal folds. The prominent patterns in the vagina are white epithelium and punctation. If there has been columnar tissue in the vagina, a feature particularly common in the diethylstilbestrol (DES)–exposed female, all the features seen on the cervix, such as mosaic structure, punctation, leukoplakia, and atypical vessels, may be present. The examination of the patient with atrophic changes in the vaginal membrane (postmenopausal or postradiation) is aided by treatment with intravaginal estrogens.

Diethylstilbestrol-Exposed Offspring

The occurrence of clear cell adenocarcinoma and cervical/vaginal anomalies in DES-exposed females provided the colposcopists with an exceptional opportunity to exercise their skills. With the naked eye, it is sometimes impossible to determine the extent of epithelial changes in the vagina and cervix in these individuals. Colposcopy can assist in the clinical evaluation, but overinterpretation of the colposcopic pattern of immature metaplasia is common by the inexperienced. Grossly, cervical hoods, ridges, and cockscombs are often visible. Colposcopically, one invariably sees a vast transformation zone, which usually covers the entire ectocervix and extends onto the vagina, occasionally down to the introitus. The metaplastic squamous epithelium of the vagina usually appears white, forming mosaic and punctation patterns resembling dysplasia. Atypical vessels are rare. As the metaplastic squamous epithelium matures, the white appearance tends to lessen. However, many years are required for the tissue to become mature enough to accept Lugol's iodine normally (see also Chapter 4.)

REFERENCES

Abdul-Karim FW, Nunez C: Cervical intraepithelial neoplasia after conization: a study of 522 consecutive cervical cones. Obstet Gynecol 65:77, 1985.

American College of Obstetricians and Gynecologists: Laser Technology. Technical Bulletin No. 146. Washington, DC, American College of Obstetricians and Gynecologists, 1990.

Andersen WA, Franquemont DW, Williams J, et al: Vulvar squamous cell carcinoma and papilloma viruses: two separate entities? Am J Obstet Gynecol 165:329, 1991.

Anderson MC: Treatment of cervical intraepithelial neoplasia with the carbon dioxide laser: report of 543 patients. Obstet Gynecol 59:720, 1982.

Anderson MC: Invasive carcinoma of the cervix following local destructive treatment for cervical intraepithelial neoplasia. Br J Obstet Gynaecol 100:657, 1993.

Baggish MS: High power density carbon dioxide laser therapy for early cervical neoplasia. Am J Obstet Gynecol 136:117, 1980.

Baggish MS, Barash F, Noel Y, Brooks M: Comparison of thermal injury zones in loop electrical and laser cervical excisional conization. Am J Obstet Gynecol 166:545, 1992.

Baggish MS, Dorsey JG: CO_2 laser for the treatment of vulvar carcinoma in situ. Obstet Gynecol 57:371, 1981.

Baggish MS, Dorsey JH: Carbon dioxide laser for combination excisional-vaporization conization. Am J Obstet Gynecol 151:23, 1985.

Baker DA, Douglas JM Jr, Buntin DM, et al: Topical podofilox for the treatment of condylomata acuminata in women. Obstet Gynecol 76:656, 1990.

Benedet JL, Miller DM, Nickerson KG: Results of conservative management of cervical intraepithelial neoplasia. Obstet Gynecol 79:105, 1992.

Benedet JL, Murphy KJ: Squamous carcinoma in situ of the vulva. Gynecol Oncol 14:213, 1982.

Berget A, Andreasson B, Bock JE, et al: Outpatient treatment of cervical intraepithelial noeplasia. Acta Obstet Gynecol Scand 66:531, 1987.

Bernstein SG, Kovacs BR, Townsend DE, Morrow CP: Vulvar carcinoma in situ. Obstet Gynecol 61:304, 1983.

Bethesda System for Reporting Cervical/Vaginal Cytologic Diagnosis. Hum Pathol 21:704, 1990.

Birch HW: Discussion of Friedrich, EG and MacLaren, NK: Genetic aspects of vulvar lichen sclerosus. Am J Obstet Gynecol 150:161, 1984.

Bjerre B, Eliasson G, Linell F, et al: Conization as only treatment of carcinoma in situ of the uterine cervix. Am J Obstet Gynecol 125:143, 1976.

Boonstra H, Aalders, JG, Koudstaal J, et al: Minimum extension and appropriate topographic position of tissue destruction for treatment of cervical intraepithelial neoplasia. Obstet Gynecol 75:227, 1990.

Bottles K, Reiter RC, Steiner AL, et al: Problems encountered with the Bethesda System: the University of Iowa experience. Obstet Gynecol 78:410, 1991.

Boyes DA, Worth AJ, Fidler HK: The results of treatment of 4389 cases of preclinical cervical squamous carcinoma. J Obstet Gynaecol Br Commonw 77:769, 1970.

Bracco GL, Carli P, Sonni L, et al: Clinical and histologic effects of topical treatments of vulval lichen sclerosus: a critical evaluation. J Reprod Med 38:37, 1993.

Broen EM, Ostergard DR: Toluidine blue and colposcopy for screening and delineating vulvar neoplasia. Obstet Gynecol 38:775, 1971.

Burger MPM, Hollema H: The reliability of the histologic diagnosis in colposcopically directed biopsies: a plea for LETZ. Int J Gynecol Cancer 3:385, 1993.

Buscema J, Woodruff JD: Progressive histologic alterations in the development of vulvar cancer. Am J Obstet Gynecol 138:146, 1980.

Capen CV, Masterson BJ, Magrina JF, Calkins JW: Laser therapy for vaginal intraepithelial neoplasia. Am J Obstet Gynecol 142:973, 1982.

Cartier R: Practical Colposcopy, 2nd Ed. Paris, Laboratorie Cartier, 1984.

Cattaneo A, Bracco GL, Maestrini G, et al: Lichen sclerosus and squamous hyperplasia of the vulva: a clinical study of medical treatment. J Reprod Med 36:301, 1991.

Chanen W, Rome RM: Electrocoagulation diathermy for cervical dysplasia and carcinoma in situ: a 15 year survey. Obstet Gynecol 61:673, 1983.

Chappatte OA, Byrne DL, Raju KS, et al: Histological differences between colposcopic-directed biopsy and loop excision of the transformation zone (LETZ): a cause for concern. Gynecol Oncol 43:46, 1991.

Cox SM, Kaufman RH, Kaplan A: Recurrent carcinoma in situ of the vulva in a skin graft. Am J Obstet Gynecol 155:177, 1986.

Creasman WT, Hinshaw WM, Clarke-Pearson DL: Cryosurgery in the management of cervical intraepithelial neoplasia. Obstet Gynecol 63:145, 1984.

Crum CP: Carcinoma of the vulva: epidemiology and pathogenesis. Obstet Gynecol 79:448, 1992.

Crum CP, Liskow A, Petras P, et al: Vulvar intraepithelial neoplasia (severe atypia and carcinoma in situ). Cancer 54:1429, 1984.

Deigan EA, Carmichael JA, Ohike ID, Karchmar J: Treatment of cervical intraepithelial neoplasia with electrocautery: a report of 776 cases. Am J Obstet Gynecol 154:255, 1986.

Demopoulos RI, Horowitz LF, Vamvakas EC: Endocervical gland involvement by cervical intraepithelial neoplasia grade III: predictive value for residual and/or recurrent disease. Cancer 68:1932, 1991.

DiPaola GR: The problem of the so-called precancerous lesions of the vulva: ten years of prospective experience. Eur J Gynecol Oncol 1:20, 1980.

Drake M: Cytological pitfalls: a review of five areas of diagnostic difficulty. Colposc Gynecol Laser Surg 1:253, 1985.

Felix JC, Muderspach LI, Duggan BD, Roman LD: The significance of positive margins in loop electrosurgical cone biopsies. Obstet Gynecol 84:996, 1994.

Ferenczy A: Comparison of cryosurgery and carbon dioxide laser therapy for cervical intraepithelial neoplasia. Obstet Gynecol 66:793, 1985.

Ferenczy A: Epidemiology and clinical pathophysiology of condylomata acuminata. Am J Obstet Gynecol 172 (suppl):1331, 1995.

Ferenczy A, Bergeron C, Richart RM: Human papillomavirus DNA in CO_2 laser generated plume of smoke and its consequences to the surgeon. Obstet Gynecol 75:114, 1990.

Fisher JC: CO_2 lasers for gynecologic surgery: how safe are they? Contemp Ob/Gyn 21:39, 1983.

Flannelly G, Anderson D, Kitchener HC, et al: The management of women with mild and moderate cervical dyskaryosis. BMJ 308:1399, 1994.

Forney JP, Morrow CP, Townsend DE: Management of carcinoma in situ of the vulva. Am J Obstet Gynecol 127:801, 1977.

Fowler JM, Davos I, Leuchter RS, Lagasse LD: Effect of CO_2 laser conization of the uterine cervix on pathologic interpretation of cervical intraepithelial neoplasia. Obstet Gynecol 79:693, 1992.

Friedrich EG: Topical testosterone for benign vulvar dystrophy. Obstet Gynecol 37:677, 1971.

Friedrich EG: Treating vulvar dystrophy. Contemp Ob/Gyn 10:19, 1977.

Friedrich EG Jr: Vulvar dystrophy. Clin Obstet Gynecol 28: 178, 1985.

Friedrich EG, Kalra PS: Serum levels of sex hormones in vulvar lichen sclerosus, and the effect of topical testosterone. N Engl J Med 310:488, 1984.

Friedrich EG, MacLaren NK: Genetic aspects of vulvar lichen sclerosus. Am J Obstet Gynecol 150:161, 1984.

Friedrich EG, Wilkinson EJ, Fu YS: Carcinoma in situ of the vulva: a continuing challenge. Am J Obstet Gynecol 36: 830, 1980.

Gall SA: Human papillomavirus infection and therapy with interferon. Am J Obstet Gynecol 172(suppl):1354, 1995.

Goff BA, Atanasoff P, Brown E, et al: Endocervical glandular atypia in Papanicolaou smears. Obstet Gynecol 79:101, 1992.

Gunasekera PC, Phipps JH, Lewis BV: Large loop excision of the transformation zone compared to CO_2 laser in the treatment of CIN: a superior mode of treatment. Br J Obstet Gynaecol 97:995, 1990.

Harrington CI, Dunsmore IR: An investigation into the incidence of autoimmune disorders in patients with lichen sclerosus et atrophicus. Br J Dermatol 104:563, 1981.

Hatch KD: Clinical appearance and treatment strategies for human papillomavirus: a gynecologic perspective. Am J Obstet Gynecol 172(suppl):1340, 1995.

Hatch KD, Shingleton HM, Austin JM Jr, et al: Cryosurgery of cervical intraepithelial neoplasia. Obstet Gynecol 57: 692, 1981.

Hørding U, Junge J, Poulsen H, Lundvall F: Vulvar intraepithelial neoplasia III: a viral disease of undetermined progressive potential. Gynecol Oncol 56:276, 1995.

Howell R, Hammond R, Pryse-Davies J: The histologic reliability of laser cone biopsy of the cervix. Obstet Gynecol 77:905, 1991.

Ireland D, Monaghan JM: The management of the patient with abnormal vaginal cytology following hysterectomy. Br J Obstet Gynaecol 95:973, 1988.

Isacson C, Kurman RJ: The Bethesda System: a new classification for managing Pap smears. Contemp Ob/Gyn June:67, 1995.

Jasionowski EA, Jasionowski PA: Further observations on the effect of topical progesterone on vulvar disease. Am J Obstet Gynecol 134:565, 1979.

Jobson WW, Homesley HD: Treatment of vaginal intraepithelial neoplasia with the carbon dioxide laser. Obstet Gynecol 62:90, 1983.

Jones RW, McLean MR: Carcinoma in situ of the vulva: a review of 31 treated and five untreated cases. Obstet Gynecol 68:499, 1986.

Jones RW, Park JS, McLean MR, Shah KV: Human papilloma virus in women with vulvar intraepithelial neoplasia III. J Reprod Med 35:1124, 1990.

Kaplan AL, Kaufman RH, Birken RA, Simkin S: Intraepithelial carcinoma of the vulva with extension to the anal canal. Obstet Gynecol 58:368, 1981.

Kaufman RH: Intraepithelial neoplasia of the vulva. Gynecol Oncol 56:8, 1995.

Kaufman RH: Atypical squamous cells of undetermined significance and low-grade squamous intraepithelial lesion: diagnostic criteria and management. Am J Obstet Gynecol 175(suppl):1120, 1996.

Kaufman RH, Gardner HL, Brown D, Beyth Y: Vulvar dystrophies: an evaluation. Am J Obstet Gynecol 120:363, 1974.

Kennedy AW, Salmieri SS, Wirth SL, et al: Results of the clinical evaluation of atypical glandular cells of undetermined significance (AGCUS) detected on cervical cytology screening. Gynecol Oncol 63:14, 1996.

Kirwan PH, Smith IR, Naftalin NJ: A study of cryosurgery and the CO_2 laser in treatment of carcinoma in situ (CIN III) of the uterine cervix. Gynecol Oncol 22:195, 1985.

Kiviat N: Natural history of cervical neoplasia: overview and update. Am J Obstet Gynecol 175(suppl):1099, 1996.

Kolstad P, Klem V: Long term followup of 1,121 cases of carcinoma in situ. Obstet Gynecol 48:125, 1976.

Korn AP: Interpretation of abnormal Pap smears. Infect Med 13:405, 1996.

Krebs HB: Treatment of vaginal intraepithelial neoplasia with laser and topical 5-fluorouracil. Obstet Gynecol 73: 657, 1989.

Krebs HB, Pastore L, Helmkamp BF: Loop electrosurgical excision procedure for cervical dysplasia: experience in a community hospital. Am J Obstet Gynecol 169:289, 1993.

Kurman RJ, Henson DE, Herbst AL: Interim guidelines for management of abnormal cervical cytology. JAMA 271: 1866, 1994.

Kurman RJ, Toki T, Schiffman MH: Basaloid and warty carcinomas of the vulva. Am J Surg Pathol 17:133, 1993.

Kwasniewski SW, Stelmachow J, Janik P: Treatment of leukoplakia of the vulva by local application of 13-cis retinoic acid [abstract]. 8th International Meeting of the European Society of Gynaecological Oncology, Barcelona, Spain, June 9–12, 1993.

Larsson G, Gullberg B, Grundsell H: A comparison of laser and cold knife conization. Obstet Gynecol 62:213, 1983.

Lavery HA, Pinkerton JHM: Vulvar dystrophy: its aetiology and classification. In Morrow CP, Bonar J (eds): Recent Clinical Developments in Gynecologic Oncology. New York, Raven Press, 1983, p 1.

Lenehan PM, Meffe F, Lickrish GM: Vaginal intraepithelial neoplasia: biologic aspects and management. Obstet Gynecol 68:333, 1986.

Leuchter RS, Townsend DE, Hacker NG, et al: Treatment of vulvar carcinoma in situ with the CO_2 laser. Gynecol Oncol 19:314, 1984.

Lifshitz S, Roberts JA: Treatment of carcinoma in situ of the vulva with topical 5-fluorouracil. Obstet Gynecol 546:242, 1980.

Lipow M: Laser physics made simple. Curr Probl Obstet Gynecol Fertil 9:25, 1986.

Luesley DM, Cullimore J, Redman CWE, et al: Loop diathermy excision of the cervical transformation zone in patients with abnormal cervical smears. Br Med J 300:1690, 1990.

Markowska J, Wiese E: Dystrophy of the vulva locally treated with 13-cis retinoic acid. Neoplasma 39:133, 1992.

Mashberg A: Re-evaluation of toluidine blue application as a diagnostic adjunct in the detection of asymptomatic oral squamous carcinoma: a continuing prospective study of oral cancer III. Cancer 46:758, 1980.

Mathevet P, Dargent D, Roy M, Beau G: A randomized prospective study comparing three techniques of conization: cold knife, laser, and LEEP. Gynecol Oncol 54:175, 1994.

McIndoe WA, McLean MR, Jones RW, Mullins PR: The invasive potential of carcinoma in situ of the cervix. Obstet Gynecol 64:451, 1984.

Meisels A, Fortin R. Condylomatous lesions of the cervix and vagina. I. Cytologic patterns. Acta Cytol 20:505, 1976.

Meisels A, Morin CM: Human papillomas and cancer of the uterine cervix. Gynecol Oncol 12:S111, 1981.

Mering JH: Some further observations on wide skin undercutting for intractable pruritus vulvae. Am J Obstet Gynecol 71:386, 1956.

Meyrick-Thomas RH, Holmes RC, Rowland-Payne CME, et al: The incidence of development of autoimmune diseases in women after the diagnosis of lichen sclerosus et atrophicus. Br J Dermatol 107:29, 1982.

Mitchell MF, Hittleman WN, Hong WK, et al: The natural history of cervical epithelial neoplasms. Cancer Epidemiol Biomarkers Prev 3:619, 1994.

Montz FJ, Monk BJ, Fowler JM, et al: Natural history of the minimally abnormal Papanicolaou smear. Am J Obstet Gynecol 80:385, 1992.

Mor-Yosef S, Lopes A, Pearson S, Monaghan JM: Loop diathermy cone biopsy. Obstet Gynecol 75:884, 1990.

Murdoch JB, Grimshaw RN, Monaghan JM: Loop diathermy excision of the abnormal cervical transformation zone. Int J Gynecol Cancer 1:105, 1991.

Nasiell K, Nasiell M, Vaclavinková V: Behavior of moderate cervical dysplasia during long-term follow-up. Obstet Gynecol 61:609, 1983.

Nasiell K, Roger V, Nasiell M: Behavior of mild cervical dysplasia during longterm followup. Obstet Gynecol 67:665, 1986.

Naumann RW, Bell MC, Alvarez RD, et al: LLETZ is an acceptable alternative to diagnostic cold-knife conization. Gynecol Oncol 55:224, 1994.

Oclassen Pharmaceuticals, Inc: Condylox. In Physicians' Desk Reference. Montvale, NJ, Medical Economics Data Production Company, 1994, p 1853.

Oyesanya OA, Amerasinghe CN, Manning EAD: Outpatient excisional management of cervical intraepithelial neoplasia: a prospective, randomized comparison between loop diathermy excision and laser excisional conization. Am J Obstet Gynecol 168:485, 1993.

Park JS, Jones RW, McLean MR, et al: Possible etiologic heterogeneity of vulvar intraepithelial neoplasia. Cancer 67: 1599, 1991.

Patterson JW, Kao GF, Graham JH, Helwig EB: Bowenoid papulosis: a clinicopathologic study with ultrastructural observations. Cancer 57:823 1986

Peters WA III, Kumar NB, Morely DW: Carcinoma of the vagina. Cancer 55:892, 1985.

Petrilli ES, Townsend DE, Morrow CP: Vaginal intraepithelial neoplasia: biological aspects and treatment with topical 5-FU and the CO_2 laser. Am J Obstet Gynecol 138:321, 1980.

Prendiville W, Cullimore J, Norman S: Large loop excision of the transformation zone (LLETZ): a new method of management for women with cervical intraepithelial neoplasia. Br J Obstet Gynaecol 96:1054, 1989.

Pride GL: Treatment of large lower genital tract condylomata acuminata with topical 5-fluorouracil. J Reprod Med 35: 384, 1990.

Purdue Frederick Company: Alferon N Injection. In Physicians' Desk Reference. Montvale, NJ, Medical Economics Data Production Company, 1997, p 2142.

Reid R: Superficial laser vulvectomy. III. A new surgical technique for appendage conserving ablation of refractory condylomas and vulvar intraepithelial neoplasia. Am J Obstet Gynecol 152:504, 1985.

Reid R, Scalzi P: Genital warts and cervical cancer. VII: An improved colposcopic index for differentiating benign papillomavirus infections from high-grade cervical intraepithelial neoplasia. Am J Obstet Gynecol 153:611, 1985.

Rodke G, Friedrich EG Jr, Wilkinson EJ: Malignant potential of mixed vulvar dystrophy (lichen sclerosus associated with squamous cell hyperplasia). J Reprod Med 33:545, 1988.

Roman LD, Felix JC, Muderspach LI, et al: Risk of residual invasive disease in women with microinvasive squamous cancer in a conization specimen. Obstet Gynecol 90:795, 1997.

Roy M: VIN: latest management approaches. Contemp Ob/ Gyn May:170, 1988.

Rusk D, Sutton GP, Look KY, Roman A: Analysis of invasive squamous cell carcinoma of the vulva and vulvar intraepithelial neoplasia for the presence of human papillomavirus DNA. Obstet Gynecol 77:918, 1991.

Rutledge F, Sinclair M: Treatment of intraepithelial carcinoma of the vulva by skin excision and graft. Am J Obstet Gynecol 102:806, 1968.

Savage EW, Matlock DL, Salem FA, Charles EH: The effect of endocervical gland involvement on the cure rates of patients with cervical intraepithelial neoplasia undergoing cryosurgery. Gynecol Oncol 14:194, 1982.

Schering Corporation: Intron A. In Physicians' Desk Reference. Montvale, NJ, Medical Economics Production Data Company, 1997, p 2506.

Schlaerth JB, Morrow CP, Nalick RH, Gaddis O Jr: Anal involvement by carcinoma in situ of the perineum in women. Obstet Gynecol 64:406, 1984.

Schmidt C, Pretorius RG, Bonin M, et al: Invasive cervical cancer following cryotherapy for cervical intraepithelial neoplasia or human papillomavirus infection. Obstet Gynecol 80:797, 1992.

Shafi MI, Dunn JA, Buxton EJ, et al: Abnormal cervical cytology following large loop excision of the transformation zone: a case controlled study. Br J Obstet Gynaecol 100: 145, 1993.

Shafi MI, Luesley DM, Byrne P, et al: Vulval intraepithelial neoplasia: management and outcome. Br J Obstet Gynaecol 96:1339, 1989.

Spirtos N, Schlaerth JB, d'Ablaing G: A critical evaluation of the endocervical curettage. Obstet Gynecol 70:729, 1987.

Stafl A, Wilbanks GD: An international terminology of colposcopy: report of the Nomenclature Committee of the International Federation of Cervical Pathology and Colposcopy. Obstet Gynecol 77:313, 1991.

Stokes IM, Sworm MJ, Hawthorne JHR: A new regimen for the treatment of vaginal carcinoma in situ using 5-fluorouracil: case report. Br J Obstet Gynaecol 87:910, 1980.

Stoler MH: A brief synopsis of the role of human papillomaviruses in cervical carcinogenesis. Am J Obstet Gynecol 175(suppl):1091, 1996.

Syrjänen K, Kataja V, Yliskoski M, et al: Natural history of cervical human papillomavirus lesions does not substantiate the biologic relevance of the Bethesda System. Obstet Gynecol 79:675, 1992.

Townsend DE, Levine RU, Crum CP, Richart RM: Treatment of vaginal carcinoma in situ with the carbon dioxide laser. Am J Obstet Gynecol 143:565, 1982a.

Townsend DE, Levine RU, Richart RM, et al: Management of vulvar intraepithelial neoplasia by carbon dioxide laser. Obstet Gynecol 60:49, 1982b.

Townsend DE, Richart RM: Cryotherapy and carbon dioxide laser management of cervical intraepithelial neoplasia: a controlled comparison. Obstet Gynecol 61:75, 1983.

Townsend DE, Richart RM, Marks E, Nielsen J: Invasive cancer following outpatient evaluation and therapy for cervical disease. Obstet Gynecol 57:145, 1981.

Ulbright TM, Stehman FB, Roth LM, et al: Bowenoid dysplasia of the vulva. Cancer 50:2910, 1982.

Wallace HJ: Lichen sclerosus et atrophicus. Trans St. John's Hosp. Dermatol Soc 54:9, 1971.

Ward GD, Sutherst JR: Pruritus vulvae: treatment by multiple intradermal alcohol injections. Br J Dermatol 93:201, 1976.

Wilkinson EJ, Friedrich EG, Fu YS: Multicentric nature of vulvar carcinoma in situ. Obstet Gynecol 58:69, 1981.

Woodruff JD, Babaknia A: Local alcohol injection of the vulva: discussion of 35 cases. Obstet Gynecol 54:512, 1979.

Wright TC, Gagnon S, Richart RM, Ferenczy A: Treatment of cervical intraepithelial neoplasia using the loop electrosurgical excision procedure. Obstet Gynecol 79:173, 1992a.

Wright TC Jr, Richart RM, Ferenczy A, Koulos J: Comparison of specimens removed by CO_2 laser conization and the loop electrosurgical excision procedure. Obstet Gynecol 79:147, 1992b.

Wright VC, Chapman WB: Colposcopy of intraepithelial neoplasia of the vulva and adjacent sites. Obstet Gynecol Clin North Am 20:231, 1993.

Wright VC, Davies E, Riopelle MA: Laser surgery for cervical intraepithelial neoplasia: principles and results. Am J Obstet Gynecol 145:181, 1983.

Wright VC, Davies E, Riopelle MA: Laser cylindrical excision to replace conization. Am J Obstet Gynecol 150:704, 1984.

Wu AY, Sherman ME, Rosenshein NB, Erozan YS: Pathologic evaluation of gynecologic specimens obtained with the Cavitron ultrasonic surgical aspirator (CUSA). Gynecol Oncol 44:28, 1992.

3

Tumors of the Vulva

■

BENIGN TUMORS OF THE VULVA

Non-neoplastic Tumors

An impressive array of non-neoplastic tumors occur on the vulva, most of which are quite unusual. These can be subdivided into cystic and solid categories. The solid lesions include nevi (discussed under melanoma of the vulva), acrochordon, breast tissue, various types of hemangioma, and hernias.

The acrochordon or fibroepithelial polyp is a small (usually less than 1 cm), soft, pedunculated tag of smooth wrinkled skin. Symptoms result from twisting or ulceration. Treatment by snip excision is indicated if the acrochordon annoys the patient, becomes symptomatic, or exceeds 1 to 2 cm in diameter.

Rarely, breast tissue develops on the vulva. The vulva is the most distal point of the mammary ridge or "milk line" in the embryo. Since the nipple is absent, clinical recognition depends on cyclic premenstrual or gestational changes. Garcia et al (1978) noted that vulvar breast tissue encountered in pregnant women was invariably normal, whereas that excised from nonpregnant women was usually neoplastic or malignant, indicating the importance of a hormonal influence on the discovery of normal ectopic breast tissue. At least 11 cases of carcinoma arising in vulvar breast tissue have been reported (Levin et al, 1995). A 1- to 3-year history of a pre-existing, asymptomatic nodule was common.

Epidermal inclusion cysts arising from the pilosebaceous apparatus occur frequently. They are commonly interpreted clinically as sebaceous cysts, which are relatively rare on the vulva. Epidermal inclusion cysts are typically multiple, seldom exceed 1 to 2 cm in diameter, and involve the labia majora. They are filled with a thick, white material that ap-

pears yellow when viewed through the skin. Epidermal inclusion cysts are invariably asymptomatic unless they become infected or rupture into the skin. The larger cysts or those that annoy the patient can be managed by simple incision and evacuation.

Bartholin duct cysts are a sequel to bartholinitis. If they are infected, large, or symptomatic, incision and marsupialization or Word's catheter drainage are the traditional treatments. Laser incision with vaporization of the cyst wall is an effective alternative (Heah, 1988). Atypical or symptomatic Bartholin cysts in the peri- and postmenopausal woman should be excised to exclude the presence of malignancy.

Cysts lined by mucinous or ciliated epithelium occur rarely on the vulva. They originate from urogenital sinus, mesonephric (Gartner's duct), or müllerian (paramesonephric) embryonic remnants. Typically less than 1 cm in diameter and located in the vestibule, they are similar to epidermal inclusion cysts. Removal is indicated for the larger or symptomatic cysts. In the newborn, embryonic cysts, mostly paraurethral in location, have been reported, but they apparently involute spontaneously and require no treatment (Merlob et al, 1978). Cysts of the canal of Nuck occur in the upper outer labium majus or the inguinal region and correspond to the male hydrocele.

Other non-neoplastic lesions of the vulva include endometriosis (episiotomy scar), Fox-Fordyce disease, and cherry (senile) and various other hemangiomas. The interested reader is referred to the textbooks by Kaufman et al (1989) and Wilkinson (1987) for additional information.

Tumors of Epithelial Origin

Hidradenoma Papilliferum

Hidradenoma papilliferum is an uncommon, benign neoplasm arising from the apocrine or

eccrine sweat glands of the vulva and perianal region. As a rule, the lesions are less than
1 cm in diameter, intradermal, freely movable,
and have an umbilicated or cystic configuration. Rarely do these tumors exceed 2 cm in
size, although an 8-cm cystic tumor has been
reported (Kaufmann et al, 1987). Hidradenomas occur in postpubertal, predominantly
white females, typically as a single lesion on
the labium majus. In two thirds of the cases,
the growths are asymptomatic at diagnosis.
Ulceration and bleeding may occur. Hidradenomas are of special importance because,
both clinically and histologically, they have
been mistakenly diagnosed as malignant.
Rarely the lesion may evert, presenting as a
red, friable papillary mass. Excision biopsy is
always indicated to confirm the diagnosis.
Malignancy arising in a hidradenoma has
been reported (Bannatyne et al, 1989).

Hidradenomas represent an intraductal adenoma, which accounts for their variable clinical appearance. If the duct is expanded so
that the skin opening dilates, the tumor fills
or even protrudes through the duct opening,
producing an umbilicated configuration. If
the duct opening is blocked, the glandular se-
cretions accumulate, producing a cystic structure (Woodworth et al, 1971).

Syringoma

The rare syringoma is an adenoma of the eccrine or appocrine sweat glands occurring
most often in adolescent and young adult
women. Intermittent vulvar pruritis is the predominant symptom. These are multiple, soft,
skin-colored to yellowish, symmetrically distributed intradermal lesions measuring up to
5 mm in diameter and occurring predominantly on the labia majora. Other commonly
affected sites are the labia minora, mons
veneris, and adjacent thighs. The lesions may
also occur around the eyelids and on the
neck, chest, and abdomen. Syringomas can
resemble Fox-Fordyce disease or multiple epidermal cysts. Symptomatic treatment is satisfactory for vulvar lesions (Young et al,
1980). Laser removal of facial lesions has produced good cosmetic results (Wheeland et al,
1986). Syringomas may occur as one component of the mixed adnexal tumor, which
also contains trichoepitheliomatous or pilar
tumor elements. The latter is a benign squamous neoplasm arising from the pilosebaceous apparatus (Guindi et al, 1974).

Verrucous Lesions

Condylomata acuminata are discussed in
Chapter 2. The seborrheic keratoses are common lesions of the skin in postmenopausal
women that occasionally occur on the vulva.
They are raised and macular to papular in
configuration, with sharp borders, and range
from gray-brown to almost black in color. The
term seborrheic refers to the often greasy appearance of the lesions. However, their origin
has no relationship to sebaceous glands.
They may be overtly papillary in configuration, constituting one variety of squamous
papilloma. Seborrheic keratoses have a limited growth potential and are not premalignant. On the vulva, they mimic bowenoid lesions, nevi, melanomas, and other significant
entities. Consequently, excision biopsy is
recommended.

Acanthosis nigricans (AN) is generally a
progressive, diffuse dermatosis. AN is characterized by pigmented, velvety, papillomatous skin and, occasionally, mucosal lesions,
which may resemble condylomata acuminata or seborrheic keratoses. Histologically
the lesions show hyperkeratosis, acanthosis,
papillomatosis, and increased pigmentation.
Three categories of this rare disorder are recognized:

1. *Malignant AN*, the most common type, is
   associated with an internal malignancy,
   usually an adenocarcinoma of the stomach
   or other abdominal organ, including the
   ovary and uterus. Uncommonly, breast or
   lung cancer is implicated. AN is itself always benign. The appearance of AN typically precedes other clinical evidence of
   the underlying malignancy, and as a rule
   the spread and progression of AN parallel
   those of the malignancy. Similarly, the lesions of AN regress with effective cancer
   therapy.
2. *Benign AN* may be present at birth or may
   appear in childhood, but most commonly
   it develops at puberty. It is not associated
   with malignant disease. Regression or stabilization occurs after puberty.
3. *Pseudo-AN* is associated with obesity, estrogen therapy, and nicotinic acid therapy
   (Mikhail et al, 1979). AN is also associated
   with several syndromes of insulin resistance and androgen excess, including polycystic ovarian disease (Barbieri and
   Ryan, 1983; Dunaif et al, 1985).

Tumors of Mesodermal Origin

Granular Cell Myoblastoma

Also known as granular cell tumor and schwannoma, granular cell myoblastoma (GCM) is an uncommon solitary, firm, infiltrative benign tumor derived from the Schwann cell of the nerve sheath. It is usually asymptomatic and slow growing, and it ranges in size from 1 to 4 cm at diagnosis. The overlying skin is sometimes depigmented. GCM most often involves the skin, tongue, and upper respiratory tract. Multifocality and multicentricity are not unusual (Majmudar et al, 1990). Vulvar GCM, which accounts for approximately 10 percent of cases, is typically located on the labia majora or the clitoris. Another important clinicopathologic feature of GCM is the tendency for the overlying skin to undergo ulceration and develop a pseudoepitheliomatous hyperplasia, which can be mistaken for squamous carcinoma (Lieb et al, 1979, Kaufman et al, 1989).

Like pelvic neurofibroma, this tumor probably contains hormone receptors. GCM occurs predominantly during the reproductive years in black women. There are two histologic variants. The uniform variety is always benign and is adequately managed by wide excision. Local recurrence, which is fairly common, should not be interpreted as a sign of malignancy. Wide re-excision is appropriate treatment. The presence of even focal pleomorphism suggests that the tumor is malignant. However, rapid infiltrative growth is more dependable evidence of malignant behavior than is the histology, unless frankly sarcomatous areas are present. Lymphatic as well as hematogenous metastases have been observed.

Other Mesodermal Tumors

Fibromas and lipomas can reach several centimeters in size, becoming pedunculated as they grow. The fibroma is characteristically firm, with a narrow stalk, whereas the typical lipoma is soft, with a broader base. Simple excision is adequate therapy. Neurofibromas (schwannomas) are generally small, soft, polyploid lesions occurring in children and young adults. On the vulva they represent a local manifestation of von Recklinghausen's disease in up to 50 percent of cases. These lesions occur singly or in groups and may be painful, but are usually discovered at routine examination. A search for lesions elsewhere should be undertaken, especially in the patient with café au lait spots, if a diagnosis of von Recklinghausen's disease has not been made previously. Rapid growth, symptoms, and large size are indications for excision. Involvement of the clitoris may mimic other causes of clitoromegaly.

Leiomyomas of the vulva are soft to firm, generally less than 5 cm in diameter, and occur predominantly during the reproductive years. Findings suspicious of malignancy are discussed in the section "Malignant Mesodermal Tumors" later in this chapter. A syndrome of multiple smooth muscle tumors of the vulva and esophagus, termed *leiomyomatosis*, has been reported in young women (Faber et al, 1991). Several cases of glomus tumor of the vulva have been described (Katz et al, 1986). They are small, benign tumors associated with pain exacerbated by palpation. Simple excision is curative.

Nodular (pseudosarcomatous) fasciitis is a benign reactive lesion of the superficial or deep fascia that histologically resembles a spindle cell sarcoma with moderate mitotic activity. Typically the lesion is less than 3 cm in diameter, rubbery, and tender and enlarges rather rapidly. The etiology is unknown. It occurs predominantly in the 20- to 40-year age group. Excision is adequate therapy (LiVolsi and Brooks, 1987). Recurrence is indicative of a misdiagnosis (Bernstein and Lattes, 1982).

Pigmented Lesions

Pigmented lesions of the vulva are fairly commonplace (12 percent of adult white women; Rock et al, 1990) and usually innocuous. Most frequent (two thirds) among them is the lentigo, clinically similar to the freckle, which occurs in otherwise normal-appearing skin and has a homogeneous light or occasionally dark brown color with distinct borders. Vulvar lentigenes may be single or multiple, but seldom exceed 1 to 2 cm, in largest diameter. Darkening may occur during pregnancy or with the use of hormonal contraceptives. Although lentigenes are generally considered to be harmless, biopsy is warranted for any change in appearance or if symptoms develop. Dark and irregularly pigmented lentigenes should be removed. Similar in appearance to lentigenes are hemosidirin deposits and reactive hyperpigmentation, although they are typically confined to the mucosa of the vulva.

The common nevus or mole is composed of nevomelanocytes that originate in the epidermis (junctional nevus) and migrate into the dermis (compound nevus). When all the nerve cells have moved into the dermis, the nevus is an intradermal or mature nevus. Nevi are normally well demarcated, brown, and slightly elevated. The junctional nevus is flat and on the vulva tends to be deeply pigmented. Nevi typically darken during pregnancy and adolescence. They should be removed if symptomatic or atypical.

Dysplastic nevi tend to be larger and darker and have irregular borders. They are associated with an increased risk of melanoma and should be excised. Some dysplastic nevi are familial.

Atypical melanocytic hyperplasia is a premalignant, pigmented lesion that can arise de novo or occur in association with a preexisting nevus. It is darker than other spots or nevi, a feature that often alarms the patient and should prompt the physician to remove it. Incomplete excision requires re-excision.

Raised, pigmented lesions of any hue, other than a typical intradermal nevus, warrant excision biopsy. The diagnostic possibilities include nevus (junctional, compound, dysplastic), seborrheic keratosis, squamous dysplasia (Bowen's disease or bowenoid papulosis), malignant melanoma, basal cell carcinoma, AN, histiocytoma, pyogenic granuloma, and dermatofibroma, among others that are discussed later in this chapter.

Erosions and Ulcers

Most vulvar problems characterized by erosions or ulcers are infectious (syphilis, chancroid, herpes genitalis, hidradenitis suppurativa), inflammatory (lichen sclerosus, lichen simplex chronicus, lichen planus, pemphigus vulgaris, Behçet's syndrome, pemphigoid, Crohn's disease), or neoplastic (Bowen's disease, carcinoma, histiocytosis X). If the clinical picture with appropriate cultures and supportive tests fails to make a specific diagnosis, biopsy is always indicated.

The vulvar vestibulitis syndrome (idiopathic vulvodynia) of dyspareunia, vulvar pain, and focal inflammation or ulceration of the vestibule is of unknown etiology, although a history of recurrent candidiasis and condylomata accuminata is common (Mann et al, 1992). Microscopically there is inflam-

mation of the minor vestibular glands and, in some cases, small adenomas (Axe et al, 1986). Surgical removal of the involved vestibular membrane and associated glands has produced satisfactory results in 60 percent of patients (Friedrich, 1987). Reid et al (1995) report 63 percent success with flash-lamp dye laser therapy in those patients without the finding of severe Bartholin's fossa pain. For this latter group they recommend excision of Bartholin's gland.

PREMALIGNANT AND RELATED DISORDERS OF THE VULVA

Premalignant and related disorders of the vulva (condylomas, vulvar dystrophies, vulvar intraepithelial neoplasia [VIN]) are discussed in Chapter 2.

SQUAMOUS CELL CARCINOMA OF THE VULVA

Malignant tumors of the vulva account for 3 to 5 percent of all female genital cancers and 1 percent of all malignancies in women. The average age at diagnosis is 65 years, and women with this disease are commonly hypertensive, obese, and of low parity. Predisposing factors include cigarette smoking, lichen sclerosus, VIN, condylomata accuminata, immunodeficiency, and northern European ancestry. Although numerous histologic varieties exist, with wide-ranging differences in biologic behavior, the great majority are squamous cell carcinomas (Table 3–1). For this reason, it is a common, although sometimes misleading, practice to use the designation *vulvar cancer* interchangeably with *squamous carcinoma of the vulva*. The importance of vulvar cancer must be measured in terms of its potential for disabling and fatal

TABLE **3–1**

Frequency of Histologic Types of Vulvar Cancer*

Histologic Type	Percent of All Cases
Squamous carcinoma	86.6
Melanoma	5.7
Bartholin's gland adenocarcinoma	3.7
Sarcoma	1.7
Paget's disease (with invasion)	0.3
Basal cell carcinoma	2.0

*Collected data from literature.

consequences, not just its relative frequency. Both the patient and the physician have been reported consistently as contributing to a delay in the diagnosis of vulvar cancer in a large proportion of advanced cases.

In the past a high rate of local failure associated with conservative surgical measures focused attention on the need for, and efficacy of, radical surgery for vulvar carcinoma (Taussig, 1940; Way, 1948), including routine bilateral groin node dissection. Today there appears to be an increasing number of early cases diagnosed in younger women. In conjunction with this trend, a renewed interest in less radical therapy has arisen, which has as its goal minimizing the anatomic deformity and psychosexual consequences of vulvar cancer treatment without compromising the cure rate. This translates into wide excision without groin dissection in the minimally invasive, small squamous cancers, and radical local excision with ipsilateral groin dissection (lateralized lesions) or bilateral groin dissection (midline lesions) for intermediate cancers. Adjuvant radiation therapy with or without chemotherapy is being utilized for locally advanced cases to reduce the radicalness of surgical therapy, to improve the resectability rate, and to provide definitive treatment for selected cases. These changes, which reflect the recent evolution of vulvar cancer therapy, are incorporated into the following sections.

Clinical Features

Symptoms

Most women with vulvar carcinoma seek medical attention because they discover a lump or ulcer or they have pruritis, the latter often related to an associated lichen sclerosus or vulvar dysplasia rather than to the invasive lesion per se (Table 3–2). *Dysuria* in this setting refers to a burning discomfort of the vulva accompanying urination. The discovery of vulvar carcinoma in the symptom-free patient is rare, exclusive of those cases of occult invasion associated with VIN. The duration of symptoms before diagnosis is difficult to evaluate because of the frequently associated symptomatic chronic vulvar dystrophy. Nevertheless, the fear of cancer causes many women to postpone seeing a physician. Thus it is not surprising that two out of three women with vulvar cancer have had symptoms for more than 6 months and one out of three for more than 12 months at diagnosis.

TABLE 3–2

Frequency of Symptoms in Vulvar Carcinoma*

Symptoms	Percent[†] of All Patients
Mass or lump	45
Pruritus	45
Pain, burning	23
Bleeding	14
Ulceration	14
Dysuria	10
Discharge	8
Groin mass	2.5
Leg edema	<0.1
None	<0.1

*Collected data from literature.
†Many patients had more than one symptom.

Physical Findings

The general physical examination seldom produces findings related to the primary vulvar malignancy. Palpation of the groin for evidence of nodal involvement is essential because groin metastases are common, and they are of overriding importance in the prognosis and management of vulvar carcinoma. The skin of the inguinal regions, the mons pubis, and the entire perineum should be inspected and palpated for cutaneous lesions and subcutaneous nodules. Most patients with vulvar cancer have a dominant lesion, which tends to distract the examiner's attention from multifocal in situ or invasive lesions. The majority of squamous carcinomas arise from the labia majora and minora (Table 3–3), but origin from any part of the vulva or posterior perineum is possible. Rarely, the skin lateral to the crests of the labia majora is a primary site. The lesion of vulvar carcinoma may be clean or necrotic; painless or tender; white, pink, or red; and dry or weeping. Early invasive carcinoma may be clinically inapparent in the presence of a vulvar dystrophy or VIN (Chafe et al, 1988).

TABLE 3–3

Location of Lesions in Clinical Stages I and II Vulvar Carcinoma*

Site	Percentage
Labium majus	40
Labium minus	20
Labia majora and minora	15
Clitoris/prepuce/mons	10
Perineum, posterior fourchette	15

*Collected data from literature.

Squamous carcinoma of the vulva is usually unifocal and varies in size from less than 1 cm to huge lesions that replace most of the organ and extend to adjacent structures (Figs. 3–1 and 3–2). Ulcerative, exophytic, and infiltrative forms exist. The predominantly infiltrative vulvar carcinoma tends to occur in the region of Bartholin's gland, the perineal body, and the ischiorectal fossa. In such cases there may be no apparent surface lesion, only deeply placed induration.

The visual and palpatory extent of the tumor needs to be carefully determined by noting the proximity to the urethra, vagina, labial–crural folds, and anus. Fixation to the pubic bone is a rare finding. Anal and rectal examinations are routine, but in cases with associated in situ disease, vulvar dystrophy, or posteriorly located cancers, they are especially informative. In light of the frequent occurrence of synchronous vaginal, cervical, and vulvar squamous neoplasia, these areas must also be carefully evaluated. Additional factors to be assessed during the physical examination are the integrity of the pelvic floor and the adequacy of the venous and arterial systems in the lower extremities.

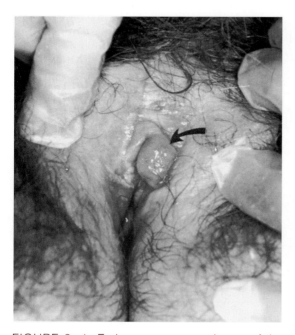

FIGURE 3–1. Early squamous carcinoma of the vulva arising from the left labium minus. There are changes involving the vulvar mucosa consistent with lichen sclerosus.

Diagnosis

Physician delay in diagnosis has been common in cases of vulvar malignancy, often because vulvar neoplasia mimics other clinical entities. Treatment for condylomata accuminata, vulvar dystrophy, and Bartholin's duct "abscess" are among the most frequent errors. A greater willingness to perform office biopsy will facilitate the correct diagnosis. When a mass lesion or ulcer is present, a Keye's punch biopsy from the center of the lesion (not the edge) is the most direct and reliable way of obtaining a diagnosis, provided that viable tissue is obtained. Lesions less than 1 cm can be removed by excision biopsy. In the case of extensive skin lesions of doubtful invasiveness, such as those that exist with lichen sclerosus and VIN (see Chapter 2), multiple biopsies are usually required. Aspiration biopsy of groin nodes is recommended only when a positive result will alter the management.

Pathophysiology

Growth

Squamous carcinoma of the vulva arises from the squamous epithelium of the skin and mucous membranes between the vaginal introitus and the lateral portions of the labia majora. It tends to be indolent, frequently arising from a background of chronic vulvar disease. Local extension to the urethra, perineal body, and vagina is common. Lesions of the posterior vulva tend to involve the vaginal introitus and to invade the anterior anorectal wall, which adheres to the vagina just proximal to the hymenal ring, as well as the anal sphincter. More advanced cases may invade the pubic bone and/or extend to the perineal region, skin of the leg, or bladder neck.

Lymphatic Drainage

A systematic, predictable pattern of lymphatic spread has traditionally been considered a hallmark of this disease. Parry-Jones (1963), in a classic study, demonstrated that the superficial and deep vulvar lymphatics course from the perineal body and labia toward the mons pubis, thence laterally to the superficial nodes in the groin. These lymphatics ordinarily do not cross the labial-crural skin crease. The superficial (inguinal) groin nodes drain into the deep (femoral) groin nodes below the cribriform fascia of the fossa ovalis.

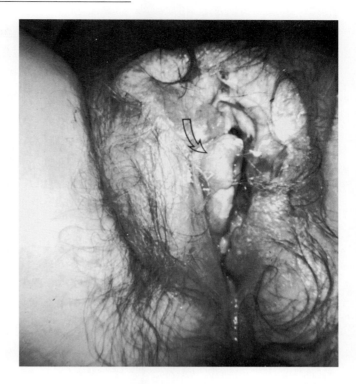

FIGURE 3–2. Extensively ulcerated and necrotic squamous carcinoma of the vulva. The mons veneris has been partly destroyed, along with the clitoris and left labium minus. The arrow points to the right labium minus. The bulge to the left of the perineal body represents tumor infiltration of the ischiorectal fossa.

The efferent lymphatics from the deep groin nodes pass under the inguinal ligament to connect with the pelvic wall lymphatics. Decussation of the vulvar lymphatics occurs in the mons pubis and the posterior fourchette. Thus it has been traditionally believed that squamous carcinoma of the vulva, which metastasizes almost exclusively via the lymphatic system, spreads first to the superficial groin nodes, followed by spread to the deep groin nodes and then to the pelvic wall lymphatics (see also Iversen and Aas, 1983). This concept needs modification in view of the recent findings of a Gynecologic Oncology Group (GOG) study in which only the superficial groin nodes were dissected in early vulvar cancer. An unexpectedly high incidence of ipsilateral groin recurrences was observed (6 of 121 [5 percent] vs. 0 of 96 historical controls), presumably because of metastases involving the lymph nodes deep to the cribriform fascia, despite the negative superficial groin nodes (Stehman et al, 1992a). These data are supported by lymphatic mapping studies (Levenback et al, 1995). Extensive involvement of the groin lymph nodes producing lymphatic obstruction is attended by retrograde movement of tumor into the subcutaneous and dermal lymphatics of the vulva, thigh, lower abdomen, buttock, and contralateral groin.

Prognostic Factors

Stage

The International Federation of Gynecology and Obstetrics (FIGO) stage grouping for vulvar carcinoma was revised in 1988 from a purely clinical to a surgical basis, retaining the tumor (T), node (N), and metastasis (M) system (Table 3–4). This stage grouping emphasizes the dominant influence of local tumor extent and regional node metastasis on prognosis. The stage grouping was modified again in 1995 to incorporate the microinvasive category into stage I.

Inguinal Node Metastasis

Node status is undoubtedly the most important prognostic determinant among operable cases of vulvar carcinoma. The unreliability of clinical assessment of the groin nodes (Table 3–5) was the obvious weakness in the old, clinically based staging system. The overall incidence of groin metastasis for all operable cases will vary with the patient population, clinical stage, thoroughness of the pathologic examination, and selection factors, but averages about 30 percent, with a range from 21 percent (Krupp and Bohm, 1978) to 42 percent (Hopkins et al, 1991) in two large series.

TABLE 3-4

FIGO Stage Grouping and TNM Classification for Vulvar Carcinoma (1995)

TNM Classification		FIGO	
Designation	Description	Stage	Description
T	Primary tumor	I	T1 N0 M0
Tis	Preinvasive carcinoma (carcinoma in situ)	Ia	T1a N0 M0
T1	Tumor confined to the vulva and/or perineum, 2 cm or less in largest diameter	Ib	T1b N0 M0
		II	T2 N0 M0
1a	≤ 1.0-mm invasion	III	T3 N0 M0
1b	> 1.0-mm invasion		T3 N1 M0
			T1 N1 M0
			T2 N1 M0
T2	Tumor confined to the vulva and/or perineum, more than 2 cm in largest diameter	IVa	T1 N2 M0
			T2 N2 M0
			T3 N2 M0
			T4 N0/N1/N2, M0
T3	Tumor of any size with (1) adjacent spread to the lower urethra and/or vagina and/or anus, and/or (2) unilateral regional lymph node metastasis	IVb	Any T, any N with M1
T4	Tumor infiltrating any of the following: upper urethra, bladder mucosa, rectal mucosa, pelvic bone and/or bilateral regional lymph node metastases		
N	Regional lymph nodes		
N0	No node metastasis		
N1	Unilateral node metastasis		
N2	Bilateral node metastases		
M	Distant metastases		
M0	No clinical metastases		
M1	Pelvic lymph node or other distant metastases		

The groin node metastasis rate in the 588-patient GOG study was 34.5 percent (Homesley et al, 1993).

The relationship of histologic groin node status to the pre-1988 FIGO (clinical) stage is presented in Table 3–6. The high incidence of groin metastases in stages III and IV is expected not only because these stages have more extensive local growth but also because they are defined in part by clinical groin node involvement. The risk of groin node metastasis correlates with numerous other clinicopathologic features, discussed in the following sections. The large body of accumulated data relative to risk of node metastasis and their predictability serve as a rational basis for the omission of groin dissection altogether or limiting the dissection to the ipsilateral groin in selected early cases, as discussed later. Nodal status overrides all other prognostic factors in stage I through III vulvar cancer, as shown in Tables 3–7 and 3–11.

Pelvic Node Metastasis

It is now generally established that the risk of pelvic node involvement is clinically insignif-icant in the absence of ipsilateral groin metastases. While the overall incidence of pelvic node metastasis reported in the literature varies from 1.9 percent (Green, 1978) to 9.4 percent (Rutledge et al, 1970), the clinically important issue is the risk of involvement in those cases with groin metastasis. Based on data from five series (Curry et al, 1980; Hacker et al, 1983; Podratz et al, 1983b; Boyce et al, 1985; Homesley et al, 1986), there were 43 patients with pelvic node metastasis (18.7 percent) among 230 patients with groin metastasis. None of 391 cases with negative groin nodes manifested evidence of pelvic metastases either histologically or on follow-up. In these reports the rate of pelvic node spread increased with the number of positive ipsilateral inguinal nodes. None of 41 patients with only one or two groin metastases had pelvic node involvement. With three-node disease, 2 of 7 patients had pelvic metastasis, and 9 of 14 with more than three-node disease had pelvic node involvement. The rate of pelvic node metastasis was 27 percent of 29 cases with bilateral groin metastasis. Histologically positive, clinically suspicious groin nodes had a higher association

TABLE **3–5**

Clinical and Histologic Correlation of Groin Node Metastasis in Operable Vulvar Carcinoma

	Clinically Not Suspicious		Clinically Suspicious or Positive	
Source	No.	% Positive Histologically	No.	% Positive Histologically
Rutledge et al (1970)	68	12	42	74
Morley (1976)	163	18	83	66
Morris (1977)*	54	20	16	69
Iversen (1981)	118	30	140	46
Homesley et al (1992)	477	24	111	80

*Includes nonsquamous cancers.

with pelvic node metastases (33 percent) than did the histologically positive, nonsuspicious nodes (5 percent). Table 3–7 gives collected survival data relative to groin and pelvic node metastases in vulvar carcinoma.

Lesion Size

Lesion size, another determinant of stage, is also a risk factor for inguinal node involvement (Table 3–8). Thus, in a collation of reports, the T1 lesions (<2 cm) were associated with inguinal node metastasis in 15 percent of cases compared with 36 percent for lesions greater than 2 cm. In a study of superficial (≤5-mm thick) vulvar squamous cancers, Sedlis et al (1987) reported a progressive increase in the rate of groin nodal involvement from 13 percent for lesions less than 1 cm in maximum diameter to 36 percent for lesions 3 to 4 cm in diameter.

Location and Configuration

Opinion is divided about the prognostic significance of the gross configuration of the tumor and its location. It is at least suspected that an infiltrative growth is more aggressive than the papillary or exophytic type. Clitoral involvement is reported to increase the risk

of nodal metastases from 25 to 40 percent (Curry et al, 1980; Boyce et al, 1985). In the report of Eriksson et al (1984), the frequencies of groin node metastasis for T1, T2, and T3 clitoral lesions were 29, 56, and 100 percent, respectively. According to these authors, clitoral lesions with groin metastases usually have pelvic node involvement.

Lymph-Vascular Space Invasion

The presence of lymph–vascular space invasion (LVSI) also correlates with the presence of node metastases. From collected data (Donaldson et al, 1981; Husseinzadeh et al, 1983; Boyce et al, 1985), the rate of groin metastasis is about 75 percent for cases of vulvar carcinoma with LVSI, in contrast to 25 percent for cases without demonstrable LVSI, although these data are undoubtedly skewed by the inclusion of the more advanced stages. The GOG data for vulvar cancers 5 mm or less in thickness are 17 percent groin node metastases without LVSI (252 cases) and 65 percent with LVSI (20 cases).

Histologic Grade

A number of studies of vulvar squamous carcinoma have demonstrated quite consistently

TABLE **3–6**

Frequency of Groin Node Metastases Related to FIGO Clinical Stage Grouping (1971)

	FIGO Stage							
	I		II		III		IV	
Source	No.	Percent*	No.	Percent	No.	Percent	No.	Percent
Donaldson et al (1981)	26	15	22	49	15	80	3	100
Hacker et al (1983)	56	11	32	25	14	71	2	100
Figge et al (1985)	55	5	61	21	31	39	6	33
Boyce et al (1985)	16	13	33	27	25	56	5	100
Total	153	10	148	26	85	56	16	75

*Percent positive for metastasis.

Pelvic and Groin Node Metastasis and Survival in Patients With Vulvar
Squamous Carcinoma*

Node Status	No.	Recurred	% NED[†]
Groin and pelvic node metastases	40	28	30
Groin metastasis only	204	74	64
Total	244	102	58

*Data from Rutledge et al (1970), Dean et al (1974), Morley (1976), Green (1978), Benedet
et al (1979), and Homesley et al (1986).
[†]NED, no evidence of disease. Not corrected for deaths from intercurrent disease. All cases
followed for at least 3 years.

that, despite variations in grading criteria, the
risk of groin node metastases increases as the
degree of differentiation decreases. Specifically, from collected data, the approximate
rate of groin node involvement is 15 percent
of G1 lesions, 35 percent for G2 lesions, and
55 percent for G3 lesions (Figge and Gaudenz, 1974; Donaldson et al, 1981; Andreasson et al, 1982; Husseinzadeh et al, 1983;
Boyce et al, 1985). Homesley et al (1993), using a system based on the proportion of the
tumor cells that is poorly differentiated, reported groin node metastasis rates of 2.8,
15.1, 41.2, and 59.7 percent for lesion grades
1 through 4, respectively, in the GOG series
of 564 patients.

Depth of Invasion

Of major importance in determining the risk
of lymphatic metastasis is the depth of invasion (Table 3–9). While there is no standard
method for measuring the depth of invasion,
several investigators have reported remarkably similar findings. Altogether, nearly 200
cases of squamous carcinoma of the vulva
with up to 1 mm of invasion have been reported in the literature, and only two have
had groin metastases. For an appropriate clin-

ical application of the data in Table 3–9, it
must be appreciated that these groin node
metastasis rates were derived entirely from lesions less than 2 cm in maximum diameter.
Thus these data may not be applicable to T2
and T3 lesions. Since there is a rather dramatic change in the rate of node metastases
from less than 1 mm to the 1- to 2-mm level,
Wilkinson (1987) recommends that the measurement be made from the epithelial-stromal
junction of the adjacent most superficial dermal papilla to the deepest point of invasion
to guard against underestimating the depth of
invasion. These data were the basis for the
1995 change in the FIGO staging system. For
further discussion of lesional thickness and
depth of invasion, see the section "T1: Microinvasion" later in this chapter.

Pattern of Invasion

The pattern of invasion is frequently viewed
as a risk factor for the spread and metastasis
of vulvar carcinoma, but no classification has
met with general acceptance. For example,
Magrina et al (1979) noted that 15 percent of
their 40 stage I patients with confluence (defined as an invasive tumor filling an area
greater than 2 mm in diameter) had inguinal
node metastasis, compared with 5 of 66 patients without confluence. Wilkinson et al
(1982) categorized invasion as confluent (a
solid mass of invading tumor with a predominant pushing margin) or diffuse, that is, a
spray pattern (multiple islands of invading tumor, often with sharp, angular prongs).
Among their 27 cases, 2 of 20 with the diffuse
pattern had metastases versus 0 of 7 in the
confluent group. Hacker et al (1984) observed that confluence (a compact mass of
tumor with a diameter greater than 1 mm)
was present in one-half of their 84 "microinvasive" cases. However, they categorized 77

Frequency of Groin Node Metastases Related to
Lesion Size in Squamous Carcinoma of the Vulva*

Lesion Size	Total Cases	% Groin Metastases
≤2 cm	341	15
≤1 cm[†]	52	4
1–2 cm[†]	99	13
2–4 cm	389	35
>4 cm	257	40

*Data from Franklin and Rutledge (1971), Krupp et al (1975), Hacker
et al (1983), Boyce et al (1985), and Homesley et al (1991).
[†]Not all authors gave results by size group under 2 cm.

TABLE 3–9

Reported Frequency of Groin Node Metastases in Clinical Stage I Squamous Carcinoma of the Vulva
Related to Depth of Invasion

Depth of Invasion (mm)	Magrina et al (1979)	Wilkinson et al (1982)	Andreasson et al (1982)	Hoffman et al (1983)	Hacker et al (1984)	Total (%)
≤1	0/19*	0/4	0/10	0/24	0/34	0/91 (0.0)
1–2	3/26	1/13	1/14	0/19	2/19	7/91 (7.7)
2–3	1/23	1/9	3/15	2/17	2/17	9/81 (11.1)
3–4	4/16	0/2	2/14	5/8	1/7	12/47 (25.5)
4–5	4/12	0/0	3/21	3/7	3/7	13/47 (27.7)

*Number of cases with groin metastases/total cases in category.

of these cases as having a broad, pushing front, of which only 6 (7.8 percent) had nodal metastasis. In contrast, two of the seven cases with a spray pattern had nodal disease. Boyce et al (1985) classified the pattern of invasion as broad front or stellate. The first pattern had a node metastasis rate of 14 percent (3 of 22), whereas the rate with the second pattern was 51 percent (27 of 53). Thus the pattern of invasion appears to be an important prognostic variable, but the terminology and definitions are inconsistent, leading at times to apparently contradictory results.

Tumor Diameter Versus Depth of Invasion

There is a relatively strong relationship between tumor diameter and depth of invasion, as the staging system implies. Thus Andreassen et al (1982) reported that average tumor diameter increased progressively from 22 mm for lesions with less than 2 mm of invasion to 31 mm for lesions with 4 to 5 mm of invasion and to 47 mm for lesions with more than 5 mm of invasion. Buscema et al (1981) found that 72.7 percent of their stage I cases had less than 3 mm of invasion, compared with 57.1 percent of their stage II cases. Correlating lesion size with penetration, Magrina et al (1979) noted that all 20 of their stage I cases with lesions less than 1 cm in diameter had less than 5 mm of stromal invasion (all were also grade 1 or 2), whereas 10 of 66 cases with lesions 1 to 2 cm in diameter had greater than 5 mm of stromal invasion. Fifteen of these 66 cases were grade 3 or 4 on the Broder scale.

Survival

Results by FIGO clinical stage reported from several institutions are collated in Table 3–10. Overall 5-year corrected survival rates are ap-

proximately 90, 80, 50, and 15 percent for stages I through IV, respectively. Within each stage, groin node status, as shown earlier, is probably the major prognostic determinant. Thus the survival of patients with a clinical stage III lesion and histologically negative groin nodes is superior (70 percent) to that of patients with a clinical stage I or II lesion and histologically positive groin nodes (45 percent; Table 3–11). Survival is also strongly influenced by the number of groin nodes involved. Combining data from these series, if only one or two groin nodes are involved, the 5-year survival rate is about 75 percent, whereas the patient with more than three node metastases has less than a 25 percent probability of 5-year survival. Bilateral groin metastasis has a similarly poor prognosis.

Homesley et al (1993), in a univariate analysis study of 588 GOG patients, reported that clinical node status, histologic grade, LVSI, tumor thickness, and patient age were statistically significant prognostic factors. Using a multivariate analysis, however, they concluded, as did Podratz et al (1983b), that there are only two significant independent prognostic variables in squamous carcinoma of the vulva: groin node status (lateralism and number) and lesion diameter. Homesley et al

TABLE 3–10

Stage Distribution and Survival for Patients With
Vulvar Carcinoma (Squamous)*

Clinical FIGO Stage	No.	Corrected 5-Year Survival (%)	Cases in Stage (%)
I	306	91.1	35.1
II	252	80.9	28.9
III	213	48.4	24.4
IV	101	15.3	11.6
Total	872	68.9	100.0

*Data from Rutledge et al (1970), Boutselis (1972), Morley (1976), Japaze et al (1977), and Hacker et al (1983).

T A B L E **3–11**

Corrected Survival by Stage and Groin Node Status in Patients With Vulvar
Carcinoma Treated by Radical Vulvectomy and Bilateral Groin Dissection*

Clinical Stage	Negative Nodes		Positive Nodes		Total	
	No.	Alive for 5 Years (%)	No.	Alive for 5 Years (%)	No.	Alive for 5 Years (%)
I, II	92	97.8	16	43.7	108	89.8
III	23	69.6	34	26.5	57	43.8
Total	115	92.2	50	32.0	165	73.9

*Data from Morley (1976).

devised a surgicopathologic staging system based on their analysis (Table 3–12). In general this system corresponds to the 1988 FIGO surgical stage system except for stage III. The discrepancy results from the fact that FIGO stage III does not take into account the number of positive groin nodes, which is a powerful prognostic determinant, and it does incorporate cases with involvement of adjacent structures, a clinical feature that does not significantly influence survival independent of lesion size. The importance of the groin node status to outcome is reflected in the GOG data listed in Table 3–13.

Treatment

Vulvar carcinoma management must be conceptualized as consisting of two separate components: treatment of the primary lesion and treatment of the regional lymph nodes. The salient themes in the recent gynecological literature on vulvar carcinoma are individualization and conservatism. It is now universally recognized that individualization of

therapy will produce the best results in terms of both patient survival and morbidity. *Individualization* means treatment will be varied with respect to both the regional nodes and the primary lesion. Some very early lesions may require only wide excision for cure, whereas extensive lesions may need more than the traditional radical vulvectomy—for example, radiation or chemoradiation therapy in addition to surgery. Regarding the regional nodes, in some cases no therapy may be warranted but in others the appropriate therapy may be ipsilateral or bilateral groin dissection with or without radiation therapy, according to the risk of tumor spread and status of the nodes.

The long-established tradition of uniformly radical surgery for even early invasive carcinoma of the vulva has been discarded. This shift to individualized more conservative therapy has been prompted by the increasing number of young women with early cancers, for whom disfiguring surgery is often unacceptable, and also by the recognition that for these early cancers such radical therapy is un-

T A B L E **3–12**

GOG Risk Groups for Vulvar Carcinoma*

Risk Group	Surgical Findings[†]	No.	Relative Survival at 5 years (%)
Minimal	Tumor ≤2 cm diameter and negative groin nodes	154	97.9
Low	Tumor 2.1–8 cm diameter and negative groin nodes Tumor ≤2 cm diameter and one positive groin node	232	87.4
Intermediate	Tumor >8 cm diameter and negative groin nodes Tumor >2 cm diameter and one positive groin node Tumor ≤8 cm diameter and two positive groin nodes[‡]	104	74.8
High	Tumor >8 cm diameter and two positive groin nodes[‡] Three or more ipsilateral positive groin nodes Bilaterally positive groin nodes	87	29.0

*Data from Homesley et al (1991).
[†]Based on surgical–pathologic status of groin nodes.
[‡]Not specified whether ipsilateral or contralateral.

TABLE 3-13

Influence of Groin Node Status on Survival in Vulvar Squamous Carcinoma[*,†]

Prognostic Feature	No.	5-Year Survival (%)	Percent of Total Group
Negative nodes	201	92	49
Ipsilateral nodes			
positive (1 or 2)	61	75	—
Bilateral nodes positive	16	30	8
Contralateral nodes			
only positive	8	27	8
>2 nodes positive	75	25	
>6 nodes positive	16	0	

[*]Data from Homesley et al (1991).
[†]Lateralized lesions only.

necessary. There are also times when conservative therapy is used not because it is thought to be optimal with respect to curing the disease, but to minimize surgical trauma in the elderly or frail patient. However, since recurrence after treatment usually occurs within 12 to 18 months, suboptimal conservative treatment must be carefully weighed against the patient's life expectancy. Radical vulvar surgery and groin node dissection are remarkably well tolerated and can be done in phases if necessitated by medical ailments.

Appropriate design of surgical therapy must consider (1) lesion size and location, (2) depth of invasion, (3) LVSI, (4) degree of histologic differentiation, (5) clinical status of the groin nodes, (6) health (and wishes) of the patient, (7) condition of the vulvar skin not involved by the cancer, (8) presence of associated problems such as genital prolapse, and (9) other sites of lower genital tract squamous neoplasia.

T1: Microinvasion

A summary of the principles of management for squamous carcinoma of the vulva is given in Figure 3–3. The 1988 FIGO staging of vulvar carcinoma was changed in 1995 to include a subgroup for microinvasion, a well-defined entity that deserves official recognition. The concept of microinvasive vulvar carcinoma—that is, vulvar carcinoma so early in its development that there is a clinically insignificant risk of metastases or local extension, making treatment of the regional lymph nodes and radical excision of the primary lesions unnecessary—was promoted by the seminal paper of Wharton et al in 1974. Reports since then have attempted to refine the data available on the risk of nodal metastasis

and local failure relative to lesion size, grade, depth of invasion, pattern of invasion, presence of LVSI, and other clinicopathologic features, as previously discussed. It is now generally agreed that for vulvar squamous carcinoma the requirements of this description of microinvasion are fulfilled by any lesion with up to 1 mm of invasion, not more than 2 cm in diameter, and with no evidence of LVSI, although the latter is not recognized in the FIGO stage definitions.

Primary Lesion. The definition of an adequate local excision of the primary lesion is not clear. Total vulvectomy for a tiny lesion is obviously excessive, but to what extent can the resection be reduced? Considering the experience with squamous carcinoma of the skin, a margin of 5 to 10 mm will probably be adequate for lesions with invasion less than 1 mm provided that the surrounding skin is normal. If the background vulvar skin is involved with dysplasia, the entire area of abnormal skin needs to be excised (or laser vaporized), with margin checks. If there is dystrophic, nondysplastic skin (lichen sclerosus) present, it may be advisable to excise or vaporize it. Although half of the patients will develop recurrence of the vulvar dystrophy after excision (Magrina et al, 1979), there is some risk of a second vulvar cancer developing from the untreated, nondysplastic vulvar dystrophy.

Regional Nodes. The rate of nodal involvement in relation to depth of invasion has been delineated by several studies (Table 3–9). It is of paramount clinical significance that the cases with lesions less than 2 cm in diameter and less than 1 mm of stromal invasion rarely have groin node metastases. Any greater degree of invasion is associated with more than a 7 percent risk of ipsilateral groin node metastasis and warrants routine groin dissection. Thus the only cases of vulvar carcinoma that do not require at least ipsilateral groin dissection are those with lesions less than 2 cm in maximum diameter, up to 1 mm of stromal invasion, no LVSI, and clinically negative groin nodes (Fig. 3–4). Failure to perform the groin dissection in circumstances other than this, as Hacker et al (1984) pointed out, is the most important cause of preventable death in early invasive vulvar cancer. While poor histologic differentiation and the spray pattern of invasion are also risk factors, they do not appear to be important when the invasion is 1 mm or less.

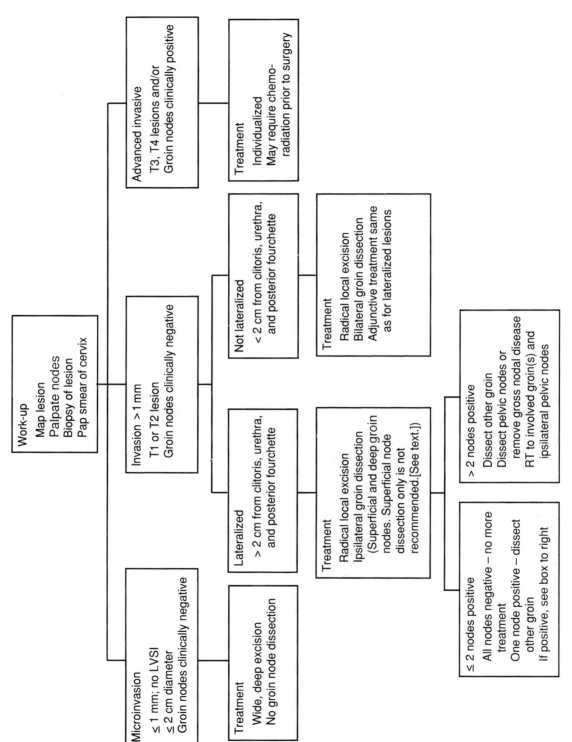

FIGURE 3–3. Management algorithm for vulvar carcinoma. LVSI = lymph–vascular space invasion.

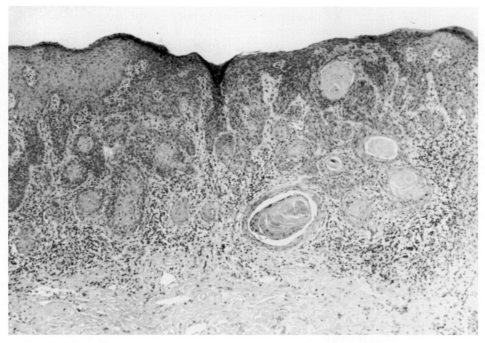

FIGURE 3–4. Histologic section of a well-differentiated microinvasive vulvar carcinoma with less than 1 mm of invasion (×80). The lesion arose on the medial aspect of the labium majus of a thin 32-year-old woman. Treatment consisted of wide local excision.

T1, T2, and T3 Lesions

Even for more deeply invasive squamous carcinomas, less than radical vulvectomy and bilateral inguinal lymph node dissection can be recommended. With anterior lesions, preservation of the mucosa over the perineal body and posterior fourchette is eminently reasonable, since the lymphatic flow is anterior and then lateral to the groin nodes. For large lesions, especially with gross nodal involvement, the risk of irregular lymphatic flow may be too great for such conservative measures. Similarly, a lesion of the posterior fourchette with clinically normal inguinal nodes may be removed with sparing of the anterior vulva, including the labia majora, clitoris, and mons veneris, since early lymphatic spread is predominantly embolic.

Primary Lesion. For clinical stage I lesions, what is an adequate margin? Hacker et al (1984) recommend at least 2 cm regardless of the depth of invasion, whereas Burke et al (1995) recommend a 2-cm margin for lesions with more than 1 mm of invasion. DiSaia et al (1979) recommend a 3-cm margin. If the lesion were 2 cm in diameter, taking a margin of 2 or 3 cm would mean excising a cylinder of tissue with a diameter of 6 to 8 cm, which

in most cases would be tantamount to a hemivulvectomy, similar to Iversen's (1981) recommendation. Except for the most superficial lesions, it is generally agreed that the deep margin should extend to the inferior fascia of the urogenital diaphragm or the aponeurosis over the public symphysis. Compiling the results of local excision from several reports in the literature, there were only two local failures (4 percent) among 49 cases. At least one of these occurred more than 3 years after treatment, suggesting that it may have been a new lesion. However, in a prospective study (Stehman et al, 1992a), the GOG reported an 8 percent local failure rate among 121 stage I patients whose lesions were resected with a 2-cm margin; Burke et al (1995) observed a 6 percent local recurrence rate at 3 years among 33 women with T1 lesions, whereas only 1 of 43 women with a T2 lesion recurred locally. Since the local failures are usually salvageable, these authors concluded that such conservative surgery is acceptable. With properly selected cases, then, "radical local excision," as it is sometimes called, is sufficiently effective to recommend it. A special case is the cancer close to or involving the clitoris. Hacker (1990) has suggested that radiation therapy as definitive treatment may provide better results in terms of psychosexual sequelae than extirpative surgery. Posttreatment biopsy should be performed to document complete resolution of the cancer.

As the primary lesion becomes progressively larger, the excision is by necessity more radical, allowing little option for vulvasparing surgery. Lesions crossing the midline obviously require bilateral therapy. Extension to the urethra, anal sphincter, rectal wall, or vagina can be treated with a combination of surgery and radiation or chemoradiation to improve local control and at the same time reduce the scope of the operative resection (Boronow, 1982; Thomas et al, 1989).

Regional Nodes. While lymph node dissection is required for cases with invasion greater than 1 mm, it is now considered acceptable to limit the dissection in stage I cases to the ipsilateral groin when the lesion is well lateralized and the contralateral groin has no clinically suspicious nodes. In this context "lateralized" has not been defined. The proximity of a lesion to the midline anteriorly is probably more critical than it is posteriorly, and the risk of contralateral node metastases is undoubtedly also influenced by the grade, LVSI, and lesion size. In general, however, if the lesion is within 2 cm of the midline, bilateral groin dissection is indicated. If the ipsilateral nodes have metastases, the contralateral groin should be treated.

Three approaches to groin node management have been studied in an attempt to downgrade the extent of surgical therapy and its attendant morbidity, particularly chronic lymphedema. First is the superficial groin (inguinal) dissection, which omits dissection of the femoral nodes in the fossa ovalis deep to the cribriform fascia (DiSaia et al, 1979). This modification was attended by an 8 percent groin recurrence rate in a GOG study (Stehman et al, 1992a) of early vulvar carcinoma, as mentioned previously. Others have reported a similar failure rate with this technique (Burke et al, 1995). These results undoubtedly reflect irregular lymphatic drainage as reported by Levenback et al (1995). In addition, the superficial node dissection has never been shown to reduce the adverse sequelae of the complete dissection. A second approach to reduce the morbidity of traditional node dissection is radiation therapy. In a randomized GOG study of radiation therapy versus surgery, the groin failure rate with radiation therapy was so much higher (5 of 27 patients) than that in the surgery arm (0 of 25

patients) that the study was terminated early (Stehman et al, 1992b). The third modification, which has been used in some clinics for many years, is a separate incision for the groin dissection (Hacker et al, 1981). This clearly reduces the risk of skin breakdown, but it does not ameliorate the incidence or severity of lymphedema, the major cause of long-term morbidity. Recurrence in the skin bridge or mons pubis is rarely seen.

In cases with more than one occult groin node metastasis or with any N2 or N3 node metastases, postoperative radiation to the involved groin and ipsilateral hemipelvis is recommended. This is based on the results of a randomized GOG study comparing postoperative radiation to surgery alone for patients with histologically documented groin node metastases (Homesley et al, 1986). Improved local control and survival were observed in the radiation therapy arm (60 vs. 30 percent 2-year survival).

These findings are in harmony with the older data of Curry et al (1980) and Hacker et al (1983). They recommended treating the pelvic nodes when a groin had clinically suspicious, histologically positive nodes or more than two occult nodal metastases. Despite the evidence that clitoral lymphatics drain directly to the pelvic wall, this has not proved to be important clinically (Piver and Xynos, 1977). Of course, if Jackson's node (the most distal iliac node) or Cloquet's node (the most proximal femoral node) is positive for cancer, pelvic node treatment should be carried out regardless of the groin node count. Treatment of the pelvic nodes can be accomplished with either surgery or radiation therapy, but if the latter is selected, large nodal metastases should be removed first.

Surgical Adverse Effects

Perhaps half of the patients undergoing radical surgery for vulvar cancer will have one or more major complications (Table 3–14), but the majority of these are temporary and not life threatening. Deaths result primarily from pulmonary embolus, myocardial infarction, and stroke. These, as well as many of the remaining complications, are largely influenced by the patient's age and the extent of the operation. A disproportionate number of deaths occur in the group undergoing pelvic lymphadenectomy, probably reflecting increased operative trauma and health factors associated with more advanced disease. Pul-

TABLE 3–14
Reported Complications After Radical Surgery for Vulvar Cancer*

Complication[†]	% of All Cases	Range of Individual Series (%)
Wound breakdown and/or infection	54	18–91
Chronic leg edema	30	8–70
Lymphocyst	10	0–31
Genital prolapse	7	0–14
Stress incontinence	5	0–12
Thrombophlebitis	3.5	0–9
Grafting of skin flaps	1.7	0–24
Hernia (femoral, inguinal)	1.5	0–5
Pulmonary embolus	1.2	0–3
Ruptured femoral artery	1.9	0–5
Hospital death	3.3	0–12

*Collected data from literature.
[†]Other complications reported are cerebral vascular accident, myocardial infarction, loss of leg, fistula, femoral nerve injury, osteitis pubis, varicosities, abscess, hematuria, introital stenosis, delayed hemorrhage, and recurrent cellulitis.

monary embolus can be reduced by using low-dose heparin and/or intermittent pneumatic calf compression. Femoral artery rupture can be avoided by transplantation of the sartorius muscle and/or the use of separate groin incisions. The most common problems are lymphocyst, lymphedema, genital prolapse (especially urinary incontinence), sexual dysfunction, and numbness or paresthesias of the anterior thigh. Lymphedema is managed by elevation, elastic hose, diuretics, and coumarin (Casley-Smith et al, 1993). Prevention of complications by conservative surgery and the use of chemoradiation when applicable is clearly the most satisfactory solution.

Radiation Therapy

There has been a resurgent interest in radiation as a treatment for vulvar squamous carcinoma, predominantly in combination with surgery or for palliation of advanced tumor. It has been a longstanding observation that this tumor is responsive to radiation therapy but that the normal tissues are not sufficiently tolerant of radiation to permit an optimal dose. When vulvar carcinoma involves the vagina extensively, traditional surgical therapy might include removal of the bladder and/or rectum (Cavanaugh and Shepherd, 1982). For selected cases, Boronow (1982) has reported a 65 to 70 percent success rate when combining radiation (usually preoperative) and surgery while preserving intact the lower urinary and intestinal tracts. However, 9 of the 33 patients in his study group devel-

oped a fistula or radiation necrosis. Radiation was administered preoperatively to two patients with N3 nodes, both of whom were among the long-term survivors in his study group. Other authors have also reported palliative and curative success using radiation therapy, with or without surgery (Prempree and Amornmarn, 1984; Fairey et al, 1985).

The success of chemoradiation for the treatment of anal carcinoma (Meeker et al, 1986) has led to the use of this combination for locally advanced vulvar cancer, both as primary therapy and as postoperative adjuvant therapy. Thomas et al (1989) observed no in-field recurrences among nine patients in the latter category and three local failures among nine cases in the primary therapy category. The chemotherapy component in their treatment group was 5-fluorouracil (5-FU) by continuous intravenous (IV) infusion over 4 to 5 days (1 gm/m^2/24 hr) at the start of radiation therapy and repeated 4 weeks later. In some cases bolus IV mitomycin C (6 mg/m^2) was also given, one injection with each course of 5-FU. Improved results for inoperable vulvar carcinoma have been reported by Nori et al (1983) when combining mitronidazole, a radiation sensitizer, with high-dose radiation (for more details, see Chapter 17).

VARIANTS OF SQUAMOUS CELL CARCINOMA

Verrucous Carcinoma

Verrucous carcinoma is a rare, indolent, invasive malignant growth that is clinically and histologically similar to the giant condyloma accuminatum. It occurs in the oral cavity as well as on the genitalia. Characteristically, it does not spread by lymphatic or vascular channels, although inflammatory enlargement of the regional lymph nodes may be present. Radiation therapy is reportedly ineffective and may be followed by more aggressive behavior. Verrucous carcinoma of the vulva is often associated with human papillomavirus (HPV) 6 and frequently occurs on the background of lichen sclerosus. It is diagnosed in women with a mean age of 58 years (Andersen and Sorensen, 1988; Brisigotti et al, 1989). Thus the presence of a giant condyloma in a postmenopausal woman should raise suspicion of a verrucous carcinoma, especially if the base of the condyloma is indurated. The recommended treatment is wide local excision. Lymph node metastasis has not been reported in unirradiated verrucous carcinoma.

Adenosquamous Carcinoma

Adenosquamous carcinoma is usually included among the squamous cancers. This tumor is composed of glandular (adenoid) and squamous cells in varying proportions and apparently arises from the skin appendages. Adenosquamous cancer of the vulva presents at a more advanced stage, is associated with a higher incidence of lymph node metastases, and may carry a poorer prognosis, stage for stage, than the more common squamous cancers. It is managed, however, in the same manner as pure squamous carcinoma.

Basal Cell Carcinoma

Basal cell carcinoma is an invasive, rarely metastasizing malignancy arising from the skin or hair follicles. It accounts for about 2 percent of all vulvar cancers (Hoffman et al, 1988). The average age at diagnosis is 58 years. It has been diagnosed as early in life as age 34 years. Nearly all patients are white. The most common complaints are pruritis, irritation, and a nodule or mass. The lesion of basal cell carcinoma may resemble a benign nevus or papilloma. An eczematoid appearance or ulceration (rodent ulcer) is also reported (Fig. 3–5). Location on the labia majora is the rule, and most of the tumors are less than 2 cm in diameter. The treatment of choice is wide excision. The reported 10 percent local recurrence rate is probably related to overly conservative excision. Regional ad-

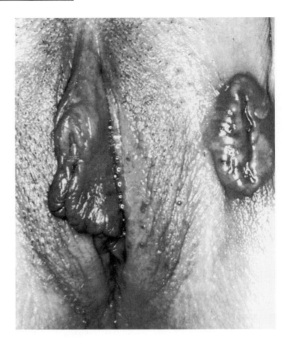

FIGURE 3–5. Basal cell carcinoma of the vulva arising on the lateral aspect of the left labium majus. This growth had been present, according to the patient, for 20 years.

enopathy needs to be assessed by fine-needle aspiration or excision biopsy. The handful of cases exhibiting regional node metastases have been 4 cm or greater in diameter (Winkelmann and Llorens, 1990). It seems reasonable that lesions of this unusual dimension would warrant routine node dissection. A histologic variant, adenoid basal cell carcinoma, should not be confused with the adenoid cystic carcinoma (cylindroma; see the section "Bartholin's Gland Carcinoma"). The latter is a fully malignant tumor, usually arising in Bartholin's gland, with a significant metastatic potential (Merino et al, 1982; Bernstein et al, 1983).

ADENOCARCINOMA

Adenocarcinoma of the vulva is one of the rarest gynecologic malignancies, accounting for only 1 percent of all vulvar cancers. Most cases arise from Bartholin's gland, but other tissues of origin include skin adnexal glands, parauretheral glands, endometriosis, ectopic breast and cloacal tissue. Because of the rarity of primary glandular cancer in the lower genital tract, an extravulvar primary carcinoma should always be considered, especially primary cancer of the rectum and upper genital tract.

Bartholin's Gland Carcinoma

Nearly as many adenocarcinomas arise from Bartholin's (greater vestibular) gland as do squamous carcinomas from Bartholin's gland duct. The affected women are nearly a decade younger, on average, than women with epidermoid cancer of the vulva, but the symptoms are in general quite similar. A history of inflammatory disease of Bartholin's gland during the reproductive years may be obtained, and all too often the cancers themselves are mistaken for a Bartholin's gland abscess, leading to misguided efforts at surgical drainage and antibiotic therapy. Inflammatory disease of Bartholin's gland is uncommon after the fourth decade and rarely occurs in the postmenopausal years. Thus excision or office biopsy is recommended in these age groups to exclude neoplastic disease. Three criteria are generally accepted as necessary to make the diagnosis of Bartholin's gland carcinoma: (1) histologically documented transition from normal Bartholin's gland to the malignant element, (2) clinical location of the tumor in the anatomic region of Bartholin's gland, and (3) absence of another primary cancer.

Malignant tumors of Bartholin's gland, as a result of their origin deep to the skin, tend to be more advanced at diagnosis than the typical epidermoid vulvar cancer that arises from the surface epithelium. Proximity to the vagina, anus, and pubic ramus also contribute to the poorer outcome. While the deep-seated location makes diagnosis more difficult than for surface growths, this problem is easily overcome by the use of fine-needle aspiration, a simple and effective office procedure.

Survival is primarily a function of the clinical stage at diagnosis. Based on four reports in the literature, seven of eight stage I patients were alive and well from 2 to 7 years later, and, of the eight stage II patients, six (all with lesions measuring 2.5 to 3.5 cm and negative nodes) were free of disease from 3 to 12 years post-treatment (Chamlian and Taylor, 1972; Wahlström et al, 1978; Leuchter et al, 1982; Copeland et al, 1986). Patients with more advanced disease have a very poor prognosis. The recommended treatment for Bartholin's gland carcinoma is radical local excision and bilateral groin dissection. Preoperative radiation may allow preservation of the anus/rectum.

Adenoid cystic carcinoma (ACC) accounts for 15 percent of cancers originating in Bartholin's gland. it occurs in women at an average age of 42 years. Like its more common parotid gland counterpart, ACC is characterized by an indolent clinical course, late recurrence, and a propensity for perineural and local invasion. These latter two features account for the high frequency of positive microscopic margins and local recurrence associated with conservative surgery. Regional lymph node recurrence is commonly reported, although Copeland et al (1986), in a review, noted that only 2 of 15 patients with node dissections had nodal involvement. Perineural invasion has been cited as the cause of the local itching and burning sensation that some patients experience long before the tumor becomes apparent. Radical excision and ipsilateral groin node dissection is the generally recommended treatment. The efficacy of adjuvant radiation therapy has been disputed (Rosenberg et al, 1989), but some authors recommend radiation therapy when the surgical margins are inadequate, and for treatment of recurrence (Rose et al, 1991).

Paget's Disease and Sweat Gland Carcinoma

Paget's disease is an intraepithelial adenocarcinoma that occurs predominantly in white women. The average age at diagnosis is 65 years, but it has occurred as early as 32 years. The patients complain of pruritis and/or soreness of the vulva, often years before the diagnosis is made. Typically, the visible lesion is well demarcated with irregular borders and an eczematoid appearance. There are frequently red and white areas representing ulceration and hyperkeratosis. Some lesions are velvety and uniformly erythematous. Extension around the anus is common, and occasionally the adjacent thigh, vagina, or urethral meatus is involved. Rarely Paget's disease extends to the vagina, cervix, or rectum. The diagnosis is frequently unsuspected before biopsy. It is generally held that Paget's disease of the vulva arises from the eccrine or apocrine sweat glands and extends to the overlying epithelium via the ducts. It may also arise in situ from the epidermal stem cells.

Histologically, the presence of the large, clear Paget's cells produces a characteristic pattern, but confusion with melanoma or Bowen's disease can occur. Unlike mammary Paget's disease, less than 20 percent of the vulvar cases have an associated invasive adenocarcinoma. The invasive component may originate from a gland or from the involved dermal epithelium. The carcinoma is more often clinically apparent than microscopic in extent. The development of invasive disease after the initial presentation is unusual. Patients with Paget's disease of the vulva, especially when the perianal region is involved, are disposed to developing extragenital, glandular cancers and need careful evaluation and follow-up from this perspective in addition to their genital problem. The major sites at risk are reported to be the rectum and breast (Stacey et al, 1986; Feurer et al, 1990).

The treatment of choice for Paget's disease, in the absence of clinical and biopsy evidence of invasion, is simple excision with a 1-cm margin. Often the disease is so extensive that primary closure is not feasible or would be disfiguring. In this situation skinning vulvectomy with split-thickness skin grafting is appropriate therapy, or local skin flaps may suffice. While the subclinical, multifocal nature of Paget's disease has been documented (Gunn and Gallagher, 1980), the common problem of local recurrence appears to be related primarily to inadequate excision of contiguous disease. The collective frequency of local recurrence in cases with a positive surgical margin was 40 percent, versus 12 percent for negative margins (Stacey et al, 1986; Bergen et al, 1989; Curtin et al, 1990). Consequently, it is recommended that intraoperative margin checks be obtained as a guide to the extent of resection. Mapping of the lesion with intravenous fluorescein and ultraviolet light has been reported (Misas et al, 1991), but in our experience it is not very reliable.

Approximately one half of the reported cases of Paget's disease with invasion have had metastases at the time of diagnosis, usually to the inguinal lymph nodes. When invasion is present, bilateral groin dissection should be done in addition to radical local excision. There is no depth of invasion known to be associated with an insignificant risk for lymph node metastases (Fine et al, 1995). The prognosis is largely determined by the initial extent of disease, but few evaluable early cases have been reported. Six of seven stage I and II patients, two of whom had groin node metastases, were well from 2 to 16 years post-therapy. The seventh patient died with disease 11 years after diagnosis (Creasman et al, 1975; Parmley et al, 1975;

Lee et al, 1977; Bergen et al, 1989; Curtin et al, 1990).

Merkel Cell Carcinoma

This small-cell, neuroendocrine tumor arises from touch-sensitive cells in the basal layer of the epidermis. Six cases have been reported to originate from the vulvar hair-bearing and non-hair-bearing surfaces (de Mola et al, 1993). These tumors are aggressive, with a high incidence of regional node metastases, local recurrence, and distant metastases. Radical local excision with intraoperative margin checks, groin lymph node dissection, and adjuvant chemotherapy is recommended.

MALIGNANT MESODERMAL TUMORS

As a group, vulvar sarcomas make up only 1 to 2 percent of all vulvar malignancies. More than a dozen histologic types have been reported, but the majority are leiomyosarcomas and malignant fibrous histiocytomas. Women with vulvar sarcoma usually present with a painful mass in the labium majus or Bartholin's gland area. There is a general tendency toward local recurrence and a protracted course.

Leiomyosarcoma

Among leiomyosarcoma (LMS) cases from three series (DiSaia et al, 1971; Davos and Abell, 1976; Tavassoli and Norris, 1979), 10 were treated by enucleation or conservative excision and 8 recurred locally. Five of these women with local recurrence died of metastatic disease at 6 months (one case) or 6 to 15 years after initial therapy. Local recurrence usually appears within 1 to 2 years. The behavior of smooth muscle tumors of the vulva is related to lesion size, mitotic activity, and the growth pattern. Although any of them may recur, the greatest risk is for lesions with a high mitosis count (>10/10 hpf), a size greater than 5 cm, and infiltrating rather than pushing margins. The recommended treatment is radical local excision. No instance of groin metastases has been reported (Moller et al, 1990).

Malignant Fibrous Histiocytoma

Malignant fibrous histiocytoma (MFH) most commonly occurs on the extremities of elderly patients. There are several histologic variants, and confusion with pleomorphic rhabdomyosarcoma, liposarcoma, and poorly differentiated sarcoma is possible. Benign and low-grade variants also exist. The average age of women with vulvar MFH is 50 years. Presentation varies from an asymptomatic lump to a painful, ulcerated mass, depending on the lesion size. Local recurrence and lymphatic and hematogenous metastases are hallmarks of its clinical behavior (Weiss and Enzinger, 1978). While relatively radiation resistant, adjuvant radiation therapy reportedly reduces the rate of local recurrence substantially (Reagan et al, 1981). Only one of several reported cases has had documented inguinal node metastases. Radical local excision is the treatment of choice. Ipsilateral groin dissection is indicated for large, deeply invading lesions (Santala et al, 1987).

Dermatofibrosarcoma Protuberans

Dermatofibrosarcoma protuberans (DFP) is a rare, low-grade sarcoma of the dermis of histiocytic or neural origin. DFP seldom produces metastases but has a high propensity for local recurrence (Agress et al, 1983; Bock et al, 1985; Barnhill et al, 1988). The few reported patients with vulvar DFP have ranged in age from 38 to 83 years. The tumor is multinodular, anteriorly located, usually slow growing, and not painful. Treatment by wide excision is adequate. However, tumor extent based on clinical assessment is not reliable.

Epithelioid Sarcoma

Epithelioid sarcoma (ES) is a malignancy of uncertain histogenesis that typically develops in the lower extremities of young adults. The few case reports of vulvar ES indicate that it is more malignant than the extragenital variant. Both local failure and distant metastases are common. Perrone et al (1989) suggest that the malignant rhabdoid tumor of the vulva has been misdiagnosed as ES, accounting for this apparent more aggressive behavior. Treatment requires at least radical local therapy (Ulbright et al, 1983).

Histiocytosis X

Histiocytosis X, or class I histiocytosis, is a malignant disease of the Langerhans-type histiocyte, predominantly affecting white children under the age of 15 years. It is charac-

terized by a variable presentation and clinical course. Included in this designation are those syndromes previously referred to as eosinophilic granuloma, Hand-Schüller-Christian disease, and Letterer-Siwe disease. The acute disseminated form is characterized by lytic bone lesions, histiocytic infiltration of the reticuloendothelial system, and an eczematoid, pruritic, sometimes ulcerating skin rash. Spontaneous remission can occur. The literature on histiocytosis X involving the vulva was reviewed by Otis et al in 1990. Only 1 of the 33 reported cases was limited to the vulva (see also Thomas et al, 1986).

Rhabdomyosarcoma

Copeland et al (1985) reported two survivors among eight cases of alveolar rhabdomyosarcoma of the vulva and perineum in females ages 13 to 20 years. This is a highly malignant tumor with a peculiar propensity for breast metastases. Unlike the embryonal variety, radiation plus vincristine, actinomycin D, and cyclophosphamide (VAC) chemotherapy seems to be of limited value for alveolar rhabdomyosarcoma. The Rhabdomyosarcoma Study Group reported 9 vulvar cases, five of which were embryonal in histology. After various combinations of chemotherapy, surgery, and radiation therapy, eight of the patients were in long-term remission (Hays et al, 1988). Thus the embryonal (botryoid) variety has an excellent prognosis (see Chapter 4).

MALIGNANT MELANOMA

Melanoma of the vulva, although a rare malignancy, is the second most common cancer occurring in this region. The tumor affects predominantly peri- and postmenopausal women with an average age at diagnosis of 57 years. The growth may arise from a pre-existing junctional nevus or the junctional component of a compound nevus, or it may originate de novo. The patient usually becomes aware of the malignancy because of pruritis, enlargement of a nevus, bleeding, or discovery of the tumor itself. More than 80 percent of vulvar melanomas arise from the labia minora and clitoris (Fig. 3–6).

Most melanomas are elevated, pigmented, and frequently ulcerated growths with an irregular border. They are often surrounded by an inflammatory margin. The differential diagnosis includes lentigo, benign nevus, dysplastic nevus, seborrheic keratosis, dermato-

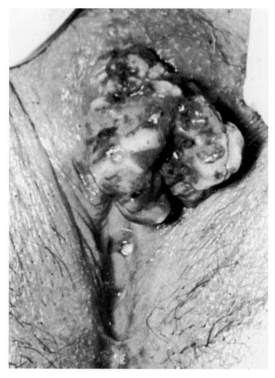

FIGURE 3–6. Exophytic vulvar melanoma arising from the clitoris and labia minora. The lesion was brown, blue, gray, and white.

fibroma, and pigmented basal cell carcinoma. The amelanotic variety may simulate a furuncle or epidermoid carcinoma. Some authorities recommend the removal of any nevus of the vulva prophylactically, because vulvar nevi are predominantly junctional and are thought to have some predisposition to becoming malignant. Acquired nevi, in contrast to melanomas and dysplastic nevi, have well-demarcated borders and are nearly always less than 1 cm in diameter.

Classification

Based on the propensity for horizontal and vertical growth, as well as on location and etiology, malignant cutaneous melanoma is characterized by several distinct clinical types. Clark et al (1975) described the three basic forms:

1. *Lentigo malignant melanoma* (LMM) is a slow-growing, relatively benign neoplasm characterized by an intraepithelial horizontal growth phase lasting for 10 or more years before invasion of the papillary der-

mis. It occurs on sun-exposed surfaces, predominantly in the elderly, and is not seen on the vulva.
2. *Superficial spreading melanoma* (SSM) similarly shows a relatively large, centrifugal growth phase before stromal invasion occurs. The superficial portion of this lesion has been clinically referred to as a pigmented flare, which typically involves the papillary dermis as well as the epidermis. Once the vertical growth phase begins, clinical progression is generally rather rapid. SSM constitutes two-thirds of vulvar melanomas.
3. Most of the remaining vulvar melanomas are of the *nodular* type (NM). This form has only a vertical growth phase. Consequently, its life history is shorter and it tends to be thicker and more deeply invasive at the time of diagnosis.

There is also a fourth type, *mucocutaneous melanoma* (MM), characterized by an LMM-like radial (horizontal) growth phase within which a vertically invasive melanoma develops. MM accounts for 10 percent of vulvar melanomas.

Stage and Prognosis

The prognosis and survival of vulvar melanoma, regardless of the clinicopathologic variety, are primarily determined by the thickness of the invasive portion of the lesion (Breslow microstaging), the depth of invasion (Clark-Mihm microstaging), the presence or absence of metastases, and extension to the urethra or vagina (Curtin and Morrow, 1992). The Clark-Mihm levels of invasion are defined in terms of the microanatomy of the skin (Fig. 3–7), while Breslow (1975) measured the vertical thickness of the lesion from the top of the granular layer to the deepest point of invasion. In cutaneous melanoma, vertical thickness is more predictive of regional node metastasis and recurrence risk than is level of invasion. The collected survival data for women with vulvar melanoma according to the FIGO, Clark-Mihm, and Breslow staging systems are presented in Table 3–15. Microstaging of vulvar melanoma is clearly superior to FIGO clinical staging for cases without clinical evidence of metastases. It cannot be concluded from the data available for vulvar melanoma which of the microstaging techniques is the better predictor of outcome. High mitotic rate (>4/10 hpf),

FIGURE 3–7. Microstaging of malignant melanoma. The Breslow system, which measures vertical thickness in millimeters, is more predictive of the prognosis. The Clark-Mihm levels of invasion are on the right. Level I is intraepithelial, level II is papillary dermis, and level III is the interface between the papillary and reticular dermis. (From Chung AF, Woodruff JM, Lewis JL Jr: Malignant melanoma of the vulva. Obstet Gynecol 45: 638, 1975, with permission.)

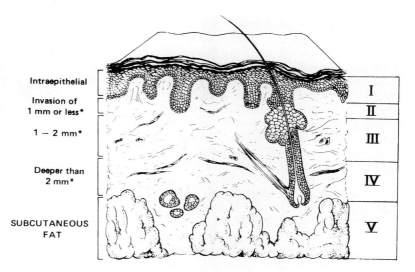

epithelioid cell type, age above 65 years, and presence of ulceration are also adverse risk factors in vulvar melanoma (Bradgate et al, 1990).

Groin node metastases, often clinically apparent, occur in about 25 percent of vulvar melanoma cases. The frequency has not been determined relative to the microstage. However, in cutaneous melanoma the risk is approximately 1 percent for lesions less than 0.76 mm thick, but rises sharply to about 25 percent for lesions 0.76 to 1.5 mm thick. The therapeutic value of routine regional node dissection in cutaneous melanoma is controversial. Dye injection and lymphoscintigraphy have been used to map the lymphatic drainage and identify "sentinel" nodes. In this approach, dissection would be done only in patients with an involved sentinel node (North and Spellman, 1996). Lymphatic mapping has been reported in vulvar melanoma, but no conclusions can be drawn at this time (Levenback et al, 1995). The local recurrence rate

is also related to lesional thickness (Sim et al, 1986; Balch et al, 1993).

In the only prospective study of surgical therapy for vulvar melanoma, the most reliable correlate of disease-free survival was the 1992 American Joint Committee on Cancer (AJCC) staging for cutaneous melanoma (Phillips et al, 1994): stage I: tumors 1.5 mm thick or less and no metastases; stage II; tumors 1.5 to 4.0 mm thick without metastases; stage III: tumors greater than 4.0 mm thick or tumors with nodal but not distant metastases; and stage IV: tumors with distant metastases. Breslow microstaging was second to the AJCC stage as an independent predictor of disease-free survival. LVSI and a centrally located primary were highly correlated with the risk for node metastases.

Treatment

The accumulated experience with microstaging cutaneous melanoma has led to a general

TABLE 3–15
Survival in Melanoma of the Vulva by Various Staging Methods*

FIGO Stage[†]		Breslow Microstage			Clark Microstage		
No.	% Alive	Thickness (mm)	No.	% Alive	Level	No.	% Alive
I	50	66	<0.76	25	96	II	22	95
II	18	11	0.76–1.50	24	71	III	29	59
III	21	38	1.51–3.0	36	58	IV	46	50
IV	7	0	>3.0	58	34	V	31	29

*Data from Chung et al (1975), Cleophax et al (1976), Jaramillo et al (1985), Phillips et al (1982), Podratz et al (1983a), Benda et al (1986), Beller et al (1986), Johnson et al (1986), Rose et al (1988), and Woolcott et al (1988).
†Clinical staging.

adoption of a conservative surgical therapy for vulvar melanoma. Melanomas that on thorough sectioning are less than 0.76 mm thick and without LVSI are adequately treated by local excision (1.0-cm margin) without regional node dissection (Sim et al, 1986), provided, of course, that the nodes are clinically negative. Thicker lesions require 2- to 3-cm margins (Balch et al, 1993) and bilateral groin node dissection. The role of pelvic lymphadenectomy has not been precisely defined, but if spread to the groin nodes has occurred, pelvic dissection should be performed. Considering the difficulty of documenting a salutary effect of excising the more proximal groin node group, however, routine pelvic lymphadenectomy is not warranted. Adjuvant therapy with alfa-2b interferon has been reported to improve survival for patients with skin melanoma more than 4 mm thick and node-positive patients (Kirkwood et al, 1996). A diagnosis of malignant melanoma is not a contraindication to replacement estrogen therapy. For information regarding melanoma and pregnancy, see Chapter 14.

From an examination of the pattern of treatment failures, the weakest point in the operation for melanoma of the vulva is the mucosal (vaginal and urethral) margin. Partial resection of the involved terminal urethra and vagina seems to be inadequate. Therefore, if the vagina is even superficially involved, the operation should be extended to include the entire vagina (and the uterus). Extension to the urethra and bladder or encroachment on the rectum is managed by exenteration. However, the effect of exenteration on survival does not appear to be large. Advanced or recurrent melanoma not amenable to surgical therapy may benefit from chemotherapy, radiation therapy, or active specific immunotherapy.

CARCINOMA OF THE URETHRAL MEATUS

Half of all malignant tumors of the urethra in women arise from the distal one third, including the meatus. Predominant symptoms are bleeding or spotting, dysuria, frequency, obstruction, and pain. Coexistence with a caruncle, or confusion with a caruncle, is relatively common. Most of the distal urethral cancers are anterior in origin and squamous in histologic type, but transitional cell carcinoma and adenocarcinoma also occur. Broadly speaking, histology does not seem to

have a strong influence on the prognosis. Large lesions may be indistinguishable from primary cancers of the vulva or vagina when extension to these organs occurs. Growth may also extend up the urethra to the bladder neck. Urethral carcinoma spreads readily by lymphatic invasion.

Antoniades (1969) reported on nine patients with lesions limited to the meatus at diagnosis and clinically negative nodes. Treatment with interstitial radiation (two patients also had simple excision) produced local control in all but one patient. No groin recurrences occurred, and no serious complications were reported. Primary urethral carcinoma with extension to the vagina, vulva, or regional nodes is attended by a poor outlook (Ampil, 1985). Radical surgery with or without irradiation may improve survival for these patients. Adenocarcinoma of the urethra with a clear cell or papillary pattern is more aggressive and more radiation resistant than

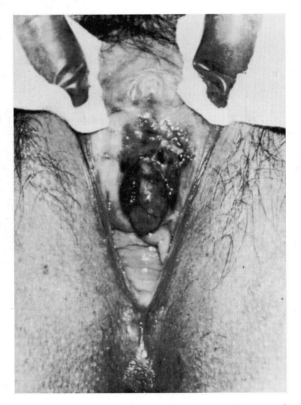

FIGURE 3–8. Polyploid malignant melanoma of the urethral meatus with a pigmented flare extending onto the surrounding mucosa. The patient was treated by anterior exenteration. She died 3 years later of breast cancer. (From Ostergard DR, Townsend DE: Malignant melanoma of the female urethra. Obstet Gynecol 31:75, 1968, with permission.)

other patterns. Anterior exenteration is recommended even when the disease is confined to the meatus. Resecting part of the symphysis may be useful (Klein et al, 1983).

The rare urethral melanoma invariably arises from the meatus in women beyond 50 years of age. These blue-black to reddish brown, pedunculated growths (Fig. 3–8) are usually advanced at the time of diagnosis. Approximately 45 cases have been reported, but there have been only three 5-year survivors. Radical surgery appears to offer the best chance to cure the early cases, especially in the absence of nodal metastases.

REFERENCES

Agress R, Figge DC, Tamimi H, Greer B: Dermatofibrosarcoma protuberans of the vulva. Gynecol Oncol 16:288, 1983.

Ampil FL: Primary malignant neoplasm of the female urethra. Obstet Gynecol 66:799, 1985.

Andersen ES, Sorensen IM: Verrucous carcinoma of the female genital tract: report of a case and review of the literature. Gynecol Oncol 30:427, 1988.

Andreasson B, Bock JE, Visfeldt J: Prognostic role of histology in squamous cell carcinoma in the vulvar region. Gynecol Oncol 14:373, 1982.

Antoniades J: Radiation therapy in carcinoma of the female urethra. Cancer 24:70, 1969.

Axe S, Parmley T, Woodruff JD, Hlopak B: Adenomas in minor vestibular glands. Obstet Gynecol 68:16, 1986.

Balch CM, Urist MM, Karakousis CP, et al: Efficacy of 2-cm surgical margins for intermediate thickness melanomas (1–4 mm): results of a multi-institutional randomized surgical trial. Ann Surg 218:262, 1993.

Bannatyne P, Elliott P, Russell P: Vulvar adenosquamous carcinoma arising in a hidradenoma papilliferum, with rapidly fatal outcome: case report. Gynecol Oncol 35:395, 1989.

Barbieri RL, Ryan KJ: Hyperandrogenism, insulin resistance, and acanthosis nigricans syndrome: a common endocrinopathy with distinct pathophysiologic features. Am J Obstet Gynecol 147:90, 1983.

Barnhill DR, Boling R, Nobles W, et al: Vulvar dermatofibrosarcoma protuberans. Gynecol Oncol 30:149, 1988.

Beller U, Demopoulos RI, Beckman EM: Vulvovaginal melanoma: a clinicopathologic study. J Reprod Med 31:315, 1986.

Benda JA, Platz CE, Anderson B: Malignant melanoma of the vulva: a clinical-pathologic review of 16 cases. Int J Gynecol Pathol 5:202, 1986.

Benedet JL, Turko M, Fairey RN, Boyes DA: Squamous carcinoma of the vulva: results of treatment, 1938 to 1976. Am J Obstet Gynecol 134:201, 1979.

Bergen S, DiSaia PJ, Liao SY, Berman ML: Conservative management of extramammary Paget's disease of the vulva. Gynecol Oncol 33:151, 1989.

Bernstein KE, Lattes R: Nodular (pseudosarcomatous) fasciitis, a nonrecurrent lesion: clinicopathologic study of 134 cases. Cancer 49:1668, 1982.

Bernstein SG, Voet RL, Lifshitz S, Buchsbaum HJ: Adenoid cystic carcinoma of Bartholin's gland: case report and review of the literature. Am J Obstet Gynecol 147:385, 1983.

Bock JE, Andreasson B, Thorn A, Holck S: Dermatofibrosarcoma protuberans of the vulva. Gynecol Oncol 20:129, 1985.

Boronow RC: Combined therapy as an alternative to exenteration for locally advanced vulvo-vaginal cancer: rationale and results. Cancer 49:1085, 1982.

Boutselis JG: Radical vulvectomy for invasive squamous cell carcinoma of the vulva. Obstet Gynecol 39:827, 1972.

Boyce J, Fruchter RG, Kasambilides E, et al: Prognostic factors in carcinoma of the vulva. Gynecol Oncol 20:364, 1985.

Bradgate MG, Rollason TP, McConkey CC, Powell J: Malignant melanoma of the vulva: a clinicopathological study of 50 women. Br J Obstet Gynaecol 97:124, 1990.

Breslow A: Tumor thickness, level of invasion and node dissection in stage I cutaneous melanoma. Ann Surg 182:572, 1975.

Brisigotti M, Moreno A, Murcia C, et al: Verrucous carcinoma of the vulva: a clinicopathologic and immunohistochemical study of five cases. Int J Gynecol Pathol 8:1, 1989.

Burke TW, Levenback C, Coleman RL, et al: Surgical therapy of T1 and T2 vulvar carcinoma: further experience with radical wide excision and selective inguinal lymphadenectomy. Gynecol Oncol 57:215, 1995.

Buscema J, Stern JL, Woodruff JD: Early invasive carcinoma of the vulva. Am J Obstet Gynecol 140:563, 1981.

Casley-Smith JR, Morgan RG, Piller NB: Treatment of lymphedema of the arms and legs with 5, 6-benzo-alpha-pyrone. N Engl J Med 329:1158, 1993.

Cavanaugh D, Shepherd JH: The place of pelvic exenteration in the primary management of advanced carcinoma of the vulva. Gynecol Oncol 13:318, 1982.

Chafe W, Richards A, Morgan L, Wilkinson E: Unrecognized invasive carcinoma in vulvar intraepithelial neoplasia (VIN). Gynecol Oncol 31:154, 1988.

Chamlian DL, Taylor HB: Primary carcinoma of Bartholin's gland: a report of 24 patients. Obstet Gynecol 39:489, 1972.

Chung AF, Woodruff JM, Lewis JL Jr: Malignant melanoma of the vulva: a report of 44 cases. Obstet Gynecol 45:638, 1975.

Clark WH Jr, Ainsworth AM, Bernardino EA, et al: The developmental biology of primary human malignant melanomas. Semin Oncol 2:83, 1975.

Cleophax JP, Pilleron JP, Durand JC, Laurent M: Le melanome malin de la vulve. Gyncologie 27:333, 1976.

Copeland LJ, Sneige N, Gershenson DM, et al: Adenoid cystic carcinoma of Bartholin gland. Obstet Gynecol 67:115, 1986.

Copeland LJ, Sneige N, Stringer CA, et al: Alveolar rhabdomyosarcoma of the female genitalia. Cancer 56:849, 1985.

Creasman WT, Gallager HS, Rutledge F: Paget's disease of the vulva. Gynecol Oncol 3:133, 1975.

Curry SL, Wharton JT, Rutledge F: Positive lymph nodes in vulvar squamous carcinoma. Gynecol Oncol 9:63, 1980.

Curtin JP, Morrow CP: Melanoma of the female genital tract. In Coppleson M (ed): Gynecologic Oncology. New York, Churchill Livingstone, 1992, p 1059.

Curtin JP, Rubin SC, Jones WB, et al: Paget's disease of the vulva. Gynecol Oncol 39:374, 1990.

Davos I, Abell MR: Soft tissue sarcomas of vulva. Gynecol Oncol 4:70, 1976.

Dean RE, Taylor ES, Weisbrod DM, Martin JW: The treatment of premalignant lesions of the vulva. Am J Obstet Gynecol 119:59, 1974.

De Mola JRL, Hudock PA, Steinetz C, et al: Merkel cell carcinoma of the vulva. Gynecol Oncol 51:272, 1993.

DiSaia PJ, Creasman WT, Rich WM: An alternate approach to early cancer of the vulva. Am J Obstet Gynecol 133:825, 1979.

DiSaia PJ, Rutledge F, Smith JP: Sarcoma of the vulva: report of 12 patients. Obstet Gynecol 38:180, 1971.

Donaldson ES, Powell DE, Hanson MB, van Nagell JR Jr: Prognostic parameters in invasive vulvar cancer. Gynecol Oncol 11:184, 1981.

Dunaif A, Hoffman AR, Scully RE, et al: Clinical, biochemical, and ovarian morphologic features in women with acanthosis nigricans and masculinization. Obstet Gynecol 66:545, 1985.

Eriksson E, Eldh J, Peterson L-E: Surgical treatment of carcinoma of the clitoris. Gynecol Oncol 17:291, 1984.

Faber K, Jones MA, Spratt D, Tarraza HM Jr: Vulvar leiomyomatosis in a patient with esophagogastric leiomyomatosis: review of the syndrome. Gynecol Oncol 41:92, 1991.

Fairey RN, MacKay PA, Benedet JL, et al: Radiation treatment of carcinoma of the vulva, 1950–1980. Am J Obstet Gynecol 151:591, 1985.

Feurer GA, Shevchuk M, Calanog A: Vulvar Paget's disease: the need to exclude an invasive lesion. Gynecol Oncol 38:81, 1990.

Figge DC, Gaudenz R: Invasive carcinoma of the vulva. Am J Obstet Gynecol 119:382, 1974.

Figge DC, Tamimi HK, Greer BE: Lymphatic spread in carcinoma of the vulva. Am J Obstet Gynecol 152:387, 1985.

Fine BA, Fowler LJ, Valente PT, Gaudet T: Minimally invasive Paget's disease of the vulva with extensive lymph node metastases. Gynecol Oncol 57:262, 1995.

Franklin EW III, Rutledge FN: Prognostic factors in epidermoid carcinoma of the vulva. Obstet Gynecol 37:892, 1971.

Friedrich EG Jr: Vulvar vestibulitis syndrome. J Reprod Med 32:110, 1987.

Garcia JJ, Verkauf BS, Hochberg CJ, Ingram JM: Aberrant breast tissue of the vulva: a case report and review of the literature. Obstet Gynecol 52:225, 1978.

Green TH Jr: Carcinoma of the vulva: a reassessment. Obstet Gynecol 52:462, 1978.

Guindi SF, Silberberg BK, Evans TN: Multifocal mixed adnexoid tumors of the vulva. Int J Gynecol Obstet 12:138, 1974.

Gunn RA, Gallagher HS: Vulvar Paget's disease: a topographic study. Cancer 46:590, 1980.

Hacker NF: Current treatment of small vulvar cancers. Oncology 4:21, 1990.

Hacker NF, Berek JS, Lagasse LD, et al: Management of regional lymph nodes and their prognostic influence in vulvar cancer. Obstet Gynecol 61:408, 1983.

Hacker NF, Berek JS, Lagasse LD, et al: Individualization of treatment for stage I squamous cell vulvar carcinoma. Obstet Gynecol 63:155, 1984.

Hacker NF, Leuchter RS, Berek JS, et al: Radical vulvectomy and bilateral inguinal lymphadenectomy through separate groin incisions. Obstet Gynecol 58:574, 1981.

Hays DM, Shimada H, Raney RB Jr: Clinical staging and treatment results in rhabdomyosarcoma of the female genital tract among children and adolescents. Cancer 61:1893, 1988.

Heah J: Methods of treatment for cysts and abscesses of Bartholin's gland. Br J Obstet Gynaecol 95:321, 1988.

Hoffman JS, Kumar NB, Morley GW: Microinvasive squamous carcinoma of the vulva: search for a definition. Obstet Gynecol 61:615, 1983.

Hoffman MS, Roberts WS, Ruffolo EH: Basal cell carcinoma of the vulva with inguinal lymph node metastases. Gynecol Oncol 29:113, 1988.

Homesley HD, Bundy BN, Sedlis A, Adcock L: Radiation therapy versus pelvic node resection for carcinoma of the vulva with positive groin nodes. Obstet Gynecol 68:733, 1986.

Homesley HD, Bundy BN, Sedlis A, et al: Assessment of current International Federation of Gynecology and Obstetrics staging of vulvar carcinoma relative to prognostic factors for survival: a Gynecologic Oncology Group study. Am J Obstet Gynecol 164:997, 1991.

Homesley HD, Bundy BN, Sedlis A, et al: Prognostic factors related to groin node metastasis in squamous cell carcinoma of the vulva: a Gynecologic Oncology Group study. Gynecol Oncol 49:279, 1993.

Hopkins MP, Reid GC, Vettrano I, Morley GW: Squamous cell carcinoma of the vulva: prognostic factors influencing survival. Gynecol Oncol 43:113, 1991.

Husseinzadeh N, Zaino R, Nahhas WA, Mortel R: The significance of histologic findings in predicting nodal metastases in invasive squamous cell carcinoma of the vulva. Gynecol Oncol 16:105, 1983.

Iversen T: The value of groin palpation in epidermoid carcinoma of the vulva. Gynecol Oncol 12:291, 1981.

Iversen T, Aas M: Lymph drainage from the vulva. Gynecol Oncol 16:179, 1983.

Japaze H, Garcia-Bunuel R, Woodruff JD: Primary vulvar neoplasia: a review of in situ and invasive carcinoma, 1935–1972. Obstet Gynecol 49:404, 1977.

Jaramillo BA, Ganjei P, Averette HE, et al: Malignant melanoma of the vulva. Obstet Gynecol 66:398, 1985.

Johnson TL, Kumar NB, White CD, Morley GW: Prognostic features of vulvar melanoma: a clinicopathologic analysis. Int J Gynecol Pathol 5:110, 1986.

Katz VL, Askin FB, Bosch BD: Glomus tumor of the vulva: a case report. Obstet Gynecol 67:43S, 1986.

Kaufman RH, Friedrich EG Jr, Gardner HL: Benign Diseases of the Vulva and Vagina, 3rd ed. Chicago, Year Book Medical Publishers, 1989.

Kaufmann T, Pawl NO, Soifer I, et al: Cystic papillary hidradenoma of the vulva: case report and review of the literature. Gynecol Oncol 26:240, 1987.

Kirkwood JM, Strawderman MH, Ernstoff MS, et al: Interferon alfa-2b adjuvant therapy of high-risk cutaneous melanoma: the Eastern Cooperative Oncology Group Trial EST 1684. J Clin Oncol 14:7, 1996.

Klein FA, Whitmore WF Jr, Herr HW, et al: Inferior pubic rami resection with en bloc radical excision for invasive proximal urethral carcinoma. Cancer 51:1238, 1983.

Krupp PJ, Bohm JW: Lymph gland metastases in invasive squamous cell cancer of the vulva. Am J Obstet Gynecol 130:943, 1978.

Krupp PJ, Lee FY, Bohm JW, et al: Prognostic parameters and clinical staging criteria in epidermoid carcinoma of the vulva. Obstet Gynecol 46:84, 1975.

Lee SC, Roth LM, Ehrlich C, Hall JA: Extramammary Paget's disease of the vulva: a clinicopathologic study of 13 cases. Cancer 39:2540, 1977.

Leuchter RS, Hacker NF, Voet RL, et al: Primary carcinoma of the Bartholin gland: a report of 14 cases and review of the literature. Obstet Gynecol 60:361, 1982.

Levenback C, Burke TW, Morris M, et al: Potential applications of intraoperative lymphatic mapping in vulvar cancer. Gynecol Oncol 59:216, 1995.

Levin M, Pakarakas RM, Chang HA: Primary breast carcinoma of the vulva: a case report and review of the literature. Gynecol Oncol 56:448, 1995.

Lieb SM, Gallousis S, Freedman H: Granular cell myoblastoma of the vulva. Gynecol Oncol 8:12, 1979.

LiVolsi VA, Brooks JJ: Nodular fasciitis of the vulva: a report of two cases. Obstet Gynecol 69:513, 1987.

Magrina JF, Webb MJ, Gaffey TA, Symmonds RE: Stage I squamous cell cancer of the vulva. Am J Obstet Gynecol 134:453, 1979.

Majmudar B, Castellano PZ, Wilson RW, Siegel RJ: Granular cell tumors of the vulva. J Reprod Med 35:1008, 1990.

Mann MS, Kaufman RH, Brown D Jr, Adam E: Vulvar vestibulitis: significant clinical variables and treatment outcome. Obstet Gynecol 79:122, 1992.

Meeker WR, Sickle-Santanello BJ, Philpott G, et al: Combined chemotherapy, radiation, and surgery for epithelial cancer of the anal canal. Cancer 57:525, 1986.

Merino MJ, LiVolsi VA, Schwartz PE, Rudnicki J: Adenoid basal cell carcinoma of the vulva. Int J Gynecol Pathol 1:299, 1982.

Merlob P, Bahari C, Liban E, Reisner SH: Cysts of the female external genitalia in the newborn infant. Am J Obstet Gynecol 132:607, 1978.

Mikhail GR, Fachnie DM, Drukker BH, et al: Generalized malignant acanthosis nigricans. Arch Dermatol 115:201, 1979.

Misas JE, Cold CJ, Hall FW: Vulvar Paget disease: fluorescein-aided visualization of margins. Obstet Gynecol 77: 156, 1991.

Moller LB, Nielsen MN, Trolle C: Leiomyosarcoma vulvae: case report. Acta Obstet Gynecol Scand 69:187, 1990.

Morley GW: Infiltrative carcinoma of the vulva: results of surgical treatment. Am J Obstet Gynecol 124:874, 1976.

Morris JM: A formula for selective lymphadenectomy: its application to cancer of the vulva. Obstet Gynecol 50:12, 1977.

Nori D, Cain JM, Hilaris BS, et al: Metronidazole as a radiosensitizer and high-dose radiation in advanced vulvovaginal malignancies: a pilot study. Gynecol Oncol 16: 117, 1983.

North JH Jr, Spellman JE: Role of sentinel node biopsy in the management of malignant melanoma. Oncology 10: 1239, 1996.

Ostergard DR, Townsend DE: Malignant melanoma of the female urethra. Obstet Gynecol 31:75, 1968.

Otis CN, Fischer RA, Johnson N, et al: Histiocytosis X of the vulva: a case report and review of the literature. Obstet Gynecol 75:555, 1990.

Parmley TH, Woodruff JD, Julian CG: Invasive Paget's disease. Obstet Gynecol 46:341, 1975.

Parry-Jones E: Lymphatics of the vulva. J Obstet Gynaecol Br Empire 70:751, 1963.

Perrone T, Swanson PE, Twiggs L, et al: Malignant rhabdoid tumor of the vulva: is distinction from epithelioid sarcoma possible? A pathologic and immunohistochemical study. Am J Surg Pathol 13:848, 1989.

Phillips GL, Bundy BN, Okagaki T, et al: Malignant melanoma of the vulva treated by radical hemivulvectomy. Cancer 73:2626, 1994.

Phillips GL, Twiggs LB, Okagaki T: Vulvar melanoma: a microstaging study. Gynecol Oncol 14:80, 1982.

Piver MS, Xynos FP: Pelvic lymphadenectomy in women with carcinoma of the clitoris. Obstet Gynecol 49:592, 1977.

Podratz KC, Gaffey TA, Symmonds RE, et al: Melanoma of the vulva: an update. Gynecol Oncol 16:153, 1983a.

Podratz KC, Symmonds RE, Taylor WF, Williams TJ: Carcinoma of the vulva: analysis of treatment and survival. Obstet Gynecol 61:63, 1983b.

Prempree T, Amornmarn R: Radiation treatment of recurrent carcinoma of the vulva. Cancer 54:1943, 1984.

Reagan MT, Clowry LJ, Cox JD, Rangala N: Radiation therapy in the treatment of malignant fibrous histiocytoma. Int J Radiat Oncol 7:311, 1981.

Reid R, Omoto KH, Precop SL, et al: Flashlamp-excited dye laser therapy of idiopathic vulvodynia is safe and efficacious. Am J Obstet Gynecol 172:1684, 1995.

Rock B, Hood AF, Rock JA: Prospective study of vulvar nevi. J Am Acad Dermatol 22:104, 1990.

Rose PG, Piver MS, Tsukada Y, Lau T: Conservative therapy for melanoma of the vulva. Am J Obstet Gynecol 159:52, 1988.

Rose PG, Tak WK, Reale FR, Hunter RE: Adenoid cystic carcinoma of the vulva: a radiosensitive tumor. Gynecol Oncol 43:81, 1991.

Rosenberg P, Simonsen E, Risberg B: Adenoid cystic carcinoma of Bartholin's gland: a report of five new cases treated with surgery and radiotherapy. Gynecol Oncol 34: 145, 1989.

Rutledge F, Smith JP, Franklin EW: Carcinoma of the vulva. Am J Obstet Gynecol 106:1117, 1970.

Santala M, Suonio S, Syrjaönen K, et al: Malignant fibrous histiocytoma of the vulva. Gynecol Oncol 27:121, 1987.

Sedlis A, Homesley H, Bundy BN, et al: Positive groin lymph nodes in superficial squamous cell vulvar cancer: a Gynecologic Oncology Group study. Am J Obstet Gynecol 156:1159, 1987.

Sim FH, Taylor WF, Pritchard DJ: Lymphadenectomy in the management of stage I malignant melanoma: a prospective randomized study. Mayo Clinic Proc 61:697, 1986.

Stacey D, Burrell MO, Franklin WE III: Extramammary Paget's disease of the vulva and anus: use of intraoperative frozen-section margins. Am J Obstet Gynecol 155:519, 1986.

Stehman FB, Bundy BN, Dvoretsky PM, Creasman WT: Early stage I carcinoma of the vulva treated with ipsilateral superficial inguinal lymphadenectomy and modified radical hemivulvectomy: a prospective study of the Gynecologic Oncology Group. Obstet Gynecol 79:490, 1992a.

Stehman FB, Bundy BN, Thomas G, et al: Groin dissection versus groin radiation in carcinoma of the vulva: a Gynecologic Oncology Group study. Int J Radiat Oncol Biol Phys 24:389, 1992b.

Taussig FJ: Cancer of the vulva. Am J Obstet Gynecol 40: 764, 1940.

Tavassoli FA, Norris HJ: Smooth muscle tumors of the vulva. Obstet Gynecol 53:213, 1979.

Thomas G, Dembo A, DePetrillo A, et al: Concurrent radiation and chemotherapy in vulvar carcinoma. Gynecol Oncol 34:263, 1989.

Thomas R, Barnhill D, Bibro M, et al: Histiocytosis-X in gynecology: a case presentation and review of the literature. Obstet Gynecol 67:46s, 1986.

Ulbright TM, Brokaw SA, Stehman FB, Roth LM: Epithelioid sarcoma of the vulva: evidence suggesting more aggressive behavior. Cancer 52:1462, 1983.

Wahlström T, Vesterinen E, Saksela E: Primary carcinoma of Bartholin's gland: a morphological and clinical study of six cases including a transitional cell carcinoma. Gynecol Oncol 6:354, 1978.

Way S: The anatomy of the lymphatic drainage of the vulva and its influence on the radical operation for carcinoma. Ann Coll Surg Engl 3:187, 1948.

Weiss SW, Enzinger FM: Malignant fibrous histiocytoma: an analysis of 200 cases. Cancer 41:2250, 1978.

Wharton JT, Gallagher S, Rutledge FN: Microinvasive carcinoma of the vulva. Am J Obstet Gynecol 118:159, 1974.

Wheeland RG, Bailin PL, Reynolds OD, Ratz JL: Carbon dioxide (CO_2) laser vaporization of multiple facial syringomas. J Dermatol Surg Oncol 12:225, 1986.

Wilkinson EJ (ed): Contemporary Issues in Surgical Pathology. Vol 9: Pathology of the Vulva and Vagina. New York, Churchill Livingstone, 1987.

Wilkinson EJ, Rico MJ, Pierson KK: Microinvasive carcinoma of the vulva. Int J Gynecol Pathol 1:29, 1982.

Winkelmann SE, Llorens AS: Metastatic basal cell carcinoma of the vulva: case report. Gynecol Oncol 38:138, 1990.

Woodworth H Jr, Dockerty MB, Wilson RB, Pratt JH: Papillary hidradenoma of the vulva: a clinicopathologic study of 69 cases. Am J Obstet Gynecol 110:501, 1971.

Woolcott RJ, Henry RJ, Houghton CR: Malignant melanoma of the vulva: Australian experience. J Reprod Med 33:699, 1988.

Young AW Jr, Herman EW, Tovell HMM: Syringoma of the vulva: incidence, diagnosis, and cause of pruritus. Obstet Gynecol 55:515, 1980.

4

Tumors of the Vagina

BENIGN TUMORS OF THE VAGINA

Vaginal cysts are usually single, small, and asymptomatic. The most common are the epidermoid inclusion cysts, which form in the superficial mucosa of the distal vagina after surgical or birth trauma. They are seldom more than 1 to 2 cm in diameter. The cheesy filling occasionally ruptures into the surrounding tissue, causing a chronic granulomatous reaction. Second in frequency are müllerian or paramesonephric cysts, usually anterolateral, with a predilection for the vaginal fornices. They average 3 cm in diameter and are lined by mucinous epithelium. The larger cysts tend to cause dyspareunia. Gartner's duct or mesonephric cysts are quite unusual, small, asymptomatic, and anterolateral in location. All large or symptomatic vaginal cysts should be excised (Evans and Paine, 1965; Deppisch, 1975; Pradhan and Tobon, 1986).

Vaginal ulcers may be benign or malignant. The benign ulcers are infectious (e.g., herpes), autoimmune (Behçet's syndrome), traumatic (tampons), or a manifestation of a dermatosis (lichen planus, pemphigoid). The history, culture, biopsy, and evidence of other cutaneous or mucosal lesions lead to the correct diagnosis in most cases (Dodson et al, 1978; Danielson, 1983; Kaufman et al, 1989).

Benign vaginal polyps are rare but important because of their similarity to malignant lesions. The benign mixed paravestibular tumor arises near the vaginal introitus, typically anterior, in the adult female. Histologically the tumor contains squamous epithelium with spindle cell and myxomatous stromal components. None of the dozen reported cases has behaved in a malignant fashion, although one local recurrence has been reported (Fowler et al, 1981). Fibroepithelial polyps resemble sarcoma botryoides grossly and microscopically. They are characteristically <2 cm in size, occasionally multiple, and are found with few exceptions in adult women. Occurrence in the postmenopausal age group may be related to estrogen use (Burt et al, 1976). On microscopic examination the polyps consist of a loose fibrovascular stroma, often with large atypical fibroblasts covered by normal vaginal mucosa. Specific mesenchymal tissue (muscle, cartilage) is absent, and mitoses are rare. The only recurrence among more than 50 reported cases was cured by local re-excision (Norris and Taylor, 1966; Chirayil and Tobon, 1981). Fibroepithelial polyps in pregnancy may be associated with vaginal bleeding (Pearl et al, 1991).

Benign rhabdomyomas are classified as cardiac and extracardiac. The former are probably hamartomas, often associated with tuberous sclerosus. The latter are of two histologic types, adult and fetal. The adult form develops almost exclusively in the head and neck region. The fetal type has a strong predilection for the vagina, cervix, and vulva of middle-aged women. These lesions are typically soft, small, and asymptomatic. Microscopically the stroma is myxoid, and some of the strap cells have cross striations or myofibrils, but there are no mitoses (Di Sant'Agnese and Knowles, 1980; Miettinen et al, 1983).

Leiomyomas (fibromyomas) are rare, but when they occur they typically involve the anterior vaginal wall of women in the fourth and fifth decades. The most frequently reported symptoms are dyspareunia and urinary dysfunction. The tumors are almost invariably less than 5 cm in diameter. There does not seem to be an association with uterine myomas. Recurrence has been reported (Ingemanson and Alfredsson, 1970).

PREMALIGNANT AND RELATED DISORDERS

For a discussion of premalignant and related disorders of the vagina (condylomas and vaginal intraepithelial neoplasia), see Chapter 2.

MALIGNANT TUMORS OF THE VAGINA

Primary malignant tumors of the vagina constitute only 1 to 2 percent of all gynecologic cancers. Although the predominant histologic type is squamous (Table 4–1), reflecting the vagina's most abundant epithelial tissue, an impressive array of nonsquamous neoplasms also occur. The cell type tends to vary with the age of the patient. Thus the botryoid embryonal rhabdomyosarcoma and endodermal sinus tumor characteristically occur in infancy. The primary vaginal malignancies of adolescence are the botryoid tumors and the diethylstilbestrol (DES)–related adenocarcinomas. Leiomyosarcoma has its peak incidence during the later reproductive years, while squamous carcinoma and melanoma are most prevalent in the seventh and eighth decades of life.

Squamous Carcinoma

Pathophysiology

Squamous carcinoma of the vagina arises from the vaginal mucous membrane, spreads locally, and invades the underlying mucosa and muscularis. Direct extension to the bladder or rectum is also an important pattern in this malignancy. Exophytic growth is the rule (Figs. 4–1 and 4–2). The most common site is in the upper one third of the vagina (40 percent), where extension to the cervix tends to obscure the actual site of origin. (Among women who have undergone previous hysterectomy, apical lesions account for 70 percent of vaginal cancers.) Similarly, distal third lesions, which are next in frequency (15 percent), may be difficult to distinguish from primary urethral or vulvar carcinomas. Growths in these areas must be regarded as possibly metastatic, especially in patients previously treated for cervical cancer. Advanced lesions involving the full length of the vagina account for 20 percent of the cases. Anterior lesions are slightly more common than posterior lesions (30 vs. 27 percent), while 23 percent arise on the lateral walls (Chyle et al, 1996).

After contiguous growth, lymphatic invasion and metastasis are the most important modes of spread. The vaginal tube is supplied with a rich network of lymph vessels, the drainage of which is related to both the anteroposterior divisions of the organ and its proximodistal sections. The distal vagina, especially the lower third, has lymphatics that drain to the inguinal nodes, whereas the upper vaginal lymphatics course mainly to the pelvic nodes. The lymphatic drainage of the vaginal fornices is essentially the same as that of the cervix (portio vaginalis). Lymphatics to the bladder and rectum, via the longitudinal pillars that connect these organs, constitute the anteroposterior-oriented drainage system. Thus the lymphatic spread of vaginal cancer is likely to be complex and may involve any of the pelvic node groups and/or the groin nodes, depending on the tumor location, size, and depth of invasion.

TABLE 4–1

Vaginal Cancer: Reported Incidence by Histology

Source	Total N	Squamous Carcinoma		Adeno- carcinoma		Melanoma/ Sarcoma	
		N	(%)	N	(%)	N	(%)
Manetta et al (1988)*	29	24	(83)	5	(17)	0	(0)
Sulak et al (1988)	48	27	(56)	11†	(23)	10	(21)
Manetta et al (1990)*	53	47	(89)	6	(11)	0	(0)
Kucera and Vavra (1991)*	110	101	(92)	9	(8)	0	(0)
Davis et al (1991)	126	93	(74)	21†	(17)	12	(0)
							(9)
Total	336	292	(80)	52	(14)	22	(6)

*Excludes melanoma and sarcoma.
†Includes DES-associated adenocarcinoma.

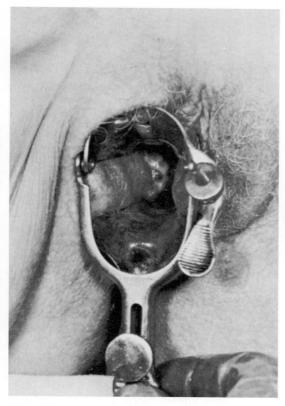

FIGURE 4–1. Stage I squamous cell carcinoma of the middle third of the vagina presented as post-menopausal bleeding.

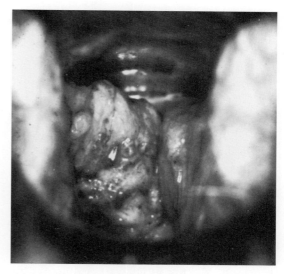

FIGURE 4–2. Stage IIb squamous cell carcinoma of the vagina. The patient was treated with radiation therapy. One year later, a total pelvic exenteration was performed for recurrent disease.

Detection, Evaluation, and Staging

Invasive carcinoma of the vagina in several series has been detected by cytology or routine examination in 20 percent of the cases. This reflects in part the continued use of cytologic screening and examination of at-risk populations. Patients with vaginal cancer frequently have had a previous hysterectomy (35 to 50 percent), and approximately 20 percent have a history of cervical and/or vulvar neoplasm (Benedet et al, 1983; Kirkbride et al, 1995; Stock et al, 1995; Sturgeon et al, 1996). Patients who are asymptomatic and are diagnosed because of an abnormal Pap smear are more likely to have a stage I cancer (Kucera and Vavra, 1991). By far the most common complaint is bleeding, which may be severe. A watery, blood-tinged, or malodorous vaginal discharge, urinary distress, and pain are also reported symptoms of vaginal cancer. Over 75 percent of patients who are symptomatic have locally advanced disease.

During the examination, of particular importance is the peripheral lymph node survey, since inguinal and supraclavicular metastases may be present at diagnosis. Before the speculum is introduced, the introitus and urethra should be inspected and palpated. A lesion in these areas can be obscured by the blades of the speculum. Mucosal redundancy makes complete examination of the vagina difficult, especially in the parous woman. With an abnormal Pap smear or local symptoms, the entire vaginal surface, inclusive of the fornices, needs to be visualized and palpated. The visual search for small lesions is greatly aided by the application of Lugol's solution if the mucosa is well estrogenized.

Vaginal squamous cancers are usually exophytic, frequently with a papillary configuration. Ulcerative and infiltrating as well as flat, superficially spreading forms are also seen. The full extent of the tumor and its relationship to the cervix, urethra, hymenal ring, and vulva must be appreciated for treatment planning. This is aided by rectovaginal palpation, at which time submucosal extension, paravaginal invasion, and the involvement of the rectum, levator muscles, or pelvic wall can be assessed. Deep invasion in the anterior or posterior direction results in bladder or rectal involvement, which, if extensive, can cause fistula formation. Urinary obstruction and renal failure can result from urethral obstruction by an anterior, distal lesion.

Tissue diagnosis can almost always be accomplished by simple office punch biopsy. In

TABLE 4-2

Diagnostic and Staging Work-up for Patients With
Vaginal Carcinoma

Tissue biopsy
Rectovaginal bimanual examination
Cystourethroscopy
Proctosigmoidoscopy
Endocervical curettage
Endometrial biopsy or curettage
Pelvic and abdominal CT scan
Chest radiograph
Serum CEA and SCA (CA-125 for adenocarcinoma)
Pretreatment staging laporotomy if medically fit

TABLE 4-3

FIGO Stages in Carcinoma of the Vagina (Clinical)

Stage	Definition
0	Carcinoma in situ, intraepithelial carcinoma
I	The carcinoma is limited to the vaginal wall
II	The carcinoma has involved the subvaginal tissue but has not extended onto the pelvic wall
III	The carcinoma has extended onto the pelvic wall
IV	The carcinoma has extended beyond the true pelvis or has clinically involved the mucosa of the bladder or rectum; bullous edema as such does not permit a case to be allotted to stage IV
IVa	Spread of the growth to adjacent organs and/or direct extension beyond the true pelvis
IVb	Spread to distant organs

the presence of a gross lesion, a Pap smear is unnecessary. The staging and metastatic work-up are presented in Table 4-2. The chest radiograph and computed tomography (CT) scan are routine. Cystourethroscopy is indicated for anterior lesions, and visualization of the rectum is recommended for posterior wall cancers. If the lesion involves the posterior fornix, the rectum and sigmoid colon should also be evaluated. A negative endocervical curettage in the absence of a cervical lesion will provide adequate assurance that the vaginal carcinoma, especially in the area of the distal urethra, is not a metastasis from a primary cervical cancer. Patients who present with bleeding or an enlarged uterus require endometrial evaluation. Pretreatment measurements of the serum tumor markers carcinoembryonic antigen CEA and squamous cell carcinoma antigen (SCA) are recommended, since these tumor markers assist in surveillance if they are elevated (Maruo et al, 1985). The serum CA-125 level may be elevated if the vaginal tumor is an adenocarcinoma.

Prognosis

The curability of vaginal squamous carcinoma is mainly a function of the stage, that is, the extent of disease at presentation as described in Tables 4-3 and 4-4. Peters et al (1985b), employing a multivariate regression analysis of 86 cases, were unable to demonstrate a statistically significant influence of grade, tumor location, size, or histology (squamous carcinoma vs. adenocarcinoma) on survival. Chu and Beechinor (1984) observed a trend toward higher local failure rates with more poorly differentiated tumors and larger tumors (<2 cm, 14 percent; >2 cm, 36 percent). A significantly lower local failure rate has been reported for cancers in the upper one

third compared with lesions in the lower two thirds (Chu and Beechinor, 1984; Ali et al, 1996). Chyle et al (1996) found that the major determinant of local control for squamous cancers was tumor bulk. The proposal by Perez and Camel (1982) to subdivide stage II vaginal carcinoma into cases without (IIa) and with (IIb) paravaginal infiltration appears to be valid, with a substantially worse survival for the patients with stage IIb.

In another study, Peters et al (1985c) suggested that very early vaginal carcinoma has an excellent prognosis. All six of their microinvasive cases arose on a background of vaginal intraepithelial neoplasia VAIN III, had less than 2.5 mm of stromal invasion, and had no vascular space invasion. The median age of the six women was 10 years less than that of the authors' other patients with stage I vaginal carcinoma. Treatment with partial or total vaginectomy was curative in every case.

Treatment

Factors to be considered in planning therapy for vaginal carcinoma are the stage, lesion

TABLE 4-4

Reported Survival by Stage of Women With
Carcinoma of the Vagina*

Stage	Total Cases	% in Stage	% 5-year Survival
I	73	16.8	76.7
II	110	25.3	44.5
III	174	40.0	31.0
IV	77	17.8	18.2

*From Kucera H, Vavra N: Primary carcinoma of the vagina: clinical and histopathological variables associated with survival. Gynecol Oncol 40:12, 1991, with permission.

TABLE 4–5

Treatment of Vaginal Carcinoma by Radiotherapy: Impact of Treatment Modality by Stage*

| | Local Failures | | | | | | | | | |
| | Stage I | | Stage II | | Stage II | | Stage IV | | Total | |
Treatment	N	(%)	N	(%)	N	(%)	N	(%)	N	(%)
External beam only	7	(14)	28	(11)	40	(33)	5	(20)	80	(23)
Brachytherapy only	24	(21)	18	(11)	0	(0)	1	(100)	43	(19)
External plus brachytherapy	28	(7)	58	(21)	15	(40)	10	(30)	111	(21)
Total	59	(8)	104	(16)	55	(34)	16	(31)	234	(20)

*Data from Chyle V, Zagars GK, Wheeler JA, et al: Definitive radiotherapy for carcinoma of the vagina: outcome and prognostic factors. Int J Radiat Oncol Biol Phys 35:891, 1996, with permission.

size, location, presence or absence of the uterus, and whether the patient has been previously irradiated (usually for cervical carcinoma). Combined external beam and internal radiation therapy is the primary mode of therapy for vaginal cancer (Table 4–5). Surgery appears to provide a similar cure rate for early lesions (Al-Kurdi and Monaghan, 1981; Ball and Berman, 1982; Rubin et al, 1985; Davis et al, 1991), but it may be less applicable than radiation therapy because the patients are often elderly and frail. Superficial growths in the posterior fornix are more suited to operative treatment, since an adequate margin of clearance relative to the bladder and rectum is easier to obtain. In addition, vaginal grafting to preserve function may not be required. Surgery should also be considered in medically suitable patients whenever coitus is an important factor if adequate radiation would necessitate treatment of more than half of the vagina, since in this situation vaginal stenosis is likely to occur (Brown et al, 1971). Apical stage I and IIa lesions should be treated by radical hysterectomy and upper vaginectomy (Davis et al, 1991).

In general terms, the treatment field for early-stage vaginal carcinoma includes the pelvic nodes, the parametrium, and the vaginal tube, including the paracolpos to a level at least 2 cm distal to the lowest extent of the growth. Surgically, this is done by a radical hysterectomy, partial or complete vaginectomy, and pelvic lymphadenectomy. Definitive radiation treatment can be accomplished by 4,000 to 5,000 cGy of whole-pelvis irradiation followed by 2,500 to 4,000 cGy of interstitial therapy (see Chapter 17). Except for small vault lesions, which may be adequately managed by a tandem and ovoid implant (or cylinder), intracavitary radiation is less effective than interstitial therapy (Stock et al,

1992). When the distal vagina is involved, the inguinal nodes are also treated. During therapy planning, it is important to bear in mind that the posterior wall and the distal vagina are less tolerant of radiation than are other areas of the vagina (Hintz et al, 1980).

No satisfactory treatment has evolved for advanced vaginal cancer (stages IIb, III, and IVa). A local failure rate of up to 50 percent and a major complication rate of 15 to 25 percent in this group of patients, in conjunction with a 5-year survival of 30 percent or less, indicate that radiation therapy alone as the first choice of treatment needs to be re-evaluated. Although there are scant data on the results of primary surgical therapy (Al-Kurdi and Monaghan, 1981), several of the patients in the reported radiation therapy series survived for 5 years after undergoing pelvic exenteration for local failure. This suggests that selected cases of advanced vaginal carcinoma might have a better chance of being cured by preoperative whole-pelvis treatment followed by radical surgery, as proposed by Perez and Camel (1982). Radiation sensitizers and neoadjuvant chemotherapy might also improve results for locally advanced vaginal carcinoma. Pretreatment lymphography, CT scan, and/or staging laparotomy should be considered in the locally advanced cases because of an expected high rate of nodal metastases.

Other Vaginal Malignancies

Adenocarcinoma

The vagina is undoubtedly the site of metastases more commonly than it is the site of a primary malignancy. Thus, when adenocarcinoma is diagnosed, the possibility that it is metastatic should always be seriously considered. In this circumstance, the patient is often known to have had cancer elsewhere, usually higher in the genital tract (endometrium, ovary, cervix), but cancers of the kidney, breast, colon, and pancreas are also capable of spreading to the vagina. Occasionally cancer arising in one of these sites becomes manifest first as a vaginal lesion.

Adenocarcinoma can arise in the vagina from residual glands of müllerian origin (adenosis). These glands are probably the source of the clear cell carcinomas in young women with a history of intrauterine DES exposure (see later). Such cases, at least until recently, have accounted for the majority of primary vaginal adenocarcinomas in young women. The rare clear cell carcinoma of the vagina reported in elderly women is also most likely of müllerian origin. Other glandular entities occurring in the vagina that are a potential source of adenocarcinoma include endometriosis (Granai et al, 1984) and Gartner's duct. The latter is a remnant of the embryonic wolffian or mesonephric duct. Four cases of vaginal adenocarcinoma have been reported in women with unilateral renal agenesis and uterine anomalies, but it is unclear if they were of mesonephric origin. Treatment of vaginal adenocarcinoma is the same as that for squamous lesions, although the prognosis may be worse. Serum CA-125 monitoring may be helpful.

Endodermal Sinus Tumor

Approximately 50 cases of vaginal endodermal sinus tumor, a rare malignancy of infancy, have been reported. Clinically it resembles sarcoma botryoides. Although surgery alone or surgery plus radiation therapy has produced a few cures, it is generally agreed today that chemotherapy plus surgery is the treatment of choice (see Chapter 11). Of the 25 patients thus treated, only three have died of cancer (Young and Scully, 1984; Anderson et al, 1985; Copeland et al, 1985).

Sarcomas

Vaginal sarcomas can be divided into two distinct groups. The most common is the rare sarcoma botryoides, which occurs in infants and children. Diagnosis usually follows the discovery of a vaginal mass, which resembles a bunch of grapes (Fig. 4–3), hence the term *botryoides* (from the Greek word *botrys*, a

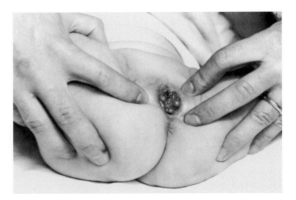

FIGURE 4–3. Sarcoma botryoides. Typical mass resembling a cluster of grapes protruding from the vagina. Differential diagnosis includes inflammatory polyps, prolapse of the urethral meatus, and endodermal sinus tumor. (From Hilgers RD, Malkasian GD, Soule EH: Embryonal rhabdomyosarcoma [botryoid type] of the vagina: a clinicopathologic review. Am J Obstet Gynecol 107:484, 1970, with permission.)

bunch of grapes). Other common symptoms are vaginal bleeding and discharge. Histologically the tumor is an embryonal rhabdomyosarcoma. The tumor may extend to the bladder and rectum, and lymphatic metastases to the pelvis and groin are frequent. Hematogenous spread also occurs. Benign vaginal polyps, which are occasionally confused with embryonal rhabdomyosarcoma, usually occur in an older age group than malignant lesions, as discussed earlier in this chapter.

Based on initial poor outcome with local excision and/or radiation therapy, the standard of therapy in the past was total pelvic exenteration (Hilgers et al., 1970). Because of the rarity of this malignancy, most of the initial reports of treatment and outcome were based on small numbers of patients. For this reason, the Intergroup Rhabdomyosarcoma Study (IRS) was organized in 1972. As a collaborative project, it has been able to accumulate the largest experience with treatment of vaginal embryonal rhabdomyosarcoma (Maurer et al, 1977). Hays et al (1988) reported on the outcome of 28 patients with vaginal embryonal rhabdomyosarcomas enrolled in either an IRS-I or an IRS-II regimen. Twenty-five of the 28 patients (mean age 2 years) were alive without disease after therapy; 5 of the 25 patients had relapses successfully treated with salvage therapy. After initial diagnosis, patients on IRS regimens I or II were treated with primary chemotherapy

TABLE 4-6

Vaginal Embryonal Rhabdomyosarcoma: Results of IRS I-II[†] Treatment in 28 Patients*

Patient Status	N	(%)
Alive	25	(89.3)
Dead of disease	2	(7.1)
Treatment death	1	(3.6)
Recurrences	7	(25.0)
Pelvic organs preserved		
Bladder	21	(75.0)
Uterus	5	(17.8)
Ovary(ies)	22	(78.5)

*Data from Hays DM, Shimada H, Raney RB Jr: Clinical staging and treatment results in rhabdomyosarcoma of the female genital tract among children and adolescents. Cancer 61:1893, 1988, with permission.
[†]Intergroup Rhabdomyosarcoma Study, regimens I and II.

(vincristine, actinomycin D, and cyclophosphamide [VAC] or VAC plus doxorubicin) or primary chemotherapy plus radiation. Exenteration was not needed to achieve these excellent results and should no longer be considered as an acceptable primary therapy (Table 4–6). The IRS III study confirmed the efficacy of conservative surgery with chemotherapy (Andrassy et al, 1995).

Malignant soft tissue sarcomas of the vagina present a spectrum of biologic activity. Leiomyosarcoma is the most common vaginal sarcoma in adults; the biologic activity is similar to that of uterine tumors (see Chapter 7). Their behavior can be predicted on the basis of mitotic counts, infiltrating versus pushing margins, and cellular atypia. Treatment is surgical, with wide local excision; the value of adjuvant radiotherapy is uncertain but should be considered for patients with a high-grade lesion. More rarely, the vagina may give rise to other unusual soft tissue sarcomas, including fibrosarcoma, angiosarcoma, and endometrial-type sarcomas (Tavasoli and Norris, 1979; Peters et al, 1985a; Curtin et al, 1995).

Malignant Melanoma

Vaginal melanoma was once considered a secondary lesion, because it had been accepted that melanocytes and nevi do not occur in the vagina. This objection is no longer valid. Not only melanocytes but also melanosis and nevi have been documented to occur in the vagina. Furthermore, of the more than 200 cases of primary vaginal melanomas reported in the world literature, many were associated with junctional activity of epidermal melanocytes, which is confirmatory of a primary lesion (Chung et al, 1980). Melanocytes, which are the presumed precursors of malignant melanoma, are found in 3 percent of adult females.

The average age at diagnosis of vaginal melanoma is 55 years, with a range from 22 to 83. Typically, the patient has vaginal bleeding or a vaginal discharge of less than 3 months' duration. The discharge is often blood tinged, foul smelling, or purulent, and the bleeding is invariably slight. Malignant melanoma may arise anywhere in the vagina, but it has a predilection for the anterior wall (45 percent) and the distal third (58 percent). It is frequently described as polypoid, pedunculated, papillary, or fungating. Ulceration and necrosis are often present. The lesion displays a variety of colors, including red and yellow, but usually it is brownish to black (Fig. 4–4). Only 5 percent are amelanotic. Satellite lesions are found in one third of the cases, but a pigmented flare is exceptional.

Vaginal melanoma is a highly malignant disease. The 5-year survival rate in collected series is 15 to 20 percent (Curtin and Morrow, 1992; Ragnarsson-Olding et al, 1993; Weinstock, 1994). Treatment modalities include conservative excision, radiation, and/or radical surgery. It is interesting to note that 80 percent of conservatively treated patients experience local recurrence. Radical surgery may reduce the risk of local recurrence but may have little effect on survival. Local excision or subtotal vaginectomy for even superficial lesions at any level of the vagina is probably inadequate. The more deeply invasive tumors invariably require extensive surgery. Whether a radical hysterectomy with total vaginectomy or anterior, posterior, or total exenteration is performed will depend on the location and extent of the lesion and the status of the regional lymph nodes. Patients who do not have an extensive growth, and patients who are not medically suited for radical surgery may benefit from a combination of limited surgery and radiation therapy. Bonner et al (1988) suggested that high-dose fractions (500 cGY to a dose of 3,000 cGY) followed by radical resection may improve locoregional control.

Vaginal melanosis is a premalignant condition characterized by intense pigmentation of the mucosa. It should be treated by vaginectomy when the diagnosis is established by representative biopsies (Bottles et al, 1984; Lee et al, 1984).

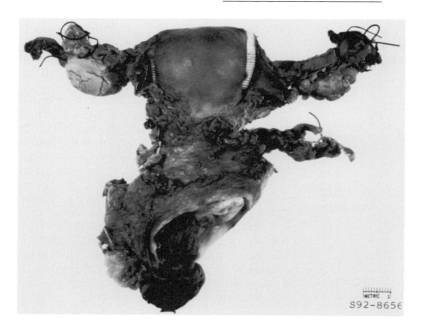

FIGURE 4–4. Malignant melanoma of the upper one third of the right vaginal wall. The pelvic nodes contained obvious pigmented metastases. Treatment was radical hysterectomy and pelvic node dissection.

VAGINAL ADENOSIS, ADENOCARCINOMA, AND DIETHYLSTILBESTROL

Duane E. Townsend

The clinical observation of an association between the maternal ingestion of DES and the subsequent development of cervical/vaginal clear cell adenocarcinoma in the exposed female offspring is one of the most important discoveries in gynecologic oncology in the past 25 years (Herbst et al, 1971). The DES-exposed female's risk of developing clear cell adenocarcinoma is relatively small, with the highest risk estimate approximately 1:1,000. The most common effects in the exposed female offspring are vaginal adenosis; structural changes in the vagina, cervix, and uterus; and infertility. The initial concern that squamous dysplasia might develop more commonly in the exposed offspring than in the unexposed population has been confirmed by the National Collaborative DES Project (Robboy et al, 1984; Borenstein et al, 1988). The exposed progeny have yet to reach the decades of life in which the most common adult cancers (e.g., breast, uterus, cervix) have their greatest incidence; consequently, the final evaluation of cancer risk must await longer follow-up.

Evaluation and Management of the Diethylstilbestrol-Exposed Patient

DES was prescribed in the United States under various trade names from approximately 1943 to 1971; the estimated number of exposed offspring ranges from 2 to 3 million. Women ages 20 to 50 years should be asked if their mothers took any medication or had any obstetric complications during the pregnancy. If a woman believes she was exposed to a hormone in utero, the gynecologic examination can often determine if the hormone was DES. The changes of the cervix and vagina characteristic of in utero DES exposure (vide infra) are occasionally found, however, in a patient with no history of DES exposure.

The initial step in the gynecologic evaluation includes careful inspection of the vagina. Cytologic specimens are taken from the endocervix and cervix; an additional swab should be obtained from the vagina. Bright red areas or sites of unusual surface contour should alert the physician to the possibility of malignancy. However, biopsies are not performed until after the colposcopic examination and staining of the tissues with iodine. Although colposcopy is not necessary for every DES examination, it is the most accurate way to assess the DES-related alterations of the cervical/vaginal tissues. Magnification helps one to recognize that the Lugol-negative tissue is adenosis, metaplasia, intraepithelial condyloma, or neoplasia. The colposcopic evaluation encompasses the cervix, the fornices, and the entire vaginal tube. Suspicious areas should be noted for subsequent biopsy. After colposcopy, the tissues are stained with a half-strength aqueous Lugol's solution. Biopsy specimens are then taken from any areas that are nodular on palpation or that have unusual gross or colposcopic findings. After removing the speculum, a bimanual examination including rectal palpation is performed. Palpation of the vagina and cervix is very important, since several clear cell adenocarcinomas have been picked up only because of palpable vaginal nodularity. Visualization and palpation are employed to assess the cervix for structural abnormalities.

Follow-up of the DES-exposed offspring depends on the findings at the initial examination. If there is no evidence of DES changes in the vagina, the patient is followed on a yearly basis. Colposcopy and iodine staining are no longer necessary in this individual un-

less the cytology becomes abnormal. Conversely, if there is evidence of adenosis (i.e., columnar tissue or squamous metaplasia in the vagina), it is recommended that the patient be evaluated every 6 months. Separate cytologic specimens are taken from the vagina and cervix at each visit. Colposcopic examination is recommended at any time the patient has an abnormal Pap smear. Examples of typical DES changes are depicted in Figures 4–5 through 4–7.

Natural History of Diethylstilbestrol Changes

The investigations of the national DES Adenosis (DESAD) Project found that vaginal adenosis is present in one third of women exposed in utero to DES, not 80 to 90 percent as was originally believed (Noller et al, 1981, 1983). Because 95 percent of the patients with vaginal clear cell adenocarcinoma have evidence of vaginal adenosis, patients with adenosis are considered to be at high risk of

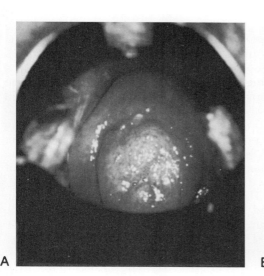

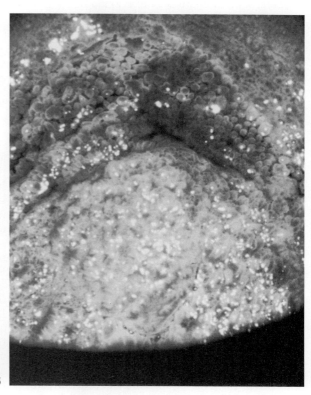

A   B

FIGURE 4–5. *A*, Gross photograph of a 19-year-old DES-exposed woman with a classic cervical collar (×16). The patient had an erythematous-appearing cervix, which extended onto the collar. *B*, Colpophotograph of the same patient as in *A* (×16). The columnar tissue has a grape-like appearance. Above the area of columnar tissue is active squamous metaplasia. The patient also had areas of adenosis and an extensive transformation zone in the vagina.

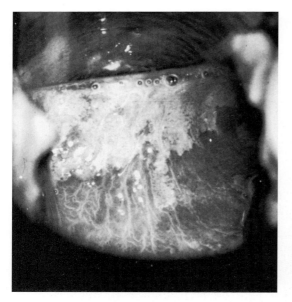

FIGURE 4–6. Colpophotograph of the midvagina in a 12-year-old girl who was exposed to DES during the first trimester (×16). The entire vagina was lined by a velvet-appearing columnar epithelium. Immature metaplastic squamous epithelium is present, with an irregular border in the upper portion of the photograph and the vertical ridges of columnar epithelium in the lower half.

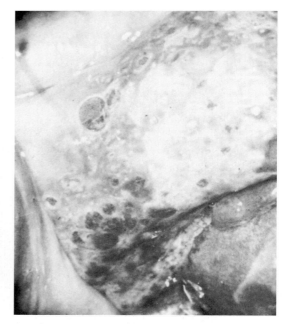

FIGURE 4–7. Colpophotograph of the upper third of the vagina in a 23-year-old woman exposed to DES during the first trimester (×16). Normal squamous epithelium is shown in the upper left-hand corner of the photograph. White metaplastic squamous epithelium is present in the right midportion of the photograph. Gland openings occur throughout the vagina, and large islands of persistent columnar tissue are present. In the lower right-hand corner of the photograph is a portion of the cervical hood, which is covered entirely by columnar epithelium.

developing clear cell adenocarcinoma. Initially the magnitude of the risk was unknown. However, the peak incidence of clear cell carcinoma related to DES exposure occurred in the late 1970s (Melnick et al, 1987), and fortunately we now know that only a small minority of women with adenosis will develop clear cell adenocarcinoma. Thus vaginal adenosis in the great majority of women is a benign tissue change, probably caused by an interference of DES with normal cervical/vaginal embryogenesis during intrauterine life.

However, the important question is not the relative prevalence of adenosis, but rather what happens to adenosis once a woman has developed this condition. Serial examination of over 2,000 exposed females revealed that adenosis (vaginal columnar tissue) behaves similarly to the columnar tissue of the cervix. Initially, the columnar tissue is replaced by immature metaplastic squamous epithelium, which colposcopically has many of the characteristics of VAIN: that is, it becomes white after the application of acetic acid and exhibits the vascular patterns of mosaicism and punctuation. The immature squamous epithelium in the DES-exposed offspring is also difficult to differentiate histologically and cyto-

logically from early VAIN. This metaplastic tissue does mature, however, and becomes less apparent as the patient ages. In fact, in a large proportion of the exposed offspring, the immature squamous epithelium has matured to a point that it cannot be detected colposcopically and in some cases iodine staining is normal. It is anticipated that most of the DES-exposed females with vaginal tissue changes will eventually have resolution of their adenosis and immature metaplasia.

The structural changes noted in the vagina and cervix—that is, transverse vaginal septum, cervical collar, cockscomb (Fig. 4–8), and hypoplastic or absent pars vaginalis—also show a substantial change over time (Jeffries et al, 1984). The most striking evolution occurs in those patients with the so-called collar or hood. In the majority of these patients, the collar tends to be absorbed as the large area of columnar tissue covering it is transformed into squamous epithelium.

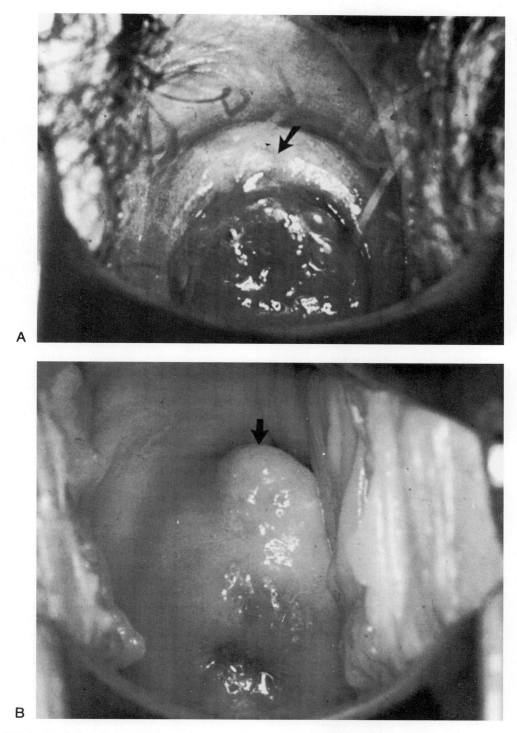

FIGURE 4–8. *A*, Cervical collar (arrow) in a DES-exposed patient encircles the cervix proper. *B*, Cocks-comb (arrow) in a DES-exposed patient.

The cockscomb becomes less prominent as well. Transverse vaginal septa tend to flatten out with sexual activity and childbirth. In summary, the majority of the cervical/vaginal changes introduced by intrauterine DES exposure tend to disappear spontaneously as the individual matures.

Clear Cell Adenocarcinoma

Following their report associating DES and clear cell adenocarcinoma, Herbst et al (1972) established a registry to study the epidemiologic, clinical, and pathologic aspects of women who developed clear cell adenocarcinoma of the cervix and/or vagina after 1940, regardless of whether maternal ingestion of the hormone could be substantiated. There was a steady rise in the number of clear cell adenocarcinomas reported per year until 1975, when a high of 32 cases were registered. Since that time, there has been a decline to a level of 5 to 15 cases per year. Exposure history reveals that approximately two thirds of the clear cell adenocarcinomas of the cervix were not preceded by maternal ingestion of DES, whereas at least two thirds of the clear cell adenocarcinomas of the vagina were associated with its use. The mean age of clear cell adenocarcinoma cases is 19 to 20 years. The youngest patient reported to the registry is 7 and the oldest is 42 years. Intrauterine exposure to DES during the first trimester of fetal life carries a fourfold increased risk of developing clear cell carcinoma compared with DES exposure after the first trimester (Herbst et al, 1986).

The clinical features of clear cell adenocarcinoma vary considerably. The vaginal lesions are usually exophytic, obvious to the naked eye, and primarily in the anterior or posterior vaginal wall (Fig. 4–9). In some patients, the lesions are entirely submucosal, and the only evidence of a neoplastic process

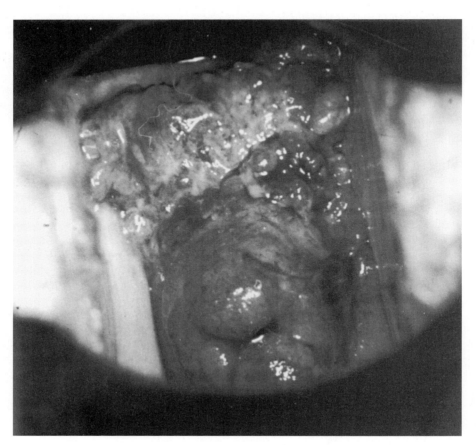

FIGURE 4–9. Clear cell adenocarcinoma of the vagina in a 20-year-old DES-exposed woman. The lesion is typically exophytic and is located in the anterior vaginal fornix. Treatment consisted of radical hysterectomy, vaginectomy, and skin graft.

is nodularity on palpation of the vagina. Occasionally, a preclinical carcinoma is first detected by cytology or colposcopy. The cervical clear cell adenocarcinomas have no unusual clinical features. Their clinical presentation is the same as that of the cervical adenocarcinomas that arise from endocervical glands (see Chapters 2 and 5).

There are three main histologic types of clear cell adenocarcinoma: tubocystic, papillary, and solid. The histologic patterns often intermix. The term *clear cell*, which has been used to identify this lesion, refers to a very characteristic cell whose cytoplasm appears clear because of the loss of glycogen during tissue processing (Fig. 4–10). The tubocystic pattern has the so-called hobnail cell, with a bulbous nucleus that protrudes beyond the apparent cytoplasmic limits of the cell (Fig. 4–11). In a 1979 study of 365 cases, Herbst et al noted that patients with the tubocystic pattern had a 5-year survival rate of 88 percent compared with 73 percent for those with papillary, solid, or combination patterns. The favorable tubocystic pattern is more common after age 19 years. This accounts for the better survival in the over-19 age group compared with the 15-year and under age group. The 5-year survival rate for patients with stage I cervical and vaginal lesions is essentially the same, that is, 90 percent. Survival with stage

III or IV disease is below 30 percent. The rate of lymph node metastasis in stage I DES-related clear cell carcinoma is 12.5 percent, but varies considerably with lesional size (<6.0 cm, 8.5 percent; >6.0, 20 percent) and depth of invasion (<6.0 mm, 8.5 percent; >6.0, 17 percent) (Herbst and Anderson, 1981).

Treatment of stages I and IIa clear cell adenocarcinoma of the cervix or vagina is primarily by radical surgery, with ovarian preservation. Pelvic lymphadenectomy is routinely performed. Partial or total vaginectomy is usually required, with reconstruction by split-thickness skin graft. Frozen section of the vaginal margins is recommended. Reviewing treatment methods and outcome from a registry of clear cell adenocarcinoma of the vagina, Senekjian et al (1987) reported that 20 percent of patients (43 of 219) with stage I neoplasms underwent local therapy. Actual survival rates at 5 and 10 years after local therapy (92 and 88 percent, respectively) were comparable with those of patients treated by standard therapy (92 and 90 percent, respectively). Based on the data from Senekjian and colleagues, we recommend that, if a patient desires future fertility and the vaginal lesion is amenable to local excision, the patient should undergo either a laparoscopic or retroperitoneal pelvic lymph

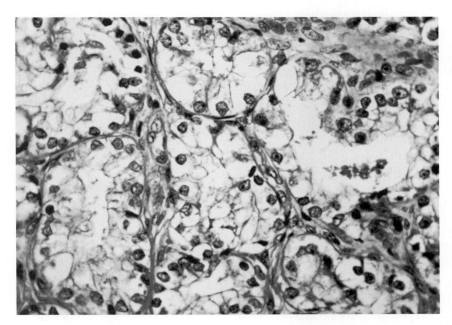

FIGURE 4–10. Photomicrograph of a clear cell carcinoma of the vagina occurring in a 14-year-old DES-exposed girl.

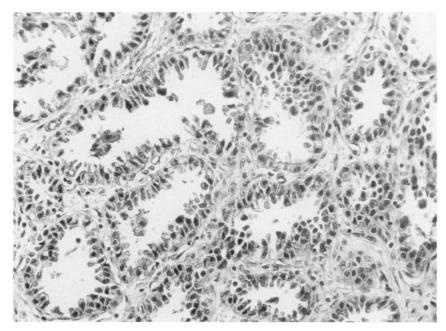

FIGURE 4–11. Tubocystic clear cell carcinoma of the vagina (×300). The hallmark of this pattern is the hobnail cell, whose nucleus protrudes into the tubular lumen.

node dissection (12 percent of stage I patients will have lymph node metastases). If there is no evidence of lymphatic spread, the lesion can be excised. Following surgery the patient is treated with local radiation. Eight of 41 patients thus treated achieved 15 pregnancies. Advanced cervical/vaginal clear cell cancer is managed in the same manner as the non–clear cell malignancies, as discussed earlier in this chapter and in Chapter 5. Late recurrences (more than 5 years after diagnosis) of clear cell adenocarcinoma have been reported (Jones et al, 1993; Fishman et al, 1996).

Squamous Cell Neoplasia

The hypothesis of Stafl and Mattingly (1974) that the DES-exposed woman has an increased risk of developing squamous cell neoplasia of the lower genital tract has been supported by data from the DESAD project (Robboy et al, 1984; Borenstein et al, 1988). If a DES-exposed woman does develop a squamous cell lesion (cervical intraepithelial neoplasia or VAIN), the area involved is often quite large, and for this reason, the treatment of the lesion is often difficult. Loop excision is recommended for cervical dysplasia in these women when preservation of fertility is important, because laser and cryosurgery are

more likely to produce significant cervical stenosis (Schmidt and Fowler, 1980; Townsend, personal communication, 1992). For extensive cervical or vaginal dysplasia, a combination of loop and laser therapy is preferable. Invasive squamous cancer of the vagina has been reported in a 34-year-old DES-exposed woman (Faber et al, 1990).

Reproductive and Other Sequelae of Diethylstilbestrol

More common sequelae to intrauterine DES exposure than cervical and vaginal neoplasia are reproductive and infertility problems secondary to anomalies of the fallopian tubes, uterus, and/or cervix (Mangan et al, 1982). In addition to the cervical anomalies (cervical hood, collar, and adenosis), the uterus is abnormal in as many as 80 percent of patients with prenatal DES exposure. Abnormalities, usually detected by hysterosalpingogram and ultrasound, include hypoplastic uterus, T-shaped endometrial cavity, and a widened lower uterine segment. The reproductive/fertility problems that are related to these changes include a higher incidence of tubal pregnancy, recurrent spontaneous abortion, and premature delivery related to incompetent cervix and premature labor (Stillman,

1982). DES-exposed women who become pregnant are more likely to undergo a surgical procedure (e.g., cervical cerclage, cesarean section) and have an increased risk of postpartum hemorrhage (Thorp et al, 1990). Herbst (1981a,b) reported that, despite these adverse outcomes, most DES-exposed women will achieve at least one successful pregnancy. A more recent report of in vitro fertilization outcome in DES-exposed women found that implantation and pregnancy outcome were impaired (Karande et al, 1990).

Males exposed in utero to DES have been reported to have an increased frequency of genital tract anomalies, including hypospadias, epididymal cysts, and testicular cancer (Gill et al, 1978). However, a large case-control study from the Mayo Clinic failed to detect an increase in genitourinary anomalies, infertility, or testicular cancer (Leary et al, 1984). In addition to the exposed progeny, the mothers who ingested DES may be at a slightly increased risk for developing breast cancer (Thomas and Chu, 1988). In a case-control cohort study, the relative risk for DES-exposed mothers was 1.4 compared with controls. The increase in breast cancer did not become statistically significant until 20 years after exposure; women who took DES should undergo screening for breast cancer on an annual basis beginning between ages 35 and 40 years. The spectrum of adverse effects of DES on both the mothers and exposed children continue to be studied. As the exposed population ages, the possibility exists that these women may experience an increased risk for the more common neoplasms of midlife, including breast, ovary, and endometrium.

REFERENCES

Ali MM, Huang DT, Goplerud DR, et al: Radiation alone for carcinoma of the vagina: variation in response related to the location of the primary tumor. Cancer 77:1934, 1996.

Al-Kurdi M, Monaghan JM: Thirty-two years experience in the management of primary tumours of the vagina. Br J Obstet Gynaecol 8:1145, 1981.

Andersen WA, Sabio H, Durso N, et al: Endodermal sinus tumor of the vagina. Cancer 56:1025, 1985.

Andrassy RJ, Hays DM, Raney RB, et al: Conservative surgical management of vaginal and vulvar pediatric rhabdomyosarcoma: a report from the Intergroup Rhabdomyosarcoma Study III. J Pediatr Surg 30:1034, 1995.

Ball HG, Berman ML: Management of primary vaginal carcinoma. Gynecol Oncol 14:154, 1982.

Benedet JL, Murphy KJ, Fairey RN, Boyes DA: Primary invasive carcinoma of the vagina. Obstet Gynecol 62:715, 1983.

Bonner JA, Perez-Tamayo C, Reid GC, et al: The management of vaginal melanoma. Cancer 62:2066, 1988.

Borenstein J, Adem E, Adler-Storthz K, Kaufman RH: Development of cervical and vaginal squamous cell neoplasia as a late consequence of in utero exposure to diethylstilbestrol. Obstet Gynecol Surv 43:15, 1988.

Bottles K, Lacey CG, Miller TR: Atypical melanocytic hyperplasia of the vagina. Gynecol Oncol 19:226, 1984.

Brown GR, Fletcher GH, Rutledge FN: Irradiation of in-situ and invasive squamous cell carcinomas of the vagina. Cancer 28:1278, 1971.

Burt RL, Prichard RW, Kim BS: Fibroepithelial polyp of the vagina. Obstet Gynecol 47:52s, 1976.

Chirayil SJ, Tobon H: Polyps of the vagina: a clinicopathologic study of 18 cases. Cancer 47:2904, 1981.

Chu AM, Beechinor R: Survival and recurrence patterns in the radiation treatment of carcinoma of the vagina. Gynecol Oncol 19:298, 1984.

Chung AF, Casey MJ, Flannery JT, et al: Malignant melanoma of the vagina: report of 19 cases. Obstet Gynecol 55:720, 1980.

Chyle V, Zagars GK, Wheeler JA, et al: Definitive radiotherapy for carcinoma of the vagina: outcome and prognostic factors. Int J Radiat Oncol Biol Phys 35:891, 1996.

Copeland LJ, Sneige N, Ordonez NG, et al: Endodermal sinus tumor of the vagina and cervix. Cancer 55:2558, 1985.

Curtin JP, Morrow CP: Melanoma of the female genital tract. In Coppleson M (ed): Gynecologic Oncology: Fundamental Principles and Clinical Practice. London, Churchill Livingstone, 1992, p 1059.

Curtin JP, Saigo P, Slucher B, et al: Soft-tissue sarcoma of the vagina and vulva: a clinicopathologic study. Obstet Gynecol 86:269, 1995.

Danielson RW: Vaginal ulcers caused by tampons. Am J Obstet Gynecol 146:547, 1983.

Davis KP, Stanhope CR, Gaton GR, et al: Invasive vaginal carcinoma: analysis of early-stage disease. Gynecol Oncol 42:131, 1991.

Deppisch LM: Cysts of the vagina. Obstet Gynecol 45:632, 1975.

Di Sant'Agnese PA, Knowles DM II: Extracardiac rhabdomyoma: a clinicopathologic study and review of the literature. Cancer 46:780, 1980.

Dodson MG, Klegerman ME, Kerman RH, et al: Behcet's syndrome. Obstet Gynecol 51:621, 1978.

Evans DMD, Paine CG: Benign cysts and tumors of developmental origin. Clin Obstet Gynecol 8:997, 1965.

Faber K, Jones M, Terraza HM: Invasive squamous cell carcinoma of the vagina in a diethylstilbestrol-exposed woman. Gynecol Oncol 37:125, 1990.

Fishman DA, William S, Small W Jr, et al: Late recurrences of vaginal clear cell adenocarcinoma. Gynecol Oncol 62:128, 1996.

Fowler WC Jr, Lawrence H, Edelman DA: Paravestibular tumor of the female genital tract. Am J Obstet Gynecol 1:109, 1981.

Gill WB, Schumacher GFB, Bibbo M: Genital and semen abnormalities in adult males two and one-half decades after in utero exposure to diethylstilbestrol. In Herbst AL (ed): Intrauterine Exposure to Diethylstilbestrol in the Human. Chicago, American College of Obstetricians and Gynecologists, 1978, p 53.

Granai CO, Walters MD, Safaii H, et al: Malignant transformation of vaginal endometriosis. Obstet Gynecol 64:592, 1984.

Hays DM, Shimada H, Raney RB Jr, et al: Clinical staging and treatment results in rhabdomyosarcoma of the female genital tract among children and adolescents. Cancer 61:1893, 1988.

Herbst AL: Diethylstilbestrol and other sex hormones during pregnancy. Obstet Gynecol 58:359, 1981a.

Herbst AL: The epidemiology of vaginal and cervical clear cell adenocarcinoma. In Herbst AL, Bern HA (eds): Developmental Effects of Diethylstilbestrol (DES) in Pregnancy. New York, Thieme-Stratton, 1981b, p 63.

Herbst AL, Anderson D: Clinical correlations and management of vaginal and cervical clear cell adenocarcinoma. In Herbst AL, Bern HA (eds): Developmental Effects of Diethylstilbestrol (DES) in Pregnancy. New York, Thieme-Stratton, 1981, p 71.

Herbst AL, Anderson S, Hubby MM, et al: Risk factors for the development of diethylstilbestrol-associated clear cell adenocarcinoma: a case-control study. Am J Obstet Gynecol 154:814, 1986.

Herbst AL, Cole P, Norusis MJ, et al: Epidemiologic aspects of factors related to survival in 384 registry cases of clear cell adenocarcinoma of the vagina and cervix. Am J Obstet Gynecol 135:876, 1979.

Herbst AL, Kurman RJ, Scully RE, Poskanzer DC: Clear cell adenocarcinoma of the genital tract in young females: registry report. N Engl J Med 187:1259, 1972.

Herbst AL, Ulfelder H, Poskanzer DC: Adenocarcinoma of the vagina: association of maternal stilbestrol therapy with tumor appearance in young women. N Engl J Med 284:878, 1971.

Hilgers RD, Malkasian GD, Soule EH: Embryonal rhabdomyosarcoma (botryoid type) of the vagina: a clinicopathologic review. Am J Obstet Gynecol 107:484, 1970.

Hintz BL, Kagan AR, Chan P, et al: Radiation tolerance of the vaginal mucosa. Int J Radiat Oncol Biol Phys 6:711, 1980.

Ingemanson CA, Alfredsson J: Recurrent fibromyoma of the vagina. Acta Obstet Gynecol Scand 49:271, 1970.

Jeffries JA, Robboy SJ, O'Brien PC, et al: Structural anomalies of the cervix and vagina in women enrolled in the Diethylstilbestrol Adenosis (DESAD) Project. Am J Obstet Gynecol 148:59, 1984.

Jones WB, Tan LK, Lewis JL Jr: Late recurrence of clear cell adenocarcinoma of the vagina and cervix: a report of three cases. Gynecol Oncol 51:266, 1993.

Karande VC, Lester RG, Muasher SJ, et al: Are implantation and pregnancy outcome impaired in diethylstilbestrol-exposed women after in vitro fertilization and embryo transfer? Fertil Steril 54:287, 1990.

Kaufman RH, Friedrich EG Jr, Gardner HL: Benign Diseases of the Vulva and Vagina, 3rd ed. Chicago, Year Book, 1989.

Kirkbride P, Fyles A, Rawlings GA, et al: Carcinoma of the vagina: experience at the Princess Margaret Hospital (1974–1989). Gynecol Oncol 56:435, 1995.

Kucera H, Vavra N: Primary carcinoma of the vagina: clinical and histopathological variables associated with survival. Gynecol Oncol 40:12, 1991.

Leary FJ, Ressaguie LJ, Kurland LT, et al: Males exposed in utero to diethylstilbestrol. JAMA 252:2984, 1984.

Lee RB, Buttoni L Jr, Dhru J, Tamimi H: Malignant melanoma of the vagina: a case report of progression from preexisting melanosis. Gynecol Oncol 19:238, 1984.

Manetta A, Gutrecht EL, Berman ML, DiSaia PJ: Primary invasive carcinoma of the vagina. Obstet Gynecol 76:639, 1990.

Manetta A, Pinto JL, Larson JE, et al: Primary invasive carcinoma of the vagina. Obstet Gynecol 72:77, 1988.

Mangan CE, Borow L, Burtnett-Rubin MM, et al: Pregnancy outcome in 98 women exposed to diethylstilbestrol in utero, their mothers and unexposed siblings. Obstet Gynecol 59:315, 1982.

Maruo T, Shibata K, Kimura A, et al: Tumor-associated antigen TA-4 in the monitoring of the effects of therapy of squamous cell carcinoma of the uterine cervix. Cancer 56:302, 1985.

Maurer HM, Moon T, Donaldson M, et al: The Intergroup Rhabdomyosarcoma Study: a preliminary report. Cancer 40:2015, 1977.

Melnick S, Cole P, Anderson D, Herbst A: Rates and risks of diethylstilbestrol-related clear-cell adenocarcinoma of the vagina and cervix: an update. N Engl J Med 316:514, 1987.

Miettinen M, Wahlstrom T, Vesterinen E, Saksela E: Vaginal polyps with pseudosarcomatous features. Cancer 51:1148, 1983.

Noller KL, Townsend DE, Kaufman RH: Genital findings, colposcopic evaluation and current management of the diethylstilbestrol-exposed female. In Herbst AL, Bern HA (eds): Developmental Effects of Diethylstilbestrol (DES) in Pregnancy. New York, Thieme-Stratton, 1981, p 81.

Noller KL, Townsend DE, Kaufman RH: Maturation of vaginal and cervical epithelium in women exposed in utero to diethylstilbestrol (DESAD Project). Am J Obstet Gynecol 146:279, 1983.

Norris JH, Taylor HB: Polyps of the vagina. Cancer 22:227, 1966.

Pearl ML, Crombleholme WR, Green JR, Bottles K: Fibroepithelial polyps of the vagina in pregnancy. Am J Perinatol 8:236, 1991.

Perez CA, Camel HM: Long-term follow-up in radiation therapy of carcinoma of the vagina. Cancer 49:1308, 1982.

Peters WA III, Kumar NB, Anderson WA, Morley GW: Primary sarcoma of the adult vagina: a clinicopathologic study. Obstet Gynecol 65:699, 1985a.

Peters WA III, Kumar NB, Morley GW: Carcinoma of the vagina. Cancer 55:892, 1985b.

Peters WA III, Kumar NB, Morley GW: Microinvasive carcinoma of the vagina: a distinct clinical entity? Am J Obstet Gynecol 153:505, 1985c.

Pradhan S, Tobon H: Vaginal cysts: a clinicopathologic study of 41 cases. Int J Gynecol Pathol 5:35, 1986.

Ragnarsson-Olding B, Johansson H, Rutqvist LE, Ringborg U: Malignant melanoma of the vulva and vagina: trends in incidence, age distribution, and long-term survival among 245 consecutive cases in Sweden 1960–1984. Cancer 71:1893, 1993.

Robboy SJ, Noller NL, O'Brien P, et al: Increased incidence of cervical and vaginal dysplasia in 3,980 diethylstilbestrol-exposed young women. JAMA 252:2979, 1984.

Rubin SC, Young J, Mikuta JJ: Squamous carcinoma of the vagina: treatment complications and long-term follow-up. Gynecol Oncol 20:346, 1985.

Schmidt G, Fowler WC Jr: Cervical stenosis following minor gynecologic procedures on DES-exposed women. Obstet Gynecol 56:333, 1980.

Senekjian ER, Frey RE, Anderson D, Herbst AL: Local therapy in stage I clear cell adenocarcinoma of the vagina. Cancer 60:1319, 1987.

Stafl A, Mattingly RF: Vaginal adenosis: a precancerous lesion? Am J Obstet Gynecol 126:666, 1974.

Stillman RJ: In utero exposure to diethylstilbestrol: adverse effects on the reproductive tract and reproductive performance and male and female offspring. Am J Obstet Gynecol 142:905, 1982.

Stock RG, Chen AS, Seski J: A 30-year experience in the management of primary carcinoma of the vagina: analysis of prognostic factors and treatment modalities. Gynecol Oncol 56:45, 1995.

Stock RG, Mychalczak B, Armstrong JG, et al: The importance of brachytherapy technique in the management of primary carcinoma of the vagina. Int J Radiat Oncol Biol Phys 24:747, 1992.

Sturgeon SR, Curtis RE, Johnson K, et al: Second primary cancers after vulvar and vaginal cancers. Am J Obstet Gynecol 174:929, 1996.

Sulak P, Barnhill D, Heller P, et al: Nonsquamous cancer of the vagina. Gynecol Oncol 29:309, 1988.

Tavasoli FA, Norris JH: Smooth muscle tumors of the vagina. Obstet Gynecol 53:689, 1979.

Thomas DB, Chu J: Nutritional and endocrine factors in reproductive organ cancers: opportunities for primary prevention. J Chronic Dis 39:1031, 1988.

Thorp JM, Fowler WC, Donehoo R, et al: Antepartum and intrapartum events in women exposed in utero to diethylstilbestrol. Obstet Gynecol 76:828, 1990.

Weinstock MA: Malignant melanoma of the vulva and vagina in the United States: patterns of incidence and population-based estimates of survival. Am J Obstet Gynecol 171:1225, 1994.

Young RH, Scully RE: Endodermal sinus tumor of the vagina: a report of nine cases and review of the literature. Gynecol Oncol 18:380, 1984.

5

Tumors of the Cervix

BENIGN TUMORS OF THE CERVIX

Endocervical Polyps

Endocervical polyps are fibroepithelial, red to pink lesions that may be associated with an abnormal Pap smear, vaginal bleeding, and/or discharge. Thus, they can mimic or mask the presence of cervical or endometrial carcinoma. Endocervical polyps, which occasionally are multiple, originate in the cervical canal, usually on a narrow stalk. They seldom exceed 1 cm in diameter, but in rare instances they are large enough to fill the vagina.

Endocervical polyps should be removed for pathologic examination and relief of the associated symptoms. The polyps themselves are rarely malignant, although the endocervical epithelium is subject to transformation to squamous metaplasia, dysplasia and, rarely, carcinoma. In postmenopausal women, an association with endometrial cancer has been reported, and endometrial evaluation is advisable for this age group.

Typically the entire stalk can be visualized. After it is cut or avulsed by twisting, the base should be cauterized to prevent recurrence. If the polyp originates high in the canal, cervical dilation under anesthesia will facilitate its removal and differentiation from an endometrial polyp.

Capillary Hemangiomas

More than 50 cases of capillary hemangioma of the cervix have been reported, often as an incidental finding. Cervical hemangiomas are thought to be of congenital origin (hamartomas). The primary significance of cervical hemangiomas is their propensity for bleeding, especially during pregnancy. Regression after each pregnancy is the usual course. Hemangiomas are recognized by their red or purple color, soft consistency, and tendency toward a polypoid configuration. Biopsy must be undertaken with circumspection because serious bleeding can occur. Most cases have been treated by hysterectomy. Successful management by CO_2 laser has been reported (Davis and Patton, 1983).

Miscellaneous Benign Conditions

Numerous other benign lesions of the cervix have been reported, including the benign mixed mesodermal tumor (see Chapter 7), papillary adenofibroma, prolapsed submucous myoma, endometriosis, and, of course, cervical leiomyoma. Of particular interest is *microglandular hyperplasia*, a small polypoid lesion that is associated with pregnancy and the use of oral contraceptives. It is important because of its histologic resemblance to certain adenocarcinomas (Young and Scully, 1989). Most cases are diagnosed during evaluation for an abnormal Pap smear (probably because of an associated immature metaplasia) or abnormal bleeding. Microglandular hyperplasia has been postulated to be an antecedent of adenocarcinoma of the cervix as related to oral contraceptive use. In a retrospective review (Jones and Silverberg, 1989), microglandular hyperplasia was not found to be a precursor of adenocarcinoma, although the power of the study was limited by small numbers. Microglandular hyperplasia is also reported to occur in women who are postmenopausal or obese, or have vaginal adenosis (Chumas et al, 1985). No treatment is required.

PREMALIGNANT AND RELATED DISORDERS

For a discussion of premalignant and related disorders of the cervix (condylomas and cervical intraepithelial neoplasia) (see Chapter 2).

SQUAMOUS CARCINOMA

Clinical Features

Symptoms

In spite of mass screening programs for cervical cancer, only 20 percent of patients with an invasive cervical cancer are asymptomatic when the diagnosis is established (Tinga et al, 1990). The two dominant symptoms of cervical carcinoma are vaginal bleeding and discharge. Perhaps 80 to 90 percent of patients experience abnormal bleeding, which can be of nearly any descriptive pattern. Contact (postcoital or postdouche) bleeding is a relatively uncommon complaint (although it is an important one), and it is not specific for cervical cancer. Most women with cervical cancer describe abnormal bleeding in terms of their menstrual periods: too long, too many, or too heavy. Among indigent populations, where endometrial cancer is relatively rare and cervical cancer is common, postmenopausal bleeding is an indication of cervical carcinoma more often than endometrial cancer. In fact, in some series, postmenopausal bleeding is the most common presenting symptom of cervical cancer (Table 5-1).

A more subtle presenting symptom of cervical malignancy is vaginal discharge, which may be watery, purulent, or mucoid in character and is not necessarily malodorous. Because vaginal discharge is a common complaint of younger women with cervical/vaginal infection, its association with malignant disease is often overlooked. A diagnosis of "severe cervicitis" based on the presence of vaginal discharge and an inflamed cervix might be reinforced by a Pap smear consistent with inflammatory atypia, a fairly common finding in the presence of overt cervical carcinoma.

Pelvic pain and urinary frequency are reported in advanced cases. Early cervical carcinoma, in contrast, is most likely to be detected by a Pap smear or by routine examination of an asymptomatic woman.

Physical Findings

The majority of patients with cervical carcinoma have a normal general physical examination. Occasionally, a patient may be found to have supraclavicular or inguinal node enlargement, a swollen leg, ascites, pleural effusion, or other evidence of metastatic disease. Vulvar, suburethral, and vaginal metastases are infrequent, but they must be specifically looked for. The vulva and vagina should also be checked for evidence of squamous dysplasia.

At speculum examination, the cervix may appear entirely normal if the cancer is very small or if it is endocervical in location. In the latter situation, which accounts for up to one third of the cases, a fairly large tumor may escape inspection. Visible disease varies greatly in appearance (Figs. 5-1 through 5-3): an ulcerative, papillary, granular, friable, bleeding, clean or necrotic appearance is common. A watery, purulent, or bloody discharge is often present. When the lesion involves the fornices or extends down the vagina, it is often appreciated best by palpation. The true extent of the cancer can be badly underestimated if the rectovaginal examination is omitted; transrectal palpation is often more revealing than vaginal palpation. Cervical carcinoma extending into the lateral parametrium or posteriorly into the uterosacral ligaments can be appreciated only on rectovaginal examination.

Parametrial involvement may be unilateral or bilateral. Fixation indicates that the tumor has extended onto the pelvic wall. Occasionally, a large, tumorous lymph node is palpable on the pelvic wall, with a free space between it and the primary carcinoma. The central lesion may achieve a size of 8 to 10 cm without fixation to the sidewall and without palpable parametrial infiltration. An enlarged uterus associated with cervical carcinoma should raise suspicion of a pyometra.

Diagnosis

Common errors that lead to a delay in the diagnosis of cervical cancer include treating

TABLE 5-1

Incidence of Symptoms Reported by 231 Consecutive Patients With Invasive Cervical Carcinoma*

Symptom	Percentage of Patients
Postmenopausal bleeding	46
Irregular menses	20
Postcoital bleeding	10
Vaginal discharge	9
Pain	6
Asymptomatic	8

*From Pardanani NS, Tischler LP, Brown WH: Carcinoma of the cervix: evaluation of treatment in a community hospital. N Y State J Med 75: 1018, 1975, with permission.

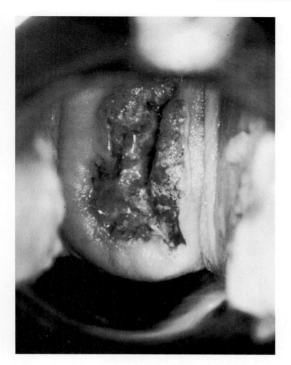

FIGURE 5–1. Ulcerating endocervical squamous carcinoma. Cone biopsy is contraindicated in cases with a target lesion.

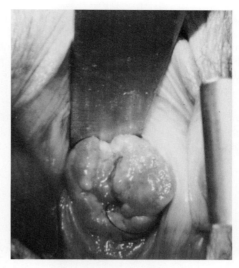

FIGURE 5–3. Clean, granular squamous carcinoma of the anterior cervical lip. An intrauterine device string is shown emerging from the cervical os.

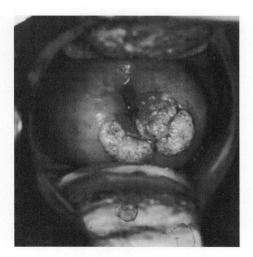

FIGURE 5–2. Small stage Ib squamous carcinoma of the ectocervix with a wart-like configuration.

patients for a menstrual disorder, complication of pregnancy, or vaginal infection without a biopsy or, in some instances, without a pelvic examination. Reliance on a Pap smear for diagnosis when a lesion is present is another frequent clinical error. The major dif-

ferential diagnoses are dysfunctional bleeding, "erosion" (columnar epithelium on the ectocervix), cervical changes secondary to oral contraceptive use (microglandular hyperplasia), "cervicitis," threatened abortion, and placenta previa. Others include cervical pregnancy, cervical fibroid, condyloma acuminatum, herpetic ulcer, chancre, and other infections such as amebiasis.

The patient who presents with symptoms and an abnormal cervix requires a directed biopsy in addition to a Pap smear. If the patient has chronic, abnormal bleeding or discharge and a normal cervix, endocervical curettage (ECC) and endometrial biopsy or ultrasound are also indicated. Biopsy specimens of an ulcerative, necrotic lesion should be taken from viable tissue at the heart of the tumor, because a biopsy at the edge often misses the cancer, causing confusion and further delay in diagnosis. Cone biopsy is contraindicated in patients with overt carcinoma; it increases the risk of hemorrhage and treatment complications. The role of the Pap smear, Lugol's staining, colposcopy, ECC, directed biopsy, and conization are discussed in Chapter 2.

Pathophysiology

Squamous carcinoma of the cervix typically arises at the active squamocolumnar junction from a pre-existing dysplastic lesion. In general, progression from mild dysplasia to invasive cancer takes several years, but wide variations exist (Fig. 5–4) (see Chapter 2).

Once the basement membrane is breached and stromal invasion occurs, the process is regarded as irreversible. Progression by local extension and lymphatic invasion predominates, but the speed with which this occurs varies considerably. The pattern of local growth may be exophytic (polypoid) if it arises from the ectocervix, or endophytic, arising in the ca-

nal. The higher the lesion is up the canal, the more likely it is to be inapparent on physical examination. The second basic growth pattern is infiltrative, which, if necrosis occurs, becomes ulcerative. The infiltrating exocervical lesion is more likely to involve the vaginal fornices and upper vagina, whereas the endocervical lesion is predisposed to invade the corpus and lateral parametrium. Combination growth patterns are common.

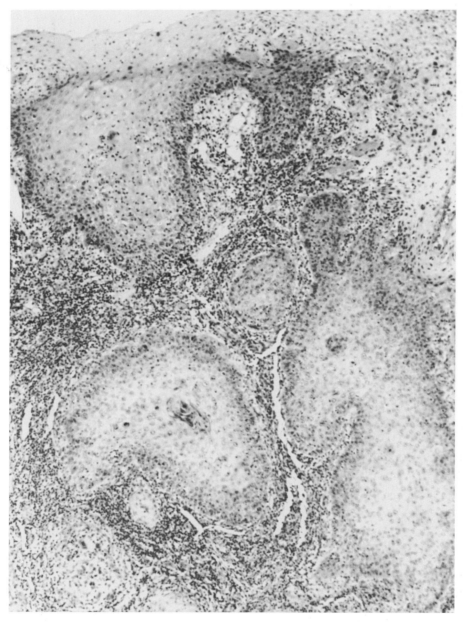

FIGURE 5–4. Squamous carcinoma arising from mildly dysplastic, keratinizing dysplasia (×80). In this case, the total depth of invasion was only 3 mm.

The cancer typically spreads by lymphatic invasion into the laterally placed cardinal ligaments before it involves the anterior or posterior parametrium. This pattern is attributable to the absence of a restraining membrane laterally (the pubovesical/cervical fascia covers the anterior and posterior cervix), and the natural drainage of the lymphatics through the lateral cervical tissue into the cardinal ligaments.

The frequency of metastasis to the parametrial and pelvic lymph nodes is governed primarily by the tumor volume. The infiltrative and endocervical growth patterns are more likely to produce lymphatic metastases than is the exophytic lesion. Nodal spread is fairly orderly and predictable. First the pelvic and parametrial nodes are involved, then the common iliac, the aortic, and, finally, the supraclavicular nodes (predominantly on the left side) via the thoracic duct. Vascular metastasis can result from lymphatic-venous anastomoses or direct invasion of the venous channels.

As the primary lesion enlarges and lymphatic involvement progresses, local invasion increases and will eventually become extensive. The bladder base, which rests on the cervix, can be invaded directly or through the vesicouterine ligaments (bladder pillars). If the ureters become surrounded by the cancerous tissue, obstruction results. Ureteral blockage also occurs at the pelvic wall, in the parametrium, and in the para-aortic region. The rectum is invaded less often because it is anatomically separated from the cervix by the posterior cul-de-sac. Extension into the uterosacral ligaments is another route of spread from which rectal involvement and spread to the lateral sacral nodes occur. Metastasis to the inguinal nodes, distal vagina, vulva, and pelvic bones results from lymphatic and vascular obstruction. Involvement of the sciatic plexus may occur in advanced cases. If the tumor penetrates through the posterior cervix or corpus, intraperitoneal spread results. Adnexal metastases are exceptional in early-stage cervical carcinoma (Brown et al, 1990; Sutton et al, 1992).

Prognostic Factors

Clinical Variables

AGE

Cervical carcinoma is relatively rare in patients under age 20, and most cases occurring before that age have been adenocarcinomas. Older women tend to have more advanced cervical cancer at the time of diagnosis, and they are also more likely to have complicating medical factors that prevent or significantly interfere with treatment. Some investigators have found that stage-corrected survival for young women (usually under 35 years) is worse than that for older women (Rutledge et al, 1992), whereas others have reported either no difference or improved survival (Carmichael et al, 1986). The largest study, and the only population-based analysis, found young age to be a significantly favorable factor (Meanwell et al, 1988).

STAGE

The more advanced a cancer is at the time of diagnosis, the poorer the prognosis; this is a universal principle of oncology. The clinical extent of cervical cancer is expressed in groups designated as stages I to IV. The International Federation of Gynecology and Obstetrics (FIGO) definitions of the four stages are presented in Table 5–2. In 1996, several key modifications were made in the classification of stage Ia and stage Ib cervical tumors. The new definition of stage Ia is similar to the 1974 Society of Gynecologic Oncologists (SGO) definition, which has been the guideline most widely accepted in the United States. The new system divides stage Ib cancers into two subgroups, reflecting the poorer prognosis associated with larger tumors (see later).

Reports from several medical centers around the world make it clear that a stepwise decrease in survival from stage I to stage IV is universally observed. However, survival rates vary considerably from institution to institution (Table 5–3). The clinical basis of cervical cancer staging has been the subject of considerable criticism related to the inevitable underreporting of lymph node metastases. Nevertheless, the staging of cervical cancer continues to be clinical, relying upon the physical examination and routine medical imaging studies. The findings obtained by surgical staging cannot be included in the reporting of data to FIGO.

Histopathologic Variables

GRADE

The numerous systems devised for the grading of squamous carcinomas of the cervix show the difficulty of correlating the micro-

T A B L E **5–2**

FIGO Stages in Carcinoma of the Cervix (Clinical)

Stage	Definition
0	Carcinoma in situ; intraepithelial carcinoma
I*	Carcinoma strictly confined to the cervix (extension to the corpus is disregarded)
Ia	Invasive cancer identified only microscopically; all gross lesions even with superficial invasion are stage Ib; invasion limited to measured stromal invasion with a maximum depth of 5.0 mm and no wider than 7.0 mm[†]
Ia1	Stromal invasion not >3.0 mm deep, not >7.0 mm wide
Ia2	Stromal invasion 3.0–5.0 mm deep, not >7.0 mm wide
Ib*	Clinical lesions confined to the cervix or preclinical lesions greater than stage Ia
Ib1	Clinical lesions not >4 cm in size
Ib2	Clinical lesions >4 cm in size
II	Carcinoma extends beyond the cervix but has not extended onto the pelvic wall; carcinoma involves the vagina but not as far as the lower third
IIa	No obvious parametrial involvement
IIb	Obvious parametrial involvement
III	The carcinoma has extended onto the pelvic wall; on rectal examination there is no cancer-free space between the tumor and the pelvic wall; the tumor involves the lower third of the vagina; all cases with a hydroureter or nonfunctioning kidney should be included unless they are due to other cause
IIIa	No extension onto the pelvic wall but involvement of the lower third of the vagina
IIIb	Extension to the pelvic wall or hydronephrosis or nonfunctioning kidney
IV	Carcinoma has extended beyond the true pelvis or has clinically involved the mucosa of the bladder or rectum
IVa	Spread of the growth to adjacent organs
IVb	Spread to distant organs

*Changed in 1995 (Creasman, 1995).
[†]The depth of invasion should not be more than 5 mm taken from the base of the epithelium, either surface or glandular, from which it originates. Vascular space involvement, either venous or lymphatic, should not alter the staging.

scopic features with outcome. The Reagan classification adopted by the World Health Organization (WHO) (Poulsen et al, 1975) has enjoyed considerable popularity. Large-cell, nonkeratinizing squamous cancers account for the majority of tumors and have the most favorable prognosis (Table 5–4). However, reported results have been inconsistent. In the series of Gauthier et al (1985), the large-cell, keratinizing type was prognostically the most favorable. Among patients with negative pelvic nodes, Inoue et al (1984) noted a substantially reduced 5-year survival rate for the small-cell type of squamous carcinoma in

comparison with the large-cell nonkeratinizing and large-cell keratinizing lesions. Nearly all grading systems take into account the presence of keratin and the size of the cells. Keratin confers some protection, whereas small cell size is prognostically disadvantageous.

LYMPH–VASCULAR SPACE INVASION

The recognition of capillary-like or lymph–vascular space invasion (LVSI) on microscopic examination is to some degree subjective, and the reported frequency as well as the prognostic significance of this finding have varied widely. It is intuitive, however, that this feature is important, and the preponderance of the data do, in fact, support this view. In the Gynecologic Oncology Group (GOG) study of operable cervical cancer (Delgado et al, 1990), LVSI was associated with a threefold increase in the incidence of lymph node involvement (25.4 vs. 8.2 percent). As expected, the disease-free survival is significantly shortened when the lymph nodes are involved with cancer (Table 5–5). It is interesting to note that several authors have distinguished between lymphatic and blood space invasion (Baltzer et al, 1982a; White et al, 1984). Baltzer et al (1982a) reported that patients with microscopic involvement of blood vessels had a significantly greater risk (70 vs. 30 percent) of dying of disease as compared to those patients with lymphatic space invasion only. More recently, studies measuring small blood vessel growth (neoangiogenesis) in the area of invasion in early-stage cervical cancer show that a higher density of microvessels is associated with an increase in pelvic lymph node metastases and a lower survival (Bremer et al, 1996). These studies are more objective and reproducible than the determination of LVSI.

DEPTH OF INVASION

It has been recognized for decades that the rate of nodal metastasis and prognosis in squamous carcinoma of the cervix are related to the depth of stromal invasion. The focus has been predominantly on lesions invading 5 mm or less, a select group categorized as microinvasive and often suited to less rigorous treatment than more deeply invasive lesions. (These superficial cancers are discussed in greater detail in the section "Stage Ia (microinvasion)" later in this chapter.) However, a rise in the incidence of pelvic node metastases with increasing depth of in-

Cervical Carcinoma: 5-Year Survival Reported From Various Treatment Centers Around the World (1982 – 1986)*

Institution	Stage I		Stage II		Stage III		Stage IV	
	N	(%)	N	(%)	N	(%)	N	(%)
Calcutta	152	(84)	238	(54)	519	(34)	0	
Cambridge	179	(80)	97	(52)	65	(23)	19	(5)
Minneapolis	126	(82)	53	(62)	17	(35)	1	(0)
Oslo	394	(81)	188	(55)	128	(25)	54	(9)
Saõ Paulo	183	(65)	260	(59)	684	(45)	86	(24)
Tokyo	134	(95)	78	(79)	54	(59)	8	(25)
Toronto	181	(72)	140	(53)	149	(34)	25	(4)
Villejuif	250	(68)	221	(55)	318	(31)	58	(12)

*From Pettersson F: Annual report on the results of treatment in gynecological cancer. Int J Gynecol Obstet 36(suppl):1, 1991. Copyright 1991, Elsevier Science, with permission.

vasion (or tumor thickness) for stage Ib cases also has been recognized. A combination of the data of Boyce et al (1984) with those of Gauthier et al (1985) shows that the rates of pelvic node metastases for lesions measuring 5 mm or less, 6 to 10 mm, 11 to 15 mm, and more than 15 mm in thickness are 2.5, 4, 26, and 44 percent, respectively. Predictably, occult parametrial extension is an adverse prognostic factor (Inoue and Okumura, 1984).

TUMOR SIZE AND VOLUME

Clinical assessment of the primary growth should have some prognostic significance because it can be used to refine the clinical stage. Understandably, interest in tumor size as a prognostic parameter has focused on the relationship of lesion size to prognosis for stage I cases. The importance of lesion size can be measured in terms of survival, recurrence, and the frequency of other established risk factors such as nodal metastasis. Based upon the independent prognostic weighting of tumor size in stage I cervical carcinoma,

Relative Frequency of Histologic Subtypes of Cervical Cancer and Survival*

Histologic Type	Total Cases	5-Year Survival (%)
Large-cell nonkeratinizing	250	61
Large-cell keratinizing	47	40
Adenocarcinoma	35	52
Small-cell	10	13

*From Randall ME, Constable WC, Hahn SS, et al: Results of the radiotherapeutic management of carcinoma of the cervix with emphasis on the influence of histologic classification. Cancer 62:48, 1988, with permission.

the FIGO staging system now discriminates between lesions that are larger or smaller than 4 cm in (presumably) transverse or anteroposterior (AP) diameter.

Delgado et al (1990), in a GOG study of 645 patients with stage Ib carcinoma of the cervix, observed a 3-year disease-free survival rate of 94.6 percent for occult cancers, an 85.5 percent disease-free survival when the primary lesion was 3.0 cm or less, and a decrease in disease-free survival to 68.4 percent when the tumor was more than 3 cm. Lesion size also correlates with the frequency of LVSI (Gauthier et al, 1985). In the study of Boyce et al (1984), only 11 percent of the lesions that involved up to two quadrants of the cervix had LVSI, compared with 55 percent of lesions that involved more than two quadrants. These results are consistent with the report of Chung et al (1981), who found a pelvic node metastasis rate of 59 percent for cervical primary cancers larger than 4 cm, whereas nodes were positive in only 20 percent of smaller tumors. Lange (1960) reported 11, 25, and 47 percent incidences of pelvic node metastasis for lesions less than 1 cm, 1 to 3 cm, and more than 3 cm, respectively. Piver and Chung (1975) noted a similar strong relationship between tumor size and lymph node metastasis.

The largest clinical diameter (transverse or AP) of a tumor and the maximum depth of invasion largely delineate the tumor volume, which, for malignancies of many organ sites, has been considered an important prognostic factor. Burghardt and Pickel (1978) examined the significance of the cross-sectional area with respect to regional node metastases in stages Ib and IIb cervical carcinomas treated by radical surgery. They reported a stepwise

TABLE 5–5

Influence of LVSI in Stage Ib Cervical Cancer on Pelvic Lymph Node Metastasis and Survival

Source	LVSI Negative			LVSI Positive		
	No.	Percent Survival	Percent Pelvic Node Metastasis	No.	Percent Survival	Percent Pelvic Node Metastasis
Boyce et al (1984)	94	97	6	41	71	32
Crissman et al (1985)	40	85	8	30	64	17
Delgado et al (1990)	360	90	8	276	78	25
Total	494	91	8	347	76	25

increase in nodal metastasis with increasing tumor cross-sectional area: less than 100 mm^2, 0 of 13 cases; 100 to 599 mm^2, 19 percent of 69 cases; 600 to 2, 100 mm^2, 46 percent of 65 cases. Using a volumetric or three-dimensional approach, Baltzer et al (1982b) found, as anticipated, that the rate of lymph node metastasis and survival correlated with increasing tumor volume (Table 5–6). None of their 66 stage Ia patients, defined as 500 mm^3 or less tumor volume (29 early stromal invasion cases) undergoing pelvic lymphadenectomy had nodal metastases (Lohe et al, 1978). Dargent et al (1985) also found nodal involvement correlated with tumor volume (<5,000 mm^3, 15 percent node metastasis; 5,000 to 10,000 mm^3, 30 percent node metastasis).

IMMUNE INCOMPETENCE

Patients with a diminished immune response have a higher risk of developing both preinvasive and invasive cancers of the cervix. Among female patients who receive immunosuppressive drugs following organ transplantation, cervical neoplasia is very common, as are other squamous neoplasias thought to be related to human papillomavirus (HPV) infection. More recently, invasive squamous cancer has been recognized as a sequel to human immunodeficiency virus (HIV) infection, but in the United States, the number of cases of invasive cervical cancer related to HIV infection probably accounts for only 1 to 2 percent of all cases. Some authors have reported that the natural history of cervical cancer in these HIV-seropositive patients is characterized by a more aggressive growth rate and higher rate of treatment failure (Maiman et al, 1993).

Multivariate Analysis

Many other histopathologic variables have been identified as potential prognostic factors in early squamous carcinoma of the cervix. Among these are the pattern of invasion (pushing versus infiltrating margins), number of mitoses, inflammatory (plasma lymphocytic) response to tumor, exocervical versus endocervical location (see the section "Stage Ib2 and IIa Tumors Larger Than 4 Centimeters ['Bulky and Barrel-Shaped' Cancers]" later in this chapter), depth of invasion relative to thickness of the cervix, stromal response, and growth pattern (papillary, solid, small cords). Clearly, many of these factors are interrelated. For example, the frequency of both LVSI and node involvement increases with the depth of invasion, a fact that may obscure other factor(s) acting as independent prognostic determinants.

Multivariate analysis attempts to identify which variables have both significant and independent impact on disease-free interval and/or survival. Several papers have statistically evaluated multiple histopathologic features of cervical carcinoma (Stendahl et al, 1983; Boyce et al, 1984; Bichel and Jakobsen, 1985; Crissman et al, 1985; Stehman et al, 1991; Kamura et al, 1992). The multifactorial analysis of Delgado et al (1990) indicated that

TABLE 5–6

Tumor Volume, Nodal Metastasis, and Survival Relationship in Cervical Squamous Carcinoma*

Tumor Volume (mm^3)	Percent with Pelvic Nodal Metastasis	5-Year Survival (% of All Cases)
<500	0	100
500–1,499	12	83
1,500–3,499	22	82
3,500–6,499	27	80
6,500–10,000	40	77

*Data from Lohe et al (1978), Zander et al (1981), Baltzer et al (1982a), and Burghardt et al (1991).

independent prognostic factors in predicting disease-free survival in early-stage cervical cancer were clinical lesion size, LVSI, and depth of invasion (both in fractional thirds and by absolute depth measured in millimeters). In more advanced cervical cancers treated with radiation therapy, factors that are significantly related to progression-free survival include para-aortic lymph node status, pelvic lymph node status, tumor size, patient age, and performance status (Stehman et al, 1991).

Regional Node Metastasis

The risk of nodal metastasis accounts largely for the prognostic importance of many clinical and histopathologic variables (stage, lesion size, depth of penetration, LVSI, grade, presence of parametrial infiltration, tumor volume) because metastases have such a powerful effect on outcome. Survival data for several series are presented in Table 5–7. In the literature, the proportion of patients with node metastases ranges from 5 to 27 percent, with a mean of 15 percent, but the reported survival of patients with negative and positive nodes is remarkably consistent, averaging 90 and 55 percent, respectively. The high survival rate reported by Delgado et al (1990) reflects the exclusion of patients with grossly positive pelvic lymph nodes, extrauterine disease, and aortic lymph node metastasis.

According to the experience of Martimbeau et al (1982), patients with bilateral pelvic node metastases have a 5-year survival (62 percent of 21 patients) similar to that of patients with unilateral pelvic node metastases (67 percent of 67 patients). Involvement of the common iliac nodes, however, carries a much worse prognosis (19 percent 5-year survival of 32 patients). The number of nodes involved also influences the outcome. Of 159 patients with stage Ib squamous carcinoma of the cervix and one to three pelvic node metastases, 72 percent survived 5 years. This compares to a 40 percent 5-year survival of 56 cases with more than three involved nodes (Morrow et al, 1980; Inoue and Morita, 1990). Positive lymph nodes less than 10 mm in diameter augur a better outcome than larger, resectable nodes. However, the number of involved nodes (>3) seems to be a more powerful determinant of outcome than the size of the nodes (Inoue and Morita, 1990; Kamura et al, 1992).

Staging and Evaluation

Clinical Staging

The FIGO staging system for cervical carcinoma is presented in Table 5–2. Its major components are as follows: stage I, the tumor is clinically confined to the cervix (and uterus); stage II, the tumor has extended to the vagina or parametrium, but not onto the pelvic wall; stage III, the tumor has extended onto the pelvic wall; and stage IV, there is tumor invasion of the bladder or rectal mucosa (IVa) or distant metastases (IVb).

Studies that are useful in the staging of cervical cancer include tissue biopsy, colposcopy, ECC, cystoscopy, chest radiograph, magnetic resonance imaging (MRI), and computed tomography (CT) scan. Within each stage, prognosis varies in relation to the tumor volume. For example, a stage Ib carcinoma 1 cm in diameter has a far better prognosis than a stage Ib carcinoma 6 cm in diameter. Similarly, a small stage IIa lesion with minimal extension onto the adjacent vaginal fornix has a more favorable prognosis than a large stage Ib lesion.

The grouping of cancer cases into stages of growth provides a means of comparing the

TABLE 5–7

Early-Stage Squamous Carcinoma of the Cervix: Reported Frequency of Pelvic Lymph Node Metastases and Survival

Source	Negative Nodes		Positive Nodes		
	No.	% Survival	No.	% Positive	% Survival
Larson et al (1987)	164	92	30	15.5	67*
Monaghan et al (1990)	392	91	102	20.6	50
Soisson et al (1990b)	271	90	49	15.3	67
Delgado et al (1990)	545	86	100	15.5	83[†]
Kamura et al (1992)	281	91	64	18.5	63

*Reported percentage of patients with recurrences.
[†]Excluded patients with grossly positive pelvic lymph nodes.

TABLE 5–8

Cervical Carcinoma: Routine Pretreatment
Evaluation

All Cases	Stage II–IV and Bulky Stage Ib Disease
Physical examination	Cystoscopy
Tissue diagnosis	Sigmoidoscopy
Chest radiograph	Liver function tests
Serum tumor marker (SCA,* CA-125, CEA)	Serum calcium
Routine laboratory tests	CT scan of abdomen and pelvis
	Stool guaiac

*Squamous carcinoma antigen.

TABLE 5–9

Cervical Carcinoma: Findings on Intravenous
Pyelography*,†

Stage	Total Cases	Ureteral Obstruction (%)
I	535	2
II	581	6.2
III	303	32.3
IV	148	48

*Data from Shingleton et al (1971), van Nagell et al (1975), and Lindell and Anderson (1987).
†Although the IVP is seldom done today when the CT scan is available, these data are applicable to the expected CT findings.

results from different institutions. Therefore, it should be done as uniformly as possible. Optimal conditions for the pelvic examination require a relaxed, cooperative patient and at least one experienced examiner. Often, staging is done jointly by the gynecologist and the radiation therapist. To improve the accuracy of the physical examination, regional or general anesthesia may be used. In this case, cystoscopy, sigmoidoscopy, and other studies are carried out at the same time. Recommendations for routine pretreatment evaluation are given in Table 5–8. The frequency of significant abnormalities on the IVP and at cystoscopy are summarized in Tables 5–9 and 5–10. The IVP today is almost invariably done in conjunction with the CT scan.

IMAGING STUDIES

As is true in other disease states, imaging studies should be obtained only when the findings may have an impact on treatment decisions. While the physical examination is the most valuable component of pretreatment staging in cervical carcinoma, two imaging studies are important: the chest radiograph and the abdominal-pelvic CT scan. Lung metastases are rarely found in early-stage disease, but routine pretreatment chest radiographs detect metastases in approximately 5 percent of patients with clinical stage III or IV cervical cancer.

The CT scan with double contrast has become an established component of the pretreatment evaluation of patients with clinical stage IIb through IVa cervical cancer. It is more accurate in the assessment of aortic than pelvic lymph nodes (Camilien et al, 1988), and unreliable for detecting parametrial infiltration. Confirmation of CT-positive

lymph nodes by fine-needle aspiration (FNA) or surgical excision is recommended because there is a 5 to 25 percent false-positive rate associated with the scan (Bandy et al, 1985; Heller et al, 1990). Routine CT scans are unlikely to provide useful clinical information on patients with early-stage cervical cancer.

MRI can provide high-resolution images of the cervix and parametrium, particularly when special coils are placed within the vicinity of the tumor. These images can provide information regarding the depth of cervical invasion as well as the status of the parametrium (Martin et al, 1994). However, the precise images created by MRI often have no impact on the clinical decision-making process or treatment. Transrectal and transvaginal probe ultrasonography have also been used to measure the primary tumor. Ultrasonography can be useful to differentiate lymphatic obstruction from venous thrombosis in the patient with leg edema.

In the past, lymphography has been widely employed to image the pelvic and aortic lymph nodes. However, this procedure is now of historical interest only. Bone scans are unproductive in the absence of clinical symptoms.

TABLE 5–10

Cervical Carcinoma: Cystoscopic Findings*

State	Total Cases	Bullous Edema (%)	Positive Biopsies (%)
I	517	0.6	—
II	562	1.7	—
III	331	8.0	19.3
IV	162	1.4	20.1

*Data from Shingleton et al (1971), Van Nagell et al (1975), and Lindell and Anderson (1987).

ENDOSCOPY

Cystoscopy and sigmoidoscopy are seldom productive in evaluating the asymptomatic patient with cervical cancer and are almost never useful in early disease (Table 5–10). The urinary cytology and stool hematest are adequate screening studies when no specific indications exist for bladder and rectosigmoid endoscopy. Shingleton et al (1971) reported that only 1 of 340 patients with stage I or II cervical carcinoma had an abnormality on barium enema because of tumor, compared to 7.5 percent of 212 patients with stage III or IV disease. Thus, colon contrast studies are warranted only for conventional indications.

LABORATORY STUDIES

As with other tests, the more advanced the disease, the more likely are laboratory studies to be abnormal. The important medical complications of cervical cancer are blood loss, renal failure, and hypercalcemia. Thus, the most common laboratory abnormalities include anemia, elevated blood urea nitrogen and serum creatinine levels, and associated electrolyte disturbances. Abnormal liver function tests should trigger an investigation to rule out metastases to that organ. Hypercalcemia usually denotes advanced disease with bone involvement, or it may represent a paraneoplastic endocrinopathy. Rarely is the bone marrow infiltrated even with widely metastatic disease.

TUMOR MARKERS

Carcinoembryonic antigen (CEA) has been used to monitor the response to therapy and follow cervical carcinoma patients. The serum level in early cases correlates with tumor volume and nodal metastasis, and patients with an elevated CEA value have a poorer prognosis regardless of the stage. A rising CEA level may precede the clinical diagnosis of recurrence (Kjorstad and Orjasaester, 1982; TeVelde et al, 1982).

Squamous carcinoma antigen (SCA) is another useful tumor marker for cervical carcinoma. Increased serum values are found in 50 to 75 percent of locally advanced cases. The serum value correlates with stage, tumor volume, and prognosis. As is true of other serum tumor markers, a rising level of SCA antigen after therapy precedes clinically detectable disease in many patients (Maruo et al, 1985; Senekjian et al, 1987; Holloway et al, 1989).

Surgical Staging

Traditionally, cervical carcinoma has been managed as if it were a disease biologically confined to the pelvis, even in its advanced stages. However, a number of investigators have challenged this concept because aortic node metastases were sometimes encountered at surgery in women with early-stage disease. Several clinical studies have now quantified the frequency of extrapelvic disease in women with cervical carcinoma (Table 5–11). The documentation of the magnitude of error in the clinical staging of cervical carcinoma provides the basis for employing pretreatment surgical staging in high-risk groups. The argument against the surgical staging of cervical carcinoma focuses on the risk/benefit trade-off. The surgery itself adds cost and morbidity and increases the normal risks of complications from radiation therapy (Moore et al, 1989).

PELVIC AND AORTIC NODE METASTASES

The rate of aortic and common iliac node metastases in stages Ib and IIa cervical carcinoma is 5 to 10 percent, although these numbers may be exaggerated by case selection (Table 5–11). Aortic node involvement is common enough in certain subgroups of stages I and IIa to warrant routine evaluation in order to avoid an underestimation of the extent of disease. For example, nearly all patients with aortic node metastasis have pelvic node metastasis, and the rate increases with the number of involved pelvic nodes (3 percent with one pelvic node, 12 percent with three or more) (Delgado et al, 1985).

The risk of aortic node involvement is also a function of tumor differentiation. Chung et al (1981) reported that 47 percent of grade 3

T A B L E **5–11**

Aortic and Pelvic Node Metastases in Cervical Carcinoma: Frequency at Staging Laparotomy*

Clinical Stage	Total Cases	Percent with Aortic Node Metastases[†]	Percent with Pelvic Node Metastases[‡]
Ib	570	6	—
IIa	174	12	—
IIb	421	21	24
III, IVa	615	31	50

*Collected data.
[†]Some authors included common iliac nodes.
[‡]Most series did not include data on pelvic nodes.

stage Ib and IIa cervical squamous carcinomas had pelvic node metastasis and 24 percent had aortic node metastasis, compared to 8 and 2 percent, respectively, for grade 1 and 2 cancers. This relationship also held for stage IIb through IVa cases (80 percent aortic node metastases for grade 3 versus 12 percent for grades 1 and 2).

The 20 to 30 percent incidence of aortic node involvement in stage IIb through IVa cervical cancer is a clear indication for assessment of these nodes on a routine basis. Imaging studies, unfortunately, are not very reliable. The most accurate and sensitive means of detecting microscopic nodal metastases is by surgery, with excision of the node-bearing tissue along the aorta.

OTHER FINDINGS

Other reasons for surgical staging exist. An additional goal is to remove bulky, presumably incurable, node metastases within the field of radiation. This technique improves the outcome for patients with large node metastases (Downey et al, 1989; Hacker, 1995). Approximately 10 percent of patients with stage II or greater disease have unsuspected intraperitoneal, adnexal, or liver metastases diagnosed at surgery. A few cases are downstaged on the basis of adnexal inflammatory disease, ovarian tumors, or endometriosis. The frequency of positive peritoneal cytology in locally advanced squamous carcinoma of the cervix may be as high as 10 percent (Kilgore et al, 1984), but this finding does not appear to affect survival (Stehman et al, 1991).

RETROPERITONEAL VERSUS
TRANSPERITONEAL STAGING

The surgical approach to evaluation of the aortic and pelvic lymph nodes has evolved from transperitoneal to retroperitoneal laparotomy to laparoscopy. The extraperitoneal method is superior to the transperitoneal method in terms of operative and radiation-related enteric morbidity (Berman et al, 1977; LaPolla et al, 1986; Weiser et al, 1989). More recently, laparoscopic lymph node sampling has been employed, either transperitoneally or retroperitoneally, further reducing morbidity. After laparoscopic staging, the patients are often ready to begin radiation therapy within 7 to 10 days of surgery, and the risk of wound infection is avoided.

EXTENDED-FIELD RADIATION

Since surgical staging is proving to be acceptable from the point of view of morbidity, it is important to look at the benefit to the patient in terms of treatment results. Evidence indicates that extended-field radiation therapy improves survival for patients with pelvic, common iliac, or aortic node metastases. Although no randomly selected, untreated control group exists for comparison, the data of Hughes et al (1980) certainly support the thesis that extended-field radiation therapy can improve survival (Fig. 5–5) over the results achieved with pelvic radiation therapy alone for patients with documented aortic node metastases (47 vs. 29 percent survival at 2 years; 32 vs. 0 percent survival at 5 years). The 5-year survival rate in the Hughes et al report is consistent with that of other investigators (Welander et al, 1981; Berman et al,

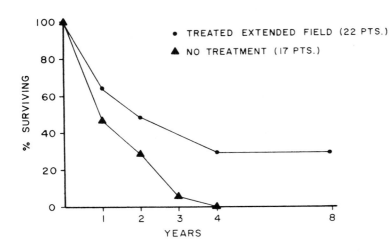

FIGURE 5–5. Carcinoma of the cervix. Life table survival of patients with aortic node metastases. (From Hughes RR, Brewington KC, Hanjani P, et al: Extended field irradiation for cervical cancer based on surgical staging. Gynecol Oncol 9:153, 1980, with permission.)

1984; Potish et al, 1985; LaPolla et al, 1986; Cunningham et al, 1991).

An alternative to surgical staging is to give "prophylactic" extended-field radiation empirically to all patients at high risk for aortic lymph node metastasis (Rotman et al, 1990). This approach, however, will not provide maximum benefit for patients with macroscopic nodal metastases, which need to be resected, and may incur more long-term morbidity than surgical staging in the large proportion of patients with negative nodes who undergo radiation therapy.

Treatment

Early-Stage Disease

STAGE Ia (MICROINVASION)

The mean age of women with microinvasive carcinoma falls within the reproductive years, intermediate between the ages of women with cervical intraepithelial neoplasia (CIN) III and women with frankly invasive cervical carcinoma. Most cases are detected by routine cytologic examination, but some patients complain of abnormal vaginal bleeding and discharge.

Definition. The diagnosis of microinvasion is based on microscopic examination of the entire dysplastic lesion from a cervical conization or hysterectomy specimen (Table 5–12). The most common criteria on which the diagnosis is based are (1) the depth of invasion, measured from the originating basement membrane; (2) the pattern of invasion; and (3) the presence or absence of LVSI.

The term *microinvasion* should refer to a degree of invasion so limited that the risk of spread beyond the cervix is negligible. In this context, microinvasive disease would be adequately treated by local, nonradical measures. Although the concept of microinvasion is almost universally recognized, it has no universally accepted definition. Consequently the term is often used loosely, leading to confusion and mismanagement.

In 1995 FIGO again revised the classification of stage Ia cervical cancer. The revision of 1985 had divided stage Ia into those tumors with "minimal stromal invasion" (stage Ia1) and those that could be measured microscopically (stage Ia2). The upper limit of invasion allowable for stage Ia2 was 5 mm in depth and 7 mm of horizontal spread. The 1995 staging system classifies those cancers with not greater than 3 mm of invasion as stage Ia1; tumors with a maximum invasion between 3 mm and 5 mm are classified as stage Ia2. Unlike the 1974 SGO definition, the current FIGO definition fails to address the issue of LVSI in microinvasive cancer (see later). Neither system limits the definition to squamous carcinomas.

Prognostic Factors. As is true for more advanced cervical cancer, the most important prognostic factors for microinvasive carcinoma of the cervix are depth of invasion, tumor volume, and LVSI (Benedet and Anderson, 1996; Maiman et al, 1988; van Nagell et al, 1983). Accurate determination of the recurrence risk and best therapy have been difficult because of the excellent outcome, the relatively small number of patients in individual series, and the variations in treatment. Confounding this problem are the differences in definitions of microinvasion that have been used over the years, as well as the various study endpoints. For example, in some series the development of vaginal dysplasia after therapy for microinvasive cervical cancer is included in the definition of "local recurrence." Despite these limitations, the recurrence and/or death rate for stage Ia1 is less than 2 percent and that for stage Ia2 is less than 5 percent. If cases with LVSI are excluded, the outcome would be almost universally favorable.

Depth of invasion has been considered to be the most accurate predictor of outcome in stage Ia squamous cancer of the cervix, but a closer look at the data indicates that LVSI is more dangerous. Although the risk of lymph node metastases is nearly zero when the tumor invades less than 3 mm (stage Ia1), we do not have data regarding the subset of cases with LVSI. The rate of pelvic node me-

TABLE **5–12**

Recommended Conditions for Diagnosis of Microinvasive Carcinoma of the Cervix Before Conservative Therapy

Diagnosis must be based on pathologic examination of a cone, trachelectomy, or hysterectomy specimen

Cone specimen must clear the lesion at the apical, ectocervical, and deep margins

Cone or cervix specimen (from the hysterectomy) should be cut into 2–3-mm slices, and three or four slides should be made from each at 100- to 200-µm steps

Invasion must not be greater than 3 mm, as measured from the basement membrane of the originating epithelium

No LVSI (capillary, blood, or lymhpatic) should be noted

Invasion of a questionable degree should be step sectioned

tastasis jumps to approximately 8 percent when the tumor invades to a depth of 3 to 5 mm, but in these patients node metastasis risk is clearly linked to LVSI. In a GOG study, 15.6 percent of stage Ia2 cases with LVSI had pelvic node involvement, compared to only 1 percent of stage Ia2 cases if there was no LVSI (Creasman, 1994). LVSI was observed in 25 percent of the study group.

Burghardt and colleagues (1991), among others, have reported that the tumor volume can be a strong predictor of outcome (Table 5–6). Determination of tumor volume is a labor-intensive analysis requiring multiple step-sections and measurement of the three greatest dimensions of the tumor. This process is rarely carried out in the routine pathologic review of a cone specimen. Nevertheless, the most recent FIGO staging definition of a stage Ia cervical cancer takes into account lateral spread, which must not exceed 7 mm. This limits stage Ia1 lesions to 150 mm^3 and Ia2 lesions to 250 mm^3. The pattern of invasion also has been used to delineate the metastatic risk of early invasive cancers. Thus, the presence of buds, tongues, or prongs of malignant epithelium breaking through the basement membrane (early stomal invasion; ESI) (Fig. 5–6), although frequently multifocal, is considered to be favorable, whereas

confluent growth characterized by anastomosing cords of invasive cancer (Fig. 5–7) is associated with a greater risk for lymph node metastases and local recurrence. Grade of tumor is rarely included in the analysis of microinvasive cancer of the cervix. However, both Kolstad (1989) and Burghardt et al (1991) reported that patients who recur after treatment for microinvasive cervical carcinoma often have either anaplastic or poorly differentiated tumors.

Treatment Plan. The overall treatment plan for microinvasive squamous cancer (stage Ia) is presented in Figure 5–8. Surgery is the standard modality, but radiation therapy is suitable for those patients considered to be medically inoperable.

Stage Ia1. This subset of stage Ia cervical carcinomas identifies those patients who can be treated with a high degree of safety in a manner similar to the treatment of CIN III. There is reasonably strong evidence in the literature corroborating the clinical perception that such management is safe. Three series report only two recurrences among 178 patients with 3 mm or less of invasion treated by simple hysterectomy (Yajima and Noda, 1979; Larsson et al, 1983; Van Nagell et al, 1983). Unfortunately, the site of recurrence

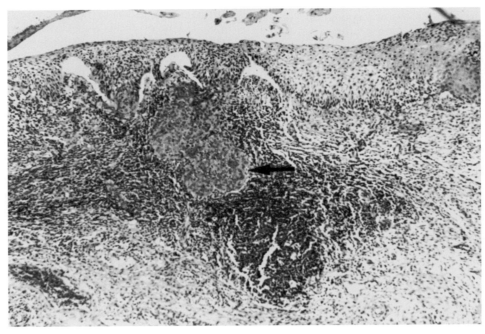

FIGURE 5–6. Bud of squamous carcinoma invading the stroma to a depth of about 0.5 mm (arrow). Note the intense inflammatory cell infiltrate. This lesion is often termed *early stromal invasion* and in selected cases can be treated by conization (see text).

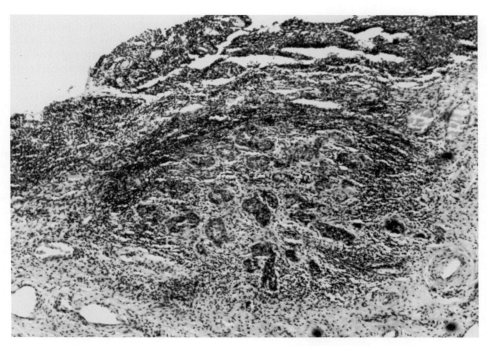

FIGURE 5–7. Squamous microcarcinoma of the cervix (< 2 mm invasion) in a 32-year-old mother of five (×80). This was one of several areas of microscopic invasion. LVSI was present in other sections. The patient had annual Pap smears since her first pregnancy.

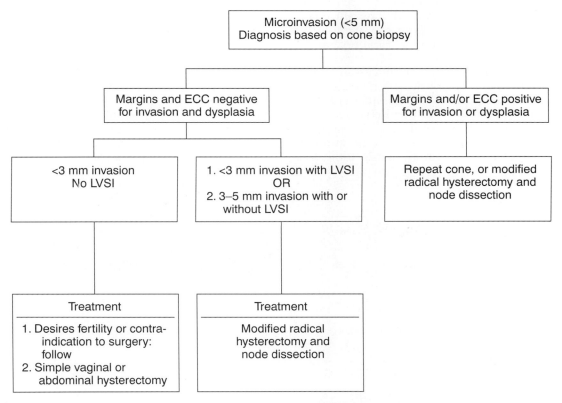

FIGURE 5–8. Algorithm for managing microinvasive carcinoma of the cervix. ECC = endocervical curettage (above cone).

was not specified in these series, but clearly simple hysterectomy is eminently successful, and probably more radical than necessary. Only 20 to 25 of the 178 cases, however, had LVSI, so further data are needed before more conservative treatment can be recommended in this circumstance.

The excellent results with simple hysterectomy suggest that, at least in selected cases, stage Ia1 cervical carcinoma can be treated safely by cone biopsy. This is supported by the findings of Boyes and Worth (1981), who reported that 7.1 percent of carcinoma in situ (CIS) lesions diagnosed by routine cone biopsy have microscopic foci of invasion (5.7 percent ESI) when the cone specimens are step sectioned. Since cone biopsy has long been accepted as adequate therapy for cervical CIS, these data demonstrate that very limited invasive cancer of the cervix has been almost universally and very successfully, albeit unwittingly, treated by conization for decades. Burghardt and colleagues (1991) reported that, after a minimum of 5 years' follow-up, only 1 of 93 patients with stage Ia1 (ESI) cervical cancer treated by conization alone recurred; this patient refused annual examination and presented 12 years after treatment with an advanced cervical cancer.

The collected data from the literature on cases with 1 to 3 mm of invasion reveals that only 2 of 77 patients treated by cone biopsy recurred. One of the recurrent cases had LVSI and the other had a positive cone margin (Table 5–13). The status of the cone tip provides important evidence for the safety of the cone procedure as definitive therapy. Roman et al (1997) reported that 23 percent of 43 apparent stage Ia1 cases with dysplasia at the cone

tip had residual invasive disease in the uterus (10 percent had more than 3 mm of invasion and LVSI). If there was dysplasia at the cone tip and also in the ECC specimen, 35 percent had residual invasion.

Based on the foregoing data, it can be recommended that the patient with stage Ia1 cervical carcinoma with a negative cone tip and no LVSI, who does not desire future fertility, be managed by simple hysterectomy. Because these patients are at greater risk for subsequent lower genital tract squamous neoplasia than the general population, they should be examined on a yearly basis, including vaginal cytology.

Conversely, if the patient has not completed childbearing, a cervical cone biopsy is the recommended definitive therapy provided that the criteria for diagnosis previously delineated are met—that is, there is no LVSI and the cone margins are negative (Fig. 5–8; Table 5–12). It is also desirable that the patient is capable of complying with a long-term follow-up program.

Kolstad (1989) reported that 40 percent of women with microinvasive carcinoma of the cervix are younger than age 40; therefore, it can be expected that many of these women will inquire about fertility-sparing treatment. The recommendation of cone biopsy is made on the presumption that this conservative procedure does carry some increased risk of tumor recurrence compared to hysterectomy, but the risk is counterbalanced by preserving the patient's reproductive integrity. From the numerous reports in the literature, it appears that most recurrences following cone biopsy will be local, indicating the importance of close follow-up. Pap smears, with emphasis

TABLE **5–13**

Treatment of Stage Ia1 (1- to 3-mm Invasion) Squamous Carcinoma of the Cervix by Conization*

Source	Total N	Invasive Recurrences N	LVSI	DOD[†]	Years Follow-up
Coppleson (1992)	17	1[‡]	1	1	>5
Morgan et al (1993)	29	0	0	0	2–9
Morris et al (1993)	13	0	0	0	2.2 (median)
Andersen et al (1993)	11[§]	0	0	0	3 (mean)
Östör et al (1994)	7	1[‖]	0	0	1–22
Total	77	2	1	1	—

*Excludes ESI (i.e., invasion <1 mm).
[†]DOD = dead of disease.
[‡]LVSI, refused hysterectomy. Pelvic wall recurrence at 3.2 years.
[§]No LVSI, negative margins.
[‖]Positive cone margin. Carcinoma of cervix at 8 years.

on adequate endocervical sampling, should be obtained every 3 months for the first 2 years after conization, and then every 6 months. Any subsequent abnormal Pap smear should be evaluated by colposcopy and directed biopsy; a second conization of the cervix would be done for the conventional indications.

Stage Ia2. Given the increased probability of lymphatic spread for squamous cancers of the cervix invading more than 3 mm, the risk of failure is deemed to be too great to routinely employ simple hysterectomy or cone biopsy alone as the only treatment for stage Ia2 cervical carcinoma. A modified radical hysterectomy (medial parametrium, 1-cm vaginal cuff) with pelvic lymphadenectomy is the recommended therapy, whether or not LVSI is identified on the cone biopsy. Nevertheless, as the GOG data indicate, in the absence of LVSI, the rate of node metastases is low enough to consider omitting the lymphadenectomy when special circumstances warrant it. If the patient is strongly motivated to retain the potential for pregnancy, an alternative to radical hysterectomy is the radical vaginal trachelectomy with uterine retention advocated by Dargent et al (1994) (see the section "Radical Vaginal Procedures" later in this chapter).

Microinvasive Adenocarcinoma. Diagnosis and treatment of microinvasive adenocarcinoma is discussed later in this chapter.

STAGES Ib1 AND IIa LESS THAN
4 CENTIMETERS

Surgery and radiation therapy are complementary as well as competitive methods of treatment in cervical cancer. Optimal results cannot be obtained for all patients with either modality alone. Surgery has the advantages of shorter treatment time, removal of the primary lesion, and less injury to normal tissue. It is the inability of the surgical approach to treat cancer in adjacent organs and at the same time preserve these organs that confines its applicability to early lesions. A recommended treatment scheme is presented in Figure 5–9.

Radiation therapy is capable of treating cervical carcinoma that has invaded adjacent tissues without loss of bladder, rectal, or coital function, although some impairment is not unusual. Furthermore, radiation therapy is applicable to tumors involving the pelvic wall, which are unresectable. Therefore, primary surgical therapy is usually reserved for the stage I and IIa lesions that are not expected to have irregular or extensive lymphatic invasion.

When either treatment is applicable, the quality of the therapy is more important than the treatment mode. This is apparent from the similar results of randomized series with evaluable intramural controls (Roddick and Greenelaw, 1971; Newton, 1975; Morley and Seski, 1976), and the Patterns of Care Studies (Coia et al, 1990). The complementary roles of surgery and radiation, which are discussed in detail in subsequent sections and in Chapter 17, include the following: (1) preoperative intracavitary therapy to shrink and inactivate the primary lesion; (2) preoperative whole-pelvis radiation therapy for resectable lesions with a cancerous rectovaginal or vesicovaginal fistula; (3) postoperative pelvic radiation for adverse features such as pelvic node metastasis or an inadequate surgical margin; (4) postsurgical pelvic recurrence; (5) adjuvant hysterectomy for cases with a large central lesion; (6) surgical treatment for radiation central failures; and (7) surgical treatment for radiation complications (fistula, bowel obstruction, proctosigmoiditis).

Radical Hysterectomy. Collective experience and randomized trials have established that radical hysterectomy with pelvic lymphadenectomy is as curative as radiation therapy in the management of stage I and IIa cervical squamous carcinoma. Radiation therapy can be used in nearly every case, however, whereas surgically treated cases must be selected, particularly with respect to medical contraindications to surgery. In practice, most patients with early disease are acceptable for operation.

Some physicians choose to reserve surgery for the young patient on the premise that ovarian preservation and better sexual function of the nonirradiated tissues justify the operative approach. However, this implies unfairly that coital function is not an important concern for older women. Postmenopausal women, in the absence of other medical problems, tolerate radical hysterectomy well and are likely to have less blood loss than younger women. Furthermore, older women often have local conditions (conical vagina) that are unfavorable to good radiation therapy. In contrast, young women usually have commodious vaginal fornices, which permit optimal radium application with large ovoids that minimize the radiation dose to the va-

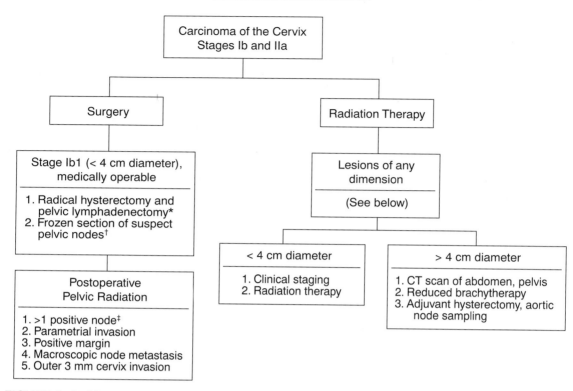

FIGURE 5–9. Management algorithm for stages Ib and IIa carcinoma of the cervix. *If the patient is peri- or postmenopausal, the adnexa should also be removed. †If the suspect node(s) is (are) positive, the common iliac and aortic nodes should be sampled because the risk of aortic node involvement is about 10 percent (Delgado et al, 1985). If these are positive, extended-field irradiation is indicated. ‡The radiation therapy for patients with pelvic node metastases should include the common iliac nodes if the latter have not been removed. Consideration should be given to chemotherapy in addition to radiation therapy.

gina. A thin habitus is desirable because it makes surgery easier, but radiation injury is more common in the thin patient than in the average-sized or obese patient. Some specific indications for primary surgical therapy are a history of diverticular, tubo-ovarian, or appendiceal abscess; fear of radiation therapy; prior radiation therapy; pelvic kidney; and the need for rapid treatment, as in the psychotic patient.

Just as the dose (or radicalism) of radiation therapy needs to be individualized, so does cancer surgery. The basic design of the radical hysterectomy is the removal of the uterus, along with adjacent portions of the vagina, cardinal ligaments, rectal pillars, uterosacral ligaments, and bladder pillars (Fig. 5–10). There are, however, numerous variations in the extent of excision available to the surgeon, which can be adapted to the extent of disease under treatment.

Some gynecologic oncologists prefer to limit operative treatment to patients with le-

sions of relatively small size (e.g., ≤4 cm) or to exophytic lesions, which are less likely to have lymphatic spread than the endocervical variety. Preoperative intracavitary therapy is used in some treatment centers to reduce the lesion size, reduce the extent of the requisite paracervical resection, and minimize the risk of operative cancer spread (Draca et al, 1980; Timmer et al, 1980).

Radical hysterectomy is almost always combined with pelvic node dissection. If the pelvic nodes are involved, the common iliac nodes should be removed in keeping with the principle that the lymph nodes should be treated one station proximal to the highest level of involvement. Removal of the ovaries is determined on the basis of patient age and other factors. Squamous carcinoma rarely metastasizes to the adnexa before it becomes locally advanced. In the premenopausal woman, transposition of the ovaries out of the pelvis at the time of radical hysterectomy in anticipation of postoperative radiation ther-

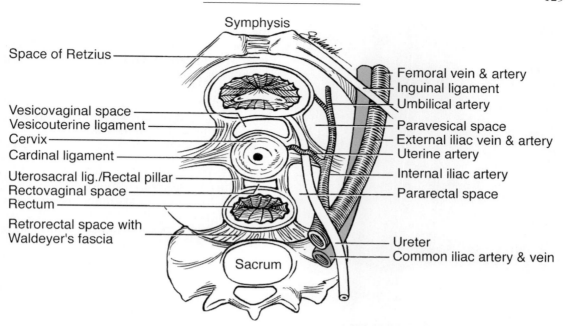

Symphysis

Space of Retzius

Vesicovaginal space
Vesicouterine ligament
Cervix
Cardinal ligament

Uterosacral lig./Rectal pillar
Rectovaginal space
Rectum

Retrorectal space with
Waldeyer's fascia

Femoral vein & artery
Inguinal ligament
Umbilical artery

Paravesical space
External iliac vein & artery
Uterine artery

Internal iliac artery

Pararectal space

Ureter
Common iliac artery & vein

Sacrum

FIGURE 5–10. The spaces and ligaments of the female pelvis. The primary route of extension for cervical carcinoma is via the cardinal ligament. The pubovesicle cervical fascia encompasses the bladder. (From Morrow P, Curtin J, de la Osa E (eds): Gynecologic Cancer Surgery. New York, Churchill Livingstone, 1996, p 111, with permission.)

apy can preserve ovarian function, but it is not recommended as a routine procedure because of the associated complications (Chambers et al, 1990; Anderson et al, 1992).

Radical Vaginal Procedures. Although radical vaginal hysterectomy was frequently done in the first half of this century, the abdominal approach to radical hysterectomy has been the standard for several decades because the nodes can be readily dissected through the same incision, and nowadays abdominal surgery is quite safe. Vaginal hysterectomy has often been reserved for the occasional patient with cervical carcinoma complicating uterovaginal prolapse (Fig. 5–11). In the past 5 years, there has been a resurgent interest in the vaginal approach because the pelvic nodes can be removed via laparoscopy, potentially reducing the overall morbidity, decreasing the length of hospitalization, and providing for a quicker recovery. Good results have been reported with this technique, but there are obvious disadvantages: it is necessary for the surgeon to learn an entirely new operative technique (laparoscopy) and a new, somewhat difficult operation (radical vaginal hysterectomy). In some reports the anticipated advantages have been outweighed by an unacceptably high rate of serious complications.

Another operation that combines a vaginal approach with laparoscopic lymph node dissection is the radical trachelectomy (Dargent et al, 1994). This procedure involves a transvaginal radical dissection of the paracervical tissue followed by amputation of the cervix just distal to the isthmus. To avoid cervical incompetence, a cerclage must be done at the same time. Radical trachelectomy with uterine preservation is applicable to the patient with a small ectocervical carcinoma that exceeds the limits of invasion considered safe for treatment by cone biopsy alone.

Surgical Adverse Effects. Ureteral complications, either fistula or stricture, were the most important adverse effects of radical hysterectomy in the past. Improvements in the technique of extricating the ureter from the parametrium and vesicouterine ligament (tunnel), with emphasis on atraumatic handling of the ureter, have reduced the injury rate from 10 to 15 percent to 1 to 3 percent (Table 5–14).

Although the potential complications of radical hysterectomy other than ureteral injury are extensive, only two occur with sufficient frequency and severity to warrant special mention. The first is bladder dysfunction, which affects nearly every patient to some degree. This results from interrupting the au-

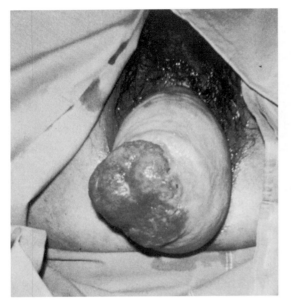

FIGURE 5–11. Cervical carcinoma. Complete procidentia with a stage IIa lesion in a 60-year-old woman. Treatment was radical vaginal hysterectomy with repair of pelvic floor defects. Retroperitoneal pelvic node dissection was carried out concurrently through a midline abdominal incision.

tonomic nerves that supply the bladder. These traverse the cardinal ligament and rectal and bladder pillars. Recovery of bladder function occurs within a few days to 3 weeks or longer depending upon the radicalness of the procedure, the preoperative status of the bladder, and individual variability. It is important to prevent overdistention of the bladder during its recovery phase. Preoperative assessment of the bladder does not help to identify the patient who will have postoperative voiding problems (Carenza et al, 1982). The operation affects the function of both

the detrussor muscle and the sphincter. Kerr-Wilson et al (1986) reported that beta-sympathomimetic agents might be beneficial. Except with the most radical operation, however, satisfactory bladder function eventually returns in nearly every case. Rectal dysfunction manifested by constipation is also common after radical hysterectomy.

Another important adverse effect of radical hysterectomy, which is also the most common life-threatening complication, is deep vein thrombosis with pulmonary embolus. Mortality from pulmonary embolus can be reduced approximately 10-fold from the expected 0.5 to 1 percent range by the use of low-dose, subcutaneous heparin or intermittent pneumatic calf compression (Collins et al, 1988). Bleeding complications may be increased by the heparin treatment, however, so the calf compression technique is preferable (National Institutes of Health Consensus Conference, 1985).

STAGE Ib2 AND IIa TUMORS LARGER THAN 4 CENTIMETERS ("BULKY AND BARREL-SHAPED" CANCERS)

One of the basic tenets of cancer therapy is that tumor volume correlates with prognosis: the more cancer cells that are present, stage for stage, at the onset of treatment, the poorer the outcome. For this reason the 1995 FIGO staging system has subdivided stage Ib cancers into those less than 4 cm in diameter (stage Ib1) and those that are larger (stage Ib2). The poorer prognosis of the larger cancers is reflected in both a higher incidence of regional lymph node metastases and a higher incidence of local (central), pelvic wall, and distant failures. This principle of cancer biology also explains the adverse effect of tumor volume on radiation therapy, because the

TABLE 5–14

Reported Incidence of Major Complications After Radical Hysterectomy for Cervical Cancer

Source	Total Cases	Vesical/ Ureteral Fistula (%)	Total Major Complications (%)	Deaths (%)
Artman et al (1987)	275	(1.5)	(22.8)	(0.7)
Lee et al (1989)	954	(2.4)	(12.3)	(0.4)
Monaghan et al (1990)	498	(1.2)	—*	(0.6)
Photopulos and Zwaag (1991)	102	(3.0)	(14.0)	(0.0)
Ayhan et al (1991)	270	(2.9)	(14.1)	(0.3)
Total	2099	(2.1)	(14.5)	(0.5)

*Not reported.

population of hypoxic, radioresistant tumor cells expands as the tumor volume increases, and therefore the probability of treatment failure increases. Since adenocarcinomas are more likely than squamous cancers to have a bulky, endocervical growth pattern, it is understandable that the glandular forms have been viewed as more radioresistant. For these reasons, large-volume (>4 to 6 cm transverse diameter) stage Ib and IIa cervical carcinomas, which account for 5 to 10 percent of cases, have been treated in many clinics by radiation therapy followed in 4 to 6 weeks by a simple, extrafascial hysterectomy to remove any residual radioresistant cancer (Rutledge et al, 1976; Gallion et al, 1985; Russell et al, 1987; Moyses et al, 1996).

The patients with bulky stage I and II cancers undergoing adjuvant hysterectomy have fewer central failures compared with a similar group of patients treated by radiation alone. For example, Durrance et al (1969) reported that only 1 of 39 such patients having adjuvant simple hysterectomy experienced central failure, versus 14 of 94 patients treated by radiation alone. Gallion et al (1985) analyzed their experience with carcinomas of the cervix greater than 5 cm in diameter. Pelvic recurrence was reduced from 19 to 2 percent in the simple hysterectomy group. There was also a drop in the extrapelvic recurrence rate from 16 to 7 percent. These authors subsequently defined the bulky lesion as greater than 3 cm in diameter (Maruyama et al, 1989). Although the central failure rate is lower in patients having good regression after the external beam therapy (50 percent failure with <25 percent regression, vs. 15 percent failure with >50 percent regression; Mendenhall et al, 1984), adjuvant hysterectomy may still be beneficial in the good-response group. Despite these data, none of the studies has demonstrated a clear survival advantage for the hysterectomy group.

Because the addition of even simple hysterectomy to full-dose external beam and intracavitary radiation incurs a substantial risk of serious complications, the standard practice for combining the two treatment modalities has been to reduce the brachytherapy component about 25 percent. Even with this modification, the rate of vault necrosis and related complications following simple hysterectomy may be 5 to 10 percent (O'Quinn et al, 1980; Gallion et al, 1985; Russell et al, 1987).

Some authors have reported that radical surgery is an equally effective method of treating bulky stage Ib cervical cancer, although the rate of complications is increased relative to the treatment of smaller lesions (Bloss et al, 1992; Alvarez et al, 1993). Twenty-five to 50 percent of these patients will receive postoperative adjunctive radiation and/or chemotherapy on the basis of surgico-pathologic features putting them at high risk for pelvic and distant recurrence (lymph node metastases, parametrial invasion, close or positive resection margin, outer one third cervical invasion). Few patients in these reports had lesions larger than 6 cm. The severe complication rate is approximately 18 percent, the pelvic failure rate is 25 percent or greater, and nearly half the patients have required blood transfusion. It is not obvious, therefore, that this is the optimal mode of treatment.

The radiation oncologists argue that appropriately aggressive radiation therapy alone (see Chapter 17) is just as effective in achieving control of the primary cancer as combination therapy. Unfortunately, the quality of radiation therapy in cervical cancer cannot be taken for granted according to the outcome of the Patterns of Care Study, which reviewed treatment trends of cervical cancer in the United States (Montana et al, 1995). From the results of this survey, it is apparent that many patients fail to receive adequate radiation therapy, most often related to inadequate utilization of brachytherapy.

Neoadjuvant chemotherapy for patients with stage Ib2 and large IIa cervical cancers is also being investigated. This treatment involves the administration of chemotherapy for one to three cycles followed by radical hysterectomy. In a GOG-sponsored pilot study, Eddy and colleagues (1995) achieved a high response rate with three cycles of cisplatin and vincristine given at 3-day intervals (total treatment time 3 weeks). The GOG is currently comparing standard therapy to neoadjuvant therapy in a prospective randomized clinical trial.

Our recommendation is to employ the adjuvant simple hysterectomy in all medically operable patients with a Ib or IIa cervical carcinoma more than 4 cm in diameter, with squamous or glandular histology (Fig. 5–9). If there is clinical evidence of residual carcinoma, a modified radical hysterectomy is performed. In the case of a thickened parametrium, resection of the involved cardinal ligament is carried out. These more extensive procedures will increase the risk of local complications, however. At the same time, the common iliac and distal aortic lymph nodes should be dissected in view of the 5 to 15 percent incidence of metastases in patients with bulky, albeit "early-stage" disease. Radiation therapy alone is a reasonable alternative provided that there is a good tumor response to external beam therapy, and adequate brachytherapy can be applied.

POSTOPERATIVE ADJUVANT THERAPY

Whole-pelvis radiation therapy is commonly recommended for patients who are at high risk for recurrence following radical hysterectomy. The risk factors have been previously discussed but include pelvic lymph node metastases, a tumor greater than 4 cm in diameter, a positive surgical margin, tumor invasion into the outer one third of the cervix, and other histologic findings. A life-sparing benefit of postoperative radiation has been difficult to demonstrate (Table 5–15); however, local recurrence rates are decreased. If the pelvic nodes contain metastases, the treatment field should be extended to include the common iliac nodes, and if these are involved the patient should receive aortic node irradiation. Radiation treatment of early-stage cervical carcinoma with positive aortic nodes carries a 5-year survival rate approaching 50 percent (Cunningham et al, 1991).

The rate of severe complications from pelvic radiation therapy following radical pelvic surgery is undoubtedly increased, with a reported incidence up to 15 percent (Alvarez et al, 1993; Monk et al, 1994). Combination chemotherapy alone or in conjunction with radiation therapy has been studied, without, however, conclusive evidence of efficacy (Tattersal et al, 1992; Curtin et al, 1996; Morton and Thomas, 1996; Wertheim et al, 1985).

For this reason we prefer to give postoperative radiation alone when patients have risk factors for local recurrence. If there is an increased risk for extrapelvic recurrence (e.g., pelvic nodal metastases), cisplatin-based chemotherapy and pelvic radiation should be considered.

RADIATION THERAPY FOR EARLY-STAGE DISEASE

When radiation is the primary treatment modality for bulky stage Ib cervical carcinoma, the retroperitoneal nodes should be evaluated by CT scan. If aortic node metastases are present and documented by FNA, a left scalene node dissection is recommended to rule out more widely disseminated disease (Vasilev and Schlaerth, 1990) before extended-field radiation therapy is administered. Large pelvic nodes should be removed prior to radiation therapy, but, if the patient is going to have an adjuvant hysterectomy, removal of these nodes can be done after the radiation has been completed. If the nodes are unresectable, intraoperative radiation therapy may be beneficial (Petrilli et al, 1986).

Stages IIb Through IV

Treatment of locally advanced cervical carcinoma is managed by radiation therapy because it works reasonably well and because adequate surgery would be impossible or would require removal of the bladder and/or rectum. In the best series, the 5-year survival for stage IIb patients is around 65 percent and that for stage III patients 45 percent (Perez et al, 1986; Hopkins and Morley, 1991; Stehman and Thomas, 1994). However, 15 to 35 percent of these cases have pelvic failures, at least half of which are central. Thus the dom-

TABLE **5–15**

Postoperative Radiation Therapy for Pelvic Node Metastasis After Radical Hysterectomy

Source	Postoperative Radiotherapy		No Postoperative Radiotherapy	
	N	(%) DFS*	N	(%) DFS
Morrow et al (1980)	30	(60)	144	(59)
Fuller et al (1982)	32	(56)	39	(61)
Larson et al (1987)	20	(75)	10	(50)
Kinney et al (1989)	60	(63)	60	(65)
Berman et al (1990)	68	(51)	26	(35)
Soisson et al (1990b)	40	(70)	7	(100)
Stock et al (1995)	108	(65)	35	(41)

*DFS = disease-free survival.

inant therapeutic problem is large central disease with the attendant substantial risk of pelvic and aortic node metastasis.

To improve the therapeutic ratio, surgical staging has been utilized to assess the extent of disease more accurately (Tables 5–11 and 5–16), and radiation sensitizers have been tested to improve the control of a bulky, hypoxic primary tumor mass (Hreshchyshyn et al, 1979; Thomas et al, 1984; Stehman et al, 1988; Runowicz et al, 1989; Heaton et al, 1990). (The staging laparotomy data were presented earlier in this chapter.) The cumulative results of these and other trials are considered to be inconclusive; however, the rationale of employing a radiation sensitizer is so compelling that we believe it is reasonable to recommend the routine use of a sensitizer with standard radiation therapy in the management of locally advanced cervical carcinoma. The most recent studies of combination therapy indicates that the agents of choice are cisplatin and/or 5-fluorouracil (5-FU) (see Chapter 17).

Figure 5–12 provides an algorithm for managing cervical carcinoma stages IIb through IVa. The basic principles are as follows: (1) exclude the presence of distant metastases; (2) remove CT-detectable aortic/common iliac node metastases prior to radiation therapy; (3) surgically evaluate the CT-negative aortic nodes; (4) give a radiation sensitizer in conjunction with radiation therapy to treat bulky disease; (5) treat aortic nodes with radiation therapy when there are no other extrapelvic metastases; (6) extend the radiation therapy field one nodal group above the highest level of known metastases; (7) use surgical salvage therapy for patients with postradiation persistent central disease; and (8) give palliative therapy to patients with extensive aortic node or more distal metastases. For the latter cases, single-fraction (1,000 rad) pelvic radiation should be considered along with systemic chemotherapy for palliation (Chafe et al, 1984).

The value of extended-field radiation in cervical carcinoma was discussed in the section "Surgical Staging" earlier in this chapter. The reported 5-year survival for these patients varies from 20 to 50 percent, depending on the stage of disease, and size and number of the nodal metastases.

Some patients with locally advanced cervical cancer have a vesicovaginal or rectovaginal fistula at presentation (Hopkins and Morley, 1991). If the tumor is resectable, treatment is instituted by administering 4,000 to 5,000 cGy of whole-pelvis radiation therapy followed by surgery. Diverting colostomy will almost always be necessary prior to radiation therapy in the presence of a rectovaginal fistula, but it is better to postpone the urinary diversion until after the radiation therapy unless the radiation port must include the perineum, in which case urinary diversion should be done before radiation therapy is instituted.

Patients presenting with distant metastases (stage IVb) are rarely suited for comprehensive radiation therapy. Local control can usually be achieved by single-pulse or rapid-course radiation therapy to the pelvis followed by systemic chemotherapy. If a urinary or fecal fistula is present, diversion is indicated for palliation unless the life expectancy is very short. Occasionally, an untreated patient will present with uremia and bilateral ureteral obstruction. Percutaneous diversion of one or both kidneys is warranted to permit full evaluation followed by the application of potentially curative therapy (Taylor and Andersen, 1981). When distant metastases or sciatic neuropathy is present, the poor prognosis should be discussed with the patient before diversion. Table 5–17 lists some of the many factors that might necessitate treatment modification for cervical carcinoma.

Special Treatment Categories

Pregnancy

(This topic is discussed in detail in Chapter 14.) The effect of pregnancy on the outcome of cervical cancer is difficult to assess with any reliability because of numerous confounding factors: (1) stage of disease; (2) histologic type; (3) patient age and parity; (4) time of diagnosis relative to pregnancy (i.e.,

TABLE 5–16

Findings at Staging Surgery That Might Influence Treatment Planning and Outcome

Para-aortic node metastasis
Common iliac node metastasis
Resectable, large nodal metastasis
Adnexal disease
  Inflammatory
  Neoplastic
Other pelvic disease
  Endometriosis
  Diverticulitis
Intraperitoneal carcinoma
Adhesions of bowel to uterus
Positive peritoneal cytology

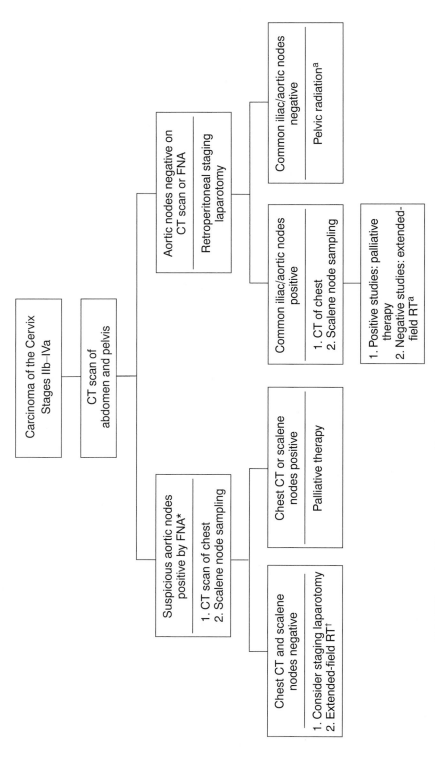

FIGURE 5–12. Management algorithm for stages IIb through IVa cervical carcinoma. RT = radiation therapy. *Aortic field RT is not given to patients with extrapelvic metastases other than aortic node. †Patients with bulky disease are treated with RT plus chemotherapy such as 5-FU or cisplatin.

TABLE 5–17

Patient Factors That Might Necessitate Treatment Modification in Cervical Carcinoma

Pregnancy	Adnexal mass
Pyometra	Fibroids
Prolapse of uterus	Cervical stump
Psychosis	Diverticulitis
Pelvic kidney	Stenotic vagina
Pelvic inflammatory disease	Advanced age
Prior radiation therapy	Bilateral ureteral obstruction
Prior surgery	Bleeding
Prior chemotherapy	Inanition

gestational age, prepartum or postpartum status, and, if postpartum, the time since the antecedent pregnancy); (5) delivery through a cancerous cervix; and (6) relative rarity of cervical cancer associated with pregnancy.

The findings from studies of cervical cancer and pregnancy can be summarized as follows:

1. The overall survival is not altered when risk factors are taken into account.
2. The proportion of stage I cases diagnosed during pregnancy is greater than expected, but the difference diminishes with the advancement of the gestational age.
3. There is a notable increase in the proportion of stage III and IV cases when cervical cancer is diagnosed within 1 year postpartum, and the prognosis is worsened for these women.
4. When the diagnosis of early-stage cervical carcinoma is made in the second half of pregnancy, delay of therapy until after fetal viability appears to be a safe policy.
5. Women with invasive cervical carcinoma should be delivered at term by classical cesarean section.

Cervical Stump

The proportion of cervical cancer cases arising in a cervical stump, compared to those in an intact uterus, has varied from 1 to 10 percent among series in the literature (Prempree et al, 1979; Miller et al, 1984). This reflects the practice regarding the indications for hysterectomy in general and supracervical (subtotal) hysterectomy in particular. The latter is most often performed today in difficult cases of pelvic inflammatory disease, cesarean hysterectomy, endometriosis, and obesity. If one excludes from analysis cases in which subtotal hysterectomy was done in the presence

of cervical carcinoma, the prognosis for patients with stump cancer is not substantially different from that of patients with cervical cancer in the intact uterus. This is somewhat surprising considering that intracavitary therapy is necessarily suboptimal, although partial compensation can be achieved by using interstitial radiation.

The difficulty of irradiating stump cancer substantially increased the complication rate in the 250-case series of Miller et al (1984). This is undoubtedly due to the emphasis on external radiation in the face of a greater likelihood for adhesions involving the bladder, sigmoid colon, and small bowel to the cervical slump, either from the surgery or from the pelvic disease that necessitated the supracervical hysterectomy.

Stage I and IIa stump carcinoma can be, and perhaps ought to be, managed surgically in patients with a history of pelvic inflammatory disease. The operation is often somewhat more difficult with the corpus absent, especially if adhesions and retroperitoneal fibrosis are present (Mikuta et al, 1977), but the overall results are similar to those for carcinoma of the cervix in the intact uterus.

Inappropriate Simple Hysterectomy

The surprise finding of invasive carcinoma of the cervix in the surgical specimen after a simple vaginal or abdominal hysterectomy usually follows incomplete evaluation of a young woman undergoing hysterectomy for a more pedestrian pathologic condition. The most common preoperative diagnosis in such cases is cervical dysplasia (Heller et al, 1986; Hopkins et al, 1990). Less frequently, patients have a condition that obscures the need for routine evaluation of the cervix, such as abnormal bleeding attributed to fibroids, perimenopausal dysfunctional bleeding, complications of pregnancy, or tubo-ovarian abscess (Roman et al, 1993b). In some instances, a false-negative Pap smear report has been obtained, or the clinician has accepted a reading of "inadequate" or "inflammatory" as a normal result.

The term *cut through* is widely used for this situation, but it should be reserved for those cases in which tumor is present at a surgical margin. In a compilation of contemporary series, true "cut throughs" accounted for only a small percentage of the cases of simple hysterectomy performed in the presence of invasive cervical cancer (Roman et al,

TABLE **5-18**

Survival After Simple Hysterectomy for Invasive
Cervical Cancer*

Histology/Extent of Disease	Total Cases	% 5-Year Survival
Squamous	64	80
Adenocarcinoma	28	41
Squamous, ≤50% invasion[†]	21	96
Squamous, >50% invasion	29	75

*From Hopkins MP, Peters WA III, Andersen W, Morley GW: Invasive cervical cancer treated initially by standard hysterectomy. Gynecol Oncol 36:7, 1990, with permission.
[†]Cervical tissue thickness measured from surface of endocervical canal.

1993a). The prognosis following simple hysterectomy correlates well with the extent of disease and the histologic subtype (Table 5–18). It is clear that survival is excellent, provided that gross tumor is not transected. The worst results follow subtotal hysterectomy. In the series of Durrance (1969), only 2 of 11 such patients were well at 3 years' follow-up.

With the exception of the patient whose lesion qualifies for conservative therapy based on microscopic findings, as discussed in the section "Stage Ia (Microinvasion)" earlier in this chapter, postoperative radiation therapy is indicated. Selected cases are suitable for definitive surgical therapy by radical proximal vaginectomy plus pelvic node dissection (Orr et al, 1986).

The overall good results of therapy after simple hysterectomy for frankly invasive cervical carcinoma must not be used to justify poor medical practice. These results are a testimony to the efficacy of adjuvant radiation therapy in a group of patients with often subclinical and, therefore, favorable disease. Not only is the risk of complications increased (Perkins et al, 1984; Hopkins et al, 1990), but the absence of the uterus precludes optimal intracavitary therapy. Furthermore, some patients having a true "cut through" operation will be doomed by intraperitoneal spread of carcinoma.

Endometrial Extension

Another measure of the risk for treatment failure related to an extensive endocervical lesion is involvement of the endometrium and uterine corpus. The presence of endometrial stromal invasion by the cervical carcinoma in uterine curettings is associated with a higher incidence of local, pelvic wall, and distant failure (Perez et al, 1981; Prempree et al,

1982). When the endometrium is involved, then, by early-stage cervical carcinoma, it is reasonable to perform an adjuvant simple hysterectomy with selective aortic node dissection after radiation therapy, in the manner of the bulky stage Ib and IIa cervical carcinomas.

Pyometra

During therapy, weekly examination permits a dynamic assessment of tumor response and vaginal capacity. Probing the uterine cavity with a sound identifies the endocervical canal, provides a measure of uterine cavity length, and also will uncover an occult pyometra. Patients with a pyometra should be followed with serial sonographic studies, have the uterine cavity sounded frequently, or have a drain inserted. Undrained, the pyometra may become a source of sepsis either during external beam therapy or at the time of intracavitary treatment. Untreated pyometra is a contraindication to placement of intracavitary brachytherapy.

Bleeding

Particularly in more advanced cases, serious bleeding from the cervical cancer may be present at the time of diagnosis. This is typically controlled within a day or two after initiation of external beam therapy. Depending upon the severity of the bleeding, the normal daily fractions can be increased up to a total of 300 to 500 cGy for 2 or 3 days. Transvaginal orthovoltage treatments have been used effectively for this purpose and have the added advantage that not all of the radiation needs to be included in the dose calculations, because most of the transvaginal dose is absorbed by the tumor. Control of the bleeding before initiation of radiation therapy can often be achieved by Monsel's solution (ferrous subsulfate) and vaginal packing. During this time, the patient is kept at bed rest, and the packing is changed every day or two. Soaking the pack in an antibiotic solution will prevent the proliferation of bacteria. The occasional patient in whom these measures fail to control the bleeding almost invariably has extensive tumor invasion of the corpus. Arteriographic embolization of the hypogastric or uterine arteries is quite successful in these cases (Harima et al, 1989; Pisco et al, 1989), although this procedure may further increase tumor hypoxia and, therefore, increase radiation resistance. If embolization is not an option, hypogastric artery ligation is indicated.

Follow-up and Recurrence

Post-treatment Surveillance

Because the majority of recurrences appear within the first 2 years after treatment, follow-up visits should be most frequent during that time. Similarly, the interval can be significantly increased after the 5-year mark because of the very low incidence of late recurrence (Table 5–19). At each visit, the patient should be asked about pain, vaginal bleeding, bowel and bladder function and have her weight recorded. Although weight loss is not a specific indicator of recurrent tumor, the maintenance of weight or weight gain in the absence of fluid accumulation provides some assurance that the patient is doing well; conversely, progressive weight loss should alert the physician to the possibility of recurrence or radiation bowel disease. Patients frequently attribute cancer-related weight loss to voluntary diet control.

Physical examination includes careful assessment of the supraclavicular and inguinal nodes for metastases, as well as the abdominal and pelvic examination. Special attention should be paid to the lower vagina and suburethral areas. The vaginal tube and cervix should be inspected and palpated. Adequate pelvic evaluation always includes bimanual rectovaginal palpation, noting the amount and character of parametrial induration (smooth or nodular) and the presence of any masses. A Pap smear is obtained at each visit. Periodic CT scan and chest radiograph are occasionally helpful in monitoring patients for recurrence after treatment for locally advanced disease. Serial serum CEA and SCA measurements are also useful in monitoring for recurrence. Unfortunately, curative treatment is seldom possible except in the case of central recurrence, a site that is most amenable to detection by the simple measures of clinical examination and screening cytology (Soisson et al, 1990a).

Recurrence

Squamous carcinoma of the cervix is one of the more curable malignancies, with an overall cure rate above 50 percent. Persistent or recurrent carcinoma of the cervix—the consequence of treatment failure—is, by comparison, a far more malignant disease, with a 1-year survival rate of 15 percent and a 5-year survival rate of less than 5 percent. In early-stage disease, the likelihood of salvage after recurrence is determined in part by the extent of disease at initial diagnosis. Fuller et al (1989), for example, reported that 18 percent of patients with stage Ib and IIa cervical carcinoma and negative lymph nodes were salvaged after recurrence, whereas no patient with recurrence after initially having positive lymph nodes was successfully treated. Treatment failure after primary surgical therapy is most suited to management by irradiation. However, most treatment failures occur in the more advanced stages of disease; consequently, the discussion here concerns recurrence or persistence after irradiation.

About 50 percent of recurrences are diagnosed during the first year of follow-up, 75 percent by 2 years, and 95 percent within 5 years. Hence, the 5-year survival rate is a reasonably accurate measure of cure. The most important recurrences to identify are those that are potentially curable. Practically speaking, the curable recurrences are local (central), that is, those of the cervix, vagina, bladder, rectum, and parametrium. Such recurrences are detected by routine physical examination or by evaluation of the patient with an abnormal Pap smear, rising serum tumor antigen level, vaginal bleeding or discharge, or hematuria. Occasionally, the first evidence of central recurrence is ureteral obstruction. The diagnosis of central recurrence is most often made by punch biopsy of a cervical or vaginal lesion, but parametrial needle biopsy, cone biopsy, or rectal or bladder biopsy may be required.

TREATMENT OF CENTRAL RECURRENCE

Surgery

Radical Hysterectomy. Occasionally the patient with a small, centrally persistent or recurrent carcinoma of the cervix after radiation

---

T A B L E **5–19**

Post-therapy Surveillance Program for Cervical Carcinoma

Examination every 3–4 months for 2 years, then every 6 months

Pap smear at every visit

Serum tumor market (SCA, CEA, and/or CA-125)

For advanced disease, periodic CT scan of the abdomen and pelvis, chest radiograph annually therapy can be treated by radical hysterectomy rather than pelvic exteneration. The literature indicates, however, that pelvic recurrence and severe complications in this situation are common. In four series totaling 132 patients, more than 50 percent experienced severe complications, including an operative death rate of 3.8 percent (Rubin et al, 1987; Terada and Morley, 1987; Coleman et al, 1994; Rutledge et al, 1994). Almost all patients with lymph node metastases at the time of salvage radical hysterectomy died of recurrent disease. The best results were achieved in those patients who had a lesion clinically confined to the cervix, 2 cm or less in diameter, and originally stage I. This group had a 95 percent survival rate and a very low rate of severe complications. Radical hysterectomy as treatment for cervical cancer after radiation therapy should be limited to this favorable group of patients unless there are circumstances justifying high-risk, suboptimal treatment.

Pelvic Exenteration. The importance of recognizing central failure after therapy for cervical carcinoma lies in the fact that 25 to 50 percent of the cases without metastases on work-up can be cured by pelvic exenteration (Table 5–20). After radiation therapy, with or without central necrosis and infection, palpatory findings become extremely unreliable. Consequently, the true extent of the pelvic recurrence is often not ascertainable without surgical exploration. A resectability rate of about 50 percent can be expected unless the only patients explored are those with small, mobile central lesions (Morley et al, 1989; Miller et al, 1993). Persistent cancer in the field of radiation is more likely to follow irregular routes of spread, which makes less radical surgery based on normal spread patterns inadequate. En bloc excision of the uterus, cervix, vagina, bladder, and rectum is, indeed, radical therapy, and it is justified only when it offers some hope for cure or sustained remission. After a thorough evaluation to exclude extrapelvic or nonresectable pelvic disease (CT scan of abdomen and pelvis), the patient is counseled regarding the extent of surgery.

At operation, careful exploration is performed for any evidence of intraperitoneal or extrapelvic spread. Aortic node sampling is routine. Pelvic node dissection is carried out after developing the pararectal and paravesical spaces and determining that the tumor is free of the side wall and the levators. Inability to obtain free margins is a general contraindication to exenteration. Close margins may benefit from intraoperative radiation therapy (Petrelli et al, 1986; Höckel and Knapstein, 1992; Selzer et al, 1995). If the pelvic nodes contain metastatic tumor, continuing the operation may be inadvisable because few patients can be cured. Anterior exenteration has a lower morbidity than total exenteration and is appropriate for cases of an anterior recurrence. Depending on the vaginal extension of cancer, the distal resection is at the level of the levators or the vaginal introitus.

The major technical advances in this operation have to do with reconstruction after the exenteration. The continent urostomy (Penalver et al, 1989), low rectal stapled anastomosis (Hatch et al, 1988), omental carpet, and rectus abdominis myocutaneous flap to reconstruct the vagina, close the perineal wound, and help fill the pelvic basin (Cain et al, 1989; Pursell et al, 1990) have markedly reduced morbidity and facilitated rehabilitation. Even with these improvements, however, the exenteration patient requires expert postoperative medical and emotional support. The latter must come from the surgeon, nursing personnel, family, and spouse.

T A B L E **5–20**

Five-Year Survival After Pelvic Exenteration

Source	Total Cases	Total Cervix Cancers	Operative Mortality (%)	5-Year Survival (%)
Rutledge et al (1977)	296	195	13.5	34
Averette et al (1984)	92	69	24	37
Kraybill et al (1988)	99	57	14	45
Morley et al (1989)	100	66	2	61
Shingleton et al (1989)	143	143	6.3	50
Lawhead et al (1989)	65	51	9.2	23
Stanhope et al (1990)	72	72	4	46
Robertson et al (1994)	83	54	4	41

Factors that predict outcome after exenteration include size of tumor, interval from initial treatment to recurrence, pelvic sidewall fixation, and margin status of the operative specimen. Operative mortality associated with pelvic exenteration today should be less than 5 percent. This risk depends to a great extent on the skill and experience of the surgeon, but patient selection is also a very important determinant. Survival statistics are, of course, strongly influenced by patient selection. If only the most favorable cases are chosen for surgery, better results will be obtained because unexplored cases are not taken into account when survival rates are assessed.

Radiation Therapy for Central Recurrence. Radiation therapy for cervical carcinoma that is recurrent in the pelvis after definitive radiation is advisable only in very select cases because normal tissues never recover fully from the radiation changes. Therefore, re-irradiation is associated with high morbidity and limited palliation. The best candidates for re-irradiation are those patients with unresectable, small volume disease that has recurred relatively late (>2 years). Technically resectable patients treated by re-irradiation for medical reasons appear to have a substantial chance for cure if the recurrence occurs 5 or more years after initial therapy.

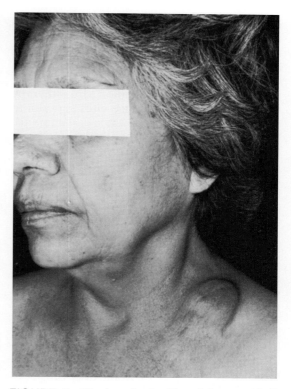

FIGURE 5–13. A patient with a left supraclavicular mass appearing 4 years after primary treatment for stage I squamous cell carcinoma of the cervix.

OTHER RECURRENCES

Metastasis or recurrence at distant sites (Fig. 5–13) is rarely curable, but patients often benefit from resection, radiation, chemotherapy, or various combinations of these modalities. Bone and brain metastases are especially suited to palliative radiation therapy. An isolated lung metastasis should be resected in the absence of other sites of involvement (Mountain et al, 1984). Because patients with cervical cancer, especially smokers, are at increased risk for second primary cancers not only of the vagina but also the lung and the head and neck region, prompt evaluation is indicated for any symptoms related to these areas.

CHEMOTHERAPY

Recurrent and disseminated squamous carcinoma of the cervix unsuitable for surgery or radiation therapy is a frequent management problem. Several features common to this group of patients can restrict the possibility of a beneficial drug response. First, nearly all of these patients have had pelvic field irradia-

tion, and many of the recurrences are in the pelvis. The bone marrow reserve in these patients is diminished, thereby reducing tolerance to cytotoxic therapy, and the inevitable loss of pelvic tissue vascularity prevents achieving optimal tissue levels of drug. Furthermore, it is not uncommon for these patients to have necrotic, infected tumor involving the upper vagina, cervix, and adjacent portions of the bladder and rectum. If sepsis and fistulas do not occur spontaneously, they may follow administration of chemotherapy. The frequent association of pelvic recurrence and bilateral ureteral obstruction limits the potential for treatment of this disease with drugs that are nephrotoxic or excreted by the kidney.

Nevertheless, the most important reason that chemotherapy has not proven to be particularly useful in cervical carcinoma is not the limitations imposed by the residual effects of radiation therapy or of renal obstruction, but the generally low level of activity displayed by the many agents tested against it. Cisplatin is one of the most active drugs, but it has a response rate of only 20 percent when used as a single agent (Bonomi et al, 1989). Cisplatin is quite nephrotoxic, however, and it use is contraindicated in the patient with bilateral ureteral obstruction or significant renal dysfunction. Combination drug therapy has proven to give response rates superior to single-agent therapy in cervical carcinoma, but the reported rates vary widely and survival is typically not improved. Because of the increased toxicity and lack of sustained remissions, the higher response rates achieved by combination therapy do not necessarily justify their use (Bonomi et al, 1989). Unless the patient is enrolled in a prospective clinical trial, cisplatin appears to be the single agent of choice. The best candidates for chemotherapy are those with an excellent performance status and recurrence outside the field of irradiation not amenable to resection or radiation therapy (see Chapter 16).

VERRUCOUS CARCINOMA

More than 30 cases of bona fide verrucous carcinoma of the cervix have been reported (de Jesus et al, 1990), but many reports inappropriately include cases of papillary, well-differentiated squamous carcinoma and giant condyloma acuminatum. Verrucous carcinoma occurs most commonly in the oral cavity, but also arises from the skin and larynx, as well as the male and female genitalia. It is characteristically an indolent, locally invasive, warty, fungating growth that rarely metastasizes. Radiation therapy is considered ineffective and may change the lesion into a rapidly growing, metastasizing, poorly differentiated squamous carcinoma (Ferlito and Recher, 1980). Histologically, anaplasia is lacking and the tumor fronds are benign in appearance, except for the presence of stromal invasion by the bulbous rete pegs.

Radical hysterectomy without node dissection is indicated for stage I and II lesions. Recurrent verrucous carcinoma may be associated with node metastasis and has a much poorer prognosis (Raheja et al, 1983).

ADENOCARCINOMA

Adenocarcinoma in Situ

The incidence of adenocarcinoma in situ (ACIS) is uncertain because it appears to be significantly underdiagnosed and underre-

ported. Some authors have found ACIS once in every 50 to 250 cone biopsies (Qizilbash, 1975; Boon et al, 1981; Ostor et al, 1984). The average age at diagnosis is 37 years, which is about 10 years less than that of women with invasive adenocarcinoma (Hopkins et al, 1988a). Progression to microinvasive and frankly invasive adenocarcinoma has been described (Poyner et al, 1995).

The differential diagnosis of ACIS includes a very well-differentiated adenocarcinoma (adenoma malignum or minimal deviation adenocarcinoma), endometriosis, mesonephric duct remnants, microglandular hyperplasia associated with oral contraceptive (OC) use, and the Arias-Stella changes of pregnancy.

ACIS and microinvasive adenocarcinoma may be identified by exfoliative cytology. The diagnosis of ACIS, however, in the great majority of cases results from the investigation of an abnormal Pap smear suspicious for squamous dysplasia, with which it has been associated in two thirds of the reported cases. Office biopsy and endocervical scraping have often failed to detect ACIS during the workup of an abnormal Pap smear, but, when ACIS is detected on office biopsy or by cytology (Fig. 5–14), conization is always required. ACIS frequently (10 percent of cases) displays a diffuse or multifocal involvement of the endocervical glands, and is sometimes associated with invasive adenocarcinoma. Hopkins et al (1988a), in a literature review of the subject, reported that 12 of 44 patients undergoing cone biopsy prior to hysterectomy had a positive cone margin. Eight of the 12 patients (67 percent) had residual ACIS compared to only 2 of 32 patients (6 percent) with negative cone margins. The findings of Muntz et al (1992) are essentially the same. These data are somewhat different, however, than those of Poyner et al (1995), who reported that 4 of 10 patients (40 percent) with ACIS and negative cone margins had residual ACIS on repeat cone or hysterectomy, versus 3 of 8 (38 percent) with a positive cone margin. Each group also had one case of invasive adenocarcinoma. The ECC was positive for ACIS in 43 percent of patients undergoing conization. Furthermore, these authors noted that 7 of 15 patients managed conservatively developed a recurrent glandular lesion, two cases of which were invasive.

The treatment of choice for ACIS is cone biopsy to exclude invasive carcinoma, followed by simple hysterectomy in the absence of invasion. For the patient who wishes to

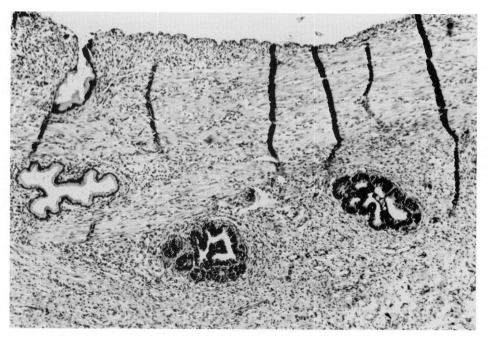

FIGURE 5–14. Section from cone biopsy of the cervix showing normal cervical glands on the left and two foci of adenocarcinoma in situ (×80). The patient had atypical glands underlying an area of squamous dysplasia on colposcopically directed punch biopsy.

retain her reproductive potential, conization only is a reasonable if somewhat risky management. When the cone margins or ECC above the cone shows ACIS, the patient should undergo repeat conization, trachelectomy, or hysterectomy to remove the residual disease.

Microinvasive Adenocarcinoma

The FIGO staging system has been based entirely on data derived from squamous microinvasive cancers. As discussed in subsequent paragraphs, frankly invasive adenocarcinoma of the cervix may be associated with a poorer prognosis than squamous carcinoma, depending upon the histologic variety and grade. Therefore, it is not intuitively obvious that microinvasive glandular lesions will behave in the same manner as the squamous cancers. Furthermore, it is more difficult to accurately determine the presence and depth of invasion of adenomatous lesions because of the variable gland configurations and the normal location of the glands within the cervical stroma. The shortage of data specific to microinvasive adenocarcinomas has led many clinicians in the past to treat all "microinvasive" adenocarcinomas by radical hys-

terectomy and pelvic node dissection. This approach is no longer tenable.

Several publications indicate that the definition of microinvasive cancer employed for squamous lesions can be applied to adenocarcinomas as well (Nakajima 1983; Berek et al, 1985; Teshima et al, 1985; Jones et al, 1993; Kaspar et al, 1993; Östör et al, 1997; Kaku et al, 1997b). Adenocarcinomas comprise 13 percent of all microinvasive lesions (<5 mm) and 8 percent of all cervical adenocarcinomas (Jones et al, 1993). Correlating the data from the previously referenced studies, 60 percent of cases had invasion of less than 3 mm. Considering tumor volume, only one of 110 cases of less than 500 mm^3 experienced tumor relapse. Volume, however, was at best marginally superior to depth of stromal invasion for predicting treatment failure. Recurrence was observed in 1 of 75 patients with less than 3 mm of invasion and 3 of 43 patients with 3 to 5 mm of invasion. One of the three recurrent tumors had a volume less than 500 mm^3. Only 1 of the 119 patients undergoing pelvic lymphadenectomy had nodal metastases. That single patient, whose lesion was more than 500 mm^3 in volume, was among approximately 90 patients with less than 3 mm of invasion. There were no reported cases with parametrial invasion, adnexal metastases, or simultaneous primary ovarian malignancy. While interpreting these data, however, it must be kept in mind that most patients were treated by radical hysterectomy with node dissection. Only 10 lesions with less than 3 mm of invasion were managed by cone biopsy alone. Eight percent of all microinvasive glandular lesions were reported to have LVSI, 6 percent were grade 3, and 27 percent were multifocal.

On the basis of these data, it seems reasonable to recommend simple hysterectomy alone as adequate therapy, at least for G1 and G2 lesions when the depth of invasion is less than 3 mm (or the volume is <500 mm^3) and there is no LVSI. The safety of cone biopsy as treatment is uncertain, especially in view of the propensity for glandular lesions to be multifocal. Nevertheless, conization of the cervix should be considered in carefully selected cases. For deeper or thicker stage Ia adenocarcinomas of the cervix and all stage Ia cases with LVSI (Fig. 5–15), our recommended treatment is a modified radical hysterectomy and pelvic node dissection.

Frankly Invasive Adenocarcinoma

Pure adenocarcinomas of the cervix account for 5 to 20 percent of all cervical carcinomas in various series, and evidence indicates that the incidence has been increasing during the past 20 to 30 years. Shingleton et al (1981), for example, reported that the proportion of cervical cancers of glandular histology increased from 7 percent in 1974 to 18 percent in 1980. In a population-based study of cervical adenocarcinoma in women under age 35, Peters et al (1986) calculated an average annual rate of increase of 8 percent from 1972 to 1982 in Los Angeles County. There is concern that this change may reflect an association with prolonged use of OCs. This thesis is supported by the case-control study of the Los Angeles County Cancer Surveillance Program, in which it was found that the use of OCs was associated with a twofold increase in risk of cervical adenocarcinoma. The risk ratio was increased to fourfold baseline when OCs were used for more than 12 years (Ursin et al, 1994). Adenocarcinoma of the cervix is commonly associated with CIN, which sug-

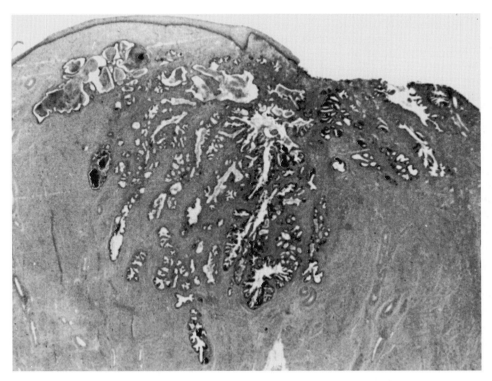

FIGURE 5–15. Adenocarcinoma of the cervix (stage Ia2). Maximum depth of invasion was 5 mm. Diagnosis was made on a hysterectomy specimen from a 48-year-old woman with abnormal bleeding. Preoperative ECC and cervical biopsy were read as negative. Upon review, both specimens contained cytologically atypical glands.

gests that in some patients these neoplastic changes may share a common etiology. Preliminary analysis of adenocarcinomas of the cervix by DNA hybridization suggest that HPV-18, a relatively uncommon HPV subtype associated with squamous cervical cancer, is found in 25 to 50 percent of these tumors (Wilczynski et al, 1988).

Epidemiologically, adenocarcinoma of the cervix shares risk factors associated with both endometrial adenocarcinoma and cervical squamous carcinoma. That is, in some reports, the obese, diabetic, nulliparous, and hypertensive woman has a two- to threefold greater risk than the average woman of developing glandular cervical carcinoma (Korhonen, 1980; Milsom and Friberg, 1983). Other authors (Hopkins et al, 1988b) found that the rates of obesity, hypertension, diabetes, smoking, and OC use were similar in patients with adenocarcinoma of the cervix as compared to the general population.

The WHO has adopted a classification of cervical adenocarcinoma that includes five subtypes: endocervical, endometrioid, clear cell, adenoid cystic, and adenosquamous. Their relative frequencies are given in Table 5–21. A special category of adenocarcinoma is the colloid (mucinous or gelatinous) carcinoma, which is characterized clinically by an increased mucous discharge and microscopically by a large volume of extracellular mucin. Similar patterns are seen in colon and breast cancer. Lesions of secondary or metastatic origin should be mentioned for completeness. Most metastases to the cervix are from the endometrium. Other sites to be considered are the ovary, bowel, and breast.

The anatomic origin of cervical adenocarcinoma is traditionally considered to be more endocervical or higher in the canal than squamous lesions, explaining the tendency for adenocarcinomas to be more extensive locally at the time of diagnosis. However, Teshima

and colleagues (1985) reported that only 3 of 22 early invasive adenocarcinomas were separate from the transformation zone. It is likely, therefore, that the lesions originate in the transformation zone but spread preferentially into the canal.

In early-stage disease, the results of colposcopy and gross examination are often negative, and the false-negative Pap smear rate is increased relative to squamous cancers (Korhonen, 1978). Because vaginal bleeding (postmenopausal, postcoital, intermenstrual) is the presenting symptom in 70 to 80 percent of cases (Eifel et al, 1991) and chronic discharge is the presenting symptom in most of the remaining cases, endocervical and endometrial curettage are essential steps in evaluating these women if the results of gross, colposcopic, and cytologic examination are negative.

Prognostic Factors

The prognosis for patients with adenocarcinoma of the cervix is related to the depth of invasion, size of the lesion, stage, differentiation, lymphatic invasion, and form of therapy. The outcome may also be related to the histologic subtype. Adenocarcinoma of the cervix may have a poorer outlook than squamous carcinoma, but the difference is determined largely by the poorly differentiated and more virulent histologic types. For example, Ireland et al (1985) reported that grades 1 and 2, stage Ib cases had an 11 percent incidence of pelvic node metastases and a recurrence rate of 20 percent, compared with 44 and 60 percent, respectively, for grade 3 cases. These figures are supported by the experience of Berek et al (1985) and Tamimi and Figge (1982). Lymph node metastases appear to be the most important prognostic factor (Matthews et al, 1993).

Management

The treatment of patients with adenocarcinoma of the cervix is for the most part similar to the treatment of squamous cancers, although there is somewhat more disagreement with regard to early-stage disease, in which some authors consider combined surgery and radiation therapy to be superior to either method alone (Prempree et al, 1985; Moberg et al, 1986; Weiss and Lucas, 1986; Brand et al, 1988). This opinion is consistent with the findings of Kjorstad and Bond (1984) and also Moyses et al (1996) that patients undergoing

TABLE **5–21**

Cervical Adenocarcinoma: Frequency of Various Histologic Types*

Cell Type	% of All Cases
Endocervical	47–69
Endometrioid	<1–17
Clear cell	0–13
Adenoid cystic	0–3
Adenosquamous	8–25

*Data from Hurt et al (1977), Korhonen (1978), Tamimi and Figge (1982), Saigo et al (1986), and Hopkins et al (1988b).

surgery after intracavitary radiation therapy for adenocarcinoma of the cervix have a much higher rate of residual carcinoma (30 percent) than patients with squamous carcinoma (11 percent). Eifel et al (1991), however, found no benefit to the addition of simple hysterectomy after radiotherapy. Conversely Hopkins and coauthors (1988b and c) reported that the addition of radiotherapy to radical hysterectomy did not improve survival when compared to radical hysterectomy alone. From several reports, the average 5-year survival for adenocarcinoma of the cervix is 75 percent for stage I and 50 percent for stage II.

The management of microinvasive adenocarcinoma is discussed in the foregoing paragraphs. For stages Ib and IIa, radical hysterectomy and pelvic node dissection are recommended. Adjuvant pelvic radiation therapy should be added for those cases with node metastasis, LVSI, an inadequate margin, and perhaps grade 3 histology. Removal of the ovaries should be considered in patients with endometrioid histology (Kaminski and Norris, 1984) and poorly differentiated adenocarcinomas based on the risk of a second primary or metastatic involvement. Peritoneal cytology is more likely to be positive, and is of greater significance with cervical adenocarcinoma than squamous carcinoma. This finding correlates with other adverse prognostic features (Abu-Ghazaleh et al, 1984).

When radiation is the primary treatment for early adenocarcinoma of the cervix, an adjuvant simple hysterectomy is recommended for all but the smallest lesions. Adjuvant hysterectomy is also recommended after radiation therapy for stage IIb cases in which the parametrium becomes palpably free of tumor. The prognosis for more advanced cases seems to be especially poor. In this situation radiation therapy is the treatment of choice, and it should be combined with a chemotherapy sensitizer. The rationale and indications for preradiation surgical staging are the same as for squamous cancers.

Follow-up with serum CEA and CA-125 tumor antigen is of value in cervical adenocarcinomas, especially those with initially elevated values (Duk et al, 1989, 1990). Tissue for hormone receptor assay should also be obtained. Gao et al (1983) have shown that two thirds of cervical adenocarcinomas are progesterone receptor positive, a finding of prognostic significance in the premenopausal age group.

Other Adenocarcinomas

MINIMAL DEVIATION ADENOCARCINOMA

Also known as *adenoma malignum*, minimal deviation adenocarcinoma of the cervix is an extremely well-differentiated mucinous or endometrioid carcinoma characterized by slow growth and almost normal-appearing glands. It occurs predominantly in women in the fourth and fifth decades of life, who usually present with vaginal bleeding or mucous discharge. Local and distant failures often occur, sometimes years after the initial treatment. This neoplasm may be more malignant in postmenopausal women. An unusual frequency of ovarian carcinoma in these patients has been noted, as well as an association with Peutz-Jeghers syndrome (Gilks et al, 1989).

The expected finding of normal-appearing glands on punch biopsy will lead to a delay in diagnosis, advancing stage, and poorer results of therapy unless the clinician continues to persue the diagnosis on the basis of the abnormal examination and the patient's symptoms. The lesion may also be suspected by findings on the Pap smear (Vogelsand et al, 1995). Cone biopsy, trachelectomy, and even hysterectomy have been required to document the extension of the normal-appearing glands to a depth that represents unequivocal invasion. Radical hysterectomy with adnexectomy is the recommended treatment for operable cases (Kaku and Enjoji, 1983; Kaminski and Norris, 1983, 1984; Michael et al, 1984).

ENDOMETRIOID CARCINOMA

The villoglandular papillary variant of cervical adenocarcinoma has been considered a less malignant variant, but conservative therapy is probably not warranted (Kaku et al, 1997a). The typical endometrioid pattern is uncommon but characteristically contains benign squamous elements (adenoacanthoma). Some authorities regard the adenosquamous cancers as variants of this group. The endometrioid pattern suggests that the origin of the lesion may be endometrial, and, for classification purposes, when the endometrium is also involved such tumors should be considered endometrial in origin. Those cancers arising at the isthmus are most difficult to classify correctly.

CLEAR CELL CARCINOMA

Clear cell carcinoma of the cervix was rare before the diethylstilbestrol (DES) era (see

Chapter 4). Adenocarcinoma of the clear cell type accounted for most of the cervical cancers in women under 20 years of age even before in utero DES exposure occurred. Hameed reviewed the literature in 1968 and found only 95 well-documented cases. Thirty-eight had the tubocystic clear cell pattern and 56 were papillary or solid. The mean ages of the two groups were 33 and 43 years, respectively, both lower than the mean age for endocervical adenocarcinoma patients of typical histology. The tubocystic clear cell pattern may have a better prognosis than the other patterns; a favorable outcome is also associated with low nuclear grade (Kaminski and Maier, 1983). Although it is probable that all patterns are predominantly müllerian in origin, at least 14 cases of clear cell cancer of the cervix arising from mesonephric remnants have been reported. They may have a more indolent behavior than the müllerian-derived lesions (Clement et al, 1995).

MIXED CARCINOMAS

Adenosquamous Carcinoma

Adenosquamous carcinoma (mixed carcinoma, adenoepidermoid carcinoma) consists of intimately admixed malignant glandular and squamous components. It is reported to comprise 5 to 25 percent of all cervical adenocarcinomas. Despite the relatively high frequency, few investigators have analyzed their data on this lesion separately from the pure adenocarcinomas.

Some reports indicate that the outcome is poorer, stage for stage, than that of cervical squamous and/or adenocarcinoma. In the series of Gallup et al (1985), the adenosquamous lesions were predominantly stage I, 30 percent had no visible lesion, and half had a negative Pap smear the year prior to diagnosis. Only 4 of 15 stage I patients survived for 5 years, compared with 93 percent of those with stage I squamous carcinomas. However, Yazigi et al (1990) reported that small (<3 cm) stage Ib adenosquamous cancers of the cervix had a 5-year survival rate of 85 percent, similar to a group of patients with stage Ib squamous cancers, and Harrison et al (1993) found that there was no statistically significant difference among patients with adenosquamous, squamous, and adenocarcinomas of the cervix with respect to patient age, tumor size, depth of invasion,

grade 3 lesions, rate of node metastases, and survival.

Adenoic Cystic Carcinoma

Adenoid cystic carcinoma (cylindroma) is a pattern of adenosquamous cancer most often exhibited in the salivary glands and upper respiratory tract. This lesion, which is rare in the cervix, has distinctive clinical and microscopic features.

More than 100 cases have been reported (Berchuck and Mullin, 1985; Musa et al, 1985), with an average age of 65 years. The predominance of cases appears to be among the black population and among women of high parity. In nearly three fourths of reported cases, either squamous carcinoma or squamous dysplasia was coexistent with the adenoid cystic carcinoma. Less often, frank adenocarcinoma accompanied the adenoid cystic pattern, which in some cases made up a minor portion of the tumor. About half of the cases have been stage I at presentation. Overall survival may be poorer than for pure squamous carcinoma, and lung metastases are more common (Fowler et al, 1978; Prempree et al, 1980). A complete response to cyclophosphamide (Cytoxan), doxorubicin (Adriamycin), and cisplatin (CAP) chemotherapy has been reported (Phillips and Frye, 1985).

Adenoid Basal Carcinoma

Some authors have not distinguished between adenoid cystic and adenoid basal carcinoma of the cervix. Van Dihn and Woodruff (1985) point out that the adenoid basal lesion behaves like a basal cell carcinoma of the skin; that is, it grows slowly and invades locally but does not metastasize, provided there is no associated invasive squamous or adenocarcinoma.

Fowler et al (1978) state that conservative therapy is appropriate if the following conditions are met: (1) diagnosis is based on a cone biopsy; (2) no solid areas of tumor are present; (3) no adenoid cystic, squamous, or adenocarcinoma component is present; (4) no LVSI has occurred; (5) there is no visible lesion; and (6) the Pap smear is concordant with the diagnosis.

Glassy Cell Carcinoma

Another variant of the adenosquamous or mixed cancer is the glassy cell carcinoma.

The average age at diagnosis is 45 years. The mode of presentation is similar to that of other cervical cancers. Collating data from several series, approximately 40 percent of cases present in clinical stage I. The 5-year survival of stage I cases is 50 to 60 percent, and for stage II cases, 30 to 40 percent (Maier and Norris, 1982; Pak et al, 1983; Ulbright and Gersell, 1983; Nunez et al, 1985).

MISCELLANEOUS CANCERS OF THE CERVIX

Small-Cell Carcinoma (APUDoma)

APUDomas are neuroendocrine tumors that originate from the neural crest and have enzymatic and amine uptake (storing) properties. APUD stands for *a*mine *p*recursor *u*ptake and *d*ecarboxylation, and refers to the ability of these cells to synthesize amines (polypeptides) from amino acids.

These neoplasms and hyperplasias tend to occur in groups designated as *multiple endocrine adenomatosis type I* (Werner's syndrome) and *type II* (Sipple's syndrome). The former is an autosomal dominant genetic disorder featuring the triad of pituitary adenoma, hyperplasia of the parathyroid glands, and a pancreatic islet cell tumor. The latter syndrome is characterized by medullary carcinoma of the thyroid, pheochromocytoma, and parathyroid hyperplasia. The APUDoma group also encompasses the paraendocrine syndromes of ectopic hormone production (e.g., oat cell carcinoma of the lung producing adrenocorticotropic hormone [ACTH]) and production of a foreign hormone by a neuroendocrine tissue (e.g., ACTH production by a carcinoid tumor).

Cervical APUDomas are of three types: carcinoids, small- (oat) cell carcinomas, and primitive neuroendocrine tumors (PNETs), but the carcinoid tumors predominate. The carcinoids constitute a specific subset of the small-cell cervical carcinomas and are characterized by neurosecretory granules and argyrophilic cells. The poorly differentiated APUDomas are histologically identical to the oat cell carcinoma of the lung. Few cervical APUDomas have been associated with any clinical evidence of endocrine activity, but carcinoid syndrome and the production of ACTH, insulin, and parathormone have been reported.

The importance of this diagnosis is the associated poor prognosis (Randall et al, 1988).

Sheets and associates (1988) reported that 14 of 14 patients with neuroendocrine small-cell cervical carcinoma recurred after surgical therapy for early disease. The well-differentiated carcinoids, however, have a better prognosis than the poorly differentiated tumors (Mullins et al, 1981; Silva et al, 1984; Yamasaki et al, 1984; Groben et al, 1985).

Sarcoma

Rotmensch et al published a review of cervical sarcomas in 1983. Among their 44 collected cases, excluding the botryoid sarcomas (see Chapter 4), there were 18 leiomyosarcomas, 12 stromal sarcomas, 9 mixed mesodermal sarcomas, 4 adenosarcomas, and 1 pure liposarcoma. Prognosis and treatment are similar to those for the analogous uterine tumors except that radical hysterectomy is sometimes applicable, with or without adjuvant radiation or chemotherapy.

Lymphoma

In 1984, Harris and Scully reported 27 cases of malignant lymphoma and granulocytic sarcoma of the uterus, cervix, and vagina. Twenty-one were cervical in origin, with a median patient age of 41 years; only four patients were past age 50. Two patients had granulocytic sarcoma, 7 had nodular lymphoma, and 12 had diffuse large-cell (histiocytic) lymphoma. Most patients presented with abnormal vaginal bleeding and an intact, enlarged, sometimes nodular cervix. Seventy-five percent of the patients were in FIGO stages I and II, of whom 80 percent were alive and well 2 to 14 years post-treatment. The majority of patients were treated by simple hysterectomy and postoperative radiation or chemotherapy. Both patients with granulocytic sarcoma died of acute leukemia.

Primary lymphoma of the cervix is undoubtedly underdiagnosed because, in the experience of Harris and Scully (1984), the referring pathologist's diagnosis was correct in only 55 percent of the cases (most often interpreted as an inflammatory lesion or a malignant undifferentiated tumor). The proper diagnosis is important, as other authors have also emphasized (Komaki et al, 1984; Perren et al, 1992), because the prognosis for patients with primary lymphoma of the cervix (and vagina) is excellent, in contrast to the prognosis for patients with undifferentiated sarcoma or undifferentiated carcinoma. Staging should be by the Ann Arbor system for lymphomas rather than the FIGO system for cervical carcinomas.

Melanoma

Primary melanoma of the cervix is rare, with only 20 to 25 cases identified in the literature (Holmquist and Torres, 1988). There are few reports of successful outcome (Krishnamoorthy et al, 1986). A logical choice for treatment of early lesions would be radical hysterectomy and pelvic lymphadenectomy. Adjuvant therapy with interferon alfa-2b is recommended because of the high risk for recurrence (Kirkwood et al, 1996). Palliative radiotherapy may diminish bleeding in more advanced stages.

Metastatic Tumors

Cervical malignant neoplasms occasionally represent a metastatic focus from another primary. Among gynecologic malignancies, endometrial cancer is commonly found to be invading the cervix. While the proper classification of the tumor is obvious in the typical case, when there is a gross cervical lesion, determining the origin can be problematic. It is an oddity when ovarian cancer involves the uterine cervix, but on rare occasions the presenting symptom of ovarian cancer is vaginal bleeding due to a cervical metastasis. Among nongynecologic cancers, colon and other primary gastrointestinal cancers are the most common source of metastatic lesions in the cervix (Lemoine and Hall, 1986). Cancer metastatic to the cervix typically occurs in the patient with a known primary cancer, but occasionally the cervical lesion is the presenting finding (Sommerville et al, 1991).

REFERENCES

Abu-Ghazaleh S, Johnston W, Creasman WT: The significance of peritoneal cytology in patients with carcinoma of the cervix. Gynecol Oncol 17:139, 1984.

Alvarez RD, Gelder MS, Gore H, et al: Radical hysterectomy in the treatment of patients with bulky early stage carcinoma of the cervix uteri. Surg Gynecol Obstet 176:539, 1993.

Andersen ES, Husth M, Joergensen A, Nielsen K: Laser conization for microinvasive carcinoma of the cervix: short-term results. Int J Gynecol Cancer 3:183, 1993.

Anderson B, Buller R, LaPolla J, et al: Ovarian transposition in cervical cancer [abstract]. Gynecol Oncol 45:81, 1992.

Artman LE, Hoskins WJ, Bibro MC, et al: Radical hysterectomy and pelvic lymphadenectomy for stage IB carcinoma of the cervix: 21 years experience. Gynecol Oncol 28:8, 1987.

Averette HE, Lichtinger M, Sevin B-U, Girtanner RE: Pelvic exenteration: a 15 year experience in a general metropolitan hospital. Am J Obstet Gynecol 150:179, 1984.

Ayhan A, Tuncer ZS, Yarali H: Complications of radical hysterectomy in women with early stage cervical cancer: clinical analysis of 270 cases. Eur J Surg Oncol 17:492, 1991.

Baltzer J, Kopcke W, Lohe KJ, et al: Age and five-year survival rates in patients with operated carcinoma of the cervix. Gynecol Oncol 14:220, 1982a.

Baltzer J, Lohe KJ, Kopcke W, Zander J: Histologic criteria for the prognosis in patients with operated squamous cell carcinoma of the cervix. Gynecol Oncol 13:184, 1982b.

Bandy LC, Clarke-Pearson Dl, Silverman PM, Creasman WT: Computed tomography in evaluation of extrapelvic lymphadenopathy in carcinoma of the cervix. Obstet Gynecol 65:73, 1985.

Benedet JL, Anderson GH: Stage Ia carcinoma of the cervix revisited. Obstet Gynecol 87:1052, 1996.

Berchuck A, Mullin TJ: Cervical adenoid cystic carcinoma associated with ascites. Gynecol Oncol 22:201, 1985.

Berek JS, Hacker NF, Fu YS, et al: Adenocarcinoma of the uterine cervix: histologic variables associated with lymph node metastasis and survival. Obstet Gynecol 65:46, 1985.

Berman ML, Bergen S, Salazar H: Influence of histological features and treatment on the prognosis of patients with cervical cancer metastatic to pelvic lymph nodes. Gynecol Oncol 39:127, 1990.

Berman ML, Keys H, Creasman W, et al: Survival and patterns of recurrence in cervical cancer metastatic to periaortic lymph nodes: a Gynecologic Oncology Group study. Gynecol Oncol 19:8, 1984.

Berman ML, Lagasse LD, Watring WD, et al: The operative evaluation of patients with cervical carcinoma by an extraperitoneal approach. Obstet Gynecol 50:658, 1977.

Bichel P, Jakobsen A: Histopathologic grading and prognosis of uterine cervical carcinoma. Am J Clin Oncol 8:247, 1985.

Bloss JD, Berman ML, Mukhererjee J, et al: Bulky stage Ib cervical carcinoma managed by primary radical hysterectomy followed by tailored radiotherapy. Gynecol Oncol 47:21, 1992.

Bonomi P, Blessing J, Ball H, et al: A phase II evaluation of cisplatin and 5-fluorouracil in patients with advanced squamous cell carcinoma of the cervix: a Gynecologic Oncology Group study. Gynecol Oncol 34:357, 1989.

Boon ME, Baak JPA, Kurver PJH, et al: Adenocarcinoma in situ of the cervix: an underdiagnosed lesion. Cancer 48:768, 1981.

Boyce JG, Fruchter RG, Nicastri AD, et al: Vascular invasion in stage I carcinoma of the cervix. Cancer 53:1175, 1984.

Boyes DA, Worth AJ: Treatment of early cervical neoplasia: definition and management of preclinical invasive carcinoma. Gynecol Oncol 12:S317, 1981.

Brand E, Berek JS, Hacker NF: Controversies in the management of cervical adenocarcinoma. Obstet Gynecol 71:261, 1988.

Bremer GL, Tiebosch ATMG, van der Putten HWHM, et al: Tumor angiogenesis: an independent prognostic parameter in cervical cancer. Am J Obstet Gynecol 174:126, 1996.

Brown JV, Fu YS, Berek JS: Ovarian metastases are rare in stage I adenocarcinoma of the cervix. Obstet Gynecol 76:623, 1990.

Burghardt E, Girardi F, Lahousen M, et al: Microinvasive carcinoma of the uterine cervix (International Federation of Gynecology and Obstetrics stage IA). Cancer 67:1037, 1991.

Burghardt E, Pickel H: Local spread and lymph node involvement in cervical cancer. Obstet Gynecol 52:138, 1978.

Cain JM, Diamond A, Tamimi HK, et al: The morbidity and benefits of concurrent gracilis myocutaneous graft with pelvic exenteration. Obstet Gynecol 74:185, 1989.

Camilien L, Gordon D, Fruchter RG, et al: Predictive value of computerized tomography in the presurgical evaluation of primary carcinoma of the cervix. Gynecol Oncol 30:209, 1988.

Carenza L, Nobili F, Giacobini S: Voiding disorders after radical hysterectomy. Gynecol Oncol 13:213, 1982.

Carmichael JA, Clarke DH, Moher D, et al: Cervical carcinoma in women aged 34 and younger. Am J Obstet Gynecol 154:264, 1986.

Chafe W, Fowler WC, Currie JL, et al: Single-fraction palliative pelvic radiation therapy in gynecologic oncology: 1,000 rads. Am J Obstet Gynecol 148:701, 1984.

Chambers SK, Chambers JT, Holm C, et al: Sequelae of lateral ovarian transposition in unirradiated cervical cancer patients. Gynecol Oncol 39:155, 1990.

Chumas JC, Nelson B, Mann WJ, et al: Microglandular hyperplasia of the uterine cervix. Obstet Gynecol 66:406, 1985.

Chung CK, Nahhas WA, Zaino R, et al: Histologic grade and lymph node metastasis in squamous cell carcinoma of the cervix. Gynecol Oncol 12:348, 1981.

Clement PB, Young RH, Keh P, et al: Malignant mesonephric neoplasms of the uterine cervix: a report of 8 cases, including four with a malignant spindle cell component. Am J Surg Pathol 19:1158, 1995.

Coia L, Won M, Lanciano R, et al: The Patterns of Care Outcome Study for cancer of the uterine cervix: results of the Second National Practice Survey. Cancer 66:2451, 1990.

Coleman RL, Keeney ED, Freedman RS, et al: Radical hysterectomy for recurrent carcinoma of the uterine cervix after radiotherapy. Gynecol Oncol 55:29, 1994.

Collins R, Scrimgeour A, Yusuf S, Petro R: Reduction in fatal pulmonary embolism and venous thrombosis by perioperative administration of subcutaneous heparin. N Engl J Med 318:1162, 1988.

Coppleson M: Early invasive squamous and adenocarcinoma of cervix (FIGO stage Ia): clinical features and management. In Coppleson M (ed): Gynecologic Oncology, 2nd ed., Melbourne, Churchill Livingstone, 1992, p 631.

Creasman WT: Early invasive carcinoma of the cervix. Presented at the 25th annual meeting of the Society of Gynecologic Oncologists, Orlando, FL, February 1994.

Creasman WT: New gynecologic cancer staging [editorial]. Gynecol Oncol 58: 157, 1995.

Crissman JD, Makuch R, Budhraja M: Histopathologic grading of squamous cell carcinoma of the uterine cervix. Cancer 55:1590, 1985.

Cunningham MJ, Dunton CJ, Corn B, et al: Extended-field radiation therapy in early-stage cervical carcinoma: survival and complications. Gynecol Oncol 43:51, 1991.

Curtin JP, Hoskins WJ, Venkatraman ES, et al: Adjuvant chemotherapy versus chemotherapy plus pelvic irradiation for high-risk cervical cancer patients after radical hysterectomy and pelvic lymphadenectomy (RH-PLND): a randomized phase III trial. Gynecol Oncol 61:3, 1996.

Dargent D, Brun JL, Roy M, Rémy I: Pregnancies following radical trachelectomy for invasive cervical cancer (abstract). Gynecol Oncol 52:105, 1994.

Dargent D, Frobert JL, Beau G: V factor (tumor volume) and T factor (FIGO classification) in the assessment of cervix cancer prognosis: the risk of lymph node spread. Gynecol Oncol 22:15, 1985.

Davis GD, Patton WS: Capillary hemangioma of the cervix and vagina: management with carbon dioxide laser. Obstet Gynecol 62:95S, 1983.

de Jesus M, Tang W, Sadjadi M, et al: Carcinoma of the cervix with extensive endometrial and myometrial involvement. Gynecol Oncol 36:263, 1990.

Delgado G, Bundy B, Zaino R, et al: Prospective surgical-pathological study of disease-free interval in patients with stage IB squamous cell carcinoma of the cervix: a Gynecologic Oncology Group study. Gynecol Oncol 38:352, 1990.

Delgado G, Stehman F, Zaino R, et al: Surgical staging in Ib cervical carcinoma: clinical and pathological findings of the Gynecologic Oncology Group. Presented at the 16th annual meeting of the Society of Gynecologic Oncologists, Miami, February 3–6, 1985.

Downey GO, Potish RA, Adcock LL, et al: Pretreatment surgical staging in cervical carcinoma: therapeutic efficacy of pelvic lymph node resection. Am J Obstet Gynecol 160: 1055, 1989.

Draca P, Tesi M, Valuh M, et al: On the value of preoperative intracavital irradiation in carcinoma of the uterus. Gynecol Oncol 9:1, 1980.

Duk JM, Aalders JG, Fleuren GJ, et al: Tumor markers CA-125, squamous cell carcinoma antigen, and carcinoembryonic antigen in patients with adenocarcinoma of the uterine cervix. Obstet Gynecol 73:661, 1989.

Duk JM, De Bruijn HW, Groenier KH, et al: Adenocarcinoma of the uterine cervix: prognostic significance of pretreatment serum CA-125, squamous cell carcinoma antigen, and carcinoembryonic antigen levels in relation to clinical and histopathologic tumor characteristics. Cancer 65: 1830, 1990.

Durrance FY: Treatment for carcinoma of the cervix following inadequate surgical therapy. In Cancer of the Uterus and Ovary. Chicago, Year Book Medical Publishers, 1969, p 229.

Eddy GL, Manetta A, Alvarez RD, et al: Neoadjuvant chemotherapy with vincristine and cisplatin followed by radical hysterectomy and pelvic lymphadenectomy for FIGO stage Ib bulky cervical cancer: a Gynecologic Oncology Group pilot study. Gynecol Oncol 57:412, 1995.

Eifel PJ, Burke TW, Delclos L, et al: Early stage I adenocarcinoma of the uterine cervix: treatment results in patients with tumors <4 cm in diameter. Gynecol Oncol 41:199, 1991.

Eifel PJ, Morris M, Wharton JT, Oswald MJ: The influence of tumor size and morphology on the outcome of patients with FIGO stage Ib squamous cell carcinoma of the uterine cervix. Int J Radiat Oncol Biol Phys 29:9, 1994a.

Eifel PJ, Thoms WW Jr, Smith TL, et al: The relationship between brachytherapy dose and outcome in patients with bulky endocervical tumors treated with radiation alone. Int J Radiat Oncol Biol Phys 28:113, 1994b.

Ferlito A, Recher G: Ackerman's tumor (verrucous carcinoma) of the larynx. Cancer 46:1617, 1980.

Fowler WC, Miles PA, Surwit EA, et al: Adenoid cystic carcinoma of the cervix: report of 9 cases and a reappraisal. Obstet Gynecol 52:337, 1978.

Fuller AF Jr, Elliott N, Kosloff C, Lewis JL, Jr: Lymph node metastases from carcinoma of the cervix, stages IB and IIA: implications for prognosis and treatment. Gynecol Oncol 13:165, 1982.

Fuller AF Jr, Elliott N, Kosloff C, et al: Determinants of increased risk for recurrence in patients undergoing radical hysterectomy for stage IB and IIA carcinoma of the cervix. Gynecol Oncol 33:34, 1989.

Gallion HH, van Nagell JR, Donaldson ES, et al: Combined radiation therapy and extrafascial hysterectomy in the treatment of stage Ib barrel-shaped cervical cancer. Cancer 56:262, 1985.

Gallup DG, Harper RH, Stock RJ: Poor prognosis in patients with adenosquamous cell carcinoma of the cervix. Obstet Gynecol 65:416, 1985.

Gao YL, Twiggs LB, Leung BS, et al: Cytoplasmic estrogen and progesterone receptors in primary cervical carcinoma: clinical and histopathologic correlates. Am J Obstet Gynecol 146:299, 1983.

Gauthier P, Gore I, Shingleton HM, et al: Identification of histopathologic risk groups in stage IB squamous cell carcinoma of the cervix. Obstet Gynecol 66:569, 1985.

Gilks CB, Young RH, Aguirre P, et al: Adenoma malignum (minimal deviation adenocarcinoma) of the uterine cervix: a clinicopathological and immunohistochemical analysis of 26 cases. Am J Surg Pathol 13:717, 1989.

Groben P, Reddick R, Askin F: The pathologic spectrum of small cell carcinoma of the cervix. Int J Gynecol Pathol 4:42, 1985.

Hacker NF: Primary surgery is optional therapy for bulky stage Ib cervical carcinoma (abstract 54). Int J Gynecol Cancer 5:175, 1995.

Hameed K: Clear cell "mesonephric" carcinoma of uterine cervix. Obstet Gynecol 32:564, 1968.

Harima Y, Shiraishi T, Harima K et al: Transcatheter arterial embolization therapy in cases of recurrent and advanced gynecologic cancer. Cancer 63:2077, 1989.

Harris NL, Scully RE: Malignant lymphoma and granulocytic sarcoma of the uterus and vagina. Cancer 53:2530, 1984.

Harrison TA, Sevin B-U, Koechli O, et al: Adenosquamous carcinoma of the cervix: prognosis in early stage disease treated by radical hysterectomy. Gynecol Oncol 50:310, 1993.

Hatch KD, Shingleton HM, Potter ME, Baker VV: Low rectal resection and anastomosis at the time of pelvic exenteration. Gynecol Oncol 32:262, 1988.

Heaton D, Yordan E, Reddy S, et al: Treatment of 29 patients with bulky squamous cell carcinoma of the cervix with simultaneous cisplatin, 5-fluorouracil, and split-course hyperfractionated radiation therapy. Gynecol Oncol 38:323, 1990.

Heller PB, Barnhill DR, Mozer A, et al: Cervical carcinoma found incidentally in uteri removed for benign conditions. Obstet Gynecol 67:187, 1986.

Heller PB, Maletano JH, Bundy BN, et al: Clinical-pathologic study of stage IIB, III, and IVA carcinoma of the cervix: extended diagnostic evaluation for paraaortic node metastasis—a Gynecologic Oncology Group study. Gynecol Oncol 38:425, 1990.

Höckel M, Knapstein PG: The combined operative and radiotherapeutic treatment (CORT) of recurrent gynecologic tumors infiltrating the pelvic wall [abstract]. Gynecol Oncol 45:79, 1992.

Holloway RW, To A, Moradi M, et al: Monitoring the course of cervical carcinoma with the squamous cell carcinoma serum radioimmunoassay. Obstet Gynecol 74:944, 1989.

Holmquist ND, Torres J: Malignant melanoma of the cervix: report of a case. Acta Cytol 32:252, 1988.

Hopkins MP, Morley GW: Squamous cell cancer of the cervix: prognostic factors related to survival. Int J Gynecol Cancer 1:173, 1991.

Hopkins MP, Peters WA III, Andersen W, Morley GW: Invasive cervical cancer treated initially by standard hysterectomy. Gynecol Oncol 36:7, 1990.

Hopkins MP, Roberts JA, Schmidt RW: Cervical adenocarcinoma in situ. Obstet Gynecol 71:842, 1988a.

Hopkins MP, Schmidt RW, Roberts JA, Morley GW: Gland cell carcinoma (adenocarcinoma) of the cervix. Obstet Gynecol 72:789, 1988b.

Hopkins MP, Schmidt RW, Roberts JA, Morley GW: The prognosis and treatment of stage I adenocarcinoma of the cervix. Obstet Gynecol 72:915, 1988c.

Hreshchyshyn MM, Aron BS, Boronow RC, et al: Hydroxyurea or placebo combined with radiation to treat stages IIIB and IV cervical cancer confined to the pelvis. Int J Radiat Oncol Biol Phys 5:317, 1979.

Hughes RR, Brewington KC, Hanjani P, et al: Extended field irradiation for cervical cancer based on surgical staging. Gynecol Oncol 9:153, 1980.

Hurt WG, Silverberg SG, Frable WJ, et al: Adenocarcinoma of the cervix: histopathologic and clinical features. Am J Obstet Gynecol 129:304, 1977.

Inoue T, Chihara T, Morita K: The prognostic significance of the size of the largest nodes in metastatic carcinoma from the uterine cervix. Gynecol Oncol 19:187, 1984.

Inoue T, Morita K: The prognostic significance of number of positive nodes in cervical carcinoma stages IB, IIA, and IIB. Cancer 65:1923, 1990.

Inoue T, Okumura M: Prognostic significance of parametrial extension in patients with cervical carcinoma stages IB, IIA, and IIB: a study of 628 cases treated by radical hysterectomy and lymphadenectomy with or without postoperative irradiation. Cancer 54:1714, 1984.

Ireland D, Hardiman P, Monaghan JM: Adenocarcinoma of the uterine cervix: a study of 73 cases. Obstet Gynecol 65:82, 1985.

Jones MW, Silverberg SG: Cervical adenocarcinoma in young women: possible relationship to microglandular hyperplasia and use of oral contraceptives. Obstet Gynecol 73:984, 1989.

Jones WB, Mercer GO, Lewis JL Jr, et al: Early invasive carcinoma of the cervix. Gynecol Oncol 51:26, 1993.

Kaku T, Enjoji M: Extremely well-differentiated adenocarcinoma ("adenoma malignum") of the cervix. Int J Gynecol Pathol 2:28, 1983.

Kaku T, Kamura T, Shigamatsu T, et al: Adenocarcinoma of the uterine cervix with predominantly villoglandular growth pattern. Gynecol Oncol 64:147, 1997a.

Kaku T, Toshiharu K, Kunihiro S, et al: Early adenocarcinoma of the uterine cervix. Gynecol Oncol 65:281, 1997b.

Kaminski PF, Maier RC: Clear cell adenocarcinoma of the cervix unrelated to diethylstilbestrol exposure. Obstet Gynecol 62:720, 1983.

Kaminski PF, Norris HJ: Minimal deviation carcinoma (adenoma malignum) of the cervix. Int J Gynecol Pathol 2:141, 1983.

Kaminski PF, Norris HJ: Coexistence of ovarian neoplasms and endocervical adenocarcinoma. Obstet Gynecol 64:553, 1984.

Kamura T, Tsukamoto N, Tsuruchi N, et al: Multivariate analysis of the histopathologic prognostic factors of cervical cancer in patients undergoing radical hysterectomy. Cancer 69:181, 1992.

Kaspar HG, Dinh TV, Doherty MG, et al: Clinical implications of tumor volume measurement in stage I adenocarcinoma of the cervix. Obstet Gynecol 81:296, 1993.

Kerr-Wilson RHJ, Orr JW Jr, Shingleton HM, et al: The effect of β-adrenergic stimulation on the bladder and urethra following radical hysterectomy. Gynecol Oncol 23:267, 1986.

Kilgore LC, Orr JW, Hatch KD, et al: Peritoneal cytology in patients with squamous cell carcinoma of the cervix. Gynecol Oncol 19:24, 1984.

Kinney WK, Alvarez RD, Reid GC, et al: Value of adjuvant whole-pelvis irradiation after Wertheim hysterectomy for early-stage squamous carcinoma of the cervix with pelvic nodal metastasis: a matched-control study. Gynecol Oncol 34:258, 1989.

Kirkwood JM, Strawderman MH, Ernstoff MS, et al: Interferon α-2b adjuvant therapy of high risk cutaneous melanoma: the ECOG trial EST 1684. J Clin Oncol 14:7 1996.

Kjorstad KE, Bond B: Stage Ib adenocarcinoma of the cervix: metastatic potential and patterns of dissemination. Am J Obstet Gynecol 150:297, 1984.

Kjorstad KE, Orjasaester H: The prognostic value of CEA determinations in the plasma of patients with squamous cell cancer of the cervix. Cancer 50:283, 1982.

Kolstad P: Follow-up study of 232 patients with stage IA1 and 411 patients with stage Ia2 squamous cell carcinoma of the cervix (microinvasive carcinoma). Gynecol Oncol 33:265, 1989.

Komaki R, Cox JD, Hansen RM, et al: Malignant lymphoma of the uterine cervix. Cancer 54:1699, 1984.

Korhonen MO: Adenocarcinoma of the uterine cervix: an evaluation of the available diagnostic methods Acta Pathol Microbiol Scand 264(Sect A, suppl):3, 1978.

Korhonen MO: Epidemiological differences between adenocarcinoma and squamous cell carcinoma of the uterine cervix. Gynecol Oncol 10:312, 1980.

Kraybill WG, Lopez MJ, Bricker EM: Total pelvic exenteration as a therapeutic option in advanced malignant disease of the pelvis. Surg Gynecol Obstet 166:259, 1988.

Krishnamoorthy A, Desai M, Simanowitz M: Primary malignant melanoma of the cervix: case report. Br J Obstet Gynaecol 93:84, 1986.

Lange P: Clinical and histological studies on cervical carcinoma: precancerous, early metastases and tubular structures in the lymph nodes. Acta Pathol Microbiol Scand 50(suppl 143):9, 1960.

LaPolla JP, Schlaerth JB, Gaddis O Jr, Morrow CP: The influence of surgical staging on the evaluation and treatment of patients with cervical carcinoma. Gynecol Oncol 24:194, 1986.

Larson DM, Stringer CA, Copeland LJ, et al: Stage IB cervical carcinoma treated with radical hysterectomy and pelvic lymphadenectomy: role of adjuvant radiotherapy Obstet Gynecol 69:378, 1987.

Larson G, Alm P, Gullberg B, Grundsell H: Prognostic factors in early invasive carcinoma of the uterine cervix: a clinical, histopathologic, and statistical analysis of 343 cases. Am J Obstet Gynecol 146:145, 1983.

Lawhead RA Jr, Clark DG, Smith DH, et al: Pelvic exenteration for recurrent or persistent gynecologic malignancies: a 10-year review of the Memorial Sloan-Kettering Cancer Center experience (1972–1981). Gynecol Oncol 33:279, 1989.

Lee YN, Wang KL, Lin MH, et al: Radical hysterectomy with pelvic lymph node dissection for treatment of cervical cancer: a clinical review of 954 cases. Gynecol Oncol 32:135, 1989.

Lemoine NR, Hall PA: Epithelial tumors metastatic to the uterine cervix. Cancer 57:2002, 1986.

Lindell LK, Anderson B: Routine pretreatment evaluation of patients with gynecologic cancer. Obstet Gynecol 69:242, 1987.

Lohe KJ, Burghardt E, Hillemanns HG, et al: Early squamous cell carcinoma of the uterine cervix: II. Clinical results of a cooperative study in the management of 419 patients with early stromal invasion and microcarcinoma. Gynecol Oncol 6:31, 1978.

Maier RC, Norris HJ: Glassy cell carcinoma of the cervix Obstet Gynecol 60:219, 1982.

Maiman MA, Fruchter RG, DiMaio TM, Boyce JG: Superficially invasive squamous cell carcinoma of the cervix. Obstet Gynecol 72:399, 1988.

Maiman M, Fruchter RA, Guy L, et al: Human immunodeficiency virus infection and invasive cervical carcinoma. Cancer 71:402, 1993.

Martimbeau PW, Kjorstad KE, Iversen T: Stage IB carcinoma of the cervix, the Norwegian Radium Hospital: II. Results when pelvic nodes are involved. Obstet Gynecol 60:215, 1982.

Martin AJ, Poon CS, Thomas GM, et al: MR evaluation of cervical cancer in hysterectomy specimens: correlation of quantitative T2 measurement and histology. J Magn Reson Imaging 4:779, 1994.

Maruo T, Shibata K, Kimura A, et al: Tumor-associated antigen, TA-4, in the monitoring of the effects of therapy for squamous cell carcinoma of the uterine cervix: serial determinations and tissue localization. Cancer 56:302, 1985.

Maruyama Y, van Nagell JR, Yoneda J, et al: Dose-response and failure pattern for bulky or barrel-shaped stage IB cervical cancer treated by combined photon irradiation and extrafascial hysterectomy. Cancer 63:70, 1989.

Matthews CM, Burke TW, Tomos C, et al: Stage I cervical adenocarcinoma: prognostic evaluation of surgically treated patients. Gynecol Oncol 49:19, 1993.

Meanwell CA, Kelly KA, Wilson S, et al: Young age as a prognostic factor in cervical cancer: analysis of population based data from 10,022 cases Br Med J 296:386, 1988.

Mendenhall WM, Thar TL, Bova FJ, et al: Prognostic and treatment factors affecting pelvic control of stage IB and IIA–B carcinoma of the intact uterine cervix treated with radiation therapy alone. Cancer 53:2649, 1984.

Michael H, Grawe L, Kraus FT: Minimal deviation endocervical adenocarcinoma: clinical and histologic features, immunohistochemical staining for carcinoembryonic antigen, and differentiation from confusing benign lesions. Int J Gynecol Pathol 3:261, 1984.

Mikuta JJ, Giuntoli RL, Rubin E, Mangan CE: The "problem" radical hysterectomy. Am J Obstet Gynecol 128:119, 1977.

Miller BE, Copeland LJ, Hamberger AD, et al: Carcinoma of the cervical stump. Gynecol Oncol 18:100, 1984.

Miller B, Morris M, Rutledge F, et al: Aborted exenterative procedures in recurrent cervical cancer. Gynecol Oncol 50:94, 1993.

Milsom I, Friberg LG: Primary adenocarcinoma of the uterine cervix: a clinical study. Cancer 52:942, 1983.

Moberg PJ, Einhorn N, Silfversward C, Soderberg G: Adenocarcinoma of the uterine cervix. Cancer 57:407, 1986.

Monaghan JM, Ireland D, Mor-Yosef S, et al: Role of centralization of surgery in stage IB carcinoma of the cervix: a review of 498 cases. Gynecol Oncol 37:206, 1990.

Monk BJ, Cha D-S, Walker JL, et al: Extent of disease as an indication for pelvic radiation following radical hysterectomy and bilateral pelvic lymph node dissection in the treatment of stage Ib and IIa cervical carcinoma. Gynecol Oncol 54:4, 1994.

Montana GS, Hanlon AL, Brickner TJ, et al: Carcinoma of the cervix: Patterns of Care Studies: review of 1978, 1983, and 1988–1989 surveys. Int J Radiat Oncol Biol Phys 32:1481, 1995.

Moore DH, Fowler WC Jr, Walton LA, Droegemueller W: Morbidity of lymph node sampling in cancers of the uterine corpus and cervix. Obstet Gynecol 74:180, 1989.

Morgan PR, Anderson MC, Buckley CH, et al: The Royal College of Obstetricians and Gynaecologists Microinvasive Carcinoma of the Cervix Study: preliminary results. Br J Obstet Gynaecol 100:664, 1993.

Morley GW, Hopkins MP, Lindenauer SM, Roberts JA: Pelvic exenteration, University of Michigan: 100 patients at five years. Obstet Gynecol 74:934, 1989.

Morley GW, Seski JC: Radical pelvic surgery versus radiation therapy for stage I carcinoma of the cervix (exclusive of microinvasion). Am J Obstet Gynecol 126:785, 1976.

Morris M, Mitchell MF, Silva EG, et al: Cervical conization as definitive therapy for early invasive squamous carcinoma of the cervix. Gynecol Oncol 51:193, 1993.

Morrow CP, Shingleton HM, Averette HE, et al: Is pelvic radiation beneficial in the postoperative management of stage IB squamous cell carcinoma of the cervix with pelvic node metastasis treated by radical hysterectomy and pelvic lymphadenectomy? A report from the Presidential Panel at the 1979 annual meeting of the Society of Gynecologic Oncologists. Gynecol Oncol 10:105, 1980.

Morton GC, Thomas GM: Does adjuvent chemotherapy change the prognosis of cervical cancer? Curr Opin Obstet Gynecol 8:17, 1996.

Mountain CF, McMurtrey MJ, Hermes KE: Surgery for pulmonary metastasis: a 20-year experience. Ann Thorac Surg 38:323, 1984.

Moyses HM, Morrow CP, Muderspach LI, et al: Residual disease in the uterus after preoperative radiation therapy and hysterectomy in stage Ib cervical cancer. J Clin Oncol 19:433, 1996.

Mullins JD, Hilliard GD: Cervical carcinoid ("argyrophil cell" carcinoma) associated with an endocervical adenocarcinoma: a light and ultrastructural study. Cancer 47:785, 1981.

Muntz HG, Bell DA, Lage JM, et al: Adenocarcinoma in situ of the uterine cervix. Obstet Gynecol 80:935, 1992.

Musa AG, Hughes RR, Coleman SA: Adenoid cystic carcinoma of the cervix: a report of 17 cases. Gynecol Oncol 22:167, 1985.

Nakajima H: A clinicopathological study of early adenocarcinoma of the uterine cervix. Nagasaki Med J 58:218, 1983.

National Institutes of Health Consensus Conference: Prevention of venous thrombosis and pulmonary embolism. JAMA 256:744, 1986.

Newton M: Radical hysterectomy of radiotherapy for stage I cervical cancer: a prospective comparison with 5 and 10-year follow-up. Am J Obstet Gynecol 123:535, 1975.

Nunez C, Abdul-Karim FW, Somrak TM: Glassy-cell carcinoma of the uterine cervix. Acta Cytol 29:303, 1985.

O'Quinn AG, Fletcher GH, Wharton JT: Guidelines for conservative hysterectomy after irradiation. Gynecol Oncol 9:68, 1980.

Orr JW, Ball GC, Soong SJ, et al: Surgical treatment of women found to have invasive cervix cancer at the time of total hysterectomy. Obstet Gynecol 68:353, 1986.

Östör AG, Pagano R, Davoren RAM, et al: Adenocarcinoma in situ of the cervix. Int J Gynecol Pathol 3:179, 1984.

Östör AG, Rome RM: Micro-invasive squamous cell carcinoma of the cervix: a clinico-pathologic study of 200 cases with long-term follow-up. Int J Gynecol Cancer 4:257, 1994.

Östör A, Rome R, Quinn M: Microinvasive adenocarcinoma of the cervix: a clinicopathologic study of 77 women. Obstet Gynecol 89:88, 1997.

Park HY, Yokota SB, Paladugu RR, Agliozzo CM: Glassy cell carcinoma of the cervix: cytologic and clinicopathologic analysis. Cancer 52:307, 1983.

Pardanani NS, Tischler LP, Brown WH: Carcinoma of the cervix: evaluation of treatment in a community hospital. NY State J Med 75:1018, 1975.

Penalver MA, Bejany DE, Averette HE, et al: Continent urinary diversion in gynecologic oncology. Gynecol Oncol 34:274, 1989.

Perez CA, Camel HM, Askin F, Breaux S: Endometrial extension of carcinoma of the uterine cervix: a prognostic factor that may modify staging. Cancer 48:170, 1981.

Perez CA, Camel HM, Kuske RR, et al: Radiation therapy alone in the treatment of carcinoma of the uterine cervix: a 20-year experience. Gynecol Oncol 23:127, 1986.

Perkins PL, Chu AM, Jose B, et al: Posthysterectomy megavoltage irradiation in the treatment of cervical carcinoma. Gynecol Oncol 17:340, 1984.

Perren T, Farrant M, McCarthy K, et al: Lymphomas of the cervix and upper vagina: a report of five cases and a review of the literature. Gynecol Oncol 44:87, 1992.

Peters RK, Chao A, Mack TM, et al: Increased frequency of adenocarcinoma of the uterine cervix in young women in Los Angeles County. J Natl Cancer Inst 76:423, 1986.

Petrilli ES, Delgado G, Goldson AL: Intra-operative radiation therapy for cervical carcinoma. In Morrow CP, Smart GE (eds): Gynaecological Oncology. New York, Springer-Verlag, 1986, p 79.

Pettersson F: Annual report on the results of treatment in gynecological cancer. Int J Gynecol Obstet 36(suppl):1, 1991.

Phillips GL Jr, Frye LP: Adenoid cystic carcinoma of the cervix: a case report with implications for chemotherapeutic treatment. Gynecol Oncol 22:260, 1985.

Photopulos GJ, Zwaag RV: Class II radical hysterectomy shows less morbidity and good treatment efficacy compared to class III. Gynecol Oncol 40:21, 1991.

Pisco JM, Martins JM, Correia MG: Internal iliac artery embolization to control hemorrhage from pelvic neoplasms. Radiology 172:337, 1989.

Piver MS, Chung WS: Prognostic significance of cervical lesion size and pelvic node metastases in cervical carcinoma. Obstet Gynecol 46:507, 1975.

Potish RA, Twiggs LB, Okagaki T, et al: Therapeutic implications of the natural history of advanced cervical cancer as defined by pretreatment surgical staging. Cancer 56:956, 1985.

Poulsen HE, Taylor CW, Sobin LH: Histologic typing of female genital tract tumours. In International Histological Classification of Tumours, No. 13. Geneva, World Health Organization, 1975.

Poyner EA, Barakat RR, Hoskins WJ: Management and follow-up of patients with adenocarcinoma in situ of the uterine cervix. Gynecol Oncol 57:158, 1995.

Prempree T, Amornmarn R, Wizenberg MJ: A therapeutic approach to primary adenocarcinoma of the cervix. Cancer 56:1264, 1985.

Prempree T, Patanaphan V, Scott RM: Radiation management of carcinoma of the cervical stump. Cancer 43:1262, 1979.

Prempree T, Patanaphan V, Viravathana T, et al: Radiation treatment of carcinoma of the cervix with extension into the endometrium: a reappraisal of its significance. Cancer 49:2015, 1982.

Prempree T, Villasanta U, Tang C-K: Management of adenoid cystic carcinoma of the uterine cervix (cylindroma): report of six cases and reappraisal of all cases reported in the medical literature. Cancer 46:1631, 1980.

Pursell SH, Day TG Jr, Tobin GR: Distally based rectus abdominis flap for reconstruction in radical gynecologic procedures. Gynecol Oncol 37:234, 1990.

Qizilbash AH: In-situ and microinvasive adenocarcinoma of the uterine cervix: a clinical, cytologic and histologic study of 14 cases. Am J Clin Pathol 64:155, 1975.

Raheja A, Katz DA, Dermer JS: Verrucous carcinoma of the endocervix. Obstet Gynecol 62:535, 1983.

Randall ME, Constable WC, Hahn SS, et al: Results of the radiotherapeutic management of carcinoma of the cervix with emphasis on the influence of histologic classification. Cancer 62:48, 1988.

Robertson G, Lopes A, Beynon G, Monaghan JM: Pelvic exenteration: a review of the Gateshead experience 1974–1992. Br J Obstet Gynaecol 101:529, 1994.

Roddick JW Jr, Greenelaw RH: Treatment of cervical cancer: a randomized study of operation and radiation. Am J Obstet Gynecol 109:754, 1971.

Roman LD, Felix JC, Muderspach LI, et al: Risk of residual invasive disease in women with microinvasive squamous cancer in a conization specimen. Obstet Gynecol 90:759, 1997.

Roman LD, Morris M, Eifel PJ, et al: Reasons for inappropriate simple hysterectomy in the presence of invasive cancer of the cervix. Obstet Gynecol 79:485, 1993a.

Roman LD, Morris M, Mitchell MF, et al: Prognostic factors for patients undergoing simple hysterectomy in the presence of invasive cancer of the cervix. Gynecol Oncol 50:179, 1993b.

Rotman M, Choi K, Guse C, et al: Prophylactic irradiation of the para-aortic lymph node chain in stage IIB and bulky stage IB carcinoma of the cervix: initial treatment results of RTOG 7920. Int J Radiat Oncol Biol Phys 19:513, 1990.

Rotmensch J, Rosenshein NB, Woodruff JD: Cervical sarcoma: a review. Obstet Gynecol Surv 38:456, 1983.

Rubin SC, Hoskins WJ, Lewis JL Jr: Radical hysterectomy for recurrent cervical cancer following radiation therapy. Gynecol Oncol 27:316, 1987.

Runowicz CD, Wadler S, Rodriguez-Rodriguez L, et al: Concomitant cisplatin and radiotherapy in locally advanced cervical carcinoma. Gynecol Oncol 34:395, 1989.

Russell et al: 1987

Rutledge FN, Carey MS, Prichard H, et al: Conservative surgery for recurrent or persistent carcinoma of the cervix following irradiation: is exenteration always necessary? Gynecol Oncol 52:353, 1994.

Rutledge FN, Mitchell MF, Munsell M, et al: Youth as a prognostic factor in carcinoma of the cervix: a matched analysis. Gynecol Oncol 44:123, 1992.

Rutledge FN, Smith JP, Wharton JT, O'Quinn AG: Pelvic exenteration: analysis of 296 patients. Am J Obstet Gynecol 129:881, 1977.

Rutledge FN, Wharton JT, Fletcher GH: Clinical studies with adjunctive surgery and irradiation therapy in the treatment of carcinoma of the cervix. Cancer 38:596, 1976.

Saigo PE, Cain JM, Kim WS, et al: Prognostic factors in adenocarcinoma of the uterine cervix. Cancer 57:1584, 1986.

Senekjian EK, Young JM, Weiser P, et al: An evaluation of squamous cell carcinoma antigen in patients with cervical squamous cell carcinoma. Am J Obstet Gynecol 157:433, 1987.

Sheets EE, Berman ML, Hrountas CK, et al: Surgically treated, early-stage neuroendocrine small-cell cervical carcinoma. Obstet Gynecol 71:10, 1988.

Shingleton HM, Fowler WC Jr, Koch GG: Pretreatment evaluation in cervical cancer. Am J Obstet Gynecol 110:385, 1971.

Shingleton HM, Gore H, Bradley DH, Soong S-J: Adenocarcinoma of the cervix. I. Clinical evaluation and pathologic features. Am J Obstet Gynecol 139:799, 1981.

Shingleton HM, Soong SJ, Gelder MS, et al: Clinical and histopathologic factors predicting recurrence and survival after pelvic exenteration for cancer of the cervix. Obstet Gynecol 73:1027, 1989.

Silva EG, Kott MM, Ordonez NG: Endocrine carcinoma intermediate cell type of the uterine cervix. Cancer 54:1705, 1984.

Soisson AP, Geszler G, Soper TJ, et al: A comparison of symptomatology, physical examination, and vaginal cytology in the detection of recurrent cervical carcinoma after radical hysterectomy. Obstet Gynecol 76:106, 1990a.

Soisson AP, Soper JT, Clarke-Pearson DL, et al: Adjuvant radiotherapy following radical hysterectomy for patients with stage IB and IIA cervical cancer. Gynecol Oncol 37:390, 1990b.

Sommerville M, Koonings PP, Curtin JP, d'Ablaing G: Gastrointestinal signet ring carcinoma metastatic to the cervix during pregnancy: a case report. J Reprod Med 36:813, 1991.

Stanhope CR, Webb MJ, Podratz KC: Pelvic exenteration for recurrent cervical cancer. Clin Obstet Gynecol 33:897, 1990.

Stehman FB, Bundy BN, DiSaia PJ, et al: Carcinoma of the cervix treated with radiation therapy: a multi-variate analysis of prognostic variables in the Gynecologic Oncology Group. Cancer 67:2776, 1991.

Stehman F, Jobson V, Bundy B, et al: A randomized trial of hydroxyurea vs. misonidazole (MI) adjunct to radiation therapy in carcinoma of the cervix: a preliminary report of a group study. Am J Obstet Gynecol 159:87, 1988.

Stehman FB, Thomas GM: Prognostic factors in locally advanced carcinoma of the cervix treated with radiation therapy. Semin Oncol 21:25, 1994.

Stelzer KJ, Koh WJ, Greer BE, et al: The use of intraoperative radiation therapy in radical salvage for recurrent cervical cancer: outcome and toxicity. Am J Obstet Gynecol 172:1881, 1995.

Stendahl U, Eklund G, Willen R: Prognosis of invasive squamous cell carcinoma of the uterine cervix: a comparative study of the predictive values of clinical staging IB–III and a histopathologic malignancy grading system. Int J Gynecol Pathol 2:42, 1983.

Stock RJ, Chen ASJ, Flickinger JC, et al: Node positive cervical cancer: impact of pelvic irradiation and patterns of failure. Int J Radiat Oncol Biol Phys 31:31, 1995.

Sutton GP, Bundy BN, Delgado G, et al: Ovarian metastases in stage IB carcinoma of the cervix: a Gynecologic Oncology Group study. Am J Obstet Gynecol 166:50, 1992.

Tamimi HK, Figge DC: Adenocarcinoma of the uterine cervix. Gynecol Oncol 13:335, 1982.

Tattersal MHN, Ramirez C, Coppleson M: A randomized trial of adjuvant chemotherapy after radical hysterectomy in stage Ib–IIa cervical cancer patients with pelvic lymph node metastasis. Gynecol Oncol 46:176, 1992.

Taylor PT, Andersen WA: Untreated cervical cancer complicated by obstructive uropathy and oliguric renal failure. Gynecol Oncol 11:162, 1981.

Terada K, Morley GW: Radical hysterectomy as salvage therapy for gynecologic malignancy. Obstet Gynecol 70:913, 1987.

Teshima S, Shimosato Y, Kishi K, et al: Early stage adenocarcinoma of the uterine cervix: histopathologic analysis with consideration of histogenesis. Cancer 56:167, 1985.

TeVelde ER, Persijn JP, Ballieux RE, Faber J: Carcinoembryonic antigen serum levels in patients with squamous cell carcinoma of the uterine cervix: clinical significance. Cancer 49:1866, 1982.

Thomas GM, Dembo AJ, Beale FA, et al: A pilot study of concurrent radiation, mitomycin C and 5-FU in poor prognosis carcinoma of the cervix [abstract]. Am J Clin Oncol 7:113, 1984.

Timmer PR, Aalders JG, Bouma J: Radical surgery after preoperative intracavitary radiotherapy for stage IB and IIa carcinoma of the uterine cervix. Gynecol Oncol 18:206, 1980.

Tinga DJ, Beentjes JA, Van de Wiel HB, et al: Detection, prevalence, and prognosis of asymptomatic carcinoma of the cervix. Obstet Gynecol 76:860, 1990.

Ulbright TM, Gersell DJ: Glassy cell carcinoma of the uterine cervix: a light and electron microscopic study of five cases. Cancer 51:2255, 1983.

Ursin G, Peters RK, Henderson BE, et al: Oral contraceptive use and adenocarcinoma of cervix. Lancet 344:1390, 1994.

Van Dinh T, Woodruff JD: Adenoid cystic and adenoid basal carcinomas of the cervix. Obstet Gynecol 65:705, 1985.

van Nagell JR Jr, Greenwell N, Powell DF, et al: Microinvasive carcinoma of the cervix. Am J Obstet Gynecol 145:981, 1983.

van Nagell JR Jr, Sprague AD, Roddick JW Jr: The effect of intravenous pyelography and cystoscopy on the staging of cervical cancer. Gynecol Oncol 3:87, 1975.

Vasilev SA, Schlaerth JB: Scalene lymph node sampling in cervical carcinoma: a reappraisal. Gynecol Oncol 37:120, 1990.

Vogelsang PJ, Nguyen GK, Honore LH: Exfoliative cytology of adenoma malignum (minimal deviation adenocarcinoma) of uterine cervix. Diagn Cytopathol 13:146, 1995.

Weiser EB, Bundy BN, Hoskins WJ, et al: Extraperitoneal versus transperitoneal selective paraaortic lymphadenectomy in the pretreatment surgical staging of advanced cervical carcinoma. Gynecol Oncol 33:283, 1989.

Weiss RJ, Lucas WE: Adenocarcinoma of the uterine cervix. Cancer 57:1996, 1986.

Welander CE, Pierce VK, Nori D, et al: Pretreatment laparotomy in carcinoma of the cervix. Gynecol Oncol 12:336, 1981.

Wertheim MS, Hakes TB, Daghestani AN, et al: A pilot study of adjuvant therapy in patients with cervical cancer at high risk of recurrence after radical hysterectomy and pelvic lymphadenectomy. J Clin Oncol 3:912, 1985.

White CD, Morley GW, Kumar NB: The prognostic significance of tumor emboli in lymphatic or vascular spaces of the cervical stroma in stage IB squamous cell carcinoma of the cervix. Am J Obstet Gynecol 149:342, 1984.

Wilczynski SP, Walker J, Liao SY, et al: Adenocarcinoma of the cervix associated with human papillomavirus. Cancer 62:1331, 1988.

Yajima A, Noda K: The results of treatment of microinvasive carcinoma (stage IA) of the uterine cervix by means of simple and extended hysterectomy. Am J Obstet Gynecol 135:685, 1979.

Yamasaki M, Tateishi R, Hongo J, et al: Argyrophil small cell carcinomas of the uterine cervix. Int J Gynecol Pathol 3: 146, 1984.

Yazigi R, Sandstad J, Munoz AK, et al: Adenosquamous carcinoma of the cervix: prognosis in stage IB. Obstet Gynecol 75:1012, 1990.

Young RH, Scully RE: Atypical forms of microglandular hyperplasia of the cervix simulating carcinoma: a report of five cases and review of the literature. Am J Surg Pathol 13:50, 1989.

Zander J, Baltzer J, Lohe KJ, et al: Carcinoma of the cervix: an attempt to individualize treatment. Results of a 20-year cooperative study. Am J Obstet Gynecol 13:752, 1981.

C H A P T E R

6

Tumors of the Endometrium

PREMALIGNANT TUMORS

Endometrial Hyperplasia

The endometrial hyperplasias (EHs) represent various morphologic and biologic alterations of the endometrial glands and stroma, ranging from an exaggerated physiologic state to in situ carcinoma. The clinically significant forms usually evolve within a background of proliferative endometrium and almost invariably have proliferative-type glands. The hyperplasias result from protracted estrogen stimulation of a susceptible endometrium in the absence of progestin influence. Occasionally EH develops in the ovulating woman, apparently from focal insensitivity of the endometrium to progesterone. The EHs are clinically important because they may (1) cause abnormal uterine bleeding, (2) cause excessive blood loss, (3) be an indication of anovulation and infertility, (4) be associated with estrogen-producing ovarian tumors, (5) result from medicinal estrogens, and (6) precede or occur simultaneously with endometrial carcinoma.

Classification

Numerous histopathologic systems have been devised to classify EHs in a clinically meaningful way with respect to their potential for evolving into carcinoma. It is now generally agreed that the most significant microscopic feature is cellular atypia. Hyperplasias with atypia are considered to be premalignant, whereas those without atypia are benign. Classifications that reliably correlate clinical behavior with histology are those of Welch and Scully (1977), Kurman et al (1985), and the Society of Gynecological Pathologists (Silverberg, 1988). The latter, which is most practical, has three categories: (1) simple, (2)

complex (adenomatous without atypia), and (3) atypical (Figs. 6–1 through 6–3).

The complex hyperplasias in this scheme are characterized by marked architectural changes in the glands, with irregular outlines and back-to-back crowding but no cytologic atypia. Nevertheless, the more important hyperplasias, which probably should be termed neoplasias, are those with cellular atypia whether the architecture is simple or complex (Fig. 6–3). Any of the hyperplasias may be focal or diffuse and may exist entirely within a polyp.

Malignant Potential

The risk of EH progressing to carcinoma is related to the severity of cytologic atypia, the chronicity of the anovulatory state, the association with exogenous estrogen use, and probably the age of the patient. In the absence of cellular atypia, it is inappropriate to designate the hyperplasias as premalignant. However, these conditions do identify an endometrium predisposed to the development of carcinoma because of an underlying pathophysiologic state, especially if that state is irreversible.

The endometrial cancer risk as defined by the study of Kurman et al (1985) is presented in Table 6–1. Among 122 patients with hyperplasia and no atypia (mean age 42 years), the hyperplasia persisted in 11 percent, and 2 patients (1.5 percent) developed carcinoma with an average of 11 years' follow-up. There were 48 patients with atypical hyperplasia, of whom 17 percent had persistence and 23 percent progressed to carcinoma, a progression rate substantially lower than the 57 percent reported by Sherman and Brown in 1979. Among 20 women in the Kurman et al study whose hyperplasias were diagnosed while they were receiving medicinal estrogen therapy, none developed carcinoma and the hy-

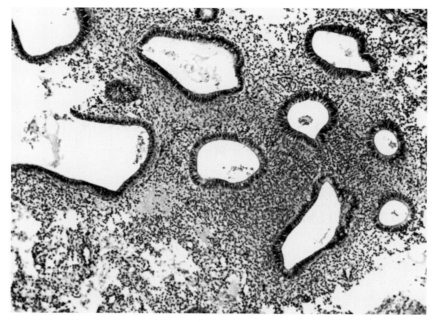

FIGURE 6–1. Photomicrograph of simple (cystic) endometrial hyperplasia. In this expression of the physiologic response to prolonged estrogen exposure, the endometrium becomes thickened by a hyperplasia of the glands and stroma. The epithelium is proliferative, and some glands are dilated.

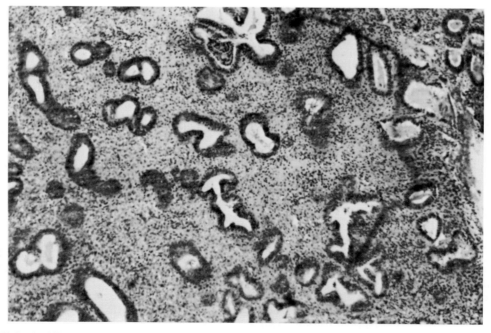

FIGURE 6–2. Microscopic features of complex hyperplasia, including bud-like projections, clustering of glands, and proliferative epithelium.

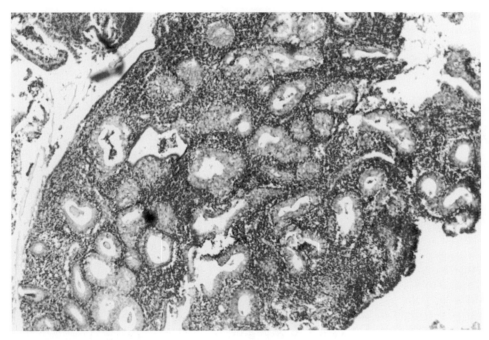

FIGURE 6-3. Atypical hyperplasia characterized by large, crowded glands and enlarged, tall columnar epithelial cells with nuclear abnormalities. Intraglandular bridging and piled-up epithelium are common. It is unlikely to revert to normal if the hormonal milieu is not altered, in which case progression to cancer is common.

perplasia persisted in only 2 (both had simple hyperplasia) after discontinuing the estrogens. The fact that 20 to 50 percent of women undergoing hysterectomy for atypical hyperplasia are found to have endometrial carcinoma provides further evidence of the malignant potential of this lesion (Janicek and Rosenshein, 1994; Widra et al, 1995).

Diagnosis

The only symptom of EH is abnormal uterine bleeding, pre- or postmenopausal. The chronically anovulatory/amenorrheic woman

may have significant EH, and rarely a normally menstruating woman, usually infertile, develops EH or even carcinoma. Diagnosis requires histologic evaluation of endometrial and endocervical tissues obtained by biopsy or fractional curettage (Fig. 6-4). When the diagnosis of complex or atypical hyperplasia in a postmenopausal woman is based on an office biopsy specimen and the planned treatment is less than a total abdominal hysterectomy (e.g., hormone therapy, vaginal hysterectomy), as a general rule a hysteroscopy and fractional curettage are indicated to ascertain that the most advanced abnormality has been

TABLE 6-1

Relationship Between Type of Endometrial Hyperplasia and Risk of
Persistence or Progression to Cancer*

Type of Hyperplasia	Total Cases	Persisted		Progressed to Carcinoma		Mean Years of Follow-Up
		No.	Percent	No.	Percent	
Simple	93	18	19	1	1	15.2
Complex	29	5	17	1	3	13.5
Atypical simple	13	3	23	1	8 }	11.4
Atypical, complex	35	5	14	10	29 }	

*Data from Kurman et al. (1985).

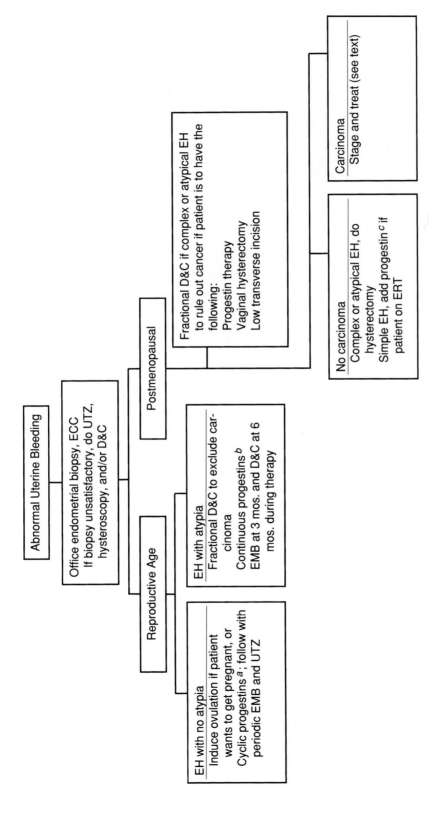

FIGURE 6–4. Management algorithm for women with endometrial hyperplasia. [a]Medroxyprogesterone acetate (MPA) or megestrol acetate, 20 mg/day orally 10 to 14 days each month. [b]MPA or megestrol acetate, 20 to 40 mg twice daily for 6 months to reverse the lesion; [c]MPA 2.5 mg/day continuously or MPA 5 mg 10 to 14 days each month. ECC = endocervical curettage; ERT = estrogen replacement therapy; UTZ = ultrasound.

identified. Premenopausal women with an office biopsy–based diagnosis of EH with cytologic atypia or marked architectural abnormalities also need evaluation by fractional curettage. Detection and assessment of EH by cytologic means is generally unsatisfactory (Yazigi et al, 1983; Meisels and Jolicoeur, 1985). Evaluation of the cervix is required in cases of abnormal uterine bleeding and postmenopausal bleeding to rule out endocervical carcinoma.

Uterine curettage may not be necessary if the patient is scheduled to undergo an abdominal hysterectomy because curettage under anesthesia is not substantially more sensitive than a well-performed office biopsy (Janicek and Rosenshein, 1994). Furthermore, the patient undergoing abdominal hysterectomy can be managed as if she had a uterine malignancy, and the uterus examined for cancer intraoperatively. The operation should entail a midline incision, careful abdominal exploration, peritoneal cytology, and removal of the adnexa. In addition, the uterine elevator should not be used, and, of course, supracervical hysterectomy and myomectomy are contraindicated.

Treatment

Numerous factors must be considered to determine the best course of management for the woman with EH. The two most common determinants are the patient's reproductive status and the specific type of EH (Fig. 6–4). In the premenopausal woman, when fertility is not desired, hysterectomy with ovarian preservation is the preferred treatment for complex and atypical hyperplasia. In the healthy peri- or postmenopausal woman, hysterectomy plus adnexectomy is recommended for hyperplasias other than simple, unless the woman is taking estrogens. In this case progestins are given or estrogens discontinued until the hyperplasia is reversed.

Progestins are used to treat those patients who have a contraindication to surgery, such as preservation of fertility or significant concurrent medical problems. Progestin therapy is very effective in reversing EH without atypia, but less effective for EH with atypia. Collating the results from three reports, 83 percent of 115 patients with simple or complex EH had complete reversal of their lesions (Kurman et al, 1985; Gal, 1986; Ferenczy and Gelfand, 1989). For these hyperplasias, ovulation induction, medroxyprogesterone acetate (MPA) 10 mg/day for 14 days per month, and continuous progestin therapy (e.g., megestrol acetate 20 to 40 mg PO daily) are effective therapies, although the latter is probably the most reliable for reversing complex hyperplasia.

The reported results of medical therapy for atypical EH are mixed and may reflect differences in progestin dose and schedule. In the study of Ferenczy and Gelfand (1989), only 10 of 20 patients in the atypical EH group remitted on MPA 20 mg PO daily, and 5 of these recurred on therapy. Five of the treatment failures eventually progressed to carcinoma. This compares to 30 remissions of 32 cases (94 percent) among the atypical EH patients receiving 20 to 40 mg megestrol acetate/day and no progressions to cancer in the Gal (1986) study. In the latter report all seven patients who discontinued hormone therapy relapsed. Thus the patient with spontaneous atypical EH is at high risk for the development of endometrial cancer as long as her uterus is present. For this reason, the progestins should be continued indefinitely. Periodic endometrial biopsy and/or transvaginal ultrasound is advisable. When pregnancy is to be undertaken, reversal of the lesion should be documented by dilatation and curettage after 6 months of therapy. It is less certain if continuous therapy and monitoring are necessary for patients with complex EH without cytologic atypia. In the young patient with this lesion, oral contraceptives or ovulation induction are reasonable options.

Hysteroscopic ablation or resection of the endometrium is not recommended for women with EH or who are epidemiologically at high risk for endometrial carcinoma since not all the endometrium is ablated. Furthermore, endometrial carcinoma can be overlooked at hysteroscopy (Colafranceschi et al, 1996).

Endometrial Polyps

Endometrial polyps are benign tumors arising from endometrial mucosa. They are attached by a pedicle and contain thick-walled blood vessels and stromal fibrosis in addition to endometrial glands. Endometrial polyps reach their highest incidence in the fifth decade of life, and 75 percent occur in women between the ages of 30 and 60 years (Van Bogaert, 1988). Endometrial polyps may be functional, inactive, or hyperplastic, and about 2 to 3 percent are of the adenomatous variety. Normal secretory changes are uncommon. Endometrial polyps are found in association with 10 to 30 percent of endometrial cancers and are not uncommonly involved secondarily by cancer, but only 0.5 percent of carcinomas arise in a polyp. Such malignancies may be endometrioid, papillary serous, or carcinosarcomatous in histology (Scully, 1982; Schlaen et al, 1988; Silva and Jenkins, 1990). A number of cases of endometrial polyps characterized by edema and cystic dilated glands were reported in women undergoing tamoxifen therapy for breast cancer (Corley et al, 1992) (see the section "Epidemiology" in Chapter 1).

Women with endometrial polyps (Fig. 6–5) present with abnormal menstrual bleeding (metrorrhagia more than menorrhagia) or postmenopausal bleeding, accounting for about 25 percent of the latter category. Occasionally an endometrial polyp is visible at the cervical os. Because of their mobility and fibrous composition, these lesions are often missed at curettage. Recurrent uterine bleeding after curettage should raise the suspicion of an endometrial polyp. Hydroultrasonography and hysterography are the preferred means of diagnosing these lesions. Hysteroscopic polyp excision is recommended for the typical benign polyp.

Endometrial Metaplasia

Hendrickson and Kempson (1980) have defined the status of non-neoplastic epithelial metaplasia of the endometrium, pointing out that the changes so produced can be misinterpreted as carcinoma or cytologically atypical hyperplasia. Their classification of the benign metaplasias includes squamous morules as well as papillary, tubal, eosinophilic, mucinous, hobnail, and clear cell types. Most cases occur in postmenopausal women who have received unopposed estrogen replacement therapy. Andersen et al (1987) report that endometrial metaplasia can occur simultaneously with carcinoma and hyperplasia, especially in younger women.

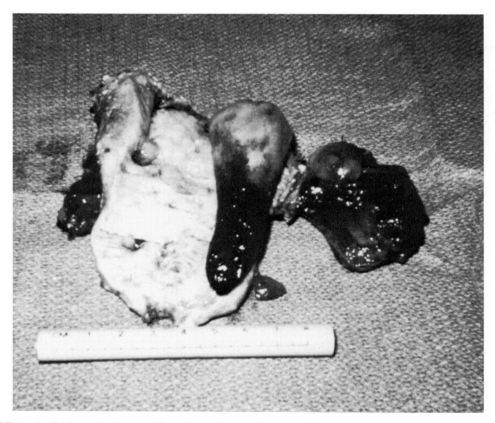

FIGURE 6–5. Endometrial polyp. Specimen from a 72-year-old woman with recurrent postmenopausal bleeding.

TABLE 6–2

Endometrial Pathology in Women With Endometrial
Cells on Cervical Cytology*

Endometrial Cells	Premenopausal				Postmenopausal			
	Total	EH	Polyps	Cancer	Total	EH	Polyps	Cancer
Normal[†]	57	3	4	0	74	9	1	1[‡]
Atypical	2	0	1	0	22	0	1	5
Malignant	2	0	0	2	31	1	0	23[§]

*Data from Yancey et al. (1990).
[†]Secretory phase only for premenopausal group.
[‡]Ovarian carcinoma.
[§]Two cervical, 1 breast, 1 ovarian, and 19 endometrial cancers.

ENDOMETRIAL CARCINOMA

Clinical Features

Symptoms

The pre-eminent symptom of endometrial carcinoma (EC) is postmenopausal bleeding. Approximately three fourths of the cases occur in this age group, and in more than 90 percent of them the initial complaint is vaginal bleeding. The importance of this symptom is recognized by most women, and they usually seek medical consultation within 3 months after the first episode. Other important initial symptoms are a purulent, sometimes blood-tinged discharge (pyometra) and pain. The latter is generally associated with metastatic disease. Only 1 to 5 percent of the cases of EC are diagnosed while the patient is asymptomatic. This usually results from investigation of a Pap smear with atypical or malignant endometrial cells (Table 6–2) or the discovery of cancer in a uterus removed for benign gynecologic indications. While Cherkis et al (1988) reported that 13 percent of postmenopausal women with normal endometrial cells on routine Pap smears had endometrial cancer, Yancey et al (1990) found none.

The causes of postmenopausal bleeding are numerous (Table 6–3), but 10 to 20 percent of patients with this complaint have a gynecologic malignancy, usually EC. Thus postmenopausal bleeding is a more important indicator of malignancy than is an abnormal Pap smear. Common physician errors in managing these patients are the assumption that the bleeding is due to medicinal estrogens or to atrophic vaginitis, that the bleeding is insufficient to warrant investigation (especially if the endocervical canal appears stenotic),

and that a normal Pap smear is adequate evaluation for postmenopausal bleeding. Although a single episode of spotting or bleeding is most likely due to causes such as an atrophic vaginal mucosa, in the study of Hawwa et al (1970), 7 percent of these patients had carcinoma, approximately the same as patients with 2 to 6 days of spotting or bleeding. Surprisingly, the amount of bleeding did not seem to be indicative of its seriousness. The older the patient with bleeding, however, the greater the risk of cancer (Table 6–4). Recurrent postmenopausal bleeding following a benign initial evaluation is frequently due to endometrial hyperplasia, polyps, or atrophy, but carcinoma is an unlikely cause (Fung et al, 1997).

Women with EC who are premenopausal invariably have abnormal uterine bleeding,

TABLE 6–3

Etiology of Postmenopausal Bleeding

Etiologic Factor	Hawwa et al. (1970)* (N = 335; %)	Pacheco and Kempers (1968)[†] (N = 401; %)
Estrogen therapy	27	27
No pathology (atrophic endometrium)	23	20
Cancer	19.5	18
Endometrium	(13)	(16)
Cervix	(4)	(1)
Other	(2.5)	(1)
Atrophic vaginitis	10	9
Endometrial polyps	7	23
Cervical polyps—cervicitis	6.5	14
Endometrial, benign[‡]	3	—
Other (myoma, caruncle, trauma, etc.)	4	9

*Lahey Clinic.
[†]Mayo Clinic.
[‡]Includes proliferative, secretory, and hyperplastic endometrium.

TABLE **6–4**

Frequency of Endometrial Carcinoma by Age Group in Women With Postmenopausal Bleeding*

| Age Group (yr) | Total Cases | Corpus Cancer | |
		No.	Percent
<50	34	0	0.0
50–59	161	15	9.3
60–69	92	15	16.3
70–79	43	12	27.9
>80	5	3	60.0

*Data from Hawwa et al (1970).

often characterized as menometrorrhagia or oligomenorrhea. A variation of this pattern is cyclic bleeding, which may persist after the expected age of the menopause. This is often misinterpreted as ovulatory bleeding. For this reason, periodic endometrial evaluation is recommended for women still "menstruating" after age 52 years. Most premenopausal women with corpus cancer are in the over-40 age group, but the disease must also be considered in younger women with abnormal bleeding that is persistent or recurrent or at any time if obesity and chronic anovulation (oligomenorrhea) are present.

There have been several articles devoted to the perception that two distinct pathogenetic forms of EC exist (Bokhman, 1983; Degligdisch and Cohen, 1985; Smith and McCartney, 1985). One type is associated with excessive, prolonged estrogen exposure, either exogenous or endogenous, and has a more favorable outcome. The estrogen-associated lesion is further characterized by coexisting EH, better differentiation, less myometrial invasion, earlier stage, and a higher hormone receptor content than the non-estrogen-related malignancy.

Physical Examination

Clues to the presence of EC are seldom found on general examination, although obesity and hypertension are commonly associated constitutional factors. Rarely, peripheral lymph gland metastases or ascites is present, the latter suggesting concomitant ovarian malignancy or papillary serous EC. During the gynecologic examination, special attention should be given to the vaginal introitus and suburethral area, fairly common sites of metastasis. The entire vagina and cervix are inspected and palpated, but findings other than bleeding from the external os are the exception. Bimanual rectovaginal palpation should

specifically evaluate the parametrium for induration and nodularity, the uterus for size and mobility, the cul de sac for nodularity, and the adnexa for masses, the last representing metastases or concurrent primary ovarian neoplasia. The uterus is frequently enlarged by fibroids, myometrial hypertrophy, tumor, hemato/pyometra, and occasionally tumor bulk; in some instances the uterus is atrophic. Consequently, uterine size does not correlate with the presence or absence of cancer. It is not unusual for the entire examination to be normal. The examiner should bear in mind that the woman with EC is epidemiologically similar to the woman at increased risk for breast, ovarian, and colorectal cancer.

Diagnosis

The more common conditions that must be considered in evaluating the patient suspected of having EC are those that cause abnormal bleeding, especially postmenopausal bleeding. Included are vaginal, cervical, tubal, and ovarian carcinoma; benign and malignant myometrial tumors; endometrial polyps; and EH. Metastasis to the endometrium causing vaginal bleeding is rarely the first sign of extrapelvic carcinoma (Kumar and Hart, 1982).

Microscopic analysis of endometrial tissue is required to make the diagnosis of EC. The classic means for obtaining the tissue specimen is the fractional curettage. This consists of a circumferential endocervical canal scrape followed by a systematic, comprehensive endometrial curettage. The two specimens are submitted to the laboratory separately. Fractionating the curettage is most important to detect an occult endocervical carcinoma, but this also serves to determine if the EC involves the cervix. Naturally, biopsy specimens should be taken from any lesion of the cervix or vagina.

Today, office endometrial biopsy (EMB) with endocervical curettage (ECC), rather than a formal curettement in the operating room, is the accepted first step in evaluating postmenopausal bleeding or whenever endometrial pathology is suspected. The EMB consists of multiple strokes with a suction or other curet, sampling as much of the uterine lining as feasible. It is generally well tolerated, accurate, and cost effective (Feldman et al, 1993). If the suspicion for cancer is high, hysteroscopy should not be employed unless it is necessary to assist in making a correct diagnosis, since cancer cells can be pushed into the peritoneal cavity (Egarter et al, 1996). When the cervical canal is stenotic or patient tolerance does not permit adequate office evaluation of the endometrium and endocervix, a curettage under anesthesia may be warranted.

Granberg et al (1991) proposed using vaginal ultrasound to screen women with postmenopausal bleeding before performing uterine curettage. They point out that fewer than 10 percent of women with postmenopausal bleeding have EC. Using a cutoff limit of 5 mm for the thickness of the normal endometrial stripe, 80 percent of curettages could be avoided. Karlsson et al (1995), in a multicenter study, reported that none of 518 women with a stripe of 4 mm or less had EC at dilatation and curettage. However, 2 of 88 women with a 5-mm stripe had EC. Thus the 4-mm mark is a safer cutoff. In view of these data, when office evaluation of the woman with postmenopausal bleeding is unsatisfactory or inconclusive, transvaginal ultrasound can be used to select patients for formal uterine curettage. An endometrial stripe up to 8 mm thick may be normal for women taking estrogens. Endometrial fluid in the absence of a thickened stripe is not a significant finding (Brooks et al, 1996). Patients with postmenopausal bleeding whose pelvic examination is unsatisfactory should also be evaluated with ultrasound, regardless of the EMB outcome.

Unless the results of these studies are negative, it is not appropriate to attribute postmenopausal bleeding to benign causes such as atrophic vaginitis, hormone therapy, or urethral caruncle. Fibroids should never be accepted as a cause of postmenopausal bleeding. Recurrent bleeding after a negative evaluation is an indication for ultrasound, hysteroscopy, and curettage (Gimpelson and Rappold, 1988; De Jong et al, 1990).

Pathophysiology

The uterus arises from the glandular component of the endometrial mucosa, usually in the upper portion of the corpus. It may evolve through the various degrees of hyperplasia and dysplasia or arise de novo in a diffuse or circumscribed pattern. Occasionally, EC arises within a polyp or from the isthmus. The initial growth tends to be slow, producing an exophytic, friable mass that manifests itself by spontaneous bleeding. As the malignancy continues to proliferate, it usually invades the underlying myometrium and advances toward the isthmus and cervix (Fig. 6–6). Spread beyond the uterus also occurs by lymphatic invasion, resulting in metastasis to the parametrial, pelvic, aortic, or inguinal lymph nodes and occasionally to the suburethral area. Blood-borne metastases are usually pulmonary; less frequently liver, brain, or bone is involved. Peritoneal implants from transtubal spread or transmural penetration of the tumor are relatively common in the more aggressive ECs, especially the papillary serous type. Once in the peritoneal cavity, EC behaves similarly to ovarian cancer.

Based on anatomic studies of uterine lymphatics and necropsy data from treated and untreated women dying with, and usually of, EC, several misconceptions regarding the behavior of this disease evolved. These misconceptions can be summarized as follows: (1) the primary route of spread is hematogenous; (2) lymphatic metastases occur preferentially to the aortic nodes; and (3) when pelvic node metastases are present, the disease has invariably spread beyond the pelvis. Several systematic, surgicopathologic investigations of operable EC have been reported that refute the aforementioned scenario of the EC spread pattern (Boronow et al, 1984; Creasman et al, 1987; Morrow et al, 1991). These studies have documented a clinically significant incidence of pelvic and aortic node metastases in clinical stage I EC (Table 6–5). The node metastasis rate increases with the depth of myoinvasion, loss of tumor differentiation, and extension to the isthmus or cervix. About one half of the patients with pelvic node metastases also have aortic node metastases, but the aortic glands are seldom a solitary site of metastasis. Thus these studies are in agreement with the long-recognized correlation between tumor grade, myoinvasion, and prognosis.

Pathology

Histologic expression of EC includes clear cell, adenosquamous, papillary serous, papillary endometrioid, mucinous, and secretory carcinoma. These are discussed later in this chapter. The common villoglandular and endometrioid ECs are typically divided into three subgroups on the basis of their histologic features, the least differentiated being designated grade 3. While histologic differentiation of EC is a major determinant of the prognosis, it has not been incorporated by

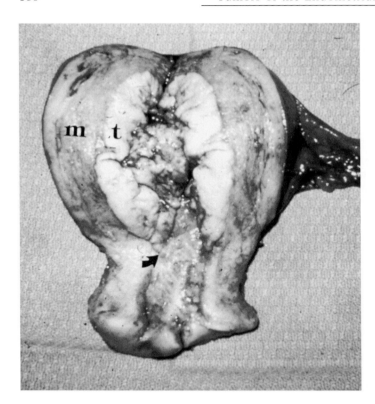

FIGURE 6-6. Adenocarcinoma with diffuse involvement of the endometrium. The margin between the tumor (t) and the myometrium (m) is distinct. Note that the tumor extends to the isthmis and stops (arrow).

the International Federation of Gynecology and Obstetrics (FIGO) into the staging of corpus carcinoma (Tables 6–6 and 6–7). For stage I cases, the distribution of grades 1, 2, and 3 approximates 45, 35, and 20 percent, respectively. Well-differentiated tumors are the most common, but wide variations are reported, reflecting different patient populations and the lack of a standardized grading

system. The new FIGO grading system is semiquantitative, which may produce greater consistency. It also introduces nuclear atypia into the grading system such that atypia inappropriate for the architectural grade raises the grade one level. Many lesions show differences in grade from area to area; thus grading must be based on thorough sampling. The influence of histologic grade on survival is apparent from the data reported in Table 6–8.

Diagnostic problems are encountered at both extremes of the differentiation scale: the very well-differentiated carcinomas are difficult to distinguish from atypical hyperplasia (Fig. 6–7), and the very poorly differentiated carcinomas may resemble sarcoma. Errors of the first type are far more common, however. It is important to distinguish well-differentiated carcinoma from atypical hyperplasia in the curettage specimen from the young woman who wishes to remain fertile. The crux of the problem, according to Kurman and Norris (1982), is identifying endometrial stromal invasion. They have proposed four criteria: (1) an irregular infiltration of glands associated with an altered fibroblastic stroma; (2) a confluent, cribriform glandular pattern; (3) an extensive glandular pattern; and (4) re-

TABLE 6-5

Frequency of Significant Factors Determined in Patients With Clinical Stage I Endometrial Carcinoma Undergoing Surgicopathologic Staging (Gynecologic Oncology Group data)*

Prognostic Factor	No.	Percent of Total
Outer one third myometrial invasion	33	14.9
Positive pelvic peritoneal cytology	26	11.7[†]
Pelvic node metastases	23	10.4
Extension to cervix/isthmus	18	8.1
Aortic node metastases	17	7.6[‡]
Adnexal metastases	16	7.2
LVSI	16	7.2
Peritoneal tumor implants	6	2.7

*Data from Boronow et al (1984).
[†]Percentage of all 222 cases. Procedure not done in 51 cases.
[‡]Percentage of all 222 cases. Procedure not done in 65 cases.

TABLE 6–6

FIGO Surgical Staging for Carcinoma of the Corpus Uteri (1988)*

Stage I
Stage Ia G123 — Tumor limited to endometrium
Stage Ib G123 — Invasion to less than one-half the myometrium
Stage Ic G123 — Invasion to or more than one-half the myometrium
Stage II
Stage IIa G123 — Endocervical glandular involvement only
Stage IIb G123 — Cervical stromal invasion
Stage III
Stage IIIa G123 — Tumor invades serosa and/or adnexa, and/or positive peritoneal cytology
Stage IIIb G123 — Vaginal metastases
Stage IIIc G123 — Metastases to pelvic and/or para-aortic lymph nodes
Stage IV
Stage IVa G123 — Tumor invasion of bladder and/or bowel mucosa
Stage IVb — Distant metastases including intra-abdominal and/or inguinal lymph nodes

*From International Federation of Gynecology and Obstetrics: Annual report on the results of treatment in gynecologic cancer. Int J Gynecol Obstet 28:189, 1989. Copyright 1991, Elsevier Science, with permission.

placement of stroma by masses of squamous epithelium. The presence of cilia does not exclude malignancy (Hendrickson and Kempson, 1983). The magnitude of discrepant diagnoses in various studies has ranged from 15 to 30 percent, usually on the overcall side (Bhagavan et al, 1984; Winkler et al, 1984). When the uterus is available for study, the presence of myometrial invasion is unequivocal evidence of malignancy. Unfortunately, because of the irregularity of the endometrial-myometrial interface, early myometrial invasion is subject to misinterpretation.

The importance of cervical extension, vascular space invasion, and depth of myoinvasion is discussed later in this chapter. It is noted here that EC can arise from, or involve secondarily, pre-existing adenomyosis, even in the outer third of the myometrium. This situation is apparently attended by a better prognosis than true myoinvasion (Jacques and Lawrence, 1990).

Clinical Staging

In recognition of the longstanding fact that nearly all patients with EC undergo surgery, in 1988 the FIGO staging for EC was changed from clinical to surgical. However, clinical staging is still important in terms of preoperative evaluation and planning for surgery, and still correlates well with prognosis (Table 6–9). The most important elements are the physical examination and the fractional curettage, as previously discussed. In more than 75 percent of the cases there is no clinical evidence of extrauterine involvement. For these patients the only additional studies re-

TABLE 6–7

FIGO Definition of Grading for Endometrial Carcinoma*

Cases of carcinoma of the corpus should be grouped with regard to the degree of differentiation of the adenocarcinoma as follows:
G1, 5% or less of a nonsquamous or nonmorular solid growth pattern
G2, 6–50% of a nonsquamous or nonmorular solid growth pattern
G3, more than 50% of a nonsquamous or nonmorular solid growth pattern

Notes on Pathologic Grading:
1. Notable nuclear atypia, inappropriate for the architectural grade, raises the grade of a grade 1 or grade 2 tumor by 1
2. In serous adenocarcinomas, clear cell adenocarcinomas, and squamous cell carcinomas, nuclear grading takes precedence
3. Adenocarcinomas with squamous differentiation are graded according to the nuclear grade of the glandular component

*From International Federation of Gynecology and Obstetrics: Annual report on the results of treatment in gynecologic cancer. Int J Gynecol Obstet 28:189, 1989. Copyright 1991, Elsevier Science, with permission.

TABLE 6–8

Actuarial 5-Year Survival of Patients With Clinical Stages Ia and Ib Endometrial Carcinoma*

Histologic Grade	Total Patients	Percent in Grade	Percent Survival Stage Ia	Percent Survival Stage Ib
1	2455	48.6	85.4	79.7
2	1863	36.9	79.5	66.3
3	729	14.4	70.9	54.0

*Data from International Federation of Gynecology and Obstetrics (1991).

TABLE 6–9

Actuarial Survival of Patients With Endometrial Carcinoma Related to Clinical Stage, 1982–1986*

Clinical Stage	Total Patients	Percent in Stage	5-Year Survival (%)
I	7,092	70.2	76.3
II	1,803	17.8	59.2
III	818	8.1	29.4
IV	364	3.6	10.3

*Data from International Federation of Gynecology and Obstetrics (1991).

quired are chest radiography and the usual preoperative chemistries. Malignant tissue in the ECC does not confirm cervical involvement unless there is cervical invasion present, since the false-positive rate is high when tumor tissue is present but cervical tissue invasion is not observed (Chen and Lee, 1986) (Table 6–10). The prognostic importance of stromal invasion in the endocervical curettings has been well documented (Table 6–11). Gross cervical involvement augurs a worse prognosis than microscopic disease (60 vs. 75 percent 5-year survival). The lesion grade, however, more strongly influences the outcome in EC than does the presence of cervical invasion (Wallin et al, 1984).

Conization should be used only when it is uncertain that a malignancy exists or whether the cancer is endometrial or cervical in origin.

Hysteroscopy and hysterography have been used to determine the extent of tumor and its proximity to the cervix, but both have the potential to push cancer cells through the fallopian tubes and into uterine vascular spaces. Their use should be limited to cases in which a diagnosis is not forthcoming by the usual procedures. Occasionally, both cervix and endometrium are overtly involved with adenocarcinoma, and it is impossible to determine whether the origin is cervical, isthmic, or fundal. This is the classic *corporis et colli* lesion and should be considered endometrial in origin.

About 20 percent of patients with clinical stage I or II EC have an elevated serum CA-125 value, a finding that correlates with the risk for extrauterine disease. In the combined reports of Duk et al (1986) and Patsner et al

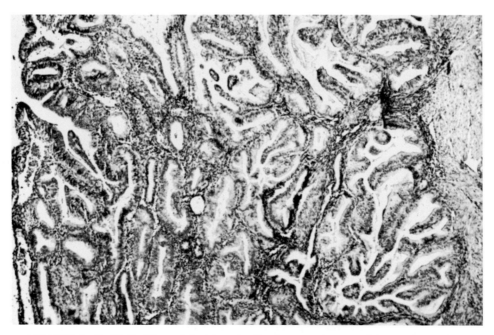

FIGURE 6–7. Well-differentiated (grade 1) adenocarcinoma of the endometrium.

TABLE **6–10**

Reliability of Endocervical Curettage (ECC) in Detecting Cervical Invasion by Endometrial Carcinoma*

| | False-Positive Rate | | | | False-Negative Rate | | | |
| | | Cervix Not Invaded[†] | | | | | Cervix Invaded[†] | |
Tumor in ECC	Total Cases	No.	Percent	No Tumor in ECC	Total Cases	No.	Percent
With normal endocervical cells	29	26	90	Normal endocervical cells	65	5	8
Tumor only	16	13	80	Inadequate specimen	13	0	0
Stroma invaded	7	0	0	No tissue in specimen	4	0	0
Total	52	39	75	Total	82	5	6

*Data from Chen and Lee (1986).
[†]Based on pathologic evaluation of hysterectomy specimen.

(1988), 80 percent of surgically upstaged patients had an elevated serum CA-125 value preoperatively, compared with 8 percent of patients without surgicopathologic evidence of extrauterine disease.

A spate of reports has appeared since 1985 concerning transvaginal ultrasound and magnetic resonance imaging (MRI) of myoinvasion. Since the probability of extrauterine metastases correlates with the depth of myoinvasion, this is potentially important information in planning surgery. In brief, it appears that both methods can measure the depth of myoinvasion in about 80 percent of cases, but the accuracy is poor for deeply invasive lesions. The studies are somewhat less reliable for detecting cervical invasion and unreliable for determining the presence of lymph node and intraperitoneal metastases (Cacciatore et al, 1989; Gordon et al, 1990; Belloni et al, 1990; Hricak et al, 1991). Since MRI is much more expensive than ultrasound, the latter is the method of choice for assessing myometrial invasion preoperatively.

TABLE **6–11**

Survival in Stage II Endometrial Carcinoma Related to Cervical Stromal Invasion on Endocervical Curettage or Hysterectomy

| | Stromal Invasion | | | |
| | Present | | Absent | |
Source	N	Survival (%)	N	Survival (%)
Surwit et al (1979)*	78[†]	47	39[‡]	74
Bigelow et al (1983)[§]	14	50	5	100

*Altogether, 47 patients received preoperative radiation and 14 were given radiation alone. The effect of radiation on the findings and survival was not given in the paper.
[†]Twenty cases were diagnosed on the basis of hysterectomy.
[‡]Twelve cases were diagnosed on the basis of hysterectomy.
[§]Hysterectomy specimens only. No patients received preoperative radiation.

More extensive preoperative evaluation is indicated for patients whose disease has features that put them at high risk for metastases. When the lesion is poorly differentiated, papillary serous, clear cell, or sarcomatous, computed tomography (CT) of the abdomen and pelvis is warranted to evaluate the liver and retroperitoneal nodes. CT scanning should also be performed on patients who have abnormal liver function tests, an elevated serum CA-125 value, clinical evidence of metastases, or parametrial or vaginal extension. Adnexal pathology is common in patients with EC, because the tubes and ovaries are frequent sites of metastases. Furthermore, EC tends to occur in conjunction with certain ovarian malignancies (endometrioid, clear cell, and granulosa tumors). Ultrasound is the study of choice to evaluate the adnexa. For locally advanced disease, cystoscopy and/or barium enema may be indicated. Bone and brain scans are not useful in the absence of symptoms.

Surgicopathologic Staging

The inherent inaccuracy of clinical staging for EC is a serious impediment to the selection of optimal therapy and over the years has resulted in both overtreatment and undertreatment. The magnitude of understaging is 15 to 25 percent (Boronow et al, 1984; Cowles et al, 1985; Creasman et al, 1987; Morrow et al, 1991; Orr et al, 1991). While node metastases, myometrial invasion, intraperitoneal implants, adnexal metastases, lymph–vascular space invasion (LVSI), and peritoneal cytology cannot be readily evaluated or are not evaluable clinically, even those data on which clinical staging has been based often cannot be assessed accurately or are of dubious prognostic significance. Up to 20 percent of tumors have a worse histologic grade based on the hysterectomy specimen than the curettings (Cowles et al, 1985; Daniel and Peters, 1988), and the false-negative rate for the ECC is 5 to 10 percent (Chen and Lee, 1986). On occasion, overstaging may also occur, especially if the interpretation of a positive ECC is not based on documented cervical invasion.

The findings of the 222-patient Gynecologic Oncology Group (GOG) pilot surgicopathologic staging study of EC are presented in Table 6–5. (This study is more representative of the frequency of these events than is the subsequent group-wide GOG study, since the latter admitted patients more selectively.) Altogether, 18 percent of the study group had demonstrable evidence of extrauterine spread, including 10 percent with pelvic and 7 percent with aortic node metastases. Some patients had multiple site involvement. The prognosis with a single adverse finding is obviously better than that for patients with multiple adverse factors. Table 6–12 correlates the frequency of pelvic and aortic node metastases with histologic grade and myometrial invasion determined by the group-wide GOG staging study. The node metastasis rate to the pelvic and aortic chains ranges from 14 to 34 percent for grade 2 and 3 lesions with outer one third myometrial invasion, a clinically substantial number. Other reports are in harmony with these findings (Piver et al, 1982; Chen and Lee, 1983; Figge et al, 1983).

The prognostic value of the surgicopathologic staging data has been quantified in the group-wide GOG study (Morrow et al, 1991). There is a recurrence risk of 60 percent at 5 years for patients with aortic node metastasis, 35 percent for LVSI, 25 percent for pelvic node or adnexal metastasis, and 22 percent for positive pelvic cytology. With two or more sites of extrauterine metastases, nearly 45 per-

cent of patients had recurrence. Involvement of the isthmus/cervix was not a statistically significant factor, but the varying degrees of cervical involvement as incorporated in the 1988 FIGO staging system were not assessed separately.

It is of interest that, after aortic node metastasis, LVSI appears to be the single most important adverse prognostic feature. Other investigators have also noted a higher recurrence rate in patients with demonstrable LVSI (Aalders et al, 1984b; Hanson et al, 1985; Sivridis et al, 1987). About 15 percent of stage I cases have LVSI. The frequency of this finding increases with advancing age, grade, and muscle invasion, and time to recurrence is shorter in patients with LVSI.

The depth of myometrial invasion and histologic grade have prognostic import even in the absence of LVSI and extrauterine disease. This is clearly demonstrated in the 390 GOG patients with all risk factors negative (aortic and pelvic nodes, adnexa, cytology, LVSI, and cervix) other than grade and myoinvasion. Altogether, 5 percent recurred. Only 3.8 percent of patients with grade 1 tumors and less than middle one third myoinvasion suffered a relapse, compared with 19 percent of patients with grade 3 cancers and middle to outer one third invasion (Table 6–13).

Other tumor factors also have prognostic importance, although their role in treatment planning remain uncertain. Schink et al (1991) reported that the rate of pelvic node metastasis correlates with tumor size in EC (<2 cm, 4 percent; >2 cm, 15 percent; entire cavity, 35 percent). They found that, for grade 2 lesions less than 2 cm in diameter, there were no patients with pelvic node involvement if myoinvasion was less than 50 percent, but with deeper myoinvasion 18 percent had node metastases. Hormone-receptor-rich EC has a better prognosis than does hormone-receptor-poor EC, even after correcting for stage and grade (Palmer et al, 1988; Ingram et al, 1989; Nyholm et al, 1995). DNA ploidy and S-phase fraction determined by flow cytometry have been studied intensely during the past decade to determine their value in predicting malignant behavior. The reported results for EC are mixed, largely because aneuploidy and tetraploidy, although associated with a poor prognosis, strongly correlate with dedifferentiation. It is still uncertain whether flow cytometry will be of value in distinguishing atypical hyperplasia from grade 1 carcinoma or in predicting which

T A B L E **6–12**

Frequency of Pelvic and Aortic Node Metastasis in Clinical Stage I Endometrial Carcinoma*

Histologic Grade	Total Cases	Maximum Myoinvasion			
		None	Inner 1/3	Mid 1/3	Outer 1/3
		Percent pelvic node metastases			
1	180	0	3	0	11
2	288	3	5	9	19
3	153	0	9	4	34
		Percent aortic node meatastases			
1	180	0	1	5	6
2	288	3	4	0	14
3	153	0	4	0	24

*Data from Creasman et al (1987).

TABLE 6–13

Recurrences in Endometrial Cancer With Negative Risk Factors[*,†]

Histologic Grade	Myoinvasion	Radiation Therapy		None	Total	Percent
		Implant Only	Pelvic	None	Total	Percent
1	<1/3	0/22	1/19°	5/116[++,°]	6/157	3.8
	>1/3	0/4	2/17[+]	0/4	2/25	8.0
2	<1/3	0/20	3/25	2/58	5/103	4.8
	>1/3	0/4	6/36[+,°]	2/9[°°]	8/49	16.3
3	<1/3	0/7	2/16[+]	3/12°	5/35	14.3
	>1/3	0/1	3/19[+]	1/1[+]	4/21	19.0

*Data from Morrow et al (1991).
†Aortic nodes, pelvic nodes, adnexa, cervix, and cytology negative for tumor. No LVSI.
°Each circle represents one vaginal recurrence.
+Each plus represents one pelvic recurrence.

grade 1 cancers will recur (Britton et al, 1990; Newbury et al, 1990; Sorbe et al, 1990; Podratz et al, 1993; Pfisterer et al, 1995). Oncogene expression (HER-2/*neu* and p53, inter alia) has not yet achieved clinical value because of the strong association with grade, myoinvasion, and other standard prognostic determinants (Hetzel et al, 1992; Kohler et al, 1996).

Treatment

It has been known for more than 50 years that most women with early EC can be cured by hysterectomy or intracavitary radiation therapy (Heyman et al, 1941). Early on, a common site of failure in the surgical series was observed to be the vaginal cuff and paracervical tissue, whereas persistent tumor in the uterus was frequent in the radiation therapy group even with use of the uterine packing technique. As hysterectomy became a safer procedure, a widespread practice evolved in the United States to treat EC with intracavitary radium therapy followed by hysterectomy after a 4- to 6-week recovery period. The incidence of local failure in stage I was reduced from the 3 to 8 percent range to 1 to 3 percent by the use of radiation. In addition, surgery eliminated uterine failures. Treatment by surgery alone in this scheme has been generally reserved for the patient with a very low risk of recurrence (grades 1 and 2 upper corpus lesions with little or no myometrial invasion), whereas radiation therapy alone is used in medically (severe pulmonary and/or heart disease) and technically inoperable cases.

The survival rate with hysterectomy is greater than that with radiation therapy alone by 15 to 25 percentage points (Varia et al, 1987; Sorbe et al, 1989; Lehoczky et al, 1991). Extending the operation to a modified or full radical hysterectomy, with or without pelvic lymphadenectomy, does not seem to improve the results (Rutledge, 1974). Simple hysterectomy alone, however, in some clinics has produced survival rates similar to those of combined radiation therapy and surgery, even with the higher incidence of cuff failures in the surgery-only group (Hording and Hansen, 1985), not because radiation therapy has no life-sparing effect but because the number of cases salvaged by the addition of radiation therapy is too small to detect in most clinical trials (Aalders et al, 1980).

The cuff or paracervical recurrences have been attributed to operative spill through the cervical canal or intraoperative squeezing of the tumor into the lymphatics at the perimeter of the uterus. A number of mechanical methods were introduced to occlude the cervix (screws, clamps, suturing the cervix closed), but they have failed to gain acceptance. Ligating the tubes at hysterectomy has also been recommended. However, it is very doubtful that these local failures are due to surgically induced implantation metastases. The risk of cuff recurrence is directly related to the degree of myometrial invasion, tumor dedifferentiation, and cervical extension. These factors are well known to be associated with the risk of lymphatic invasion. Preoperative irradiation customarily treats the cervix, upper vagina, and paracervical tissue in addition to the uterine tumor, and it is just as reasonable to accept the idea that the local recurrence rate is diminished because tumor already existing in lymphatic channels is eradicated by the radiation.

With the development of high-energy radiation therapy machines, there has been a rapid shift from intracavitary, preoperative irradiation to whole-pelvis external beam therapy, without any measurable change in results except, perhaps, a small increase in complications. Teletherapy has the attractive advantage of delivering a homogeneous dose of radiation to the uterus and the tissues at its perimeter in an outpatient setting. Postoperative radiation therapy has also become a common practice in the management of operable EC. While it lacks the potential of preventing intraoperative spread of cancer, in practice it has proved to be as effective as preoperative radiation therapy in eliminating local or pelvic failures while permitting a more accurate assessment of the extent of disease, both intra- and extrauterine. With this information, individualization of treatment can be optimized. Nevertheless, it is probably true that postoperative whole-pelvis radiation, especially following extended surgical staging, carries a slightly higher risk of complications than does preoperative whole-pelvis radiation. Some treatment centers use one preoperative intracavitary implant followed by hysterectomy within 3 to 5 days so that accurate surgicopathologic staging is still possible (Sause et al, 1990). This approach also takes advantage of the uterus for brachytherapy insertion, permitting a higher parametrial dose to be given more safely.

During the past decade, the focal point of EC management has shifted from refinements in radiation therapy technique, measured against extramural and historical controls, to randomized clinical studies and surgicopathologic staging. The latter permits the surgeon to define the population at risk for recurrence more accurately and to tailor treatment to the needs of the individual patient. The following paragraphs contain the authors' recommendations for managing EC. Algorithms for operative and postoperative management of stages I and II (occult) are presented in Figures 6–8 and 6–9, respectively. The permutations of this treatment plan in use today are numerous.

Stage I and Occult Stage II

After the work-up is completed, the patient with clinical stage I or occult stage II (positive ECC with no clinical evidence of cervical involvement) EC of any grade or histology is subjected to an exploratory laparotomy as the

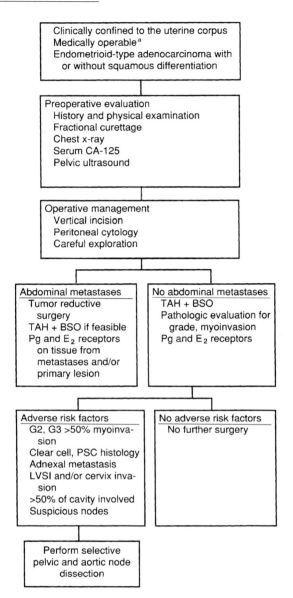

FIGURE 6–8. Algorithm for operative management of clinical stages I and II (occult) endometrial carcinoma. [a]Vaginal hysterectomy is feasible when patient is medically unsuitable for abdominal surgery. BSO = bilateral salpingo-oophorectomy; PSC = papillary serous carcinoma; TAH = total abdominal hysterectomy.

first step in the treatment program. This approach reflects the generally accepted evidence that most patients with EC do not need adjuvant radiation therapy, that preoperative radiation therapy can obscure important surgicopathologic information about the cancer, and that postoperative radiation therapy is as effective as preoperative radiation therapy in

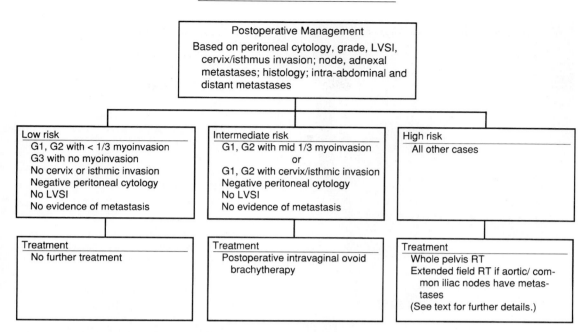

FIGURE 6–9. Postoperative management algorithm for endometrial carcinoma. RT = radiation therapy.

reducing the risk for local/regional recurrence. The objective is to obtain, as accurately as feasible, the surgicopathologic staging data concurrent with the hysterectomy. These staging data provide the information base for the selection of postoperative adjuvant therapy. Pertinent details of the operative procedure are described in the following paragraphs. It is important to recognize that additional surgery of any magnitude adds to the operative risk. Consequently, the indications for selective lymph node dissection must always be evaluated in light of the risk to the patient. Operative death attributable to surgical staging has been reported, but in general, when performed by trained personnel, the procedure adds little morbidity to the basic surgery (Moore et al, 1989; Orr et al, 1991). Preoperative indications that extended surgical staging may be necessary are cervical invasion, high-risk histology, and elevated serum CA-125.

The abdomen is opened with a vertical, lower abdominal incision, and peritoneal washings are taken of the pelvis and abdomen. Careful exploration is then carried out looking and feeling for evidence of omental, liver, peritoneal, cul de sac, and adnexal metastases. The aortic and pelvic areas are palpated for nodal metastases. An extrafascial, total hysterectomy with bilateral salpingo-oophorectomy is then performed in the least

traumatic fashion. No instruments should be placed on the uterus itself. Removal of the adnexa, even if they appear normal, is part of the therapy, since the adnexa may contain microscopic metastases or a primary ovarian tumor. This is true even for premenopausal women with EC (Gitsch et al, 1995). Furthermore, the ovaries may be the source of estrogen production that could stimulate residual, occult EC. It is not necessary to remove a margin of vaginal cuff, nor does there appear to be any benefit from excising parametrial tissue in the usual case. The entire cervix, however, needs to be removed.

The uterus is opened off the field to determine the extent of the growth. If there is obvious adnexal involvement or grossly suspicious pelvic or aortic node involvement, regardless of histologic grade, or evidence of greater than 50 percent myoinvasion with a grade 2 or 3 lesion (Fig. 6–10), a selective left and right aortic/common iliac node dissection is performed (Fig. 6–8). (In the group-wide GOG study, 47 of 48 patients with aortic node involvement had one or more of these findings at staging laparotomy.) If the depth of invasion is not grossly evident, it should be determined by frozen section analysis (Fig. 6–11). Gross evaluation of myoinvasion becomes less reliable with decreasing grade of lesion. Frozen section analysis is about 95 percent reliable compared with 80 percent for

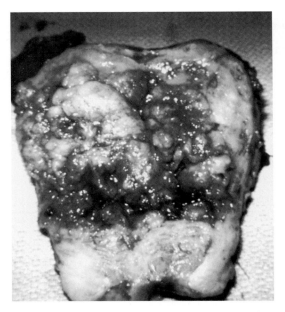

FIGURE 6–10. The uterus has been opened on one side and laid flat, exposing a polypoid endometrial carcinoma. Since the tumor extends to the isthmus, a fractional curettage (two fractions) will probably contain carcinoma in the endocervical component. While this might be considered a false-positive finding, the implications of tumor at the isthmus are similar to those of cervical extension (stage II).

gross inspection (Goff and Rice, 1990; Noumoff et al, 1991). Node sampling is also recommended for all patients with a papillary serous or clear cell carcinoma. The node-bearing retroperitoneum should first be evaluated with the peritoneum opened to identify enlarged or suspicious lymph nodes. If these are positive on frozen section, selective node dissection (Fig. 6–12) is unnecessary, but all enlarged nodes should be removed. About 25 percent or fewer EC patients will have an indication for aortic node sampling.

An alternative approach is the laparoscopic-assisted vaginal hysterectomy and adnexectomy. The pelvic and aortic nodes can be removed as indicated, the peritoneal cavity scrutinized, and the cytology obtained. This method has the advantage of reduced patient recovery time (Childers et al, 1993).

The pathologist's intra- and postoperative evaluations of the specimen are extremely important if optimal results are to be obtained. The least differentiated area of the tumor, the greatest depth of myometrial invasion, the presence of LVSI, the histologic subtype, and the proximity of the tumor to

the isthmus and cervix need to be defined. Each of these factors has prognostic as well as therapeutic implications. In addition, accurate study of the peritoneal cytology, lymph nodes, and adnexa is necessary. Hormone receptor analysis of the primary and metastatic tumor is recommended to assist in the selection of postoperative treatment and to advise the patient with regard to estrogen replacement therapy.

Postoperatively, patients can be divided into three groups based on the risk for recurrence (Fig. 6–9):

1. *Low risk* (<5 percent): patients with grade 1 or 2 endometrioid/adenosquamous lesions confined to the upper two thirds of the corpus, no evidence of extrauterine spread, no LVSI, and no or superficial myoinvasion. These patients require no further treatment.
2. *Intermediate risk* (5 to 10 percent): grade 1 or 2 EC confined to the upper two thirds of the corpus, no evidence of extrauterine spread, with middle one third myoinvasion and no LVSI. Grade 1 or 2 lesions with no or superficial myoinvasion and extension to the cervix or isthmus also fall into this group. These patients should have postoperative intravaginal ovoid brachytherapy.
3. *High risk* (>10 percent): adnexal metastases, grade 3 with any degree of myoinvasion, grade 1 or 2 with greater than two thirds myoinvasion, grade 2 with middle one third invasion, and isthmic/cervix involvement; pelvic node metastases; and LVSI. These patients are candidates for postoperative pelvic radiation (4,000 to 5,000 cGy at 170 to 180 rad/daily fraction).

If metastases to the aortic nodes are documented, extended-field radiation therapy is recommended in the absence of more widespread metastases, because 40 percent of these patients are expected to survive 5 years or longer (American College of Obstetricians and Gynecologists [ACOG], 1991; Potish et al, 1985b; Morrow et al, 1991).

In this scheme 50 to 75 percent of patients receive no postoperative therapy. Patients with aortic node metastases should have a postoperative CT scan of the liver and thorax prior to initiating radiation therapy. If the aortic node metastases are large or multiple, a scalene fat pad dissection is warranted, since node metastasis at this level would be a con-

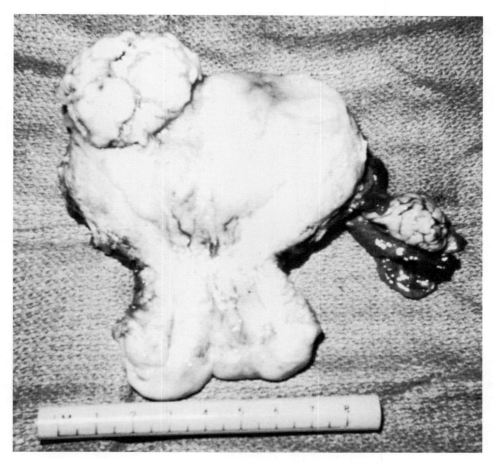

FIGURE 6–11. Endometrial carcinoma. Specimen from a 53-year-old overweight female. Frozen section evaluation revealed a grade 3 lesion with 50 percent myometrial invasion. Clinically occult aortic node metastases were documented by removing the precaval fat pad. The patient is alive and well 10 years after extended-field radiation therapy.

traindication to aortic field radiation therapy. The morbidity of extended-field therapy after surgery, in our view, precludes the use of aortic radiation therapy solely on the basis of uterine risk factors (e.g., grade 3 lesions with outer one third myometrial invasion). Thus the emphasis in this protocol is on surgical documentation of nodal involvement.

Vaginal cuff radiation adds little to the local control benefit of external beam therapy and clearly increases the risk of complications, especially after the extra dissection required by the surgical staging procedure. Therefore, vaginal cuff radiation therapy is not recommended in conjunction with external beam radiation therapy. Treatment of the entire vagina in early EC is unwarranted.

Modifications of the optimal therapy are permissible or even necessary at times. For instance, there are situations in which the low transverse incision is a reasonable choice, especially in the young obese woman with a well-differentiated adenocarcinoma. However, the surgeon who selects this incision should be prepared to make a separate vertical incision if it is required to carry out the proper surgical procedure. The incision must not determine which operation is performed. In EC, the probability that a low transverse incision will prove to be inadequate is substantial if the patient has a moderately to poorly differentiated malignancy, an enlarged uterus, deep myoinvasion, cervical extension, adnexal tumor, adverse histology, advanced age, or elevated serum CA-125 value.

Vaginal hysterectomy for EC is another compromise that is useful in certain cases even though the adnexa may not be remov-

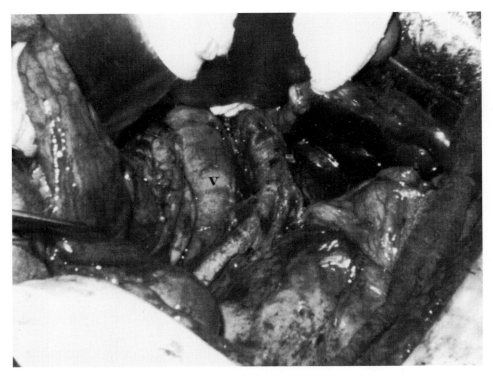

FIGURE 6–12. Selective aortic node dissection for endometrial carcinoma. Photograph taken after removal of the precaval fat pad and the left aortic nodes. V = vena cava.

able and exploration of the pelvis and abdomen not possible (Peters et al, 1983; Bloss et al, 1991). The most frequently cited indication for vaginal hysterectomy in EC is morbid obesity. However, vaginal hysterectomy is often a more imposing procedure in the obese woman, especially if she is nulliparous, than is abdominal hysterectomy. Consequently, the vaginal approach is often not an easy solution to this problem. Furthermore, most obese women are in generally good health, so they should get optimal therapy. The most convincing indication for vaginal hysterectomy as definitive surgical therapy for EC is the existence of a medical problem that is a contraindication to an abdominal operation but would be an acceptable risk for vaginal surgery. Thus the vaginal approach becomes a choice intermediate between optimal surgery and no surgery.

Adjuvant therapy with progestins, cytotoxic chemotherapy, and radiation therapy have all been tested in early-stage EC (the latter two modalities for patients at high risk for recurrence), with no obvious patient benefit in the trials reported to date (Martinez et al, 1989; Vergote et al, 1989; Stringer et al, 1990; Moore et al, 1991).

Stage II

Patients with clinically occult stage II EC (a clinically normal cervix with microscopic cervical invasion on the ECC) are managed the same as stage I patients, except that no intraoperative frozen section is needed to document the indication for selective pelvic and aortic node dissection. A modified radical hysterectomy would also be appropriate since microscopic parametrial disease is found in 10 percent of these patients (Yura et al, 1996). The reported survival of stage II patients varies widely, but there is considerable agreement that patients with occult involvement have a substantially better 5-year survival than do those with overt cervical invasion.

When the cervix is clinically involved by tumor, whole-pelvis radiation therapy, intracavitary brachytherapy, plus adjunctive simple hysterectomy with selective aortic/common iliac node dissection is the traditional treatment of choice (see also Chapter 17). As in stage I EC, the addition of hysterectomy substantially improves the survival in stage II disease (Cox et al, 1980). In selected cases primary surgical therapy may be appropriate.

Optimal surgical treatment requires a Wertheim radical hysterectomy with bilateral pelvic lymphadenectomy and selective aortic node dissection. If the pelvic and aortic nodes, surgical margins, and washings are negative, no further treatment is needed. Otherwise, pelvic or extended-field radiation therapy may be appropriate, especially for hormone-receptor-poor tumors.

Stage III

Patients who have clinical stage III EC as a result of vaginal or parametrial extension are given pelvic radiation therapy after a thorough metastatic survey. When the therapy is complete, exploratory laparotomy is recommended for those patients whose disease seems to be resectable. Along with the hysterectomy and adnexectomy, surgicopathologic staging is carried out to determine the extent of residual disease. Extended-field radiation therapy or systemic therapy with cytotoxic drugs or hormones is warranted in the presence of extrapelvic metastases. If tumor tissue is obtained for hormone receptor analysis, the choice between chemotherapy and hormone therapy can be facilitated.

Patients placed in the clinical stage III category on the basis of an adnexal mass should, after proper evaluation, undergo surgery without preoperative radiation therapy to determine the nature of the mass (inflammatory, primary ovarian cancer, metastasis), to perform surgicopathologic staging, and to carry out tumor-reductive surgery. If the uterus is resectable, hysterectomy and adnexectomy should also be done.

The current FIGO stage III is surgicopathologic and includes those patients with disease involving the adnexa, pelvic lymph nodes, aortic lymph nodes, vagina, and pelvic peritoneum and with malignant peritoneal cytology—a very heterogeneous prognostic group (e.g., pelvic lymph node metastasis as the only adverse feature is associated with a 75 percent 5-year survival rate). Although parametrial disease is not mentioned in the new staging system, presumably this would also qualify a patient for stage III grouping. Patients with microscopic stage III disease have a 40 to 80 percent 5-year survival compared with the 10 to 30 percent rate for those with gross extrauterine pelvic extension. Survival in the latter group, however, correlates strongly with resectability (Aalders et al, 1984a; Mackillop and Pringle, 1985; Genest et al, 1987). A large proportion of the current FIGO stage III cases are otherwise stage I patients who have a positive cytology. The treatment of these patients is discussed later in this chapter. The recommended treatment of patients with pelvic and/or aortic node metastases was discussed earlier in this chapter.

Stage IV

EC patients with clinical evidence of extrapelvic metastasis are usually most suitable for systemic hormonal therapy or chemotherapy. Local radiation, however, is often beneficial, particularly to brain or bone metastases (Fig. 6–13). Occasionally, pelvic radiation therapy or hysterectomy will be indicated to provide local tumor control (Aalders et al, 1984c) and prevent bleeding or complications such as

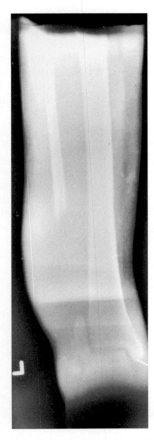

FIGURE 6–13. Roentgenogram of the lower leg. The patient presented with an enlarged, painful ankle and uterine bleeding. She refused therapy, but biopsy of the endometrium and leg documented the diagnosis of endometrial adenocarcinoma with metastases to the fibula.

pyometra, especially in the patient who is to undergo chemotherapy. The efficacy of whole-abdomen radiation therapy in EC involving the peritoneal cavity is uncertain. Some authors report that macroscopic metastases cannot be cleared with whole-abdomen radiation (Potish et al, 1985a), whereas others report good success in patients with residual disease less than 2 cm (Greer and Hamberger, 1983). Nevertheless, it is good practice to reserve whole-abdomen therapy for those patients having no macroscopic abdominal disease or more distant metastases at the time of laparotomy (Loeffler et al, 1988). The remaining cases are managed the same as ovarian cancer: tumor-reductive surgery and chemotherapy, unless the metastases contain a high level of hormone receptor protein, in which case progestin or antiestrogen therapy is indicated.

Follow-Up

Surveillance of patients after treatment for clinical stage I EC has been critically evaluated in several studies (Berchuck et al, 1995; Reddock et al, 1995). The physical examination is most likely to be productive in the patient without symptoms, whereas the serum CA-125 and chest radiograph are the most useful tests in the patients who are asymptomatic and have a normal physical examination. From 75 to 95 percent of recurrences occur within 36 months of treatment, and 95 percent of the recurrences will be detected by evaluation of the symptomatic patient, routine physical examination, and routine serum CA-125 determination. The recommended follow-up schedule consists of an abdominal, pelvic, and peripheral lymph node examination, vaginal cytology studies, and serum CA-125 level determination at each visit. The interval between visits should be 3 to 6 months during the first 2 to 3 years, depending on the degree of risk for recurrence, and every 6 to 12 months thereafter. Periodic chest radiography and perhaps CT scanning of the abdomen might also be informative, the latter in patients with known nodal disease.

Estrogen Replacement Therapy

Many women after treatment for EC will suffer the effects of estrogen deficiency, including vasomotor instability, dyspareunia, vaginal dryness, and the risks of osteoporosis and atherosclerotic heart disease. Nevertheless, estrogen replacement therapy (ERT) has tra-

ditionally been proscribed because of the concern that residual, dormant EC might be activated by the hormone. While the magnitude of this risk has never been quantified, it is a logical concern. During the past decade a flood of data documenting the adverse effects of estrogen deficiency have renewed interest in giving estrogens to this group of women on the basis that the proven risks of not taking estrogen far outweigh the presumed risks of taking estrogen. The ACOG (1990) Committee Opinion on the issue follows this line of reasoning. It states that

> estrogens could be used for the same indications as for any other woman, except that the selection of appropriate candidates should be based upon prognostic indicators and the risk the patient is willing to assume. . . . For some women, the sense of well-being afforded by amelioration of menopausal symptoms or the need to treat atrophic vaginitis or osteoporosis may outweigh the risk of stimulating tumor growth.

Nevertheless, the ACOG (1986) Technical Bulletin on ERT lists EC as a contraindication to ERT.

When the tumor is negative for estrogen and progestin receptors, or there is no myometrial invasion, the administration of estrogens is clearly appropriate since the risk of recurrent cancer is nearly nil or the tumor would be insensitive to the hormone. For most women, however, an intermediate position would seem to provide the greatest benefit with the least risk. Since 75 percent or more of recurrences appear within 3 years after treatment, withholding ERT during this time period would minimize the chance of administering the hormone to patients with residual carcinoma. In the interim, satisfactory subjective improvement with respect to hot flashes can be obtained by prescribing MPA, 10 mg daily PO or 150 mg IM every 3 months. Bellergal and clonidine, both nonhormonal agents that are used to treat vasomotor symptoms in breast cancer patients, are alternatives to estrogen for relief of vasomotor symptoms. The recent availability of raloxifene, a selective estrogen receptor modulator, to a large degree solves the dilemma of administering estrogens to women with endometrial (and breast) cancer. This agent has an agonist-like effect on bone tissue and serum lipids, but an antagonist-like effect on endometrial and breast tissue (Draper et al, 1996).

Should nonestrogenic remedies prove ineffective, the balance of risks to benefits for ERT should be reviewed. The addition of progestin might diminish the potential growth-enhancing effect of the estrogen should there be any residual hormone-dependent carcinoma. However, an adequate antitumor dose would undoubtedly abrogate some of the beneficial effects of estrogen on the serum lipoproteins. Having receptor data on the patient's EC can assist in the decision to prescribe estrogens.

It is interesting to note that the patients most at risk for recurrence are least likely to have hormone-dependent tumors. Furthermore, the grade 1 lesions are most likely to be hormone responsive, but tend to recur late. Thus the administration of estrogens to women who have been treated for EC can never be considered absolutely safe with respect to the cancer.

RECURRENT ENDOMETRIAL CARCINOMA

The distribution of recurrences in early EC is strongly influenced by the type of treatment, that is, whether the patient receives local/regional radiation therapy in addition to surgery. In the surgery-only group, local/pelvic failure occurs more often than after combination therapy. For example, in the GOG study of 390 surgical stage I patients, vaginal/pelvic recurrences accounted for 53 percent of all recurrent cases in the surgery-only group, but only 30 percent in the surgery plus radiation therapy group (Morrow et al, 1991). Thus after radiation therapy 70 percent or more of patients who fail treatment will have distant metastases, and the majority of these will be without evidence of pelvic/local recurrence. The most common sites of extrapelvic metastases are lung, abdomen, aortic and supraclavicular nodes, brain, liver, and bone. Inguinal node and distal vaginal (suburethral) metastases also occur with sufficient frequency to be mentioned. In nonirradiated patients, the pelvic wall, parametrium/paracolopos, and vaginal apex are more important sites of treatment failure (Aalders and Abeler, 1982; Mandell et al, 1985; SK Chambers et al, 1987; Burke et al, 1990; Lurain et al, 1991).

Early-stage disease, especially grade 1, tends to relapse late, with as many as 20 percent of all recurrences appearing 5 years or more after initial therapy. Overall, however, as previously stated, 75 percent or more of the failures are diagnosed within the first 3 years after treatment (Aalders et al, 1984b; Greven and Olds, 1987; Kuten et al, 1989). Isolated local/regional recurrence after surgery has a much better prognosis than does a similar recurrence after radiation therapy but is also more common. The most favorable recurrence is the isolated proximal or distal vaginal recurrence. Five-year survival rates in the 25 to 50 percent range are usually reported. Outcome is better for late recurrence (>3 years) and for lesions less than 2 cm in diameter (Phillips et al, 1982; Greven and Olds, 1987; Kuten et al, 1989).

Local recurrences are preferably managed by radiation, surgery, or a combination of the two. In particular, large lesions should be excised whenever feasible. If the area has not been previously treated, the tumor bed can be irradiated postoperatively. An isolated pelvic recurrence of any grade is potentially curable, especially when it appears more than 1 or 2 years after initial therapy. In this setting, extended or radical surgery, including exenteration, may be justified if the patient has already received radiation. The results of pelvic exenteration, in properly selected cases, are similar to those obtained in cervical cancer (Morris et al, 1996). The best results with exenteration in endometrial carcinoma are obtained in patients with recurrence in the central pelvis at least 1 year post-therapy, grade 1 or 2, not amenable to curative radiation or hormonal therapy, with no evidence of extrauterine/central pelvic disease.

Hormonal Therapy

Background

In 1961, Kelly and Baker described objective regression of metastatic EC lasting for 9 to 54 months in 6 of 21 patients receiving high-dose progesterone or 17-alpha-hydroxyprogesterone acetate (Delalutin) therapy. Many of the patients also reported an improved sense of well-being and appetite. Since this landmark report, worldwide experience has consistently documented the efficacy of progestational drugs in treating recurrent or advanced EC. More recent reports, however, are discordant with the 20 to 40 percent response rates noted by earlier investigators (Table 6–14). Combining the results of the GOG and Mayo Clinic studies, among 474 pa-

TABLE **6–14**

Reported Response of Metastatic Endometrial Carcinoma to Progestin Therapy

Source	Progestin*	Dose	Total Cases	Objective Response[†] CR (%)	PR (%)	Stable (%)
Thigpen et al (1991)	MPA	200 mg/day PO	138	17	9	—
		1,000 mg/day PO	140	10	8	—
Thigpen et al (1986)	MPA	50 mg t.i.d. PO	331	10	8	50
Podratz et al (1985)	Megestrol	320 mg/day PO	81 ⎫			
	MPA	1–3 gm/week IM	33 ⎬	6	5	40
	Medrogestrone	800 mg/day PO	26 ⎭			
Piver et al (1980)	HPC	1 gm/week IM	51	14[‡]		20
	MPA	1 gm/week IM	37	19[‡]		30

*MPA = medroxyprogesterone acetate (Provera); megestrol = Megace; medrogestrone = Colprone; HCP = 17-alpha-hydroxyprogesterone caproate (Delautin).
[†]CR = complete response; PR = partial response.
[‡]Complete plus partial response.

tients with measurable disease, the complete and partial response rates were only 8.6 and 7.0 percent, respectively. Stabilization of disease was observed in 47 percent of patients. Consistent with the older literature, there was no apparent difference in the efficacy of the three agents. The median duration of survival for complete response patients was 57 months, for partial response patients 13 months, and for stable disease patients 5 months. The overall 5-year survival rate was 8 percent. A good response correlated with histologic differentiation (94 percent with grade 1, 15 percent with grade 2, and 1.5 percent with grade 3). Favorable prognostic factors included smaller tumor burden (<10 cm³) and longer duration since primary therapy (>36 months).

Regarding the duration of disease, Reifenstein (1974) observed, in a 308-patient study group, that the response rate ranged from 6 percent for patients whose cancer had been diagnosed 2 to 5 months before starting progestin therapy to 65 percent for patients with disease of more than 5 years' duration. The patient's age is also a prognostic factor, although it may not be an independent variable. Women who develop endometrial carcinoma at an early age tend to have less aggressive, better differentiated lesions that are prone to recur late. Disease that is widespread or within the field of radiation also appears to be less susceptible to progestin control than unirradiated or less extensive disease. The survival curves for responders and nonresponders are shown in Figure 6–14.

There is no convincing evidence in the literature of a dose-response effect of proges-

tational agents in EC, although it has been reported for breast cancer (160 vs. 800 mg/day megestrol acetate [Muss et al, 1990]; 1,000 mg MPA IM daily vs. 500 mg MPA IM twice weekly [Cavalli et al, 1984]). In fact, the GOG data comparing 200 mg/day to 1,000 mg/day of oral MPA in a randomized study showed better, but not statistically significant, results with the lower dose (16.7% vs. 10.0% CR) (Thigpen et al, 1991). There is also no evidence that one progestin is superior to another or that one route of administration is more therapeutic, despite the somewhat erratic absorption of progestins from the gastrointestinal tract.

Several studies of tamoxifen therapy in EC have been reported. It appears that the agent may be as effective against EC as progestin therapy, but it is quite inactive in patients refractory to progestins (Slavik et al, 1984; Edmonson et al, 1986; Quinn and Campbell, 1989). Gonadotropin-releasing hormone analogs have also been reported to have an antitumor effect in endometrial cancer, presumably by a direct effect on the tumor cells, even in patients with tumors refractory to progestin therapy (Jeyarajah et al, 1996).

Hormone Receptors

In the past two decades, important discoveries have been made about the modus operandi of the steroid hormones. Pre-eminent among these discoveries are the hormone receptor proteins. Normal endometrial growth is initiated by estradiol, which enters the cytoplasm by simple diffusion through the cell membrane. Specific cytoplasmic proteins (receptors) bind the hormone, and the complex

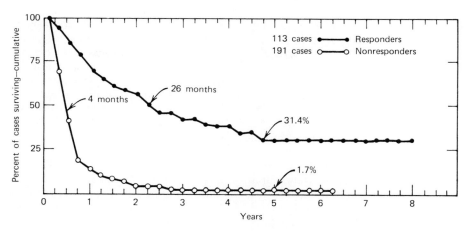

FIGURE 6–14. Survival curves for progestin responders and nonresponders among patients with advanced or recurrent endometrial carcinoma. (From Reifenstein EC Jr: The treatment of advanced endometrial cancer with hydroxyprogesterone caproate. Gynecol Oncol 2:377, 1974, with permission.)

enters the nucleus, where it binds to an acceptor protein at a specific locus on the DNA. This initiates protein synthesis, which leads to cell growth and division. Two of the proteins synthesized in response to estradiol modulation are estrogen receptor (ER) and progesterone receptor (PR). The latter complexes with progestin, enters the nucleus, binds with DNA, and, among other effects, inhibits the production of ER (and therefore also itself), promotes cell differentiation, and inhibits mitosis.

Since 1985 many investigators have published data on the relationship of receptor content in EC with traditional prognostic factors, response to hormone therapy, and outcome. The reports are most notable for their contradictory or inconsistent results. The major reasons for the divergent findings are probably the lack of a standard cutoff value for receptor positivity and assay variations resulting from the presence of receptor-containing nontumor tissue (stroma and myometrium). Nevertheless, some general conclusions can be made.

About 85 percent of primary ECs contain ER and/or PR levels greater than 5 to 10 fmol, and 50 to 60 percent are positive for both receptors (Chambers et al, 1988; Kleine et al, 1990). The majority of ECs have lower levels of ER and PR than normal endometrium. PR levels are more important prognostically than ER levels. PR levels are substantially higher in well-differentiated than poorly differentiated lesions. There is, however, great variance in the concentration of both receptors among

carcinomas of the same grade. Stage, survival, and tumor-free survival are all correlated with tumor PR levels, and in some reports receptor status is an independent prognostic factor based on multivariate analysis (Palmer et al, 1988; Ingram et al, 1989; Nyholm et al, 1995). The clinically most significant PR level has not been determined, but it is surely more than 50 fmol and may be more than 100 fmol (Ingram et al, 1989; Nyholm et al, 1995). While much of the prognostic value of PR receptor undoubtedly proceeds from its association with grade 1 tumors, Chambers et al (1988) reported a 5-year survival rate of 48 percent for patients with grade 3 receptor-rich tumors compared with 20 percent for patients with grade 3 receptor-poor tumors.

The cumulative data indicate that the receptor content of EC is a more reliable predictor of the response to progestin therapy than is the histologic grade of the tumor. From 15 to 30 percent of grade 3 primary lesions, compared with 90 to 95 percent of grade 1 lesions, have measurable levels of PR. The probability of objective response to progestin therapy of any EC that contains both PR and ER is about 75 percent compared with less than 5 percent for carcinomas that are negative for both receptors. Since chemotherapy will be more effective than hormonal therapy against receptor-poor tumors, obtaining receptor data from the metastases will facilitate determining the best therapy.

Tissue retrieved by fine-needle aspiration can be analyzed for PR and ER by immunocytochemical techniques, providing a practical means of obtaining tissue from relatively inaccessible recurrence sites without major surgery (Tani et al, 1989). It is less reliable to choose between hormone and cytotoxic therapy on the basis of receptor data from the primary lesion than from the metastasis. For example, Runowicz et al (1990) reported that only 25 percent of metastatic tumors were PR positive versus 60 percent of primary tumors from the same patients. When fresh tissue is not available for standard hormone receptor bioassay, immunohistochemical determination of receptor content for both ER and PR from formalin-fixed, paraffin-embedded tissue is possible. In fact, some authors believe that the immunohistochemical method may be more valid than the traditional assay, because a false reading caused by receptor-containing nontumor tissue is avoided (Chambers et al, 1990; Soper et al, 1990).

Chemotherapy

Chemotherapy of EC is reviewed in Chapter 16. Briefly, doxorubicin, cisplatin, and paclitaxel are the most active agents. They produce objective responses in about 30 percent of patients, although the complete remission rate is only 5 to 10 percent. There are now numerous studies of doxorubicin plus cisplatin with or without cyclophosphamide in advanced/recurrent EC (Burke et al, 1991; Fung et al, 1991; Moore et al, 1991). In sum, these studies indicate that doxorubicin/cisplatin-based chemotherapy induces a complete remission in 15 percent of patients and a partial response in 25 percent. The response is not significantly influenced by the site of disease, prior radiation therapy, prior progestin therapy, patient age, time to recurrence, or histologic grade. As expected, good performance status is associated with a superior rate of response.

Recommended Management

Surgery and/or radiation therapy should be used whenever feasible for recurrent but localized (pelvic, suburethral, bone, peripheral node) EC. Patients with nonlocalized, PR-rich (>50 fmol), recurrent tumors are candidates for progestin therapy, MPA 50 to 100 mg three times a day, or megestrol acetate 80 mg two to three times a day. The progestin therapy is continued as long as the disease is static or in remission. The maximum clinical response may not be apparent for 3 or more months after initiating therapy. Failure to respond to standard-dose progestin therapy is an indication to initiate chemotherapy, as discussed previously. All patients with recurrent or metastatic EC treated by surgery and/or radiation therapy should also be placed on long-term progestin therapy unless they are known to have a PR-negative tumor. In the presence of a relative contraindication to high-dose progestin therapy (e.g., prior deep vein thrombosis, pulmonary embolus, severe heart disease, breast cancer), tamoxifen 20 mg b.i.d. is preferred. Chemotherapy is indicated for patients with advanced/recurrent disease that is not amenable to treatment by surgery, radiation therapy, or hormone therapy.

SPECIAL TREATMENT CATEGORIES

Preoperative Radiation

Physicians who employ preoperative radiation in the management of early-stage EC should be familiar with the indications for performing surgery first. The most common one is the presence of a stage I, grade 1 lesion, which seldom requires adjuvant therapy. Other contraindications to preoperative radiation are the presence of an adnexal mass; a history of, or concurrent, pelvic abscess (tubo-ovarian, appendiceal, diverticular); and pelvic kidney. The presence of pyometra, numerous prior abdominal surgeries, and previous abdominal-perineal resection are also relative contraindications to preoperative radiation therapy. The patient who fears radiation, who is unable to cooperate during a prolonged treatment course, who is very thin (Potish and Twiggs, 1986), or who has had prior pelvic radiation is not a candidate for pre- or postoperative radiation treatment.

Radiation-Hysterectomy Interval

If a course of preoperative radiation therapy is undertaken, it is a common practice to wait several weeks before hysterectomy is carried out. The usual reasons cited in favor of waiting are (1) resolution of radiation "reaction," (2) regression of a large carcinomatous mass, and (3) eradication of the uterine cancer ("sterilization" of the uterus). The first two are presumed to facilitate the surgical procedure, while the last is thought to provide maximum, if not absolute, protection against intraoperative tumor spread. None of these reasons is supported by any substantive data. Immediate hysterectomy is not associated with a clinically significant increase in morbidity (Chambers et al, 1985). Delay may be deleterious, since it provides additional time for a residual viable uterine tumor, present in 25 to 50 percent of cases, to involve extrauterine sites. Since there is no way to identify preoperatively those cases that have total eradication of the uterine tumor, individualization of the radiation-hysterectomy time interval would not be reliable. The waiting policy is probably most unsuited to high-grade cancers, since they are the most rapidly growing and most aggressive. The poorly differentiated tumors also appear to be the most difficult to destroy by preoperative radiation (Table 6–15).

In summary, it can be said of the radiation-hysterectomy interval that delay has no therapeutic effect, that the risk of spread persists during the waiting period, that the highest grade lesions are the most likely to persist after radiation, and that there is seldom a technical advantage in delaying surgery. Waiting is indicated to permit the patient to recuperate from the acute effects of the radiation. While the "empty" uterus has prognostic value, this is not a sufficient reason to postpone hysterectomy, which is, after all, the most important element in the treatment of EC.

Radical Hysterectomy

Radical hysterectomy at first glance seems to be well suited to encompass the known spread pattern of stage I and II EC. However, the patient population tends to be obese, elderly, and diabetic, and to suffer from cardiovascular disease—all conditions that increase the risks of extended pelvic surgery. Even in well-selected cases, there are problems with the use of radical hysterectomy for EC therapy. Many, if not most, patients would be seriously overtreated by such surgery. Identifying the patients who require more than a simple hysterectomy is not readily done preoperatively, even after excluding grade 1 cases, although ultrasound testing can identify some of the patients with deep myoinvasion. Furthermore, many of the patients who may benefit from radical hysterectomy and pelvic lymphadenectomy on the basis of the risk of lymphatic spread will already have extrapelvic spread, as evidenced by positive peritoneal cytology or aortic node metastases. Intensifying regional therapy in patients with extraregional metastases is not likely to improve survival.

Therefore, the role of radical hysterectomy must remain a minor one in EC management. The most frequent candidates are (1) the cervical cancer patient who, subsequent to radiation therapy, develops EC (unfortunately, these patients usually have extrauterine disease [Kwon et al, 1981]); (2) the occasional patient who exhibits appropriate risk factors and refuses radiation therapy; (3) the patient who has a contraindication to radiation therapy; and (4) the patient with gross cervical involvement who is physically and medically suited to radical hysterectomy.

Diagnosis Posthysterectomy

The posthysterectomy diagnosis of EC can present a difficult management problem, especially if the adnexa have not been removed. This situation, which usually arises following vaginal hysterectomy for pelvic relaxation, can be averted by opening the excised uterus routinely in the operating room. Recommendations for postoperative treatment (Table 6–16) are based on the known risk of extrauterine and extrapelvic disease related to histologic grade and myometrial penetration. Removal of the adnexa and sur-

---

TABLE **6–15**

Relationship Between Histologic Grade and Frequency of Residual Tumor in the Uterus After Preoperative Radiation

Source	Percent Residual	
	Grades 1–2	Grade 3
Silverberg and DeGiorgi (1974)*	60	88[†]
Macasaet et al (1980)	45.2	85.7

*Study group of 76 cases.
[†]Values are 88% for poorly differentiated adenocarcinomas and 82% for adenosquamous carcinomas.

TABLE **6–16**

Recommended Management of Patients With Endometrial Carcinoma Diagnosed on the Postoperative Hysterectomy Specimen*

Grade 1 or 2 confined to upper two thirds of corpus, less than one third myometrial invasion, and no LVSI: no further treatment

Grade 1 or 2 confined to upper two thirds of corpus, middle one third myometrial invasion, no LVSI, no evidence of metastasis: vaginal cuff or pelvic irradiation

All others: reoperate to remove adnexa and surgically stage

*If a supracervical hysterectomy was done, reoperation to remove the cervix and adnexa is recommended.

gical staging by laparoscopy provides a means of obtaining the missing information without performing a laparotomy (Childers et al, 1993).

The Medically Inoperable Patient

Severe cardiopulmonary disease and morbid obesity are the primary reasons a patient with EC is deemed to be medically inoperable. Clinical judgment varies a great deal in these cases. Nevertheless, in every gynecologist's experience, there will be patients for whom the risks of anesthesia and surgery are judged to exceed the likely benefits of even vaginal hysterectomy. For patients with grade 1 lesions and a temporary contraindication to general anesthesia, or for those who are al-together unsuited to radiation therapy or surgery, high-dose progestins or tamoxifen is the treatment of choice. All other patients should be treated with radiation. If the uterus is small, tandem and ovoid intracavitary therapy alone may be appropriate. Patients with a large uterus probably stand a better chance of being cured using the Heyman packing technique (Fig. 6–15), but few therapists are familiar with this technique today. Whenever radiation or hormonal therapy is administered as definitive treatment, the uterine lesion can be monitored with ultrasound and serum CA-125 determinations. Endometrial biopsy or curettage should be performed after 3 months. If the tumor persists, the contraindications to surgery must be reassessed.

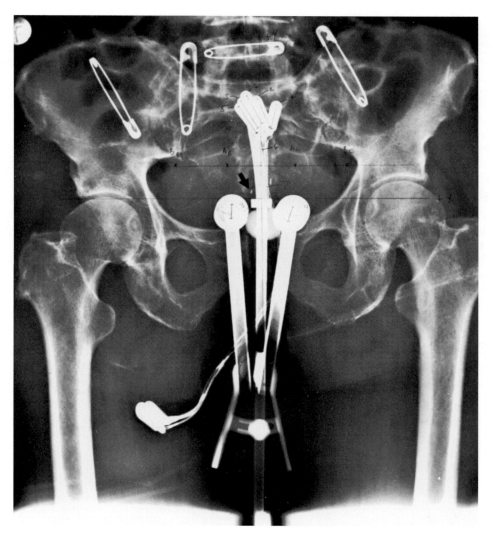

FIGURE 6–15. Anteroposterior view of the pelvis, illustrating six Heyman capsules, a short cervical tandem, and vaginal ovoids in place. Silver seeds (arrow) are embedded 0.5 cm in the cervix.

The Young Woman

The diagnosis of EC during the reproductive years should always be viewed with skepticism, since the malignancy is uncommon and frequently confused with hyperplasia (Crissman et al, 1981; Silverberg, 1988; Lee and Scully, 1989). The histologic distinction between atypical hyperplasia, which can be treated successfully with progestins, and well-differentiated carcinoma, which should be treated surgically, is to some extent subjective. When preservation of fertility is a significant clinical factor, the diagnosis of well-differentiated carcinoma should be based on endometrial curettings, not an office biopsy, and consultation with a recognized authority in the field of endometrial pathology is recommended. Equivocal lesions are managed in the same manner as atypical hyperplasia (see the section "Endometrial Hyperplasia" earlier in this chapter). When a diagnosis of EC is confirmed, however, hysterectomy with removal of the adnexa is the treatment of choice.

Studies suggest that the majority of women under age 40 who develop EC do not fit the stereotypical phenotype. Less than half are obese, nulliparous, or hypertensive. Few are diabetic, and only 10 to 30 percent have evidence of Stein-Leventhal syndrome or chronic anovulation. Normal-weight patients tend to have more severe disease (Ramzy and Nisker, 1979; Gallup and Stock, 1984; Quinn et al, 1985).

Pelvic Relaxation

The woman with EC who has concurrent symptomatic pelvic relaxation should have the corrective surgery done before external radiation therapy, because postradiation fibrosis may cause fixation of the paravaginal tissues, including the urethral-vesicle angle, preventing satisfactory repair. A combined vaginal and abdominal approach is employed unless a retropubic suspension will solve the problem. Repair at the time of hysterectomy is not attended by a significant risk for implantation metastases according to the data of Cliby et al (1995). They reported only four recurrences among 53 patients having vaginal hysterectomy with anterior and posterior repair.

Malignant Peritoneal Cytology

Since the original report of Dahle (1956), numerous investigators have recovered malignant cells from the pelvis at the time of surgery for early EC. The reported yield ranges from 5 to 25 percent, with the low figure most applicable to surgical stage I cases and the high figure to clinical stage I cases with extrauterine spread (adnexa, nodes). For clinical stages III and IV, positive peritoneal cytology is reported in 65 to 85 percent of cases (Harouny et al, 1988). In addition to stage, the frequency of positive cytology is influenced by the histologic grade and depth of myoinvasion. In the GOG staging study, the positive cytology rates were 5.5, 12, and 17 percent for grades 1 through 3, respectively. The rates for less than one third, middle third, and outer one third myoinvasion, respectively, were 8, 12, and 17 percent (Morrow et al, 1986). Overall, recurrence was noted in 18 percent of surgical stage I cases having positive peritoneal cytology, and the effect on survival was statistically significant by multivariate analysis (Morrow et al, 1991). These data should dispel the perception that EC cells in the pelvic washings are a harmless consequence of uterine curettage.

The presence of malignant cells in the peritoneal washings following preoperative radiation therapy probably has even greater adverse prognostic significance than in the nonirradiated patient (Turner et al, 1989). The prognosis is worse for patients with numerous tissue fragments or sheets of carcinoma cells than for those with a sparse yield of malignant cells (Szpak et al, 1981).

The interpretation of peritoneal cytology is often difficult because reactive mesothelial cells take on the appearance of malignancy. Thus treatment of EC for positive peritoneal cytology should not be undertaken without a cytopathology review. Even then, the management is controversial because there are insufficient data regarding recurrence risk and treatment results. Success has been reported with both intraperitoneal radionuclides (Fountain and Malkasian, 1981; Soper et al, 1985) and whole-abdomen radiation (Greer and Hamberger, 1983; Potish et al, 1985a). A major disadvantage of the intraperitoneal treatment is that the preponderance of patients with positive washings have other surgicopathologic risk factors that require pelvic or even extended-field radiation. The use of intraperitoneal radionuclides with external beam radiation necessitates lowering the external beam dose to suboptimal levels to avoid severe intestinal complications (Soper et al, 1985). We recommend that patients with lesions of histologic grade 2 or 3 and copious malignant cells on peritoneal cytology be managed by progestins if the tumor is PR positive. Otherwise, whole-abdomen radiation therapy or chemotherapy is advised.

HISTOLOGIC SUBTYPES OF ENDOMETRIAL CARCINOMA

Adenocarcinoma With Squamous Differentiation

EC frequently exhibits areas of squamous epithelium, which may be benign, malignant, or indeterminant. When benign squamous epithelium is present, the lesion has traditionally been termed *adenoacanthoma* or adenocarcinoma with squamous metaplasia; EC with malignant squamous epithelium has by custom been called *adenosquamous carcinoma* (ASC) or mixed-cell carcinoma. In the general population of EC patients, adenoacanthoma accounts for about 15 percent of EC and ASC for 5 percent. A few cases of glassy cell EC, which may be a variant of ASC, have been reported (Hachisuga et al, 1990).

The contribution of squamous differentiation to the biologic behavior of EC has been disputed but, after a thorough study of this topic, Zaino and Kurman (1988) concluded that there was no prognostic significance attributable to the presence of benign or malignant squamous elements. This largely reflected their finding that the differentiation of the squamous component paralleled the grade of the adenocarcinoma. Some studies report that ASC tends to occur in older women, is more often associated with LVSI, and has a higher incidence of deep myoinvasion and lymph node metastases than the pure adenocarcinomas. However, these differences diminish when corrected for histologic grade, since ASC more often has a poorly differentiated glandular component. Certainly squamous differentiation is a weak determinant of the outcome compared with clinical stage and the histologic grade of the adenocarcinoma component.

Squamous Cell Carcinoma

Thirty-six cases of primary squamous cell carcinoma (SCC) of the endometrium have been published (Glaubitz et al, 1994; Im et al, 1995). The average age at diagnosis (62 years) is similar to that of the general population of women with EC. In the earlier reports, association with pyometra, uterine in-

version, and prior radiation was noted. Since the diagnosis is inappropriate if any malignant glandular foci are present or if the cervix is involved, most of the reported cases are clinical stage I and none stage II. Nine of 25 clinical stage I patients with follow-up died within 36 months, suggesting that the disease has a poorer prognosis than the common endometrioid variety of corpus carcinoma. In situ squamous carcinoma, verrucous carcinoma, and condyloma of the endometrium have also been reported (Ryder, 1982; Venkateseshan and Woo, 1985; Radhika et al, 1993).

Clear Cell Carcinoma

Clear cell carcinoma (CCC) of the endometrium occurs in women who are, on average, a few years older than women with the endometrioid variety, and it accounts for 3 to 5 percent of all corpus carcinomas. CCC is believed to be of müllerian rather than mesonephric origin. Abeler and Kjorstad (1991) reported their experience with 97 cases of CCC, which constituted 4.9 percent of all corpus carcinomas at the Norwegian Radium Hospital between 1970 and 1977. Two thirds were pure CCC. Only 59 percent of stage I cases and 27 percent of stage II cases survived 5 years. Myoinvasion and LVSI were important prognostic indicators. Of the 17 patients with intramucosal tumors, 90 percent survived 5 years. Others have reported a 5-year survival of 70 percent for patients with stage I and II CCC (Carcangiu et al, 1995; Malpica et al, 1995). Thus, the prognosis for patients with CCC appears to be worse than that for other histologic variants of EC (Table 6–17). Association with papillary serous carcinoma is common. Surgical staging and postoperative adjuvant radiation is recommended. CCC is

TABLE **6–17**

Five-Year Status of Patients With Endometrial Cancer Subtypes: Clinical Stage I Only*

Histologic Subtype	Of 819 Cases	
	Percent Alive	*Percent Dead of Cancer*
Adenoacanthoma	87.5	6.3
Adenocarcinoma	79.8	6.3
Papillary carcinoma[†]	69.7	21.2
Adenosquamous carcinoma	53.1	32.7
Clear cell carcinoma	44.2	51.2

*Data from Christopherson et al (1983).
[†]Includes those with and without serous epithelium.

not known to be responsive to progestin or antiestrogen therapy.

Papillary Serous Carcinoma

Papillary serous carcinoma (PSC) of the endometrium is a variant of EC (Hendrickson et al, 1982) characterized histologically by features resembling papillary serous carcinoma of the ovary, often with psammoma bodies. Areas of CCC may be seen. More than half of the clinical stage I cases have deep myoinvasion, three fourths manifest LVSI, and 50 percent have extrauterine disease at surgery. Positive peritoneal cytology, spread by peritoneal implantation, and lymphatic metastasis are common (Jeffrey et al, 1986; JT Chambers et al, 1987; Christman et al, 1987; O'Hanlan et al, 1990). The 5-year survival for surgical stage I patients is about 60 percent. PSC arising in an endometrial polyp has been reported, sometimes associated with a concurrent primary lesion in the tube or ovary, suggesting that PSC may be a variant of ovarian surface PSC (Silva and Jenkins, 1990). PSC should not be confused with papillary (villoglandular) endometrial carcinoma, which apparently has a behavior and prognosis similar to the common, endometrioid type of EC (see next section).

Surgery with extended staging should be the first step in management, and nearly all patients will be candidates for postoperative therapy. Platinum-based chemotherapy produced complete responses in only 1 of 19 recurrent cases in the combined series of Gallion et al (1989) and JT Chambers et al (1987). PSC obviously does not respond to cytotoxic therapy as well as ovarian serous carcinoma, and the efficacy of cytotoxic therapy in an adjuvant setting for PSC is unknown. Pelvic radiation alone is recommended for patients with negative surgical staging, negative LVSI, and superficial myoinvasion. For patients with more advanced disease, cisplatin, cyclophosphamide, and doxorubicin chemotherapy or whole-abdomen radiation therapy may be of value (Christman et al, 1987). The tumor is devoid of hormone receptors (Umpierre et al, 1994).

Miscellaneous Subtypes

According to Sutton et al (1987) and Ward et al (1990), *papillary carcinoma** of the en-

dometrium without serous features is not more aggressive than the common EC, but at least one study found it to occupy a position intermediate between EC and PSC in terms of surgical upstaging, depth of myoinvasion, and upper abdominal recurrences (O'Hanlan et al, 1990). *Mucinous EC* is a rare variant that tends to be well differentiated with a good prognosis (Melhem and Tobon, 1987). The prognosis for patients with *secretory EC* is predictably good since this lesion probably represents a well-differentiated carcinoma with progestin effect. In the series of Christopherson et al (1982), 3 of 15 stage I patients experienced recurrence, 1 before and 2 after 5 years of follow-up. This lesion has been mistaken for CCC. Four cases of primary *endodermal sinus tumor* of the endometrium have been reported in women ages 24 to 42 years. The tumors are histologically identical to endodermal sinus tumor from other sites, produce alpha-fetoprotein, and respond well to chemotherapy. Many cases of *small-cell carcinoma* of the endometrium have been reported. It is often mixed with other histologies, tends to be bulky, and tends to present with extrauterine metastases. The small cells stain for neuron-specific enolase. Like neuroendocrine tumors of other organs, the uterine version appears to be aggressive, with a reduced prognosis (Huntsman et al, 1994; van Hoeven et al, 1995). Surgical staging is indicated for patients with apparent early disease. Adjuvant chemotherapy with cisplatin and doxorubicin is recommended on the basis of results obtained in small-cell carcinoma of the lung.

REFERENCES

Aalders JG, Abeler V: Recurrent adenocarcinoma of the endometrium: a clinical and histopathological study of 379 patients. In Prognostic Factors and Treatment of Endometrial Carcinoma: A Clinical and Histopathological Study. Groningen, Drukkerij Dijkstra Niemeyer BV, 1982, p 78.

Aalders JG, Abeler V, Kolstad P: Clinical (stage III) as compared to subclinical intrapelvic extrauterine tumor spread in endometrial carcinoma: a clinical and histopathological study of 175 patients. Gynecol Oncol 17:64, 1984a.

Aalders JG, Abeler V, Kolstad P: Recurrent adenocarcinoma of the endometrium: a clinical and histopathological study of 379 patients. Gynecol Oncol 17:85, 1984b.

Aalders JG, Abeler V, Kolstad P: Stage IV endometrial carcinoma: a clinical and histopathological study of 83 patients. Gynecol Oncol 17:75, 1984c.

Aalders JG, Abeler V, Kolstad P, Onsrud M: Postoperative external irradiation and prognostic parameters in stage I endometrial carcinoma. Obstet Gynecol 56:419, 1980.

Abeler V, Kjorstad KE: Clear cell carcinoma of the endometrium: a histopathological and clinical study of 97 cases. Gynecol Oncol 40:207, 1991.

---

*Most of these are of the villoglandular type, which resemble the villous adenoma of the intestine.

American College of Obstetricians and Gynecologists: Estrogen Replacement Therapy. Technical Bulletin No. 93. Washington, DC, American College of Obstetricians and Gynecologists, 1986.

American College of Obstetricians and Gynecologists: Estrogen Replacement Therapy and Endometrial Cancer. Committee Opinion No. 80. Washington, DC, American College of Obstetricians and Gynecologists, 1990.

American College of Obstetricians and Gynecologists: Carcinoma of the Endometrium. Technical Bulletin No. 162. Washington, DC, American College of Obstetricians and Gynecologists, 1991.

Andersen WA, Taylor PT Jr, Fechner RE, Pinkerton JV: Endometrial metaplasia associated with endometrial adenocarcinoma. Am J Obstet Gynecol 157:597, 1987.

Belloni C, Vigano R, del Maschio A, et al: Magnetic resonance imaging in endometrial carcinoma staging. Gynecol Oncol 37:172, 1990.

Berchuck A, Anspach C, Evans AC, et al: Postsurgical surveillance of patients with FIGO stage I/II endometrial adenocarcinoma. Gynecol Oncol 59:20, 1995.

Bhagavan BS, Parmley TH, Rosenshein NB, et al: Comparison of estrogen-induced hyperplasia to endometrial carcinoma. Obstet Gynecol 64:12, 1984.

Bigelow B, Vekstein V, Demopoulos RI: Endometrial carcinoma stage II: route and extent of spread to the cervix. Obstet Gynecol 62:363, 1983.

Bloss JD, Berman ML, Bloss LP, Buller RE: Use of vaginal hysterectomy for the management of stage I endometrial cancer in the medically compromised patient. Gynecol Oncol 40:74, 1991.

Bokhman JV: Two pathogenetic types of endometrial carcinoma. Gynecol Oncol 15:10, 1983.

Boronow RC, Morrow CP, Creasman WT, et al: Surgical staging in endometrial cancer: clinicopathologic findings of a prospective study. Obstet Gynecol 63:825, 1984.

Britton LC, Wilson TO, Gaffey TA, et al: DNA ploidy in endometrial carcinoma: major objective prognostic factor. Mayo Clin Proc 65:643, 1990.

Brooks SE, Yeatts-Peterson M, Baker SP, Reuter KL: Thickened endometrial stripe and/or endometrial fluid as a marker of pathology: fact or fancy? Gynecol Oncol 63:19, 1996.

Burke TW, Heller PB, Woodward JE, et al: Treatment failure in endometrial carcinoma. Obstet Gynecol 75:96, 1990.

Burke TW, Stringer CA, Morris M, et al: Prospective treatment of advanced or recurrent endometrial carcinoma with cisplatin, doxorubicin and cyclophosphamide. Gynecol Oncol 40:264, 1991.

Cacciatore B, Lehtovirta P, Wahlström T, Ylöstalo P: Preoperative sonographic evaluation of endometrial cancer. Am J Obstet Gynecol 160:133, 1989.

Carcangiu ML, Chambers JT: Early pathologic stage clear cell carcinoma and uterine papillary serous carcinoma of the endometrium: comparison of clinicopathologic features and survival. Int J Gynecol Pathol 14:30, 1995.

Cavalli F, Goldhirsch A, Jungi F, et al: Randomized trial of low- versus high-dose medroxyprogesterone acetate in the induction treatment of postmenopausal patients with advanced breast cancer. J Clin Oncol 2:414, 1984.

Chambers JT, Carcangiu ML, Voynick IM, Schwartz PE: Immunohistochemical evaluation of estrogen and progesterone receptor content in 183 patients with endometrial carcinoma. Am J Clin Pathol 94:255, 1990.

Chambers JT, Kapp DS, Lawrence R, et al: Immediate versus delayed hysterectomy for endometrial carcinoma: surgical morbidity and hospital stay. Obstet Gynecol 65:245, 1985.

Chambers JT, MacLusky N, Eisenfield A, et al: Estrogen and progestin receptor levels as prognosticators for survival in endometrial cancer. Gynecol Oncol 31:65, 1988.

Chambers JT, Merino M, Kohorn EI, et al: Uterine papillary serous carcinoma. Obstet Gynecol 69:109, 1987.

Chambers SK, Kapp DS, Peschel RE, et al: Prognostic factors and sites of failure in FIGO stage I, grade 3 endometrial carcinoma. Gynecol Oncol 27:180, 1987.

Chen SS, Lee L: Retroperitoneal lymph node metastases in stage I carcinoma of the endometrium: correlation with risk factors. Gynecol Oncol 16:319, 1983.

Chen SS, Lee L: Reappraisal of endocervical curettage in predicting cervical involvement by endometrial carcinoma. J Reprod Med 31:50, 1986.

Cherkis RC, Patten SF Jr, Andrews TJ, et al: Significance of normal endometrial cells detected by cervical cytology. Obstet Gynecol 71:242, 1988.

Childers JM, Brzechffa PR, Hatch KD, Surwit EA: Laparoscopically assisted surgical staging (LASS) of endometrial cancer. Gynecol Oncol 51:33, 1993.

Christman JE, Kapp DS, Hendrickson MR, et al: Therapeutic approaches to uterine papillary serous carcinoma: a preliminary report. Gynecol Oncol 26:228, 1987.

Christopherson WM, Alberhasky RC, Connelly PJ: Carcinoma of the endometrium: 1. A clinicopathologic study of clear-cell carcinoma and secretory carcinoma. Cancer 49:1511, 1982.

Christopherson WM, Connelly PJ, Alberhasky RC: Carcinoma of the endometrium: V. An Analysis of prognosticators in patients with favorable subtypes and stage I disease. Cancer 51:1705, 1983.

Cliby WA, Dodson MK, Podratz KC: Uterine prolapse complicated by endometrial cancer. Am J Obstet Gynecol 172:1675, 1995.

Colafranceschi M, Bettocchi S, Mencaglia L, van Herendael BJ: Missed hysteroscopic detection of uterine carcinoma before endometrial resection: report of three cases. Gynecol Oncol 62:298, 1996.

Corley D, Rowe J, Curtis MT, et al: Postmenopausal bleeding from unusual endometrial polyps in women on chronic tamoxifen therapy. Obstet Gynecol 79:111, 1992.

Cowles TA, Magrina JF, Masterson BJ, Capen CV: Comparison of clinical and surgical staging in patients with endometrial carcinoma. Obstet Gynecol 66:413, 1985.

Cox JD, Komaki R, Wilson JF, Greenberg M: Locally advanced adenocarcinoma of the endometrium: results of irradiation with and without subsequent hysterectomy. Cancer 45:715, 1980.

Creasman WT, Morrow CP, Bundy BN, et al: Surgical pathologic spread patterns of endometrial cancer: a Gynecologic Oncology Group study. Cancer 60:2035, 1987.

Crissman JD, Azoury RS, Barnes AE, Schellhas HF: Endometrial carcinoma in women 40 years of age or younger. Obstet Gynecol 57:699, 1981.

Dahle T: Transtubal spread of tumor cells on carcinoma of the body of the uterus. Surg Gynecol Obstet 103:332, 1956.

Daniel AG, Peters WA III: Accuracy of office and operating room curettage in the grading of endometrial carcinoma. Obstet Gynecol 71:612, 1988.

Degligdisch L, Cohen C: Histologic correlates and virulence implications of endometrial carcinoma associated with adenomatous hyperplasia. Cancer 56:1452, 1985.

De Jong P, Doel F, Falconer A: Outpatient diagnostic hysteroscopy. Br J Obstet Gynaecol 97:299, 1990.

Draper MW, Flowers DE, Huster WJ: A controlled trial of raloxifene (LY139481) HCl: impact on bone turnover and serum lipid profile in healthy postmenopausal women. J Bone Miner Res 11:835, 1996.

Duk JM, Aalders JG, Fleuren GJ, deBruijn HWA: CA-125: a useful marker in endometrial carcinoma. Am J Obstet Gynecol 155:1097, 1986.

Edmonson JH, Krook JE, Hilton JF, et al: Ineffectiveness of tamoxifen in advanced endometrial carcinoma after failure of progestin treatment. Cancer Treat Rep 70:1019, 1986.

Egarter C, Krestan C, Kurz C: Abdominal dissemination of malignant cells with hysteroscopy. Gynecol Oncol 63:143, 1996.

Feldman S, Berkowitz R, Tosteson A: Cost-effectiveness of strategies to evaluate postmenopausal bleeding. Obstet Gynecol 81:968, 1993.

Ferenczy A, Gelfand M: The biologic significance of cytologic atypia in progestogen-treated endometrial hyperplasia. Am J Obstet Gynecol 160:126, 1989.

Figge DC, Otto PM, Tamimi HK, Greer BE: Treatment variables in the management of endometrial cancer. Am J Obstet Gynecol 146:495, 1983.

Fountain KS, Malkasian GD Jr: Radioactive colloidal gold in the treatment of endometrial cancer: Mayo Clinic experience, 1952–1976. Cancer 47:2430, 1981.

Fung MFK, Burnett M, Faught W: Does persistent postmenopausal bleeding justify hysterectomy? Eur J Gynaecol Oncol 18:26, 1997.

Fung MFK, Krepart GV, Lotocki RJ, Heywood M: Treatment of recurrent and metastatic adenocarcinoma of the endometrium with cisplatin, doxorubicin, cyclophosphamide, and medroxyprogesterone acetate. Obstet Gynecol 78:1033, 1991.

Gal D: Hormonal therapy for lesions of the endometrium. Semin Oncol 13:33, 1986.

Gallion HH, van Nagell JR, Powell DF: Stage I serous papillary carcinoma of the endometrium. Cancer 63:2224, 1989.

Gallup DG, Stock RJ: Adenocarcinoma of the endometrium in women 40 years of age or younger. Obstet Gynecol 64:417, 1984.

Genest P, Drouin P, Girard A, Gerig L: Stage III carcinoma of the endometrium: a review of 41 cases. Gynecol Oncol 26:77, 1987.

Gimpelson RJ, Rappold HO: A comparative study between panoramic hysteroscopy with directed biopsies and dilation and curettage: a review of 276 cases. Am J Obstet Gynecol 158:489, 1988.

Gitsch G, Hanzal E, Jensen D, Hacker NF: Endometrial cancer in premenopausal women 45 years and younger. Obstet Gynecol 85:504, 1995.

Glaubitz M, Kupsch E, Günter HH, et al: Primary squamous cell carcinoma of the endometrium. Eur J Gynaecol Oncol 15:37, 1994.

Goff BA, Rice LW: Assessment of depth of myometrial invasion in endometrial adenocarcinoma. Gynecol Oncol 38:46, 1990.

Gordon AN, Fleischer AC, Reed GW: Depth of myometrial invasion in endometrial cancer: preoperative assessment by transvaginal ultrasonography. Gynecol Oncol 39:321, 1990.

Granberg S, Wikland M, Karlsson B, et al: Endometrial thickness as measured by endovaginal ultrasonography for identifying endometrial abnormality. Am J Obstet Gynecol 164:47, 1991.

Greer BE, Hamberger AD: Treatment of intraperitoneal metastatic adenocarcinoma of the endometrium by the whole-abdomen moving-strip technique and pelvic boost irradiation. Gynecol Oncol 16:365, 1983.

Greven K, Olds W: Isolated vaginal recurrences of endometrial adenocarcinoma and their management. Cancer 60:419, 1987.

Hachisuga T, Sugimori H, Kaku T, et al: Glassy cell carcinoma of the endometrium: case report. Gynecol Oncol 36:134, 1990.

Hanson MB, van Nagell JR Jr, Powell DE, et al: The prognostic significance of lymph-vascular space invasion in stage I endometrial cancer. Cancer 55:1753, 1985.

Harouny VR, Sutton GP, Clark SA, et al: The importance of peritoneal cytology in endometrial carcinoma. Obstet Gynecol 72:394, 1988.

Hawwa ZM, Nahhas WA, Copenhaver EH: Postmenopausal bleeding. Lahey Clin Foundation Bull 19:61, 1970.

Hendrickson MR, Kempson RL: Endometrial epithelial metaplasia: proliferations frequently misdiagnosed as adenocarcinoma. Am J Surg Pathol 4:525, 1980.

Hendrickson MR, Kempson RL: Ciliated carcinoma—a variant of endometrial adenocarcinoma: a report of 10 cases. Int J Gynecol Pathol 2:1, 1983.

Hendrickson M, Ross J, Eifel PJ, et al: Adenocarcinoma of the endometrium: analysis of 256 cases with carcinoma limited to the uterine corpus. Gynecol Oncol 13:373, 1982.

Hetzel DJ, Wilson TO, Keeney GL, et al: HER-2/neu expression: a major prognostic factor in endometrial cancer. Gynecol Oncol 47:179, 1992.

Heyman J, Reuterwall O, Benner S: The Radiumhemmet experience with radiotherapy in cancer of the corpus of the uterus. Acta Radiol 22:114, 1941.

Hording U, Hansen U: Stage I endometrial carcinoma: a review of 140 patients primarily treated by surgery only. Gynecol Oncol 22:51, 1985.

Hricak H, Rubinstein LV, Gherman GM, Karstaedt N: MR imaging evaluation of endometrial carcinoma: results of an NCI cooperative study. Radiology 179:829, 1991.

Huntsman DG, Clement PB, Gilks CB, Scully RE: Small cell carcinoma of the endometrium: a clinicopathological study of sixteen cases. Am J Surg Pathol 18:364, 1994.

Im DD, Shah KV, Rosenshein NB: Report of three new cases of squamous carcinoma of the endometrium with emphasis on the HPV status. Gynecol Oncol 56:464, 1995.

Ingram SS, Rosenman J, Heath R, et al: The predictive value of progesterone receptor levels in endometrial cancer. Int J Radiat Oncol Biol Phys 17:21, 1989.

International Federation of Gynecology and Obstetrics: Annual report on the results of treatment in gynecologic cancer. Int J Gynecol Obstet 28:189, 1989.

International Federation of Gynecology and Obstetrics: Annual report on the results of treatment in gynecologic cancer. Int J Gynecol Obstet 36(suppl):1, 1991.

Jacques SM, Lawrence WD: Endometrial adenocarcinoma with variable-level myometrial involvement limited to adenomyosis: a clinicopathologic study of 23 cases. Gynecol Oncol 37:401, 1990.

Janicek MF, Rosenshein NB: Invasive endometrial cancer in uteri resected for atypical endometrial hyperplasia. Gynecol Oncol 52:373, 1994.

Jeffrey JF, Krepart GV, Lotocki RJ: Papillary serous adenocarcinoma of the endometrium. Obstet Gynecol 67:670, 1986.

Jeyarajah AR, Gallagher CJ, Blake PR, et al: Long-term follow-up of gonadotrophin-releasing hormone analog treatment for recurrent endometrial cancer. Gynecol Oncol 63:47, 1996.

Karlsson B, Granberg S, Wikland M, et al: Transvaginal ultrasonography of the endometrium in women with postmenopausal bleeding: a Nordic multicenter study. Am J Obstet Gynecol 172:1488, 1995.

Kelly RM, Baker WH: Progestational agents in the treatment of carcinoma of the endometrium. N Engl J Med 264:216, 1961.

Kleine W, Maier T, Geyer H, Pfleiderer A: Estrogen and progesterone receptors in endometrial cancer and their prognostic relevance. Gynecol Oncol 38:59, 1990.

Kohler MF, Carney P, Dodge R, et al: p53 overexpression in advanced-stage endometrial adenocarcinoma. Am J Obstet Gynecol 175:1246, 1996.

Kumar NB, Hart WR: Metastases to the uterine corpus from extragenital cancers: a clinicopathologic study of 63 cases. Cancer 50:2163, 1982.

Kurman RJ, Kominski PF, Norris HJ: The behavior of endometrial hyperplasia: a long-term study of "untreated" hyperplasia in 170 patients. Cancer 56:403, 1985.

Kurman RJ, Norris HJ: Evaluation of criteria for distinguishing atypical endometrial hyperplasia from well differentiated carcinoma. Cancer 49:2547, 1982.

Kuten A, Grigsby PW, Perez CA, et al: Results of radiotherapy in recurrent endometrial carcinoma: a retrospective analysis of 51 patients. Int J Radiat Oncol Biol Phys 17:29, 1989.

Kwon TH, Prempree T, Tang C-K, et al: Adenocarcinoma of the uterine corpus following irradiation for cervical cancer. Gynecol Oncol 11:102, 1981.

Lee KR, Scully RE: Complex endometrial hyperplasia and carcinoma in adolescents and young women 15 to 20 years of age: a report of 10 cases. Int J Gynecol Pathol 8:201, 1989.

Lehoczky O, Bôsze P, Ungar L, Töttössy B: Stage I endometrial carcinoma: treatment of nonoperable patients with intracavitary radiation therapy alone. Gynecol Oncol 43:211, 1991.

Loeffler JS, Rosen EM, Niloff JM, et al: Whole abdominal irradiation for tumors of the uterine corpus. Cancer 61:1332, 1988.

Lurain JR, Rice BL, Rademaker AW: Prognostic factors associated with recurrence in clinical stage I adenocarcinoma of the endometrium. Obstet Gynecol 78:63, 1991.

Macasaet M, Brigati D, Boyce J, et al: The significance of residual disease after radiotherapy in endometrial carcinoma: clinicopathologic correlation. Am J Obstet Gynecol 138:557, 1980.

Mackillop WJ, Pringle JF: Stage III endometrial carcinoma: a review of 90 cases. Cancer 56:2519, 1985.

Malpica A, Tornos C, Burke TW, Silva EG: Low stage clear cell carcinoma of the endometrium. Am J Surg Pathol 19:769, 1995.

Mandell LR, Nori D, Hilaris B: Recurrent stage I endometrial carcinoma: results of treatment and prognostic factors. Int J Radiat Oncol Biol Phys 11:1103, 1985.

Martinez A, Schray M, Podratz K, et al: Postoperative whole abdomino-pelvic irradiation for patients with high risk endometrial cancer. Int J Radiat Oncol Biol Phys 17:371, 1989.

Meisels A, Jolicoeur C: Criteria for the cytologic assessment of hyperplasias in endometrial samples obtained by the Endopap endometrial sampler. Acta Cytol 29:297, 1985.

Melhem MF, Tobon H: Mucinous adenocarcinoma of the endometrium: a clinico-pathological review of 18 cases. Int J Gynecol Pathol 6:347, 1987.

Moore DH, Fowler WC Jr, Walton LA, Droegemueller W: Morbidity of lymph node sampling in cancers of the uterine corpus and cervix. Obstet Gynecol 74:180, 1989.

Moore TD, Phillips PH, Nerenstone SR, Cheson BD: Systemic treatment of advanced and recurrent endometrial carcinoma: current status and future directions. J Clin Oncol 9:1071, 1991.

Morris M, Alvarez RD, Kinney WK, Wilson TO: Treatment of recurrent adenocarcinoma of the endometrium with pelvic exenteration. Gynecol Oncol 60:288, 1996.

Morrow CP, Bundy BN, Kurman RJ, et al: Relationship between surgical-pathological risk factors and outcome in clinical stage I and II carcinoma of the endometrium: a Gynecologic Oncology Group study. Gynecol Oncol 40:55, 1991.

Morrow CP, Creasman WT, Homesley H, et al: Carcinoma as a function of extended surgical staging data. In Morrow CP, Smart G (eds): Gynaecological Oncology: Proceedings of the 2nd International Conference on Gynaecological Cancer, Edinburgh, September 1983. New York, Springer-Verlag, 1986, p 147.

Muss HB, Case LD, Capizzi RL: High- versus standard-dose megestrol acetate in women with advanced breast cancer: a phase III trial of the Piedmont Oncology Association. J Clin Oncol 8:1797, 1990.

Newbury R, Schuerch C, Goodspeed N, et al: DNA content as a prognostic factor in endometrial carcinoma. Obstet Gynecol 76:251, 1990.

Noumoff JS, Menzin A, Mikuta J, et al: The ability to evaluate prognostic variables on frozen section in hysterectomies performed for endometrial carcinoma. Gynecol Oncol 42:202, 1991.

Nyholm HCJ, Christensen IJ, Nielson AL: Progesterone receptor levels independently predict survival in endometrial adenocarcinoma. Gynecol Oncol 59:347, 1995.

O'Hanlan KA, Levine PA, Harbatkin D, et al: Virulence of papillary endometrial carcinoma. Gynecol Oncol 37:112, 1990.

Orr JW Jr, Holloway RW, Orr PF, Holimon JL: Surgical staging of uterine cancer: an analysis of perioperative morbidity. Gynecol Oncol 42:209, 1991.

Pacheco JC, Kempers RD: Etiology of postmenopausal bleeding. Obstet Gynecol 32:40, 1968.

Palmer DC, Muir IM, Alexander AI, et al: The prognostic importance of steroid receptors in endometrial carcinoma. Obstet Gynecol 72:388, 1988.

Patsner B, Mann WJ, Cohen H, Loesch M: Predictive value of preoperative serum CA 125 levels in clinically localized and advanced endometrial carcinoma. Am J Obstet Gynecol 158:399, 1988.

Peters WA III, Andersen WA, Thornton N Jr, Morley GW: The selective use of vaginal hysterectomy in the management of adenocarcinoma of the endometrium. Am J Obstet Gynecol 146:285, 1983.

Pfisterer J, Kommoss F, Sauerbrei W, et al: Prognostic value of DNA ploidy and S-phase fraction in stage I endometrial carcinoma. Gynecol Oncol 58:149, 1995.

Phillips GL, Prem KA, Adcock LL, Twiggs LB: Vaginal recurrence of adenocarcinoma of the endometrium. Gynecol Oncol 13:323, 1982.

Piver MS, Barlow JJ, Lurain JR, Blumenson LE: Medroxyprogesterone acetate (Depo-Provera) vs hydroxyprogesterone caproate (Delalutin) in women with metastatic endometrial adenocarcinoma. Cancer 45:268, 1980.

Piver MS, Lele SB, Barlow JJ, Blumenson L: Paraaortic lymph node evaluation in stage I endometrial carcinoma. Obstet Gynecol 59:97, 1982.

Podratz KC, O'Brien PC, Malkasian GD Jr, et al: Effects of progestational agents in treatment of endometrial carcinoma. Obstet Gynecol 66:106, 1985.

Podratz KC, Wilson TO, Gaffey TA, et al: Deoxyribonucleic acid analysis facilitates the pretreatment identification of high-risk endometrial cancer patients. Am J Obstet Gynecol 168:1206, 1993.

Potish RA, Twiggs LB: A decision theory analysis of radiotherapeutic and chemotherapeutic toxicity in the management of ovarian cancer. In Morrow CP, Smart GE (eds): Gynaecologic Oncology: Proceedings of the 2nd International Conference on Gynaecologic Cancer, Edinburgh, September 1983. New York, Springer-Verlag, 1986, p 201.

Potish RA, Twiggs LB, Adcock LL, Prem KA: Role of whole abdominal radiation therapy in the management of endometrial cancer: prognostic importance of factors indicating peritoneal metastases. Gynecol Oncol 21:80, 1985a.

Potish RA, Twiggs LB, Adcock LL, et al: Paraaortic lymph node radiotherapy in cancer of the uterine corpus. Obstet Gynecol 65:251, 1985b.

Quinn MA, Campbell JJ: Tamoxifen therapy in advanced/recurrent endometrial carcinoma. Gynecol Oncol 32:1, 1989.

Quinn MA, Kneale BJ, Fortune DW: Endometrial carcinoma in premenopausal women: a clinicopathological study. Gynecol Oncol 20:298, 1985.

Radhika S, Dey P, Gupta SK: Primary squamous cell carcinoma in situ of the endometrium: a case report. Indian J Cancer 30:92, 1993.

Ramzy I, Nisker JA: Histologic study of ovaries from young women with endometrial adenocarcinoma. Am Soc Clin Pathol 71:253, 1979.

Reddock JM, Burke TW, Morris M, et al: Surveillance for recurrent endometrial carcinoma: development of a follow-up scheme. Gynecol Oncol 59:221, 1995.

Reifenstein EC Jr: The treatment of advanced endometrial cancer with hydroxyprogesterone caproate. Gynecol Oncol 2:377, 1974.

Runowicz CD, Nuchtern LM, Braunstein JD, Jones JG: Heterogeneity in hormone receptor status in primary and metastatic endometrial cancer. Gynecol Oncol 38:437, 1990.

Rutledge F: The role of radical hysterectomy in adenocarcinoma of the endometrium. Gynecol Oncol 2:331, 1974.

Ryder DE: Verrucous carcinoma of the endometrium—a unique neoplasm with long survival. Obstet Gynecol 59: 78S, 1982.

Sause WT, Fuller DB, Smith WG, et al: Analysis of preoperative intracavitary cesium application versus postoperative external beam radiation in stage I endometrial carcinoma. Int J Radiat Oncol Biol Phys 18:1011, 1990.

Schink JC, Rademaker AW, Miller DS, Lurain JR: Tumor size in endometrial cancer. Cancer 67:2791, 1991.

Schlaen I, Bergeron C, Ferenczy A, et al: Endometrial polyps: a study of 204 cases. Surg Pathol 1:375, 1988.

Scully RE: Definition of endometrial carcinoma precursors. Clin Obstet Gynecol 25:39, 1982.

Sherman AI, Brown S: The precursors of endometrial carcinoma. Am J Obstet Gynecol 135:947, 1979.

Silva EG, Jenkins R: Serous carcinoma in endometrial polyps. Mod Pathol 3:120, 1990.

Silverberg SG: Hyperplasia and carcinoma of the endometrium. Semin Diagn Pathol 5:135, 1988.

Silverberg SG, DeGiorgi LS: Histopathologic analysis of preoperative radiation therapy in endometrial carcinoma. Am J Obstet Gynecol 119:698, 1974.

Sivridis E, Buckley CH, Fox H: The prognostic significance of lymphatic vascular space invasion in endometrial adenocarcinoma. Br J Obstet Gynaecol 94:991, 1987.

Slavik M, Petty WM, Blessing JA, et al: Phase II clinical study of tamoxifen in advanced endometrial adenocarcinoma: a Gynecologic Oncology Group study. Cancer Treat Rep 68:809, 1984.

Smith M, McCartney AJ: Occult, high-risk endometrial cancer. Gynecol Oncol 22:154, 1985.

Soper JT, Creasman WT, Clarke-Pearson DL, et al: Intraperitoneal chromic phosphate P-32 suspension therapy of malignant peritoneal cytology in endometrial carcinoma. Am J Obstet Gynecol 153:191, 1985.

Soper JT, Segreti EM, Novotny DB, et al: Estrogen and progesterone receptor content of endometrial carcinomas: comparison of total tissue versus cancer component analysis. Gynecol Oncol 36:363, 1990.

Sorbe B, Frankendal B, Risberg B: Intracavitary irradiation of endometrial carcinoma stage I by a high dose-rate afterloading technique. Gynecol Oncol 33:135, 1989.

Sorbe B, Risberg B, Frankendal B: DNA ploidy, morphometry, and nuclear grade as prognostic factors in endometrial carcinoma. Gynecol Oncol 38:22, 1990.

Stringer CA, Gershenson DM, Burke TW: Adjuvant chemotherapy with cisplatin, doxorubicin, and cyclophosphamide (PAC) for early-stage high-risk endometrial cancer: a preliminary analysis. Gynecol Oncol 38:305, 1990.

Surwit EA, Fowler WC Jr, Rogoff EE: Stage II carcinoma of the endometrium. Int J Radiat Oncol Biol Phys 5:323, 1979.

Sutton GP, Brill L, Michael H, et al: Malignant papillary lesions of the endometrium. Gynecol Oncol 27:294, 1987.

Szpak CA, Creasman WT, Vollmer RT, Johnston WW: Prognostic value of cytologic examination of peritoneal washings in patients with endometrial carcinoma. Acta Cytol 25:640, 1981.

Tani E, Borregon A, Humla S, Skoog L: Estrogen receptors in fine-needle aspirates from metastatic lesions of gynecologic tumors. Gynecol Oncol 32:365, 1989.

Thigpen T, Blessing J, DiSaia P, Ehrlich C: Oral medroxyprogesterone acetate in advanced or recurrent endometrial carcinoma: results of therapy and correlation with estrogen and progesterone receptor levels. The Gynecologic Oncology Group experience. In Baulieu E, Iacobelli S, McGuire W (eds): Endocrinology and Malignancy. Park Ridge, NJ, Parthenon, 1986, p 446.

Thigpen T, Blessing J, Hatch K, et al: A randomized trial of medroxyprogesterone acetate (MPA) 200 mg versus 1000 mg daily in advanced or recurrent endometrial carcinoma: a Gynecologic Oncology Group study. Proc ASCO 10:185, 1991.

Turner DA, Gershenson DM, Atkinson N, et al: The prognostic significance of peritoneal cytology for stage I endometrial cancer. Obstet Gynecol 74:775, 1989.

Umpierre SA, Burke TW, Tornos FC, et al: Immunocytochemical analysis of uterine papillary serous carcinomas for estrogen and progesterone receptors. Int J Gynecol Pathol 13:127, 1994.

Van Bogaert LJ: Clinicopathologic findings in endometrial polyps. Obstet Gynecol 71:771, 1988.

Van Hoeven KH, Hudock JA, Woodruff JM, Suhrland MJ: Small cell neuroendocrine carcinoma of the endometrium. Int J Gynecol Pathol 14:21, 1995.

Varia M, Rosenman J, Halle J, et al: Primary radiation therapy for medically inoperable patients with endometrial carcinoma—stage I–II. Int J Radiat Oncol Biol Phys 13:11, 1987.

Venkataseshan VS, Woo TH: Brief communication: diffuse viral papillomatosis (condyloma) of the uterine cavity. Int J Gynecol Pathol 4:370, 1985.

Vergote I, Kjorstad K, Abeler V, Kolstad P: A randomized trial of adjuvant progestagen in early endometrial cancer. Cancer 64:1011, 1989.

Wallin TE, Malkasian GD Jr, Gaffey TA, et al: Stage II cancer of the endometrium: a pathologic and clinical study. Gynecol Oncol 18:1, 1984.

Ward BG, Wright RG, Free K: Papillary carcinomas of the endometrium. Gynecol Oncol 39:347, 1990.

Welch WR, Scully RE: Precancerous lesions of the endometrium. Hum Pathol 8:503, 1977.

Widra EA, Dunton CJ, McHugh M, Palazzo JP: Endometrial hyperplasia and the risk of carcinoma. Int J Gynecol Cancer 5:233, 1995.

Winkler B, Alvarez S, Richart RM, Crum CP: Pitfalls in the diagnosis of endometrial neoplasia. Obstet Gynecol 64: 185, 1984.

Yancey M, Magelssen D, Demaurez A, Lee RB: Classification of endometrial cells on cervical cytology. Obstet Gynecol 76:1000, 1990.

Yazigi R, Sanchez J, Duarte I, Verni J: Cytologic detection of endometrial carcinoma by the Endocyte technique. Gynecol Oncol 16:346, 1983.

Yura Y, Tauchi K, Koshiyama M, et al: Parametrial involvement in endometrial carcinomas: its incidence and correlation with other histological parameters. Gynecol Oncol 63:114, 1996.

Zaino RJ, Kurman RJ: Squamous differentiation in carcinoma of the endometrium: a critical appraisal of adenoacanthoma and adenosquamous carcinoma. Semin Diagn Pathol 5:154, 1988.

7

Uterine Sarcomas and Related Tumors

CLASSIFICATION

Uterine sarcomas arise from either the myometrium or the endometrium. Although their histologic and biologic expressions vary considerably, for practical purposes all myometrial sarcomas are leiomyosarcomas. The endometrial sarcomas, in contrast, are usually composed of one or more types of malignant connective tissue with glandular carcinoma abundantly intermixed. Ober and Tovell (1959) credit Zenker for dividing uterine sarcomas into pure (only one cell type present) and mixed categories. These were subdivided into homologous (all tissue elements represented in the tumor are native to the uterus) or heterologous. The most frequent heterologous tissues are striated muscle, cartilage, and bone. Different authors have designated these endometrial sarcomas as mesenchymal, mesodermal, or müllerian, since the tissue of origin (endometrium) is a derivative of the müllerian apparatus, which in turn is a product of mesodermal celomic epithelium and its subjacent mesenchyme.

It has been generally agreed that the sarcomatous and carcinomatous elements are both expressions of an undifferentiated malignant stem cell. Immunochemical studies, however, suggest that the sarcomatous element in many of these mixed tumors represents metaplasia of the carcinomatous component (Meis and Lawrence, 1990; Silverberg et al, 1990), a perception that is reinforced by the finding that the metastases are usually composed entirely of carcinoma (Bitterman et al, 1990; Silverberg et al, 1990). Such malignant mixed tumors could be considered variants of endometrial carcinoma.

Some authors use the term *carcinosarcoma* to designate only those malignant mixed tumors containing stromal sarcoma and adenocarcinoma (homologous tissues), whereas others (e.g., the International Society of Gynecologic Pathologists) apply it to all tumors composed of malignant epithelial tissue mixed with homologous or heterologous sarcoma. Those who refer only to the homologous mixed tumors as carcinosarcomas often designate the heterologous mixed forms as *mixed mesodermal sarcomas* or *malignant mixed mesodermal (müllerian) tumors*. The latter term is used in this chapter, conforming to the World Health Organization (WHO) classification (Table 7–1).

From a clinical point of view, the uterine sarcomas can be divided into four major groups: (1) endometrial stromal sarcomas (ESSs), (2) leiomyosarcomas (LMSs), (3) carcinosarcoma or malignant mixed mesodermal tumors (MMMT), and (4) adenosarcomas. This is a practical working classification that encompasses the great majority of uterine sarcomas and avoids the cumbersome, sometimes confusing, albeit more specific histogenetic system. Stage for stage, the prognoses of patients with heterologous and homologous tissues are similar, limiting the usefulness of these subcategories. Carcinosarcomas account for 50 percent of uterine sarcomas; LMSs, 40 percent, and ESSs, about 8 percent. Adenosarcomas, pure heterologous sarcomas, and other even rarer variants make up the remaining 1 to 2 percent. The interested reader is referred to the articles by Ober (1959), Taylor and Norris (1966), Lauchlan (1968), Kempson and Hendrickson (1988), Silverberg et al (1990), and Clement and Scully (1991) for more detailed information about the pathogenesis of these tumors.

ENDOMETRIAL STROMAL TUMORS

There are three variants of stromal tumors described by Norris and Taylor (1966a) on the basis of morphologic features, mitosis count,

TABLE 7–1

Classification of Mesenchymal and Related Tumors of the Uterus*

Nonepithelial tumors
　Endometrial stromal tumors
　　Stromal nodule
　　Stromal sarcoma
　　　Low grade (endolymphatic stromal myosis)
　　　High grade
　Smooth muscle tumors
　　Leiomyoma and variants
　　　Cellular
　　　Epithelioid
　　　Bizarre
　　　Lipoleiomyoma
　　Smooth muscle tumor of uncertain malignant potential
　　Leiomyosarcoma and variants
　　　Epithelioid
　　　Myxoid
　　Others
　　　Intravenous leiomyomatosis
　　　Diffuse leiomyomatosis
　　　Disseminated peritoneal leiomyomatosis
　　　Benign metastasizing leiomyoma
Mixed epithelial/stromal tumors
　Benign
　　Adenofibroma
　　Adenomyoma
　Malignant
　　Malignant mixed mesodermal tumor
　　　Homologous
　　　Heterologous
　　Adenosarcoma
　　　Homologous
　　　Heterologous
　　Carcinofibroma
Miscellaneous

*Adapted from Clement PB, Scully RE: Pathology of uterine sarcomas, In Coppleson M (ed): Gynecologic Oncology. Edinburgh, Churchill Livingstone, 1991, p 803, with permission.

and biologic behavior. These are the stromal nodule (benign), low-grade stromal sarcoma or endolymphatic stromal myosis (a low-grade, infiltrating sarcoma), and high-grade stromal sarcoma (a frankly malignant tumor). The first two neoplasms characteristically have recognizable proliferative phase endometrial stromal differentiation, while the third is composed of anaplastic cells like the stromal component of malignant mixed mesodermal tumors (Norris and Taylor, 1966a; Evans, 1982; Chang et al, 1990).

Endometrial Stromal Nodule

Norris and Taylor (1966a) concluded, after reviewing the pathologic findings and clinical course of 18 patients (ages not specified) with a well-circumscribed myometrial nodule of pure neoplastic endometrial stroma, that the lesions were benign. All had pushing margins, were solitary, and were devoid of vascular and lymphatic space invasion. Although the mitosis count in one instance was 15/10 hpf, 16 of the 18 cases had counts of 3/10 hpf or less. None of the patients experienced recurrence, but the length of follow-up was not stated. Fekete and Vellios (1984) reported 12 cases of endometrial stromal nodule, with a median patient age of 53 years. The usual presentation was with vaginal bleeding and an enlarged uterus. The nodules varied in size from 2 to 9 cm. One woman had a mitosis count of 11/10 hpf, the only count above 3/10 hpf. No recurrences were noted. Because so few cases of this entity with a high mitosis count have been observed, it would be prudent to restrict the diagnosis to those lesions with three or fewer mitoses per 10 hpf. Hysterectomy is adequate therapy. Successful treatment of a 12-cm stromal nodule by "myomectomy" has been reported (Chang et al, 1990).

Low-Grade Endometrial Stromal Sarcoma (Endolymphatic Stromal Myosis)

Clinicopathologic Features

Low-grade endometrial stromal sarcoma (LGESS) occurs predominantly in premenopausal women. It arises from the endometrial stroma, from adenomyosis, or, rarely, from endometriosis. The patients usually present with abnormal vaginal bleeding. Pelvic and abdominal pain are also frequent complaints. The diagnosis is seldom made preoperatively. This may in part reflect the predominantly intramural rather than intracavitary growth pattern (Fig. 7–1). Typically, the patient undergoes surgery for "uterine fibroids" or a pelvic mass. The physician should be alert to this diagnosis when uterine curettings yield hyperplastic stroma with few glands.

In a literature review of 138 cases of LGESS, Bohr and Thomsen (1991) found that one third had extended beyond the uterus at the time of diagnosis, but, in the series of Chang et al (1990), 84 percent of 92 cases had stage I disease. Table 7–2 gives the stage distributions in several reports from the literature. The extrauterine extensions usually consist of pale yellow, worm-like, rubbery growths extending through the myometrium into the lymphatic and venous channels of the broad ligament, adnexa, and cardinal ligament.

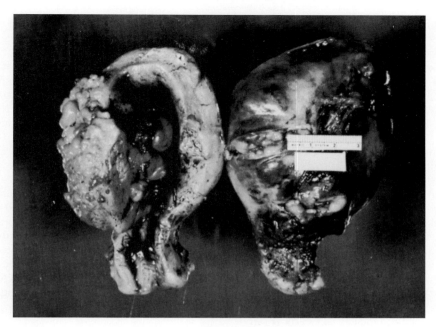

FIGURE 7–1. Low-grade endometrial stromal sarcoma. Gross specimen with deep invasion of the my-ometrium and extension into the parametrium on the right. The patient had negative pelvic nodes.

Intra-abdominal spread and pulmonary me-tastases also occur. Microscopically, LGESS is characterized by pushing or infiltrating mar-gins and lymphatic or vascular invasion. There is minimal cytologic atypia and usually fewer than 5 to 10 mitoses per 10 hpf. Within this range, however, the mitosis count does not identify which stage I cases will behave aggressively (Chang et al, 1990). For exam-ple, in Kempson's (1994) series of 73 stage I patients, 4 of 15 with grade 2 or 3 cytologic atypia and a mitotic index (MI = mitoses/10 hpf) greater than 10 relapsed, compared with 22 of 54 patients with grade 1 atypia and a MI of less than 10. Among the 17 stage III and IV patients, 5 of 6 with grade 2 or 3 cy-tologic atypia and a MI greater than 10 re-lapsed. Thus, stage is a more important de-terminant of relapse than cytologic atypia or MI (Chang et al, 1990). LGESS that contains benign endometrial glands should not be in-terpreted as adenosarcoma or uterine MMMT.

The clinical behavior of LGESS is not that of a low-grade malignancy in terms of the fre-quency of recurrence, since 30 to 50 percent of stage I cases relapse. However, the recur-rences do tend to appear late (median 36 months) and progress slowly. Sites of recur-rence are predominantly pelvic, parametrial, vaginal, and bladder. The abdomen and lung are the most common sites of distant metas-tasis. Long-term survival is the rule, but cure

TABLE 7–2

Uterine Sarcomas: Distribution by Stage and Cell Type*

Stage	LGESS†		HGESS‡		LMS		MMMT§	
	No.	Percent	No.	Percent	No.	Percent	No.	Percent
I	132	78	47	63	151	65	118	50
II	7	4	4	5	13	6	33	14
III	21	12	14	19	25	11	41	17
IV	9	5	9	12	42	18	43	18
Total	169		74		231		235	

* Data from Chang et al (1990), Covens et al (1987), Echt et al (1990), Kahanpää et al (1986), Olah et al (1991), and Piver et al (1984).
† LGESS = low-grade endometrial stromal sarcoma.
‡ HGESS = high-grade endometrial stromal sarcoma.
§ MMMT = malignant mixed mesodermal tumor.

rates are difficult to calculate since recurrences after 5 or 10 years are common and reports in the literature vary widely. For example, in Kempson and Bari's (1970) series, nine stage I and II patients were all free of recurrence 3 to 15 years posthysterectomy. Norris and Taylor (1966a) reported on 15 stage I and II patients, 3 of whom recurred locally at 4, 10, and 15 years (all 3 had been treated by supracervical hysterectomy). These compare with Hart and Billman's four patients (1978) with disease confined to the uterus, of whom three recurred (at 2, 2, and 14 years).

Piver et al (1984) collated data on 55 cases of LGESS from several institutions. The patients' ages ranged from 20 to 79 years, but 70 percent were younger than 50 years. The percentage of cases in surgicopathologic stages I to IV were 65.6, 5.7, 21.1, and 7.6, respectively. Recurrence was diagnosed in 55 percent of the stage I cases: 12 pelvis, 4 pelvis plus extrapelvic, and 3 with distant metastases only. The median time to recurrence was 36 months, with a range from 3 to 274 months. None of five stage I patients who received postoperative pelvic radiation developed pelvic recurrence, although two manifested distant metastases. The status of all recurrent stage I patients is given in Table 7–3. Seven are free of disease with further therapy, including three of four patients receiving pelvic radiation therapy.

Overall, in the Piver et al (1984) series 13 patients received progestins for recurrent or advanced disease. There were three complete, three partial, and six stable disease responses lasting 2 to 104 months (median >48 months). Nine patients were still responding, while three progressed at 60, 36, and 30 months. In the review of Bohr and Thomsen (1991), 5 of 15 patients with recurrent LGESS exhibited a complete response to progestin therapy.

Chemotherapy was given to 12 patients in the Piver series, 9 of whom received regimens incorporating doxorubicin. There were two responders, both continuing at 19 and 27 months. It is of interest that the 5- and 10-year survival rates did not seem to be greatly influenced by the stage (88, 66, 100, and 75 percent for stages I to IV, respectively). From the papers of Yoonessi and Hart (1977) and Norris and Taylor (1966a), six of eight cases (75 percent) with extrauterine extension recurred.

The reports of Gloor et al (1982), Baker et al (1984), and Sutton et al (1986) document that LGESS frequently contains significant levels of estrogen (21 to 72 fmol) and progesterone (71 to 803 fmol) receptor protein, which probably correlate with hormone responsiveness and prognosis. DNA ploidy is reported to have only minor prognostic significance (Nordal et al, 1996).

Treatment

The spread and recurrence patterns of LGESS suggest that primary therapy by radical hysterectomy should improve local control (Krieger and Gusberg, 1973). Since nodal involvement is unusual, lymphadenectomy is of dubious value. The applicability of radical hysterectomy is limited, however, because the diagnosis is usually made during or after surgery. It may be prudent to remove the adnexa, which can be a site of occult involvement by tumor. Furthermore, the ovaries are a source of estrogen, which may stimulate residual LGESS. Removing the ovaries has been reported to be either beneficial or neutral with respect to the cancer (Berchuck et al, 1990; Norris and Taylor, 1966a). While the overall rate of recurrence in stage I cases is 50 percent, recurrence is more likely with tumors greater than 5 cm or that have vascular space invasion or parametrial extension. Post-

TABLE 7–3

Low-Grade Endometrial Stromal Sarcoma: Treatment of Recurrence and Survival of 19 Surgicopathologic Stage I Cases*

Status	Progestin		Chemotherapy		Pelvic Radiation		Pelvic Radiation Plus Progestin	
	No.	Months	No.	Months	No.	Months	No.	Months
Alive, no evidence of disease	3	2, 76, 104	1	19	2	73, 74	1	80
Alive, with cancer	2	4, 112	1	121	1	172	—	—
Dead with cancer	3	84, 113, 143	5	3, 3, 8, 36, 38	—	—	—	—

*Data from Piver et al (1984).

operative therapy is warranted routinely in these cases (Fig. 7–2). Both high-dose progestogen (e.g., medroxyprogesterone acetate 100 mg/day orally) and pelvic radiation seem to be effective. The absence of hormone receptors would favor the use of radiation, while slender stature and other features increasing the risk of radiation complications would favor hormone therapy if progestin receptor proteins are present. Because hormone therapy is generally considered to be cytostatic, once a response is achieved, the progestin should be continued for life unless progression intervenes. Chemotherapy can be recommended only for those cases of LGESS that progress or are symptomatic after the standard measures fail. Follow-up with determination of serial serum CA-125 levels may be helpful (Patsner and Mann, 1988).

High-Grade Endometrial Stromal Sarcoma (HGESS)

Clinicopathologic Features

High-grade endometrial stromal sarcoma, a pure, homologous uterine sarcoma, occurs predominantly in postmenopausal women, although it can develop during the reproductive years or even in childhood. The patient seeks treatment most commonly because of postmenopausal bleeding or menometrorrhagia, but a significant number complain of pelvic pain. The diagnosis is usually made by uterine curettage (Fig. 7–3).

Survival data in the literature seldom take into account the histologic variants of HGESS. In fact, LGESS with a high mitosis count and HGESS are often reported together. Further-

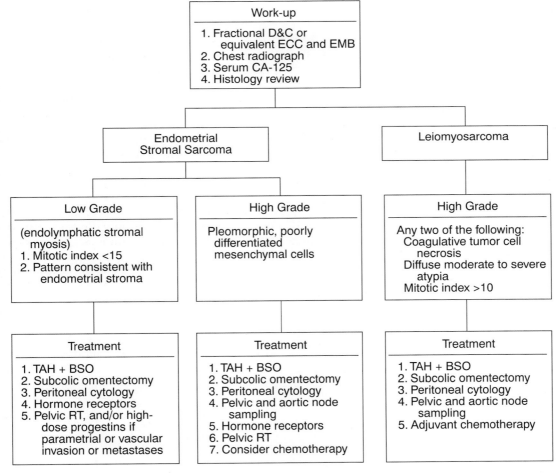

FIGURE 7–2. Management algorithm for uterine stromal sarcoma and leiomyosarcoma. BSO = bilateral salpingo-oophorectomy; D&C = dilatation and curettage; ECC = endocervical curettage; EMB = endometrial biopsy; RT = radiation therapy; TAH = total abdominal hysterectomy.

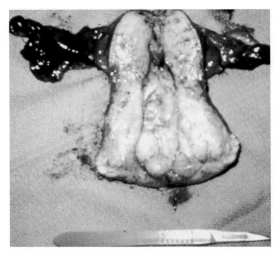

FIGURE 7–3. High-grade endometrial stromal sarcoma arising from the lower corpus and protruding through the external cervical os. Diagnosis was made from tissue removed during office examination.

more, the extent of disease at the time of diagnosis is commonly ignored, and both surgical and clinical staging systems are employed. Nevertheless, it can be concluded that the two most important prognostic factors are the histology and the surgical stage of disease (Table 7–4). Evans (1982) reported on seven patients with poorly differentiated stromal sarcoma. Although none had gross tumor beyond the uterus at hysterectomy, six experienced recurrence and died within 3 years.

Treatment

Total abdominal hysterectomy and bilateral salpingo-oophorectomy is the first step in

TABLE 7–4

Uterine Sarcoma: Survival by Histology and Clinical Stage[*,†]

Histology	Total Cases	Stage I N	Stage I (%)	Stage II N	Stage II (%)	Stage III N	Stage III (%)	Stage IV N	Stage IV (%)
LGESS	65	55	(89)	4	(75)	6	(67)	0	(—)
HGESS	100	90	(78)	1	(0)	7	(14)	2	(0)
LMS	108	91	(48)	3	(67)	5	(0)	9	(0)
MMMT	399	245	(36)	55	(22)	69	(10)	30	(6)

[*] Data from Berchuck et al (1988, 1990), Covens et al (1987), De Fusco et al (1989), Doss et al (1984) Kahanpää et al (1986), Larson et al (1990a, 1990b), Macasaet et al (1985), Mantravadi et al (1981), Norris and Taylor (1966a,b), Norris et al (1966), Piver et al (1984), Spanos et al (1984), Wheelock et al (1985), and Yoonessi and Hart (1977).

[†] Not all patients were followed for 5 years.

therapy. Surgical staging is also warranted. (In the autopsy study of Fleming et al [1984], four of six patients had nodal metastases and all six had intraperitoneal metastases). Pelvic irradiation undoubtedly improves local control and is recommended for all stage I patients, but it appears that local/regional therapy may be inadequate, especially if the myometrium is deeply invaded. High receptor content would make progestins the first choice for adjuvant therapy. For receptor-negative tumors, doxorubicin-based combination chemotherapy would be appropriate. Follow-up with serum CA-125 determinations may be of value.

TUMORS OF THE MYOMETRIUM

For the past decade or more, the clinical behavior of uterine smooth muscle tumors (USMTs) has been predicated on the MI, i.e. the number of mitoses counted per 10 hpf. It has been clear, however, that some USMTs with a low MI (<5) were clinically malignant, whereas some USMTs with a high MI (>10) were clinically benign. Furthermore, mitosis counting is subject to substantial interobserver variability. The dilemma of predicting the clinical behavior of USMTs on the basis of their histopathologic features has been largely solved by Bell et al (1994) in a study of 213 USMTs that they termed problematic. The authors excluded neoplasms with a myxoid or epithelioid component, and also neoplasms with a MI less than 5 that lacked cellular atypia. To discriminate between the benign and malignant tumors, three criteria were employed: MI greater than 10, diffuse moderate to severe cytologic atypia, and coagulative tumor cell necrosis (CTCN). USMTs with any two of these three features were associated with a 63 percent relapse rate (32 of 51 cases). Other investigators have shown that DNA ploidy and proliferative activity of these tumors is of little or no value in predicting clinical behavior (Peters et al, 1992).

Variants of Leiomyoma

Lipoleiomyoma

In 1978, Willén et al were able to find more than 150 instances of this tumor reported in the world's literature, although it seems to be rarely encountered in clinical practice today.

Lipoleiomyomas are simply myomas containing adipose tissue, and clinically they are indistinguishable from the ordinary leiomyoma. The pattern of fat within the tumor may be focal, intermixed, or predominant. In the latter case the neoplasm resembles a lipoma. Not unexpectedly, the lipoleiomyoma is more likely to occur in obese women and women with gallbladder disease. The fat is thought to arise from metaplasia of the smooth muscle or normal connective tissue of the myoma. Some authorities have classified these tumors as benign mixed mesodermal tumors. None of these tumors has been reported to exhibit malignant behavior.

Cellular Leiomyoma

The cellular leiomyoma is relatively common but has no clinical significance in the absence of increased mitotic activity, cytologic atypia, or CTCN provided that it is not misdiagnosed as a leiomyosarcoma. Uterine myomas may grow in response to ovarian steroid hormones, raising the suspicion of malignancy. Clinically this occurs in reproductive-age women, especially during pregnancy, while taking oral contraceptives, or during clomiphene therapy. These events are associated with a slightly increased MI in the normal myometrium and benign myomas. Kawaguchi et al (1989) quantified the variability of the MI in myomas in relation to patient age and phase of the menstrual cycle. The average MI was 2 in myomas from women less than 35 years of age, compared with an average MI of 1 in women older than 35. They also reported that, during the secretory phase of the menstrual cycle, the average MI of myomas was 1.3 versus 0.4 during the proliferative phase. Thus it seems that the mitotic activity of uterine myomas is promoted more by the combined effect of estrogen and progesterone than by estrogen alone. Of particular interest is the finding that 5 percent of myomas examined during the secretory phase had a MI of 4 to 5.

Considering the findings of Kawaguchi and colleagues, the MI of the garden-variety uterine leiomyoma in a favorable hormonal milieu could overlap the low-end mitosis count considered to be of low malignant potential when employing MI as the only criterion for malignancy. This stresses the importance of the work of Bell et al (1994) in using the three histopathologic criteria of MI, cytologic atypia, and CTCN for separating the benign from the malignant smooth muscle tumors.

Smooth Muscle Tumors of Uncertain Malignant Potential

As indicated in the preceding paragraphs, prior to the report of Bell et al (1994), USMTs with an MI of 5 to 10 were viewed as having an uncertain or low degree of malignant potential. This problem has largely been resolved by basing the diagnosis of benignity or malignancy upon the absence or presence of cytologic atypia and CTCN in addition to the MI, as discussed previously. However, in the Bell study there were two groups of USMTs that did not qualify as leiomyosarcomas but that exhibited a low level of malignant behavior. One group of 46 USMTs had no CTCN and a MI less than 10, but moderate to severe diffuse cytologic atypia. One of these tumors recurred, but the patient was alive, albeit with disease, at 60 months' follow-up. The authors designated this group of tumors as "atypical leiomyomas with a low risk of recurrence." The other group, designated "leiomyomas with increased mitotic activity," consisted of 89 USMTs with an MI of 5 to 20 but with no more than mild cellular atypia and no coagulative necrosis. The single recurrence in this group resulted in a fatal outcome 96 months after diagnosis. The authors point out that, by combining their cases in this group with those in the literature, only 1 in 200 has recurred. The benign behavior of mitotically active, bland UTSMs has been reported by others (Perrone and Dehner, 1988; O'Connor and Norris, 1990; Prayson and Hart, 1992).

Epithelioid Leiomyomas

Included in this diagnosis are the leiomyoblastoma, clear cell leiomyoma, and plexiform tumorlet. The epithelioid leiomyoma is characterized by round or polygonal epithelial-like cells with a clear or eosinophilic cytoplasm, in contrast to the typical cigar-shaped cells of the classic leiomyoma. Kurman and Norris (1976) reported on 26 cases of these atypical USMTs. The patient ages ranged from 27 to 67 years with a mean of 48 years. The most frequent presenting complaints were common to all uterine myomas: vaginal bleeding, pelvic-abdominal pain, and enlargement of the abdomen.

On gross pathology the epithelioid leiomyoma is not different than the conventional uterine myoma. Microscopically 18 had infiltrating margins, 4 had evidence of LVSI, and 3 had a MI greater than 10 in the Kurman and

Norris report. Only one of the 26 cases had marked cytologic atypia. There were a total of three recurrences. Malignant behavior was associated with CTCN, size greater than 6 cm, and a MI greater than 2. Kempson (1994) considers epithelioid USMTs with a MI greater than 2 combined with either CTCN or cytologic atypia to be malignant.

The plexiform variant results from extensive ischemic necrosis with hyalinization. The pattern may be multifocal, at times with extensive involvement of the tumor. None has been known to recur (Kaminski and Tavassoli, 1984).

USMTs Diagnosed at Myomectomy

Van Dinh and Woodruff (1982) reviewed the outcome of six patients undergoing myomectomy whose myomas were found to have a MI from 4 to 9. One of the six recurred with metastases 2 years later. In the series of O'Connor and Norris (1990), 14 of 73 women with mitotically active leiomyomas had been managed by myomectomy. The single patient with recurrence was cured by hysterectomy. Bell et al (1994) reported that 56 of their 213 problematic USMTs were initially managed by myomectomy. None of the 27 with a MI greater than 5, no significant cytologic atypia, and no CTCN persisted or recurred. Among the 21 tumors with significant cytologic atypia but no CTCN and a MI less than 10 that were removed by myomectomy, 3 had a histologically identical tumor in the hysterectomy specimen. All 21 of these patients were alive and well.

On the basis of these reports, myomectomy seems to be a reasonable treatment alternative to hysterectomy for the patient with a uterine myoma having only one of the three histopathologic criteria for malignancy who desires reproductive preservation. This does not apply to the epithelioid and myxoid leiomyomas, which, despite a low mitosis count and benign appearance, have a substantial malignant potential.

The Uterine Leiomyomatoses

Intravenous Leiomyomatosis

Intravenous leiomyomatosis (IVL) is a rare neoplastic disorder that occurs predominantly in premenopausal women. The clinical presentation is characterized by pain, abnormal uterine bleeding, and an irregular, enlarged uterus. At surgery the presence of yellow, worm-like, fibrous extensions of the myoma into the uterine veins is pathognomonic. These intravenous protrusions may also grow into the broad ligament and vaginal veins. The pelvic veins are involved in 80 percent of cases, and in 30 percent the tumor extends into the vena cava and right heart. The origin of IVL may be directly from the vein wall or from a myoma, and the tumor may be densely adherent or easily removed from the veins. Histologically, IVL may represent any of the variants of myoma, including cellular, epithelioid, and myxoid types (Clement et al, 1988).

According to the review of Clement (1988), 17 of 75 collected cases recurred from 0.6 to 15 years posthysterectomy. The sites of recurrence were almost exclusively intravenous: pelvis, vena cava, and right heart. There is reasonable evidence that, as with leiomyomas, the behavior of these tumors is influenced by female sex steroids. For examples, all six recurrences among the 45 cases reported by Norris and Parmley (1975), Evans et al (1981), and Bahary et al (1982) had residual functioning ovarian tissue, and regression of pulmonary metastases during pregnancy has been reported (Horstmann et al, 1977). It is also known that IVL contains estrogen and progesterone receptors. Thus it seems prudent to remove both ovaries in addition to the uterus, especially if the tumor cannot be completely excised. In the presence of densely adherent, unresectable intravenous tumor, ligation of the vein proximal to the tumor has been recommended (Heinonen et al, 1984). While response to tamoxifen has been reported (Tierney et al, 1980), the first line of therapy for recurrent tumor should be surgical.

More than 22 cases of IVL with extension into the vena cava and right heart have been reported in the literature, of which 15 have been successfully treated with surgery (Suginami et al, 1990). These patients present with cardiac symptoms attributable to impaired tricuspid valve function. The finding of a right atrial mass on echocardiography in a patient with a pelvic mass or prior hysterectomy for fibroids should lead to the suspicion of IVL rather than atrial myxoma (Kaszar-Siebert et al, 1988).

Benign Metastasizing Leiomyoma

Benign metastasizing leiomyoma (BML), another rare biologic expression of uterine smooth muscle behavior, does not have the intravascular extensions of IVL, but produces pulmonary metastases that may appear many years after hysterectomy for typical myomas. Other sites of involvement include the retroperitoneal and mediastinal lymph nodes, soft tissue, and bone. Histologically the lesions appear benign. Cho et al (1989) suggest that at least some instances of BML might be multifocal in origin. This theory is supported by cases with an unusual distribution of metastases and also by the occurrence of multifocal smooth muscle gastrointestinal and cutaneous tumors, the latter represented by familial leiomyomatosis cutis (piloleiomyomas) et uteri (Reed syndrome). BML, which occurs predominantly during the reproductive years, has been reported to regress during pregnancy and at menopause, suggesting that it is hormone dependent (Hortsmann et al, 1977). The treatment of choice is antiestogen therapy (e.g., gonadotropin-releasing hormone analog, progestogen, tamoxifen, or ovariectomy). Patients with pulmonary insufficiency may be candidates for lung transplantation.

A possibly related disorder that occurs only in women is pulmonary lymphangioleiomyomatosis (LAM), characterized by proliferation of the smooth muscle along the thoracic and pulmonary lymphatics and causing interstitial and obstructive lung disease. The patients present with spontaneous pneumothorax, chylothorax, hemoptysis, and dyspnea (Taylor et al, 1990). Like BML, LAM is more likely to progress before menopause than after. The two entities can occur simultaneously, presenting additional evidence of an etiologic-biologic relationship.

Disseminated Peritoneal Leiomyomatosis

Also known as *leiomyomatosis peritonealis disseminata*, disseminated peritoneal leiomyomatosis (DPL) is a rare, usually benign hyperplastic disorder featuring multiple smooth muscle, subperitoneal nodules involving the parietal and visceral peritoneum, the uterus, and the omentum. The nodules are firm, grey-white, and usually under 3 cm in diameter, although much larger masses have been reported. In 1988, Fujii collected 61 cases of DPL from the literature. The patients' ages ranged from 22 to 69 years, 42 percent were black, 23 percent had been using oral contraceptives, and 40 percent of the cases were associated with pregnancy. The average age of the hormone-associated cases (pregnancy, oral contraceptives) was 33, versus 41 for the others. A single case had a concomitant granulosa tumor of the ovary. The 37 nonpregnant patients presented with pelvic discomfort or pain, with or without abnormal bleeding. Coexisting uterine myomas were present in 33 of these patients. Occasionally, DPL was an incidental finding at laparotomy for unrelated reasons.

During follow-up, most cases manifested regression that was spontaneous or related to bilateral oophorectomy, withdrawal of hormones, or resolution of a pregnancy. Tumor progression has been reported with subsequent pregnancy, and persistence with or without subsequent pregnancy can occur even after many years. Because of the predominantly benign course, no specific treatment is required. Hysterectomy is occasionally necessitated because of extensive involvement of the uterus by multiple leiomyomatous nodules. Although no deaths from DPL have been reported, at least one case has converted to LMS (Akkersdijk et al, 1990).

Leiomyosarcoma

Clinical Features

LMSs comprise 15 to 40 percent of all uterine sarcomas. The average age at diagnosis is 53 years. Women with cellular or bizarre leiomyomas are on the average 10 years younger. Twenty percent of women with LMS are nulliparous. The initial symptom in three fourths of the cases is either menometrorrhagia or postmenopausal bleeding. Other first symptoms include pelvic-abdominal pain or pressure, the awareness of a mass, and a vaginal discharge. Pap smears are rarely of any value. Diagnosis at uterine curettage is made in only 15 to 30 percent of cases, even though 50 percent have submucous lesions. Most cases are diagnosed incidental to surgery for "fibroids." In a study by Leibsohn et al (1990), approximately 1 percent of women over age 40 years who underwent surgery with a preoperative diagnosis of uterine leiomyoma proved to have LMS. Most of these LMS patients had abnormal bleeding and a single uterine tumor, findings that should increase the suspicion of sarcoma. Parker et al (1994) have addressed the validity of a rapidly enlarging myomatous uterus as a clinical sign of sarcoma. Among 371 women in their study operated on for a rapidly growing leiomyoma, only one had a uterine sarcoma. These authors also noted that there is scant evidence in the literature to support the common teaching that rapid uterine enlargement heralds the onset of LMS. Obvious clinical extension beyond the uterus at the time of presentation is unusual, but when it occurs the most common site is the lung (Goff et al, 1993). Rarely, LMS arises in the broad ligament or other extrauterine pelvic sites (Todd et al, 1995).

Spread Pattern

Uterine LMS spreads by local extension, peritoneal implantation, and lymph–vascular space invasion (LVSI). The reported frequency of nodal metastases associated with clinical stage I and II cases varies from less than 5 percent to 75 percent, with an average of about 15 percent (Chen, 1989). In the Gynecologic Oncology Group (GOG) study, 83 percent of 59 clinical stage I and II LMS patients were surgical stage I. Only 2 of the 59 patients had lymph node metastases, 2 had adnexal involvement, and 3 had a positive peritoneal cytology. However, because the GOG surgical staging procedure used node sampling rather than a clean node dissection, it is expected that the frequency of nodal metastases was underestimated in their study. In the series of Goff et al (1993), 4 of 15 cases (27 percent) had lymph node involvement, but all 4 of these patients also had intraperitoneal metastases. That lymph node spread occurs commonly as a late manifestation of LMS is further supported by the data of Fleming et al (1984). In a collected series of 34 autopsies on patients dying of LMS, 44 percent had lymph node metastases which, in some reports, were predominantly aortic. Fifty-five percent of the cases had disease above the diaphragm. Sites of distant metastasis included the lung, liver, brain, kidney, and bone.

Pathology

Malignant as well as benign USMTs are thought to arise from either the myometrium itself or the smooth muscle of the myometrial veins. LMS invariably contains no type of malignant cell other than smooth muscle. For many years the diagnostic criteria for malignancy were controversial, but, as previously noted, this issue has been largely resolved by the studies of Bell et al (1994). Malignant behavior is almost exclusively limited to USMTs

with any two of the sentinel histopathologic features: CTCN, diffuse moderate to severe cytologic atypia, and MI greater than 10. These diagnostic criteria do not apply to the epithelioid and myxoid LMSs (Salm and Evans, 1985; Buscema et al, 1986). Rarely USMTs may exhibit malignant behavior without meeting these diagnostic criteria, but they are almost invariably indolent and have at least one of the sentinel histologic features. LMSs may be located anywhere in the uterus but are predominantly intramural. The size varies in the extreme, but 50 percent are between 6 and 10 cm (Major et al, 1993). Origin in a benign myoma (5 to 10 percent of cases), premenopausal patient status, and size less than 5 cm are reported to be favorable prognostic features (Evans et al, 1988).

Treatment

Surgery. LMS of the uterine corpus is treated by total abdominal hysterectomy and bilateral salpingo-oophorectomy. Because the cervix is often involved, a supracervical hysterectomy must be considered inadequate therapy. Intraoperative diagnosis based on frozen section of a suspicious myoma is reported to be accurate in only 20 percent of cases (Schwartz et al, 1993). This fact adds weight to the importance of performing a fractional dilatation and curettage (D&C) before hysterectomy in the patient with a myomatous uterus and abnormal bleeding. Not only is the clinician able to detect important causes of bleeding unrelated to the myomas (cervical or endometrial cancer), but 15 to 30 percent of LMSs can be diagnosed by uterine curettage. With a known diagnosis of LMS, aortic and pelvic node sampling, partial omentectomy, and peritoneal cytology are recommended as part of the surgical procedure. When the diagnosis is made after myomectomy, reoperation should be undertaken to remove the residual internal genitalia and perform surgical staging.

Radiation Therapy. Two studies suggest that radiation has little value in the treatment of uterine LMS. In a GOG report (Hornback et al, 1986), 2 of 6 recurrences in the pelvic radiation group were vaginal/pelvic compared with 2 of 17 recurrences in the no-radiation-therapy group. Berchuck et al (1988) observed no responses to radiation therapy among 10 patients with recurrent LMS. In another GOG report (Major et al, 1993), however, there were no pelvic recurrences among 13 patients receiving postoperative pelvic radiation therapy compared with 8 of 46 (17 percent) in the no-radiation-therapy group. It is the authors' opinion, considering the predominance of distant metastases and the lack of, or inconsistent, evidence that LMS is radiation sensitive, the role of radiation therapy in the management of uterine LMS should be restricted to special situations such as treating bone metastases.

Chemotherapy. The relatively high rate of recurrence (50 to 75 percent) in patients with clinical stage I and II uterine LMS, and the preponderance of distant metastases (40 to 80 percent) make patients with this malignancy excellent candidates for adjuvant chemotherapy. Unfortunately, evidence for the efficacy of such therapy is not conclusive. In a GOG randomized study of postoperative adjuvant doxorubicin, fewer patients in the treatment arm developed distant metastases (27 percent) than in the control arm (55 percent), although there was no significant difference in survival (Omura et al, 1985). That doxorubicin may be useful in the adjuvant setting is also supported by the findings of another GOG study in which 25 percent of patients with advanced or recurrent LMS exhibited an objective response to doxorubicin (Omura et al, 1983). Agents reported to be active against LMS in addition to doxorubicin are ifosfamide (Sutton et al, 1993) and oral etoposide (Chantarawiroj et al, 1995).

On the basis of these considerations, and recognizing that it is an area of reasonable disagreement, we recommend doxorubicin-based adjuvant chemotherapy for patients with high-grade uterine LMS, that is, those with malignant tumors based upon the criteria of Bell et al (1994). Certainly when extrauterine extension is documented, chemotherapy is indicated. Follow-up with serum CA-125 values, gynecologic examination, and chest radiograph is recommended. Surgical resection of pulmonary or other metastases, especially those temporally remote from the original therapy, may be indicated in the absence of widespread disease. Five-year survival rates of up to 43 percent have been reported in this circumstance (Levenback et al, 1992).

Outcome

The most informative survival data derive from the GOG surgical staging study, even though postoperative therapy was not pre-scribed in the protocol. The 3-year progression-free survival for al 59 clinical stage I and II patients (49 surgical stage I) was 31 percent; the figure was only 21 percent with tumors having a MI greater than 20 (Major et al, 1993). In the series of Goff et al (1993), none of eight patients with surgical stage I disease limited to the inner 50 percent of the myometrium relapsed. Major et al (1993) studied the recurrence pattern in 42 patients. The first site of recurrence in 57 percent was lung, whereas only 20 percent recurred first in the pelvis. These data are consistent with the findings of other authors (Omura et al, 1985; Van Dinh et al, 1982). Late-developing, isolated lung metastases are unusual.

OTHER SOFT TISSUE TUMORS

Adenomatoid Tumor

The adenomatoid tumor, a variant of benign mesothelioma, also occurs in the uterus. Clinically it resembles a subserous myoma, measuring up to 8 cm in diameter (Grunebaum and Sedlis, 1982). Simple removal is adequate therapy (see also Chapter 10).

Hemangiopericytoma

Wilbanks and coauthors (1975) collected 42 cases of uterine hemangiopericytoma (HPC) from the literature, and in 1987 Buscema et al reported 21 additional cases. The age at diagnosis has varied from 19 to 81 years, with an average of 42 years. Patients with uterine HPC present with abnormal vaginal bleeding and an irregular, enlarged uterus usually thought to contain leiomyomas. The lesions range up to 25 cm in maximum diameter, are firm unless necrotic, and vary in color. Most are yellow on cross-sectioning. Uterine HPC should be considered a low-grade malignancy. Eight of 56 patients followed for 2 years or longer experienced recurrence. Two of the eight were apparently cured with further treatment. The reported time to recurrence was 2 to 26 years. No clinical or pathologic feature predictive of recurrence has been identified. Extrauterine, pelvic HPC is evidently more malignant. In the review of Wilbanks et al (1975), only three of seven patients were alive and well after 2 years of follow-up.

Treatment of uterine HPC is primarily surgical. If complete resection cannot be carried out, radiation therapy or chemotherapy may be indicated. For pelvic HPC, preoperative angiography can be diagnostic. Because of the vascularity of extrauterine HPC, embolization has been used to facilitate surgical excision (Smullens et al, 1982).

Angiosarcoma

Twelve cases of angiosarcoma (hemangioendothelioma) of the uterus have been reported (Quinonez et al, 1991) in women ages 17 to 76 years. Of the eight patients with more than 6 months' follow-up, six experienced recurrence and two were alive and well at 18 and 48 months. The latter received adjuvant doxorubicin/cisplatin chemotherapy. Of the patients with recurrence, one was apparently cured by radiation therapy. Another patient had three recurrences over 8 years and died of cancer.

Rhabdomyosarcoma

Pure pleomorphic rhabdomyosarcoma of the endometrium is a rare form of corpus sarcoma. In a literature review, Donkers et al (1972) found only 51 cases. Patient ages ranged from 36 to 90 years, with only a few under age 50 years. Many of the patients died within 1 year of diagnosis, and it has been generally accepted that the prognosis is grave. Nearly all adult uterine rhabdomyosarcomas are pleomorphic. These patients are candidates for posthysterectomy adjuvant therapy, but the value of either radiation or chemotherapy is dubious. A doxorubicin-containing drug regimen may be preferable to vincristine, actinomycin D, and cyclophosphamide (VAC) chemotherapy.

In contrast, the prognosis for early-stage embryonal rhabdomyosarcoma of the uterus (Fig. 7–4) is generally excellent. All six of the patients reported by Montag et al (1986) were alive and well 24 to 144 months after diagnosis. The recommended treatment is modified radical hysterectomy, pelvic lymphadenectomy, and VAC chemotherapy for six cycles. If there is microscopic parametrial disease or node metastases, pelvic radiation is also advisable. Advanced disease treated initially with chemotherapy may permit subsequent curative surgical extirpation (Hays et al, 1988; Ghavimi, 1991).

Osteosarcoma

Crum and co-workers (1980) and Piscioli et al (1985) have reviewed the literature on pure

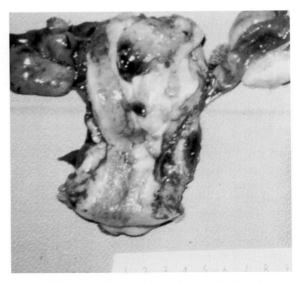

FIGURE 7–4. Botryoid embryonal rhabdomyosarcoma. Surgical specimen from a 26-year-old woman showing extension to the cervix. The patient is alive and well 8 years after radical hysterectomy (modified), bilateral pelvilymphadenectomy, and VAC chemotherapy.

osteogenic sarcoma of the uterus. Only nine cases have been documented. The youngest patient was 41 years and the oldest 82 years at diagnosis. All but one presented with vaginal bleeding. In four patients the tumor was extending beyond the uterus (stages III and IV). Of the five patients with disease confined to the uterus, two survived beyond 1 year but died at 20 and 38 months with distant metastases. Patients with osteogenic sarcomas are clearly candidates for adjuvant postoperative therapy.

Chondrosarcoma

The literature on uterine chondrosarcoma was reviewed by Clement in 1978. Including his own patient, he was able to identify 13 patients with this rare malignant neoplasm. They were 36 to 66 years of age and presented with vaginal bleeding, abdominal pain, dysuria, vaginal discharge, and an enlarged uterus. Several had tumor protruding through the cervical os. Despite the absence of clinical metastases at diagnosis, seven of eight patients with more than 6 months follow-up died of disease 4 to 23 months postoperation. The other patient was alive and well at 8 months. Recurrences were abdominal, pelvic, and pulmonary.

Lymphoma

Involvement of the uterus, cervix, and ovaries is relatively common in disseminated lymphoma and leukemia, but primary lymphoma (non-Hodgkin's) is rare. The patients present with vaginal bleeding, pain, and uterine enlargement. The endometrial biopsy/curettings may be misdiagnosed as poorly differentiated carcinoma. In one report, all cases were of the B-cell variety (Aozasa et al, 1993). The prognosis is excellent for early-stage primary uterine lymphoma. The treatment of choice is hysterectomy followed by radiation therapy (see the section on "Lymphoma" in Chapter 5).

MIXED TUMORS OF THE ENDOMETRIUM

Benign Mixed Tumors

Adenofibroma of the endometrium occurs in pre- and postmenopausal women, presenting with vaginal bleeding, an enlarged uterus, and frequently tissue protruding through the cervical os in the manner of adenosarcoma and carcinosarcoma. The glandular component is usually of the proliferative endometrial type (Clement and Scully, 1988). No case of endometrial adenofibroma has recurred outside the uterus, but incomplete removal by D&C may be followed by regrowth within the uterus. Differentiation from endometrial müllerian adenosarcoma is important. Hysterectomy is recommended to ensure adequate histologic evaluation and definitive therapy.

A papillary variant of the endometrial adenofibroma was reported by Vellios and co-workers in 1973. They described five cases with a papillary glandular component, which they considered a benign mixed mesodermal tumor of müllerian origin. An additional nine cases were described by Zaloudek and Norris in 1981. The patients were 40 to 84 years of age (median 62 years), and nearly all presented with vaginal bleeding. The largest tumor was 10 cm in diameter. Microscopically there was squamous, mucinous, and endometrial epithelium; papillae within or without cystic spaces; and a fibrous or endometrial stroma. One tumor had a focus of well-differentiated adenocarcinoma. Atypia of the mesenchymal cells was never more than moderate, and mitoses were not in excess of 3/10 hpf. An identical tumor has also been observed to arise from the cervix.

Occasionally an endometrial polyp has a smooth muscle rather than endometrial or fibrous stroma. This entirely benign lesion is termed *adenomyoma* and presents no diagnostic problems. In 1986 Young et al reported 26 cases of *atypical polypoid adenomyoma* (APA), a neoplasm that can be mistaken for carcinoma. APAs are composed of smooth muscle and atypical endometrial glands. They occur in premenopausal women (average age 39 years), cause abnormal vaginal bleeding, and arise from the lower uterine segment. Histologically the glands may exhibit any degree of cytologic or architectural atypia up to carcinoma in situ. Squamous metaplasia is usually present, and at times it is extensive. The smooth muscle stroma occasionally has mild to moderate atypia, but the mitosis count is less than 2/10 hpf. The treatment should be hysterectomy. Although the efficacy of conservative therapy (D&C or hysteroscopic resection) is not known, it should be considered when fertility is an important issue.

Proliferating glial tissue, occasionally with islands of cartilage and bone, presenting as a cervical polyp months to years after a pregnancy (usually ended by an induced vaginal abortion), has been reported by many authors. The phenomenon is not well understood but is believed to result from the implantation of fetal tissue. Glia is the most common tissue encountered, probably because it is the least antigenic. The endometrium may also be involved. Apparently none of these has been mistaken for a malignancy (Grönroos et at, 1983).

Uterine Adenosarcoma

More than 150 cases of uterine adenosarcoma have been reported since the original description in 1974 (Clement and Scully, 1990). Uterine adenosarcoma is a distinctive mixed müllerian tumor arising in the endometrium of predominantly postmenopausal women (median age 58 years), although it also occurs in adolescent and reproductive-age women. These women present with abnormal vaginal bleeding and, less commonly, with pelvic pain. Tissue protruding from the external os is found in about one half of the cases, and an enlarged uterus is also a frequent finding. Misdiagnosis as recurring endometrial polyps has been reported in a few cases.

Grossly the tumor arises from the endometrium in a sessile or pedunculate, polypoid or papillary form, with a mean size of 5 cm.

Microscopically the adenosarcoma is composed of an admixture of stromal sarcoma or fibrosarcoma and usually benign, neoplastic glands lined by endometrial, mucinous, or other müllerian epithelium. However, cytologic and architectural atypia may be present. Myometrial invasion greater than 2 mm was present in only 17 percent of cases. About one fifth contain heterologous elements, most commonly embryonal rhabdomyosarcoma. The mitosis count and degree of atypia of the sarcomatous component vary widely. About one third of the cases have more than 10 mitoses/10 hpf, and a similar proportion have grade 3 cytologic atypia.

Recurrence was diagnosed in 25 percent of the Clement and Scully series, with an average follow-up of 5.9 years and an average time to recurrence of 3.4 years. However, nearly 40 percent of the recurrences were diagnosed 5 or more years after hysterectomy. Kaku et al (1992) reported recurrence in 2 of 17 stage I cases. Recurrence in two thirds of cases are vaginal or pelvic and tend to be more cellular than the primary. The only clinicopathologic features clearly associated with recurrence risk are sarcomatous overgrowth and deep myoinvasion. More than 10 mitoses/10 hpf tend to occur with a similar frequency in the recurrent and nonrecurrent groups.

The recommended treatment is removal of the uterus, tubes, and ovaries, followed by whole-pelvis radiation therapy for patients with deep myoinvasion. Although it is uncertain if the radiation will significantly reduce the pelvic recurrence rate, it is useful in the histologically similar MMMTs and ESSs. Adjuvant chemotherapy may be more appropriate for cases with sarcomatous overgrowth, especially embryonal rhabdomyosarcoma (Fig. 7–5). In these cases the lymph nodes should also be dissected, and a modified radical hysterectomy performed.

Malignant Mixed Mesodermal Tumors (Carcinosarcomas)

Clinicopathologic Features

Also referred to as carcinosarcomas, *malignant mixed mesodermal tumors* (MMMT), account for 3 to 6 percent of all uterine cancers. The average age at diagnosis is during the seventh decade of life. Women with uterine MMMT have a number of characteristics in common with the endometrial adenocarci-

noma population. On the average, 25 percent are nulliparous, 40 percent obese, and 15 percent diabetic, although individual reports vary widely. Postmenopausal estrogen use has not been implicated in the etiology of this form of endometrial cancer, although uterine MMMT has been reported to occur during estrogen replacement therapy (Schwartz et al, 1989, 1991). Based on several papers, 10 percent of the patients give a history of prior radiation therapy to the pelvis, but individual series vary from 0 to 30 percent (Norris and Taylor, 1965; Meredith et al, 1986). Rarely, MMMT originates in pelvic endometriosis.

When patients seek medical attention, the most frequent complaints are vaginal bleeding (85 percent), and vaginal discharge. In advanced cases, weight loss is also common. The most notable physical finding is, in 30 to 50 percent of the cases, tumor tissue protruding through the cervical os. The uterus is usually enlarged and soft to palpation. Lung, abdominal, peripheral node, or aortic node metastases are found in 10 to 20 percent of the cases at diagnosis (stage IV).

Pathology. In most instances, the endometrium is diffusely involved and the myometrium is deeply invaded. The uterine cavity typically is filled with a polypoid, fungating mass of tumor with areas of hemorrhage and necrosis (Figs. 7–6 and 7–7). Microscopically, either carcinoma or sarcoma may be the predominant component. The carcinoma is usually endometrial in pattern and grade 2 or 3. Clear cell, tubal, and mucinous glandular patterns also occur. The malignant endometrial stroma is often expressed as an undifferentiated spindle cell or fusiform sarcoma. When differentiation produces a recognizable pattern, it is usually composed of malignant endometrial stromal cells. Other types include LMS and malignant fibrous histiocytoma. The frequencies of the various heterologous components are presented in Table 7–5. Immunoperoxidase staining is often useful in identifying the tissues represented in poorly differentiated endometrial tumors so they can be classified as carcinoma or sarcoma, homologous or heterologous.

Surgical Staging. From various reports, 25 to 50 percent of clinical stage I cases are understaged according to surgicopathologic findings (Table 7–6). More specifically, these studies indicate that 15 to 40 percent of patients with uterine MMMT clinically confined to the uterus and cervix (stage I/II) have node

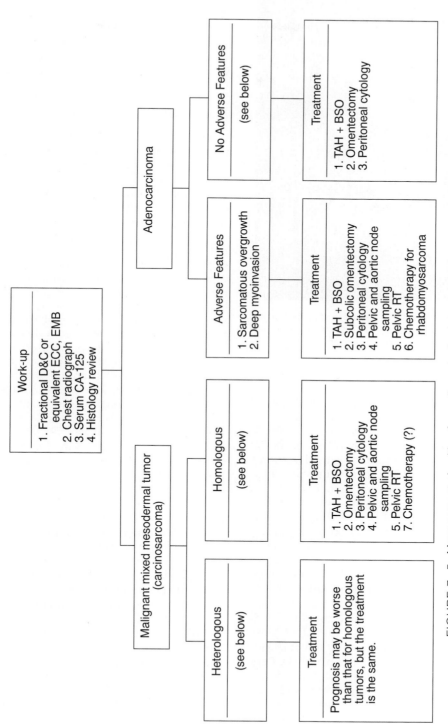

FIGURE 7–5. Management algorithm for malignant mixed mesodermal tumor and adenosarcoma. BSO = bilateral salpingo-oophorectomy; ECC = endocervical curettage; EMB = endometrial biopsy; RT = radiation therapy; TAH = total abdominal hysterectomy.

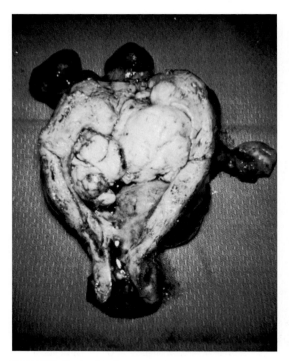

FIGURE 7–6. Malignant mixed mesodermal tumor. The endometrial cavity is distended by bulky tumor. Myometrial invasion is evident.

metastases. The risk is related to the depth of myometrial invasion and cervical extension, but not the presence or absence of heterologous elements. The distribution of nodal metastases in 91 surgically staged patients was pelvic only in 19 percent and pelvic plus aortic in 16 percent. Only one patient had aortic node involvement with negative pelvic nodes (DiSaia et al, 1978; Gallup and Cordray, 1979; Chen, 1989; Podczaski et al, 1989). In the 301-patient GOG study of uterine MMMT, the risk of metastasis was related to depth of myoinvasion (<50 percent invasion, 10 percent; >50 percent invasion, 34 percent). Only 37 percent of patients had greater than 50 percent myoinvasion. LVSI was present in two thirds of the cases with, and one third of the cases without metastases (Silverberg et al, 1990; Major et al, 1993). Peritoneal/omental implants and adnexal metastases are reported in 3 to 5 percent of clinical stage I/II cases and positive peritoneal cytology in 15 to 22 percent. Pretreatment evaluation consists of tumor marker determination (CA-125, carcinoembryonic antigen) chest radiograph, and other routine tests. If the liver function studies are abnormal, ultrasound or computed tomography evaluation of that organ is indicated.

Collected survival data for patients with endometrial MMMT by clinical stage at diagnosis are presented in Table 7–4. The 5-year survival rate reported for surgical stage I cases is usually about 50 percent. Long-term survival with more advanced disease is unusual.

Treatment

In the management of endometrial MMMT, surgery should be performed as the initial step when the tumor appears to be confined to the uterus clinically, because of the high incidence of extrauterine spread found at laparotomy (see Fig. 7–5). The recommended operative procedure is exploratory laparotomy via a vertical incision, total abdominal hysterectomy, and bilateral salpingo-oophorectomy. Peritoneal cytology, infracolic omentectomy, and selective pelvic and aortic node dissection should also be carried out because they are important in assessing prognosis and treatment planning. Extrauterine tumor masses should be removed if feasible.

The recurrence pattern reported for clinical stage I/II cases is about 16 percent pelvic, 16 percent pelvic plus distant metastasis, and 67 percent distant metastasis only. This is substantially influenced by adjuvant radiation therapy. For example, in the GOG study of stage I/II uterine MMMTs, 54 percent of first recurrences were pelvic in the no-radiation group versus 23 percent in the pelvic radiation therapy group (Hornback et al, 1986). Thus all patients with tumor apparently confined to the pelvis should be given whole-pelvis irradiation postoperatively. Radiation alone is indicated for patients who are medically inoperable, but the outcome is much poorer (Larson et al, 1990b). Follow-up with CA-125 serum value determination is recommended (Peters et al, 1986).

The chemotherapeutic agents known to have significant activity against uterine MMMT are doxorubicin, cisplatin, and ifosfamide (Sutton et al, 1989; Thigpen et al, 1991). These drugs have induced a complete remission in 8 to 18 percent of patients with advanced/recurrent carcinosarcoma. Cyclophosphamide and vincristine may also have a significant effect. Combination drug therapy should be more effective than single-agent therapy, but there are very few documentary data (Seltzer et al, 1984; Andersen et al, 1989). It is uncertain whether adjuvant therapy is ef-

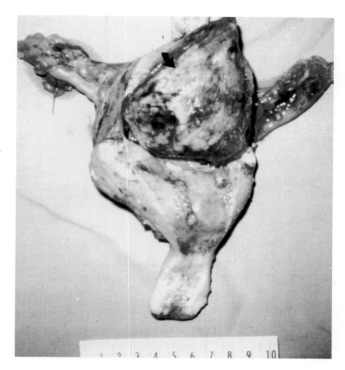

FIGURE 7–7. Malignant mixed mesodermal tumor. The uterus has been opened in the frontal plane and the halves spread apart to expose the large polypoid tumor. Its configuration reflects the shape of the uterine cavity. Light areas of the tumor (arrow) were necrotic.

fective for this type of malignancy, but there is some supportive evidence. In the randomized GOG adjuvant doxorubicin study, the number of distant metastases was greater, recurrences were more frequent, and the survival rate was worse (but the differences were not statistically significant) in the no-doxorubicin arm (Omura et al, 1985). Furthermore, Peters et al (1989) reported that 10 of 15 patients receiving adjuvant doxorubicin plus cis-

platin were free of disease with an average follow-up of 34 months. On the basis of these data, it is reasonable to treat all MMMT patients with adjuvant chemotherapy in addition to the pelvic radiation if there is any extrauterine disease at surgery (e.g., adnexal or nodal metastasis, malignant peritoneal cytology) or if the primary lesion has outer-50-percent myoinvasion or LVSI. Combination chemotherapy with cisplatin and ifosfamide with or without doxorubicin is recommended. All patients with metastatic/advanced disease are candidates for combination chemotherapy.

Sutton et al (1986) have measured hormone receptor proteins in uterine sarcomas.

TABLE 7–5

Histologic Expression of 96 Malignant Mixed Mesodermal Tumors of the Endometrium Containing at Least One Malignant Heterologous Tissue*

Malignant Tissue Type	Percentage of Total Cases
Sarcoma	
Striated muscle	36
Cartilage	27
Bone	7
Fat	5
Combinations with muscle	17
Combinations without muscle	7
Carcinoma	
Endometrioid	60
Adenosquamous	26
Serous	11
Clear cell	2.5

*Data from Silverberg et al (1990).

TABLE 7–6

Comparison of Clinical and Surgical Staging of Uterine Malignant Mixed Mesodermal Tumors (228 Cases)*

Stage	Clinical No.	Clinical Percent	Surgical No.	Surgical Percent
I	145	64	106	46
II	38	17	27	5
III	23	10	37	16
IV	22	10	58	25

*Data from Dinh et al (1989), Doss et al (1984), Macasaet et al (1985), Podczaski et al (1989), and Spanos et al (1984).

In their study, the median progesterone and estrogen receptor levels in homologous tumors were 36 and 20 fmol, respectively. The corresponding values for heterologous tumors were 0 and 7 fmol. That some uterine MMMTs may be responsive to hormone manipulation is further supported by the work of Tseng et al (1986), who demonstrated in vitro that the growth rate of uterine MMMT was slowed by progestin and that progesterone could induce aromatase activity in receptor-positive tumors. Clinically, however, only occasional, usually transient, responses may be seen with high-dose progestin or tamoxifen in patients with advanced uterine MMMT.

Outcome

Collected survival data for patients with endometrial MMMT by clinical stage at diagnosis are in Table 7–4. The 5-year survival reported for surgical stage I uterine MMMT cases is about 50 percent. Long-term survival with more advanced disease is unusual. The most comprehensive survival information has been published by the GOG. Progression-free survival at 3 years for 167 clinical stage I/II homologous MMMT patients was 55 percent, substantially better than the 43 percent for the 134-patient heterologous tumor group. The difference at 5 years was 53 percent versus 35 percent. If the patient was surgical stage I/II, the progression-free survival was 65 percent at 3 years for the homologous group and 55 percent for the heterologous group. With metastatic disease (surgical stages III and IV), these progression-free survival rates dropped to less than 20 percent. An interesting observation regarding uterine MMMT is that the carcinomatous component accounts for most of the LVSI and the metastases (Sreenan and Hart, 1995).

REFERENCES

Akkersdijk GJM, Flu PK, Giard RWM, et al: Malignant leiomyomatosis peritonealis disseminata. Am J Obstet Gynecol 163:591, 1990.

Andersen WA, Young DE, Peters WA, et al: Platinum-based combination chemotherapy for malignant mixed mesodermal tumors of the ovary. Gynecol Oncol 32:319, 1989.

Aozasa K, Saeki K, Ohsawa M, et al: Malignant lymphoma of the uterus: report of seven cases with immunohistochemical study. Cancer 72:1959, 1993.

Bahary CM, Gorodeski IG, Nilly M, et al: Intravascular leiomyomatosis. Obstet Gynecol 59:73s, 1982.

Baker VV, Walton LA, Fowler WC Jr, Currie JL: Steroid receptors in endolymphatic stromal myosis. Obstet Gynecol 63:72S, 1984.

Bell SW, Kempson RL, Hendrickson MR: Problematic uterine smooth muscle neoplasms: a clinicopathologic study of 213 cases. Am J Surg Pathol 18:535, 1994.

Berchuck A, Rubin SC, Hoskins WJ, et al: Treatment of uterine leiomyosarcoma. Obstet Gynecol 71:845, 1988.

Berchuck A, Rubin SC, Hoskins WJ, et al: Treatment of endometrial stromal tumors. Gynecol Oncol 36:60, 1990.

Bitterman P, Chun B, Kurman RJ: The significance of epithelial differentiation in mixed mesodermal tumors of the uterus: a clinicopathologic and immunohistochemical study. Am J Surg Pathol 14:317, 1990.

Bohr L, Thomsen CF: Low-grade stromal sarcoma: a benign appearing malignant uterine tumour; a review of current literature; differential diagnostic problems illustrated by four cases. Eur J Obstet Gynecol Reprod Biol 39:63, 1991.

Buscema J, Carpenter SE, Rosenshein NB, Woodruff JD: Epithelioid leiomyosarcoma of the uterus. Cancer 57:1192, 1986.

Buscema J, Klein V, Rotmensch J et al: Uterine hemangiopericytoma. Obstet Gynecol 69:104, 1987.

Chang KL, Crabtree GS, Lim-Tan SK, et al: Primary uterine endometrial stromal neoplasms: a clinicopathologic study of 117 cases. Am J Surg Pathol 14:415, 1990.

Chantarawiroj P, Tresukosol D, Kudelka AP, et al: Prolonged oral etoposide for refractory advanced uterine leiomyosarcoma. Gynecol Oncol 58:248, 1995.

Chen SS: Propensity of retroperitoneal lymph node metastasis in patients with stage I sarcoma of the uterus. Gynecol Oncol 32:215, 1989.

Cho KR, Woodruff D, Epstein JI: Leiomyoma of the uterus with multiple extrauterine smooth muscle tumors: a case report suggesting multifocal origin. Hum Pathol 20:80, 1989.

Clement PB: Chondrosarcoma of the uterus: report of a case and review of the literature. Hum Pathol 9:726, 1978.

Clement PB: Intravenous leiomyomatosis of the uterus. Pathol Ann 23:153, 1988.

Clement PB, Scully RE: Uterine tumors with mixed epithelial and mesenchymal elements. Semin Diagn Pathol 5:199, 1988.

Clement PB, Scully RE: Müllerian adenosarcoma of the uterus; a clinicopathologic analysis of 100 cases with a review of the literature. Hum Pathol 21:363, 1990.

Clement PB, Scully RE: Pathology of uterine sarcomas. In Coppelson M (ed): Gynecologic Oncology. Edinburgh, Churchill Livingstone, 1991, p 803.

Clement PB, Young RH, Scully RE: Intravenous leiomyomatosis of the uterus: a clinicopathological analysis of 16 cases with unusual histologic features. Am J Surg Pathol 12:932, 1988.

Covens AL, Nisker JA, Chapman WB, Allen HH: Uterine sarcoma: an analysis of 74 cases. Am J Obstet Gynecol 156:370, 1987.

Crum CP, Rogers BH, Andersen W: Osteosarcoma of the uterus: case report and review of the literature. Gynecol Oncol 9:256, 1980.

De Fusco PA, Gaffey TA, Malkasian G, et al: Endometrial stromal sarcoma: review of Mayo Clinic experience, 1945–1980. Gynecol Oncol 35:8, 1989.

Dinh TV, Slavin RE, Bhagavan BS, et al: Mixed müllerian tumors of the uterus: a clinicopathologic study. Obstet Gynecol 74:388, 1989.

DiSaia PJ, Morrow CP, Boronow R, et al: Endometrial sarcoma: lymphatic spread pattern. Am J Obstet Gynecol 130:104, 1978.

Donkers B, Kazzaz BA, Meijering JH: Rhabdomyosarcoma of the corpus uteri. Am J Obstet Gynecol 114:1025, 1972.

Doss LL, Llorens AS, Henriquez EM: Carcinosarcoma of the uterus: a 40-year experience from the State of Missouri, Gynecol Oncol 18:43, 1984.

Echt G, Jepson J, Steel J, et al: Treatment of uterine sarcoma. Cancer 66:35, 1990.

Evans AT III, Symmonds RE, Gaffey TA: Recurrent pelvic intravenous leiomyomatosis. Obstet Gynecol 56:260, 1981.

Evans HL: Endometrial stromal sarcoma and poorly differentiated endometrial sarcoma. Cancer 50:2170, 1982.

Evans HL, Chawla SP, Simpson C, Finn KP: Smooth muscle neoplasms of the uterus other than ordinary leiomyoma: a study of 46 cases, with emphasis on diagnostic criteria and prognostic factors. Cancer 62:2239, 1988.

Fekete PS, Vellios F: The clinical and histologic spectrum of endometrial stromal neoplasms: a report of 41 cases. Int J Gynecol Pathol 3:198, 1984.

Fleming WP, Peters WA III, Kumar NB, Morley GW: Autopsy findings in patients with uterine sarcoma. Gynecol Oncol 19:168, 1984.

Fujii S: Leiomyomatosis peritonealis disseminata. In Williams CJ, Krikorian JG, Green MR, Raghavan D (eds): Textbook of Uncommon Cancer. New York, John Wiley & Sons, 1988, p 133.

Gallup DG, Cordray DR: Leiomyosarcoma of the uterus: case reports and a review. Obstet Gynecol Surv 34:300, 1979.

Ghavimi F: Genitourinary rhabdomyosarcoma. In Maurer HM, Ruymann FB, Pochedly C (eds): Rhabdomyosarcoma and Related Tumors in Children and Adolescents. Boca Raton, FL, CRC Press, 1991, p 347.

Gloor E, Schnyder P, Cikes M, et al: Endolymphatic stromal myosis. Cancer 50:1888, 1982.

Goff BA, Rice LW, Fleischhacker D, et al: Uterine leiomyosarcoma and endometrial stromal sarcoma: lymph node metastases and sites of recurrence. Gynecol Oncol 50: 105, 1993.

Grönroos M, Meurman L, Kahra K: Proliferating glia and other heterotopic tissues in the uterus: fetal homografts? Obstet Gynecol 61:261, 1983.

Grunebaum AN, Sedlis A: Adenomatoid tumor of the uterus simulating interstitial pregnancy. Obstet Gynecol 59:87S, 1982.

Hart WR, Billman JK Jr: A reassessment of uterine neoplasms originally diagnosed as leiomyosarcomas. Cancer 41:1902, 1978.

Hays DM, Shimada H, Raney RB Jr, et al: Clinical staging and treatment results in rhabdomyosarcoma of the female genital tract among children and adolescents. Cancer 61: 1993, 1988.

Heinonen PK, Taina E, Nerdrum T, et al: Intravenous leiomyomatosis. Ann Chir Gynaecol 73:100, 1984.

Hornback NB, Omura G, Major FJ: Observations on the use of adjuvant radiation therapy in patients with stage I and II uterine sarcoma. Int J Radiat Oncol Biol Phys 12:2127, 1986.

Hortsmann JP, Pietra GG, Harman JA, et al: Spontaneous regression of pulmonary leiomyomas during pregnancy. Cancer 39:314, 1977.

Kahanpää KV, Wahlström T, Gröhn P, et al: Sarcomas of the uterus: a clinicopathologic study of 119 patients. Obstet Gynecol 67:417, 1986.

Kaku T, Silverberg SG, Major FJ: Adenosarcoma of the uterus: a Gynecologic Oncology Group study of 31 cases. Int J Gynecol Pathol 11:75, 1992.

Kaminski PF, Tavassoli FA: Plexiform tumorlet: a clinical and pathologic study of 15 cases with ultrastructural observations. Int J Gynecol Pathol 3:124, 1984.

Kaszar-Siebert DJ, Gauvin GP, Rogoff PA, et al: Intracardiac extension of intravenous leiomyomatosis. Radiology 168: 409, 1988.

Kawaguchi K, Fujii S, Konishi I, et al: Mitotic activity in uterine leiomyomas during the menstrual cycle. Am J Obstet Gynecol 160:637, 1989.

Kempson RL: Uterine mesenchymal neoplasms. In the Annual Review Course on Gynecologic Oncology and Pathology, Matsumoto, Japan, November 22–23, 1994.

Kempson RL, Bari W: Uterine sarcomas: classification, diagnosis, and prognosis. Hum Pathol 1:331, 1970.

Kempson RL, Hendrickson MR: Pure mesenchymal neoplasms of the uterine corpus: selected problems. Semin Diagn Pathol 5:712, 1988.

Krieger PD, Gusberg SB: Endolymphatic stromal myosis: a grade I endometrial sarcoma. Gynecol Oncol 1:299, 1973.

Kurman RJ, Norris HJ: Mesenchymal tumors of the uterus. VI. Epithelioid smooth muscle tumors including leiomyoblastoma and clear-cell leiomyoma. Cancer 37:1853, 1976.

Larson B, Silfverswärd C, Nilsson B, Pettersson F: Endometrial stromal sarcoma of the uterus: a clinical and histopathological study. The Radiumhemmet series 1936–1981. Eur J Obstet Gynecol Reprod Biol 35:239, 1990a.

Larson B, Silfverswärd C, Nilsson B, Pettersson F: Mixed müllerian tumours of the uterus—prognostic factors: a clinical and histopathologic study of 147 cases. Radiat Oncol 17:123, 1990b.

Lauchlan SC: Conceptual unity of the müllerian tumor group: a histologic study. Cancer 22:601, 1968.

Leibsohn S, d'Ablaing G, Mishell DR Jr, Schlaerth JB: Leiomyosarcoma in a series of hysterectomies performed for presumed uterine leiomyomas. Am J Obstet Gynecol 162: 968, 1990.

Levenback C, Rubin SC, McCormack PM, et al: Resection of pulmonary metastases from uterine sarcomas. Gynecol Oncol 45:202, 1992.

Macasaet MA, Waxman M, Fruchter RG, et al: Prognostic factors in malignant mesodermal (müllerian) mixed tumors of the uterus. Gynecol Oncol 20:32, 1985.

Major FJ, Blessing JA, Silverberg SG, et al: Prognostic factors in early-stage uterine sarcoma. Cancer 71:1702, 1993.

Mantravadi RVP, Bardawil WA, Lochman DJ, et al: Uterine sarcomas: an analysis of 69 patients. Int J Radiat Oncol Biol Phys 7:917, 1981.

Meis JM, Lawrence D: The immunohistochemical profile of malignant mixed müllerian tumor: overlap with endometrial adenocarcinoma. Am J Clin Pathol 94:1, 1990.

Meredith RF, Eisert DR, Kaka Z, et al: An excess of uterine sarcomas after pelvic irradiation. Cancer 58:2003, 1986.

Montag TW, d'Ablaing G, Schlaerth JB, et al: Embryonal rhabdomyosarcoma of the uterine corpus and cervix. Gynecol Oncol 25:171, 1986.

Nordal RR, Kristensen GB, Kaern J, et al: The prognostic significance of surgery, tumor size, malignancy grade, menopausal status, and DNA ploidy in endometrial stromal sarcoma. Gynecol Oncol 62:254, 1996.

Norris HJ, Parmley T: Mesenchymal tumors of the uterus. V. Intravenous leiomyomatosis. Cancer 36:2164, 1975.

Norris HJ, Roth E, Taylor HB: Mesenchymal tumors of the uterus. II. A clinical and pathologic study of 31 mixed mesodermal tumors. Obstet Gynecol 28:57, 1966.

Norris HJ, Taylor HB: Postirradiation sarcomas of the uterus. Obstet Gynecol 26:689, 1965.

Norris HJ, Taylor HB: Mesenchymal tumors of the uterus. I. A clinical and pathological study of 53 endometrial stromal tumors. Cancer 19:755, 1966a.

Norris HJ, Taylor HB: Mesenchymal tumors of the uterus. III. A clinical and pathologic study of 31 carcinosarcomas. Cancer 19:1459, 1966b.

Ober WB: Uterine sarcomas: histogenesis and taxonomy. Ann N Y Acad Sci 75:568, 1959.

Ober WB, Tovell HMM: Mesenchymal sarcomas of the uterus. Am J Obstet Gynecol 77:246, 1959.

O'Connor DM, Norris HJ: Mitotically active leiomyomas of the uterus. Hum Pathol 21:223, 1990.

Olah KS, Blunt S, Dunn JA, et al: Retrospective analysis of 318 cases of uterine sarcoma. Eur J Cancer 27:1095, 1991.

Omura GA, Blessing JA, Lifshitz S, et al: A randomized clinical trial of adjuvant adriamycin in uterine sarcomas: a Gynecologic Oncology Group study. J Clin Oncol 3:1240, 1985.

Omura GA, Major FJ, Blessing JA, et al: A randomized study of Adriamycin with and without dimethyl triazenoimidazole carboxamide in advanced uterine sarcomas. Cancer 52:626, 1983.

Parker WH, Fu YS, Berek JS: Uterine sarcoma in patients operated on for presumed leiomyoma and rapidly growing leiomyoma. Obstet Gynecol 83:414, 1994.

Patsner B, Mann WJ: Use of serum CA-125 in monitoring patients with uterine sarcoma: a preliminary report. Cancer 62:1355, 1988.

Perrone T, Dehner LP: Prognostically favorable "mitotically active" smooth-muscle tumors of the uterus. Am J Surg Pathol 12:1, 1988.

Peters WA III, Bagley CM, Smith MR: CA-125: use as a tumor marker with mixed mesodermal tumors of the female genital tract. Cancer 58:2625, 1986.

Peters WA III, Howard DR, Andersen WA, Figge DC: Deoxyribonucleic acid analysis by flow cytometry of uterine leiomyosarcomas and smooth muscle tumors of uncertain malignant potential. Am J Obstet Gynecol 166:1646, 1992.

Peters WA III, Rivkin SE, Smith MR, Tesh DE: Cisplatin and Adriamycin combination chemotherapy for uterine stromal sarcomas and mixed mesodermal tumors. Gynecol Oncol 34:323, 1989.

Piscioli F, Govoni E, Polla E, et al: Primary osteosarcoma of the uterine corpus: report of a case and critical review of the literature. Int J Gynaecol Obstet 23:377, 1985.

Piver MS, Rutlege FN, Copeland L, et al: Uterine endolymphatic stromal myosis: a collaborative study. Obstet Gynecol 64:173, 1984.

Podczaski ES, Woomert CA, Stevens CW Jr, et al: Management of malignant mixed mesodermal tumors of the uterus. Gynecol Oncol 32,240, 1989.

Prayson RA, Hart WR: Mitotically active leiomyomas of the uterus. Am J Clin Pathol 97:14, 1992.

Quinonez GE, Paraskevas MP, Diocee MS, Lorimer SM: Angiosarcoma of the uterus: a case report. Am J Obstet Gynecol 164:90, 1991.

Salm R, Evans DJ: Myxoid leiomyosarcoma. Histopathology 9:159, 1985.

Schwartz LB, Diamond MP, Schwartz PE: Leiomyosarcomas: clinical presentation. Am J Obstet Gynecol 168:180, 1993.

Schwartz SM, Thomas DB, The World Health Organization Collaborative Study of Neoplasia and Steroid Contraceptives: a case-control study of risk factors for sarcomas of the uterus. Cancer 64:2487, 1989.

Schwartz SM, Weiss NS, Daling JR, et al: Incidence of histologic types of uterine sarcoma in relation to menstrual and reproductive history. Int J Cancer 49:362, 1991.

Seltzer V, Kaplan B, Vogl S, Spitzer M: Doxorubicin and cisplatin in the treatment of advanced mixed mesodermal uterine sarcoma. Cancer Treat Rep 68:1389, 1984.

Silverberg SG, Major FJ, Blessing JA, et al: Carcinosarcoma (malignant mixed mesodermal tumor) of the uterus: a Gynecologic Oncology Group pathologic study of 203 cases. Int J Gynecol Pathol 9:1, 1990.

Smullen SN, Scotti DJ, Osterholm JL, Weiss AJ: Preoperative embolization of retroperitoneal hemangiopericytomas as an aid in their removal. Cancer 50:1870, 1982.

Spanos WJ Jr, Wharton JT, Gomez L, et al: Malignant mixed müllerian tumors of the uterus. Cancer 53:311, 1984.

Sreenan JJ, Hart WR: Carcinosarcomas of the female genital tract: a pathologic study of 29 metastatic tumors. Further evidence for the dominant role of the epithelial component and the conversion theory of histogenesis. Am J Surg Pathol 19:666, 1995.

Suginami H, Kaura R, Ochi H, Matsuura S: Intravenous leiomyomatosis with cardiac extension: successful surgical management and histopathologic study. Obstet Gynecol 76:527, 1990.

Sutton GP, Blessing JA, Malfetano JH: A phase II trial of doxorubicin, ifosfamide and mesna in patients with advanced or recurrent uterine leiomyosarcomas. Proc Am Soc Clin Oncol 12:A870, 1993.

Sutton GP, Blessing JA, Rosenshein N, et al: Phase II trial of ifosfamide and mesna in mixed mesodermal tumors of the uterus: a Gynecologic Oncology Group study. Am J Obstet Gynecol 161:309, 1989.

Sutton GP, Stehman FB, Michael H, et al: Estrogen and progesterone receptors in uterine sarcomas. Obstet Gynecol 68:709, 1986.

Taylor HB, Norris HJ: Mesenchymal tumors of the uterus. IV. Diagnosis and prognosis of leiomyosarcomas. Arch Pathol 82:40, 1966.

Taylor JR, Ryu J, Colby TV, Raffin TA: Lymphangioleiomyomatosis: clinical course in 32 patients. N Engl J Med 323:1254, 1990.

Thigpen JT, Blessing JA, Beecham J, et al: Phase II trial of cisplatin as first-line chemotherapy in patients with advanced or recurrent uterine sarcomas: a Gynecologic Oncology Group study. J Clin Oncol 9:1962, 1991.

Tierney WM, Ehrlich CE, Bailey JC, et al: Intravenous leiomyomatosis of the uterus with extension into the heart. Am J Med 69:471, 1980.

Todd CS, Michael H, Sutton G: Retroperitoneal leiomyosarcoma: eight cases and a literature review. Gynecol Oncol 59:333, 1995.

Tseng L, Tseng JK, Mann WJ, et al: Endocrine aspects of human uterine sarcoma: a preliminary study. Am J Obstet Gynecol 155:95, 1986.

Van Dinh T, Woodruff JD: Leiomyosarcoma of the uterus. Am J Obstet Gynecol 144:817, 1982.

Vellios F, Ng AB, Reagan JW: Papillary adenofibroma of the uterus: a benign mesodermal mixed tumor of müllerian origin. Am J Clin Pathol 60:543, 1973.

Wheelock JB, Krebs H-B, Schneider V, Goplerud DR: Uterine sarcoma: analysis of prognostic variables in 71 cases. Am J Obstet Gynecol 151:1016, 1985.

Wilbanks GD, Szmanska Z, Miller A: Pelvic hemangiopericytoma: report of 4 patients and review of the literature. Am J Obstet Gynecol 123:555, 1975.

Willén R, Gad A, Willén H: Lipomatous lesions of the uterus. Virchows Arch 377:315, 1978.

Yoonessi M, Hart WR: Endometrial stromal sarcomas. Cancer 40:898, 1977.

Young RH, Treger T, Scully RE: Atypical polypoid adenomyoma of the uterus: a report of 27 cases. Am J Clin Pathol 86:136, 1986.

Zaloudek CJ, Norris HJ: Adenofibroma and adenosarcoma of the uterus: a clinicopathologic study of 35 cases. Cancer 48:354, 1981.

C H A P T E R

8

Tumors of the Fallopian Tube and Broad Ligament

■

BENIGN TUMORS AND TUMOR-LIKE CONDITIONS

Although the fallopian tube is commonly involved in non-neoplastic "tumor" formations such as tubal pregnancy, pyosalpinx, and hydrosalpinx, it is rarely the primary site of true neoplasia. Benign tumors occur but are reported with less frequency than malignant tumors. Of the reported benign tumors, the most common are cystic teratomas, which are histopathologically the same as ovarian dermoid cysts. Neurilemmoma, adenomatoid tumor, serous cystadenoma, hemangioma, and leiomyoma have also been reported to arise in the fallopian tube.

Atypical epithelial proliferations of the fallopian tube are relatively common. Moore and Enterline (1975) found areas consistent with ademomatous hyperplasia or carcinoma in situ in the tubes in 18 percent of 124 non-selected hysterectomy specimens. These epithelial abnormalities were more common in cases of salpingitis or endometrial carcinoma. Because these lesions occur so frequently and tubal carcinoma is so rare, the authors concluded that tubal epithelial proliferations are not premalignant. Stern et al (1981) echoed this opinion after a review of 39 cases of proliferative tubal epithelial lesions, nearly all of which were associated with a benign or malignant neoplasm of the ovary or endometrium. Others have reported similar findings (Bartnik et al, 1989; Robey and Silva, 1989).

It also appears that further treatment is not needed for the postpartum patient with the *metaplastic papillary tumor* of the fallopian tube described by Saffos et al (1980). Although the metaplastic papillary tumor had all the features of a serous papillary borderline tumor, based on their analysis of four cases diagnosed from postpartum tubal sterilization specimens, Saffos et al believed the lesion to be a reversible, proliferative lesion peculiar to pregnancy.

Paratubal cysts or *hydatid cysts of Morgagni* are of paramesonephric or mesothelial origin. They are commonplace, incidental findings at surgery, especially during the reproductive years, that are located predominantly near the fimbria. Rarely, a neoplasm of serous histology arises within a paratubal cyst. In a review of 79 cases of paratubal cyst by Samaha and Woodruff (1985), only 3 were symptomatic, all were mesothelial, and the size varied from 6 to 20 cm. Torsion of the smaller hydatid cysts has been reported.

■

MALIGNANT TUMORS OF THE FALLOPIAN TUBE

Epidemiology

Primary cancer of the fallopian tube accounts for 0.1 to 0.5 percent of all gynecologic malignancies. It has a predilection for women of low parity, with 25 to 30 percent of reported cases nulliparous (Nordin, 1994). The average age at diagnosis is about 56 years. Although the great majority of cases occur between the ages of 40 and 60 years, the malignancy has been reported at the age extremes of 14 and 87 years. Chronic salpingitis of a tuberculous or nontuberculous nature was formerly considered a predisposing factor in the genesis of tubal malignancy. It appears, however, that a history of pelvic tuberculosis is no more common in these women than in the general population. The incidence of nontuberculous salpingitis is more difficult to evaluate because there is often an inflammatory response to the malignancy itself.

Clinicopathologic Features

Symptoms

Tubal carcinoma typically causes lower abdominal or pelvic pain, sometimes colicky in nature; vaginal bleeding; and discharge (Latzko's triad). As expected, considering the prevailing age group of these patients, postmenopausal bleeding is the single most frequent symptom. When an adnexal mass is present in conjunction with these symptoms and a negative uterine curettage, the likelihood of tubal carcinoma is substantial. According to the review by Nordin (1994), the classic syndrome of *hydrops tubae profluens*, consisting of colicky lower abdominal pain relieved by the discharge of a serous fluid from the vagina, is present in less than 10 percent of patients with tubal carcinoma and is therefore of limited clinical value. More common is a rather profuse yellow or amber, watery discharge suggestive of serum or urine. Vaginal-cervical cytology is positive in 5 to 10 percent of the reported cases but seldom leads to the diagnosis.

Diagnosis

The diagnosis of tubal carcinoma is made preoperatively in less than 5 percent of cases, partly because it is rare and partly because of associated pathologic conditions. In most cases the preoperative diagnosis is fibroids, tubo-ovarian abscess, hydrosalpinx, ovarian cancer, or ovarian endometriosis. Ultrasonography, a relatively recent but extremely useful diagnostic technique for evaluating the female pelvis, may improve the identification of tubal carcinoma preoperatively. Cervical cytology is positive in 5 to 10 percent of the reported cases but seldom leads to the diagnosis. Recurrent postmenopausal bleeding or a Pap smear suggestive of adenocarcinoma in a patient with a negative fractional curettage is very suspicious for occult tubal (or ovarian) carcinoma. The tubes and ovaries need to be visualized or removed in these cases (Ryan and Mehmi, 1985). The serum CA-125 value is frequently elevated in patients with tubal carcinoma, as it is with most adenocarcinomas of the female genital tract, and it should be measured whenever tubal cancer is in the differential diagnosis. However, the CA-125 provides no basis for distinguishing tubal cancer from other causes of a pelvic mass, ascites, or vaginal bleeding.

Pathology

The dominant histologic variant of primary tubal cancer is papillary serous carcinoma, histologically identical to ovarian serous carcinoma. Bilateralism is reported in 10 to 25 percent of cases, with the lower rate in stage I patients, and concurrent müllerian primaries (endometrium, ovary) are not uncommon. Glandular and solid patterns also exist, and mixtures are common. The reported degree of differentiation varies widely, but on average about half the cases are considered to be grade 3. Adenosquamous, endometrioid, clear cell, transitional, glassy cell, and squamous carcinomas arising in the fallopian tube have been observed, as have MMMTs (vide infra), leiomyosarcoma, and immature teratoma. An alpha-fetoprotein–producing hepatoid carcinoma of the oviduct has also been reported (Aoyama et al, 1996). Gestational choriocarcinoma following tubal pregnancy is a well-known but rarely encountered cause of tubal malignancy. Isolated instances of tubal epithelium involved by severe squamous dysplasia concurrent with endometrial and endocervical squamous dysplasia have been reported. In addition to uterine leiomyomata, endometrial hyperplasia, endometrial carcinoma, and endometriosis are frequent incidental findings in patients with tubal cancer. Because metastases to the tube are relatively more common than primary tubal carcinoma, several authors have proposed criteria to assure uniformity in diagnosing primary tubal cancer. Those of Hu et al (1950) are as follows: (1) grossly, the main tumor is in the tube; (2) microscopically, the mucosa should be chiefly involved and should exhibit a papillary pattern; and (3) if the tubal wall is involved to a great extent, the transition between benign and malignant tubal epithelium should be demonstrated.

Spread Pattern

Fallopian tube carcinoma behaves somewhat like ovarian carcinoma, but there are several notable differences: (1) in tubal carcinoma, lymphatic spread appears to be a more important route of dissemination; (2) distant metastases, predominantly lymphatic, are a more common feature of recurrent tubal carcinoma; and (3) tubal carcinoma tends to be more indolent, with late relapse not uncommon among patients with early-stage disease, or advanced disease after platinum-based chemotherapy. The initial growth, invariably

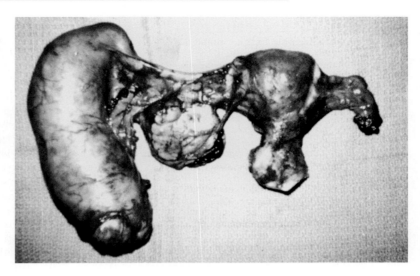

FIGURE 8–1. Tubal carcinoma. Sausage-shaped right fallopian tube. The tumor was predominantly intraluminal.

in the distal two thirds of the tube, is typically exophytic, expanding the lumen and producing a fusiform mass that may resemble a hydrosalpinx or tubo-ovarian abscess if the fimbriae are closed (Fig. 8–1). Both intraperitoneal and lymphatic spread are common, but ascites is less often reported in advanced tubal cancer (22 percent) than in ovarian cancer (Tamimi and Figge, 1981; Rose et al, 1990). Peritoneal metastasis evidently occurs via the tubal lumen, and some authors have stated that the prognosis is better if the fimbriated end of the tube is occluded.

The perception that lymphatic dissemination is important in tubal carcinoma has been documented by Klein et al (1994), who performed pelvic and aortic node dissections on 21 women with tubal carcinoma. None of six patients with apparent International Federation of Gynecology and Obstetrics (FIGO) stage I disease had lymph node metastases, while three of seven stage II patients had nodal metastases and all but two of the eight patients with more advanced disease had nodal involvement. There was a slight dominance of pelvic node metastasis (nine cases) over aortic node metastasis (seven cases). Tamimi and Figge (1981) found that five of their 15 sampled patients had aortic node metastases, 2 of whom had no other extratubal disease. Peters et al (1989) reported on 10 women with isolated recurrent tubal cancer in supraclavicular, pelvic, aortic, groin, or axillary lymph nodes. Others have noted that one third to one half of recurrences involve the lymph nodes (McMurray et al, 1986; Semrad et al, 1986; Maxson et al, 1987). Inguinal node metastases are also common. Frigerio et

al (1993) noted that 3 of 11 stage I, 2 of 10 stage II, and 7 of 8 stage III patients had positive peritoneal cytology. Naturally, local extension to involve the ovary, uterus, sigmoid colon, and other pelvic tissues is also an important mode of spread.

Prognostic Factors

Extent of disease at diagnosis is the major predictor of outcome. The FIGO system for staging tubal carcinoma is presented in Table 8–1, and the stage distribution from several series is summarized in Table 8–2. The depth of invasion into the muscular wall of the tube in early-stage disease is also an important prognostic indicator. In one report the five-year survival for stage I patients was 80 percent when muscular invasion was less than 50 percent, compared to 40 percent for patients with deeper mural invasion (Peters et al, 1988). In most of the reported series, neither histologic pattern nor grade has had an obvious impact on prognosis; nevertheless, poor differentiation is probably unfavorable (Rose et al, 1990). Lymph–vascular space invasion is associated with an increased risk of metastasis (Tamini and Figge, 1981), and advancing age may also be unfavorable. In one series no correlation was found between DNA ploidy, histologic grade, and FIGO stage, nor did progesterone or estrogen receptor content correlate with outcome (Rosen et al, 1994a, 1994b). Endometrioid carcinoma of the fallopian tube may have a better prognosis than the more common serous type. According to Navani et al (1996), in a study of 26 cases, the lesions were more often early

TABLE 8–1

FIGO Stage Grouping for Carcinoma of the Fallopian Tube*

Stage	Definition
0	Carcinoma in situ (limited to tubal mucosa)
I	Growth limited to the fallopian tubes
Ia	Growth limited to one tube with extension into the submucosa and/or muscularis but not penetrating the serosal surface; no ascites
Ib	Same as Ia except growth limited to both tubes
Ic	Ia or Ib with tumor extension through or onto the tubal serosa, or with ascites containing malignant cells or with positive peritoneal washings
II	Growth involving one or both fallopian tubes with pelvic extension
IIa	Extension and/or metastasis to the uterus and/or ovaries
IIb	Extension to other pelvic tissues
IIc	IIa or IIb with ascites containing malignant cells or positive peritoneal washings
III	Tumor involves one or both fallopian tubes with peritoneal implants outside the pelvis and/or retroperitoneal or inguinal lymph node metastases; superficial liver metastasis equals stage III
IIIa	Tumor is grossly limited to the true pelvis, with negative nodes but with histologically confirmed seeding of abdominal peritoneal surfaces
IIIb	Histologically confirmed gross implants of the abdominal peritoneal surfaces, ≤2 cm in diameter; lymph nodes negative
IIIc	Abdominal implants >2 cm in diameter and/or retroperitoneal or inguinal lymph node metastasis
IV	Distant metastases present; pleural effusion with malignant cells equals stage IV; parenchymal liver metastases equal stage IV

* Staging for fallopian tube cancer is by the surgicopathologic system. Operative findings designating stage are determined before tumor debulking.

stage, noninvasive, or superficially invasive, and the survival was better than that reported for the serous histology.

Survival

Data from the literature regarding survival of patients with tubal carcinoma are difficult to assess with accuracy because of the numerous staging systems used over the years, the relatively small number of cases, and the total lack of any standard management scheme. Denham and MacLennan (1984) calculated the following 5-year actuarial survival rates from several reported series using the FIGO stage system for ovarian carcinoma: stage I, 72 percent; stage II, 38 percent; stage III, 18 percent; and stage IV, 0 percent. In a collaborative retrospective study of 115 patients from three institutions, the 5-year survival

rates for stages I through IV were 61, 29, 17, and 0 percent, respectively (Peters et al, 1988). In the series of Podratz et al (1986), stages I and II had a nearly identical survival rate (65 percent at 5 years). These authors also noted that 5 of 10 patients with stage Ia and IIa disease treated by surgery only, or surgery plus pelvic radiation therapy, relapsed. By comparison, only one of six patients who received postoperative chemotherapy or whole-abdomen radiation therapy relapsed. Conversely, Rosen and colleagues (1994c) found that therapy did not influence outcome in stages I and II, and that patients with tubal carcinoma had a poorer prognosis than patients with ovarian carcinoma. In one study, patients with stage III or IV disease by virtue of nodal metastasis had a better prognosis than those with intra-abdominal metastases (Eddy et al, 1984b). Patients with advanced but completely resectable disease have a significantly increased 5-year survival compared to patients with any amount of gross residual disease (Peters et al, 1988; Barakat et al, 1991).

Management

The preoperative evaluation of the patient with tubal carcinoma will be determined largely by the presenting symptoms and findings. Those patients having vaginal bleeding should undergo evaluation of the cervix and uterine curettage. Nearly all patients will need a pelvic ultrasound and measurement of the serum CA-125 level (Rosen et al, 1994d). When carcinoma is high on the list of preoperative diagnoses, a mechanical and antibiotic bowel prep is indicated, and the abdomen should be opened with a vertical midline incision. During surgery for "benign" tubal disease, particularly hydrosalpinx or chronic salpingitis, the tube should be opened intraoperatively to exclude the presence of tubal carcinoma.

Initial Surgical Therapy

In view of the high frequency of occult nodal disease, it is clear that the traditional surgicopathologic evaluation of tubal carcinoma has been inadequate. Peritoneal cytology, selective pelvic and aortic lymph node dissection, and infracolic omentectomy should be routinely performed for accurate staging. The aortic node dissection must include the proximal nodes since the tubal lymphatics, like the ovarian lymphatics, drain along the ter-

TABLE **8–2**

Stage Distribution of 409 Cases of Tubal Carcinoma

Source	Stage I		Stage II		Stage III		Stage IV	
	N	(%)	N	(%)	N	(%)	N	(%)
Podratz et al (1986)	12		14		17		4	
McMurray et al (1986)	9		11		7		3	
Peters et al (1988)	39		26		25		4	
Rose et al (1990)*	6		11		19		1	
Morris et al (1990)*	3		5		9		1	
Gurney (1990)	5		12		10		3	
Barakat et al (1991)*	3		4		27		4	
Rosen (1993)	47		20		34		14	
Total	124	(30.3)	103	(25.2)	148	(36.2)	34	(8.3)

* Staged according to the FIGO tubal cancer system.

minus of the ovarian vein. It is important in the absence of intraperitoneal spread to know intraoperatively whether the disease is unilateral or bilateral, and, therefore, whether the node dissections need to be uni- or bilateral. Tumor-reductive surgery is carried out just as it would be for ovarian cancer. Complete hysterectomy with bilateral adnexectomy and omentectomy is the standard therapy, although conservative surgery with retention of the ovaries and uterus has been reported in a patient with stage Ib disease (Fedele et al, 1989). In all cases tumor tissue should be assayed for hormone receptor content, and postoperative surveillance by serial CA-125 measurement is recommended.

Radiation Therapy

The results of treatment for advanced-stage tubal cancer by radiation therapy have been uniformly poor (Brown et al, 1985; Podratz et al, 1986), while the reported results of treating early-stage disease are inconsistent. In a retrospective study of stage I patients, Klein et al (1994) found that patients receiving postoperative pelvic radiation therapy had a significantly better survival rate than patients receiving chemotherapy. By way of contrast, in an older study, Roberts and Lifshitz (1982) reported no difference in survival among stage I and II patients (their own patients combined with series from the literature) treated with and without postoperative pelvic radiation therapy. Jareczek et al (1996) observed that only 2 of 13 tubal cancer patients receiving postoperative radiation therapy relapsed in the pelvis, compared to 6 of 12 patients not receiving postoperative radiation therapy. Overall, two thirds of the patients with recurrence relapsed in the abdomen, one half re-

lapsed in the pelvis, and one third developed extra-abdominal disease after treatment. In view of these facts, radiation therapy seems to be a reasonable choice as aduvant therapy only for early-stage disease. The treatment field should encompass the entire abdomen.

Chemotherapy

The drug sensitivity of tubal cancer has almost uniformly proved to follow that of ovarian carcinoma. Thus for many years the chemotherapy of choice has been platinum based. Peters et al (1989), for example, reported on 47 patients with measurable disease. Thirteen of 16 patients (80 percent) treated with cisplatin-based chemotherapy had an objective tumor response. By way of comparison, only 2 of 7 patients (28 percent) treated with multiagent chemotherapy without cisplatin, and 2 of 23 patients (9 percent) receiving single-agent chemotherapy, had an objective tumor response. Median survival for the cisplatin-treated patients was 36 months, three times that of the patients treated with other regimens. Morris et al (1990) achieved an overall response rate of 53 percent among 18 patients treated with cisplatin, doxorubicin, and cyclophosphamide. The median survival for stages II through IV was 44 months. None of the 3 stage I patients experienced relapse, 2 of 5 stage II patients relapsed, and 5 of the 10 stage III and IV patients relapsed. Among 11 patients with measurable disease, Pectasides et al (1994) reported eight complete responses and two partial responses. Of the five patients undergoing second-look laparotomy, four had pathologically confirmed complete responses. The median survival of their 11 patients was 33 months. It is probable that paclitaxel will improve outcome in tubal cancer just as it has in ovarian carcinoma. However, there are only anecdotal data available regarding its activity (Tresukosol et al, 1995).

Second-Look Laparotomy

In the largest series reported in the literature, Barakat et al (1993) reviewed the Memorial Sloan-Kettering Hospital experience with 35 cases. Twenty-one of 35 patients undergoing second-look staging laparotomy after platinum-based chemotherapy had no evidence of disease. Gross residual disease after primary surgery correlated with a positive second look, but neither stage nor grade did. With a mean follow-up of 50 months, only 4 of 21 patients with a negative second-look operation relapsed. All 4 were among the 24 stage III patients. The 5-year survival of the negative second-look patients was 85 percent compared to 30 percent for patients with a positive second-look operation. All stage I ($N = 3$) and grade 1 ($N = 1$) patients had a negative second-look operation.

In a literature review, Barakat et al (1993) found that only 16 percent of 310 patients with tubal cancer had been subjected to a second-look laparotomy. Sixty-three percent of the patients were surgicopathologic complete responders, of whom 22 percent subsequently relapsed, often at a late interval, suggesting that the disease is less aggressive than the corresponding ovarian carcinomas.

Treatment Recommendations

All cases of tubal carcinoma except the in situ form should receive postoperative treatment because of the high risk for recurrence. Chemotherapy is the preferred treatment in all stages because it seems to be at least as effective as radiation therapy, and it causes less long-term morbidity. Furthermore metastases outside the abdomen are relatively common and cannot be addressed with radiation therapy alone. The drug therapy of choice is logically the same as that used for epithelial ovarian malignancies: a platinum plus paclitaxel regimen. A second-look operation is recommended for all stage IIb through IV cases and for stage I and IIa cases not fully evaluated at initial surgery (Eddy et al, 1984a), as discussed earlier. Because high levels of progesterone receptor protein may be found in tubal carcinoma, progestins may have a therapeutic benefit (Deppe et al,

1980), and should be considered in treatment planning.

Malignant Mixed Mesodermal Tumor

At least 46 cases of mixed malignant mesodermal tumor carcinosarcoma of the fallopian tube have been reported, accounting for 4 percent of tubal malignancies on the average (Carlson et al, 1993). The average age at diagnosis is 55 years, with a range of 14 to 87 years. The majority are advanced at diagnosis, and the mean survival time is only 17 months. The 5-year survival rate for patients with stage I and II tubal MMMT has improved according to reports published since 1987. Carlson et al (1993) noted that, among stage I patients, 8 of 12 were alive at 2 years and 50 percent at 3 years. A benefit from adjuvant therapy was not obvious. Among 11 stage III patients, 7 were alive at 2 years and 5 at 3 years. Three of 10 patients with stage III disease survived 3 years or longer. Five of the 6 patients who received combination radiation and chemotherapy survived 5 or more years. However, all but one of these were stage I or II. Of the eight stage III patients treated with chemotherapy, three survived more than 2 years and two more than 4 years.

We recommend that patients with MMMT of the oviduct undergo surgical staging, tumor-reductive surgery, and postoperative chemotherapy in the manner of ovarian MMMT. It is unclear whether the addition of pelvic radiation as recommended by Carlson and coauthors (1993) will improve outcome.

TUMORS OF THE BROAD LIGAMENT

Although relatively rare, a wide variety of epithelial and nonepithelial neoplasms arise within the broad ligament. The origin of these tumors can be ectopic ovarian tissue, invasion or insinuation from adjacent tissues or organs, or embryonic remnants, especially from the mesonephric and paramesonephric systems.

Parovarian Cysts

Parovarian cysts arise in the broad ligament from embryonic müllerian (paramesonephric) remnants, embryonic mesonephric (wolffian duct) remnants, or peritoneal inclusions.

TABLE **8–3**

Incidence of Malignancy in Parovarian Cysts

Source	Total N	LMP* N	Carcinoma N	Total Malignant N (%)
Genadry et al (1977)	140	3	1	4 (2.8)
Stein et al (1990)	168	2	1	3 (2.0)
Total	308	5	2	7 (2.3)[†]

*LMP = low-malignant-potential tumor.
[†]All malignancies were greater than 5 cm in diameter.

Genadry et al (1977) found that the majority of parovarian cysts were of mesothelial (peritoneal inclusion) origin. The incidence of bilaterality ranges from 3 to 20 percent, and 2 to 3 percent are malignant (Genadry et al, 1977; Stein et al, 1990). All of the malignant tumors in these two series were larger than 5 cm in diameter and occurred in women of reproductive age. Combining the two series, five of the seven malignancies were serous tumors of low malignant potential, and two were invasive serous adenocarcinomas (Table 8–3).

Small parovarian cysts are nearly always asymptomatic and are discovered by pelvic ultrasound or at laparoscopy or laparotomy performed for other indications. Larger cysts (>5 cm) may be clinically detectable and may cause symptoms. The diagnostic and therapeutic approach to these larger cysts should be similar to that for ovarian cysts of equal size. Any parovarian cyst with ultrasonic findings of internal papillations should be considered a neoplasm, potentially malignant, requiring removal intact. Discovery of a malignancy confirmed by intraoperative frozen section is an indication for surgical staging.

Other Broad Ligament Neoplasms

Leiomyoma is the most common neoplasm of the uterine broad ligament. Nearly all the other true neoplasms in this region are epithelial, and the majority are tumors of low malignant potential. Aslani and Scully (1989) reported four cases of primary carcinoma of the broad ligament, as well as eight cases previously published in the literature. Three of the four patients reported had endometriosis, which suggests an origin in endometriotic tissue. Twenty-eight cases of *female adnexal tumor* of probable wolffian origin have been reported (Brescia et al, 1985). They are solid tumors, usually 10 to 12 cm in diameter, that occur in the broad ligament of women at an average age of 50 years. Seven have recurred or metastasized, most after a tumor-free interval of several years. Increased mitotic activity and nuclear atypicality are suggestive of malignant potential.

Other neoplasms found to arise in the broad ligament include mucinous cystadenoma, granulosa cell and other ovarian stroma tumors, leiomyosarcoma, and malignant fibrous histiocytoma.

REFERENCES

Aoyama T, Mizuno T, Andoh K, et al: Alpha-fetoprotein producing (hepatoid) carcinoma of the fallopian tube. Gynecol Oncol 63:261, 1996.

Aslani M, Scully, RE: Primary carcinoma of the broad ligament. Cancer 64:1540, 1989.

Barakat RE, Rubin SC, Saigo PE, et al: Cisplatin based combination chemotherapy in carcinoma of the fallopian tube. Gynecol Oncol 42:156, 1991.

Barakat RR, Rubin SC, Saigo PE, et al: Second-look laparotomy in carcinoma of the fallopian tube. Obstet Gynecol 32:748, 1993.

Bartnik J, Powell WS, Moriber-Katz S, et al: Metaplastic papillary tumor of the fallopian tube. Arch Pathol Lab Med 113:545, 1989.

Brescia RJ, Cardoso de Almeida PC, Fuller AF, et al: Female adnexal tumor of probable Wolffian origin with multiple recurrences over 16 years. Cancer 56:1456, 1985.

Brown MD, Kohorn EI, Kapp DS, et al: Fallopian tube carcinoma. Int J Radiat Oncol Biol Phys 11:583, 1985.

Carlson JA Jr, Ackerman BL, Wheeler JE: Malignant mixed mullerian tumor of the fallopian tube. Cancer 71:187, 1993.

Denham JW, MacLennan KA: The management of primary carcinoma of the fallopian tube. Cancer 53:166, 1984.

Deppe G, Bruckner HW, Cohen CJ: Combination chemotherapy for advanced carcinoma of the fallopian tube. Obstet Gynecol 56:530, 1980.

Eddy GL, Copeland LJ, Gershenson DM: Second-look laparotomy in fallopian tube carcinoma. Gynecol Oncol 19: 182, 1984a.

Eddy GL, Copeland LJ, Gershenson DM, et al: Fallopian tube carcinoma. Obstet Gynecol 64:546, 1984b.

Fedele G, Cittadini E, Gortolozzi G, et al: Successful in vitro fertilization and embryo transfer after limited surgical treatment for tubal adenocarcinoma. Cancer 64:1546, 1989.

Frigerio L, Pirondini A, Pileri MI: Primary carcinoma of the fallopian tube. Tumori 79:40, 1993.

Genadry R, Parmley T, Woodruff JD: The origin and clinical behavior of the paraovarian tumor. Am J Obstet Gynecol 129:873, 1977.

Gurney H, Murphy D, Crowther D: The management of primary fallopian tube carcinoma. Br J Obstet Gynaecol 97: 822, 1990.

Hu CY, Taymor ML, Hertig AT: Primary carcinoma of the fallopian tube. Am J Obstet Gynecol 59:58, 1950.

Jareczek B, Jassem J, Kobierska A: Primary cancer of the fallopian tube: report of 26 patients. Acta Obstet Gynecol Scand 75:281, 1996.

Klein M, Rosen A, Lahousen M, et al: Lymphogenous metastasis in primary carcinoma of the fallopian tube. Gynecol Oncol 55:336, 1994.

Maxson WZ, Stehman FB, Ulbright TM, et al: Primary carcinoma of the fallopian tube: evidence of activity of cisplatin combination therapy. Gynecol Oncol 26:305, 1987.

McMurray EH, Jocobs AJ, Perez CA, et al: Carcinoma of the fallopian tube. Cancer 58:2070, 1986.

Moore SW, Enterline HT: Significance of proliferative epithelial lesions of the uterine tube. Obstet Gynecol 45:385, 1975.

Morris M, Gershenson DM, Burke TW, et al: Treatment of fallopian tube carcinoma with cisplatin, doxorubicin and cyclophosphamide. Obstet Gynecol 76:1020, 1990.

Navani SS, Alvarado-Carrero I, Young RH, Scully RE: Endometrioid carcinoma of the fallopian tube: a clinicopathologic analysis of 26 cases. Gynecol Oncol 63:371, 1996.

Nordin AJ: Primary carcinoma of the fallopian tube: a 20 year literature review. Obstet Gynecol Surv 49:349, 1994.

Pectasides D, Barbounis V, Sintila A, et al: Treatment of primary fallopian tube carcinoma with cisplatin-containing chemotherapy. Am J Clin Oncol 17:68, 1994.

Peters WA III, Andersen WA, Hopkins MP: Results of chemotherapy in advanced carcinoma of the fallopian tube. Cancer 63:836, 1989.

Peters WA III, Anderson WA, Hopkins MP, et al: Prognostic features of carcinoma of the fallopian tube. Obstet Gynecol 71:757, 1988.

Podratz KC, Podczaski ES, Gaffey TA, et al: Primary carcinoma of the fallopian tube. Am J Obstet Gynecol 154: 1319, 1986.

Roberts JA, Lifschitz S: Primary adenocarcinoma of the fallopian tube. Gynecol Oncol 13:301, 1982.

Robey SS, Silva EG: Epithelial hyperplasia of the fallopian tube: its association with serous borderline tumors of the ovary. Int J Gynecol Pathol 8:214, 1989.

Rose PG, Piver MS, Tsukada Y: Fallopian tube cancer. Cancer 66:2661, 1990.

Rosen AC, Klein M, Lahousen M, et al: Primary fallopian tube carcinoma: a retrospective analysis of 115 patients. Austrian Cooperative Study Group for Fallopian Tube Carcinoma. Br J Cancer 68:605, 1993.

Rosen AC, Graf AH, Klein M, et al: DNA ploidy in primary fallopian tube carcinoma using image cytometry. Int J Cancer 58:362, 1994a.

Rosen AC, Reiner A, Klein M, et al: Prognostic factors in primary fallopian tube carcinoma: Austrian Cooperative Study Group for Fallopian Tube Carcinoma. Gynecol Oncol 53:307, 1994b.

Rosen AC, Sevelda P, Klein M, et al: A comparative analysis of the management and prognosis in stage I and II fallopian tube carcinoma and epithelial ovarian carcinoma. Br J Cancer 69:577, 1994c.

Rosen AC, Klein M, Rosen HR, et al: Preoperative and postoperative CA 125 serum levels in primary fallopian tube carcinoma. Arch Gynecol Obstet 255:65, 1994d.

Ryan EAJ, Mehmi SA: A case report of primary adenocarcinoma of the fallopian tube. Am J Obstet Gynecol 151: 211, 1985.

Saffos RO, Rhatigan R, Scully RE: Metaplastic papillary tumor of the fallopian tube: a distinctive lesion of pregnancy. Am J Clin Pathol 74:232, 1980.

Samaha M, Woodruff JD: Paratubal cysts: frequency, histogenesis, and associated clinical features. Obstet Gynecol 65:691, 1985.

Semrad N, Watring W, Fu YS, et al: Fallopian tube adenocarcinoma: common extraperitoneal recurrence. Gynecol Oncol 24:230, 1986.

Stein AL, Koonings PP, Schlaerth JB, et al: Relative frequency of malignant parovarian tumors: should parovarian tumors be aspirated? Obstet Gynecol 75:1029, 1990.

Stern J, Buscema J, Parmley T, et al: Atypical epithelial proliferations in the fallopian tube. Am J Obstet Gynecol 140: 309, 1981.

Tamimi HK, Figge DC: Adenocarcinoma of the uterine tube: potential for lymph node metastases. Am J Obstet Gynecol 141:132, 1981.

Tresukosol D, Kudelka AP, Edwards CL, et al: Primary fallopian tube adenocarcinoma: clinical complete response after salvage treatment with high-dose paclitaxel. Gynecol Oncol 58:258, 1995.

9

Tumors of the Ovary: Classification; The Adnexal Mass

CLASSIFICATION OF OVARIAN TUMORS

Background

A universally acceptable, clinically functional classification of ovarian neoplasms has been slow in evolving for many reasons. First, the ovary gives rise to more varieties of neoplasms with a greater diversity of histologic appearance and biologic behavior than any other organ. Second, the ovary is subject to numerous non-neoplastic, tumorous conditions such as pregnancy luteoma, sclerocystic disease, and physiologic cysts. Third, the ovary is often the target for metastases from malignant tumors of other organs, especially the gastrointestinal tract, the genital tract, and the breast, that can simulate primary ovarian cancer clinically and histologically. Fourth, native ovarian tumors seldom resemble the parent tissue histologically. Finally, primary or secondary ovarian tumors can be associated with the production of biologically active hormones, evoking clinical syndromes of an endocrine nature. While standard nomenclature is important for precise communication among the pathologists, clinicians, and researchers, it is nevertheless not surprising that no classification has been devised that considers all the diverse features of ovarian tumors.

The simplest and most clinically oriented classification merely divides ovarian neoplasms into benign or malignant. This is clearly unsatisfactory because of the wide variation in the malignant behavior of ovarian neoplasms even among tumors of the same general histologic type. In addition, there are critical differences in the spread pattern and response to treatment among the malignant tumors. Even the benign tumors have important clinical differences, such as the variable frequency of bilateralism, the differences in endocrine activity, and the association of certain tumors with genetic disorders. The shortcomings of the benign-malignant division of ovarian tumors are even more apparent if the neoplastic-like ovarian enlargements are to be incorporated into the classification of ovarian tumors. While the designation of benign or malignant is useful and important, it is not enough.

Classifications emphasizing the gross composition of ovarian tumors have also been employed and are currently important in estimating the probability of malignancy based upon ultrasound evaluation of a pelvic mass. Clinically, a solid tumor is always considered to be neoplastic, whereas the cystic, spherical tumor in a premenopausal woman could be a self-limited physiologic follicle or a corpus luteum cyst not requiring surgical intervention. The solid or cystic-solid composition of teratomas and epithelial ovarian tumors suggests malignancy, whereas the cystic configuration is more consistent with a benign diagnosis. Thus the cystic-solid classification parallels the benign-malignant classification. It also suffers from similar deficiencies. These gross features may be important to the clinician and surgeon with respect to certain management decisions, but they do not provide the basis for diagnosis and treatment.

The stromal tumors in particular have been subdivided on the basis of their hormonal activity, that is, feminizing and masculinizing effects. This system is seriously flawed by the inconsistent association of hormone activity with tumor type. Granulosa tumors can be inert, or they can produce estrogen, progesterone, or androgen. Furthermore, nonstromal ovarian tumors and tumors metastatic to the ovary can exhibit endocrine effects through the non-neoplastic ovarian stroma. Certain ovarian tumors (e.g., lipoid cell) have the ability to produce corticosteroids and Cushing's syndrome, presumably because ovarian celomic epithelium arises near the adrenal gland in the so-called steroid ridge of the embryo.

Histogenetic Classification

There is now general agreement that the most useful classification of ovarian tumors is based on the presumed cell of origin. Thus the best contemporary classifications are histogenetic. In this scheme there are three major categories:

1. Tumors arising from the *celomic epithelium* or *mesothelium* covering the ovary (also termed *germinal, surface, paramesonephric,* and *müllerian* epithelium). This category includes the common, and some uncommon, predominantly glandular tumors that resemble the müllerian-derived epithelia of the genital tract. The serous tumors correspond to tubal epithelium, endometrioid tumors to the endometrial epithelium, and mucinous tumors to the endocervical epithelium (although the malignant mucinous tumors are usually of the intestinal type). Also in this group are the clear cell tumors, poorly differentiated adenocarcinomas, mixed mesodermal neoplasms, and endometrial stromal sarcomas.
2. Tumors arising from the *specialized gonadal stroma* (sex cord stromal tumors), that is, the theca and granulosa cells, the Sertoli-Leydig cells, and their precursors. Some authors also include the lipoid cell tumors in this category.
3. Tumors arising from the *germ cells*. The neoplasms in this category arise from an unfertilized ovum and are composed of tissue representing the cell of origin (dysgerminoma), extraembryonic tissue (yolk sac, trophoblast), embryonic tissue (polyembryoma, immature teratoma), or adult tissue (dermoid cyst, monodermal teratoma). The gonadoblastoma can also be included in this category.

The classification is completed by several minor groups of ovarian neoplasms. The lipoid cell tumors, often incorporated with the tumors of sex cord stromal origin, are in some instances clearly of nonstromal origin (e.g., the hilus cell tumor, which may arise from the

cells of the same name in the hilum of the ovary). There are also tumors arising from nonspecialized ovarian stroma (fibromas, angiomas, lymphomas) and tumors that involve the ovary but arise in other organs, that is, metastatic or secondary ovarian tumors. This last category accounts for only a small percentage of ovarian tumors that present as primary ovarian cancer. Prognosis and treatment of tumors metastatic to the ovary depend on the site of origin. Many secondary ovarian malignancies are associated with androgenic effects and may simulate other ovarian tumors histologically.

When ovarian tumors are grouped into this histogenetic schema, it is generally observed that 60 to 70 percent of all ovarian neoplasms are derived from the celomic epithelium, while 15 to 20 percent are of germ cell origin. The ovarian stromal groups, specialized and nonspecific, each account for 5 to 10 percent of ovarian tumors. About 5 percent of ovarian tumors are secondary or metastatic in origin if only clinically significant ovarian metastases are included.

The World Health Organization (WHO) has adopted a comprehensive classification of ovarian tumors that incorporates the widely accepted International Federation of Gynecology and Obstetrics (FIGO) classification of epithelial ovarian neoplasms. The WHO classification is too complex to be a functional instrument for the clinician, but it can serve as a useful reference guide to the oncologist, pathologist, and researcher. An abbreviated version is presented in Table 9–1.

OVARIAN NEOPLASIA

Every woman at birth has a 5 to 7 percent lifetime risk of developing an ovarian neoplasm and a 1 to 2 percent lifetime risk for developing a malignant ovarian tumor. Because the ovary has the capacity to produce such a wide variety of tumors with respect to both histologic structure and biologic behavior, the clinical manifestations are protean and constitute one of the most remarkable features of these neoplasms. Ovarian tumors may be associated with the production of estrogenic, androgenic, progestational, and adrenal steroid hormones, as well as the clinical manifestations reflecting the physiologic function of these agents. The elaboration of the polypeptide human chorionic gonadotropin may mimic early pregnancy or induce iso-

TABLE 9–1

Modified World Health Organization Comprehensive Classification of Ovarian Tumors*

I. Common "epithelial" tumors
  Serous ⎫
  Mucinous ⎪
  Endometrioid ⎬ Benign, borderline, or malignant
  Clear cell ⎪
  Brenner ⎭
  Mixed epithelial
  Undifferentiated
  Mixed mesodermal tumors
  Unclassified
II. Sex cord stromal tumors
  A. Granulosa stromal cell
    1. Granulosa cell
    2. Thecoma-fibroma
  B. Androblastomas; Sertoli-Leydig cell tumors
    1. Well-differentiated (Pick's adenoma, Sertoli cell tumor)
    2. Intermediate differentiation
    3. Poorly differentiated
    4. With heterologous elements
  C. Lipid cell tumors
  D. Gynandroblastoma
  E. Unclassified

III. Germ cell tumors
  A. Dysgerminoma
  B. Endodermal sinus tumor
  C. Embryonal carcinoma
  D. Polyembryoma
  E. Choriocarcinoma
  F. Teratomas
    1. Immature
    2. Mature (dermoid cyst)
    3. Monodermal (struma ovarii, carcinoid)
  G. Mixed forms
  H. Gonadoblastoma
IV. Soft tissue tumors not specific to the ovary
V. Unclassified tumors
VI. Secondary (metastatic) tumors
VII. Tumor-like conditions (pregnancy luteoma, etc.)

*Modified from International Histologic Classification of Tumors, No. 9. Geneva, World Health Organization, 1973.

sexual precocity. A hyperthyroid state can result from functioning teratomatous thyroid tissue, and such paraendocrine disorders as hypercalcemia, hypertension, and hypoglycemia have been reported. Rarely autoimmune hemolytic anemia is caused by the common dermoid cyst. Ascites and hydrothorax, suggestive of advanced malignancy, can be manifestations of the generally harmless ovarian fibroma, and peritoneal implants occasionally develop from benign epithelial tumors and benign teratomas. Although an ovarian neoplasm is often silent or productive of only minor symptoms, it may present as a surgical emergency secondary to torsion, infarction, rupture, or hemorrhage. Thus ovarian tumors cause a wide spectrum of clinical conditions that can readily mask the underlying disease.

Symptoms

The majority of ovarian tumors manifest themselves in a similar manner. As enlargement occurs, there is progressive compression of the surrounding pelvic structures, producing such common symptoms as urinary frequency, constipation, pelvic discomfort, and a feeling of heaviness. Dyspareunia is reported in some instances. When the diameter of the mass exceeds 12 to 15 cm in the adult, it begins to rise out of the pelvis, which can

no longer accommodate it. At this stage of development the patient is likely to notice abdominal enlargement, which she may attribute to weight gain or pregnancy. During the late reproductive years the coincidental occurrence of menopausal amenorrhea and abdominal swelling may also be misinterpreted as a pregnancy. Pain of various degrees is one of the most common initial symptoms of ovarian tumors, whether neoplastic or function. Persistent, unexplained pelvic pain is an indication for laparoscopy to determine the cause and exclude malignancy. (Rapid enlargement producing capsular stretching, twisting of the tumor on its vascular pedicle, intracystic hemorrhage, and rupture are all mechanisms of pain production.) Occasionally, such an event initiates severe pain and the clinical features of a surgical emergency (Fig. 9–1; Table 9–2). In childhood and the early reproductive years, torsion of an ovarian tumor may simulate acute appendicitis. Menstrual irregularity, often associated with a functional cyst, is an uncommon symptom of benign ovarian neoplasia.

Malignant ovarian tumors seldom are discovered in asymptomatic patients, a fact attributable to their rapid growth. Abdominal pain and swelling are consistently the two most frequent complaints reported. In the presence of ascites or metastases to the upper abdomen, bloating, heartburn, nausea, ano-

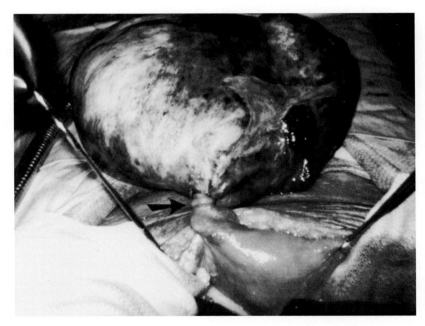

FIGURE 9–1. Mucinous cystadenoma manifesting as a surgical emergency. The neoplasm has infarcted and contains a hemorrhagic, viscid fluid. The twisted vascular pedicle is marked by an arrow.

rexia, and abdominal discomfort are common. It is understandable that the patient frequently seeks advice from an internist, because these symptoms suggest cholecystitis, peptic ulcer, and other gastrointestinal disturbances. When ascites is clinically apparent, liver disease is often a tentative diagnosis. Abnormal vaginal bleeding is more commonly a symptom of ovarian cancer than of benign ovarian neoplasia. In the reproductive years the bleeding abnormality may take the form of absent, irregular, or excessive menses. Some women, before seeking medical attention, will have noticeable weight loss because of chronic anorexia and nausea. Uncommon or rare paraneoplastic manifestations of ovarian cancer are dermatomyositis, migratory thrombophlebitis, and cerebellar degeneration (Hall et al, 1985; Sigurgeirsson et al, 1992). Longstanding symptoms are attended by a better prognosis, reflecting the less aggressive nature of the neoplasm.

The relative frequencies of the various complaints in ovarian cancer are given in Table 9–3. Since the woman with ovarian carcinoma has no unique appearance or characteristic symptoms that distinguish her from the numerous patients with the ordinary problems encountered in everyday office practice, the physician must exercise constant vigilance.

Physical Findings

An adequate pelvic examination is important to the diagnosis of ovarian neoplasms. Prerequisites include an empty bladder and rectum, with relaxed pelvic and abdominal muscles. Even under optimal conditions a small ovarian mass may not be detected, particu-

TABLE 9–2

Operative Findings in 128 Women With
Adnexal Torsion*,†

Diagnosis	No.	Percent
Benign neoplasm		
Dermoid	38	29.7
Serous	12	9.4
Mucinous	6	4.7
Fibroma-thecoma	4	3.1
Other	2	1.6
Serous carcinoma	2	1.6
Cyst, non-neoplastic		
Parovarian	24	18.7
Corpus luteum	7	5.5
Serous	6	4.7
Endometrioma	2	1.6
Normal adnexa	27	21.1

* Data from Hibbard (1985).
† A total of 2.7% of 3,772 operations performed for surgical emergencies. The probabilities of torsion are as follows: parovarian cyst, 1:5; solid benign neoplasm, 1:6; serous cyst, 1:7; dermoid cyst, 1:9; and mucinous cyst, 1:13.

TABLE 9-3

Main Initial Symptoms in Early and Advanced Ovarian Carcinoma*

Symptom	Stages Ia to IIa		Stages IIb to IV	
	No.	Percent	No.	Percent
Abdominal swelling	46	26.8	46	24.3
Abdominal pain	29	16.9	20	10.6
Gastrointestinal symptoms	25	14.5	46	24.2
Vaginal bleeding/discharge	21	12.2	22	11.6
Dysuria	17	9.9	9	4.7
Fatigue/fever	7	4.1	28	14.6
Tenesmus	3	1.8	—	—
Breast swelling	3	1.8	—	—
Dyspnea/back pain	3	1.8	15	7.9
No symptoms	18	10.2	4	2.1
Total	172		190	

*Data from Flam et al (1988).

larly in the obese patient. In the face of an equivocal or negative examination in a symptomatic patient, ultrasound is indicated. As a rule, the lower genital tract is normal in the patient with an ovarian neoplasm, but the cervix and vagina may be displaced by extrinsic pressure. Although an adnexal mass may be palpable on vaginoabdominal bimanual examination, the rectovaginal bimanual palpation of the pelvic organs is of greater value. This maneuver permits an assessment of the posterior uterine surface, the uterosacral ligaments, the pouch of Douglas, and the parametrium. Small ovarian tumors, cul-de-sac nodularity, and neoplastic disease involving the rectovaginal septum, which might otherwise not be appreciated on physical examination, may be detected in this manner. The uterus is often distinctly separate from an adnexal mass, but at times such discrimination is impossible. Most ovarian tumors lie posterior to the uterus, but they may have an anterior position or ascend into the abdomen.

It is not possible on physical examination to determine with certainty whether an ovarian mass is benign or malignant, but if the mass is unilateral, cystic, mobile, and less than 10 cm in diameter, a benign diagnosis is favored (see the section "Solitary Functional Cysts [Follicle and Corpus Luteum Cysts]" in Chapter 12), whereas solid, bilateral, fixed masses, and those greater than 10 cm are more likely to be malignant. Paradoxically, a huge cystic tumor filling the abdomen is usually a benign or borderline (low-malignant-potential) mucinous cystadenoma. Although the presence of ascites is a strong indication of a malignant tumor, even with an adnexal mass it is not a pathognomonic sign (see the section "Fibroma" in Chapter 12). Ascites can be associated with liver disease, endometriosis (even bloody ascites), pancreatitis, tuberculous peritonitis, theca-lutein cysts, heart failure, and prior abdominal radiation, in addition to certain benign ovarian neoplasms, especially fibromas, thecomas, and Brenner tumors. The delineation of a large ovarian mass on abdominal examination is frequently a simple matter, particularly in a thin subject with a solid or semisolid tumor, but differentiation of ascites from a large ovarian cyst may be exceedingly difficult (Figs. 9-2 and 9-3). A fluid wave can be elicited in either condition. However, the tympanitic note of the small intestine should be central in a supine patient with ascites and lateral when the distension is secondary to a tumor. Furthermore, ascites will cause an umbilical hernia to balloon, but a neoplastic mass within the abdomen will not. Ultrasound examination can readily differentiate ascites from a large ovarian neoplasm.

The physical examination must not be limited to the pelvis in the patient with a gynecologic tumor. The peripheral lymph nodes need to be carefully assessed. Both the supraclavicular and inguinal nodes are frequent sites of metastases from ovarian cancer, and even the axillary nodes may be clinically involved. The breast and rectum are more common sites of primary cancer in women than any of the genital organs, and they should always be examined. Other features to be looked for include pleural effusion, leg edema, and the stigmata of abnormal hormone production.

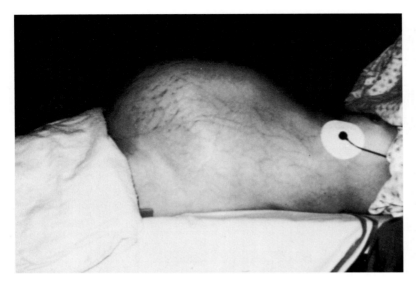

FIGURE 9–2. Marked abdominal distention in a 45-year-old mother of three. She delayed seeking medical attention for more than a year because her husband was terminally ill. A close-up view of the ovarian neoplasm is shown in Figure 9–3.

THE ADNEXAL/PELVIC MASS

Fundamentally, the clinical evaluation and management of ovarian neoplasms fall under the more general heading of the adnexal/pelvic mass. The algorithm for the differential diagnosis of these masses can be very complex, as Figure 9–4 suggests. On the basis of the patient's medical history, physical examination, laboratory tests, and imaging studies, the gynecologist must make several critical decisions to determine the most appropriate plan of management. Is the problem gynecologic? Is the patient pregnant? Is the mass uterine or adnexal? Is the mass neoplastic? Is it malignant? Is surgery required? Is surgery urgent?

Table 9–4 presents the operative diagnoses as reported in two series after excluding surgical emergencies, pregnancy-related conditions, overt infectious/inflammatory processes, and clinically obvious leiomyomata uteri. Nearly all the remaining adnexal/pelvic masses fall into two categories: the obvious adnexal mass and the poorly defined pelvic mass. The latter often extends across the midline to the pelvic wall and is irregular in outline, not clearly cystic, and more or less fixed. The poorly defined mass is most likely to be cancer, a tubo-ovarian abscess, a large (often broad ligament) leiomyomatous uterus, or severe endometriosis with endometriomas. The cancers may be genital, gastrointestinal, or even retroperitoneal. The proportion of each diagnosis varies with age group. For example, in Table 9–4 nearly one-half of the patients older than 50 years had malignant tumors, but none in this age group had a chronic adnexal abscess. In the under-30 age group, only 5 percent had a malignant tumor and 13 percent had a chronic adnexal abscess.

The Clinically Obvious Adnexal Mass

Cystic Ovarian Tumors

Most of the clinical decisions regarding the obvious adnexal cyst are based upon the history, physical examination, pregnancy testing, pelvic ultrasound, and a serum CA-125 determination. The ultrasound imaging can determine the size, the internal consistency (number of locules, wall thickness, papillations, mural nodules, solid components), and the character of the fluid contents. Thus dermoid cysts, endometriomas, and benign cystomas, can often be recognized on ultrasound with a reasonable level of confidence (Schwartz and Seifer, 1992). During the reproductive years functional cysts are fairly common. Simple, unilateral adnexal cysts up to 10 cm in diameter should be followed for 4 to 6 weeks, even if the patients is taking oral contraceptives, especially triphasics or low-dose monophasics (Holt et al, 1992), to avoid operative intervention for a physiologic follicular or corpus luteum cyst, the majority of which will involute spontaneously during this short period of observation (see Chapter 12). Other cysts, including persistent simple cysts, need to be managed surgically. Whether open laparotomy or laparoscopy is performed will depend upon the situation and

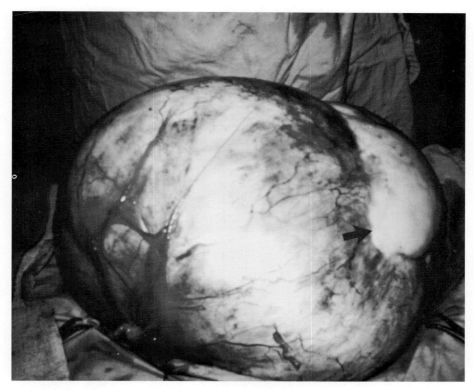

FIGURE 9–3. The major portion of this 35-lb mucinous tumor was a single cyst. The ovarian pole contained a 10-cm multilocular mass that had histologic features of a borderline mucinous cystadenoma. The arrow points to an area of necrosis that was adherent to the upper abdominal wall and transverse colon.

the experience of the operator. This is discussed in the section "Operative Management" later in this chapter.

Solid Ovarian Tumors

A solid adnexal mass may be a pedunculated or broad ligament myoma, a stromal tumor, or a malignant epithelial tumor. The myoma is readily identified by ultrasound unless it is degenerating, in which case it may have a cystic or cystic-solid configuration suggestive of a malignant ovarian tumor. Solid stromal tumors are typically fibrothecomas or Brenner tumors. These often have a rock-hard consistency on pelvic examination, and areas of calcification are common. Each of these three groups of tumors may be associated with an elevation of the serum CA-125 value, but this is more frequently seen with the solid carcinoma, particularly if the value is above 200 U/ml. The major exception to this general rule is the solid, benign tumor with clinical ascites. In this case the CA-125 value may be in the thousands.

Benign or Malignant: Clinical Differentiation

Numerous investigations have been carried out to test the ability of ultrasound and serum CA-125 to distinguish preoperatively between benign and malignant ovarian tumors. Combining the results of two retrospective studies, ultrasound has a positive predictive value of 38 percent and a negative predictive value of 96 percent in both pre- and postmenopausal women (Luxman et al, 1991; Sassone et al, 1991). In the Luxman study of postmenopausal women, 2 of 33 simple cysts (6 percent; both <5 cm), 5 of 17 solid tumors (29 percent), and 22 of 52 complex tumors (42 percent) proved to be malignant.

In a prospective study of 226 women with an adnexal mass, Roman et al (1997) found that 99 percent in the premenopausal and 100 percent in the postmenopausal age groups had a benign tumor when the clinical examination (mobile, regular contour), tumor markers, and transvaginal ultrasound (<25 percent solid, no papillations) were nonsuspicious. If all three indicators were suspi-

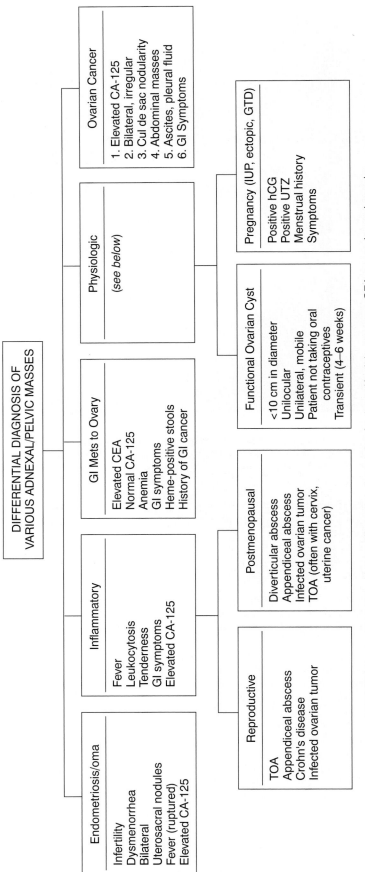

FIGURE 9–4. Algorithm of the differential diagnosis of adnexal/pelvic masses. CEA = carcinoembryonic antigen; GI = gastrointestinal; GTD = gestational trophoblastic disease; hCG = human chorionic gonadotropin; IUP = intrauterine pregnancy; Mets = metastases; TOA = tubo-ovarian abscess; UTZ = ultrasound.

TABLE 9–4

Causes of Adnexal/Pelvic Mass in Various Age Groups*

Postoperative Diagnosis	Percent by age group in years		
	<30 (N = 108)	30–50 (N = 175)	>50 (N = 81)
Cancer[†]	5	10	45
Dermoid cyst	34	8	6
Endometriosis	12	20	2
Cystoma[‡]	30	36	34
TOA/PID (chronic)[§]	13	13	0
Leiomyomata[‖]	5	13	12
Miscellaneous	7	9	9

*Data from Killackey and Neuwirth (1988) and Hernandez and Miyazawa (1988).
[†]Altogether there were 61 cancers: 40 ovarian, 3 tubal, 3 uterine, 3 cervical, 6 colonic, 1 jejunal, 1 bladder, and 4 other.
[‡]Includes a few functional cysts.
[§]Tubo-ovarian abscess with pelvic inflammatory disease.
[‖]Not preoperative diagnosis. Some were pedunculated.

cious, 77 percent of the masses in the premenopausal women and 83 percent in the postmenopausal women were malignant. In the younger group the ultrasound findings alone were predictive of malignancy in 65 percent of the cases versus 1 percent for the nonsuspicious cases. However, 5 percent of masses were malignant in the postmenopausal age group despite the findings of a normal

CA-125 and ultrasound, while 60 percent were malignant if either or both were suspicious. Others have reported similar findings (Finkler et al, 1988; Vasilev et al, 1988).

The value of transvaginal color flow imaging relative to gray scale ultrasound in discriminating between benign and malignant tumors is controversial (Caruso et al, 1996; Roman et al, 1997). The serum CA-125 measurement is of very limited benefit in identifying ovarian malignancy in premenopausal women because elevations, although rarely over 100 to 200 U/ml, can be associated with endometriosis, adenomyosis, leiomyomata uteri, pregnancy, and pelvic inflammatory disease (Table 9–5). The CA-125 predictive value is enhanced if the platelet count is higher than $400,000/mm^3$ (Chalas et al, 1992).

The Clinically Indeterminate Adnexal/Pelvic Mass

The clinical differentiation of less clearly defined adnexal/pelvic masses is more complicated. The first order of business is to define which are gynecologic and then which are malignant. Table 9–6 lists the most common nongynecologic diseases found at pelvic laparotomy for a presumed gynecologic problem. These are predominantly gastrointesti-

TABLE 9–5

Serum CA-125 Values Reported for Various Conditions Other Than Advanced Ovarian Carcinoma*

Condition	Total	No. Elevated[†]	Mean ± SEM	Highest Value
Endometrioma >4 cm	19	19[‡]	53 ± 2	110[‖]
Endometriosis	7	0	15 ± 1	—
Nonendometriotic cyst	20	0	11 ± 1	—
Liver cirrhosis				
No ascites	16		43.5 ± 14.2	225
Ascites	24	24	291 ± 29.0	800
Pregnancy (IUP)	17	7[§]	27 ± 6.7	150
Ectopic, intact	10	9	97 ± 9.6	275
Ectopic, ruptured	17	13	84.4 ± 9.4	360
Systemic lupus				
Active	28	10	48	272
Inactive	9	2	32	132
Meigs' syndrome	1	1	—	226
Stage I ovarian carcinoma	13	3	54	70
Pelvic inflammatory disease	30	10	—	550

*Data from Bergmann et al (1987), Halila et al (1986), Jones and Surwit (1989), Mann et al (1988), Moncayo and Moncayo (1991), Pittaway et al (1987), and Sadovsky et al (1991).
[†]Greater than 35 U/ml except where specified.
[‡]Normal less than 20 U/ml.
[§]Normal less than 18 U/ml.
[‖]In the authors experience serum values of ~1000 μ/ml can be found in patients who have endometriosis with ascites.

TABLE 9–6

Nongynecologic Causes of an Apparent Adnexal Mass*

Neoplastic	Non-neoplastic
Tumors of the colon, appendix	Diverticular abscess
Small bowel tumor	Appendiceal abscess
Mesothelial tumor	Crohn's disease
Retroperitoneal tumor	Pelvic kidney
Lymphoma	Anterior sacral meningocele
Cancer metastatic to the ovary or cul-de-sac	

*Data from Schnur et al (1969) and Kajanoja and Procopé (1975).

nal. Evidence supporting the diagnosis of a gastrointestinal primary other than gastrointestinal symptoms include iron-deficiency anemia, elevated carcinoembryonic antigen (CEA) level, normal CA-125 level, and occult blood in the stool. Endoscopic and/or radiologic studies of the stomach and colon are indicated for these patients. A firm, fixed, lateralized mass is suggestive of a retroperitoneal tumor such as a sarcoma or lymphoma, especially if it extends into the paravaginal or pararectal space. In this instance a computed tomographic (CT) scan of the abdomen and pelvis is helpful. Findings on physical examination, other than bilateralism, favoring a diagnosis of malignancy are, in the main, manifestations of metastatic disease. Such findings include cul-de-sac nodularity, ascites, pleural effusion, lymphadenopathy, and a palpable abdominal mass. The differential diagnosis of ascites is presented in Table 9–7.

TABLE 9–7

Differential Diagnosis of Ascites

Malignant	Benign*
Gynecologic	Gynecologic
Ovary, tube, uterus,[†] peritoneum, cervix	Ovarian fibroma, thecoma, Brenner tumor
GTD[‡]	Endometriosis[§]
	Prior abdominal radiotherapy
Nongynecologic	Nongynecologic
Colon,[∥] stomach, breast, pancreas, gallbladder	Heart failure
	Liver failure
	Pancreatitis
	Tuberculous peritonitis

*Ascites can be mimicked by an obese abdominal wall or a large ovarian cyst.
[†]Usually papillary serous carcinoma.
[‡]GTD, gestational trophoblastic disease with theca-lutein cysts.
[§]May be bloody.
[∥]Usually right colon.

THE SUBCLINICAL OVARIAN CYST

Because of the widespread use of ultrasound, CT, and magnetic resonance imaging (MRI) as adjuncts to the physical examination for a variety of clinical situations, a frequent problem that has evolved lately is the subclinical ovarian cyst. This cyst is particularly common in premenopausal women because of the physiologic nature of the ovulatory cycle, but such cysts are found with surprising frequency also in postmenopausal women, an age group in which concern for malignancy in small cysts is more realistic. In the study of Wolf et al (1991), the observed prevalence of simple ovarian cysts less than 3 cm in diameter in postmenopausal women was 13 percent. Since malignancy is rare in simple cysts of this size, the recommended management is observation if the CA-125 value is normal. The regression/persistence rates are unknown, but the 13 percent prevalence rate in the Wolf et al study far exceeds the known incidence of benign and malignant ovarian tumors. An algorithm for managing these patients is given in Figure 9–5. A subclinical, clearly defined, solid or cystic-solid adnexal mass on ultrasound in a postmenopausal woman should be evaluated laparoscopically and removed.

PREOPERATIVE EVALUATION

The diagnosis and management of a suspected ovarian neoplasm, benign or malignant, are ultimately dependent on surgical removal and pathologic examination. After excluding the diagnosis of a functional cyst (Fig. 9–4), the preoperative work-up is begun. It should be tailored to the physical findings, the patients' symptomatology, and her general medical condition. The most common mistaken preoperative diagnosis in patients with ovarian cancer is uterine fibroids. While the ultrasound examination has become the primary diagnostic study in the work-up of the patient with a presumed ovarian mass, occasionally the plain abdominal radiograph can often provide a clue to the nature of the mass. For example, about one-half of dermoid cysts can be positively identified because of their characteristic radiographic features (Fig. 9–6). Papillary serous tumors, gonadoblastomas, fibrothecomas, fibroadenomas, and Brenner tumors (benign

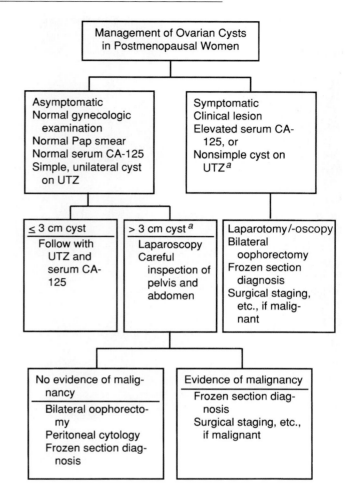

FIGURE 9–5. Algorithm for managing subclinical ovarian cysts in postmenopausal women. [a]No specific upper size limit. Cyst should be removed without rupture or spill. UTZ = ultrasound.

or malignant) may contain sufficient calcifications to be visible radiographically. Metastases from borderline or malignant serous tumors with psammoma bodies similarly may be visualized (Fig. 9–7).

Intravenous urography has fallen into disfavor because of the widespread use of CT scanning with contrast. Nevertheless, it can give the surgeon valuable information about renal function, urinary tract anomalies, ureteral obstruction, and retroperitoneal involvement by tumor. The chest radiograph provides important information about the status of the heart and lungs. It may also detect clinically silent metastases or a pleural effusion. The indications for upper and lower gastrointestinal studies have already been discussed. In general, however, in the absence of specific indications, the CT scan, MRI, intravenous pyelogram, and barium enema are not helpful in the work-up of the patient with ovarian carcinoma (Guidozzi and Sonnen-

decker, 1991). Liver function studies are essential in the evaluation of a patient with ascites or whenever malignancy is suspected. If they are abnormal, the liver needs to be evaluated for metastases. Paracentesis for cytologic, bacteriologic, or biochemical studies is seldom warranted in the patient with a pelvic mass and ascites (see the section "Serous Effusions" in Chapter 10).

Cytology and/or colposcopy should be performed to evaluate the cervix for neoplasia if this has not been done recently. Endometrial biopsy and endocervical curettage are indicated in the patient with abnormal uterine bleeding or endometrial stripe on ultrasound consistent with neoplasia. Levels of the germ cell tumor markers lactic dehydrogenase, beta-human chorionic gonadotropin, and alpha-fetoprotein should be obtained preoperatively in the young patient with a cystic-solid or solid adnexal mass. Serum CA-125 and CEA levels should be determined in all

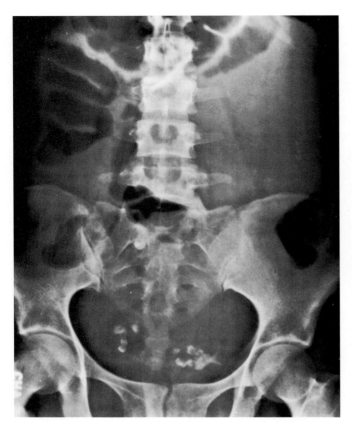

FIGURE 9–6. Dermoid cyst. Anteroposterior film of the abdomen and pelvis. The two sets of calcifications in the pelvis represent teeth in bilateral ovarian dermoids. The teeth on the patient's right occupy a radiolucent shadow cast by the lipidic fluid in the cyst. (From Morrow CP, Hart WR. The ovaries. In Romney S (ed): Textbook of Obstetrics and Gynecology: The Healthcare of Women. New York, McGraw-Hill, 1981, with permission.)

patients undergoing surgery for a potentially malignant gynecologic tumor. As previously discussed, an elevated serum CA-125 level is reasonably good evidence that the postmenopausal patient has a malignant ovarian tumor, especially a nonmucinous epithelial carcinoma, while a high CEA level suggests that a gastrointestinal cancer may be present.

Ultrasound, examination under anesthesia, and laparoscopy can be very helpful in defining an ovarian enlargement that is suspected but uncertain on pelvic examination. These studies are also helpful in evaluating the patient with persistent symptoms and a normal pelvic examination. In addition to identifying an ovarian mass and providing useful information about its characteristics, ultrasound can image an early intrauterine or tubal pregnancy, detect preclinical ascites, and disclose unsuspected metastases. Whenever there is reason to evaluate the retroperitoneum, however, the CT scan is clearly superior to ultrasound. Both tests have serious limitations in evaluating the abdominal contents, as does MRI. It should be mentioned, in the interest of completeness, that radionuclide bone scanning in the absence of localizing symptoms is fruitless in patients with ovarian cancer.

Indications to prepare the patient for radical cytoreductive surgery include gastrointestinal symptoms, weight loss, a fixed or nodular mass, ureteral or rectosigmoid obstruction, nodularity on rectal examination, and clear evidence of malignancy, such as ascites or metastases. These patients need preoperative mechanical and antibiotic bowel preparation, a vertical incision, and detailed discussion regarding the possibility of sterilizing surgery, bowel resection, colostomy, blood transfusion, and so on. If an antibiotic bowel preparation has been done, colostomy is seldom required even when a low rectosigmoid resection is performed.

OPERATIVE MANAGEMENT

Laparoscopy

Although laparoscopic surgery is unlikely to be as suitable for the management of ovarian tumors as its most ardent proponents claim, it can be safe and beneficial to the patient

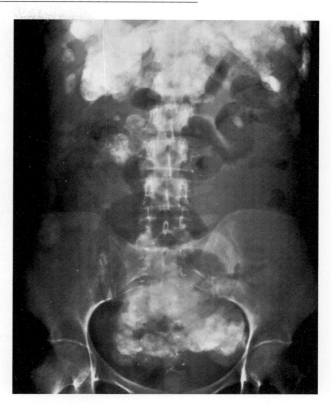

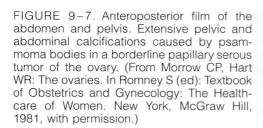

FIGURE 9–7. Anteroposterior film of the abdomen and pelvis. Extensive pelvic and abdominal calcifications caused by psammoma bodies in a borderline papillary serous tumor of the ovary. (From Morrow CP, Hart WR: The ovaries. In Romney S (ed): Textbook of Obstetrics and Gynecology: The Healthcare of Women. New York, McGraw Hill, 1981, with permission.)

depending upon the circumstance and the skill of operator (Parker and Berek, 1990; Childers et al, 1996). The main issues are the appropriateness of the surgical procedure, avoiding spill, and patient safety. Considerations regarding the surgical procedure include cystectomy versus oophorectomy, removal of the tumor intact (i.e., without spill or morcellation), determining intraoperatively whether or not the tumor is malignant, and establishing the correct stage if the tumor is malignant.

Spill and malignancy are perhaps the most important issues. Decompression is essential prior to the removal of most ovarian cysts, and large cysts cannot be decompressed within a laparoscopically placed container. Especially in women for whom fertility is an important issue, uncontrolled rupture of a dermoid cyst or endometrioma may result in a local inflammatory reaction and severe adhesions, while spill of a mucinous neoplasm might result in pseudomyxoma. With regard to malignant cysts, cancer cells may be introduced into the peritoneal cavity during the process of decompression or if rupture occurs. Many authors discount the potential for spreading ovarian cancer by intraoperative spill, citing the lack of supportive evidence in

the literature (Childers et al, 1996). However, such an event would have to be very dangerous indeed to significantly alter the survival curves of patients with a stage I cancer while taking into account the grade, histology, treatment, and other factors known to influence outcome. Retrospective reviews are simply not sensitive enough to detect small changes in mortality rates. The risk of spill is increased not only by the size of the tumor, but also by fixation (adherence) and type of procedure (cystectomy vs. adnexectomy).

Malignancy is also an issue because implantation metastases frequently develop at laparoscopy trocar puncture sites in patients with ascites or peritoneal implants (Kruitwagen et al, 1996). Because cytology of ascitic fluid is not always positive in patients with intra-abdominal metastases, this problem may not be completely averted by paracentesis cytology. Furthermore, it is uncertain whether surgicopathologic staging is as accurate at laparoscopy as it is at laparotomy. Certainly digital palpation at laparotomy is superior to instrument palpation at laparoscopy, and the examination of the small bowel, Morison's pouch, and the suprahepatic space is probably more reliable at laparotomy than at laparoscopy.

General principles that should be followed in performing laparoscopy for ovarian tumors are as follows:

1. Potentially physiologic cysts should be observed for 4 to 6 weeks before laparoscopic intervention.
2. Cysts that are potentially neoplastic should be removed, not fenestrated or needled and left in situ.
3. No cyst should be drained into the peritoneal cavity.
4. Cysts with clinical or ultrasonic evidence of malignancy should be managed by laparotomy if they cannot be removed laparoscopically without spill of the cyst contents.
5. The entire abdomen and pelvis must be inspected for evidence of metastases.
6. In postmenopausal women, laparoscopic bilateral oophorectomy is the recommended procedure for a persistent ovarian cyst that can be removed intact.
7. If surgical staging is indicated and the staging can be accomplished laparoscopically, laparotomy may not be necessary.

8. A solid ovarian mass that is small enough to be removed intact via colpotomy or minilaparotomy is properly evaluated by laparoscopy. Morcellation is not acceptable unless its benignity is a certainty.
9. The patient should be prepared for laparotomy.

Laparotomy

The abdominal incision selected must be adapted to the operative procedures that the surgeon envisions considering the diagnostic possibilities. A vertical midline incision permits the greatest flexibility, but will not always be necessary. Nevertheless, the surgeon who selects a low transverse incision must recognize the limitations of that incision. The operation must be dictated by the clinical situation, the operative findings, and the surgeon's best judgment—not the incision. Premenopausal women with an uncomplicated ovarian cystoma not eligible for laparoscopic removal are the best candidates for surgery through a low transverse incision.

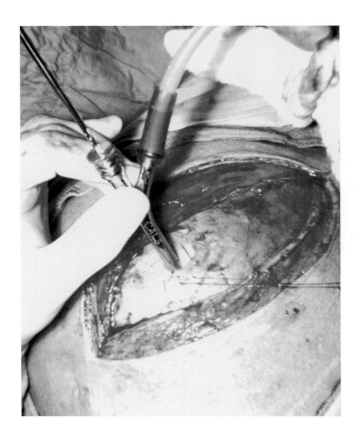

FIGURE 9–8. One method of decompressing a large, unilocular ovarian cystoma to avoid intraoperative rupture. Lap sponges are placed around the trocar to absorb any fluid that might leak out. Before inserting the pursestring suture, some fluid is removed by needle aspiration to relax the cyst wall.

TABLE 9-8

Frequent Gross Features Favoring a Diagnosis of Benign or Malignant Ovarian Tumor

Benign	Malignant*
Unilateral	Bilateral
Capsule intact	Capsule ruptured
Freely mobile	Adherent to adjacent organs
Smooth surface	Excrescences on surface
No ascitic fluid	Ascites, especially hemorrhagic
Smooth peritoneal surfaces	Peritoneal implants
Entire tumor viable	Areas of hemorrhage and necrosis
Cystic	Solid or partly solid
Smooth cyst lining	Intracystic papillations
Uniform appearance	Variegated

*None of these findings is pathognomonic of malignancy.

There is a natural reluctance, especially in young women, to extend an incision in order to facilitate the intact removal of a cystic ovarian tumor. Although such a tumor is likely to be benign, the critical issue is whether rupture of a malignant cyst might be harmful to the patient. To assume that the spillage of fluid from a malignant cyst is innocuous is insupportable, since exfoliated malignant cells are often present in the fluid of malignant cysts. Incurring the risk of seeding the peritoneal cavity with cancer cells by unnecessarily rupturing an ovarian cyst is contrary to the most fundamental principles of cancer surgery and patient care. Controlled decompression of a unilocular cyst in these young women is a reasonable approach, since the risk of malignancy is very low (Fig. 9–8), and the likelihood of spill miniscule.

Frequently, at the time of surgery, the preservation or sacrifice of the reproductive and endocrine functions of the genital tract depends on recognition of the malignant potential of the ovarian neoplasm. Although in most cases absolute identification must await histopathologic studies, several gross features that suggest malignancy may be observed at surgery (Table 9–8). None of these findings per se is diagnostic of malignancy, but hemorrhagic ascites, excrescences on the external surface of the tumor, and peritoneal implants (Fig. 9–9; see also Table 9–9) are seldom found with benign neoplasms. Additional information can be obtained by sectioning the neoplasm after it has been removed. Areas of hemorrhage and necrosis, numerous

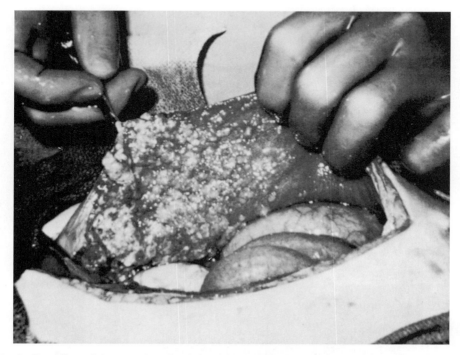

FIGURE 9–9. Studding of the anterior parietal peritoneum from serous carcinoma of the ovary. Distended loops of small bowel are in the right foreground.

TABLE 9–9

Differential Diagnosis of Benign Peritoneal Implants: "Carcinomatosis"

Foreign body granulomas (suture, starch, talc, Avitene, ruptured dermoid)
Infectious granulomas (tuberculosis, pinworms, ecchinococcosis, actinomycosis)
Hyperplasia—neoplasia (endosalpingosis, endometriosis, splenosis, benign mesothelioma, leiomyomatosis peritonealis, gliomatosis peritonei)

intracystic papillary growths, and a cystic-solid composition are highly suggestive of malignancy (Fig. 9–10). By contrast, when a tumor is composed of one or more smooth, thin-walled cysts, is free of papillary excrescences, and has no solid areas, it is in all likelihood benign. The finding of hair, teeth, and sebaceous material identifies the tumor as a cystic teratoma, and a chocolate filling in a premenopausal woman denotes an endometrioma, which, with few exceptions, is benign.

In a child or young woman of reproductive age, for whom conservative surgical management is a major consideration, or whenever doubt exits about the nature of the neoplasm, microscopic examination of the tumor by frozen section analysis should be obtained to guide the surgeon in selection of therapy. If the diagnosis of malignancy is certain or probable and the tumor is confined to one ovary (stage Ia), a careful, systematic search for evidence of extraovarian disease is indicated to allow a more informed recommendation for management postoperatively. This process is called *extended surgical staging.* The intraoperative algorithm for decision making is presented in Figure 9–11. As a general rule, when a putative malignant tumor does not involve both ovaries or the uterus, a sterilizing procedure is contraindicated during the reproductive years. Even in the presence of bilateral ovarian cystadenomas of low malignant potential, cystectomy is the treatment of choice. This conservative approach is indicated because it is usually adequate treatment, final pathology too often differs significantly from the limited intraoperative frozen section, and the patient can be fully counseled only after all the results are available. More detailed discussion of the surgical management of ovarian carcinoma, including operative staging, tumor reductive surgery, and second-look operation, is given in Chapters 10 and 11.

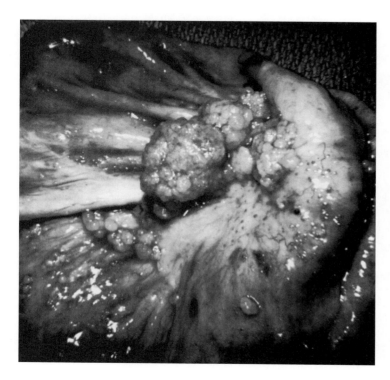

FIGURE 9–10. Unilocular serous ovarian neoplasm. Wart-like intra-cystic growths are suggestive of malignancy. This case proved to be a papillary serous tumor of border-line malignant potential.

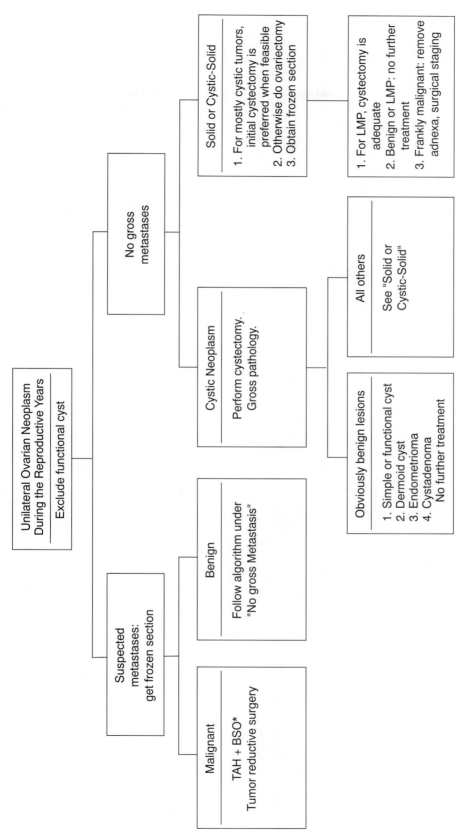

FIGURE 9–11. Algorithm for operative management of a unilateral ovarian tumor in the reproductive-age female. *In the case of a unilateral germ cell or epithelial tumor with limited metastases, reproductive conservation may still be feasible. BSO = bilateral salpingo-oophorectomy; LMP = low malignant potential tumor; TAH = total abdominal hysterectomy.

REFERENCES

Bergmann J, Bidart J, George M, et al: Elevation of CA-125 in patients with benign and malignant ascites. Cancer 59: 213, 1987.

Caruso A, Caforio L, Testa AC, et al: Transvaginal color Doppler ultrasonography in the presurgical characterization of adnexal masses. Gynecol Oncol 63:184, 1996.

Chalas E, Welshinger M, Engellener W, et al: The clinical significance of thrombocytosis in women presenting with a pelvic mass. Am J Obstet Gynecol 166:974, 1992.

Childers JM, Nasseri A, Surwit EA: Laparoscopic management of suspicious adnexal masses. Am J Obstet Gynecol 175:1451, 1996.

Finkler NJ, Benacerraf B, Lavin PT, et al: Comparison of serum CA-125, clinical impression, and ultrasound in the preoperative evaluation of ovarian masses. Obstet Gynecol 72:659, 1988.

Flam F, Einhorn N, Sjovall K: Symptomatology of ovarian cancer. Eur J Obstet Gynecol Reprod Biol 27:53, 1988.

Guidozzi F, Sonnendecker WW: Evaluation of preoperative investigations in patients admitted for ovarian primary cytoreductive surgery. Gynecol Oncol 40:244, 1991.

Halila H, Stenman U, Seppala M: Ovarian cancer antigen CA-125 levels in pelvic inflammatory disease and pregnancy. Cancer 57:1327, 1986.

Hall DJ, Dyer ML, Parker JC Jr: Ovarian cancer complicated by cerebellar degeneration: a paraneoplastic syndrome. Gynecol Oncol 21:240, 1985.

Hernandez E, Miyazawa K: The pelvic mass: patients' age and pathologic findings. J Reprod Med 33:361, 1988.

Hibbard LT: Adnexal torsion. Am J Obstet Gynecol 152:456, 1985.

Holt VL, Daling JR, McKnight B, et al: Functional ovarian cysts in relation to the use of monophasic and triphasic oral contraceptives. Obstet Gynecol 79:529, 1992.

International Histologic Classification of Tumors, No. 9. Geneva, World Health Organization, 1973.

Jones OW III, Surwit EA: Meigs syndrome and elevated CA-125. Obstet Gynecol 73:520, 1989.

Kajanoja P, Procopé BJ: Nongenital pelvic tumors found at gynecologic operations. Surg Gynecol Obstet 140:605, 1975.

Killackey MA, Neuwirth RS: Evaluation and management of the pelvic mass: a review of 540 cases. Obstet Gynecol 71:319, 1988.

Kruitwagen RFPM, Swinkels BM, Keyser KGG, et al: Incidence and effect on survival of abdominal wall metastases at trocar or puncture sites following laparoscopy or paracentesis in women with ovarian cancer. Gynecol Oncol 60:233, 1996.

Luxman D, Bergman A, Sagi J, David MP: The postmenopausal adnexal mass: correlation between ultrasonic and pathologic findings. Obstet Gynecol 77:726, 1991.

Mann WJ, Patsner B, Cohen H, Loetsch M: Preoperative serum CA-125 levels in patients with surgical stage I invasive ovarian adenocarcinoma. J Natl Cancer Inst 80:208, 1988.

Moncayo R, Moncayo H: Serum levels of CA-125 are elevated in patients with active systemic lupus erythematosus. Obstet Gynecol 77:932, 1991.

Morrow CP, Hart WR: The ovaries. In Romney S (ed): Textbook of Obstetrics and Gynecology: The Healthcare of Women. New York, McGraw-Hill, 1981.

Parker WH, Berek JS: Management of selected cystic adnexal masses in postmenopausal women by operative laparoscopy: a pilot study. Am J Obstet Gynecol 163:1574, 1990.

Pittaway DE, Fayez JA, Douglas JW: Serum CA-125 in the evaluation of benign adnexal cysts. Am J Obstet Gynecol 157:1426, 1987.

Roman LD, Muderspach LI, Stein SM, et al: Pelvic examination, tumor marker level, and gray-scale and Doppler sonography in the prediction of pelvic cancer. Obstet Gynecol 89:493, 1997.

Sadovsky Y, Pineda J, Collins JL: Serum CA-125 levels in women with ectopic and intrauterine pregnancies. J Reprod Med 36:875, 1991.

Sassone AM, Timor-Tritsch IE, Artner A, et al: Transvaginal sonographic characterization of ovarian disease: evaluation of a new scoring system to predict ovarian malignancy. Obstet Gynecol 78:70, 1991.

Schnur PL, Symmonds RE, Williams TJ: Intestinal disorders masquerading as gynecologic problems. Surg Gynecol Obstet 128:1016, 1969.

Schwartz LB, Seifer DB: Diagnostic imaging of adnexal masses: a review. J Reprod Med 37:63, 1992.

Sigurgeirsson B, Lindelof B, Edhag O, Allander E: Risk of cancer in patients with dermatomyositis or polymyositis: a population-based study. N Engl J Med 326:363, 1992.

Vasilev SA, Schlaerth JB, Campeau J, Morrow CP: Serum CA-125 levels in preoperative evaluation of pelvic masses. Obstet Gynecol 71:751, 1988.

Wolf SI, Gosink BB, Feldesman MR, et al: Prevalence of simple adnexal cysts in postmenopausal women. Radiology 180:65, 1991.

10

Tumors of the Ovary: Neoplasms Derived from Celomic Epithelium

Ovarian neoplasms of celomic epithelial origin constitute the largest subgroup in the histogenetic classification scheme. These tumors are believed to arise from the ovarian surface (germinal) epithelium, which is of paramesonephric (müllerian) derivation and is closely related to the lining cells of the peritoneal (celomic) cavity. Most neoplasms in this group contain epithelium histologically similar to the endocervix, endometrium, or endosalpinx and are designated as *mucinous*, *endometrioid*, and *serous tumors*, respectively. Mixtures of these cell types are not uncommon, and the tumors are categorized according to the dominant cell type. Less common varieties of ovarian neoplasms derived from the celomic epithelium include the transitional cell and clear cell carcinomas. Most epithelial neoplasms can be further classified according to their histologic and cytologic features as benign, borderline, or malignant. The degree of histologic differentiation may vary widely within the same neoplasm, but each tumor is graded according to the least differentiated region. Occasionally, the benign stromal component of an epithelial tumor predominates. The neoplasm is then referred to as a *cystadenofibroma* or *adenofibroma*.

The reported frequencies of benign and malignant ovarian tumors and the various subtypes range widely in the literature. Table 10–1 presents data from two population-based studies dealing with cases that underwent pathology review. The proportion of malignant tumors increases from 4 percent before age 20 to 40 percent after age 50. Dermoid cysts constitute one third to one half of benign ovarian neoplasms from ages 20 to 50, after which only 10 percent of the benign tumors are dermoids. Fibromas and fibrothecomas account for 5 to 10 percent of cases,

with the higher figure applicable to the postmenopausal period. The remaining tumors are predominantly serous and mucinous, the combination of which account for one half to two thirds of the benign neoplasms prior to menopause and 80 percent afterward. The split between the two is perhaps 60:40 in favor of the serous type.

BENIGN EPITHELIAL NEOPLASMS

Characteristics of the Histologic Subtypes

Serous Cystadenomas

Serous cystadenomas account for approximately 25 percent of all benign ovarian neoplasms. They occur predominantly during the reproductive years and are rare before puberty. The incidence of bilateralism is reported to be 15 percent, but this varies with age. Russell (1979a) found no bilateral cases in women under age 35. Serous tumors have a smooth outer surface (Fig. 10–1), a smooth lining, and one or more locules. Papillary serous cystadenomas are characterized by warty growths protruding into the lumen of the tumor. They are frequently multilocular. About one quarter of papillary serous tumors contain microscopic calcospherites (psammoma bodies), which may be extensive enough to be detected by pelvic roentgenogram. Papillations are more characteristic of borderline (see Fig. 9–10) and malignant serous tumors.

ENDOSALPINGOSIS

The term *endosalpingosis* refers to benign ectopic, tubal-type epithelium, usually involv-

TABLE **10–1**

Frequency of Ovarian Tumors by Histologic Type and Patient Age*

| | Patients by Age (Years) | | | | | | | | | |
| | <20 | | 20–39 | | 40–49 | | ≥50 | | Total | |
Tumor type	N	%	N	%	N	%	N	%	N	%
Benign†										
Epithelial	26	30.2	169	27.0	86	33.2	95	34.8	376	30.2
Nonepithelial	54	62.8	383	61.3	77	29.7	48	17.5	562	45.2
Borderline	0	0.0	24	3.8	16	6.2	9	3.3	49	3.9
Malignant‡										
Epithelial	0	0.0	29	4.6	77	29.7	119	43.6	225	18.1
Nonepithelial	6	7.0	20	3.2	3	1.1	2	0.7	31	2.5
Total	86	100	625	100	259	100	273	100	1,243	100

*Data from Katsube et al (1982) and Koonings et al (1989).
†There were 480 dermoid cysts and 235 serous cystadenomas.
‡Most common malignant tumor was serous carcinoma (N = 104).

ing the pelvic parietal or visceral peritoneum, the ovarian surface, or the omentum. It is a relatively common, incidental pathologic finding, but gross lesions do occur. Unlike its endometrial counterpart, endometriosis, it is almost invariably asymptomatic. In common with endometriosis, the tubal epithelial lining of these microscopic cysts has the potential for malignant transformation. The natural history of endosalpingosis is prolonged inactivity or regression. The etiology of endosalpingosis, like that of endometriosis, is unknown. Metaplasia of celomic epithelium and/or implantation of endotubal epithelium are the preferred theories. At times, endosalpingosis and endometriosis occur together.

Mucinous Cystadenomas

Mucinous cystadenomas account for 15 percent of benign ovarian tumors. Only 5 percent are bilateral. In a series of 688 mucinous ovarian tumors confined to one or both ovaries, 80 percent were benign, 14 percent were borderline, and only 7 percent were malignant (Hart and Norris, 1973). These neoplasms are generally multilocular and are lined with simple, mucus-secreting columnar epithelium of the endocervical type, sometimes mixed with intestinal-type mucinous epithelium. The occasional coexistence of mucinous with endometrioid or serous epithelium supports an origin from surface ce-

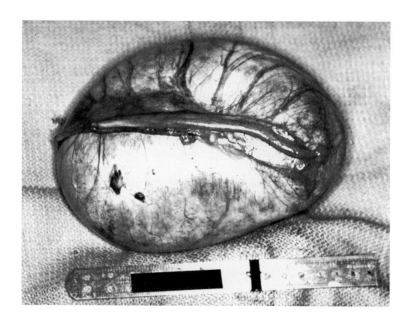

FIGURE 10–1. Gross appearance of a simple serous cystadenoma. The neoplasm is composed of a unilocular, smooth-walled cyst entirely free of papillary growths on the outer and inner surfaces. The fallopian tube crosses the outer surface of the cyst.

lomic epithelium; however, some mucinous cystadenomas have goblet cells, argentaffin cells, and occasionally Paneth's cells, suggesting a teratomatous origin. Dermoid cysts and Brenner tumors have been frequently found in association with mucinous cystadenomas (Fig. 10–2). The majority of the so-called giant tumors of the ovary are of the mucinous variety (Fig. 10–3), and, in general, benign serous tumors tend to be smaller than benign mucinous tumors. Mucinous cystadenomas may develop papillary excrescences that protrude from the cyst lining, but this is less common than in serous tumors. Mucinous ascites is reported to occur with histologically benign ovarian mucinous tumors, although in most cases the tumor has a small perforation. When peritoneal "implants" are present, the condition is known as *pseudomyxoma peritonei*. This is, however, more commonly associated with a malignant or borderline malignant mucinous neoplasm (see later).

Endometrioid and Clear Cell Tumors

It is uncertain if the ovarian endometrioma is a true neoplasm. If these lesions are excluded, endometrioid cysts are an extremely rare form of benign ovarian tumor, as is the benign clear cell variety (Czernobilsky, 1982). Occasionally, endometrioid and clear cell epithelium may be found in cystadenofibromas (Kao and Norris, 1979).

Endometriosis refers to the presence of ectopic, endometrial-like epithelium and stroma outside the uterus. It is found predominantly on the pelvic peritoneum and the ovaries. Any of the endometrioid-type malignancies (e.g., endometrioid carcinoma, clear cell carcinoma, carcinosarcoma, stromal sarcoma) can arise from endometriosis (Heaps et al, 1990).

Brenner Tumors

In 1907, Brenner described a tumor composed of nests of transitional-like epithelial cells embedded in an abundant fibrous stroma. He believed the tumor to be related to the granulosa tumor and designated it *oophoroma folliculare*. (According to Shevchuk et al [1980], this tumor was first recognized by MacNaughton-Jones in 1898. It was named after Brenner by Robert Meyer in 1932.) It is now generally accepted that Brenner tumors arise by metaplasia from celomic epithelium.

Brenner tumors account for less than 1 percent of all ovarian tumors; over half occur in the postmenopausal age group. Many of the reported Brenner tumors were discovered only incidentally on microscopic examination of the ovary. Extensive calcification may be

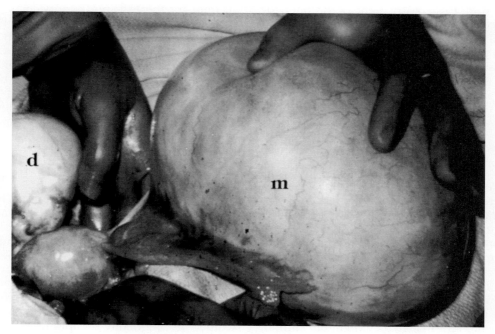

FIGURE 10–2. Synchronous mucinous cystadenoma (m) and a dermoid cyst (d).

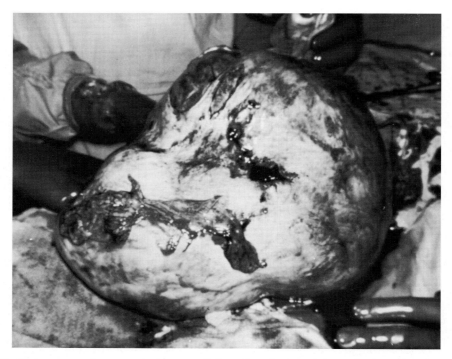

FIGURE 10–3. Large mucinous cystadenoma. Cut section disclosed the typical multilocular composition. The locules were lined with an entirely smooth epithelium, and no solid areas were found. Slightly viscous mucoid fluid filled the locules.

present, which is a diagnostic clue that can be found on abdominal x-ray films. Bilateralism is uncommon, and less than 5 percent of Brenner tumors are proliferative or malignant. From 10 to 20 percent of Brenner tumors occur mixed with, or in conjunction with, a mucinous cystadenoma or dermoid cyst in the same or opposite ovary. The typical histologic features are shown in Figure 10–4. A few Brenner tumors in postmenopausal women have been associated with evidence of estrogen or androgen production.

Cystadenofibromas and Adenofibromas

Cystadenofibromas and adenofibromas are characterized grossly by a predominantly solid fibrous component. Approximately 20 percent are bilateral. Occasionally in a cystadenofibroma, the epithelium covering the ovarian surface has a papillary character, with warty excrescences. On cut section, the cystadenofibroma has prominent cystic spaces, often with thick papillae. This configuration makes it one of the more common lesions to be mistaken for malignancy on ultrasound. In contrast, the adenofibroma on cut section has

faintly visible or microscopic cysts. In 80 to 90 percent of cases, the cystic spaces of these neoplasms are lined with serous epithelium. Endometrioid, clear cell, and mixed varieties account for the rest, but they occur in older women (mean age 57 years) than the typical serous type (Kao and Norris, 1979). Borderline and malignant cystadenofibromas of all cell types have been described (Roth et al, 1981, 1984). Cystadenofibroma with benign peritoneal implants has been reported (Hafiz and Toker, 1986).

Benign Mesotheliomas

There are two varieties of tumor derived from the mesothelium that, on rare occasion, may be encountered by the gynecologist. The *adenomatoid tumor* is almost invariably a small, firm, gray-white nodule on the posterior uterus, fallopian tube, or ovary found incidentally at laparotomy or on pathologic examination of these organs. Its behavior is invariably benign.

The *benign cystic mesothelioma* (Fig. 10–5) occurs predominantly in reproductive-age women, is frequently symptomatic, and recurs in 25 to 50 percent of cases, although

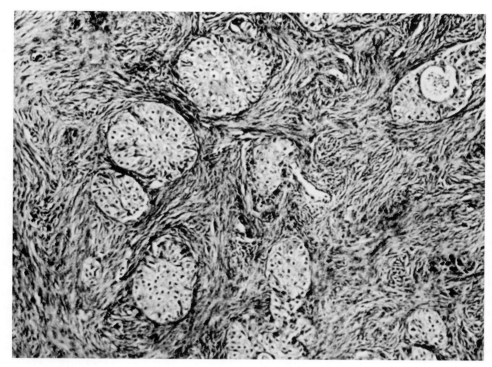

FIGURE 10–4. Brenner tumor of the ovary. Anastomosing cords of transitional-like epithelium embedded in an abundant fibrous stroma. The epithelial "islands" tend to form central cavities, which may be lined with mucinous epithelium. Malignant forms are rarely encountered.

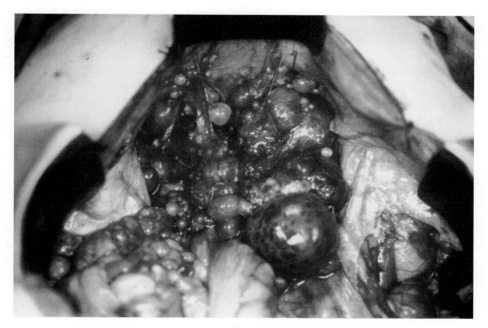

FIGURE 10–5. Benign cystic mesothelioma, recurrent in a 68-year-old woman. The bladder blade is visible at the top center of the picture and the sigmoid colon at the bottom center. (Courtesy of Laila Muderspach, MD.)

none has been fatal. The characteristic findings are multiple or multiocular cystic masses involving the pelvic organs and peritoneum. The cysts are transparent, filled with a clear fluid, and lined with a simple cuboidal epithelium. Exfoliated papillary clusters in the cyst lumina and cellular atypicality are seen occasionally (Miles et al, 1986).

Management of Benign Ovarian Tumors

Surgical removal is adequate therapy for any benign ovarian neoplasm, but factors other than excision of the tumor enter into the treatment decisions. During the reproductive years, preservation of the childbearing and hormonal functions of the reproductive tract is of major importance in the treatment of benign ovarian tumors; consequently, conservative surgery is the rule. The risk of preserving the contralateral ovary has been examined by Randall et al (1962), who studied the outcome of 213 women after unilateral oophorectomy for a benign serous or mucinous cystadenoma. On long-term follow-up, these women did not show any increase or decrease in the risk of developing a benign ovarian tumor as compared with the general population. The number of cases was too small to confirm either an increase or a decrease in the risk of malignancy developing in the retained ovary (Table 10–2).

Enucleation of a benign-appearing, unilateral, cystic ovarian neoplasm is generally recommended to conserve ovarian tissue. This maneuver is essential in the young patient with bilateral benign cysts or with a single ovary. In Randall et al's study, 4 of 42 patients with an enucleated benign neoplasm subsequently developed a second neoplasm in the same ovary. None of the four neoplasms was malignant, and none was of the same cell type as the original lesion.

Because ovarian tumors tend to be bilateral, surgical incision of the normal appearing, contralateral ovary has been suggested in the past to uncover an occult neoplasm. There is no doubt that an otherwise inapparent tumor can be discovered in this manner, but neither the rate of discovery nor the morbidity to the bivalved ovary has been determined. This practice has proved to be unnecessary in the case of dermoid cysts (Doss et al, 1977), and is not recommended for any benign neoplasm.

When a benign ovarian cyst is discovered in a peri- or postmenopausal woman, the established practice has been to remove the uterus (inclusive of the cervix), tubes, and ovaries, which are relatively common sites for cancer. It has become established practice to remove these organs when pelvic surgery is required after the menopause. The rationale for not performing a cystectomy is that the higher incidence of malignancy in ovarian cysts after age 40, and the risk of rupture, potentially seeding the peritoneal cavity, exceed the benefit of ovarian preservation. From a physiologic perspective these organs are considered to be expendable, although the ovaries continue to function many years after the menopause. From a psychologic perspective, preserving the normal reproductive organs may be very important to the individual. Hysterectomy incidental to bilateral salpingo-oophorectomy has been reported to be cost effective (Grover et al, 1996).

TABLE **10–2**

Frequency of Neoplasia Developing in the Preserved Ovary After
Unilateral Oophorectomy[*,†]

First Neoplasm	Total Cases	Subsequent Neoplasm			
		Benign		Malignant[‡]	
		N	%	N	%
Mucinous	73	3	4.1	2	2.7
Serous, simple	107	7	6.5	1	0.9
Serous, papillary	33	2	6.1	1	3.0
Dermoid	132	8	6.1	0	—
Total	345	20	5.8	4	1.2

*Data from Randall et al (1962).
†Forty-two patients had an ovarian cystectomy.
‡Average follow-up 15 years; range 5 to 30 years.

EPITHELIAL TUMORS OF LOW MALIGNANT POTENTIAL (TUMORS OF BORDERLINE MALIGNANCY)

For many years, the existence of a group of epithelial ovarian tumors that have histologic and biologic features occupying a position between those of the clearly benign and frankly malignant ovarian epithelial neoplasms has been recognized (Taylor, 1929). Clinically, these tumors are characterized by a predominantly early stage at diagnosis, infrequent and late recurrence, and long survival with residual or recurrent malignancy. The International Federation of Gynecology and Obstetrics (FIGO) accorded these tumors official status in its 1971 classification of epithelial ovarian tumors and designated them as *cystadenomas of low potential malignancy* characterized by proliferating activity of the epithelial cells and nuclear abnormalities with no infiltrative destructive growth (Table 10–3). These borderline malignancies, which account for approximately 15 percent of all epithelial ovarian cancers, are also referred to as *proliferative cystadenomas.* Nearly three quarters of borderline tumors are stage I, and the average of age of occurrence is between that of women with frankly malignant ovarian carcinomas and benign cystomas.

Characteristics of the Histologic Subtypes

Serous Low Malignant Potential Tumors

Approximately three fourths of the serous tumors of low malignant potential (LMP) are confined to the ovaries at the time of diagnosis (Table 10–4), and one fourth of the stage I cases involve both ovaries. Ascites is uncommon, and bilateralism is the rule in more advanced stages. Surface papillations are found frequently, even in stage I, with occasional tumors composed predominantly of an exophytic growth pattern (*surface papilloma*). This configuration apparently does not correlate with the risk for peritoneal implants (Kennedy and Hart, 1996). The typical LMP serous lesion, however, is a unilocular cyst with intracystic, warty growths that cannot be readily distinguished grossly from benign or even some malignant serous tumors.

Histologically, the characteristic features are (1) no stromal invasion and (2) complex, branching papillae covered by (3) stratified, atypical serous epithelium that forms tufts without a connective tissue core (Figs. 10–6 through 10–8). The degree to which these tufts are formed has been used by Russell (1979b) to divide the borderline tumors into four grades that tend to correlate with their behavior. Psammoma bodies are common and may be extensive. Serous cystadenomas with focal epithelial atypia should be classified with the serous cystadenomas. They do not have epithelial tufting (Colgan and Norris, 1983).

Although the serous borderline tumors characteristically have a homogeneous histologic composition, thorough study is important. A few cases will have foci of microscopic stromal invasion. These should be graded according to the invasive component, although it appears that the prognosis is not altered by this finding (Bell and Scully, 1990; Kennedy and Hart, 1996; Nayar et al, 1996). Some of these microinvasive cases may represent a variant termed *micropapillary serous carcinoma* by Burks et al (1996). Discordance between the ovarian primary and peritoneal implants has been reported. Thus resection of the implants for histologic study is highly desirable for purposes of staging and treatment planning. Ten to 20 percent of implants associated with serous LMP tumors are invasive; the effect on survival, however, is uncertain (Bell et al, 1988; Gershenson and Silva, 1990). Spontaneous regression of peritoneal implants from borderline serous tumors has been documented, but it is probably uncommon and usually incomplete. Benign glandular inclusions are not infrequent findings in pelvic and aortic nodes in women with ovarian neoplasia, but these must not be interpreted as metastases (Ehrmann et al, 1980).

Genadry et al (1981) have proposed the term *primary papillary peritoneal neoplasia* for serous tumors involving the peritoneal

TABLE **10–3**

FIGO Histologic Classification of the Common Primary Epithelial Tumors of the Ovary

Benign cystadenomas

Cystadenomas with proliferative activity of the epithelial cells and nuclear abnormalities, but with no infiltrative destructive growth (borderline cases; low potential malignancy)

Cystadenocarcinomas

T A B L E **10-4**

Stage Distribution of Ovarian LMP[†] Tumors by Histology[*]

	Serous		Mucinous		Other	
Stage	N	%	N	%	N	%
I						
a	222	46	247	71	15	62
b	91	19	9	3	0	
c	33	7	29	8	3	
II						
a	15	3	6	2	1	
b & c	42	8	18	5	3	
III	71	15	31	9	2	
IV	4	<1	6	2	0	
Total	478		346		24	

*Data from Pettersson (1988).
†LMP = low malignant potential.

surfaces as well as the ovarian surface epithelium since, in their opinion, this represents a multicentric origin rather than implantation metastases. This theory would be more attractive if the disease were not so rare in women who have had their ovaries removed for unrelated causes.

Among 314 stage I cases from seven series (Julian and Woodruff, 1972; Katzenstein et al, 1978; Russell, 1979b; Nikrui, 1981; Barnhill et al, 1985, 1995; Kliman et al, 1986), there were two "recurrences" (0.6 percent), both in the preserved ovary. (The great majority of these cases had bilateral ovariectomy.) However, Tazelaar et al (1985) observed five "recurrences" in their series of 42 stage Ia, borderline serous tumors. Of these five recurrences, three were in the residual ovary 2 to 3 years after the initial surgery. It is interesting to note that surgical staging of LMP serous tumors apparently confined to the ovaries will disclose evidence of extraovarian disease in some patients (Yazigi et al, 1988; Leake et al, 1991; Snider et al, 1991). Thus the fact that none of the 314 cases mentioned previously recurred outside the ovary may reflect the very indolent nature of the disease, the insensitivity of clinical examination, and a limited duration of

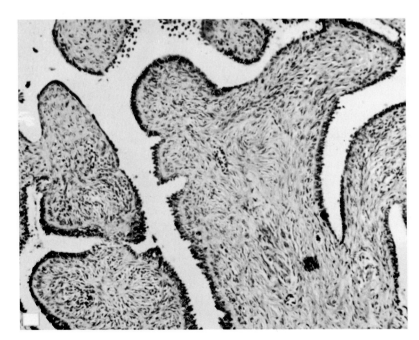

FIGURE 10-6. Benign serous cystadenoma. The papillary growths are composed of a broad connective tissue core covered by a simple tubal-type epithelium free of nuclear aberrations.

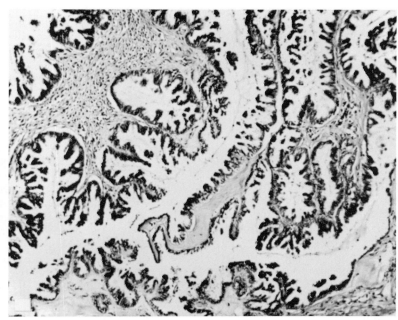

FIGURE 10–7. Serous tumor of low malignant potential. The papillary growths are more extensive, with secondary and tertiary branching. The epithelial proliferation results in a piling up of cells. The individual cells have the cytologic features of malignancy, but there is no evidence of infiltrative, destructive growth.

follow-up. It is quite clear from the reports of Bostwick and associates (1986) and Silva et al (1995) that stage I serous LMP tumors can recur outside the ovary, although such an event is not necessarily fatal.

In these same series, the recurrence or progression rate for stages II and III serous LMP tumors was about 30 percent. However, many of the stage III patients with recurrence were well, without clinical evidence of cancer. In one study patients not cured of their malignancy had a mean life expectancy of about 10 years after diagnosis (Katzenstein et al, 1978). Silva et al (1995) reported on 39 patients with recurrence after surgery. The 10 cases with recurrence of LMP histology, remained clinically free of disease, while only 5 of the 29 cases recurring as invasive serous

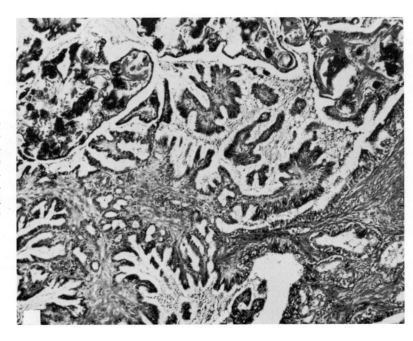

FIGURE 10–8. Serous carcinoma. The epithelium is anaplastic, and the orderly papillary branching is lost. There is invasion of the stroma, unequivocal evidence of malignancy. Numerous psammoma bodies can be seen at the top of the picture.

cancer were free of disease at the time of their report. The average time to recurrence of the 11 cases originally stage I was 20.4 years. Time to recurrence was longer for patients less than 45 years of age.

Mucinous Low Malignant Potential Tumors

In Russell and Merkur's (1979) series of 144 ovarian LMP neoplasms, 36 percent were mucinous and 49 percent were serous. Other authors have reported that the mucinous LMP tumors occur with equal or greater frequency than the serous LMP tumors (Kaern et al, 1993a; Buttini et al, 1997). Mucinous borderline tumors are three times as common as mucinous carcinomas. Eighty to 90 percent of the mucinous LMP tumors are stage I at diagnosis (Table 10–4), and less than 5 percent are bilateral. An entirely benign neoplasm is found with the same frequency as another LMP tumor in the contralateral ovary. Characteristically, mucinous borderline tumors are multilocular; solid areas, nodules, papillations, hemorrhage, and necrosis may be seen, although ascites is unusual. Mucinous tumors often exhibit a wide variation in histologic composition, requiring very thorough sampling to avoid missing areas of borderline or frank malignancy. LMP mucinous tumors composed of intestinal type epithelium are much more common than the müllerian type. The LMP lesions are characterized by secondary cyst formation exhibiting stratified, atypical mucinous epithelium with papillary infolding. Occasionally, a predominant papillary pattern is found. By definition, stromal invasion is absent. However, it is common to find mucin dissecting through the stroma, a condition designated *pseudomyoxoma ovarii*. This should not be interpreted as stromal invasion. As in the case of the serous LMP neoplasms, an occasional ovarian LMP mucinous tumor will have foci of true microinvasion (Nayar et al, 1996).

Mucinous LMP tumors appear to have a greater malignant potential than their serous counterparts. Although only 9 of 264 stage I patients (8 of 247 stage Ia) from collected series recurred, all died of disease: 4 within 2 years and 3 between 4 and 10 years after diagnosis. Of 20 stage III patients, 8 were dead with disease (7 within 3 years) and 2 were alive with disease less than 2 years after diagnosis (Hart and Norris, 1973; Russell, 1979b; Nikrui, 1981; Barnhill et al, 1985; Chai-

tin et al, 1985; Tazelaar et al, 1985; Bostwick et al, 1986; Kliman et al, 1986). Death typically results from peritoneal implants causing uncontrolled mucinous ascites, as discussed in the following paragraphs.

PSEUDOMYXOMA PERITONEI

Pseudomyxoma peritonei (PMP), as named and described by Werth in 1884, referred to a complication of mucinous neoplasms characterized by extracellular gelatinous material filling the peritoneal cavity, partly free and partly attached to the peritoneal surfaces, forming masses contained within a connective tissue membrane (Ries, 1924). This viscid, mucinous "ascites" cannot be drained by paracentesis; repeated laparotomy is required to remove the free and/or encysted mucin for palliation of discomfort, distention, and bowel obstruction.

PMP is nearly always associated with a ruptured mucinous tumor of the ovary or appendix, although the defect may be microscopic in dimension. If the mucin originates in the peritoneal cavity, the mucin itself will contain the cells of origin. It may also be produced by mucinous epithelium growing on the visceral and parietal peritoneum. Removing the ruptured ovarian and/or appendiceal lesion along with the mucin and all the involved peritoneum can be anticipated to cure the patient. However, if the primary and/or the peritoneal lesions cannot be removed in toto, the outcome is continued production of mucin eventuating in repeated small bowel obstruction and death.

There are two theories of histogenesis. The more likely is that preoperative, chronic spillage of neoplastic, mucinous epithelium from an ovarian or appendiceal neoplasm implants on the peritoneal surfaces (Ronnett et al, 1995). The second theory postulates that the mucinous epithelium results from metaplasia of the mesothelial cells of the peritoneum in response to an irritant effect of the spilled mucin (Sandenbergh and Woodruff, 1977).

The reported association of PMP with benign or malignant mucinous tumors varies widely, but the majority of cases are associated with lesions of low malignant potential. There appear to be well-documented, cytologically benign primary ovarian lesions associated with pseudomyxoma, but these have shown evidence, nevertheless, of stromal invasion or manifested pools of apparently acellular mucin in the ovarian stroma (pseudomyxoma ovarii, vide supra). Concomitant ovarian and appendiceal lesions are frequent, the latter potentially occult with a microscopic rupture. For this reason, the appendix should be removed routinely in cases of mucinous ovarian tumor. The appendiceal lesion (mucocele) may be a simple retention cyst or a benign, borderline, or malignant neoplasm (Aho et al, 1973). In one series of 25 cases in which there were concomitant ovarian and appendiceal lesions with PMP, the lesion in the appendix was occult in only 2 instances. In half of the cases both ovaries were involved; when only one ovary was involved, it was more often the right ovary (Seidman et al, 1993a).

Treatment of PMP associated with ovarian neoplasia consists of hysterectomy, bilateral salpingo-oophorectomy, and removal of the mucin, the peritoneal implants, and the appendix. PMP has been reported to be completely resectable in about one third of cases (Gough et al, 1994). If the implants cannot be entirely removed, recurrence is probable. Repeat laparotomy with evacuation of the mucin, resection of encysted masses, and relief of bowel obstruction are recommended as clinical conditions require. Platinum-based chemotherapy has been reported to be ineffective (Mann et al, 1990), while the efficacy of intraperitoneal therapy, such as 5-fluorouracil, has been given mixed reviews (Nasr et al, 1993; Gough et al, 1994; Look et al, 1995).

Reported survival of patients with PMP varies widely. In the combined series of Limber et al (1973) and Sandenbergh and Woodruff (1977), 13 of 15 patients died. Only four women survived more than 3 years, two of whom survived longer than 5 years. However, in a literature review of PMP with concomitant ovarian and appendiceal lesions, Campbell et al (1973) reported only 7 deaths, with a mean survival of 6 years, among 26 patients. More recently, Wertheim et al (1994) reported on 19 patients with PMP and a median of 2.5 years' follow-up. Recurrence was observed from 3 months to 19 years after the initial diagnosis and treatment. Seven of 10 patients with an ovarian mucinous LMP tumor were clinically free of disease; 2 patients had died of disease and 1 was alive with PMP. Of the nine patients with invasive mucinous ovarian tumors, three were alive and well, five were dead of disease, and one was alive with PMP. Gough and associates (1994) reported that 76 percent of PMP cases progress, with a 5-year survival rate of 53 percent and

a 10-year survival rate of 32 percent. Survival is related to the degree of malignancy and the extent of disease (resectability) at the time of diagnosis. Thus cases with a noninvasive primary lesion and noninvasive implants have a much better prognosis (Costa, 1994). Total parenteral nutrition may prolong survival in patients who are not candidates for surgical management of their bowel obstruction (Mann et al, 1990).

Endometrioid Low Malignant Potential Tumors

In Russell's series (1979b), the endometrioid variety of LMP ovarian neoplasia accounted for only 7 percent of all cases. These tumors are associated with pelvic endometriosis (30 to 50 percent of cases) and endometrial carcinoma. Histologically, the endometrial-like glandular epithelium recapitulates the usual variations of endometrial hyperplasia, including atypia and squamous metaplasia (Norris, 1993). Peritoneal implants are distinguished from endometriosis by the absence of both endometrial stroma and evidence of hemorrhage. Snyder and colleagues (1988) divided these intermediate endometrioid neoplasms into three subsets: (1) proliferative endometrioid tumors (predominately adenofibromas); (2) endometrioid tumors of low malignant potential (adenofibromas and papillary tumors); and (3) endometrioid tumors of low malignant potential with microinvasion.

Clear Cell Low Malignant Potential Tumors

Clear cell tumors of borderline malignancy accounted for 2 percent of Russell's (1979b) series. All were cystadenofibromas. Bell and Scully (1985) classified 25 clear cell adenofibromatous lesions (21.3 percent of 122 adenofibromas) as benign in 3 cases, borderline in 11, malignant in 7, and as clear cell carcinoma arising in an adenofibroma in 4. All borderline and all malignant lesions were stage I. Ten of the 11 women with LMP tumors were postmenopausal. Bilateralism was observed once. Three of the entire group of 25 cases were associated with endometriosis. Of the tumors classified as malignant, three were stage Ia predominantly borderline tumors with several foci of microinvasion. One of these recurred locally at 3.3 years of follow-up. Roth et al (1984) reported one tumor death (after 5.2 years) among two patients with an LMP clear cell cancer exhibiting areas of microinvasion.

Brenner and Transitional Cell Low Malignant Potential Tumors

More than 60 cases of the intermediate forms of Brenner tumor have been reported. They occur in women with a mean age of 60 years. Grossly the tumors are typically composed of one or more large cysts with solid components. Although they have been subdivided into proliferating tumors and tumors of borderline malignancy on the basis of histologic criteria, none of either type has behaved in a malignant fashion. The former is histologically similar to low-grade papillary neoplasms of the bladder. The LMP Brenner tumors are characterized by cystic lesions with papillary epithelium; nuclear atypia, which may be severe; and increased mitotic activity. Stromal invasion is absent by definition. The epithelium of these tumors resembles a grade III papillary transitional cell carcinoma of the bladder or papillary squamous cell carcinoma in situ. The occurrence of an intermediate transitional or squamous cell tumor without Brenner elements has not been described (Czernobilsky, 1985; Kempson and Hendrickson, 1993).

Management of Low Malignant Potential Tumors

The majority of ovarian neoplasms in the borderline malignant category occur in women of reproductive age and are stage I at the time of diagnosis. These cases are adequately managed by cystectomy or oophorectomy. In general, cystectomy is the procedure of choice when fertility is desired by the patient (Lim-Tan et al, 1988). However, cystectomy is essential when the patient has bilateral ovarian cystic neoplasms or a single ovary. The opposite ovary should be carefully evaluated for evidence of bilateralism. If the patient is beyond or near the menopause, a hysterectomy with bilateral adnexectomy is recommended. For younger women with no interest in future fertility, bilateral adnexectomy should be considered in the case of serous and endometrioid tumors. Appendectomy should accompany pelvic surgery for mucinous tumors.

The role of surgical staging of LMP tumors is controversial. Although microscopic lesions have been reported in the omentum and the pelvic and aortic lymph nodes in apparent stage I cases (Yazigi et al, 1988; Leake et al, 1991; Snider et al, 1991), this information appears to be of little clinical value because postoperative treatment has had no measurable effect on outcome. It is the authors' practice to limit surgical staging to biopsy or removal of suspicious lesions, partial omentectomy, and peritoneal cytology. Although an intraoperative diagnosis of LMP tumor of the ovary is relatively accurate, some patients will have a frankly invasive, albeit well-differentiated lesion of the ovary after review of the permanent histologic sections (Robinson et al, 1992; Menzin et al, 1995). Semiannual monitoring is recommended; a suspicious mass or ovarian enlargement during follow-up is an indication for surgical evaluation (Hopkins and Morley, 1989).

In those unusual cases of ovarian borderline malignancy more advanced than stage I, the cornerstone of therapy is surgery. Whenever feasible, complete excision should be done, recognizing that if the preliminary diagnosis is right, the patient stands to benefit little from life-threatening surgery because these tumors typically have an indolent course. Careful pathologic evaluation of the primary tumor and its "metastases" is essential, even for serous tumors, to exclude areas of frank invasion and dedifferentiation. If a tumor has a purely borderline histology, there is no convincing evidence that postoperative chemotherapy or radiation therapy alters in any beneficial way the course of this disease (Nikrui, 1981; Creasman et al, 1982; Barnhill et al, 1985; Kliman et al, 1986; Chambers et al, 1988; Fort et al, 1989). Lately many investigators have attempted to identify by genetic markers the subset of LMP tumors that will behave in an aggressive manner. The majority of these studies have measured the DNA content. Although the results are inconclusive, it does appear that aneuploidy confers some increased risk of progression. Mucinous LMP tumors are more frequently aneuploid than serous tumors, and the rate of aneuploidy increases with stage (Padberg et al, 1992; Harlow et al, 1993; Kaern et al, 1993b; Seidman et al, 1993b; Guerrieri et al, 1994; Diebold et al, 1996; Link et al, 1996). LMP tumors of the ovary have also been shown to have p53 and HER-2/neu overexpression, as well as alterations in DNA methylation intermediate between benign and frankly malignant ovarian tumors of similar histology (Koshiyama et al, 1995; Cheng et al, 1997; Eltabbakh et al,

1997). These findings suggest a relationship in the evolution of LMP neoplasms and that of ovarian carcinoma.

In the face of clinical progression, further tumor-reductive surgery followed by chemotherapy seems reasonable. Some authors (Barakat et al, 1995; Hopkins and Morley, 1989) have documented response to cisplatin-based chemotherapy at second-look laparotomy. For this reason platinum-based chemotherapy is recommended. One common regimen would be carboplatin plus paclitaxel. The leukemia risk of long-term alkylating-agent therapy argues against prolonged treatment with these agents (e.g., cisplatin). Remission of an LMP ovarian serous tumor with tamoxifen has also been reported (Llerena et al, 1997). It must be kept in mind, however, that borderline ovarian carcinoma can be a progressive, fatal disease. At least for the serous tumors, the distribution of metastases in fatal cases includes liver, lymph nodes, and even bone, similar to that of the frankly malignant tumors, although the disease course is more protracted. Thus regional therapy has intrinsic shortcomings.

OBVIOUSLY MALIGNANT EPITHELIAL NEOPLASMS

Malignant tumors of the ovary derived from celomic epithelium account for 85 percent of all ovarian cancers. They demonstrate a broad variation in biologic behavior that correlates rather well with the degree of histologic differentiation. The cell type of the epithelial component can usually be identified as serous, mucinous, endometrioid, transitional cell, clear cell, or a mixture of these types. Approximately 15 percent of the cases are too poorly differentiated to allow classification by cell type.

Characteristics of the Histologic Subtypes

Serous Carcinomas

Serous carcinoma accounts for 50 percent of all epithelial malignancies of the ovary. It is the most common ovarian cancer in the adult female. Typically, the tumor is partly cystic and partly solid, with areas of extensive papillary growths. Similar to the benign and borderline forms, psammoma bodies are encountered in approximately 30 percent of malignant serous tumors. Bilateral involvement occurs in approximately one third of the stage I cases (Fig. 10–9) and is more common in the advanced stages of the disease.

Histologically, papillary, glandular, and solid patterns of growth are observed, the last being typical of the poorly differentiated serous carcinomas. Growth tends to be rapid, with early spread throughout the peritoneal cavity, as the stage distribution indicates (Table 10–5). The prognosis is related to the stage, grade, and operability. Whether or not ascites with or without malignant cells, or

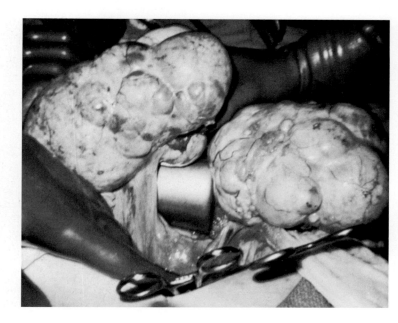

FIGURE 10–9. Bilateral serous cystadenocarcinomas before removal at laparotomy. The posterior surface of the uterus is visible between the bladder blade and the clamp. Ascites and peritoneal seeding were absent. The irregular bosselations reflect the multilocular, partially solid structure and suggest that the neoplasms are malignant.

T A B L E 10–5

Stage Distribution of True Carcinomas of the Ovary by Histologic Subtype*

Stage	Serous N	Serous (%)	Mucinous N	Mucinous (%)	Endometrioid N	Endometrioid (%)	Clear Cell N	Clear Cell (%)	Undifferentiated N	Undifferentiated (%)
I	687	(17.0)	452	(49.5)	338	(29.1)	134	(39.9)	170	(12.7)
a	334		301		189		92		90	
b	131		29		34		7		25	
c	222		142		115		35		55	
II	587	(14.5)	132	(14.4)	290	(24.9)	76	(22.6)	180	(13.4)
a	114		29		67		11		43	
b & c	473		103		223		65		137	
III	2,007	(49.6)	213	(23.3)	387	(33.3)	82	(24.4)	622	(46.4)
IV	762	(18.8)	97	(10.6)	148	(12.7)	44	(13.1)	369	(27.5)
Total	4,043	(51.8)	914	(11.7)	1,163	(14.9)	336	(4.3)	1,341	(17.2)

*Data from Pettersson (1988).

peritoneal washings with malignant cells, is an independent prognostic variable remains unsettled (Pettersson, 1988; Dembo et al, 1990). The importance of grade as a determinant of survival in patients with serous tumors is documented by survival data. For example, among 400 stage Ia cases in the 1988 FIGO Annual Report (Pettersson, 1988), the 5-year survival rates for grades 1, 2, and 3 were 92.5, 86, and 62.8 percent, respectively (Table 10–6). This influence is manifested throughout the various stages, such that stage IIIa, grade 1 cases have a survival similar to stage Ia, grade 3 cases.

Primary papillary serous carcinoma of the peritoneum ("normal-sized ovary syndrome") accounts for 5 to 10 percent of all advanced epithelial ovarian carcinomas. This entity is characterized by an exophytic growth pattern, normal-sized to moderately enlarged ovaries, bilateralism, moderate to poor differentiation, and extensive intra-abdominal spread of disease with ascites. Some instances of this condition may arise in a multifocal fashion from the ovarian and peritoneal surfaces, although in some cases the ovary is completely replaced by tumor. A small proportion of cases may represent primary papillary mesothelioma (Fromm et al, 1990; Rothacker and Mobius, 1995; Liapis et al, 1996). Since the ovaries may not be enlarged or the malignancy may involve only the ovarian surface, there is a tendency to attribute the carcinomatosis to other than an ovarian primary, especially clinically when the pelvic examination, ultrasound, and computed tomography (CT) scan disclose no evidence of ovarian enlargement. Cytology of the ascitic fluid is almost invariably consistent with a papillary serous tumor, however. The treatment and survival for patients with this syndrome are similar to those for the classic serous carcinoma of the ovary, provided that stage and grade are taken into consideration (Mulhollan et al, 1994).

T A B L E 10–6

Influence of Stage and Histologic Grade on Survival of Patients With Obviously Malignant Serous Carcinoma of the Ovary*

Stage	Percentage 5-Year Survival (Corrected) All Grades	G1	G2	G3
I				
a	85.3	92.5	86	62.8
b	69.0	85	90	79
c	59.0	78	49	51
II				
a	62.0	64	65	39
b	51.0	79	43	42
c	43.0	68	46	20
III				
a	31.4	58	38	20
b	38.0	73	42	21
c	18.0	46	22	14
IV	8.0	14	8	6

*Data from Pettersson (1988).

Mucinous Carcinomas

Mucinous carcinomas comprise only 10 to 15 percent of ovarian carcinomas. Approximately 50 percent are diagnosed before evidence of extrapelvic spread occurs. Bilateralism in stage I occurs 5 to 10 percent of the time. Grossly, mucinous carcinomas are multilocular and commonly contain nodules or solid areas. Intracystic or surface papillations are uncommon. The cysts may contain fluid varying in consistency from watery to gelati-

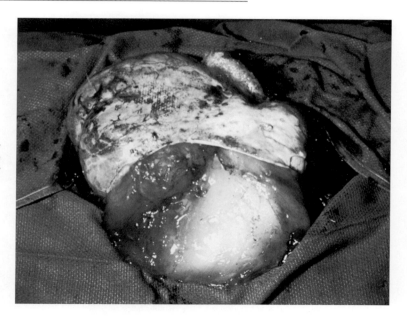

FIGURE 10–10. Mucinous ovarian neoplasm. In this case, the mucinous contents are unusually gelatinous.

nous (Fig. 10–10). Mucinous neoplasms tend to be larger than their serous counterparts. Like the benign and borderline mucinous tumors, ovarian mucinous carcinomas may be of the endocervical or intestinal-type epithelium, but the fully malignant tumors are predominantly of the intestinal type, and their behavior is more aggressive than those composed of müllerian mucinous epithelium (Kikkawa et al, 1996). Metastasis from an intestinal primary tumor should be considered when an ovarian mucinous cancer is predominantly solid. Furthermore, appendiceal primaries tend to relapse in the ovary (Merino et al, 1985). Microscopically, great variability within the same tumor is characteristic. Consequently, frank malignancy may be missed if adequate sampling is not carried out. Stage for stage, the prognosis for mucinous carcinomas is the same as that for serous carcinomas.

Mucinous tumors containing large, circumscribed, sarcomatous or poorly differentiated carcinomatous mural nodules have been reported (Prat et al, 1982). The latter appear to be associated with a poor prognosis. Concomitant ovarian and endocervical mucinous carcinomas have been reported (Young and Scully, 1988).

Endometrioid Malignancies

CARCINOMAS

Endometrioid carcinoma of the ovary was first described by Sampson in 1925, but only in the past 30 years has it become generally accepted as a distinct variant of ovarian epithelial carcinoma. It accounts for 10 to 15 percent of the common ovarian malignancies. Concomitant endometrial carcinoma is reported in 15 to 30 percent of cases, while less than 5 percent of all ovarian cancers are associated with endometrial cancer. The reported association of endometrioid carcinoma with ovarian endometriosis is around 10 percent, although in a well-documented study of stage I cases, 40 percent were associated with endometriosis, one third of which arose in the endometriosis (Sainz de la Cruz et al, 1996). Fifteen percent of stage I endometrioid carcinomas are bilateral. Endometrioid carcinomas are typically cystic, with solid areas that may be papillary in nature. The cysts are filled with a mucoid or chocolate-like fluid. Microscopically, the epithelial component is indistinguishable from primary endometrial carcinoma. Squamous metaplasia is common (Fig. 10–11). Endometrioid histology may be a favorable prognostic factor independent of stage and grade, since patients with advanced endometrioid ovarian carcinoma have a longer median survival as compared to patients with serous or mucinous carcinoma (Kline et al, 1990).

ENDOMETRIOID SARCOMAS

The ovary is capable of reproducing all the histologic subtypes of malignancy that arise from the endometrial glands or stroma of the

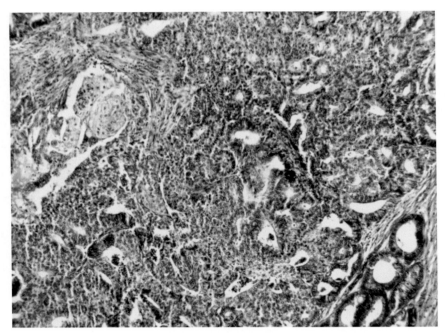

FIGURE 10-11. Endometrioid ovarian carcinoma. A focus of squamous metaplasia can be seen in the left upper quadrant of the photomicrograph.

uterus. In addition to the common adenocarcinoma with or without benign squamous components, adenosquamous carcinoma, pure squamous carcinoma, low-grade and high-grade endometrial stromal sarcoma, adenosarcoma, and malignant mixed mesodermal tumors (MMMT) have been reported. Origin from the celomic epithelium or endometriosis is postulated. According to the World Health Organization (WHO) classification, MMMT of the ovary is a subset of endometrioid carcinoma and is therefore considered an epithelial tumor.

The MMMT is by far the most frequently encountered ovarian "sarcoma." It occurs at an average patient age of 65 years, and the preponderance of cases have pelvic as well as abdominal metastases at the time of diagnosis (Dinh et al, 1988; Le et al, 1997). Malignant epithelial components are typically represented by endometrioid and serous carcinoma of moderate to poor differentiation, often papillary; the stromal component is frequently heterologous (cartilage, striated muscle) intermixed with a malignant spindle cell stroma. Areas of keratinizing squamous carcinoma are also common. Rarely areas of osteosarcoma or liposarcoma are present. Several instances of pure ovarian rhabdomyosarcoma have been reported (Guerard et al, 1983).

Outcome does not seem to be influenced by the presence of heterologous elements as strongly as it is by stage and resectability (Muntz et al, 1995). Five-year survival of all stages is typically lower than for other histologic types of epithelial ovarian cancer. For stage I patients survival may be 30 percent at 5 years, while few stage III patients live longer than 2 years (Hernandez et al, 1977; Morrow et al, 1984; Dictor, 1985; Dinh et al, 1988). Postoperative treatment with platinum and doxorubicin has been reported to improve outcome (Anderson et al, 1989; Le et al, 1997). Pelvic or whole-abdomen radiation therapy may also be of value in properly selected cases.

Benign (cellular adenofibroma) and low-grade (adenosarcoma) variants of ovarian mixed mesodermal tumors have also been reported. The *adenosarcomas* occur in women at an average age of 46 years. Typically, they are cystic-solid growths, often with surface or intracystic papillations. In these tumors, the epithelial component is benign (characteristically endometrioid). The histology of the malignant stroma varies considerably but most often resembles endometrial stroma. The number of mitoses per 10 hpf has ranged from 2 to 30, with no obvious relationship to stage or outcome. About half of the reported patients have suffered local recurrences

(Clement and Scully, 1978; Kao and Norris, 1978).

Pure *endometrioid stromal sarcoma* of the ovary occurs at an average patient age of 54 years. The majority are low grade. Bilateralism, association with endometriosis, and extension beyond the ovary are common. Indolent clinical behavior, local recurrence, and long survival are typical of the low-grade lesions (Young et al, 1984).

Clear Cell Carcinomas

Clear cell carcinoma is considered by some authorities to be properly classified as a subtype of the endometrioid malignancies of the ovary. The average age at discovery is similar to that of patients with other ovarian carcinomas. Two to 5 percent of the ovarian epithelial malignancies are of the clear cell variety. Association with endometriosis is reported in more than 25 percent of cases, compared to 8 percent for all ovarian cancers (Crozier et al, 1989; Sainz de la Cruz et al, 1996). Endometrial carcinoma found in association with clear cell ovarian cancer is more likely to be less well differentiated and more invasive than that accompanying endometrioid ovarian carcinoma. Bilateralism is reported in 5 to 10 percent of stage I cases, which comprise over 50 percent of all clear cell carcinomas.

Typically these tumors are cystic on gross examination, often unilocular (sometimes within an endometriotic cyst), with one or more solid tumor nodules protruding into the cavity. Areas of hemorrhage and necrosis are common. Microscopically, glycogen-filled clear cells found in sheets or lining tubules (Fig. 10–12), hobnail cells lining tubules or cysts, and a papillary configuration are characteristic. Mixtures with endometrioid patterns are also common (Scully, 1979; Shevchuk et al, 1981; Czernobilsky, 1982).

The prognosis, stage for stage, appears to be worse than that for the more common varieties of ovarian carcinoma. Most patients with clear cell carcinoma of the ovary are stage I at diagnosis (Jenison et al, 1989; Goff et al, 1996). Hypercalcemia, the most frequent paraendocrine disorder associated with ovarian carcinoma, is encountered propor-

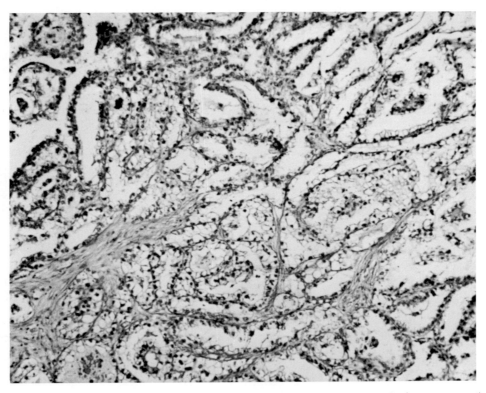

FIGURE 10–12. Clear cell carcinoma of the ovary. Characteristic microscopic features are the small cystic spaces lined with large cells that have a clear cytoplasm. This neoplasm probably arises from the paramesonephric, celomic epithelium and not from embryonic rests of mesonephric origin.

tionately more often in cases of clear cell carcinoma than in the other epithelial cell types. Patients with clear cell cancer of the ovary may also be at increased risk for thromboembolic complications (Goff et al, 1996).

Malignant Brenner and Transitional Cell Tumors

The malignant Brenner tumor is a rare variety of ovarian carcinoma that occurs in women at an average age of 60 years. Among the 37 cases reported by Woodruff et al (1981), 3 of 16 stage I tumors were bilateral. As with other ovarian tumors containing large amounts of stroma, abnormal uterine bleeding is common. Grossly, the Brenner carcinomas are characterized by one or more cysts, which may have a velvety lining with papillomatous, solid, or nodular masses. Microscopically, the malignant epithelium is transitional or squamous, occurring in nests or lining cysts embedded in the rubbery, benign fibromatous or thecomatous stroma (Scully, 1979; Haid et al, 1983). The stroma frequently contains calcifications. Benign Brenner elements must be present to distinguish the malignant Brenner tumor from the transitional cell carcinoma of the ovary. The latter presents more often in a high stage and has a worse prognosis (Austin and Norris, 1987).

In the series of Woodruff et al (1981), the outcome for patients with a malignant Brenner tumor was almost uniformly fatal except for those with stages Ia and Ib lesions, of whom only 25 percent were dead of disease after 5 years of follow-up. Roth and Czernobilsky (1985) reported on nine patients, eight of whom were stage I. Two of these died of late recurrence.

In two studies, retrospective pathology review of advanced epithelial ovarian carcinomas has found that 20 to 25 percent were composed of 50 percent or more malignant transitional-type epithelium. One of the studies reported that the transitional cell cancers were more chemosensitive and had a better outcome than the serous cancers (Gershenson et al, 1993), while in the other study there was no difference in outcome (Hollingsworth et al, 1996).

Small-Cell Carcinomas

Small-cell carcinoma of the ovary is a rare epithelial malignancy that occurs in young women (average age 24 years) and, in two thirds of patients, is associated with hypercalcemia. Nearly all reported cases have been unilateral, and 50 percent have had extraovarian metastases at diagnosis. Among 42 patients with stage Ia disease, 33 percent were alive and well at an average follow-up of 5.7 years (Young et al, 1994). A poorer prognosis in stage I cases is associated with hypercalcemia, large tumor, and age over 30 years. Advanced-stage disease is rarely curable.

Multiple Primary Müllerian Carcinomas

Most commonly the endometrium and ovary are involved when multiple müllerian carcinomas occur. Because the prognosis and treatment may be quite different if this combination represents two separate primaries, or one primary and one metastatic lesion, it is important to distinguish between the two conditions. When the lesions are histologically different, the answer is clear, but the most common situation involves an endometrioid ovarian carcinoma with an endometrioid carcinoma of the endometrium. The features typical of coexistent primary lesions are (1) identical histology, usually well-differentiated; (2) absent or minimal myometrial invasion; (3) absence of other metastases; and (4) an ovarian lesion with gross features typical of a primary tumor, often bilateral. These patients also tend to be younger than the average woman with primary ovarian or endometrial carcinoma. As expected, the prognosis for synchronous stage I, grade 1 endometrioid carcinomas of the ovary and uterus is excellent (Eifel et al, 1982; Woodruff et al, 1985). When the disease is more advanced, it becomes less important whether the lesions are separate primaries or not (Zaino et al, 1984).

Pathophysiology

Ovarian carcinoma can spread by (1) local extension, (2) lymphatic invasion and metastasis, (3) intraperitoneal implantation, (4) hematogenous dissemination, (5) field carcinogenesis, and (6) transdiaphragmatic passage.

Local Extension

Once capsular invasion takes place, direct involvement of adjacent structures by ovarian carcinoma can occur in a manner similar to that for other cancers. The most common sites directly involved by ovarian carcinoma are the pelvic peritoneum, posterior cul-de-sac, sigmoid colon, and adherent omentum. Involvement of these structures is often superficial, permitting a plane to be safely developed at surgery, but this is by no means always the case. For example, full-thickness invasion and obstruction of the pelvic colon is rather common. Occasionally, ovarian carcinoma assumes a retroperitoneal growth pattern via the uterosacral and cardinal ligaments, with encasement of the ureters.

Lymphatic Invasion and Metastasis

The spread of ovarian cancer occurs via the lymphatics of the infundibulopelvic and broad ligaments to the pelvic and aortic lymph nodes. The retroperitoneal nodes may also be involved via the peritoneal lymphatic drainage, and the mediastinal lymph nodes via the diaphragmatic lymphatics. Supraclavicular and inguinal node metastasis are relatively common, and rarely the axillary nodes are clinically involved by ovarian carcinoma (Hockstein et al, 1997).

Lymphatic invasion is clearly an important mode of spread of ovarian carcinoma, but its frequency has only lately been systematically studied (see the section "Lymph Node Involvment" later in this chapter). Lymphatic spread has been appreciated microscopically in the tumor itself, the mesovarium, and the oviduct. Data derived from autopsy studies of patients dying of advanced ovarian cancer convincingly document the frequent widespread involvement of the lymphatic system (Table 10–7). It is reasonable to assume that lymphatic extension also occurs in less advanced cases. This issue is discussed in the section "Surgical Staging" later in this chapter.

Intraperitoneal Implantation

The most common and most widely recognized behavior characteristic of ovarian cancer is that, after breaching its capsule, it seeds the peritoneal cavity with nests of tumor cells. These tumor particles have the potential for implanting anywhere on the peritoneum, but their distribution tends to follow sites of stasis along the circulatory pathway of the peritoneal fluid. Thus the preferred sites seem to be the posterior cul-de-sac, the paracolic gutters, the right hemidiaphragm, hernia sacs (including the umbilical recess), and, of course,

TABLE 10–7

Sites of Metastases in Advanced Epithelial Ovarian Carcinoma: Autopsy Findings*

Site Involved	Patients	
	N	%
Peritoneum	316	83
Lymph nodes		
Abdominal	221	58
Pelvic	182	48
Thoracic	108	28
Neck	52	14
Small intestine	166	44
Large intestine	190	50
Liver	181	48
Lung	130	30
Pleura	108	28
Brain, pericardium		<5
Urinary tract		<5

*Data from Rose et al (1989).

the omentum. This pattern helps direct the surgeon in the search for extraovarian spread.

Implantation metastasis of ovarian carcinoma is one of its hallmarks, and accounts for a common method of manifestation and death. Failure to eradicate the disease inevitably leads to the familiar clinical course related to progressive encasement of intra-abdominal organs, especially the digestive tract. The patient develops intractable anorexia, nausea, vomiting, and inanition. This picture may be modified by bowel strangulation, uncontrolled effusions, or pulmonary embolus. Rarely is death in a patient with ovarian cancer the result of distant metastasis without abdominal disease.

Another hallmark of ovarian cancer is ascites, which occurs in patients with and without peritoneal metastases. The etiology of the fluid is not clear, but it may involve increased production by the normal parietal and visceral peritoneum, or decreased clearance as a result of obstruction of peritoneal lymphatics, or both. The development of ascites is a common precipitating factor in events leading to the diagnosis of ovarian cancer. It produces abdominal distention and contributes to gastrointestinal and respiratory dysfunction. The ascites may also facilitate the peritoneal spread of ovarian cancer.

Hematogenous Dissemination

Hematogenous spread of ovarian carcinoma is clinically an unusual phenomenon, but the data of Rose et al (1989) show that it is not infrequent in advanced disease. Clinically, the more common sites are the lung and liver; the brain, skin, and bone are rarely involved. Perhaps the most important implication of this information is that, while advanced disease is not often cured, regional treatment may be doomed to failure from the outset.

Peritoneal Carcinogenesis and Multifocal Müllerian Malignancy

Parmley (1982) as well as Woodruff and TeLinde (1976) have emphasized that, at least in some instances, ovarian carcinoma conceivably could evolve simultaneously from the ovarian surface epithelium and the peritoneum as the result of a carcinogenic field effect. There is no doubt that the peritoneum, especially the pelvic and omental peritoneum, has the capacity for transforming into any of the various müllerian epithelia, particularly tubal (serous) and endometrial, which can cause confusion about the malignant potential of a coexistent ovarian neoplasm (Fox, 1993). Multifocal extraovarian serous carcinoma has been reported (Genadry et al, 1981; August et al, 1985; Chen and Flam, 1986). These may be tumors of low malignant potential or frankly malignant, invasive carcinomas (Rothacker and Mobius, 1995). The possibility that pelvic peritoneum can be a site of malignant transformation plays a particularly important role in patients with familial/hereditary ovarian carcinoma. Primary papillary serous carcinoma of the peritoneum, which is histologically and biologically similar to serous carcinoma of the ovary, has been reported to occur following prophylactic oophorectomy in patients with a family history of breast/ovarian cancer. Tobachman et al (1982) reported 3 of 28 patients who developed "ovarian cancer" after prophylactic oophorectomy. More recently, Piver et al (1993) reported 6 cases among a cohort of 324 women who had undergone prophylactic oophorectomy. Of these 324 women, 102 had two or more first-degree relatives with ovarian cancer, five of whom developed primary papillary serous carcinoma of the peritoneum.

Another interesting and important feature of "müllerian" neoplasia is its tendency to evolve simultaneously or sequentially in more than one organ (Axelrod et al, 1984). This is manifested in two forms. First, it is seen in the widely recognized tendency toward bilateralism of ovarian neoplasms. Although metastasis can occur from one ovary to the other, it is generally recognized that independent primary tumors of the ovaries frequently occur both simultaneously and sequentially. Data from two studies place the risk of occult bilateralism in stage I cases at 5 to 10 percent (Munnell, 1969; Williams and Dockerty, 1976). For stages II to IV, bilateral tumors are reported in 30 to 60 percent of cases.

A second, less common manifestation of the propensity of the müllerian epithelium toward multifocal neoplasia is the association of endometrial and ovarian carcinoma (vide supra). In endometrioid and clear cell ovarian cancers, simultaneous development of endometrial carcinoma is reported to occur in 15 to 30 percent of the cases. Occasionally, the ovary, tube, endometrium, and even the endocervix simultaneously exhibit primary cancers. This phenomenon has important therapeutic implications.

Transdiaphragmatic Passage

Meigs et al (1943) demonstrated the movement of ascitic fluid through the right hemidiaphragm into the right pleural cavity. If the ascitic fluid contains malignant cells, at least in some instances the cells are able to traverse the diaphragm and enter the pleural space, with the potential for implanting on the pleura. Left-sided effusions also occur, but are more likely to be independent of ascites. The finding of malignant cells in a pleural effusion is the most common criterion for classifying a patient as having stage IV ovarian cancer.

Prognostic Factors

Surgicopathologic stage, histologic grade, DNA content, and residual disease are all significant factors in the prognosis of ovarian cancer. Other prognostic variables also have an impact on survival in advanced ovarian carcinoma. In a review of two Gynecologic Oncology Group (GOG) protocols for patients with advanced (stages III and IV) disease, favorable prognostic factors, as determined by multivariate analysis, included cell type other than mucinous or clear cell, cisplatin-based chemotherapy, good performance status, young age, and absence of ascites (Omura et al, 1991).

Surgicopathologic Stage

The extent of the tumor growth and spread at the time of diagnosis is the most important

TABLE 10-8

FIGO Staging of Ovarian Carcinoma (Surgicopathological)*

Stage I	Growth limited to the ovaries
Stage Ia	Growth limited to one ovary; no ascites
	No tumor on the external surface; capsule intact
Stage Ib	Growth limited to both ovaries; no ascites
	No tumor on the external surfaces; capsules intact
Stage Ic[†]	Tumor either Stage Ia or Ib, but with tumor on surface of one or both ovaries; or with capsule ruptured; or with ascites present containing malignant cells or with positive peritoneal washings
Stage II	Growth involving one or both ovaries with pelvic extension
Stage IIa	Extension and/or metastases to the uterus and/or tubes
Stage IIb	Extension to other pelvic tissues
Stage IIc[†]	Tumor either Stage IIa or IIb, but with tumor on surface of one or both ovaries; or with capsule(s) ruptured; or with ascites present containing malignant cells or with positive peritoneal washings
Stage III	Tumor involving one or both ovaries with peritoneal implants outside the pelvis and/or positive retroperitoneal or inguinal nodes. Superficial liver metastasis equals Stage III
	Tumor is limited to the true pelvis but with histologically proven malignant extension to small bowel or omentum
Stage IIIa	Tumor grossly limited to the true pelvis with negative nodes but with histologically confirmed microscopic seeding of abdominal peritoneal surfaces
Stage IIIb	Tumor involving one or both ovaries with histologically confirmed implants of abdominal peritoneal surfaces none exceeding 2 cm in diameter. Nodes are negative
Stage IIIc	Abdominal implants greater than 2 cm in diameter and/or positive retroperitoneal or inguinal nodes
Stage IV	Growth involving one or both ovaries with distant metastases. If pleural effusion is present there must be positive cytology to allot a case to Stage IV
	Parenchymal liver metastasis equals Stage IV

*From Pettersson F (ed): FIGO annual report on the results of treatment in gynecological cancer. Int J Gynecol Obstet 36(suppl): 1, 1991. Copyright 1991, Elsevier Science, with permission.

[†]In order to evaluate the impact on prognosis of the different criteria for allotting a case to Stage Ic or IIc, it would be of value to know (1) if the source of malignant cells detected was (a) peritoneal washings or (b) ascites; and (2) if rupture of the capsule was (a) spontaneous or (b) caused by the surgeon.

variable influencing the prognosis in ovarian carcinoma. For purposes of comparing treatment results among different institutions, the extent of the disease is usually expressed in terms of stages. Although many staging systems have been devised, the FIGO system (Table 10–8) should be uniformly used for reporting purposes. This is a surgicopathologic system and not purely clinical, such as that used in cervical carcinoma. The basic divisions of this system are as follows: stage I—tumor is confined to the ovaries; stage II—tumor is confined to the pelvis; stage III—tumor is confined to the abdomen; and stage IV—tumor extends outside the abdominal cavity. Nearly one fourth of all true carcinomas are confined to the ovaries and 40 percent are confined to the pelvis at the time of diagnosis (Table 10–9).

Referring to Table 10–6, the 5-year survival gradient is apparent for all four stages as exemplified by the serous carcinomas. The prognosis for stages Ia, Ib, and Ic are significantly different, with survival rates of 85, 69, and 59 percent, respectively. For stages IIa, b, and c the survival rates are 62, 51, and 43 percent, respectively. Survival curves for the stage III subgroups are presented in Figure 10–13. The stage is assigned on the basis of all clinical, surgical, and pathologic findings, together with cytologic studies of peritoneal fluid and serous effusions.

Histologic Grade

Accurate knowledge of the histologic types of ovarian malignancy is indispensable in assessing the prognosis and in planning treatment, but for epithelial tumors, the degree of tissue differentiation and the stage are typi-

TABLE 10-9

Percentage Stage Distribution of 8,082 Cases of Obviously Malignant and 1,217 Cases of Borderline Malignant Ovarian Tumors*

Stage	Obviously Malignant	Borderline Malignant
I (all)	22.7	74.1
a	12.4	55.4
b	2.9	12.0
c	7.4	6.7
II	15.4	9.4
III	40.9	10.5
IV	17.5	1.4
Unstaged	3.5	4.6

*Data from Pettersson (1988).

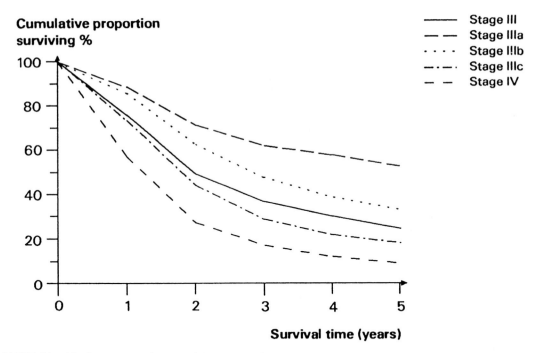

FIGURE 10–13. Serous carcinoma of the ovary: life table survival for stage III and IV obviously malignant cases. (From Pettersson F: FIGO annual report on the results of treatment of gynecological cancer. Int J Gynecol Obstet 36(suppl):250, 1991. Copyright 1991, Elsevier Science, with permission.)

cally of greater prognostic importance than is the cell type. The biologic growth potential is far more limited for borderline tumors than for true carcinomas, and grade 1 carcinomas are less aggressive than the more undifferentiated forms (Table 10–6). Currently, grade is not incorporated into the staging, except for separation of the LMP group.

DNA Content

Friedlander et al (1983, 1988) studied the nuclear DNA content of ovarian carcinomas and found a significant association of ploidy with stage, but not grade, for obviously malignant tumors. All diploid tumors were early stage, and all late-stage (III and IV) tumors were aneuploid. However, 40 percent of early-stage tumors were also aneuploid. In a study of the DNA content of early-stage serous tumors, Erhardt et al (1985) found that the DNA content of well-differentiated invasive cancers resembled that of the borderline tumors, while the grade 2 and 3 tumors generally had a high, scattered DNA content. Nevertheless, no clear-cut demarcation was possible between borderline and benign or obviously malignant serous tumors. Zanetta and associates (1996) measured the DNA

content in 282 advanced ovarian carcinomas and found that 80 percent were nondiploid. Diploidy was associated with a significantly better prognosis than the nondiploid state. This was true even among patients with a pathologically confirmed complete response to chemotherapy.

Residual Disease

Residual disease status after primary tumor-reductive surgery is of pre-eminent prognostic importance in advanced ovarian cancer. Patients are categorized as having microscopic disease only (all gross tumor resected), optimal cytoreduction (no single mass >1 cm in diameter), or suboptimal cytoreduction (residual tumor masses >1 cm). The effect on outcome is demonstrated in Figure 10–14. This topic is discussed in detail in subsequent paragraphs.

Management

Surgery

The basic principle of surgical therapy for ovarian carcinoma is to remove the primary lesion and all metastases without putting the

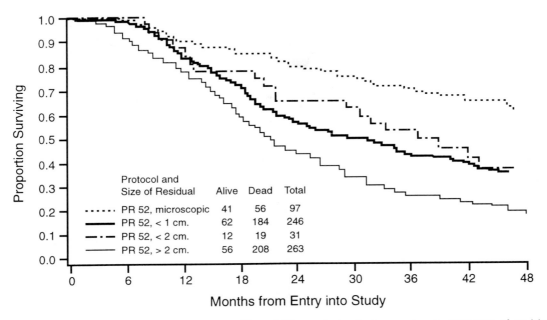

FIGURE 10–14. Ovarian carcinoma stages III and IV: survival rate by maximum diameter of residual disease. (From Hoskins WJ, McGuire WP, Brady F, et al: The effect of diameter of largest residual disease on survival after primary cytoreductive surgery in patients with suboptimal residual epithelial ovarian carcinoma. Am J Obstet Gynecol 170:974, 1994, with permission.)

patient's life in jeopardy. When fertility is not a consideration, both adnexa and the uterus are removed, although exceptions can be made in patients with early disease. The contralateral ovary is excised because it is expendable, occult metastatic or primary carcinoma may be present, and there is an increased risk of carcinoma eventually developing in the uninvolved ovary, especially if the involved ovary contains a serous or endometrioid neoplasm. Removal of the uterus also has its controversial aspects, but it is generally recommended as part of the treatment in resectable ovarian cancer because (1) it may be involved by lymphatic metastasis; (2) there may be a coexistent endometrial primary tumor; (3) there may be serosal implants; (4) the organ is dispensible when fertility is not a consideration; (5) it can usually be removed with little additional risk; and (6) patients with ovarian cancer have a propensity to develop subsequent müllerian primaries, particularly endometrial. (In 1976, Obel found that, of 103 women with ovarian carcinoma who survived for 10 or more years and who had their uterus preserved, 10 developed endometrial carcinoma and 6 cervical carcinoma.) It is also easier to assess the pelvis on follow-up examination with the uterus absent, and estrogen replacement therapy is simplified (no bleeding, no risk of endometrial neoplasia). Management of early ovarian cancer with reproductive conservation is discussed later in this chapter.

SURGICAL STAGING

Several studies (Piver et al, 1976; Young et al, 1983; McGowan et al, 1985) have documented that the initial evaluation of women with early ovarian carcinoma is often inaccurate because of an inadequate work-up, inadequate surgical exploration, or an inadequate operative staging procedure. According to McGowan et al (1985), operative staging is most likely to be deficient (65 percent of cases) when performed by a general surgeon, compared to an incomplete staging score of 48 percent for gynecologists and 3 percent for gynecologic cancer specialists. Staging procedures are most important for early ovarian cancer, especially when the disease is, at first glance, limited to one ovary. It is these patients who are most likely to suffer from undertreatment. For advanced cases, the major surgical issue is not staging but the optimal extent of tumor-reductive surgery.

Exploration in every case requires a systematic visual and palpatory examination of the pelvic and abdominal peritoneum, especially the pouch of Douglas, the right hemi-diaphragm, Morison's pouch, the retroperi-toneal nodes (pelvic and aortic), and the omentum. Any suspicious area should be biopsied. In the absence of target lesions, the GOG study of extended surgical staging in early ovarian cancer (Buchsbaum et al, 1989) provides important information regarding the yield of routine selective biopsies (Table 10–10). The two procedures most likely to yield positive results for apparent stage I cases were peritoneal cytology (15 percent) and di-agnostic aortic node dissection (4.2 percent). Random biopsies of clinically normal parietal and diphragmatic peritoneum seldom yielded evidence of disease. Pelvic node sampling was negative in all 93 cases. This study dem-onstrates that careful exploration by a trained and experienced gynecologic cancer special-ist provides a very accurate assessment of early-stage disease. This is in contrast to the findings of Young et al (1983) in which 22 percent of 58 patients reported to have stage I disease after initial laparotomy by nongy-necologic oncologists were upstaged at re-operation. Of the cases with poorly differen-tiated histology, 46 percent were upstaged, compared with 34 percent of grade 2 cases and 16 percent of grade 1 cases. Faught et al (1996) reported an identical rate of upstaging (11 of 51 cases). Based on these data, surgical staging of early ovarian carcinoma should generally include the procedures listed in Ta-ble 10–11. The therapeutic ratio of repeat laparotomy on inadequately staged patients may be unfavorable because of a fairly high complication rate (Stier et al, 1996); obtaining the missing data laparoscopically, however, would be justified if chemotherapy could be averted.

Although some authors recommend surgi-cal staging for all cases, it certainly is indi-cated in the patients at higher risk for metas-tasis and recurrence. This includes those patients whose epithelial ovarian malignancy appears to be completely resectable and con-fined to the pelvis or is histologic grade 2 or 3, or in whom there are dense adhesions or high-risk histology (clear cell, carcinosar-coma, small cell). All cases of apparent stage II disease are candidates for surgical staging. The patient must be a good operative candi-date for the procedure, and consideration must be given to the potential effect of the procedure on fertility in women of reproduc-tive age. Patients with more advanced disease without macroscopic nodal involvement can

TABLE 10–10

Results of Surgical Staging of Obviously Malignant Ovarian Tumors; Gynecologic Oncology Group Data*

Biopsy Site	Apparent Stage I	Apparent Stage II
Cytology	14/96[†]	Not available
Omentum	0/96	7/36[†]
Diaphragm	1/95	2/35
Peritoneum	2/87	11/35
Pelvic nodes	0/93	8/41
Aortic nodes	4/95	8/41

*Modified from Buchsbaum HJ, Brady MF, Delgado G, et al: Surgical staging of ovarian carcinoma: stage I, II, and III (optimal): a Gyneco-logic Oncology Group study. Surg Gynecol Obstet 169:226, 1989, with permission.
[†]Number positive/total cases.

have the aortic and pelvic nodes evaluated at the second-look staging procedure following chemotherapy.

LYMPH NODE INVOLVEMENT

An important question is the likelihood of retroperitoneal node metastases in early ovar-ian cancer. Burghardt et al (1986, 1991) have championed the concept of complete pelvic and aortic lymphadenectomy for all stages of ovarian cancer, even when there is unresect-able, bulky intra-abdominal disease. As doc-umented in numerous studies, there is a high rate of retroperitoneal nodal involvement in ovarian carcinoma (Table 10–12). It is of in-terest, however, that the limited dissection in the GOG staging study (Buchsbaum et al, 1989) yielded a rate of aortic node metastasis similar to that reported by Burghardt's group (4 of 95 vs. 1 of 20). The pelvic node metas-atis rate was lower in the GOG study (0 of 93 vs. 3 of 20). Complete or radical node dissec-tion for early ovarian carcinoma remains of unproven benefit and therefore more limited staging is recommended (Hacker, 1995). The

TABLE 10–11

Recommended Surgical Staging Procedure for Cases of "Early" Ovarian Carcinoma (Stages I to IIIa)

Abdominal cytology (washings or ascites)
Meticulous exploration
Total abdominal hysterectomy and bilateral salpingo-oophorectomy*
Excisional biopsy of target lesions
Infracolic omentectomy
Appendectomy
Selective pelvic and aortic lymph node sampling

*See discussion in the section "Reproductive Conversation" later in this chapter.

TABLE **10–12**

Early-Stage Ovarian Carcinoma: Incidence of Lymph Node Metastases
(Aortic and Pelvic)

Source	Stage I		Stage II	
	N	%	N	%
DiRe et al (1990)	16/134*	12	—†	—
Chen and Lee (1984)	2/11	18	2/10	20
Averette et al (1983)	1/11	9	5/17	29
Pickel et al (1989)	7/28	23	4/13	31
Buchsbaum et al (1989)	4/95	4	8/41	20
Burghardt et al (1991)	3/20	15	5/7	71
Total	33/289	11	24/88	27

*Numerator is the number of cases with nodal metastases; denominator is the number of cases examined.
†Not reported.

frequency and distribution of nodal metastasis in ovarian carcinoma are undoubtedly related also to the stage, histologic grade, and perhaps cell type. Thus, Chen and Lee (1984) observed a much higher frequency of node metastases associated with grade 3 lesions and lymph–vascular space invasion. Later Petru et al (1994) reported that node metastasis risk in stage I cases correlated with substage Ic (dense adhesions, surface excrescences) as well as poor differentiation. While the retroperitoneal lymph nodes may be, on occasion, the only site of extraovarian spread, this does not appear to be responsible for any large portion of the treatment failures even in advanced stages. Thus node sampling may occasionally reveal the only evidence of persistent disease after treatment for ovarian carcinoma, but the great majority of patients failing treatment have intraperitoneal disease.

On the average, three fourths of patients with advanced ovarian carcinoma have retroperitoneal node metastases (Burghardt et al, 1991; Scarabelli et al, 1995; Spirtos et al, 1995). The rate of nodal metastases to the aortic zone is nearly identical to that in the pelvic zone (60 percent), with two thirds of patients having metastases to both areas. In one study the ratio of macroscopic to microscopic nodal involvement was 2:1 regardless of whether the metastases were to the aortic or pelvic nodes (Spirtos et al, 1995). In the case-control study of Scarabelli and associates (1995), the estimated survival of the 30 patients undergoing complete aortopelvic node dissection as part of the primary surgical therapy was significantly better than that of the no-lymphadenectomy group (median survival 30 months vs. 6 months, respectively). With a median follow-up of 30 months, Spirtos and co-workers (1995) observed that 46

percent of 13 patients with microscopic node metastases, 43 percent of 23 patients with macroscopic node metastases, and 50 percent of 20 patients with negative nodes were alive. They suggest these data are consistent with a therapeutic effect of node dissection.

CYTOREDUCTIVE SURGERY

It is a general principle that the more extensive ovarian cancer is at the time of diagnosis, the poorer the prognosis. It is also true, in general, that survival correlates with the amount of ovarian carcinoma remaining after surgery. This has been demonstrated in many studies, including randomized studies (Tables 10–13 and 10–14). Griffiths (1975; Griffiths et al, 1979) showed, by multivariate analysis of stage III ovarian carcinoma, that survival was the same for patients with residual metastases of less than 1.5 cm in diameter after resection of larger metastases as it was for patients with residual metastasis of less than 1.5 cm who did not have larger metastases. Griffiths' data also indicate that the smaller the residual under the less-than-1.5-cm mark, the better the prognosis. The validity of these data was supported by the study of Wharton and Herson (1981), who distinguished "simple tumor removal" from tumor-reductive surgery and "inoperable" cases (residual >2 cm regardless of the extent of tumor removal). Their patients undergoing tumor-reductive surgery had the same survival as those undergoing simple tumor removal provided that the residual disease was 2 cm or less. Conversely, patients undergoing partial tumor removal with residual greater than 2 cm had no better survival than patients who had biopsy only. Hoskins et al (1992), in their analysis of GOG data, made a related observation that patients

TABLE **10–13**

Effect of Primary Tumor Reductive Surgery on Survival in Advanced Ovarian Carcinoma

| | <2 cm Residual | | >2 cm Residual | |
Source	N	Median Survival (months)	N	Median Survival (months)
Vogl et al (1983)	32	>40	68	16
Pohl et al (1984)	37	45	57	16
Delgado et al (1984)	21	45	54	16
Conte et al (1986)	37	>40	38	16
Seifer et al (1988)	35	30	44	12
Hoskins et al (1992)	31*	32*	263	20
Curtin et al (1997)†	40	40	52	18

*One- to 2-cm residual tumor.
†Stage IV cases.

whose only large metastases were omental had a superior survival to patients with large abdominal metastases at other sites, even when reduced to less than 1 cm. Thus cytoreductive surgery that fails to achieve optimal levels of residual malignancy will have no measurable impact on median survival. Surgical cytoreduction has even been shown to improve survival in patients with stage IV ovarian carcinoma (Curtin et al, 1997; Lui et al, 1997; Munkarah et al, 1997). There are certain clinical situations in which it may be desirable to postpone surgery for patient safety. This is discussed later in the section "Neoadjuvant Chemotherapy."

The most common procedures required for successful tumor-reductive surgery in ovarian carcinoma, in addition to removal of the uterus, tube, and ovaries, are infracolic or total omentectomy; resection of large pelvic disease, often with a segment of the rectosigmoid colon; removal of peritoneal implants; and removal of disease on the right hemidiaphragm. Lymphadenectomy, splenectomy, and segmental small or large bowel resection occasionally will convert a patient to the optimal treatment category. Extensive tumor involvement of the liver, mesenteric or celiac lymph nodes, and small intestine most frequently accounts for the failure to render the patient "optimal" with respect to residual tumor. Seldom is the pelvic tumor unresectable, but the surgeon is often required to judge whether the extent of the requisite pelvic surgery can be justified relative to the resectability of the abdominal disease. Certainly, if there are no abdominal metastases or if there is fully resectable abdominal disease, every effort should be made to excise completely the pelvic portion of the carcinoma. This is often facilitated by a retroperitoneal approach, elevating the rectum from the sacral hollow and performing a retrograde hysterectomy as described by Hudson and Chir in 1973 (Fig. 10–15).

The morbidity from ovarian radical tumor-reductive surgery can be significant. The reported average operating time by various investigators is 3.5 to 4.0 hours, blood loss 950 to 1,600 ml, hospital stay 13 to 19 days, major complication rate 6.7 to 58 percent, and collective operative mortality 1 to 2 percent.

TABLE **10–14**

Randomized Studies of Tumor Reductive Surgery (TRS) in Ovarian Carcinoma

| | Chemotherapy | | Chemo + TRS | | |
Source*	N	Survival†	N	Survival†	P value
Redman et al (1994)	34	12 mos	37	15 mos	NS
Fiorentino et al (1993)	27	36%‡	24	72%‡	0.07
van der Burg et al (1995)	138	20 mos	140	26 mos	0.012

*The study of Redman et al concerned secondary tumor reductive surgery. The other two studies involved interval tumor reductive surgery.
†Median survival.
‡Survival at 2 years.

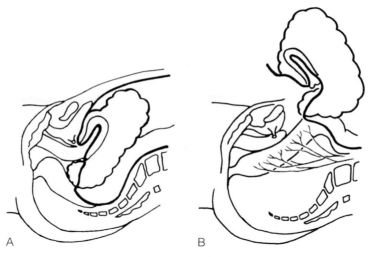

FIGURE 10–15. Radical oophorectomy. *A,* The heavy line indicates the path of dissection: beginning anteriorly, the peritoneum is stripped from the bladder, the vesicovaginal space developed, and the vagina entered through the anterior fornix. The posterior fornix is incised, entering the posterior cul-de-sac or rectovaginal space. Laterally, the peritoneum is dissected from the ureters. The pararectal and retrorectal spaces are developed. *B,* The retrograde hysterectomy has been carried out and the rectosigmoid elevated from the sacral hollow. The ovarian cancer can now be dissected from the rectosigmoid under direct vision or a segmental resection done. (From Hudson CN, Chir M: Surgical treatment of ovarian cancer. Gynecol Oncol 1:370, 1973, with permission.)

Overall, about 25 percent of patients undergoing tumor-reductive surgery have required bowel resection, usually a segmental rectosigmoid or sigmoid resection (Blythe and Wahl, 1982; Hacker et al, 1983; Delgado et al, 1984; Chen and Bochner, 1985). The success rate for rendering patients optimal in terms of residual disease (<1.5 to 3 cm) in these studies varied from 28 to 98 percent; the impact on survival appears to be clinically significant (Fig. 10–14).

When optimal cytoreductive surgery is not possible, the removal of an omental "cake," the ovarian primary, and any other large tumor masses may provide palliation in terms of reduced discomfort and less ascites. Removal of all or part of an involved ovary will assist in establishing the correct diagnosis. Patients with advanced-stage ovarian carcinoma, whether optimally resectable or not, are candidates for chemotherapy following surgery. A general treatment plan is presented in Fig. 10–16, and discussed in the following paragraphs. Those patients not optimally cytoreduced may benefit from reoperation to remove any residual tumor after two to four cycles of chemotherapy. This was shown to improve survival in a randomized trial (van der Burg et al, 1995).

LAPAROSCOPIC STAGING

It is inevitable that an ovarian malignancy will occasionally be encountered in the patient undergoing laparoscopic surgery for the management of what is presumed to be a benign adnexal mass. In most series this occurs in only 1 to 2 percent of cases. The surgeon should have a plan for this contingency included in the preoperative consent. The authors recommend laparotomy in this event with definitive staging and complete tumor removal according to the extent of the disease. However, if the laparoscopist is not trained in the surgical management of ovarian carcinoma, the procedure should be terminated and the patient referred to a gynecologic oncologist. Expert laparoscopic surgeons have reported successful staging of early ovarian carcinoma via laparoscopy (Childers et al, 1995). The use of laparoscopy for evaluating patients with ascites is ill advised because of the high incidence of trocar site implantation metastases.

Neoadjuvant Chemotherapy

Patients in poor medical condition are often better served by the administration of two to

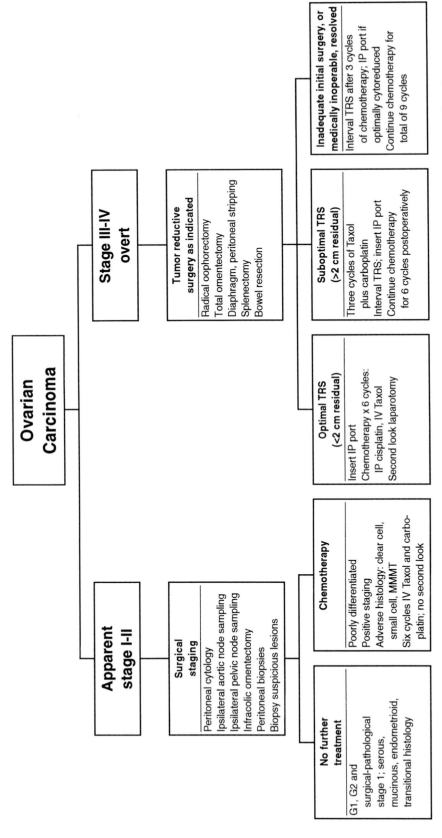

FIGURE 10–16. General algorithm for management of ovarian carcinoma. TRS = tumor reductive surgery; Taxol = paclitaxel.

three cycles of chemotherapy prior to surgery. In this category would be included patients with large ascites, severe malnutrition (serum albumin <2.8 gm/dl, weight loss >10 to 15 percent of total body weight) and concurrent serious medical problems, such as chronic obstructive pulmonary disease, myocardial ischemia, or age over 75 years. These patients are at high risk for pulmonary, renal, cardiac, and intestinal complications, as well as intraoperative or postoperative coagulopathy (JV Brown et al, 1993). In these cases diagnosis of malignancy can be achieved by examination of pleural or peritoneal effusions or fine-needle aspiration of a supraclavicular or inguinal lymph node metastasis prior to initiating chemotherapy. In our experience as well as that of others, this "neoadjuvant" chemotherapy not only allows the patient's condition to be much improved for tumor-reductive surgery, but the surgery necessary to achieve optimal tumor reduction is invariably less extensive and, therefore, attended by fewer complications (Schwartz et al, 1994; Onnis et al, 1996; Surwit et al, 1996). In general, the standard chemotherapy should be used in the neoadjuvant setting; however, patients in poor medical condition may be better served by starting treatment with a well-tolerated single agent such as carboplatin.

Postoperative Treatment

STAGES I AND II

Indications. In general, all patients with stage Ia and Ib, grade 3 or other adverse histology (e.g., clear cell, small cell, aneuploid), and stage Ic cases, other than those based upon intraoperative rupture, should have adjuvant therapy (Fig. 10–16). The grade 2 lesions are on the edge, and probably do not warrant further therapy unless the staging has been unsatisfactory. In this instance, however, the best management may be laparoscopic staging (NIH Consensus Development Conference, 1994). These recommendations are based upon the following data. Dembo et al (1990), in a combined report from the Princess Margaret Hospital and the Norwegian Radium Hospital, found histologic grade, dense adherence of tumor, and ascites to be independent prognostic factors for apparent stage I ovarian carcinoma (Table 10–15). Of these three factors, differentiation was the most powerful predictor of disease-free survival, followed by dense adhesions and ascites. Unfortunately, peritoneal cytology was

TABLE **10–15**

Percent Recurrence in Stage I Ovarian Carcinoma Related to Certain Prognostic Factors*

Risk Factor	Grade 1		Grades 2 & 3	
	N	%	N	%
Adherence				
None/minor	189	3	245	25
Dense	16	30	45	42
Ascites				
<250 ml	182	5	230	28
>250 ml	7	28	35	37

*Modified from Dembo AJ, Davy M, Stenwig AE, et al: Prognostic factors in patients with stage I epithelial ovarian cancer. Obstet Gynecol 75:263, 1990, with permission.

not available for these patients, and no standard surgical procedure was performed. In the 1991 FIGO Annual Report (Pettersson, 1991), the 5-year survival of patients with stage Ic ovarian carcinoma was 71 percent if the peritoneal cytology was positive, 68 percent if there was ascites with malignant cells, 62 percent for cases with spontaneous (preoperative) rupture, and 80 percent if rupture of the tumor was intraoperative. This histology and grade of these tumors was not given, however, so this information is of dubious value. DNA content and mitotic index may also be prognostic (Schueler et al, 1993; Vergote et al, 1993). Vergote et al (1993) analyzed for prognostic factors 290 patients with invasive stage I ovarian carcinoma and found that DNA ploidy was more predictive of relapse than dense adhesions, ascites, rupture, or extracystic growth. Among patients with diploid tumors, the disease-free survival was 90 percent, compared to 70 percent for aneuploid and 57 percent for tetraploid tumors. None of 77 patients with grade 1 diploid tumors relapsed, while 13.6 percent of the 44 patients with nondiploid grade 1 tumors relapsed.

External Beam Radiation Therapy. In the past decade, several randomized clinical trials employing postoperative radiation therapy in early-stage ovarian carcinoma have been reported (Hreshchyshyn et al, 1980; Dembo et al, 1979a,b, 1984). These studies indicate that pelvic radiation therapy after surgery in stage I ovarian carcinoma is no better, and possibly worse, than no further treatment. Only 2 of 51 stage Ia, grade 1 malignancies (3.9 percent) recurred. This supports the long-held opinion that these patients need no treatment as an adjunct to surgery. However, approximately 25 percent of the stage Ia, grade 2 and

3 cases experienced recurrence after 3 to 5 years of follow-up. There have been no randomized studies comparing whole-abdomen radiation (WAR) to no further treatment, nor has there been a valid comparison of WAR with adjuvant chemotherapy.

Intraperitoneal Radionuclide Therapy. In selected stage I cases, intraperitoneal ^{32}P has been used as postoperative adjuvant therapy, but mediocre results and serious complications have discouraged continued use of this treatment (Young et al, 1990; Soper et al, 1992). Like its predecessor, radioactive colloidal gold (Kolstad et al, 1977), intraperitoneal ^{32}P therapy should not be used in combination with whole-pelvis radiation therapy because of the very high serious complication rate (Pezner et al, 1978; Klaassen et al, 1988; Tharp and Hornback, 1994). Young et al (1990) reported on a study of 143 patients with higher risk stage I plus stage II resectable ovarian cancer who were randomized to receive melphalan or intraperitoneal ^{32}P. With a median follow-up of 6 years, the relapse rate in each treatment arm was 19 percent. Six percent of the ^{32}P patients experienced severe abdominal complications, while two patients in the melphalan arm died of leukemia. Two randomized trials comparing intravenous (IV) cisplatin (50 mg/m^2 for six cycles) to intraperitoneal ^{32}P found that disease-free survival was similar or worse for the ^{32}P patients, and that the intraperitoneal ^{32}P was associated with a high incidence of late bowel complications (Vergote et al, 1992; Pecorelli et al, 1994). In an analysis of the recurrence pattern in 12 patients with apparent stage I and II ovarian carcinoma (not surgically staged) managed by intraperitoneal ^{32}P, Soper et al (1991) found that the first recurrence in 7 was lymphatic, indicating that the radionuclide therapy was ineffective against lymph node metastases.

In summary, intraperitoneal ^{32}P is at best equivalent to systemic chemotherapy as adjunctive treatment of early-stage ovarian carcinoma, its use has a higher serious complication rate than chemotherapy, and it is not applicable to the patient who desires reproductive preservation.

Chemotherapy. Ahmed et al (1996) from the United Kingdom, in a retrospective study of 194 stage I ovarian carcinoma patients who received no adjuvant therapy, reported an overall survival for substage Ia of 93.7 percent, substage Ib 92 percent, and substage Ic

84 percent. The effect of grade on survival was, however, more important than the substage, as shown in Figure 10–17. Patients with recurrence were treated with cisplatin. The authors concluded that adjuvant therapy for early-stage ovarian cancer was unnecessary. Nevertheless, it has generally been recommended that only patients with stage Ia, grade 1 ovarian carcinoma do not need postoperative chemotherapy, although the patient with a nondiploid grade 1 tumor might benefit from therapy. There are two studies that indicate that patients with stage I, grade 2 ovarian carcinoma also do not need postoperative chemotherapy (Young et al, 1990; Monga et al, 1991). Unfortunately, in the two studies combined there were only 21 patients with grade 2 histology, of which at least one recurred (stage Ic). It is of interest to note that 5 of 25 patients with clear cell carcinoma relapsed. Others have observed that nearly all treatment failures of stage I ovarian carcinoma are among the grade 3 and stage Ic cases (Lentz et al, 1991; Petru et al, 1994). The Italian Collaborative Study Group has reported preliminary results of a randomized study that adds further concern about the value of adjuvant chemotherapy for early ovarian cancer (Pecorelli et al, 1994). Comparing IV cisplatin to observation in surgically staged patients with grade 2 and 3, stage Ia and Ib ovarian carcinoma, the relapse-free survival in the control arm at 5 years was 61 percent versus 81 percent for the cisplatin arm. However, salvage chemotherapy of relapsing patients was more effective in the control arm, resulting in a nearly identical 5-year survival in the two treatment arms (85 percent).

Treatment Recommendations. In view of these data, it is clear that the optimal postoperative management of early-stage ovarian carcinoma has not been determined. Our recommendation (Fig. 10–16) is to follow patients with grade 1, stage Ia and Ib serous, mucinous, and endometrioid tumors provided the surgical staging has been optimal. Patients with adequately staged grade 2 tumors also might be managed by observation, but those with grade 3, high-risk histology, or stage Ic tumors should receive six cycles of adjuvant chemotherapy. Judging from the randomized trials in advanced ovarian carcinoma discussed elsewhere in this chapter, the most efficacious treatment should be a combination of IV carboplatin (or cisplatin) and paclitaxel. Second-look surgery is not rec-

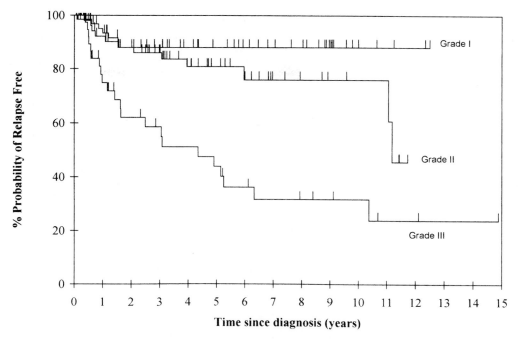

FIGURE 10–17. Ovarian carcinoma stage I: relapse-free survival by histologic grade for women with no postoperative therapy. (From Ahmed FY, Wiltshaw E, A'Hern RP, et al: Natural history and prognosis of untreated stage I epithelial ovarian cancer. J Clin Oncol 14:2968, 1996, with permission.)

ommended for the asymptomatic patient with a normal serum CA-125 level and no evidence of disease on physical examination. Probably less than 5 percent of patients who are surgically staged and receive chemotherapy would have a positive result (Walton et al, 1987; Lentz et al, 1991; Rubin et al, 1993).

STAGES III AND IV

Chemotherapy. Unlike many solid tumors, epithelial ovarian cancer is very sensitive to chemotherapy. During the past few decades there has been a series of clinical trials, often randomized and multi-institutional), documenting the activity of melphalan, doxorubicin, cyclophosphamide, cisplatin, carboplatin, and paclitaxel, among others, in the treatment of ovarian carcinoma. Multiagent regimens have generally provided higher response rates than single-agent therapy. Dose intensity analysis has demonstrated that the most effective regimens are multiagent and contain platinum (Levin and Hryniuk, 1987). The progress in chemotherapy has been characterized by incremental improvements in outcome resulting in an overall small increase in cure rates for patients with advanced disease.

Our overall scheme for the management of stages III and IV ovarian carcinoma is pre-

sented in Fig. 10–16. Two studies have established a new standard for chemotherapy in advanced-stage ovarian carcinoma (Table 10–16). One of these studies was conducted by the GOG on 385 patients with suboptimal (>1 cm residual) ovarian carcinoma. It compared cyclophosphamide 750 mg/m^2 IV plus cisplatin (Platinol) 75 mg/m^2 IV (CP) to paclitaxel (Taxol) 135 mg/m^2 IV (24-hour infusion) plus cisplatin 75 mg/m^2 IV (TP) (McGuire et al, 1966). Patients receiving TP had a superior progression-free and overall survival (Fig. 10–18). Each regimen was given for six cycles every 3 weeks. Among the 218 measurable disease patients, the clinical complete response rate was 31 percent for the CP arm and 51 percent for the TP arm ($p = 0.025$). The rate of pathologic complete response for the two treatment arms was 19 and 26 percent, respectively ($p = 0.08$). Combining the measurable and nonmeasurable disease patients, the median survival was 24.4 months for the CP group and 37.5 months for the TP group. Severe alopecia, neutropenia, febrile neutropenia, and allergic reactions were more common in the TP arm. Altogether, the deaths of 10 patients (6 CP and 4 TP) may have been related to the chemotherapy.

TABLE 10–16

Benchmark Randomized Studies of Chemotherapy in Suboptimal Stage III and IV Ovarian Carcinoma

Source	Regimen*	N	Response Rate[†]		Median Survival (months)
			% CCR	% SPCR	
Omura et al (1983)[‡]	MEL	64	20	—	12.3
	MEL + HMM	97	28	—	14.2
	ADR + CTX	72	32[§]	—	13.5
Omura et al (1986)[‡]	ADR + CTX	120	26	4	15.7
	ADR + CTX + CDDP	107	51	17	17.7
GICOA (1987)	CDDP	(total cases	54	17	—
	CDDP + CTX	392)	74	28	—
	CDDP + CTX + ADR		81	31	—
McGuire et al (1996)	CDDP + CTX	116	31	20	24.4
	CDDP + TAX	100	51	26[¶]	37.5
Alberts et al (1996)	IV CDDP + CTX	279	n/a[‖]	36	41
	IP CDDP + CTX	267	n/a	47	49[#]

*MEL = melphan; HMM = hexamethylmelamine; ADR = adriamycin (doxorubicin); CTX = cytoxan (cyclophosphamide); CDDP = cisplatin; TAX = taxol.
[†]CCR = complete clinical response; SPCR = surgicopathologic complete response.
[‡]Gynecologic Oncology Group studies.
[§]$p = 0.04$ comparing CCR rate for ADR + CTX to MEL.
[‖]All patients had less than 2 cm residual disease.
[¶]$p = 0.08$.
[#]$p = 0.02$.

The other standard-setting study involving 539 optimal disease patients was carried out jointly by the Southwest Oncology Group, the GOG, and the Eastern Cooperative Oncology Group (Alberts et al, 1996). Patients were randomized to receive either IV or intraperitoneal (IP) cisplatin 100 mg/m² for six cycles at 3 week intervals. Both treatment arms also received cyclophosphamide 600 mg/m² IV. Estimated median survival of patients on the IP arm was 49 months versus 41 months on the IV arm ($p = 0.03$). The rate of pathologic complete response was 40 percent on the IP arm and 31 percent on the IV arm ($p = 0.10$). Clinical hearing loss and neutropenia were significantly more severe and frequent on the IV treatment arm. There were only two treatment-related deaths, both on the IP arm. This is the only randomized study evaluating the efficacy of IP chemotherapy, the enthusiasm for which, until this report, had been waning. The rationale of IP therapy is based upon the very high concentrations of drug that can be achieved in the peritoneal cavity without increased toxicity compared to the maximum tolerable serum levels. The principles and prospects of the IP method have been reviewed by Markman (1991) (see also Chapter 16).

While the use of IV paclitaxel with platinum has been widely accepted as the standard drug therapy for advanced ovarian carcinoma, there are differences of opinion with respect to the specific regimen. The definitive studies establishing the efficacy of paclitaxel in the treatment of ovarian cancer have employed a dose of 135 mg/m² given as a 24-hour infusion. This regimen, as in the aforementioned GOG study, has been typically followed by IV cisplatin 75 mg/m² and hydration. This regimen requires a 1- to 2-day hospital admission. A European-Canadian randomized trial compared a 3-hour IV infusion of paclitaxel at a dose of 175 mg/m² to the 24-hour, 135-mg/m² infusion in 382 patients with relapsed ovarian carcinoma (Eisenhauer et al, 1994). There was no difference in the rates of hypersensitivity reactions (1.5 percent) or the response rates (16 vs 19 percent). The high-dose taxol group, however, had less leukopenia and a longer progression-free survival ($p = 0.02$). Because the high-dose, short-infusion-time schedule appears to be as effective and is suitable to outpatient administration, it has become the most commonly used schedule for the paclitaxel treatment of ovarian carcinoma. In addition, because it is generally believed that carboplatin is equivalent to cisplatin (Alberts, 1995), the former has become the preferred agent in most clinics, avoiding the neurotoxicity and renal toxicity of cisplatin. The optimal dose of this drug combination has not been determined, but paclitaxel is typically given at a dose of 175 to 225 mg/m², and carboplatin at a dose of 6 to 9 mg AUC, calculated by the Calvert formula, every 3 to 4

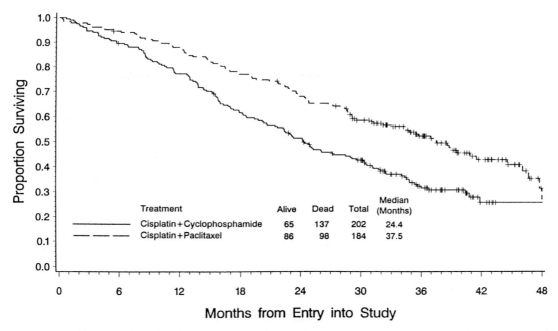

FIGURE 10–18. Ovarian carcinoma, suboptimal residual tumor. Survival of patients treated with IV cisplatin plus Taxol (paclitaxel) versus IV cisplatin plus Cytoxan (cyclophosphamide) in a randomized study. There is a significant survival advantage for the cisplatin plus Taxol treatment arm. (From McGuire WP, Hoskins WJ, Brady MF, et al: Cyclophosphamide and cisplatin compared with paclitaxel and cisplatin in patients with stage III and IV ovarian cancer. N Engl J Med 334:1, 1996, with permission.)

weeks (ten Bokkel Huinink et al, 1997). The carboplatin/paclitaxel combination at doses of 175 mg/m² and an AUC of 7 mg, respectively, can be given every 3 weeks in the great majority of patients (< 10 percent of cycles delayed). The combination seems to have a platelet-sparing effect. Neutropenia is the dose-limiting toxicity, a problem that can be managed by granulocyte cell–stimulating factor administration (Coleman et al, 1997). It must be pointed out that the 3-hour paclitaxel infusion cannot be given with cisplatin because of a high incidence of severe neurotoxicity (Connelly et al, 1996).

Based on these considerations, we recommend that patients with optimal residual disease undergo six cycles of 24-hour IV paclitaxel (135 mg/m²) and IP cisplatin (100 mg/m²) chemotherapy; patients with suboptimal tumor-reductive surgery are given the 3-hour IV paclitaxel (175 mg/m²) plus IV carboplatin (AUC 7) regimen. A second-look procedure to assess the status of the disease is also recommended after completion of the six cycles, except for those patients with a suboptimal response to chemotherapy (vide infra).

Monitoring Patients During Chemotherapy.
After initial surgical staging and debulking, frequent follow-up is indicated in patients receiving chemotherapy. Close monitoring for chemotherapy-induced side effects and early recurrence or progression of disease is required in all patients. Prior to each cycle of chemotherapy (typically given at 3-week intervals), a physical examination should be carried out with emphasis on the lymph node survey, abdominal palpation, and the rectovaginal bimanual pelvic examination. Progression of disease during chemotherapy is an indication to change treatment. The prognosis in these cases is extremely poor. Serial serum CA-125 levels are very important in assessing the response to chemotherapy, and the rapidity of decline or normalization has prognostic value. Several authors have described half-life curves based on serum clearance of CA-125 (e.g., van der Burg et al, 1988). A persistently elevated serum CA-125 level after two to three cycles of chemotherapy is highly predictive of treatment failure (Levin and Hryniuk, 1987; Mogensen et al, 1990).

Radiation Therapy. The value of radiotherapy in advanced ovarian cancer is quite limited. This is evident when it is realized that the treatment field must encompass the entire peritoneal cavity, and that the optimal dose required to achieve tumor control of even microscopic disease (4,000 to 4,500 cGy) is substantially greater than the maximum dose tolerated by the liver and kidneys (2,500 cGy).

There have been two randomized trials of WAR that included patients with optimally resected stage III ovarian carcinoma. The M.D. Anderson Hospital trial found melphalan to be as effective as, and less toxic than, strip WAR therapy in the postoperative treatment of women with stage I, II, or III optimal (<3 cm residual masses) ovarian carcinoma (Smith et al, 1975). The Princess Margaret study of optimal stage I, II, and III cases found WAR therapy to be superior to pelvic RT plus chlorambucil (Dembo et al, 1979b). These studies suggest at least a therapeutic equivalence between chemotherapy and WAR in the treatment of optimally resected ovarian carcinoma. However, both of these relatively old studies understandably employed a type of chemotherapy that is less effective than contemporary regimens. Today chemotherapy is the standard adjuvant treatment for ovarian carcinoma regardless of stage or residual disease status. WAR is applicable to patients with no residual disease, and is recommended by some authorities (Thomas, 1994). Consolidation WAR after chemotherapy does not appear to enhance survival and is associated with significant morbidity, typically small bowel injury (Fuks et al, 1988; Rothenberg et al, 1992; Lambert et al, 1993).

The Second-Look Procedure

INDICATIONS

There are many reasons for reoperating on the patient with ovarian carcinoma (Table 10–17), but the term *second look* applies specifically to a laparotomy undertaken after several (most commonly six) courses of chemotherapy to determine whether the patient with a complete clinical response is surgically and pathologically free of disease. In the absence of gross tumor, the second-look laparotomy involves multiple biopsies and peritoneal cytology in a concerted effort to detect any residual microscopic disease (Table 10–18). A second-look procedure provides the most accurate assessment of response to

TABLE **10–17**

Indications for "Second-Look" Laparotomy

A sustained clinical complete response to chemotherapy

Postoperative nonmeasurable residual disease exhibiting no evidence of progression on chemotherapy

Stable disease or a partial response to chemotherapy if residual disease might be resectable*

Cases other than stage I, grade I that were not optimally staged at initial surgery

*Surgery for known residual disease is considered not to be, by definition, a second-look laparotomy by some authors.

chemotherapy and, therefore, prognosis (Podratz and Cliby, 1994; Muderspach et al, 1995). It is more specific and sensitive than any nonoperative method of measuring residual tumor, including CT scan, ultrasound, magnetic resonance imaging, positron emission tomography (PET) scan, and clinical examination. The CT scan does not readily detect disease less than 2 cm in diameter, and it also has a significant false-positive rate (sensitivity in the study of DeRosa et al [1995] was 0.47 and specificity was 0.87).

Perhaps the most dependable measure of disease status in patients with ovarian carcinoma is the serum CA-125 value, and the time to normalization during chemotherapy correlates with survival. Several authors have reported on the relationship of serum CA-125 and the findings at second-look laparotomy. The test appears to have a positive predictive value of nearly 100 percent, but a sensitivity of only 40 percent (Hording et al, 1994; Folk et al, 1995; Kierkegaard et al, 1995; Frasci et al, 1996). An elevated serum CA-125 level im-

TABLE **10–18**

Operative Procedure for Second-Look Laparotomy in Ovarian Carcinoma

Methodical, meticulous exploration of the abdomen and pelvis

Peritoneal cytology specimens from the abdomen and pelvis

Biopsy of all target lesions

Removal of residual omentum

Resection of ovarian pedicles with peritoneum

Resection of cul-de-sac peritoneum, bowel adhesions, and peritoneal patches from paracolic gutters

Selective dissection of pelvic and aortic lymph nodes

Appendectomy

Removal of residual uterus, tubes, and ovaries*

Resection of residual carcinoma

Determination of hormone receptors on residual tumor

*In some instances, preservation of the uterus and residual adnexa is feasible (see text).

mediately prior to second-look laparotomy has the highest predictive value for residual cancer of all available clinical studies. Nearly 100 percent of these patients will have a positive second-look laparotomy (Table 10–19). A normal CA-125 value (<35 U/ml) is, however, not highly predictive of a negative second look following treatment for advanced ovarian carcinoma. Small-volume residual tumor is commonly found in this circumstance; these patients constitute a subset who may well benefit from secondary cytoreductive surgery and second-line IP chemotherapy. The site of subclinical carcinoma—that is, disease in patients with a normal physical examination and a normal CT scan of the abdomen and pelvis—in some cases can be determined by PET scan (Conti et al, 1997).

The second-look operation provides the treating physician in many cases with the only reliable data upon which to base decisions with regard to continuing, changing, or discontinuing chemotherapy. Another argument in favor of the second-look operation is the toxicity of continuing chemotherapy that has already induced a complete remission or has proven to be ineffective. Thus the second-look operation should not be considered a procedure appropriate for research studies only; rather, it should be considered a standard of practice for appropriately selected patients.

The indications for second-look surgery for patients with early ovarian carcinoma will depend upon the extent of disease and adequacy of the initial staging. As mentioned previously, second-look operations in patients with well-documented stage I disease are positive less than 5 percent of the time following chemotherapy, and are not recommended (Lentz et al, 1991; Walton et al, 1987; Rubin et al, 1993). All stage II and IIIa patients with incomplete initial staging are candidates for second-look surgery after completing six

cycles of chemotherapy. All patients with more advanced disease at initial laparotomy, especially those with postoperative residual disease, are candidates for second-look laparotomy at the completion of planned chemotherapy. Exceptions would be patients who are medically unsuitable; who have unresponsive, unresectable cancer; or who decline to continue therapy if the second staging procedure is positive. In some of these advanced cases secondary staging by laparoscopy may be indicated—for example, when the patient is believed to have residual, unresectable intraperitoneal cancer that can be documented by laparoscopy.

FINDINGS

The probability of finding residual carcinoma at second-look surgery is inversely related to the extent and resectability of the disease at the first operation, the histologic grade, the response to chemotherapy, the number of drug courses, time elapsed before second-look, and the thoroughness of the second-look staging procedure. Similarly, the relapse rate after a negative second-look procedure will be influenced to a degree by all of these factors. Collating data from the larger reported series, it can be concluded that the probability of having a surgically and/or pathologically negative second-look operation in patients with stage III or IV ovarian carcinoma after six or more cycles of chemotherapy and no clinical evidence of disease is 25 to 40 percent. Another 15 to 20 percent of cases will have microscopic disease only, and perhaps one third of the cases with macroscopic residual will be resectable (Schwartz and Smith, 1980; Greco et al, 1981; Copeland et al, 1985; Gershenson et al, 1985; Podratz et al, 1985, 1988; Smirz et al, 1985; Luesley et al, 1988; Miller et al, 1992; Potter et al, 1992; Rogers et al, 1993; McGuire et al, 1996).

TABLE **10–19**

Preoperative Serum CA-125 Levels Related to Positive Second-Look Laparotomy (SLL)

Sources	Normal CA-125 (+) SLL/Total Patients	Elevated CA-125 (+) SLL/Total Patients
Berek et al (1986)	19/43	12/12
Rubin et al (1989b)	18/29	66/67*
Patsner et al (1990)	56/102	19/23
Total	93/174 (53.4%)	97/102 (95.0%)

*One patient with negative laparotomy and elevated CA-125 level relapsed shortly after surgery.

SECOND-LOOK LAPAROSCOPY

Laparoscopy has been both recommended and condemned as a tool for staging and re-staging selected patients with ovarian carci-noma. Most of the surgical procedures, in-cluding the retroperitoneal node dissection, can be done by the laparoscopic technique, and laparoscopy provides magnification for inspecting the peritoneal surfaces and the di-aphragm. Furthermore, target biopsies and peritoneal cytology are readily obtained. In one report comparing laparoscopic second-look staging to laparotomy, the laparoscopic procedure was found to be associated with less morbidity and a shorter hospital stay (Abu-Rustum et al, 1996). For early cases, the major shortcomings, other than the technical difficulty, are the examination of the bowel and palpation of the retroperitoneum. While laparoscopy with or without node dissection is not as accurate or thorough as a full lapa-rotomy when no disease is identified, it is su-perior to no second look and is the procedure of choice when laparotomy is rejected by the patient and when residual, unresectable intra-peritoneal disease is anticipated.

RESULTS

Unfortunately, a negative second-look lapa-rotomy does not correlate well with cure or even sustained remission. The reported re-lapse rate for this group of patients ranges from 5 to 50 percent depending upon the ex-tent of the initial disease. Bolis et al (1996), for example, reported on 140 patients with a negative second-look laparotomy (out of 311 second-looks and 632 total patients) after treatment for advanced ovarian carcinoma. The overall survival rates at 3, 5, and 8 years were 76, 66, and 51 percent, respectively. The 5-year disease-free survival rate was 50 per-cent. A poorer outcome correlated with large residual disease after initial surgery (>1 cm), high grade, and lymph node positivity. Simi-larly, Maggino et al (1994) observed that 45 percent of 83 patients with advanced ovarian carcinoma relapsed at a mean interval of 27 months after a negative second-look laparot-omy. With only microscopic residual disease at second-look surgery, 30 to 60 percent of patients relapse, while 70 percent or more of patients whose disease is reduced to micro-scopic dimensions or who have small mac-roscopic residual disease after second-look surgery recur within 5 years of follow-up. Long-term survival among patients with in-vasive ovarian cancer and residual tumor greater than 2 cm after second-look surgery is uncommon.

Factors other than the amount of residual disease at second-look surgery are prognos-tic. Considering negative second-look cases, Gershenson et al (1985) reported that 32 per-cent of grade 3 cases recurred compared to 17 percent of grade 2 and no grade 1 cases. They also observed a higher relapse rate (46 vs. 19 percent) in cases with 10 or fewer bi-opsy specimens, compared to those with more than 10. It has not been demonstrated that a pathologic complete response to mul-tidrug therapy is more likely to be sustained than a pathologic complete response to single-agent therapy. Naturally the predictive value of second-look laparotomy is improved by in-creasing the interval between initiation of therapy and second-look surgery, but this may simply reflect the natural history of the disease.

Randomized clinical trials conducted by Luesley et al (1988) and Nicoletto et al (1997) indicated that patients undergoing second-look laparotomy for epithelial ovarian carci-noma did not enjoy any survival benefit when compared to patients who did not undergo second-look laparotomy. It is probable, how-ever, that the number of patients who benefit in terms of prolonged survival may be insuf-icient to affect the survival of the entire treat-ment group. There is no question that some patients with residual disease at second-look surgery have been cured by secondary cyto-reduction and additional chemotherapy. As noted elsewhere in this chapter, we continue to recommend this procedure whenever it is anticipated that the findings may alter man-agement. Thus consolidation and salvage treatment based upon the findings at second look become a key issue. For many patients this second operation should be viewed as the midpoint of the total planned treatment, with the final phase to be determined by the operative findings.

MANAGEMENT AFTER A NEGATIVE
SECOND-LOOK PROCEDURE

Patients with stage IIIb, IIIc, or IV ovarian cancer are probably not optimally treated by six cycles of chemotherapy. It is our opinion that a negative second look in these patients should be followed by an additional three cy-cles of chemotherapy. Improved survival compared to historical controls was reported by Barakat et al (1997) in a Phase II trial of

IP cisplatin plus VP-16 in patients with a negative second-look procedure.

MANAGEMENT AFTER A POSITIVE SECOND-LOOK PROCEDURE

A treatment plan for patients after second-look laparotomy is presented in Table 10–20. The value of secondary surgical debulking of gross disease discovered at second-look laparotomy is controversial, largely because of the lack of effective second-line chemotherapeutic regimens. Several authors (Lippman et al, 1988; Podratz et al, 1988; Hoskins et al, 1989; Miller et al, 1992; Potter et al, 1992); however, reported a significant improvement in survival for patients who underwent complete secondary cytoreduction at second-look laparotomy. The benefit of interval cytoreduction (van der Burg et al, 1995) is further evidence that, in appropriately selected cases, secondary cytoreduction can be salutary. Patients most likely to benefit are those whose residual tumor is completely resected. Patients with progression of disease during initial chemotherapy (approximately 10 percent of cases) rarely benefit from secondary debulking (Morris et al, 1989).

As mentioned, there is no proven, effective salvage regimen for patients with a positive second look, although several reports (Copeland et al, 1985; Miller et al, 1992; Potter et al, 1992) indicate that the prognosis for cases with only microscopic residual disease is excellent (40 to 70 percent alive at 5 years) if chemotherapy is given postoperatively. Continuing the same systemic chemotherapy after a positive second-look laparotomy is not recommended unless the amount of residual disease represents a significant reduction from the start of chemotherapy. For patients with minimal residual intraperitoneal disease IP cisplatin or floxuridine have modest efficacy

(Markman et al, 1992; Alberts et al, 1996; Muggia et al, 1996). New agents such as liposomal doxorubicin (Doxil), the taxanes, topotecan, and gemcitabine are also promising for this group of patients; high-dose chemotherapy with autologous bone marrow support may also prove to be therapeutic (Christian and Trimble, 1994; Stiff et al, 1995; Muggia et al, 1997) (see Chapter 16).

Intraperitoneal ^{32}P and WAR are conceptually appropriate for patients with microscopic residual disease, but they do not appear to be as effective or as safe as chemotherapy (Hacker et al, 1985; Smirz et al, 1985; Peters et al, 1986; Bruzzone et al, 1990; Lambert et al, 1993), although Rogers et al (1993) in a nonrandomized study reported improved survival with intraperitoneal ^{32}P in patients with a negative second-look laparatomy. The randomized study of Bruzzone et al (1990) should lay to rest the use of WAR in this situation. They compared continuing the same chemotherapy for three cycles after positive second look (microscopic or minimal residual disease) to WAR. With a median follow-up of 22 months, 55 percent of the 20 patients on the WAR treatment arm had progressed compared to 28 percent of the 21 patients on the chemotherapy arm. No serious toxicity was noted in this study, but many authors have reported a high rate (25 to 50 percent) of grade 3 or 4 gastrointestinal injury with WAR in ovarian carcinoma patients who have undergone multiple laparotomies and extensive cytoreductive surgery. Nevertheless, if the resected residual disease at second-look laparotomy is limited to the retroperitoneal lymph nodes, radiation therapy may be effective.

Tumor *hormone receptor* measurements should be obtained at second-look surgery because high-dose progestin, tamoxifen, or gonadotropin-releasing hormone analog therapy may provide some measure of tumor control, especially in cases of ovarian carcinoma with significant levels of cytosol-receptor protein (Hatch et al, 1991).

IN VITRO CHEMOSENSITIVITY ASSAY

Although in vitro testing of tumor sensitivity to chemotherapeutic agents remains largely an investigational tool, the clonogenic assay may be useful for excluding drugs from second-line chemotherapy because there is a high correlation between the in vitro and in vivo results of inactive drugs (Federico et al, 1994).

TABLE **10–20**

Treatment of Epithelial Ovarian Cancer After Second-Look Laparotomy

Tumor Status	Treatment Options
Negative second look	
1. Stages I, II	Observation
2. Stages III, IV	Consolidation chemotherapy: IP or IV
Positive second look	
1. Minimal residual	Intraperitoneal chemotherapy
2. Bulky residual	Investigational protocol; tamoxifen

High-Dose Chemotherapy

Many drugs are known to have a steep dose-response curve, but their efficacy is restricted by bone marrow toxicity. The administration of normally fatal doses of these agents has been made possible by harvesting bone marrow stem cells either from the marrow itself or from the peripheral blood. The stem cells are then given back to the patient after the administration of the drugs to repopulate the bone marrow. In Phase I and II studies, paclitaxel and carboplatin have been successfully administered in doses two to three times the maximum tolerable dose without stem cell rescue with enough responses to support continued studies, but clinical efficacy in terms of improved survival has not yet been demonstrated (Fennelly et al, 1997).

Follow-Up

After a negative second-look laparotomy, patients should be followed by serial physical examinations, radiography, and serum tumor markers (Table 10–21). Since most recurrences after negative second-look laparotomy occur within 2 years, patients should be examined every 3 months during this critical time. Symptoms of recurrence are similar to the initial presenting complaints related to ovarian carcinoma. Any rise in serum CA-125 to abnormal levels should be confirmed by repeat or serial determinations, and considered recurrent disease until proven otherwise.

If the site of recurrence cannot be identified by physical examination and CT scan, strong consideration should be given to laparoscopy or laparotomy. Another nonoperative technique is the PET scan, which we have found to be helpful in the patient with a rising CA-125 level and a negative work-up

(Conti et al, 1997). Early identification of recurrent disease may result in improved response to re-induction chemotherapy. Should recurrent disease develop after treatment with platinum-based chemotherapy, retreatment with platinum-based chemotherapy should be instituted. In one series, 18 of 18 patients so managed for recurrent ovarian cancer exhibited a clincial response (Gershenson et al, 1989). Patients are more likely to respond if the interval from initial therapy to recurrence is greater than 1 year (Reichman et al, 1989). The possibility of surgical management should be kept in mind for patients with localized recurrent disease, especially if the tumor is not poorly differentiated and there has been a tumor-free interval of more than 12 months (Morris et al, 1989; Williams, 1992; Segna et al, 1993; Pecorelli et al, 1994).

SPECIAL MANAGEMENT PROBLEMS

Reproductive Conservation

The occurrence of ovarian cancer in a young woman threatens not only her reproductive faculties but also her life. When the tumor has achieved an advanced stage, the danger to life is so great that restricting therapy to preserve the childbearing potential is rarely a reasonable alternative. However, the risk-benefit ratio of conservative surgery is usually considered acceptable when the tumor is a low-grade malignancy or is confined to one ovary (Table 10–22). Five-year survival for patients with a stage Ia borderline or grade 1 cancer managed conservatively is expected to be 95 percent or better. Thus, for patients in this category based upon proper evaluation, unilateral adnexectomy is adequate therapy.

T A B L E **10–21**

Follow-Up Schedule for Patients With Ovarian Carcinoma

Procedure	Early Stage	Advanced Stage
Physical exam	Quarterly × 2 yr, then q 6 mo	Every 3 mo × 2 yr, then q 6 mo
Tumor markers	Each visit	Each visit
CT of abdomen, pelvis	prn	Every 6 mo × 2 yr
Chest radiograph	prn	Annually
Pap smear	Every 2–3 yr*	Every 2–3 yr*
Mammogram	Annually†	Annually†

*Annually if the cervix is present.
†After age 40.

TABLE 10-22

Optimal Requirements for Conservative Surgical Management of Patients With Ovarian Cancer

Stage Ia carcinoma
Favorable histologic type
  Borderline or well-differentiated epithelial ovarian
    carcinoma
  Pure dysgerminoma, granulosa tumor, or
    arrhenoblastoma*
Young women of low parity
Cancer encapsulated and unruptured
No surface excrescences or adhesions
No invasion of capsule or mesovarium
Negative peritoneal washings
Negative ovarian biopsy and omentum
Reliable follow-up

*Well differentiated, with no heterologous elements (see Chapter 11).

The recurrence rate may be higher for patients treated conservatively, but most recurrences are in the preserved ovary and probably do not affect survival (Tazelaar et al, 1985). Furthermore, surgery and chemotherapy for the few patients who do recur will salvage some patients. Thus it is not entirely clear which strategy produces the best overall results even for high-risk stage I cases (Pecorelli et al, 1994).

The reported frequency of overt bilateralism for stage I borderline and true serous carcinomas is approximately 25 percent, and that of endometrioid lesions 15 percent. It is not clear that a biopsy of the normal-appearing ovary in these cases is warranted. The yield of the procedure is unknown but, based on the ovariectomy data, it could be 5 percent or more (Munnell, 1969; Williams and Dockerty, 1976). The frequency of bilateralism tends to increase with dedifferentiation. We do not advise routine biopsy of the normal-appearing ovary because infertility may result from adhesions or ovarian failure (Eddy et al, 1980). If ovarian biopsy is performed, the ovary should be protected by antiadhesion measures such as wrapping the ovary in Interceed.

In attempting to preserve the reproductive potential of young women with early ovarian cancer, an alternative to conservative surgery alone is conservative surgery with adjuvant chemotherapy. This therapy is applicable to all cases of high-risk histology, such as clear cell, small-cell, and grade 3 lesions. The most efficacious chemotherapy protocol has not been established, but six cycles of paclitaxel and carboplatin is recommended. The risk of gonadal damage from these agents is not known but is believed to be low. Gonadotropin-releasing hormone agonist therapy may be advisable to suppress ovarian function during chemotherapy, as discussed in Chapter 14. A second-look procedure may be indicated if the initial evaluation was inadequate, but pelvic dissection should be kept to a minimum to avoid causing infertility due to adhesions.

Bowel Obstruction

Progressive ovarian cancer often remains confined to the peritoneum and is the cause of significant gastrointestinal morbidity. The so-called tumor ileus results from encasement of the bowel and its mesentery by confluent plaques of tumor, which do not necessarily produce an obstructive narrowing of the bowel lumen but prevent peristalsis. Initial therapy of the patient with advanced ovarian cancer and a partial or complete bowel obstruction is conservative, combining tube decompression with parenteral nutrition unless there is evidence of bowel vascular compromise or perforation requiring immediate surgical intervention. Occasionally obstruction can be relieved by second-line chemotherapy. Selection of patients for operative management is subjective. The majority of patients with an intestinal obstruction resulting from advanced ovarian carcinoma have their obstruction successfully relieved by surgery, and 30 percent survive a year or longer (Clark-Pearson et al, 1987; Fernandes et al, 1988; Rubin et al, 1989a). When obstruction is due to unresectable carcinomatosis, the technique of percutaneous endoscopic gastrostomy (PEG) often allows for relief of symptoms, avoiding a nasogastric tube. However, many patients are not candidates for the PEG procedure because of tumor in the region of the stomach or the presence of abundant ascites.

Large bowel obstruction accounts for one fourth to one third of the cases of bowel obstruction caused by ovarian carcinoma (Clarke-Pearson et al, 1987; Fernandes et al, 1988). This is important to keep in mind because large bowel obstruction cannot be managed by nasogastric intubation, and it not infrequently occurs simultaneously with small bowel obstruction. It is recommended, therefore, that the surgeon evaluate at least the distal colon prior to surgery for small bowel obstruction.

Serous Effusions

Ascites

Clinically apparent ascites is associated with ovarian carcinoma in about one third of the cases and constitutes one of the more common problems in the management of this disease. Voluminous effusions are often clinically obvious, but a large ovarian cyst, distended loops of bowel, and obesity can mimic the clinical picture of ascites. Ascites itself may be a manifestation of diseases other than intra-abdominal malignancy, including cirrhosis of the liver, heart failure, pancreatitis, pelvic inflammatory disease, tuberculous peritonitis, and Meigs' syndrome. Bloody ascites is occasionally associated with endometriosis and a CA-125 value of 1,000 U or more (Iwasaka et al, 1985). Chylous ascites occurs rarely and is usually due to carcinoma obstructing lymphatics. It can also result from pelvic or abdominal radiation therapy (Sipes et al, 1985), or from malignancy (e.g., lymphoma). When the cause of abdominal distention is unclear, radiologic and ultrasound studies are helpful.

Patients with ascites should not be routinely subjected to abdominal paracentesis or laparoscopy. If the patient has a large malignant cyst rather than ascites, rupture and seeding of the peritoneal cavity may occur. In addition, malignant cells often seed the paracentesis and trocar tracts (Kruitwagen et al, 1996). The value of paracentesis in the presence of a pelvic or abdominal tumor is limited in any event. Results of cytologic examination of the fluid may be negative in the presence of malignancy, but even a positive finding may not provide a clue to the origin of the tumor. Withdrawal of the abdominal fluid should be carried out to relieve symptoms: respiratory embarrassment, pain, nausea, vomiting, and so on. Removing ascites preoperatively to avert the complications of sudden decompression of the abdomen at surgery is unnecessary and may be harmful if the fluid reforms rapidly, further depleting the patient's intravascular volume, serum proteins, and electrolytes. Slow removal of ascites at surgery, while the anesthesiologist monitors the patient's cardiovascular response, is the preferred means of decompression in the relatively asymptomatic patient. Patients with advanced ovarian carcinoma and clinical ascites are at increased operative risk because of problems with intraoperative and postoperative fluid replacement and coagulopathy (JV Brown et al, 1993).

The reaccumulation of ascites after surgery is invariably associated with residual carcinoma. However, in the great majority of these cases systemic chemotherapy is indicated, and control of ascites is one of the earliest and most sensitive indicators of tumor response. Chemotherapy can be initiated in the early postoperative period if rapid ascites formation is a problem.

Excessive production of ascites postoperatively results in fluid and electrolyte imbalance with hypovolemia, oliguria, and protein depletion. In this circumstance, with low urine output and a large third space, the administration of nephrotoxic agents, especially cisplatin or methotrexate, is hazardous. In the occasional case in which ascites cannot be adequately controlled by systemic chemotherapy, intraperitoneal chemotherapy has been used with modest success. Otherwise repeat paracentesis may be required for palliation. Peritoneovenous shunting has been utilized in the management of intractable, symptomatic ascites, but the complication rate is high (Zervos et al, 1997).

Pleural and Pericardial Effusions

Pleural effusion represents the spread of ovarian cancer to the lung and pleural surfaces, or simply a movement of ascitic fluid through the diaphragmatic lymphatics into the pleural cavity. Patients with respiratory or cardiovascular embarrassment from pleural effusion need immediate thoracentesis (and, perhaps, paracentesis). Refractory or recurrent pleural effusion during drug therapy may respond to an intrapleural sclerosing agent such as doxycycline (Fenton and Richardson, 1995). Pleural effusion refractory to these therapies may need to be management by thoracotomy tube drainage and chemical pleurodesis (Walker-Renard et al, 1994).

Occasionally ovarian cancer involves the pericardial surface, producing a symptomatic effusion that sometimes necessitates an emergency pericardiocentesis. Doxycycline appears to be an especially effective sclerosing agent in this situation, although some authorities prefer the pericardial window.

Ovarian Tumors in Children

Ovarian neoplasms in children are quite unusual, although they account for two thirds of genital tract cancers in this age group. They

TABLE **10-23**

Relative Frequency of Ovarian Tumors from Children's Hospitals*

Category	Total Cases	Germ Cell	Stromal	Epithelial	Other
Non-neoplastic	95	—	—	—	—
Neoplastic					
Benign	167	128	6	23	10
Malignant	57	35	10	9	3
Total	224	163	16	32	13

*Data from Ein et al (1970), Adelman et al (1975), Towne et al (1975), and MF Brown et al (1993).

are of special importance, however, since the malignancy rate may be as high as 50 percent. In the newborn period, nearly all ovarian enlargements are functional or non-neoplastic cysts (Carlson et al, 1972). Ovarian neoplasms of any type are decidedly rare before puberty; in a 20-year, population-based survey, only 10 of approximately 600 cancers in young girls were ovarian malignancies (Mosso et al, 1992).

The reported frequency of the different types of ovarian tumor varies widely. Considering those series from children's hospitals, usually with patient ages of 15 years and under, one third are non-neoplastic, predominantly follicular cysts (Table 10–23). Of the neoplasms, 85 percent are germ cell, but only one in six is malignant. This malignancy rate differs substantially from that of the reported pathology series (Lindfors, 1971; Norris and Jensen, 1972), in which 50 to 75 percent of the germ cell tumors are malignant. In adults, only 15 to 20 percent of ovarian neoplasms

are germ cell in origin, and more than 95 percent of these are benign cystic teratomas.

Ovarian neoplasms of epithelial histology are exceedingly rare before puberty, and the preponderance of them are benign. In the series of Norris and Jensen (Table 10–24), less than 5 percent of the neoplasms in females under 15 years of age were epithelial. Between the ages of 15 and 20, however, the proportion jumped to 28 percent. In the children's hospital series (Table 10–23), less than 20 percent of ovarian neoplasms were epithelial.

Stromal tumors comprise about 15 percent of ovarian neoplasms reported in childhood and adolescence. However, they may be reported more frequently than other neoplasms, because their hormonal effects make them especially interesting. It is estimated that 2 to 5 percent of all cases of isosexual precocious puberty are due to ovarian tumors (Adelman et al, 1975). A few well-documented examples of isosexual precocity

TABLE **10-24**

Relative Frequency of Ovarian Neoplasms in Childhood Accessioned at the Armed Forces Institute of Pathology*

	Patient Age (Years)								Total	
	0–4		5–9		10–14		15–19			
Histology	N	(%)	N	(%)	N	(%)	N	(%)	N	%
Benign										
Germ cell	2		3		14		52		71	20.1
Stromal	4		7		3		22		36[†]	10.2
Epithelial	0		1		4		54		59	16.7
Malignant										
Germ cell	5		22		52		57		136	38.5
Stromal	5		1		3		17		26	7.4
Epithelial	0		0		1		7[‡]		8	2.3
Other	2		2		5		8		17	4.9
Total	18	(5.1)	36	(10.2)	82	(23.2)	217	(61.5)	353	100.0

*Data from Norris and Jensen (1972).
[†]Includes 13 cases listed as "nonspecific," which were not designated benign or malignant.
[‡]Five of seven were borderline malignant tumors.

occurring secondary to a follicular cyst have been reported in the literature, but precocious puberty of ovarian origin is more commonly associated with a true neoplasm: granulosa cell tumor, Sertoli cell tumor, and choriocarcinoma. The granulosa cell tumors, like other non–germ cell neoplasms, are less inclined to manifest malignant behavior in this age group than in older individuals. The diagnosis of thecoma and arrhenoblastoma is extremely rare before puberty.

Ovarian Tumors in Pregnancy

For a discussion of ovarian tumors in pregnancy, see Chapter 14.

REFERENCES

Abu-Rustum NR, Barakat RR, Siegel PL, et al: Second-look operation for epithelial ovarian carcinoma: laparoscopy or laparotomy? Obstet Gynecol 88:549, 1996.

Adelman S, Benson CD, Hertzler JH: Surgical lesions of the ovary in infancy and childhood. Surg Gynecol Obstet 141:219, 1975.

Ahmed FY, Wiltshaw E, A'Hern RP, et al: Natural history and prognosis of untreated stage I epithelial ovarian cancer. J Clin Oncol 14:2968, 1996.

Aho AJ, Heinonen R, Lauren P: Benign and malignant mucocele of the appendix. Acta Chir Scand 139:392, 1973.

Alberts DS: Carboplatin versus cisplatin in ovarian cancer. Semin Oncol 22(suppl):88, 1995.

Alberts DS, Liu PY, Hannigan EV, et al: Intraperitoneal cisplatin plus intravenous cyclophosphamide versus intravenous cisplatin plus intravenous cyclophosphamide for stage III ovarian cancer. N Engl J Med 335:1950, 1996.

Andersen WA, Young DE, Peters WA III, et al: Platinum-based combination chemotherapy for malignant mixed mesodermal tumors of the ovary. Gynecol Oncol 32:319, 1989.

August CZ, Murad TM, Newton M: Multiple focal extraovarian serous carcinoma. Int J Gynecol Pathol 4:11, 1985.

Austin RM, Norris HJ: Malignant Brenner tumor and transitional cell carcinoma of the ovary: a comparison. Int J Gynecol Pathol 6:29, 1987.

Averette HE, Lovecchio JL, Townsend PA, et al: Retroperitoneal lymphatic involvement by ovarian carcinoma. In Grundmann E (ed): Cancer Campaign: Carcinoma of the Ovary. Stuttgart, Gustav Fischer Verlag, 1983.

Axelrod JH, Fruchter R, Boyce JG: Multiple primaries among gynecologic malignancies. Gynecol Oncol 18:359, 1984.

Barakat RB, Almadrones L, Venkatraman E, Spriggs R: A phase II trial of intraperitoneal (IP) cisplatin (CDDP) and etoposide (VP-16) as consolidation therapy in patients with stage III–IV epithelial ovarian cancer (EOC) following negative surgical assessment [Abstract No. 1264]. Proc ASCO 16:354a, 1997.

Barakat RB, Benjamin I, Lewis JL Jr, et al: Platinum-based chemotherapy for advanced stage serous ovarian carcinoma of low malignant potential. Gynecol Oncol 59:390, 1995.

Barnhill D, Heller P, Brzozowski P, et al: Epithelial ovarian carcinoma of low malignant potential. Obstet Gynecol 65:53, 1985.

Barnhill DR, Kurman RJ, Brady MF, et al: Preliminary analysis of the behavior of stage I ovarian serous tumors of low malignant potential: a Gynecologic Oncology Group study. J Clin Oncol 13:2752, 1995.

Bell DA, Scully RE: Benign and borderline clear cell adenofibromas of the ovary. Cancer 56:2922, 1985.

Bell DA, Scully RE: Ovarian serous borderline tumors with stromal microinvasion: a report of 21 cases. Hum Pathol 21:397, 1990.

Bell DA, Weinstock MA, Scully RE: Peritoneal implants of ovarian serous borderline tumors. Cancer 62:2212, 1988.

Berek JS, Knapp RC, Malkasian GD, et al: CA 125 serum levels correlated with second-look operations among ovarian cancer patients. Obstet Gynecol 67:685, 1986.

Blythe JG, Wahl TP: Debulking surgery: does it increase the quality of survival? Gynecol Oncol 14:396, 1982.

Bolis G, Columbo N, Peccorelli S, et al: Adjuvant treatment for early epithelial ovarian cancer. Ann Oncol 6:887, 1995.

Bolis G, Villa A, Guarnerio P, et al: Survival of women with advanced ovarian cancer and complete pathologic response at second-look laparotomy. Cancer 77:128, 1996.

Bostwick DG, Tazelaar HD, Ballon SC, et al: Ovarian epithelial tumors of borderline malignancy. Cancer 58:2052, 1986.

Brown JV, Karlan BY, Greenspoon JS, et al: Perioperative coagulopathy in patients undergoing primary cytoreduction. Cancer 71:2557, 1993.

Brown MF, Hebra A, McGeehin K, Ross AJ: Ovarian masses in children: a review of 91 cases of malignant and benign masses. J Pediatr Surg 28:930, 1993.

Bruzzone M, Repetto L, Chiara S, et al: Chemotherapy versus radiotherapy in the management of ovarian cancer patients with pathological complete response or minimal residual disease at second look. Gynecol Oncol 38:392, 1990.

Buchsbaum HJ, Brady MF, Delgado G, et al: Surgical staging of ovarian carcinoma: stage I, II and III (optimal): a Gynecologic Oncology Group study. Surg Gynecol Obstet 169:226, 1989.

Burghardt E, Girardi F, Lahousen M, et al: Patterns of pelvic and paraaortic lymph node involvement in ovarian cancer. Gynecol Oncol 40:103, 1991.

Burghardt E, Pickel H, Lahousen M, Stettner H: Pelvic lymphadenectomy in operative treatment of ovarian cancer. Am J Obstet Gynecol 155:315, 1986.

Burks RT, Sherman ME, Kurman RJ: Micropapillary serous carcinoma of the ovary: a distinctive low-grade carcinoma related to serous borderline tumors. Am J Surg Pathol 20:1319, 1996.

Buttini M, Nicklin JL, Crandon A: Low malignant potential ovarian tumors: a review of 175 consecutive cases. Aust N Z J Obstet Gynaecol 37:100, 1997.

Campbell JS, Lou P, Ferguson JP, et al: Pseudomyxoma peritonei et ovarii with occult neoplasms of appendix. Obstet Gynecol 42:897, 1973.

Carlson DH, Griscom NT: Ovarian cysts in the newborn. Am J Roentgenol Radiat Ther Nucl Med 116:664, 1972.

Chaitin BA, Gershenson DM, Evans HL: Mucinous tumors of the ovary. Cancer 55:1958, 1985.

Chambers JT, Merino MJ, Kohorn EI, Schwartz PE: Borderline ovarian tumors. Am J Obstet Gynecol 159:1088, 1988.

Chen KTK, Flam MS: Peritoneal papillary serous carcinoma with long-term survival. Cancer 58:1371, 1986.

Chen SS, Bochner R: Assessment of morbidity and mortality in primary cytoreductive surgery for advanced ovarian carcinoma. Gynecol Oncol 20:190, 1985.

Chen SS, Lee L: Prognostic significance of morphology of tumor and retroperitoneal lymph nodes in epithelial carcinoma of the ovary. Gynecol Oncol 18:87, 1984.

Cheng P, Schmutte C, Cofer KF, et al: Alterations in DNA methylation are early, but not initial events in ovarian tumorigenesis. Br J Cancer 75:396, 1997.

Childers JM, Lang J, Surwit EA, Hatch KD: Laparoscopic surgical staging of ovarian cancer. Gynecol Oncol 59:25, 1995.

Christian MC, Trimble EL: Salvage chemotherapy for epithelial ovarian carcinoma. Gynecol Oncol 55:S143, 1994.

Clarke-Pearson DL, Chin NO, DeLong ER, et al: Surgical management of intestinal obstruction in ovarian cancer. Gynecol Oncol 26:11, 1987.

Clement PB, Scully RE: Extrauterine mesodermal (Mullerian) adenosarcoma. Am J Clin Pathol 69:276, 1978.

Coleman RL, Bagnell KG, Townley PM: Carboplatin and short-infusion paclitaxel in high-risk and advanced-stage ovarian carcinoma. Cancer J Sci Am 3:246, 1997.

Colgan TJ, Norris HJ: Ovarian epithelial tumors of low malignant potential: a review. Int J Gynecol Pathol 1:367, 1983.

Connelly E, Markman M, Kennedy A, et al: Paclitaxel delivered as a 3-hr infusion with cisplatin in patients with gynecologic cancers: unexpected incidence of neurotoxicity. Gynecol Oncol 62:166, 1996.

Conte PF, Bruzzone M, Chiara S, et al: A randomized trial comparing cisplatin plus cyclophosphamide versus cisplatin, doxorubicin and cyclophosphamide in advanced ovarian cancer. J Clin Oncol 4:965, 1986.

Conti PS, Horwich T, Roman L, et al: Use of F-18 FDG and PET in assessment of minimal disease after treatment of epithelial ovarian cancer. Presented at the Society of Nuclear Medicine 44th Annual Meeting, San Antonio TX, June 1–5, 1997.

Copeland LJ, Gershenson DM, Wharton JT, et al: Microscopic disease at second-look laparotomy in advanced ovarian cancer. Cancer 55:472, 1985.

Costa MJ: Pseudomyxoma peritonei: histologic predictors of patient survival. Arch Pathol Lab Med 118:1215, 1994.

Creasman WT, Park R, Norris H, et al: Stage I borderline ovarian tumors. Obstet Gynecol 59:93, 1982.

Crozier MA, Copeland LJ, Silva EG, et al: Clear cell carcinoma of the ovary: a study of 59 cases. Gynecol Oncol 35:199, 1989.

Curtin JP, Malik R, Venkatraman E, et al: Stage IV ovarian cancer: impact of surgical debulking. Gynecol Oncol 64:9, 1997.

Czernobilsky B: Endometrioid neoplasia of the ovary: a reappraisal. Int J Gynecol Pathol 1:203, 1982.

Czernobilsky B: Common epithelial tumors of the ovary. In Roth LM, Czernobilsky B (eds): Contemporary Issues in Surgical Pathology: Tumors and Tumorlike Conditions of the Ovary. New York, Churchill Livingstone, 1985, p 11.

Delgado G, Oram DH, Petrilli ES: Stage III epithelial ovarian cancer: the role of maximal surgical reduction. Gynecol Oncol 18:293, 1984.

Dembo AJ, Bush RS, Beale FA, et al: A randomized clinical trial of moving strip versus open-field whole abdominal irradiation in patients with invasive epithelial cancer of ovary. Proc ASCO 3:212, 1984.

Dembo AJ, Bush RS, Beale FA, et al: Ovarian carcinoma: improved survival following abdominopelvic irradiation in patients with a completed pelvic operation. Am J Obstet Gynecol 134:793, 1979a.

Dembo AJ, Bush RS, Beale FA, et al: The Princess Margaret Hospital study of ovarian cancer: Stages I, II, and asymptomatic III presentations. Cancer Treat Rep 63:249, 1979b.

Dembo AJ, Davy M, Stenwig AE, et al: Prognostic factors in patients with stage I epithelial ovarian cancer. Obstet Gynecol 75:263, 1990.

DeRosa V, Mangoni di Stefano ML, Brunetti A, et al: Computed tomography and second-look surgery in ovarian cancer patients: correlation, actual role and limitations of CT scan. Eur J Gynaecol Oncol 16:123, 1995.

Dictor M: Malignant mixed mesodermal tumor of the ovary: a report of 22 cases. Obstet Gynecol 65:720, 1985.

Diebold J, Deisenhofer I, Baretton GB, et al: Interphase cytogenetic analysis of serous ovarian tumors of low malignant potential: comparison with serous cystadenomas and invasive serous carcinomas. Lab Invest 75:473, 1996.

Dinh TV, Slavin RE, Bhagavan BS, et al: Mixed mesodermal tumors of the ovary: a clinicopathologic study of 14 cases. Obstet Gynecol 72:409, 1988.

DiRe F, Fontanelli R, Raspagliesi F, DiRe EM: The value of lymphadenectomy in the management of ovarian cancer. In Sharp CF, Mason WP, Leake R (eds): Ovarian Cancer: Biologic and Therapeutic Challenges. London, Chapman and Hall, 1990.

Doss N Jr, Forney JP, Vellios F, Nalick RH: Covert bilaterality of mature ovarian teratomas. Obstet Gynecol 50:651, 1977.

Eddy CA, Asch RH, Balmaceda JP: Pelvic adhesions following microsurgical and macrosurgical wedge resection of the ovaries. Fertil Steril 33:557, 1980.

Ehrmann RL, Federschneider JM, Knapp RC: Distinguishing lymph node metastases from benign grandular inclusions in low-grade ovarian carcinoma. Am J Obstet Gynecol 136:737, 1980.

Eifel P, Hendrickson M, Ross J, et al: Simultaneous presentation of carcinoma involving the ovary and the uterine corpus. Cancer 50:163, 1982.

Ein SH, Darte JMM, Stephens CA: Cystic and solid ovarian tumors in children: a 44-year review. J Pediatr Surg 5:148, 1970.

Eisenhauer EA, ten Bokkel Huinink WW, Swenerton KD, et al: European-Canadian randomized trial of paclitaxel in relapsed ovarian cancer: high dose versus low dose and long versus short infusion. J Clin Oncol 12:2654, 1994.

Eltabbakh GH, Belinson JL, Kennedy AW, et al: p53 and HER-2/neu overexpression in ovarian borderline tumors. Gynecol Oncol 65:218, 1997.

Erhardt K, Auer G, Bjorkholm E, et al: Combined morphologic and cytochemical grading of serous ovarian tumors. Am J Obstet Gynecol 151:356, 1985.

Faught W, Lotocki R, Heywood M, Krepart GV: Early ovarian cancer: value of a negative staging laparotomy. Eur J Gynaecol Oncol 17:200, 1996.

Federico M, Alberts DS, Garcia DJ, et al: In vitro drug testing of ovarian cancer using the human tumor colony-forming assay: comparison of in vitro response and clinical outcome. Gynecol Oncol 55(suppl):S156, 1994.

Fennelly DW, Aghajanian C, Shapiro F, et al: Dose escalation of paclitaxel with high-dose carboplatin using peripheral blood progenitor cell support in patients with advanced ovarian cancer. Semin Oncol 24(suppl 2):26, 1997.

Fenton KN, Richardson JD: Diagnosis and management of malignant pleural effusion. Am J Surg 170:69, 1995.

Fernandes JR, Seymour RJ, Suissa S: Bowel obstruction in patients with ovarian cancer: a search for prognostic factors. Am J Obstet Gynecol 158:244, 1988.

Fiorentino MV, Brigato G, Cima G, et al: Randomized study of redebulking in epithelial ovarian cancer (OC). Proc ASCO 12:267, 1993.

Folk JJ, Botsford J, Musa AG: Monitoring cancer antigen 125 levels in induction chemotherapy for epithelial ovarian carcinoma and predicting outcome of second-look procedure. Gynecol Oncol 57:178, 1995.

Fort MG, Pierce VK, Saigo PE, et al: Evidence for the efficacy of adjuvant therapy in epithelial ovarian tumors of low malignant potential. Gynecol Oncol 32:269, 1989.

Fox H: Primary neoplasia of the female peritoneum. Histopathology 23:103, 1993.

Frasci G, Conforti S, Zullo F, et al: A risk model for ovarian carcinoma patients using CA 125: time to normalization renders second-look laparotomy redundant. Cancer 77:1122, 1996.

Friedlander ML, Hedley DW, Swanson C, Russell P: Prediction of long-term survival by flow cytometric analysis of cellular DNA content in patients with advanced ovarian cancer. J Clin Oncol 6:282, 1988.

Friedlander ML, Taylor IW, Russell P, et al: Ploidy as a prognostic factor in ovarian cancer. Int J Gynecol Pathol 2:55, 1983.

Fromm G-L, Gershenson DM, Silva EG: Papillary serous carcinoma of the peritoneum. Obstet Gynecol 75:89, 1990.

Fuks Z, Rizel S, Biran S: Chemotherapeutic and surgical induction of pathological complete remission and whole abdominal irradiation for consolidation does not enhance the cure of stage III ovarian carcinoma. J Clin Oncol 6: 509, 1988.

Genadry R, Poliakoff S, Rotmensch J, et al: Primary, papillary peritoneal neoplasia. Obstet Gynecol 58:730, 1981.

Gershenson DM, Copeland LJ, Wharton JT, et al: Prognosis of surgically determined complete responders in advanced ovarian cancer. Cancer 55:1129, 1985.

Gershenson DM, Kavanagh JJ, Copeland LJ, et al: Re-treatment of patients with recurrent epithelial ovarian cancer with cisplatin-based chemotherapy. Obstet Gynecol 73: 798, 1989.

Gershenson DM, Silva EG: Serous ovarian tumors of low malignant potential with peritoneal implants. Cancer 65: 578, 1990.

Gershenson DM, Silva EG, Mitchell MF, et al: Transitional cell carcinoma of the ovary: a matched control study of advanced stage patients treated with cisplatin-based chemotherapy. Am J Obstet Gynecol 168:1178, 1993.

GICOA (Gruppo Interegionale Cooperativo Oncologico Ginecologia): Randomized comparison of cisplatin with cyclophosphamide/cisplatin and with cyclophosphamide/doxorubicin/cisplatin in advanced ovarian cancer. Lancet 2:353, 1987.

Goff BA, Sainz de la Cuesta R, Muntz HG, et al: Clear cell carcinoma of the ovary: a distinct histologic type with poor prognosis and resistance to platinum-based chemotherapy in stage III disease. Gynecol Oncol 60:412, 1996.

Gough DB, Donohue JH, Schutt AJ, et al: Pseudomyxoma peritonei: long term patient survival with an aggressive regional approach. Ann Surg 219:112, 1994.

Greco FA, Julian GC, Richardson RL, et al: Advanced ovarian cancer: brief intensive combination chemotherapy and second-look operation. Obstet Gynecol 58:199, 1981.

Griffiths CT: Surgical resection of tumor bulk in the primary treatment of ovarian carcinoma. In: Symposium on Ovarian Carcinoma. National Cancer Institute Monograph No. 42. Reston, VA, National Cancer Institute, 1975, p 101.

Griffiths CT, Parker LM, Fuller AF Jr: Role of cytoreductive surgical treatment in the management of advanced ovarian cancer. Cancer Treat Rep 63:235, 1979.

Grover CM, Kuppermann M, Kahn JG, Washington AE: Concurrent hysterectomy at bilateral salpingo-oophorectomy: benefits, risks, and costs. Obstet Gynecol 88:907, 1996.

Guerard MJ, Arguelles MA, Ferenczy A: Rhabdomyosarcoma of the ovary: ultrastructural study of a case and review of literature. Gynecol Oncol 15:325, 1983.

Guerrieri C, Hogberg T, Wingren S, et al: Mucinous borderline and malignant tumors of the ovary: a clinicopathologic and DNA ploidy study of 92 cases. Cancer 74:2329, 1994.

Hacker NF: Systematic pelvic and paraaortic lymphadenectomy for advanced ovarian cancer: therapeutic advance or surgical folly? Gynecol Oncol 56:325, 1995.

Hacker NF, Berek JS, Burnison CM, et al: Whole abdominal radiation as salvage therapy for epithelial ovarian cancer. Obstet Gynecol 65:60, 1985.

Hacker NF, Berek JS, Lagasse LD, et al: Primary cytoreductive surgery for epithelial ovarian cancer. Obstet Gynecol 61:413, 1983.

Hafiz MA, Toker C: Multicentric ovarian and extraovarian cystadenofibroma. Obstet Gynecol 68:948, 1986.

Haid M, Victor TA, Weldon-Linne M, Danforth DN: Malignant Brenner tumor of the ovary. Cancer 51:498, 1983.

Harlow BL, Fuhr JE, McDonald TW, et al: Flow cytometry as a prognostic indicator in women with borderline epithelial ovarian tumors. Gynecol Oncol 50:305, 1993.

Hart WR, Norris HJ: Borderline and malignant mucinous tumors of the ovary. Cancer 31:1031, 1973.

Hatch KD, Beecham JB, Blessing JA, Creasman WT: Responsiveness of patients with advanced ovarian carcinoma to tamoxifen: a Gynecologic Oncology Group study of second-line therapy in 105 patients. Cancer 68: 269, 1991.

Heaps JM, Nieberg RK, Berek JS: Malignant neoplasms arising in endometriosis. Obstet Gynecol 75:1023, 1990.

Hernandez W, DiSaia PJ, Morrow CP, Townsend DE: Mixed mesodermal sarcoma of the ovary. Obstet Gynecol 49:59, 1977.

Hockstein S, Keh P, Lurain JR, Fishman DA: Ovarian carcinoma initially presenting as metastatic axillary lymphadenopathy. Gynecol Oncol 65:543, 1997.

Hollingsworth HC, Steinberg SM, Silverberg SG, Merino MJ: Advanced stage transitional cell carcinoma of the ovary. Hum Pathol 27:12367, 1996.

Hopkins MP, Morley GW: Second-look operation and surgical reexploration in ovarian tumors of low malignant potential. Obstet Gynecol 47:375, 1989.

Hording U, Toftager-Larsen K, Lund B, et al: The value of CA 125 measurement before second-look laparotomy in patients with ovarian carcinoma. Eur J Gynaecol Oncol 15:217, 1994.

Hoskins WJ, Bundy BN, Thigpen JT, et al: The influence of cytoreductive surgery on recurrence-free interval and survival in small-volume stage III epithelial ovarian cancer: a Gynecologic Oncology Group Study. Gynecol Oncol 47:159, 1992.

Hoskins WJ, McGuire WP, Brady MF, et al: The effect of diameter of largest residual disease on survival after primary cytoreductive surgery in patients with suboptimal residual epithelial ovarian carcinoma. Am J Obstet Gynecol 170:974, 1994.

Hoskins WJ, Rubin SC, Dulaney E, et al: Influence of secondary cytoreduction at the time of second-look laparotomy on the survival of patients with epithelial ovarian carcinoma. Gynecol Oncol 34:265, 1989.

Hreshchyshyn MW, Park RC, Blessing JA, et al: The role of adjuvant therapy in stage I ovarian cancer. Am J Obstet Gynecol 138:139, 1980.

Hudson CN, Chir M: Surgical treatment of ovarian cancer. Gynecol Oncol 1:370, 1973.

Iwasaka T, Okuma Y, Yoshimura T, et al: Endometriosis associated with ascites. Obstet Gynecol 66:72s, 1985.

Jenison EL, Montag AG, Griffiths CT, et al: Clear cell adenocarcinoma of the ovary: a clinical analysis and comparison with serous carcinoma. Gynecol Oncol 32:65, 1989.

Julian CG, Woodruff JD: The biologic behavior of low-grade papillary serous carcinoma of the ovary. Obstet Gynecol 40:860, 1972.

Kaern J, Trope CG, Abeler VM: A retrospective study of 370 borderline tumors of the ovary treated at the Norwegian Radium Hospital from 1970 to 1982. Cancer 71:1810, 1993a.

Kaern J, Trope CG, Kristensen GB, et al: DNA ploidy: the most important prognostic factor in patients with borderline tumors of the ovary. Int J Gynecol Cancer 3:349, 1993b.

Kao GF, Norris HJ: Benign and low grade variants of mixed mesodermal tumor (adenosarcoma) of the ovary and adnexal region. Cancer 42:1314, 1978.

Kao GF, Norris HJ: Unusual cystadenofibromas: endometrioid, mucinous, and clear cell types. Obstet Gynecol 54:729, 1979.

Katsube Y, Berg JW, Silverberg SG: Epidemiologic pathology of ovarian tumors: a histopathologic review of primary ovarian neoplasms diagnosed in the Denver Standard Metropolitan Statistical Area, 1 July–31 December 1969, and 1 July–31 December 1979. Int J Gynecol Pathol 1:3, 1982.

Katzenstein ALA, Mazur MT, Morgan TE, Kao MS: Proliferative serous tumors of the ovary. Am J Surg Pathol 2:339, 1978.

Kempson RL, Hendrickson MR: Miscellaneous types of surface epithelial neoplasms. In Hendrickson MR (ed): State of the Art Reviews: Surface Epithelial Neoplasms of the Ovary. Hanley & Belfus, Philadelphia, 1993, p 335.

Kennedy AW, Hart WR: Ovarian papillary serous tumors of low malignant potential (serous borderline tumors): a long-term follow-up study including patients with microinvasion, lymph node metastasis, and transformation to invasive serous carcinoma. Cancer 78:278, 1996.

Kierkegaard O, Mogensen O, Mogensen B, Jakobsen A: Predictive and prognostic values of cancer-associated serum antigen (CASA) and cancer antigen 125 (CA 125) levels prior to second-look laparotomy for ovarian cancer. Gynecol Oncol 59:251, 1995.

Kikkawa F, Kawai M, Tamakoshi K, et al: Mucinous carcinoma of the ovary: clinicopathologic analysis. Oncology 53:303, 1996.

Klaassen D, Shelley W, Starreveld A, et al: Early stage ovarian cancer: a randomized clinical trial comparing whole abdomen radiotherapy, melphalan, and intraperitoneal chromic phosphate. A National Cancer Institute of Canada Clinical Trials Group report. J Clin Oncol 6:1254, 1988.

Kliman L, Rome RM, Fortune DW: Low malignant potential (LMP) tumors of the ovary: a clinical and pathological study of 76 cases. Obstet Gynecol 68:338, 1986.

Kline RC, Wharton JT, Atkinson EN, et al: Endometrioid carcinoma of the ovary: retrospective review of 145 cases. Gynecol Oncol 39:337, 1990.

Kolstad P, Davy M, Hoeg K: Individualized treatment of ovarian cancer. Am J Obstet Gynecol 128:617, 1977.

Koonings PP, Campbell K, Mishell DR, Grimes DA: Relative frequency of primary ovarian neoplasms: a 10-year review. Obstet Gynecol 74:921, 1989.

Koshiyama M, Konishi I, Mandai M, et al: Immunohistochemical analysis of p53 protein and 72 kDa heat shock protein (HSP72) expression in ovarian carcinomas: correlation with clinicopathology and sex steroid receptor status. Virchows Arch 425:603 1995.

Kruitwagen RFPM, Swinkels BM, Keyser KGG, et al: Incidence and effect on survival of abdominal wall metastases at trocar puncture sites following laparoscopy of paracentesis in women with ovarian cancer. Gynecol Oncol 60:233, 1996.

Lambert HE, Rustin GJC, Gregory WM, Nelstrop AE: A randomized trial comparing single-agent carboplatin with carboplatin followed by radiotherapy for advanced ovarian cancer: a North Thames Ovary Group study. J Clin Oncol 11:440, 1993.

Le T, Krepart GV, Lotocki RJ, Heywood MS: Malignant mixed mesodermal ovarian tumor treatment and prognosis: a 20 year experience. Gynecol Oncol 65:237, 1997.

Leake JF, Rader JS, Woodruff JD, Rosenshein NB, Retroperitoneal lymphatic involvement with epithelial ovarian tumors of low malignant potential. Gynecol Oncol 42:124, 1991.

Lentz SS, Cha SS, Wiegand HS, et al: Stage I ovarian epithelial carcinoma: survival analysis following definitive treatment. Gynecol Oncol 43:198, 1991.

Levin L, Hryniuk WM: Dose intensity analysis of chemotherapy regimens in ovarian carcinoma. J Clin Oncol 5:756, 1987.

Liapis A, Condi-Paphiti A, Pyrgiotis E, Zourlas PA: Ovarian surface serous papillary carcinomas: a clinicopathologic study. Eur J Gynaecol Oncol 17:79, 1996.

Limber GK, King RE, Silverberg SG: Pseudomyxoma peritonei: a report of ten cases. Ann Surg 178:587, 1973.

Lim-Tan SK, Cajigas HE, Scully RE: Ovarian cystectomy for serous borderline tumors: a follow-up study of 35 cases. Obstet Gynecol 72:775, 1988.

Lindfors O: Primary ovarian neoplasms in infants and children. Ann Chir Gynaecol Fenn Suppl 177:1, 1971.

Link CJ Jr, Kohn E, Reed E: The relationship between borderline ovarian tumors and epithelial ovarian carcinoma: epidemiologic, pathologic, and molecular aspects. Gynecol Oncol 60:347, 1996.

Lippman SM, Alberts DS, Slymen DJ, et al: Second-look laparotomy in epithelial ovarian carcinoma. Cancer 61:2571, 1988.

Llerena E, Kudelka AP, Tornos C, et al: Remission of a chemotherapy resistant tumor of low malignant potential with tamoxifen. Eur J Gynaecol Oncol 18:23, 1997.

Look KY, Stehman FB, Moore DH, Sutton GP: Intraperitoneal 5-fluorouracil for pseudomyxoma peritonei. Int J Gynecol Cancer 5:361, 1995.

Luesley D, Lawton F, Blackledge G, et al: Failure of second-look laparotomy to influence survival in epithelial ovarian cancer. Lancet 1:599, 1988.

Lui PC, Benjamin I, Morgan MA, et al: Effect of surgical debulking in stage IV ovarian cancer. Gynecol Oncol 64:4, 1997.

Maggino T, Gadducci A, Romagnolo C, et al: Times and sites of relapse after negative second-look in advanced epithelial ovarian cancer. Eur J Surg Oncol 20:146, 1994.

Mann WJ Jr, Wagner J, Chumas J, Chalas E: The management of pseudomyxoma peritonei. Cancer 66:1636, 1990.

Markman M: Intraperitoneal chemotherapy. Semin Oncol 18:248, 1991.

Markman M, Reichman B, Hakes T, et al: Impact on survival of surgically defined favorable responses to salvage intraperitoneal chemotherapy in small-volume residual ovarian cancer. J Clin Oncol 10:1479, 1992.

McGowan L, Lesher LP, Norris HJ, Barnett M: Misstaging of ovarian cancer. Obstet Gynecol 65:568, 1985.

McGuire WP, Hoskins WJ, Brady MF, et al: Cyclophosphamide and cisplatin compared with paclitaxel and cisplatin in patients with stage III and IV ovarian cancer. N Engl J Med 334:1, 1996.

Meigs JF, Armstrong SH, Hamilton HH: A further contribution to the syndrome of fibroma of the ovary with fluid in the abdomen and chest: Meigs' syndrome. Am J Obstet Gynecol 46:19, 1943.

Menzin AW, Rubin SC, Noumoff JS, LiVolsi VA: The accuracy of a frozen section diagnosis of borderline ovarian malignancy. Gynecol Oncol 859:183, 1995.

Merino MJ, Edmonds P, LiVolsi V: Appendiceal carcinoma metastatic to the ovaries and mimicking primary ovarian tumors. Int J Gynecol Pathol 4:110, 1985.

Miles JM, Hart WR, McMahon JT: Cystic mesothelioma of the peritoneum: report of a case with multiple recurrences and review of the literature. Cleve Clin Q 53:109, 1986.

Miller DS, Spirtos NM, Ballon SC, et al: Critical reassessment of second-look exploratory laparotomy for epithelial ovarian carcinoma. Cancer 69:502, 1992.

Mogensen O, Mogensen B, Jacobsen A: Predictive value of CA 125 during early chemotherapy of advanced ovarian cancer. Gynecol Oncol 37:44, 1990.

Monga M, Carmichael JA, Shelly WE, et al; Surgery without adjuvant chemotherapy for early epithelial ovarian carcinoma after comprehensive surgical staging. Gynecol Oncol 43:195, 1991.

Morris M, Gershenson DM, Wharton JT: Secondary cytoreductive surgery in epithelial ovarian cancer: non-responders to first-line therapy. Gynecol Oncol 33:1, 1989.

Morrow CP, d'Ablaing G, Brady LW, et al: A clinical and pathologic study of 30 cases of malignant mixed Mullerian epithelial and mesenchymal ovarian tumors: a Gynecologic Oncology Group study. Gynecol Oncol 18:278, 1984.

Mosso ML, Colombo R, Giordano L, et al: Childhood cancer registry of the province of Torino, Italy: survival, incidence and mortality over 20 years. Cancer 69:1300, 1992.

Muderspach L, Muggia FM, Conti PS: Second look laparotomy for stage III epithelial ovarian cancer: rationale and current issues. Cancer Treat Issues 21:499, 1995.

Muggia FM, Hainsworth JD, Jeffers S, et al: Phase II study of liposomal doxorubicin in refractory ovarian cancer: antitumor activity and toxicity modification by liposomal encapsulation. J Clin Oncol 15:987, 1997.

Muggia FM, Liu PY, Alberts DS, et al: Intraperitoneal mitoxantrone or floxuridine: effects on time-to-failure and survival in patients with minimal residual ovarian cancer after second-look laparotomy. A randomized phase II study by the Southwest Oncology Group. Gynecol Oncol 61:395, 1996.

Mulhollan TJ, Silva EG, Tornos C, et al: Ovarian involvement by serous surface papillary carcinoma. Int J Gynecol Pathol 13:120, 1994.

Munkarah AR, Hallum AV, Morris M, et al: Prognostic significance of residual disease in patients with stage IV epithelial ovarian cancer. Gynecol Oncol 64:13, 1997.

Munnell EW: Is conservative therapy ever justified in stage I (Ia) cancer of the ovary? Am J Obstet Gynecol 103:641, 1969.

Muntz HG, Jones MA, Goff BA, et al: Malignant mixed müllerian tumors of the ovary: experience with surgical cytoreduction and combination chemotherapy. Cancer 76:1209, 1995.

Nasr MF, Kemp GM, Given FT Jr: Pseudomyxoma peritonei: treatment with intraperitoneal 5-fluorouracil. Eur J Gynaecol Oncol 14:213, 1993.

Nayar R, Siriaunkgul S, Robbins KM, et al: Microinvasion in low malignant potential tumors of the ovary. Hum Pathol 27:521, 1996.

Nicoletto MO, Tumolo S, Talamini R, et al: Surgical second-look in ovarian cancer: a randomized study in patients with laparoscopic complete remission. A Northeastern Oncology Cooperative Group–Ovarian Cancer Cooperative Group Study. J Clin Oncol 15:994, 1997.

NIH Consensus Development Conference statement: Ovarian cancer: screening, treatment, and follow-up. Gynecol Oncol 55(suppl):S4, 1994.

Nikrui N: Survey of clinical behavior of patients with borderline epithelial tumors of the ovary. Gynecol Oncol 12:107, 1981.

Norris HJ: Proliferative endometrioid tumors and endometrioid tumors of low malignant potential of the ovary. Int J Gynecol Pathol 12:134, 1993.

Norris HJ, Jensen RD: Relative frequency of ovarian neoplasms in children and adolescents. Cancer 30:713, 1972.

Obel EB: A comparative study of patients with cancer of the ovary, who have survived more or less than 10 years. Acta Obstet Gynaecol Scand 55:429, 1976.

Omura GA, Blessing JA, Ehrlich CE, et al: A randomized trial of cyclophosphamide and Adriamycin with or without cisplatin in advanced ovarian carcinoma: a Gynecologic Oncology Group study. Cancer 57:1725, 1986.

Omura GA, Brady MF, Homesley HD, et al: Long term follow-up and prognostic factor analysis in advanced ovarian carcinoma: the Gynecologic Oncology Group experience. J Clin Oncol 9:1138, 1991.

Omura GA, Morrow CP, Blessing JA, et al: A randomized comparison of melphalan versus melphalan plus hexamethylmelamine versus Adriamycin plus cyclophosphamide in ovarian carcinoma. Cancer 51:783, 1983.

Onnis A, Marchetti M, Padovan P. Castellan L: Neoadjuvant chemotherapy in advanced ovarian cancer. Eur J Gynaecol Oncol 176:393, 1996.

Padberg B-C, Arps H, Franke U, et al: DNA cytophotometry and prognosis in ovarian tumors of borderline malignancy. Cancer 69:2510, 1992.

Parmley T: Papillary tumors of the ovary [Editorial comments]. Int J Gynecol Pathol 1:313, 1982.

Patsner B, Orr JW, Mann WJ Jr, et al: Does serum CA-125 level prior to second-look laparotomy for invasive ovarian adenocarcinoma predict size of residual disease? Gynecol Oncol 38:373, 1990.

Pecorelli S, Sartori E, Santin A: Follow-up after primary therapy: management of the symptomatic patient—surgery. Gynecol Oncol 55:S138, 1994.

Peters WA, Blasko JC, Bagley CM, et al: Salvage therapy with whole-abdominal irradiation in patients with advanced carcinoma of the ovary previously treated by combination chemotherapy. Cancer 58:880, 1986.

Petru E, Lahousen M, Tamussino K, et al: Lymphadenectomy in stage I ovarian cancer. Am J Obstet Gynecol 170:656, 1994.

Pettersson F (ed): Annual Report of the Results of Treatment in Gynecologic Cancer, Vol. 20, International Federation of Gynecology and Obstetrics. Stockholm, Panoramic Press, 1988.

Pettersson F (ed): FIGO annual report on the results of treatment in gynecological cancer. Int J Gynecol Oncol 36(suppl):1, 1991.

Pezner RD, Stevens KR Jr, Tong D, Allen CV: Limited epithelial carcinoma of the ovary treated with curative intent by the intraperitoneal installation of radiocolloids. Cancer 42:2563, 1978.

Pickel H, Lahousen M, Stettner H, Girardi F: The spread of ovarian cancer. Bailliere's Clin Obstet Gynecol 3:3, 1989.

Piver MS, Jishi MF, Tsukada Y, Nava G: Primary peritoneal carcinoma after prophylactic oophorectomy in women with a family history of ovarian cancer. Cancer 71:2751, 1993.

Piver MS, Lele SB, Barlow JJ: Preoperative and intraoperative evaluation in ovarian malignancy. Obstet Gynecol 48:312, 1976.

Podratz KC, Cliby WA: Second look surgery in the management of epithelial ovarian carcinoma. Gynecol Oncol 55(suppl):128, 1994.

Podratz KC, Malkasian GD Jr, Hilton JF, et al: Second-look laparotomy in ovarian cancer: evaluation of pathologic variables. Am J Obstet Gynecol 152:230, 1985.

Podratz KC, Schray MF, Wieand HS, et al: Evaluation of treatment and survival after positive second-look laparotomy. Gynecol Oncol 31:9, 1988.

Pohl R, Dallenback-Hellweg G, Plugge T, et al: Prognostic parameters in patients with advanced ovarian malignant tumors. Eur J Gynaecol Oncol 3:160, 1984.

Potter ME, Hatch KD, Soong S-J, et al: Second-look laparotomy and salvage therapy: a research modality only? Gynecol Oncol 44:3, 1992.

Prat J, Young RH, Scully RE: Ovarian mucinous tumors with foci of anaplastic carcinoma. Cancer 50:300, 1982.

Randall CL, Hall DW, Armenia CS: Pathology in the preserved ovary after unilateral oophorectomy. Am J Obstet Gynecol 84:1233, 1962.

Redman CWE, Warwick J, Luesley DM, et al: Intervention debulking surgery in advanced epithelial ovarian cancer. Br J Obstet Gynaecol 101:142, 1994.

Reichman B, Markman M, Hakes T, et al: Intraperitoneal cisplatin and etoposide in the treatment of refractory/recurrent ovarian cancer. J Clin Oncol 7:1327, 1989.

Ries E: Pseudomyxoma peritonei. Surg Gynecol Obstet 39: 569, 1924.

Robinson WR, Curtin JP, Morrow CP: Operative staging and conservative surgery in the management of low malignant potential ovarian tumors. Int J Gynecol Cancer 2:118, 1992.

Rogers L, Varia M, Halle J, et al: ^{32}P following negative second-look laparotomy for epithelial ovarian cancer. Gynecol Oncol 50:141, 1993.

Ronnett BM, Kurman RJ, Zahn CM, et al: Pseudomyxoma peritonei in women: a clinicopathologic analysis of 30 cases with emphasis on site of origin, prognosis, and relationship to ovarian mucinous tumors of low malignant potential. Hum Pathol 26:509, 1995.

Rose PG, Piver S, Tsukada Y, Lau T: Metastatic patterns in histologic variants of ovarian cancer: an autopsy study. Cancer 64:1508, 1989.

Roth LM, Czernobilsky B: Ovarian Brenner tumors: II. Malignant. Cancer 56:592, 1985.

Roth LM, Czernobilsky B, Langley FA: Ovarian endometrioid adenofibromatous and cystadenofibromatous tumors: benign, proliferating, and malignant. Cancer 48:1838, 1981.

Roth LM, Langley FA, Fox H: Ovarian clear cell adenofibromatous tumors. Cancer 53:1156, 1984.

Rothacker D, Mobius G: Varieties of serous surface papillary carcinoma of the peritoneum in northern Germany: a thirty-year autopsy study. Int J Gynecol Pathol 14:310, 1995.

Rothenberg ML, Ozols RF, Glatstein E, et al: Dose-intensive induction therapy with cyclophosphamide, cisplatin, and consolidative abdominal radiation in advanced-stage epithelial ovarian cancer. J Clin Oncol 10:727, 1992.

Rubin SC, Hoskins WJ, Benjamin I, Lewis JL Jr: Palliative surgery for intestinal obstruction in advanced ovarian cancer. Gynecol Oncol 34:16, 1989a.

Rubin SC, Hoskins WJ, Hakes TB, et al: Serum CA-125 levels and surgical findings in patients undergoing secondary operations for epithelial ovarian cancer. Am J Obstet Gynecol 160:667, 1989b.

Rubin SC, Jones WB, Curtin JP, et al: Second-look laparotomy in stage I ovarian cancer following comprehensive surgical staging. Obstet Gynecol 82:139, 1993.

Russell P: The pathological assessment of ovarian neoplasms. I. Introduction to the common 'epithelial' tumours and analysis of benign 'epithelial' tumours. Pathology 11:5, 1979a.

Russell P: The pathological assessment of ovarian neoplasms. II. The proliferating 'epithelial' tumours. Pathology 11:251, 1979b.

Russell P, Merkur H: Proliferating ovarian "epithelial" tumours: a clinico-pathological analysis of 144 cases. Aust N Z J Obstet Gynaecol 19:45, 1979.

Sainz de la Cruz R, Eichorn JH, Rice LW, et al: Histologic transformation of benign endometriosis to early epithelial ovarian cancer. Gynecol Oncol 60:238, 1996.

Sampson JA: Endometrial carcinoma of ovary arising in endometrial tissue in that organ. Arch Surg 10:1, 1925.

Sandenbergh HA, Woodruff JD: Histogenesis of pseudomyxoma peritonei. Obstet Gynecol 49:339, 1977.

Scarabelli C, Gallo A, Zarrelli Z, et al: Systematic pelvic and para-aortic lymphadenectomy during cytoreductive surgery in advanced ovarian cancer: potential benefit on survival. Gynecol Oncol 56:328, 1995.

Schueler JA, Cornelisse CJ, Hermans J, et al: Prognostic factors in well-differentiated early-stage epithelial ovarian cancer. Cancer 71:787, 1993.

Schwartz PE, Chambers J, Makuch R: Neoadjuvant chemotherapy for advanced ovarian cancer. Gynecol Oncol 53: 33, 1994.

Schwartz PE, Smith JP: Second-look operations in ovarian cancer. Am J Obstet Gynecol 138:1124, 1980.

Scully RE: Tumors of the ovary and maldeveloped gonads. In: Atlas of Tumor Pathology, Second Series, Fascicle 16. Washington, DC, Armed Forces Institute of Pathology, 1979.

Segna RA, Dottino PR, Mandeli JP, et al: Secondary cytoreduction for ovarian cancer following cisplatin therapy. J Clin Oncol 11:434, 1993.

Siedman JD, Elsayed AM, Sobin LH, Tavassoli FA: Association of mucinous tumors of the ovary and appendix: a clinicopathologic study of 25 cases. Am J Surg Pathol 17: 22, 1993a.

Seidman JD, Norris HJ, Griffin JL, Hitchcock CL: DNA flow cytometric analysis of serous ovarian tumors of low malignant potential. Cancer 71:3947, 1993b.

Seifer DB, Kennedy AW, Webster KD, et al: Outcome of primary cytoreduction surgery for advanced epithelial ovarian carcinoma. Cleve Clin J Med 55:555, 1988.

Shevchuk MM, Fenoglio CM, Richart RM: Histogenesis of Brenner tumor: I. Histology and ultrastructure. Cancer 46: 2607, 1980.

Shevchuk MM, Winkler-Monsanto B, Fenoglio CM, Richart RM: Clear cell carcinoma of the ovary: a clinicopathologic study with review of the literature. Cancer 47:1344, 1981.

Silva EG, Tornos C, Malpica A, Gershenson DM: Recurrence in ovarian serous tumor of low malignant potential [Abstract No. 75]. Gynecol Oncol 56:129, 1995.

Sipes SL, Newton M, Lurain JR: Chylous ascites: a sequel of pelvic radiation therapy. Obstet Gynecol 66:832, 1985.

Smirz LR, Stehman FB, Ulbright TM, et al: Second-look laparotomy after chemotherapy in the management of ovarian malignancy. Am J Obstet Gynecol 152:661, 1985.

Smith JP, Rutledge FN, Delclos L: Postoperative treatment of early cancer of the ovary: a random trial between postoperative irradiation and chemotherapy. Natl Cancer Inst Monogr 42:149, 1975.

Snider DD, Stuart GC, Nation JG, Robertson DI: Evaluation of surgical staging in stage I low malignant potential ovarian tumors. Gynecol Oncol 40:129, 1991.

Snyder RR, Norris HJ, Tavassoli F: Endometrioid proliferative and low malignant potential tumors of the ovary: a clinicopathologic study of 46 cases. Am J Surg Pathol 12: 661, 1988.

Soper JT, Berchuck A, Clarke-Pearson DL: Adjuvant intraperitoneal chromic phosphate therapy for woman with apparent early ovarian carcinoma who have not undergone comprehensive surgical staging. Cancer 68:725, 1991.

Soper JT, Berchuck A, Dodge R, Clarke-Pearson DL: Adjuvant therapy with intraperitoneal chromic phosphate (^{32}P) in women with early ovarian carcinoma after comprehensive surgical staging. Obstet Gynecol 79:993, 1992.

Spirtos NM, Gross GM, Freddo JL, Ballon SC: Cytoreductive surgery in advanced epithelial cancer of the ovary: the impact of aortic and pelvic lymphadenectomy. Gynecol Oncol 56:345, 1995.

Stier EA, Barakat RR, Curtin JP, et al: Laparotomy to complete staging of presumed early ovarian cancer. Obstet Gynecol 87:737, 1996.

Stiff P, Bayer R, Camarda M, et al: A phase II trial of high-dose mitoxantrone, carboplatin, and cyclophosphamide with autologous bone marrow rescue for recurrent epithelial ovarian carcinoma: analysis of risk factors for clinical outcome. Gynecol Oncol 57:278, 1995.

Surwit E, Childers J, Atlas I, et al: Neoadjuvant chemotherapy for advanced ovarian cancer. Int J Gynecol Cancer 6: 356, 1996.

Taylor HC Jr: Malignant and semimalignant tumors of the ovary. Surg Gynecol Obstet 48:204, 1929.

Tazelaar HD, Bostwick DG, Ballon SC, et al: Conservative treatment of borderline ovarian tumors. Obstet Gynecol 66:417, 1985.

ten Bokkel Huinink W, Veenhof C, Huizing M, et al: Carboplatin and paclitaxel in patients with advanced ovarian cancer: a dose finding study. Semin Oncol 24(suppl 2): 31, 1997.

Tharp M, Hornback NB: Complications associated with intraperitoneal ^{32}P. Gynecol Oncol 53:170, 1994.

Thomas GM: Radiotherapy in early ovarian cancer. Gynecol Oncol 55(suppl):S73, 1994.

Tobachman JK, Tucker MA, Kane R: Intraabdominal carcinomatosis after prophylactic oophorectomy in ovarian cancer-prone families. Lancet 2:795, 1982.

Towne BH, Mahour GH, Wooley MW, Isaacs H Jr: Ovarian cysts and tumors in infancy and childhood. J Pediatr Surg 10:311, 1975.

van der Burg ME, Lammes FB, van Putten LJ, Stoter G: Ovarian cancer: the prognostic value of the serum half-life of CA-125 during induction chemotherapy. Gynecol Oncol 30:307, 1988.

van der Burg ME, van Lent M, Buyse M, et al: The effect of debulking surgery after induction chemotherapy on the prognosis in advanced epithelial ovarian cancer. N Engl J Med 332:629, 1995.

Vergote IB, Kaern J, Abeler VM, et al: Analysis of prognostic factors in stage I epthelial ovarian carcinoma: importance of degree of differentiation and deoxyribonucleic acid ploidy in predicting relapse. Am J Obstet Gynecol 169:40, 1993.

Vergote IB, Vergote-De Vos LN, Abeler VM, et al: Randomized trial comparing cisplatin with radioactive phosphorus or whole-abdomen irradiation as adjuvant treatment of ovarian cancer. Cancer 69:741, 1992.

Vogl SE, Pagano M, Kaplan BH, et al: Cisplatin based combination chemotherapy for advanced ovarian cancer: high overall response rate with curative potential only in women with small tumor burdens. Cancer 51:2024, 1983.

Walker-Renard PB, Vaughan LM, Sahn SA: Chemical pleurodesis for malignant pleural effusions. Ann Intern Med 120:56, 1994.

Walton L. Ellenberg SS, Major FJ, et al: Results of second-look laparotomy in patients with early-stage ovarian carcinoma. Obstet Gynecol 70:770, 1987.

Wertheim I, Fleischhacker D, McLachlin CM, et al: Pseudomyxoma peritonei: a review of 23 cases. Obstet Gynecol 84:17, 1994.

Wharton JT, Herson J: Surgery for common epithelial tumors of the ovary. Cancer 48:582, 1981.

Williams L: The role of secondary cytoreductive surgery in epithelial ovarian malignancies. Oncology 6:25, 1992.

Williams TJ, Dockerty MB: Status of the contralateral ovary in encapsulated low grade malignant tumors of the ovary. Surg Gynecol Obstet 143:763, 1976.

Woodruff JD, Dietrich D, Genadry R, Parmley TH: Proliferative and malignant Brenner tumors. Am J Obstet Gynecol 141:118, 1981.

Woodruff JD, Solomon D, Sullivan H: Multifocal disease in the upper genital canal. Obstet Gynecol 65:695, 1985.

Woodruff JD, TeLinde RW: The histology and histogenesis of ovarian neoplasia. Cancer 37:411, 1976.

Yazigi R, Sandstad J, Munoz AK: Primary staging in ovarian tumors of low malignant potential. Gynecol Oncol 31:402, 1988.

Young RC, Decker DG, Wharton JT, et al: Staging laparotomy in early ovarian cancer. JAMA 250:3072, 1983.

Young RC, Walton LA, Ellenberg SS, et al: Adjuvant therapy in stage I and stage II epithelial ovarian cancer. N Engl J Med 322:1021, 1990.

Young RH, Oliva E, Scully RE: Small cell carcinoma of the ovary, hypercalcemic type: a clinicopathological analysis of 150 cases. Am J Surg Pathol 18:1102, 1994.

Young RH, Prat J, Scully RE: Endometrioid stromal sarcomas of the ovary. Cancer 53:1143, 1984.

Young RH, Scully RE: Mucinous ovarian tumors associated with mucinous adenocarcinomas of the cervix. Int J Gynecol Pathol 7:99, 1988.

Zaino RJ, Unger ER, Whitney C: Synchronous carcinomas of the uterine corpus and ovary. Gynecol Oncol 19:329, 1984.

Zanetta G, Keeney GL, Cha SS, et al: Flow-cytometric analysis of deoxyribonucleic acid content in advanced ovarian carcinoma: its importance in long-term survival. Am J Obstet Gynecol 175:1217, 1996.

Zervos EE, McCormick J, Goode SE, Rosemurgy AS: Peritoneovenous shunts in patients with intractable ascites: palliation at what price? Am Surg 63:157, 1997.

CHAPTER

11

Tumors of the Ovary: Sex Cord Stromal Tumors and Germ Cell Tumors

SEX CORD STROMAL TUMORS

Approximately 5 percent of all ovarian neoplasms are derived from the specialized gonadal stroma. These were formerly referred to as *functioning* tumors because many of them synthesize steroidal hormones such as estrogen, progesterone, testosterone, other androgenic compounds, and certain corticosteroids. However, hormone production is not a feature unique to gonadal stromal tumors. Any ovarian neoplasm, primary or metastatic, may stimulate the non-neoplastic ovarian stroma to synthesize and secrete sex steroids (Aiman et al, 1986a,b). Since not all ovarian sex cord stromal tumors secrete hormones, and since it is not rare for non–sex cord stromal tumors to do so, these tumors are no longer categorized as "functioning."

The anlagen of the adrenal gland and gonad develop in adjacent areas of the embryo. Together, they have been called the steroid ridge. This proximity of embryologic origin probably accounts for the fact that some ovarian stromal tumors resemble adrenal neoplasms, although origin from adrenal rests may also occur. The embryonic gonad is sexually bipotential, and the parenchyma of the ovary and the testicle are derived from the same primitive gonadal stroma. Teilum (1977) has pointed out that granulosa and Sertoli cells are homologous, as are theca and Leydig cells. It is not too surprising, then, that both ovarian and testicular tumors can reproduce the histologic and hormonal features of male and female gonadal stroma. Gonadal or sex cord stromal tumors are classified according to their differentiation toward ovarian follicles, testicular tubules, Leydig cells, and adrenal cortical cells. The majority are tumors of "female-directed" cells, classified as

granulosa-theca tumors. A smaller percentage belong in the Sertoli-Leydig cell category and are considered to be tumors of "male-directed" cells. The gynandroblastoma contains elements of both male- and female-directed cells.

The lipid cell tumors encompass a group of neoplasms consisting primarily of Leydig (hilus)-like cells or adrenocortical-like cells, or both. Not infrequently, sex cord stromal tumors are insufficiently differentiated to allow exact classification. As mentioned earlier, hormone production by sex cord stromal tumors is not consistent and has not proven to be a reliable means of classifying this group of neoplasms. Paradoxically, a tumor composed of apparently female-directed cells (granulosa or theca) is occasionally associated with evidence of androgen production, and tumors of male-directed cells may produce estrogen. In addition, 15 percent of stromal tumors are apparently hormonally inert. Sex cord stromal tumors have also been variously classified as gonadal-stromal tumors and mesenchymomas. For the most part, sex cord stromal tumors are either benign or of low malignant potential.

Approximately 10 percent of gonadal stromal tumors cannot be readily classified as either granulosa or Sertoli-Leydig cell tumors. In a study of 32 such cases from the Armed Forces Institute of Pathology, the stage and survival were similar to those of the better differentiated sex cord stromal tumors (Seidman, 1996).

Granulosa Stromal Tumors

Granulosa cell and theca cell tumors occur with approximately equal frequency. Not uncommonly, there is an admixture of granulosa and theca elements, but these cases should be classified as granulosa cell tumors, which are malignant, and the term *thecoma* or *theca cell tumor* should be reserved for neoplasms consisting entirely of theca cells. Both granulosa cell and theca cell tumors are frequently associated with estrogen production. The clinical effects of estrogen secretion depend to a certain degree on the patient's age. The most dramatic alterations occur in girls, who may develop isosexual precocious puberty in response to the estrogen stimulation. During the reproductive years, menorrhagia and irregular bleeding are the most common symptoms, although amenorrhea is experienced by some patients. In the postmenopausal age group, resumption of vaginal bleeding, breast enlargement and tenderness, vaginal cornification, and other evidence of estrogen stimulation can be sequelae of functioning granulosa and theca tumors.

Granulosa Cell Tumors

About 50 percent of granulosa cell tumors (GCTs) occur in postmenopausal women, while less than 5 percent develop in prepubertal girls. The mean age at diagnosis is 53 years. An unusual feature of GCT is its propensity to rupture, causing pain and intraperitoneal bleeding, which can be of major proportions. Pregnancy and labor apparently increase the predisposition of GCTs to rupture. Such an event may simulate abruptio placentae. In the nonpregnant woman, hemorrhage from a GCT may mimic a ruptured tubal pregnancy. Adenocarcinoma of the endometrium is associated with granulosa (and theca) cell tumors in 5 to 15 percent of the cases, and 50 percent have associated endometrial hyperplasia or polyps. The association is twice as common in the postmenopausal age group. For this reason any postmenopausal woman with endometrial hyperplasia who is not receiving medicinal estrogen and is not obese should be suspected of having a functioning ovarian tumor of the granulosa-theca cell type. Such tumors may be too small to be readily palpated on pelvic examination; in these cases ultrasound and serum estradiol measurement may be helpful. A serum estradiol value of greater than 30 pg/ml in a postmenopausal woman not taking estrogens should raise suspicion of an estrogen-producing tumor.

Several hormones other than estrogen can be elaborated by GCTs. Among these are inhibin and follicle-regulating protein, both peptide hormones secreted by the normal granulosa cell (Lappohn et al, 1989; Rodgers et al, 1990). Inhibin testing is available commercially to use as a tumor marker. Rarely, GCTs secrete androgens, and virilization may be seen.

The prognostic clinicopathologic features of GCTs have been investigated in several large series (Norris and Taylor, 1968; Fox et al, 1975; Stenwig et al, 1979; Evans et al, 1980; Bjorkholm and Silfversward, 1981). Survival is most strongly affected by the stage at presentation. The 5- and 10-year corrected survival rates for stage I cases are greater than 95 and 95 percent, respectively, compared with 55 and 25 percent for stages II and III (Fig. 11-1).

Fortunately, 85 percent or more of the cases at diagnosis are stage Ia. The cases of bilateral ovarian involvement seem to have an unexpectedly poor outlook. In the series of Fox et al (1975), all seven stage Ib cases eventually recurred, suggesting that involvement of the second ovary may have been metastatic. It must be borne in mind that the GCTs tend to recur late. Thus the total recurrence risk is obscured by deaths from intercurrent disease and short follow-up. From these various reports, the average time to recurrence is between 5 and 10 years, with some recurrences taking place as late as 20

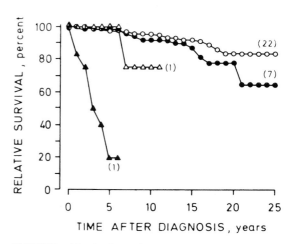

FIGURE 11-1. Granulosa cell tumor. Relative survival for clinical stage I patients with a low mitosis count ($\circ$, $n = 112$) or a high mitosis count ($\bullet$, $n = 67$) and stages II through IV with low ($\triangle$, $n = 4$) or high ($\blacktriangle$, $n = 12$) mitosis counts. Numbers in parentheses indicate patients still under observation. (From Bjorkholm E, Silfversward C: Prognostic factors in granulosa-cell tumors. Gynecol Oncol 11:261, 1981, with permission.)

years after the initial diagnosis. Fox et al estimated that 50 percent of women with a GCT would die of recurrence within 20 years if other causes of death were eliminated. However, this does not appear to be applicable to stage I cases, for which Stenwig et al (1979) and also Bjorkholm and Silfversward (1981) observed a death rate due to disease of only 15 to 20 percent at 20 years.

Another important prognostic factor of GCTs seems to be size and the associated feature of rupture. The long-term outcome is almost uniformly good with a stage I lesion less than 5 cm in diameter, compared with a recurrence rate of 20 percent for lesions 5 to 15 cm, and of more than 30 percent for lesions more than 15 cm in diameter. The prognosis is also adversely affected by a high mitosis count (>2/10 hpf), and perhaps by atypia. Most investigators observed a better prognosis for GCTs in women less than 40 years of age and also in children (Zaloudek and Norris, 1982). This may reflect, in part, the representation of the more favorable juvenile and cystic GCTs in these age groups (see later). Lymphatic space invasion and capsular invasion probably increase the risk of recurrence.

Histochemical analysis of granulosa cell tumors has detected large amounts of progesterone and cytoplasmic progesterone receptor protein (Meyer et al, 1982). It is unknown if this has prognostic or therapeutic implications, although response to progestin therapy is reported. High S-phase fraction and aneuploidy as measured by flow cytometry may be associated with a poorer prognosis (Klemi et al, 1990; Roush et al, 1995). The finding of trisomy 12 in granulosa tumors is consistent with their generally indolent behavior (Fletcher et al, 1991).

On gross examination, GCTs are usually solid and cystic, with areas of hemorrhage. They occasionally consist wholly of single or multiple thin-walled cysts. Microscopically, GCTs typically exhibit a mixture of patterns, including the microfollicular, macrofollicular, trabecular, insular, and diffuse (formerly and unfortunately referred to as sarcomatoid) types. Theca cells are often present, and luteinization is not uncommon. The pathognomonic Call-Exner bodies (Fig. 11−2) are present in the microfollicular arrangement. No pattern or combination of patterns is predictive of a better or worse outcome. Poorly differentiated adenocarcinoma, carcinoid, other stromal tumors, and breast cancer metastatic to the ovary have been confused with GCT. Obviously, such an error would badly misrepresent the patient's prognosis and lead to mismanagement.

Juvenile Granulosa Cell Tumors

The juvenile variant of GCT, originally described by Scully (1977), accounts for 85 percent of the granulosa category in prepubertal females, and 7 to 12 percent of all ovarian tumors in children (Vassal et al, 1988). It rarely occurs in older women. In Scully's updated series of 125 cases (Young et al, 1984), the juvenile GCT was associated with isosexual precocity in 70 percent of the prepubertal cases, was almost always palpable on pelvic or rectal examination, and proved to be bilateral in less than 5 percent of cases. Three fourths were stage Ia at diagnosis.

Grossly, the tumors express great variability in composition, ranging from solid to multicystic, with or without areas of hemorrhage and necrosis. The characteristic microscopic features include nodules of granulosa cells, frequently luteinized, which are solid or have a central cavity containing mucin. The nuclei of the granulosa cells appear less mature than in the adult forms of GCT. Confusion with the more malignant endodermal sinus tumor and embryonal carcinoma is possible. There appears to be an association with Ollier's disease (multiple endochondromatosis). Only 1 of 70 stage Ia cases recurred, compared to 3 of 20 stage Ic cases. All three patients with more advanced disease died. Except in the stage Ia group, malignant behavior seemed to correlate with size, mitosis count, and nuclear atypia.

Cystic Granulosa Cell Tumors

An occasional GCT is composed entirely of one or more thin-walled cysts filled with a clear, yellow fluid, grossly resembling a serous cystadenoma. These occur predominantly in young women and adolescent females. Several have been associated with virilization. Microscopically, the cysts are lined with thin layers of granulosa cells containing numerous Call-Exner bodies. In general, the prognosis for these cases appears to be better than that for solid and cystic-solid GCTs.

Thecomas-Fibromas

The thecoma-fibroma tumors represent a spectrum of neoplastic growths derived from

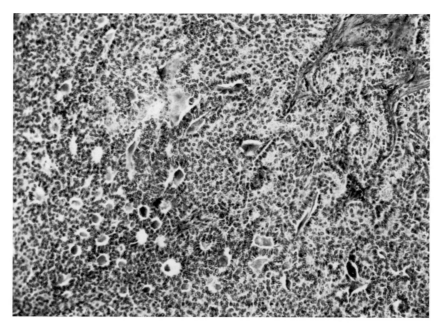

FIGURE 11–2. Granulosa cell tumor. Microfollicular pattern with characteristic Call-Exner bodies on the left side of the photograph.

ovarian stromal cells, ranging from tumors composed entirely of collagen-producing fibroblasts (fibromas) to tumors containing a predominance of lipid-rich theca cells (thecomas). All of these tumors share many similar clinical characteristics and frequently cannot be readily assigned to either the thecoma or fibroma category on the basis of clinical or microscopic examination.

Fibromas

Fibromas are typically unilateral, benign neoplasms that do not elaborate clinically significant amounts of sex steroids. The mean age at diagnosis is 48 years. Fibromas account for 1 to 5 percent of all ovarian tumors, 10 percent are bilateral, and a similar proportion are found to have a twisted pedicle at exploratory surgery. Fibromas are slow-growing tumors that present with a mass, pelvic heaviness, or pelvic pain. Calcification, which occurs in about 5 percent of cases, is occasionally extensive. These tumors are typically solid and heavy. On cut section they are white, and degenerative cystic cavities are not uncommon. The average size is 6 cm; however, the average size increases with the age at diagnosis. Also associated with tumor size is the presence of stromal edema and intraperitoneal fluid.

Ascites (>200 ml of peritoneal fluid) is reported in one third of patients with ovarian fibromas greater than 6 cm in diameter (Dockerty and Masson, 1944). While the volume is usually less than 500 ml, when ascites is clinically detectable and associated with hydrothorax, the condition is popularly known as *Meigs' syndrome* (Meigs et al, 1943). In Dockerty and Masson's series, this was found in only 2 of 283 patients with an ovarian fibroma (51 had "ascites"). Nevertheless, the syndrome is important because, as Meigs pointed out, some women with ascites, hydrothorax, and pelvic tumor (especially those with body wasting) have not been offered surgery because of the mistaken impression that they had far-advanced malignancy. Similarly, it would be an error to treat such a patient with chemotherapy without cytologic or histologic documentation that the patient has cancer.

The hydrothorax in Meigs' syndrome undoubtedly results from ascitic fluid entering the pleural space through the diaphragm, usually on the right side. The etiology of the ascites is unsettled. The prevailing hypothesis, that the fluid is a transudate from the ovarian tumor resulting from venous and lymphatic obstruction, is based upon the common findings of interstitial edema, evidence of torsion, and the absence of a true capsule enveloping the tumor (Dockerty and Masson, 1944; Samanth and Black, 1970).

While ovarian fibromas are rare in children and adolescents, they occur commonly in young women with the multiple basal cell nevus (Gorlin's) syndrome. This autosomal dominant disorder is characterized by basal cell nevi and carcinomas, dental cysts, and skeletal and other abnormalities. In these cases the ovarian fibromas are typically bilateral, multinodular, and calcified. Resection with ovarian preservation can sometimes be accomplished, although recurrence may be expected (Raggio et al, 1983).

Cellular Fibromas and Fibrosarcomas

Cellular fibromas of the ovary, which must be considered low-grade malignancies, and fibrosarcomas account for less than 1 percent of ovarian fibromatous neoplasms. Prat and Scully (1981) have distinguished these two lesions on the basis of mitosis counts, the low-grade malignancies having 1 to 3 mitoses/10 hpf and the overt sarcomas more than 3 mitoses/10 hpf. The size of these tumors averages two to three times that of benign fibromas. At surgery, malignancy is suggested by rupture, adhesions, hemorrhage, necrosis, and a soft consistency.

Thecomas

Thecomas are distinguishable clinically from fibromas by their estrogenic activity. It is common for women with thecomas to present with postmenopausal bleeding, menometrorrhagia, or amenorrhea, depending upon the functional status of their ovaries. An occasional patient will have evidence of androgen production. The age at diagnosis, incidence of bilateralism, malignancy, and tumor size are very similar to that of fibromas. Thecomas appear, however, to be less commonly associated with ascites. While breast changes are unusual, uterine pathology is the rule. Uterine myomas (30 percent), endometrial polyps (20 percent), all forms of endometrial hyperplasia (50 percent), and endometrial carcinoma (10 percent) occur with frequencies similar to those reported for GCTs (Norris and Taylor, 1968; Anikwue et al, 1978).

Grossly, the thecoma is usually firm and heavy, with a white to yellow to orange color on cut surface, depending upon the amount of lipid material within the cells. Nests of lutein or, rarely, Leydig cells are present on microscopic examination (Zhang et al, 1982).

Very rarely, thecomas are malignant. When this occurs, loss of differentiation results in a predominant cell pattern of primitive ovarian stromal cells or fibroblasts. Scully recommends the same criteria to define both malignant thecoma and ovarian fibrosarcoma (Young and Scully, 1982).

Sclerosing Stromal Tumors

A sclerosing stromal tumor of the thecomafibroma group has been described by Chalvardjian and Scully (1973). More than 60 cases have now been reported in the literature. The average patient age is 25 years. All cases have been unilateral and benign. The characteristic microscopic features are pseudolobulation, cellular areas alternating with areas of edema or collagenization (sclerosis), and a prominent vascular network.

Sertoli-Leydig Cell Tumors

Also known as androblastomas, the Sertoli-Leydig cell tumors (SLCTs) are characterized by differentiation toward testicular structures. They constitute less than 1 percent of all ovarian tumors and are characterized by the presence of Sertoli cells, Leydig cells, and fetal-like testicular tissue. Many SLCTs are masculinizing, although estrogen production may predominate.

Sertoli Cell Tumors

Pure Sertoli cell tumors (Pick's adenoma; folliculome lipidique) are rare. They manifest the range of histologic differentiation exhibited by other SLCTs. The average age at diagnosis is about 27 years. Sixty-five percent of these patients have clinical signs of estrogen production, usually metrorrhagia. The tumors are unilateral, solid, and often lobulated, with a yellow to tan appearance on cut section. The presence of androgen excess is evidence against the diagnosis of a pure Sertoli cell tumor, since androgen production is the province of Leydig cells. Malignant behavior is uncommon but can be predicated on the findings of increased mitotic activity, poor differentiation, hemorrhage, and necrosis (Tavassoli and Norris, 1980; Young and Scully, 1984a,b).

Arrhenoblastomas (Androblastomas)

The most frequently encountered SLCT is best known by its trivial name, *arrhenoblastoma* (from the Greek *arrhenos*, male). In addition to the mixture of Sertoli and Leydig cells, it also contains tissues similar to those of the fetal testis. The arrhenoblastoma, or androblastoma, is the prototype of the primary, virilizing ovarian neoplasm. However, it is occasionally associated with estrogenic or progestational manifestations (Stegner and Lisboa, 1984; Tracy et al, 1985), and approximately 15 percent demonstrate no clinical evidence of hormonal activity. Familial occurrence of the SLCT and an association with thyroid disease have been reported.

The average age at diagnosis is 25 to 30 years. Clinical hormonal effects are not as age dependent in masculinizing tumors as they are in estrogenic tumors, although the changes are less obtrusive in the postmenopausal woman. During the reproductive years, defeminization usually precedes virilization, but these two features may occur in a disorderly fashion. The former process includes oligomenorrhea with atrophy of the breast and genital tissues. The more reliable indicators of excess androgen production are the signs (Fig. 11–3) and symptoms of virilization: clitoromegaly, hirsutism, acne, hoarseness, and increased libido. Less often, the body muscle mass increases and temporal balding occurs. These changes frequently develop over a period of several years before diagnosis. While a rapid onset of virilization is considered characteristic of a neoplastic etiology, even in young women the symptoms and signs of an androgenic tumor are often insidious. With an average size of 10 cm, the arrhenoblastoma is not always palpable on clinical examination, even when there is overt evidence of endocrine activity. Only 3 percent are bilateral. An elevated alpha-fetoprotein (AFP) level has been reported (Mann et al, 1986).

The analysis by Young and Scully (1985) has clarified the malignant potential of the SLCTs. There are four categories, based on the microscopic features: (1) well differentiated: tubules of Sertoli cells separated by variable numbers of Leydig cells (Young and Scully, 1984b); (2) intermediately differentiated: cords and sheets of immature Sertoli cells separated by stroma, usually containing Leydig cells; (3) poorly differentiated: tumors predominantly composed of spindleoid Sertoli cells; and (4) SLCTs with heterologous elements. Sertoli-Leydig cell tumors with a retiform pattern accounted for 15 percent of SLCTs with heterologous elements in the series of Young and Scully.

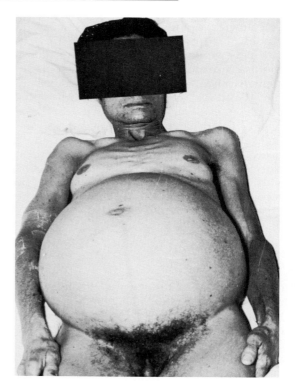

FIGURE 11–3. Arrhenoblastoma. This 45-year-old woman is obviously masculinized. In addition to clitoromegaly and facial hirsutism, she developed hoarseness. The male body habitus is partially obscured by the abdominal distension resulting from ascites. Arrhenoblastoma usually occurs in younger women and seldom manifests overt malignant behavior.

These rare tumors are often misdiagnosed as either a serous adenocarcinoma or endodermal sinus tumor (Young and Scully, 1985; Talerman, 1987). About 60 percent of all cases are clinically androgenic, but malignant behavior is exhibited only by less well-differentiated tumors and tumors with immature muscle or cartilage (Prat et al, 1982). These variants occur, on the average, in younger women and are larger at the time of diagnosis than the better differentiated benign lesions. Heterologous components such as mucinous epithelium and carcinoid appear to augur a better prognosis than muscle and cartilage (Young et al, 1982a). Malignancy is suggested by mitotic activity, hemorrhage, necrosis, and poor differentiation. Overall, perhaps 50 percent of the poorly differentiated tumors recur in spite of early stage at diagnosis. Those with immature muscle or cartilage may have an even worse prognosis, but these elements are found with poorly differentiated, homologous elements 90 percent of the time.

Sex Cord Tumor with Annular Tubules

The sex cord tumor with annular tubules (SCTAT), described by Scully (1970), is associated one third of the time with the Peutz-Jeghers syndrome: gastrointestinal polyposis with oral and cutaneous melanin pigmentation. When associated with this syndrome, SCTATs are more often bilateral, multifocal, and small, with areas of calcification. In addition, 15 percent of these cases are reported to have adenoma malignum of the cervix (see Chapter 5). While SCTATs in women with Peutz-Jeghers syndrome are invariably benign, about 20 percent of the gross tumors not associated with this syndrome have developed metastases (Young and Scully, 1982; Young et al, 1982b). Evidence of estrogen excess is found in about one half of the cases. Focal differentiation toward Sertoli or granulosa cells may be found.

Leydig and Hilus Cell Tumors

Leydig cell tumors are composed entirely of Leydig cells. The designation *hilus cell tumor* is reserved for Leydig cell tumors located in the ovarian hilum. Leydig cell tumors characteristically produce testosterone; are unilateral, usually not palpable, yellow-orange in color, and almost invariably benign; and occur predominantly after age 50. They are distinguished from lipid or lipoid cell tumors primarily by the presence of Reinke crystals, the pathognomonic microscopic feature of Leydig cells (Table 11–1). Clinically, Leydig cell

TABLE 11–1

Characteristics of Leydig (Hilus) Cell and Lipid (Lipoid) Cell Tumors

Feature	Leydig (Hilus) Cell	Lipid (Lipoid) Cell
Crystals of Reinke	Present	Absent
Age	Postmenopausal	Premenopausal
Androgen production	Testosterone (T)	Androstenedione and T
Size	Nonpalpable	Palpable
Malignancy	None	20%
Virilization	Often mild, protracted	Tends to be more rapid, severe

tumors must be distinguished from adrenal causes of androgen excess, especially adrenal adenoma. High testosterone values are generally considered to indicate an ovarian tumor, while high dehydroepiandrosterone sulfate (DHEAS) levels point to an adrenal tumor. Stimulation-suppression tests are unreliable in discriminating neoplastic from non-neoplastic ovarian lesions (see "Evaluation of Androgen Excess" later in this chapter).

Lipid (Lipoid) Cell Tumors

Lipid cell tumors are characterized by large rounded or polyhedral cells resembling Leydig (or hilus) cells, luteinized ovarian stromal cells, and adrenocortical cells. Crystals of Reinke are absent. These testosterone-producing tumors, unlike Leydig cell tumors and SLCTs, are often associated with a substantial increase in serum androstenedione. Lipid cell tumors can also produce estrogens and progesterone. Cushingoid features have been reported, as have two well-documented cases of ovarian lipid cell tumor with elevated serum cortisol (Chetkowksi et al, 1985).

Lipid cell tumors are typically unilateral but, unlike the Leydig cell tumors, perhaps as many as 20 percent are malignant. On the average, the patients with lipid cell tumors are younger and their tumors larger than what is reported for Leydig cell tumors. Those with pleomorphism, increased mitoses, or large size (>8 cm) should be considered malignant.

Gynandroblastomas

Very rarely a gonadal stromal tumor contains unequivocal granulosa cell elements combined with tubules and Leydig cells characteristic of the arrhenoblastoma (Chalvardjian and Derzko, 1982). These tumors are designated gynandroblastomas, and may be associated with either androgen or estrogen production. They can be expected to behave according to the nature of the individual components.

Evaluation of Androgen Excess

The differential diagnosis of androgen excess (Table 11–2) primarily involves discriminating between adrenal and gonadal hyperplasia and neoplasia (Lobo, 1994). The presence of a unilateral adnexal mass is very good evidence of an ovarian neoplastic source of ex-

TABLE 11-2

Differential Diagnosis of Androgen Excess

Androgen Source	Clinical Data	Laboratory Data*
Adrenal—non-neoplastic		
Congenital hyperplasia (adult onset)	Short, anovulatory	Serum 17-OH-progesterone >3.3 ng/ml
Bilateral hyperplasia (Cushing's)	Striae, hump, obese, diabetic	↑ Serum cortisol
Androgen excess		DHEAS 2.5–8 μg/ml
Adrenal—neoplastic		
Adenoma	Computed tomography scan	DHEAS > 8.0 μg/ml or T > 150 ng/dl
Carcinoma	Usually palpable	DHEAS > 8.0 μg/ml
Ovary—non-neoplastic		
Polycystic ovary	Ovaries up to three times normal size; infertility; oligomenorrhea	T < 150 ng/dl
Hyperthecosis	Ovaries up to three times normal size; obesity; hypertension; glucose intolerance	T 150–200 ng/dl
Nodular, theca-lutein hyperplasia	Patient pregnant; discovered at cesarean section; resolves postpartum	T up to 450 ng/dl
Ovary—neoplastic		
Sertoli-Leydig cell		↑ T†
Leydig-hilus cell	Often not palpable	↑ T
Lipid (lipoid) cell		DHEAS normal; ↑ urinary 17-ketosteroids; ↑ A; ↑ T
Granulosa, theca cell		↑ T
Brenner, dermoid, mucinous, Krukenberg		↑ T

*↑ = increased; DHEAS, dehydroepiandrosterone sulfate; T, testosterone; A, androstenedione.
†Serum testosterone value considered to be increased when greater than 200 ng/dl.

cess androgen, whereas bilateral ovarian enlargement points more to a stromal hyperplasia if the ovaries are less than 6 cm in diameter. In the presence of ovaries not perceptibly enlarged on pelvic examination, neoplasia and hyperplasia are both reasonable possibilities.

The work-up of androgen excess (Table 11-3) includes pelvic and transvaginal ultrasound plus measurement of serum DHEAS and testosterone levels. Since 90 percent of serum DHEAS is derived from the adrenal gland, a high value points to the adrenal gland as the source of excess androgen production. Conversely, an elevated serum testosterone level points to the ovary, which normally accounts for two thirds of the serum

TABLE 11-3

Work-up of Patients With Androgen Excess

Physical examination
Ultrasound examination of ovaries
Computed tomography (CT) scan of adrenals
Serum DHEAS, testosterone (T), luteinizing hormone, 17-OH-progesterone, cortisol
Repeat T, selective ovarian vein catheterization or radionuclide scan in reproductive age group if ultrasound and CT scan are normal and T > 150 ng/dl

testosterone content. (The free testosterone measurement is more sensitive than the total testosterone since excess androgens often suppress the production of sex hormone–binding globulin.) A DHEAS level greater than 8 μ/ml is consistent with an adrenal neoplasm. If an adrenal mass is suspected, confirmation can be obtained by computed tomography (CT) scan. With a serum testosterone level greater than 150 ng/dl, an ovarian, not adrenal, neoplasm is the more likely diagnosis, whereas testosterone values in the 80- to 150-ng/dl range are more consistent with polycystic ovaries and hyperthecosis. However, Gabrilove et al (1981), in a review of 36 virilizing adrenal adenomas, reported that serum testosterone was more often elevated than DHEAS. Only five adenomas measured less than 3 cm, and eight patients were initially treated by surgery for ovarian androgen excess.

Preoperatively, the tumor should be localized by ultrasound in cases with a nonpalpable mass. If the ultrasound is negative, ovarian vein catheterization studies may be required to detect the tumor (Friedman et al, 1985). This technique can also identify the side of the lesion. However, an occult neoplasm is more likely to be a hilus (Leydig) cell or lipid cell tumor, both of which are found predominantly in older women, in whom lateralization is not important.

Management of Sex Cord Stromal Tumors

Because the preponderance of ovarian stromal tumors are unilateral and solid, the surgical management will follow the algorithm presented in Figure 9–11. For women beyond reproductive age, removal of the uterus, tubes, and ovaries has been traditionally recommended whether the tumor is benign or malignant, stromal, germ cell, or epithelial. However, it is dubious that removal of the normal uterus and normal contralateral adnexa has any therapeutic value, and many women prefer, even after the menopause, to retain these organs if they are not diseased. Discussion of the risks and benefits is clearly indicated in this situation. The proper operation in the young woman is a unilateral ovariectomy or adnexectomy. In either case, fractional uterine curettage should be done before surgery in patients with abnormal uterine bleeding to rule out cervical and endometrial cancer. Preservation of the uterus cannot be recommended in the presence of either disease. Occasionally laparoscopic ovariectomy would be appropriate therapy.

Stromal tumors are frequently difficult to identify histologically, but frozen section analysis can be helpful in certain instances. If the tumor is predominantly solid and not deeply pigmented (orange or brown, which indicates a high lipid content), dysgerminoma and mixed germ cell tumors need to be ruled out intraoperatively. For these tumors, the retroperitoneal nodes and opposite ovary should be evaluated because occult bilateralism and lymph node involvement are common. Otherwise, peritoneal washings for cytology (abdomen and pelvis), careful exploration for evidence of intra- and retroperitoneal metastases with biopsy of suspicious lesions, subtotal omentectomy, and biopsy of any suspect areas in the opposite ovary should be carried out.

Postoperatively, adjunctive therapy should be considered for those patients who have (1) a SLCT (arrhenoblastoma) with poor differentiation or heterologous elements; (2) a lipid cell tumor with pleomorphism, increased mitosis count, or large size, and (3) a sarcoma. The value of adjuvant therapy for stage Ia GCTs with poor prognostic factors (high-mitosis-count, lesion >10 cm in diameter, preoperative rupture) is uncertain, and such therapy is not recommended given the indolent nature of this neoplasm and the overall good prognosis for these cases. Cisplatin-based combination chemotherapy is recommended for patients with positive peritoneal cytology and disease more advanced than stage I. Radiation therapy is an optional choice for patients who are sterile or who do not desire reproductive conservation. Its efficacy is, however, unproven (Segal et al, 1995).

Optimal treatment of patients with advanced or recurrent stromal tumors is unknown, but responses have been reported to both radiation and combination chemotherapy. Cisplatin (Platinol) appears to be the most active agent and has been combined with doxorubicin (Adriamycin) and cyclophosphamide (Cytoxan) (PAC), bleomycin and vinblastine (VBP), and bleomycin and etoposide (BEP) with some success. For example, Gershenson et al (1987) reported that three of eight patients with measurable metastatic ovarian sex cord stromal tumors had a complete response to PAC. Colombo et al (1986) used VBP to treat 11 patients with advanced GCTs, of whom 6 had a complete response. A 33 percent complete response rate has been attributed to BEP in six patients with measurable disease (Gershenson et al, 1996).

Follow-up

After removal of an androgenic tumor in the premenopausal patient, menses usually resume within 1 to 2 months and the breasts rapidly return to normal. The acne is reversible but the hirsutism, clitoromegaly, and hoarseness may be permanent or may resolve only slowly. Fertility seems to be unimpaired. When a stromal tumor produces measurable levels of steroid hormones, quantitative serial assays can be useful in surveillance for recurrence. Determination of testosterone levels in serum or urine after therapy for Sertoli-Leydig cell and other androgenic tumors would seem to be the most promising. AFP production by SLCTs has also been reported (Mann et al, 1986). Serial estradiol levels have revealed recurrent granulosa tumor before the disease was apparent clinically. Inhibin, a peptide hormone produced by granulosa cells, also can be used as a serum tumor marker in the management of ovarian GCTs (Lappohn et al, 1989). It is always worth checking for an elevated serum CA-125 level in patients with ovarian cancer regardless of the cell type.

GERM CELL TUMORS

Germ cell tumors constitute 15 to 20 percent of all primary ovarian neoplasms and are second only to epithelial tumors in frequency of occurrence. No other group of neoplasms encompasses such a wide range of biologic, pathologic, and clinical diversity. Their occurrence predominantly in young women (mean and median age 19 years) is another feature that serves to intensify the interest in this group of ovarian neoplasms. Familial occurrence of ovarian germ cell tumors is reported (Mendel et al, 1994). In order of decreasing frequency, the malignant ovarian germ cell tumors are dysgerminoma, endodermal sinus tumor (EST), immature teratoma, embryonal carcinoma, choriocarcinoma, and polyembryoma. Mixtures of these types account for 10 to 15 percent of cases. On the average, 60 to 75 percent of malignant germ cell tumors are stage I at diagnosis despite their general reputation as highly malignant tumors. Gonadoblastoma is included among the germ cell tumors because of its close structural relationship and its propensity to give rise to germ cell tumors. The proposed derivation of germ cell tumors is depicted in Fig. 11–4.

Benign Germ Cell Tumors (Teratomas)

Teratomas presumably arise from a single germ cell and are usually composed of elements from all three germ layers: ectoderm, mesoderm, and endoderm. Benign cystic teratomas in the vast majority of cases have a normal 46, XX karyotype; the remaining cases are mosaic, trisomic, or triploid. Three postulated mechanisms of derivation are (1) from a germ cell after meiosis I by suppression of meiosis II or by fusion of polar body II with an oocyte; (2) failure of meiosis I; and (3) duplication of a mature ovum (Ohama et al, 1985). Teratomas are cystic or solid and are composed of immature (embryonal, fetal) or mature (adult) tissues. The malignant potential of these neoplasms is related to the presence of immature or partially differentiated tissues rather than to their morphologic cystic or solid composition.

Mature "Solid" Teratomas

The rare mature, solid teratoma is composed entirely of mature or adult tissues. Thorough histologic study of the tumor is required to ensure that no immature tissue or other malignant germ cell element, such as endodermal sinus tumor or choriocarcinoma, is present before rendering this diagnosis. Such a tumor composed entirely of adult tissues is

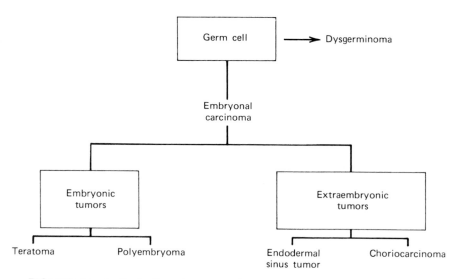

FIGURE 11–4. Derivation of germ cell tumors. (Data from Teilum [1977].)

benign. Peritoneal implants of benign tissue, usually glia, may be present. Although predominantly solid, they almost invariably contain numerous cystic areas.

Benign Cystic Teratomas

The benign cystic teratoma, or *dermoid cyst*, accounts for over 95 percent of all ovarian teratomas and 25 to 40 percent of all ovarian neoplasms (see Table 10–1). About 10 to 20 percent of benign cystic teratomas are discovered in postmenopausal women, and 50 percent occur between the ages of 30 and 50. It is the most common ovarian neoplasm of childhood.

Benign cystic teratomas are composed entirely of mature (adult) tissues, usually representing all three germ layers. Typically, there is a prominent unilocular cavity lined with skin and filled with hair and a sebaceous, oily liquid. Teeth, occasionally embedded in a rudimentary jawbone, are present in nearly one third of dermoid cysts. Rarely, parts of extremities such as fingers and caricatures of fetuses called *homunculi* (little men) are formed. The cyst wall typically has one or more nodular thickenings known as a *dermoid process*, or *Rokitansky's protuberance*. It is within this area that the greatest variety of tissues is found. Although overt bilateralism is reported in 12 percent of cases, it is exceptional to find an occult dermoid in the contralateral ovary (Doss et al, 1977).

Perhaps 25 percent of dermoid cysts are discovered in asymptomatic women on routine pelvic examination, at the time of surgery for other disease, or on abdominal x-ray films. Torsion, which is reported in 10 percent of cases, and rupture are more frequent during pregnancy. Menstrual abnormalities are unusual. Spontaneous rupture can lead to granulomatous peritonitis resembling cancer (especially immature teratoma) or tuberculosis (Stern et al, 1981; Stuart and Smith, 1983). If rupture is sudden and extensive, the clinical picture is that of acute peritonitis from a ruptured viscus. Rarely, dermoids become infected, rupture into a hollow viscus, or cause virilization. Several instances of autoimmune hemolytic anemia associated with benign cystic teratoma are recorded in the literature. Clinically and hematologically, this syndrome is indistinguishable from other causes of autoimmune hemolytic anemia but does not respond to steroids or splenectomy. The anemia is apparently cured by removal of the tumor (Payne et al, 1981).

Malignancy Arising in Dermoid Cysts

Malignancy is reported in 1 to 2 percent of otherwise benign cystic teratomas. For this reason, every dermoid cyst should be thoroughly examined histologically. At surgery, findings suspicious of malignancy are adhesions, rupture, necrosis, and nodular areas in the cyst wall. In nearly all cases, the dermoid cyst is 10 cm or greater in diameter. While secondary malignant transformation can occur in any of the mature tissues found in dermoid cysts, as might be expected, the perponderance of these malignancies are *squamous carcinomas*. In situ, microinvasive, frankly invasive, and verrucous carcinomas have been reported. Squamous carcinoma has also been observed to derive from respiratory tissues in a dermoid cyst. Perhaps half of these cases of squamous carcinoma are stage Ia, with a cure rate in the 75 percent range. Apparently adhesions, capsular invasion, and rupture (stage Ic) can worsen the prognosis substantially. Nearly all of the more advanced-disease patients die within 1 year. It is of more than passing interest that 70 percent of dermoid cysts complicated by squamous carcinoma occur in women 50 years or older (85 percent beyond the age of 40 years), although only 5 to 25 percent of all dermoids are diagnosed in this age group (Gordon et al, 1980).

Carcinoid is the second most common malignancy arising in dermoid cysts. In the review of Climes and Heath (1968), three of nine patients manifested the carcinoid syndrome at presentation. Only two recurred, both from the carcinoid syndrome group. Among the other malignancies encountered in dermoids are adenocarcinoma, sarcoma, melanoma, and, as noted in the next section, thyroid carcinoma.

Highly Specialized Teratomas

STRUMA OVARII

About 10 percent of benign cystic teratomas contain thyroid tissue. When the thyroid tissue predominates (one third of the cases), the tumor is properly designated struma ovarii. Clinically, histologically, and biologically, the entire range of thyroid pathology is encountered, including thyroid adenoma, chronic thyroiditis, and follicular as well as papillary carcinoma.

These tumors occur predominantly in the fifth decade of life, with an average age of 50 years at diagnosis. Ascites, sometimes with pleural effusion (Meigs' syndrome) is reported with uncommon frequency (5 to 10 percent) in association with benign and malignant struma ovarii (Kempers et al, 1970). Devaney et al (1993) reported on 54 cases of struma ovarii (culled from a total of 126 cases) that diverged from the normal pattern of benign thyroid tissue. Of these, 41 cases were called proliferative and 13 malignant. Three of the proliferative and one of the malignant strumas were associated with clinical and laboratory evidence of hyperthyroidism that remitted after surgery. One of the proliferative cases had Meigs' syndrome. The diagnosis of struma ovarii can be suspected at surgery by finding on cut section a predominantly solid, gelatinous, red-brown or green-brown tumor. Usually hair, sebum, teeth, or bone is also present. Bilateralism is rare, but occasionally a dermoid cyst is present in the opposite ovary.

As the series of Devaney et al (1993) documents, malignancy complicates struma ovarii in 10 percent of cases, even taking into account the strumal carcinoids (18 percent of their series), a benign variant that in the past has been misinterpreted as malignant (Scully, 1979). According to Yannopoulos et al (1976), most ovarian thyroid carcinomas arise not from an ovarian struma but from a focus of thyroid tissue in an otherwise ordinary dermoid cyst. Unlike the thyroid gland, the prevailing carcinoma in ovarian thyroid tissue is follicular, although papillary forms, mixed forms, and even the embryonal varieties occur. About one third of histologically malignant cases have exhibited clinical evidence of malignancy. These are typically low-grade carcinomas, and recurrence of malignancy may not appear until years later. Peritoneal, lymphatic, and hematogenous metastases are characteristic. According to Scully (1979), the presence of papillary or embryonal components or vascular invasion is more likely to be associated with clinically malignant behavior. Evaluation by ^{131}I scanning may be helpful in detecting metastasis. Treatment with thyroid hormone prophylactically and ^{131}I for metastases has been suggested (Yannopoulos et al, 1976; Scully, 1979).

CARCINOIDS

Over 200 cases of primary carcinoid tumor of the ovary have been recorded in the literature. They probably arise from argentaffin cells associated with gastrointestinal or bronchial mucosa occurring in teratomas. Altogether less than 10 percent of ovarian carcinoids are complicated by carcinoid heart disease (tricuspid insufficiency, pulmonary stenosis), but approximately one half of primary, insular ovarian carcinoids (midgut) larger than 4 cm are associated with the carcinoid syndrome; the trabecular (foregut, hindgut) form, which is less common, seldom exhibits this behavior. In contrast to intestinal carcinoids, metastases are not required with an ovarian primary tumor for the occurrence of the carcinoid syndrome. Apparently the syndrome is not found in nonmetastatic intestinal carcinoids because the vasoactive amines are inactivated in the liver before entering the systemic circulation. The syndrome results from the secretion of serotonin, tachykinins, substance P, and histamine, which produce episodic cutaneous flushing, diarrhea, facial cyanosis, evidence of right-sided heart failure, and bronchospasm, either in combination or alone (Kvols et al, 1986). Pedal edema and low serum albumin also are common. The heart disease can progress after removal of the tumor (Wilkowske et al, 1994).

The great majority of ovarian carcinoids are confined to one ovary at the time of diagnosis, although the contralateral ovary often contains a dermoid cyst or mucinous cystadenoma (Robboy et al, 1974, 1975, 1977). The prognosis is excellent for patients with primary carcinoids; only 5 percent recur, and these tend to be slowly progressive. In the collected series of Robboy et al, only 1 of 18 trabecular carcinoids recurred (1 of 7 greater than 3 cm in diameter), and only 2 of 48 insular carcinoids recurred (2 of 15 with carcinoid syndrome and a tumor greater than 3 cm in diameter).

Metastasis to the ovary from gastrointestinal carcinoid is less common than a primary ovarian carcinoid. These neoplasms have a variable prognosis and, if completely resected, may not require additional therapy. Characteristic features of carcinoid metastatic to the ovary are bilateralism, multiple nodules throughout the ovary and no associated teratomatous elements (Robboy et al, 1974).

STRUMAL CARCINOIDS

Strumal carcinoid is a highly specialized teratoma characterized by an intimate mixture of thyroid tissue and carcinoid, predominantly trabecular. In the series of Robboy and Scully

(1980), all fifty cases were unilateral, none had carcinoid syndrome, one recurred, and five had a contralateral dermoid cyst. In most cases there are recognizable teratomatous elements present. On the average, women with strumal carcinoid are age 47, those with ovarian stuma 49, and those with trabecular carcinoids 45, while women with ovarian insular carcinoid average 57 years of age.

Management of Benign Cystic Teratoma With and Without Malignant Degeneration

The great majority of germ cell tumors are benign cystic teratomas. As with other cystic ovarian tumors, it is desirable to remove dermoid cysts intact, since benignity is established only by adequate microscopic examination. In addition, the sebaceous and keratin contents of dermoid cysts are irritating to the peritoneum and are capable of producing a chronic granulomatous inflammatory response. Cystectomy with careful reconstruction of the ovary and anti-adhesion measures is the treatment of choice for all reproductive-age women. "Shelling out" a dermoid does not always result in complete removal, and recurrences in the preserved ovary have been reported (Engle et al, 1965). Synchronous overt bilateralism occurs in 12 percent of the cases. In this circumstance, bilateral cystectomy is indicated when preservation of ovarian function is an important consideration. Bivalving the apparently normal contralateral ovary in search of an occult dermoid frequently has been recommended, but the discovery rate of covert bilateralism is too low (Doss et al, 1977) and the risk of infertility (adhesions, ovarian failure) is too high to justify the procedure routinely. Small cysts can be aspirated to identify the sebaceous content of a dermoid as an alternative to incising the ovary.

Squamous carcinoma is the most common malignancy arising in a dermoid cyst, and the prognosis is largely contingent upon the extent of disease at the time of diagnosis. If the cyst wall is intact and free of adhesions, and if there is no evidence of extraovarian spread, surgical excision of the involved adnexa seems to be adequate therapy. In the presence of rupture, ascites, positive cytology, or other evidence of spread, however, whole-abdomen irradiation, intraperitoneal ^{32}P, or chemotherapy (cisplatin) should be adminis-

tered postoperatively. The prognosis in such cases is poor.

Primary ovarian *carcinoid* has been reported to metastasize rarely. if a detailed search for evidence of extraovarian metastasis is negative, surgical excision is sufficient treatment for this malignancy. Periodic determinations of urinary 5-hydroxyindole acetic acid (5-HIAA), a metabolite of serotonin, are of limited value in the post-treatment surveillance program but may detect clinically occult disease. If the carcinoid is unresectable or recurrent, the value of chemotherapy is debated; symptomatic relief from elevated levels of 5-HIAA may be possible using a somatostatin analog (Kvols et al, 1986).

Malignant Germ Cell Tumors

Immature Teratomas

About 20 percent of malignant germ cell tumors are pure immature teratomas (ITs). This malignancy is characterized histologically by immature tissues reminiscent of tissues normal to the human embryo. IT has formerly been designated as a partially differentiated, malignant, embryonal, or solid teratoma. The most frequently encountered immature tissues are neuroepithelium, glia, neuroblastoma, cartilage, various types of non-neural epithelia (respiratory, gut), and mesenchyme, representing all three germ layers (Fig. 11–5). Usually mature (adult) tissues are also present, and they may predominate. When other malignant germ cell elements are found (EST, embryonal carcinoma, choriocarcinoma, dysgerminoma), the diagnosis should specify their presence. The finding of mature tissue, especially one or more "dermoid cysts," in an immature teratoma has led to the mistaken diagnosis of a benign cystic teratoma. Grossly, the tumors average 18 cm in diameter and have a bossellated configuration. Although a cystic-solid composition is the rule (Fig. 11–6), an occasional immature teratoma consists of a solid mass in an otherwise uni- or multilocular cyst. Areas of hemorrhage and necrosis are not unusual.

The malignant potential of IT, as documented in the classic paper by Norris et al (1976), is related to the stage at presentation and the histologic grade (Table 11–4). A confounding feature of IT is its capacity for spontaneous maturation, as evidenced by the occasional presence of peritoneal implants consisting of grade 0 (mature) nodules of glial tissue, sometimes with ascites. This situation,

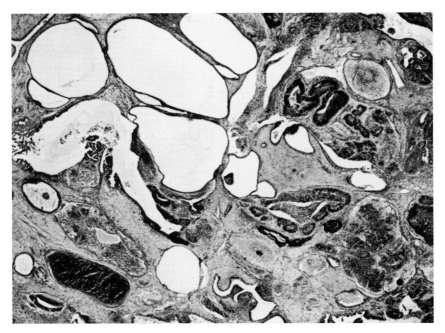

FIGURE 11–5. Immature teratoma (×20). The immature or partially differentiated character of the abundant neural tissue (right half of photograph) identifies the malignant potential of the tumor. Choroid plexus and cartilage can also be seen. No endodermal sinus tumor or choriocarcinoma was present.

referred to as *gliomatosis peritonei*, resembles carcinomatosis. These mature glial implants may be found at second-look surgery even though none was present at the initial operation. The implants tend to concentrate in the pelvis, the omentum, and other sites close to the tumor. They may be found with any grade

of teratoma, even the fully mature, benign (grade 0), solid teratoma. Since implants in any one case may vary with respect to grade and composition (pure glia or heterogeneous, i.e., composed of various tissues), the diagnosis of gliomatosis peritonei should be based on numerous biopsies, all of which show mature glia (Nielson et al, 1985). In this situation, the presence of implants bears no adverse prognostic implication. In fact, the opposite may be true. In the review of

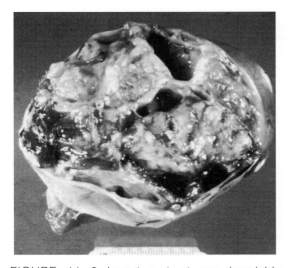

FIGURE 11–6. Immature teratomas invariably manifest a cystic and solid composition with areas of hemorrhage. Typical dermoid structures with teeth and hair may be present.

TABLE **11–4**

Recurrence in Immature Teratoma of the Ovary Before the Chemotherapy Era*

Stage	Grade	Total Cases	No Evidence of Disease at 3 years	
			No.	%
I	1	13	13	100
	2	18	9	50
	3	6	2	33
II	1	4	2	50
	2	2	1	50
	3	2	0	0.0
III	1	4	2	50
	2	2	0	0.0
	3	2	1[†]	50

*Data from Norris et al (1976).
[†]Received actinomycin D.

TABLE **11–5**

Immature Teratoma: Histopathologic Grading

Grade	Definition of Robboy and Scully (1970)	Definition of Norris et al (1976)
0	All tissues mature; no mitotic activity	All tissues mature; mitoses rare or absent
1	Minor foci of abnormally cellular or embryonal tissue mixed with mature elements; rare mitoses	Some immaturity, but neuroepithelium absent or limited to a rare low-power (×40) field; no more than one such focus in any slide
2	Moderate quantities of embryonal tissue mixed with mature elements; moderate mitotic activity	Immaturity and neuroepithelium present to a greater degree than with grade 1; neuroepithelium common, but does not exceed three low-power fields in any one slide
3	Large quantities of embryonal tissue present	Immaturity and neuroectoderm prominent; neuroectoderm occupies four or more low-power fields within individual sections

Truong et al (1982), the patients with mature glial implants did better than expected, considering the grade of the ovarian IT. Residual benign peritoneal implants, usually of a heterogeneous nature, even after many years can develop into dermoid cysts, simulating malignant progression. Almost all patients with gliomatosis peritonei have been under 23 years of age at diagnosis, with an average age of 15 years. Of further interest is the finding of entirely mature tissue at postchemotherapy second-look surgery in patients who had immature residual tissues after their first operation (Aronowitz et al, 1983).

The clinical behavior of an IT is determined by (1) the grade of the tumor (Table 11–5); (2) the presence of more malignant elements, such as endodermal sinus tumor; and (3) the surgicopathologic stage. Because immature tissue has a great capacity for implantation, recurrences in the abdominal incision were relatively common prior to the era of effective chemotherapy. The opposite ovary rarely, if ever, is involved in stage I cases, but it is not unusual to find a dermoid cyst there. Synchronous immature ovarian and immature presacral teratomas have been reported (Nielson et al, 1986). In metastatic cases the disease is generally confined to the abdomen, but intrahepatic and lung metastases have been reported. Involvement of pelvic and aortic nodes has been noted in several cases, even when the disease otherwise appeared to be confined to the primary tumor (Robboy and Scully, 1970; diZerega et al, 1975; Block et al, 1984). Although it is widely accepted that pure immature teratoma does not produce human chorionic gonadotropin (hCG) or AFP, in two series 4 of 12 patients with apparently pure IT had elevated serum AFP levels up to 3,490 ng/ml (Ihara et al, 1984; Taylor et al, 1985). Origin of AFP from a variety of endodermal and ectodermal cells in pure IT has been suggested by immunochemical studies (Burrus et al, 1985). Serum lactate dehydrogenase (LDM) (Table 11–6) and serum CA-125 may also serve as tumor markers for immature teratoma (Liu et al, 1984).

Dysgerminomas

Dysgerminoma is the most common malignant germ cell tumor, accounting for 40 percent of cases in the series of Kurman and Norris (1977). Seventy-five percent occur in the early reproductive years, and 10 percent are accounted for by prepubertal girls. The most frequently occurring malignancy associated with intersex states and gonadoblastoma is the dysgerminoma. Perhaps more than any other malignant ovarian neoplasm, dysgerminoma is detected on routine pelvic examination. Diagnosis after age 35 should be questioned because of its rarity. Confusion

TABLE **11–6**

Tumor Markers in Ovarian Germ Cell Tumors[*,†]

Tumor	hCG	AFP	LDH
Mixed	+	+	+
EC	+	+	±
EST	−	+	±
DYS	±	−	+
IT	−	±	±

[*] Some tumors produce CA-125.

[†] hCG = human chorionic gonadotropin; AFP = alpha-fetoprotein; LDH = lactate dehydrogenase; EC = embryonal carcinoma; EST = endodermal sinus tumor; DYS = dysgerminoma; IT = immature teratoma.

with poorly differentiated adenocarcinoma, lymphoma, clear cell carcinoma, carcinoid, and other malignancies is possible.

Areas of more malignant germ cell elements are found in 10 to 15 percent of dysgerminomas. The diagnosis should stipulate if the tumor is pure or contains EST, choriocarcinoma, embryonal carcinoma, or IT (including the grade). Even after thorough evaluation, however, apparently pure dysgerminoma has recurred as EST or choriocarcinoma. Pure dysgerminoma does not elaborate AFP, but elevated serum hCG levels (up to several thousand units) can be a reflection of syncytiotrophoblast-like giant cells rather than the presence of choriocarcinoma. The former situation has no prognostic significance (Knapp et al, 1985).

In common with other germ cell malignancies, two thirds of dysgerminomas are apparently confined to the ovaries (stage I) at diagnosis. However, dysgerminoma does have several unusual features:

1. The incidence of overt bilateralism in stage I is 10 to 15 percent.
2. The reported frequency of covert bilateralism approximates 15 percent.
3. There is occasional recurrence or a second primary in the residual ovary even many years later.
4. There is a much greater propensity for lymphatic spread than for intraperitoneal metastases. The latter risk is associated primarily with tumor rupture. In the series of DePalo et al (1982), among 44 cases (all stages), 12 had only retroperitoneal nodal involvement, 4 had peritoneal and nodal disease, and only 2 had extraovarian disease limited to peritoneal metastases. Of five "stage Ia" cases with nodal involvement, four were aortic only, one was aortic plus pelvic, and none was pelvic only.
5. Dysgerminoma is remarkably radiation sensitive; a tumor dose of 3,000 rad is curative in most cases.

Grossly, the tumors are lobulated, solid, and soft to firm (Fig. 11–7). The gray-white or cream-colored cut surface may have areas of hemorrhage or necrosis that suggest that EST is present. Calcification indicates that the dysgerminoma is arising from a gonadoblastoma. Microscopically, the tumor is composed of germ cells with fibrous trabeculae infiltrated by lymphocytes and, in some cases, sarcoid-like granulomas (Fig. 11–8). Syncytiotrophoblastic giant cells are unusual (Scully, 1979).

Serum LDH is a useful tumor marker in dysgerminoma (Sheiko and Hart, 1982; Awais, 1983; Schwartz and Morris, 1988). Although LDH is often elevated in the epithelial ovarian malignancies, the values tend to be higher in dysgerminoma. Furthermore, it is the two fast fractions of LDH that are increased with dysgerminoma, in contrast to the elevated slow fractions in other ovarian cancers (Pode et al, 1984; Fujii et al, 1985).

The 5-year survival for pure dysgerminoma, stage Ia, is in the 95 percent range, although the recurrence rate in some series approaches 15 percent. Most recurrences in early cases have been in the residual ovary. More advanced-stage dysgerminomas historically have an overall survival prognosis of 65 percent; the prognosis is worsened by intraperitoneal metastases (DePalo et al, 1982).

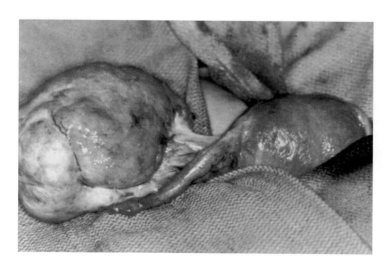

FIGURE 11–7. Dysgerminoma. The tumor is solid and lobulated, and has a "brain-like" gross appearance. It retains the general configuration of the ovary. The top of the uterus can be seen in the right half of the photograph.

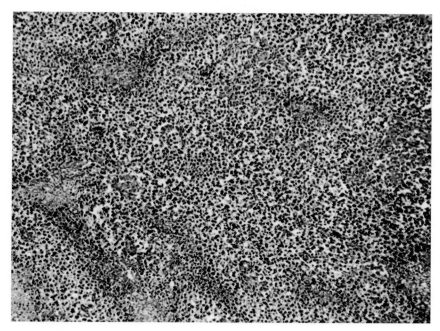

FIGURE 11–8. Microscopically, the dysgerminoma is composed of large polygonal germ cells. The fibrous trabeculae are not prominent in this section but are marked by the characteristic infiltration with lymphocytes (×75).

Endodermal Sinus Tumors

EST is one of the most malignant neoplasms arising in the ovary. Despite the fact that over half of the cases appear to be confined to the ovary at diagnosis, the 2-year mortality was 80 percent before the chemotherapy era. EST was originally described by Schiller, who mistakenly combined it with clear cell (formerly mesonephroid) carcinoma and designated the two as mesonephroma ovarii. We are indebted to Teilum (1959) for recognizing EST as a distinct entity. He noted the histologic similarity of this tumor (Fig. 11–9) and the endodermal sinus of Duval in the rodent placenta. For this reason, he preferred the term *endodermal sinus tumor.* This designation, as well as the name *yolk sac tumor,* have become generally accepted, although the former is more popular.

Like other germ cell tumors, EST occurs almost exclusively in children and young women with an average age of approximately 20 years. Most cases are confined to one ovary at the time of diagnosis, but rupture and ascites are common. Bilateralism does not occur in stage I cases, although the opposite ovary may contain a dermoid cyst. Intraperitoneal metastases are reported much more frequently than lymph node involve-

ment (Gershenson et al, 1983). Often, EST is a portion of a mixed germ cell tumor containing dysgerminoma, IT, and/or choriocarcinoma. These cases may have a better prognosis than pure EST. Frequently, hemorrhagic ascitic fluid is present at the time of surgery, reflecting the friable nature of the tumor and its tendency toward necrosis.

AFP, an alpha-globulin, is detectable in the serum of most patients with EST (Romero and Schwartz, 1981). AFP is the dominant serum protein in the early embryo. It is initially produced by the yolk sac and later by the liver, thus providing a developmental explanation for the production of AFP by ESTs and hepatomas in adults. Elevated levels of AFP also have been reported with benign and malignant SLCTs (Mann et al, 1986) and IT (Burrus et al, 1985). Serum AFP levels may be elevated by various liver diseases and by tumors of endodermally derived organs. Detection of an IT in pregnancy by maternal serum AFP testing has been reported (Montz et al, 1989). Serum hCG will be elevated if areas of trophoblastic differentiation are present. AFP and hCG values should be obtained routinely in all cases of suspected EST.

Grossly, the external surface of the intact EST is smooth and glistening (Fig. 11–10). Tears from spontaneous rupture are fre-

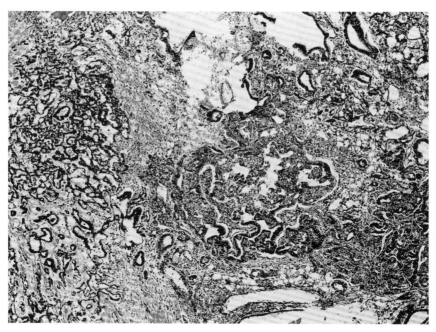

FIGURE 11–9. Endodermal sinus tumor (×35). Section from a different area of the same tumor shown in Figure 11–8. The typical microcystic pattern appears at the left of the photomicrograph. The presence of endodermal sinus tumor alters the generally good prognosis of pure dysgerminoma.

quently encountered. The cut surface characteristically has a cystic-solid composition, with extensive hemorrhage and necrosis. Microscopically, EST has three predominant features: (1) a reticular growth pattern; (2) intracellular and extracellular hyaline (periodic acid–Schiff [PAS]-positive) droplets; and (3)

Schiller-Duval bodies, which are formed by simple papillae with a central capillary. This structure projects into a space in the reticular tissue, producing a glomerulus-like appearance, which led Schiller to include these with the mesonephric tumors. The PAS-positive hyaline droplets consist of alpha$_1$-antitrypsin.

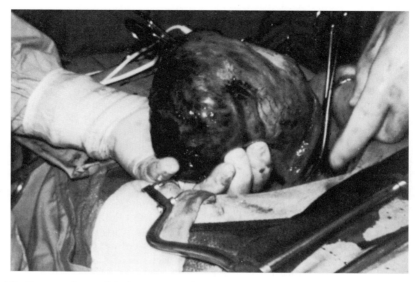

FIGURE 11–10. Pure endometrial sinus tumor. Irregular, solid growth with a smooth, glistening surface. The left portion of the tumor is hemorrhagic and necrotic.

Other growth patterns are solid, papillary, and polyvesicular vitelline (Scully, 1979). Rarely, ESTs with a pure polyvesicular vitelline pattern have been reported. They apparently have a better prognosis and are AFP negative (Nogales et al, 1978). Differentiating an EST from either a high-grade adenocarcinoma or a clear cell carcinoma may be difficult.

Embryonal Carcinomas

Kurman and Norris (1976a) reported 15 cases of an ovarian tumor that histologically resembles the embryonal carcinoma of the testis. It is composed of embryonal cells, gland-like clefts (embryoid bodies), and syncytiophoblastic giant cells. The median patient age is 15 years, somewhat younger than that of the patients with EST. The tumor produces both hCG and AFP. In Kurman and Norris' series, only four of eight stage I patients survived. Embryonal carcinomas should not be considered a variant of EST.

Choriocarcinomas

Teratomatous choriocarcinoma arising in the ovary is extremely rare and usually occurs as part of a mixed germ cell tumor (Axe et al, 1985). Documentation of the teratomatous or gestational origin in a postpubertal woman is not possible in the absence of other germ cell elements or intersex status. Choriocarcinoma in prepubertal girls is often associated with isosexual precocity. Like the gestational variety, teratomatous choriocarcinoma produces measurable levels of hCG, which may serve as an aid to diagnosis, treatment, and follow-up. The excellent therapeutic achievements with antineoplastic drugs in gestational choriocarcinoma have not to the same extent, been realized in choriocarcinoma of germ cell origin. It is postulated that gestational choriocarcinoma, which develops from fetal, not maternal, tissue, is more curable because it incites a more intense immunologic host response than nongestational choriocarcinoma. Nevertheless, several cases of prolonged remission, induced with chemotherapeutic agents, have been reported for the teratomatous variety.

Polyembryomas

Also known as *polyembryonic embryoma*, this is a very rare malignant germ cell tumor composed of embryoid bodies in various stages of presomite development. Elaboration of AFP, hCG, and human placental lactogen has been reported (Takeda et al, 1982). The degree of malignancy is not well established because of its rarity. Most reported cases have had other malignant germ cell elements.

Mixed Germ Cell Tumors

Two or more malignant germ cell components are found in 10 to 15 percent of all germ cell malignancies. These mixed tumors occur at an average age of 16 years, somewhat earlier in life than the pure lesions, except for the embryonal carcinoma. The majority are composed of dysgerminoma or IT with areas of EST. About one fourth contain areas of embryonal carcinoma and 10 percent have identifiable choriocarcinoma. Serum AFP and hCG levels are frequently elevated (Gershenson et al, 1984). Although more than half of the cases contain EST, survival appears to be better than that of the cases of pure EST (Kurman and Norris, 1976b).

Gonadoblastomas

The gonadoblastoma is an unusual tumor of the ovary, described first by Scully in 1953. It is characterized by germ cells intimately mixed with indifferent sex cord elements resembling immature granulosa and Sertoli cells. In about two thirds of the cases, Leydig-like cells are present in the stroma. Gonadoblastomas are usually small tumors, with the largest reported example achieving a diameter of only 8 cm. Bilateral involvement occurs in about one third of the cases. Gonadoblastomas occur almost exclusively in genetically abnormal individuals, who can usually be classified as having pure gonadal dysgenesis, mixed gonadal dysgenesis, or male pseudohermaphroditism. Nearly 90 percent of the cases are sex chromatin negative. The most common karyotypes are 46,XY and 45,X/46,XY. About one quarter of the cases are phenotypic males. Ambiguous genitalia are common, and patients who are phenotypic females frequently show some evidence of masculinization. Calcifications often develop in gonadoblastomas and may be demonstrable by pelvic roentgenogram.

The importance of gonadoblastoma, in addition to its almost universal association with intersex states, lies in its propensity for producing malignant germ cell tumors. Approximately half of the gonadoblastomas reported in the literature have been associated with dysgerminoma. Occasional cases of choriocarcinoma, embryonal carcinoma, and mixed germ cell tumors arising in gonadoblastomas have been reported. Although the gonadoblastoma itself is benign, the frequency with which malignant germ cell neoplasms arise from this tumor justifies its being considered as a premalignant lesion. Germ cell malignancy has developed in a gonadoblastoma as early as the first decade of life.

This strong tendency to produce malignant tumors is sufficient reason for removal of gonadoblastomas as soon as they are discovered. Bilateral excision of the gonads should be done except in the rare patient who has a normal ovary on the contralateral side. A streak enlarged to the size of an ovary by gonadoblastoma or tumor must not be mistaken for a normal ovary (Hart and Burkons, 1979). Prophylactic bilateral gonadectomy prior to puberty is recommended for intersex patients with a Y chromosome, except those with testicular feminization, in which case delay can be considered up to age 30 since the risk of malignancy prior to that age is less than 4 percent (Manuel et al, 1976). Any patient with a germ cell tumor should be examined for evidence of gonadal dysgenesis because of the common association of these two conditions. Where doubt exists, a karyotype is indicated.

Management of Malignant Germ Cell Tumors

Although the various types of malignant germ cell tumors have important biologic differences, there are many similarities with respect to their management. The possibility of a germ cell malignancy should be included in the differential diagnosis of any young woman with an ovarian mass. This is especially true when the mass is predominately solid or there are clinical signs of advanced disease (e.g., ascites or cul-de-sac nodularity). Preoperative measurement of serum tumor markers (hCG, AFP, LDH, CA-125) will aid in the diagnosis and allow for appropriate management.

Most germ cell malignancies are stage I at the time of diagnosis. The initial surgery should consist of a unilateral oophorectomy, peritoneal cytology, and meticulous exploration of the abdomen, including palpatory assessment of the retroperitoneal lymph nodes. The removed ovary should be sent for frozen section diagnosis. If the opposite ovary contains a cystic lesion, the cyst should be enucleated. Such cysts are almost invariably benign dermoids and never represent bilateral germ cell malignancy. Biopsy of a normal-appearing ovary is not indicated if the patient has a nondysgerminomatous malignancy. In the absence of clinically evident extraovarian spread of the tumor, a partial omentectomy, biopsy of adhesions, and a retroperitoneal lymph node sampling should be performed.

There is rarely an indication for total hysterectomy and bilateral salpingo-oophorectomy when managing ovarian germ cell malignancies. Since these tumors may mimic epithelial tumors histologically, and frozen section diagnosis is difficult, the surgeon should err on the conservative side and preserve fertility and ovarian function in a reproductive-age patient. As is true of epithelial tumors, many patients with germ cell cancer are inadequately staged at their initial operation. Because almost all of these patients will require additional therapy, the value of immediate re-exploration is uncertain, and it probably should not be done unless consideration is being given to conservative management.

Serum tumor marker levels should be obtained postoperatively if these tests were not done before surgery. As is true for testicular germ cell tumors, combination chemotherapy has had a remarkable impact on the survival of patients with ovarian germ cell tumors. When chemotherapy is required, the first treatment should be given as soon after surgery as the patient can tolerate it, usually before discharge from the hospital. Ovarian germ cell tumors can grow very rapidly, and a delay may adversely influence outcome.

One of the potential adverse effects of chemotherapy in this population is damage to the ovaries, which may result in immediate or delayed premature ovarian failure, the risk being dependent upon the agents used, the duration and intensity of therapy, and the age of the patient. In the past some experts have recommended that oral contraceptives (OCs) be prescribed during chemotherapy, not only to prevent pregnancy (which is important) but also to suppress ovarian function, which might protect against ovarian damage (Chapman and Sutcliffe, 1981). However, it is more likely that the administration of a gonadotropin-releasing hormone (GnRH) agonist would be protective, as the study of Blumenfeld et al (1996) suggests, because GnRH

TABLE 11–7

Combination Chemotherapy Used to Treat Patients With Ovarian Germ
Cell Malignancy*

Drug	Dosage	Schedule
BEP		
Bleomycin	20 U/m², not to exceed 30 U	IV weekly × 9 weeks
Etoposide (VP-16)	100 mg/m²	IV days 1–5 every 3 weeks
Cisplatin	20 mg/m²	IV days 1–5 every 3 weeks
VAC		
Vincristine	1.5 mg/m², not to exceed 2 mg	IV every 2 weeks × 12 weeks
Actinomycin D	350 μg/m²	IV days 1–5 every 4 weeks
Cytoxan	150 mg/m²	IV days 1–5 every 4 weeks
VIP		
Etoposide (VP-16)	75 mg/m²	IV days 1–5 every 3 weeks
Ifosfamide†	1.2 g/m²	IV days 1–5 every 3 weeks
Cisplatin	20 mg/m²	IV days 1–5 every 3 weeks

*Data from Loehrer et al (1988) and Williams et al (1989a,b).
†Must give mesna (uroprotector) when administering ifosfamide.

agonists are more suppressive of ovarian function than are OCs. These investigators administered a depot GnRH agonist for up to 6 months to 18 menstruating women during chemotherapy for lymphoma, most of whom received the MOPP/ABV regimen plus mantle irradiation. Of the 16 surviving patients, 15 resumed ovulation and menses within 3 to 8 months of the last chemotherapy cycle. This compares to a 61 percent rate of ovarian failure among a matched historical control group.

NONDYSGERMINOMATOUS MALIGNANCIES

Postoperative Chemotherapy. All cases of nondysgerminomatous germ cell malignancies require postoperative chemotherapy, with the exception of stage Ia, grade 1 IT. There are many reports in the literature documenting the activity of various drug regimens. The two most widely used are VAC, and BEP (Table 11–7). Chemotherapy is pre-scribed both as adjuvant treatment for the patient with no clinically measurable disease because of the high relapse rates, and as curative therapy for the patient with measurable or bulk disease remaining after the initial surgery.

The Gynecologic Oncology Group (GOG) has conducted several trials in the treatment of both early- and advanced-stage ovarian germ cell malignancy. According to the results of two nonrandomized, sequential prospective studies of stage I through III patients with completely resected tumor, VAC, which had been the standard treatment, is clearly inferior to BEP (Table 11–8). Only two patients failed treatment on BEP during an average follow-up of 38.6 months. Treatment with etoposide carries some risk of a second malignancy, particularly leukemia, which is dose related. In one testicular cancer study, 5 of 82 men (6 percent) receiving more than 2,000 mg/m² of etoposide developed leukemia, compared with none of 130 patients receiving

TABLE 11–8

Adjuvant Chemotherapy for Ovarian Germ Cell Malignancies — Gynecologic
Oncology Group Trials

	VAC*			BEP†		
	Treated	Disease-Free Survival		Treated	Disease-Free Survival	
Tumor	N	N	(%)	N	N	(%)
Endodermal sinus tumor	48	35	(73)	25	24	(96)
Immature teratoma	50	42	(84)	42	41	(98)
Mixed germ cell tumor	2	1	(50)	24	24	(100)

*VAC = vincristine, actinomycin-D, and cyclophosphamide (Cytoxan); data from Williams et al (1989b).
†BEP = bleomycin, etoposide, and cisplatin; data from Williams et al (1994).

a lower dose (Williams et al, 1994). Of the 91 GOG study patients, 1 developed leukemia and a second was diagnosed with a lymphoma. BEP is now considered the standard of care. In good-prognosis testicular germ cell tumors, further reduction in toxicity without decrease in efficacy has been reported in patients treated by etoposide and cisplatin without bleomycin (EP) (Bajorn et al, 1991). In a randomized trial of BEP versus EP in testicular cancer patients, however, Loehrer et al (1995) reported a significantly higher survival rate among patients treated with BEP (95 vs. 86 percent). Thus bleomycin appears to be essential to achieve maximum benefit.

Because most ovarian germ cell tumors are diagnosed at a relatively early stage, there are few studies of patients with residual, unresectable disease. The results of one such study by the GOG employing VBP are presented in Table 11–9. It is important to note that 37 percent of these patients had prior chemotherapy, the majority VAC, as adjuvant treatment of early disease.

Response to therapy is monitored by physical examination and serial measurement of serum tumor markers. Evidence of recurrence—a new mass and/or a rising serum tumor marker—is an indication for clinical staging, reoperation if the disease is potentially resectable, and further chemotherapy.

Second-Look Laparotomy. The role of second-look laparotomy in ovarian germ cell malignancies is controversial. Several authors have suggested that patients who have early-stage disease and normal serum tumor marker measurements after completion of therapy do not require second-look surgery (Schwartz, 1984; Gershenson et al, 1986a; Culine et al, 1996). In advanced cases, however, residual disease may be documented in spite of normal levels of previously elevated serum tumor markers (Curtin et al, 1989). In the GOG trial of VBP in advanced-stage germ cell cancer, 14 of 56 patients undergoing second-look laparotomy had residual tumor after completion of chemotherapy. The argument against second-look laparotomy is that early detection of subclinical residual germ cell malignancy may not affect overall survival. However, since additional therapy is capable of a significant salvage rate for patients with persistent tumor (Loehrer et al, 1988), early diagnosis will probably be of benefit to some patients. Cytoreductive surgery at the time of second look or recurrence, especially in patients with IT, appears to improve the salvage

rate (Munkarah et al, 1994). Current criteria for selection of patients for second-look laparotomy include (1) advanced (International Federation of Gynecology and Obstetrics stages II through IV), nondysgerminatous tumors; (2) unstaged or recurrent tumors; and (3) patients with stage I tumors and positive serum tumor markers after completion of chemotherapy. Patients with stage I tumors and normal levels of serum tumor markers, who were adequately staged at initial surgery, do not require a second-look laparotomy. Patients who undergo second-look laparotomy after combination chemotherapy with bleomycin should be monitored closely during anesthesia; high levels of oxygen may induce acute pulmonary decompensation (Waid-Jones and Coursin, 1991).

Outcome. After completion of therapy, all patients should be followed by serial complete physical examination and serum tumor marker measurements. Most patients will have or will resume normal menstrual function within a few months of completing chemotherapy. As discussed previously, the ovarian toxicity of the chemotherapy may be reduced by administering a GnRH agonist during treatment. Numerous reports of normal pregnancies after VAC as well as cisplatin-based chemotherapy have appeared in the literature. Gershenson et al (1988), for example, evaluated menstrual and reproductive function in 40 patients after combination chemotherapy for malignant germ cell tumors. Twenty-seven of the 40 patients (68 percent) had resumed menses. Twelve of 16 patients who attempted pregnancy became pregnant, and 11 women delivered a total of 22 healthy infants.

DYSGERMINOMAS

Most patients with dysgerminoma have stage I disease, and surgery is adequate therapy provided that serial sectioning of the tumor proves that it is a pure dysgerminoma, and all other biopsies and cytologic specimens are negative. If the tumor is not pure dysgerminoma, treatment is dictated by the most malignant element present (e.g., EST). Surgical therapy in the typical case entails careful exploration, pelvic cytology, and unilateral salpingo-oophorectomy with biopsy (a thin slice, not a wedge) of the opposite ovary to rule out occult bilaterality. The residual biopsied ovary should be wrapped in an antiadhesion agent to protect against mechanical in-

TABLE 11–9

Treatment of Advanced and Recurrent Ovarian Germ Cell Malignancies With VBP*

Tumor Type	Total Treated N	Disease-Free Survival N	(%)
Endodermal sinus tumor	29	16	(55)
Immature teratoma	26	14	(54)
Mixed germ cell tumor	27	14	(52)
Dysgerminoma	8	7	(88)
Other	7	3	(43)

*VBP = bleomycin, vinblastine, and cisplatin; data from Williams et al (1989a).

fertility. If both ovaries are involved with tumor, the smaller ovary has been preserved and successfully treated with systemic chemotherapy (DePalo et al, 1987).

Indications for surgical staging include size greater than 10 cm, preoperative elevation of the tumor markers, the presence of hemorrhage or necrosis in the tumor, or stage higher than Ia. In these situations the ipsilateral pelvic and aortic nodes should be dissected. Postoperatively, patients should be closely monitored by physical examination and serum LDH measurement. Intersex states must be excluded by karyotyping, as previously mentioned.

Dysgerminoma is unique among the ovarian germ cell malignancies in that it is a radiosensitive tumor. Consequently, radiation therapy for many years was the standard therapy for patients with advanced and/or recurrent disease. Unilateral pelvic or aortic nodal disease could be managed by giving radiation therapy to the affected side only. In most instances this will preserve ovarian function and fertility (DePalo et al, 1987; Bjorkholm et al, 1990).

Nevertheless, in spite of the radiosensitivity of dysgerminoma, most clinicians now prefer to treat high risk patients and those having metastatic disease with platinum-based chemotherapy (Gershenson et al, 1986b, 1990; Williams et al, 1989a; Gershenson, 1994). The regimen of choice is BEP. In two clinical trials involving stage III and IV patients, 25 of 26 were alive and well with a median follow-up of 26 months after BEP therapy (Gershenson et al, 1990; Williams, 1994).

REFERENCES

Aiman J, Forney JP, Parker CR Jr: Androgen and estrogen secretion by normal and neoplastic ovaries in premenopausal women. Obstet Gynecol 68:327, 1986a.

Aiman J, Forney JP, Parker CR Jr: Secretion of androgens and estrogens by normal and neoplastic ovaries in postmenopausal women. Obstet Gynecol 68:1, 1986b.

Anikwue C, Dawood MY, Kramer E: Granulosa and theca cell tumors. Obstet Gynecol 51:214, 1978.

Aronowitz J, Estrada R, Lynch R, Kaplan AL: Retroconversion of malignant immature teratomas of the ovary after chemotherapy. Gynecol Oncol 16:414, 1983.

Awais GM: Dysgerminoma and serum lactic dehydrogenase levels. Obstet Gynecol 61:99, 1983.

Axe SR, Klein VR, Woodruff JD: Choriocarcinoma of the ovary. Obstet Gynecol 66:111, 1985.

Bajorn DF, Geller NL, Weisen SF, Bosl GJ: Two-drug therapy in patients with metastatic germ cell tumors. Cancer 67:29, 1991.

Bjorkholm E, Lundell M, Gyftodimos A, Silfversward C: Dysgerminoma: the Radiumhemmet series 1927–1984. Cancer 65:38, 1990.

Bjorkholm E, Silfversward C: Prognostic factors in granulosa-cell tumors. Gynecol Oncol 11:261, 1981.

Block M, Gilbert E, Davis C: Metastatic neuroblastoma arising in an ovarian teratoma with long-term survival. Cancer 54:590, 1984.

Blumenfeld A, Avivi I, Linn S, et al: Prevention of irreversible chemotherapy induced ovarian damage in young women with lymphoma by a gonadotrophin releasing hormone agonist in parallel to chemotherapy. Hum Reprod 11:1620, 1996.

Burrus DR, Okagaki T, Twiggs LB, Brooker DC: Immunochemical evidence of heterogeneous origin of α-fetoprotein in immature teratoma of the ovary. Gynecol Oncol 21:73, 1985.

Chalvardjian A, Derzko C: Gynandroblastoma: its ultrastructure. Cancer 50:710, 1982.

Chalvardjian A, Scully RE: Sclerosing stromal tumors of the ovary. Cancer 31:664, 1973.

Chapman RM, Sutcliffe SB: Protection of ovarian function by oral contraceptives in women receiving chemotherapy for Hodgkin's disease. Blood 58:849, 1981.

Chetkowski RJ, Judd HL, Jagger PI, et al: Autonomous cortisol secretion by a lipoid cell tumor of the ovary. JAMA 254:2628, 1985.

Climes ARW, Heath LP: Malignant degeneration of benign cystic teratomas of the ovary. Cancer 22:824, 1968.

Colombo N, Sessa C, Landoni F, et al: Cisplatin, vinblastine, and bleomycin combination chemotherapy in metastatic granulosa cell tumor of the ovary. Obstet Gynecol 67:265, 1986.

Culine S, Lhomme C, Michel G, et al: Is there a role for second look laparotomy in the management of malignant germ cell tumors of the ovary? J Surg Oncol 62:40, 1996.

Curtin JP, Rubin SC, Hoskins WJ, et al: Second-look laparotomy in endodermal sinus tumor: report of two patients with normal levels of alpha-fetoprotein with residual tumor at reexploration. Obstet Gynecol 137:893, 1989.

DePalo G, Lattuada A, Kenda R, et al: Germ cell tumors of the ovary: the experience of the National Cancer Institute of Milan. I. Dysgerminoma. Int J Radiat Oncol Biol Phys 13:853, 1987.

DePalo G, Pilotti S, Kenda R, et al: Natural history of dysgerminoma. Am J Obstet Gynecol 143:799, 1982.

Devaney K, Snyder R, Norris HS, Tavassoli FA: Proliferative and histologically malignant struma ovarii: a clinicopathologic study of 54 cases. Int J Gynecol Pathol 12:333, 1993.

diZerega G, Acosta A, Kaufman RH, Kaplan AL: Solid teratoma of the ovary. Gynecol Oncol 3:93, 1975.

Dockerty MB, Masson JC: Ovarian fibromas: a clinical and pathological study of 283 cases. Am J Obstet Gynecol 47:741, 1944.

Doss N Jr, Forney JP, Vellios F: Covert bilaterality of mature ovarian teratomas. Obstet Gynecol 50:651, 1977.

Engel T, Greeley AV, Sweeney WE III: Recurrent dermoid cysts of the ovary. Obstet Gynecol 26:757, 1965.

Evans AT III, Gaffey TA, Malkasian GD Jr: Clinicopathologic review of 118 granulosa and 82 theca cell tumors. Obstet Gynecol 55:231, 1980.

Fletcher JA, Gibas Z, Donovan K, et al: Ovarian granulosa-stromal cell tumors are characterized by trisomy 12. Am J Pathol 138:515, 1991.

Forney JP: Pregnancy following removal and chemotherapy of ovarian endodermal sinus tumor. Obstet Gynecol 52:360, 1978.

Fox H, Agrawal K, Langley FA: A clinicopathologic study of 92 cases of granulosa cell tumor of the ovary with special reference to the factors influencing prognosis. Cancer 35:231, 1975.

Friedman CI, Schmidt GE, Kim MH, Powell J: Serum testosterone concentrations in the evaluation of androgen-producing tumors. Am J Obstet Gynecol 153:44, 1985.

Fujii S, Konishi I, Suzuki A, et al: Analysis of serum lactic dehydrogenase levels and its isoenzymes in ovarian dysgerminoma. Gynecol Oncol 22:65, 1985.

Gabrilove JL, Seman AT, Sabet R, et al: Virilizing adrenal adenoma with studies on the steroid content of the adrenal venous effluent and a review of the literature. Endocrinol Rev 2:462, 1981.

Gershenson DM: Menstrual and reproductive function after treatment with combination chemotherapy for malignant ovarian germ cell tumors. J Clin Oncol 6:270, 1988.

Gershenson DM: Management of early ovarian cancer: germ cell and sex cord stromal tumors. Gyencol Oncol 55(suppl):S62, 1994.

Gershenson DM, Copeland LJ, Del Junco G, et al: Second-look laparotomy in the management of malignant germ cell tumors of the ovary. Obstet Gynecol 67:789, 1986a.

Gershenson DM, Copeland LJ, Kavanagh JJ, et al: Treatment of metastatic stromal tumors of the ovary with cisplatin, doxorubicin and cyclophosphamide. Obstet Gynecol 70:765, 1987.

Gershenson DM, Del Junco G, Copeland LJ, Rutledge FN: Mixed germ cell tumors of the ovary. Obstet Gynecol 64:200, 1984.

Gershenson DM, Del Junco G, Herson J, Rutledge FN: Endodermal sinus tumor of the ovary: the M.D. Anderson experience. Obstet Gynecol 61:194, 1983.

Gershenson DM, Morris M, Burke TW, et al: Treatment of poor prognosis sex cord stromal tumors of the ovary with the combination of bleomycin, etoposide, and cisplatin. Obstet Gynecol 87:527, 1996.

Gershenson DM, Morris M, Cangir A, et al: Treatment of malignant germ cell tumors of the ovary with bleomycin, etoposide, and cisplatin. J Clin Oncol 8:715, 1990.

Gershenson DM, Wharton JT, Kline RC, et al: Chemotherapeutic complete remission in patients with metastatic ovarian dysgerminoma. Cancer 58:2594, 1986b.

Gordon A, Rosenshein N, Parmley T, Bhagavan B: Benign cystic teratomas in postmenopausal women. Am J Obstet Gynecol 138:1120, 1980.

Hart WR, Burkons DM: Germ cell neoplasms arising in gonadoblastomas. Cancer 43:669, 1979.

Ihara T, Ohama K, Satoh H, et al: Histologic grade and karyotype of immature teratoma of the ovary. Cancer 54:2988, 1984.

Kempers RD, Dockerty MD, Hoffman DL: Struma ovarii—ascitic, hyperthyroid, and asymptomatic syndromes. Ann Intern Med 72:883, 1970.

Klemi PJ, Joensuu H, Salmi T: Prognostic value of flow cytometric DNA content analysis in granulosa cell tumor of the ovary. Cancer 65:1189, 1990.

Knapp DS, Kohorn EI, Merino MJ, LiVolsi VA: Pure dysgerminoma of the ovary with elevated serum human chorionic gonadotropin: diagnostic and therapeutic considerations. Gynecol Oncol 20:234, 1985.

Kurman RJ, Norris HJ: Embryonal carcinoma of the ovary. Cancer 38:2420, 1976a.

Kurman RJ, Norris HJ: Malignant mixed germ cell tumors of the ovary: a clinical and pathologic analysis of 30 cases. Obstet Gynecol 48:579, 1976b.

Kurman RJ, Norris HJ: Malignant germ cell tumors of the ovary. Human Pathol 8:551, 1977.

Kvols LK, Moertel CG, O'Connell MJ, et al: Treatment of the malignant carcinoid syndrome: evaluation of a long-acting somatostatin analogue. N Engl J Med 315:663, 1986.

Lappohn RE, Burger HG, Bouma J, et al: Inhibin as a marker for granulosa-cell tumors. N Engl J Med 321:790, 1989.

Liu TL, Lian IJ, Deppe G: Serum lactic dehydrogenase (SLDH) in germ cell malignancies of the ovary. Gynecol Oncol 19:355, 1984.

Lobo RA: Androgen excess: differential diagnosis and evaluation. In Mishell DR, Brenner PF (eds): Management of Common Problems in Obstetrics and Gynecology. Oradell, NJ, Medical Economics Books, 1994, p 619.

Loehrer PJ Sr, Johnson D, Elson P, et al: Importance of bleomycin in favorable-prognosis disseminated germ cell tumors: an Eastern Cooperative Oncology Group trial. J Clin Oncol 13:470, 1995.

Loehrer PJ Sr, Lauer R, Roth BJ, et al: Salvage therapy in recurrent germ cell cancer: ifosfamide and cisplatin plus either vinblastine or etoposide. Ann Intern Med 109:540, 1988.

Mann WJ, Chumas J, Rosenwaks Z, et al: Elevated serum α-fetoprotein associated with Sertoli-Leydig cell tumors of the ovary. Obstet Gynecol 67:141, 1986.

Manuel M, Katayama KP, Jones HW: The age of occurrence of gonadal tumors in intersex patients with a Y chromosome. Am J Obstet Gynecol 124:293, 1976.

Meigs JV, Armstrong SH, Hamilton HH: A further contribution to the syndrome of fibroma of the ovary with fluid in the abdomen and chest, Meigs' syndrome. Am J Obstet Gynecol 46:19, 1943.

Mendel M, Toren A, Kende G, et al: Familial clustering of malignant germ cell tumors and Langerhans' histiocytosis. Cancer 73:1980, 1994.

Meyer JS, Rao BR, Valdes R Jr, et al: Progesterone receptor in granulosa cell tumor. Gynecol Oncol 13:252, 1982.

Montz FJ, Hornstein J, Platt LD, et al: The diagnosis of immature teratoma by maternal serum alpha-fetoprotein screening. Obstet Gynecol 73:522, 1989.

Munkarah A, Gershenson DM, Levenback C, et al: Salvage surgery for chemorefractory ovarian germ cell tumors. Gynecol Oncol 55:217, 1994.

Nielson SN, Gaffey TA, Malkasian GD: Immature ovarian teratoma: a review of 14 cases. Mayo Clin Proc 61:110, 1986.

Nielsen SNJ, Scheithauer BW, Gaffey TA: Gliomatosis peritonei. Cancer 56:2499, 1985.

Nogales FF Jr, Matilda A, Nogales-Ortiz F, Galera-Davidson HL: Yolk sac tumors with pure and mixed polyvesicular vitelline patterns. Human Pathol 9:553, 1978.

Norris HJ, Taylor HB: Prognosis of granulosa-theca tumors of the ovary. Cancer 21:255, 1968.

Norris HJ, Zirkin HJ, Benson WL: Immature (malignant) teratoma of the ovary. Cancer 37:2359, 1976.

Ohama K, Nomura K, Okamoto E, et al: Origin of immature teratoma of the ovary. Am J Obstet Gynecol 152:896, 1985.

Payne D, Muss HB, Homesley HD, et al: Autoimmune hemolytic anemia and ovarian dermoid cysts: case report and review of the literature. Cancer 48:721, 1981.

Pode D, Kopolovic S, Gimmon Z: Serum lactic dehydrogenase: a tumor marker of ovarian dysgerminoma in a female pseudohermaphrodite. Gynecol Oncol 19:110, 1984.

Prat J, Scully RE: Cellular fibromas and fibrosarcomas of the ovary: a comparative clinicopathologic analysis of seventeen cases. Cancer 47:2663, 1981.

Prat J, Young RH, Scully RE: Ovarian Sertoli-Leydig cell tumors with heterologous elements. II. Cartilage and skeletal muscle. Cancer 50:2465, 1982.

Raggio M, Kaplan AL, Harberg JF: Recurrent ovarian fibromas with basal cell nevus syndrome (Gorlin syndrome). Obstet Gynecol 61:95S, 1983.

Robboy SJ, Norris HJ, Scully RE: Insular carcinoid primary in the ovary: a clinicopathologic analysis of 48 cases. Cancer 36:404, 1975.

Robboy SJ, Scully RE: Ovarian teratoma with glial implants on the peritoneum. Human Pathol 1:643, 1970.

Robboy SJ, Scully RE: Strumal carcinoid of the ovary: an analysis of 50 cases of a distinctive tumor composed of thyroid tissue and carcinoid. Cancer 46:2019, 1980.

Robboy SJ, Scully RE, Norris HJ: Carcinoid metastatic to the ovary: a clinicopathologic analysis of 35 cases. Cancer 33:798, 1974.

Robboy SJ, Scully RE, Norris HJ: Primary trabecular carcinoid of the ovary. Obstet Gynecol 49:202, 1977.

Rodgers KE, Marks JF, Ellefson DD, et al: Follicle regulatory protein: a novel marker for granulosa cell cancer patients. Gynecol Oncol 37:381, 1990.

Romero R, Schwartz PE: Alpha fetoprotein determinations in the management of endodermal sinus tumors and mixed germ cell tumors of the ovary. Am J Obstet Gynecol 141:126, 1981.

Roush GR, El-Naggar AK, Abdul-Karim FW: Granulosa cell tumor of ovary: a clinicopathologic and flow cytometric DNA analysis. Gynecol Oncol 56:430, 1995.

Samanth KK, Black WC: Benign ovarian stromal tumors associated with free peritoneal fluid. Am J Obstet Gynecol 107:538, 1970.

Schwartz PE: Combination chemotherapy in the management of ovarian germ cell malignancies. Obstet Gynecol 64:564, 1984.

Schwartz PE, Morris JM: Serum lactic dehydrogenase: a tumor marker for dysgerminoma. Obstet Gynecol 72:511, 1988.

Scully RE: Gonadoblastoma: a gonadal tumor related to the dysgerminoma (seminoma) and capable of sex hormone production. Cancer 6:455, 1953.

Scully RE: Sex cord tumor with annular tubules: a distinctive ovarian tumor of the Peutz-Jeghers syndrome. Cancer 25:1107, 1970.

Scully RE: Ovarian tumors: a review. Am J Pathol 87:686, 1977.

Scully RE: Tumors of the ovary and maldeveloped gonads. In Atlas of Tumor Pathology, Fascicle 16. Bethesda, MD, Armed Forces Institute of Pathology, 1979.

Segal R, DePetrillo AD, Thomas G: Clinical review of adult granulosa cell tumors of the ovary. Gynecol Oncol 56:338, 1995.

Seidman JD: Unclassified ovarian gonadal stromal tumors: a clinicopathologic study of 32 cases. Am J Surg Pathol 20:699, 1996.

Sheiko MC, Hart WR: Ovarian germinoma (dysgerminoma) with elevated serum lactic dehydrogenase: case report and review of literature. Cancer 49:994, 1982.

Stegner H-E, Lisboa BP: Steroid metabolism in an androblastoma (Sertoli-Leydig cell tumor): a histopathological and biochemical study. Int J Gynecol Pathol 2:410, 1984.

Stenwig JT, Hazekamp JT, Beecham JB: Granulosa cell tumors of the ovary: a clinicopathological study of 118 cases with long-term follow-up. Gynecol Oncol 7:136, 1979.

Stern JL, Buscema J, Rosenshein NB, Woodruff JD: Spontaneous rupture of benign cystic teratomas. Obstet Gynecol 57:363, 1981.

Stuart GC, Smith JP: Rupture of benign cystic teratomas mimicking gynecologic malignancy. Gynecol Oncol 16:139, 1983.

Takeda A, Ishizuka T, Goto T, et al: Polyembryoma of ovary producing alpha-fetoprotein and hCG: immunoperoxidase and electron microscopic study. Cancer 49:1878, 1982.

Talerman A: Ovarian Sertoli-Leydig cell tumor (androblastoma) with retiform pattern: a clinicopathologic study. Cancer 60:3056, 1987.

Tavassoli FA, Norris HJ: Sertoli tumors of the ovary: a clinicopathologic study of 28 cases with ultrastructural observations. Cancer 46:2281, 1980.

Taylor MH, De Petrillo AD, Turner AR: Vinblastine, bleomycin, and cisplatin in malignant germ cell tumors of the ovary. Cancer 56:1341, 1985.

Teilum G: Endodermal sinus tumors of the ovary and testis: comparative morphogenesis of the so-called mesonephroma ovarii (Schiller) and extraembryonic (yolk sac allantoic) structures of the rat placenta. Cancer 12:1029, 1959.

Teilum G: Special Tumors of Ovary and Testis and Related Extragonadal Lesions: Comparative Pathology and Histological Identification, ed. 2. Philadelphia, JB Lippincott, 1977.

Tracy SL, Askin FB, Reddick RL, et al: Progesterone secreting Sertoli cell tumor of the ovary. Gynecol Oncol 22:85, 1985.

Truong LD, Jurco S III, McGavran MH: Gliomatosis peritonei: report of two cases and review of literature. Am J Surg Pathol 6:443, 1982.

Vassal G, Flamant F, Caillaud JM, et al: Juvenile granulosa cell tumor of the ovary in children: a clinical study of 15 cases. J Clin Oncol 6:990, 1988.

Waid-Jones MI, Coursin DB: Perioperative considerations for patients treated with bleomycin. Chest 99:993, 1991.

Wilkowske MA, Hartmann LC, Mullany CJ, et al: Progressive carcinoid heart disease after resection of primary ovarian carcinoid. Cancer 73:1889, 1994.

Williams SD: Current management of ovarian germ cell tumors. Oncology 8:53, 1994.

Williams S, Blessing JA, Liao S-Y, et al: Adjuvant therapy of ovarian germ cell tumors with cisplatin, etoposide, and bleomycin: a trial of the Gynecologic Oncology Group. J Clin Oncol 12:701, 1994.

Williams SD, Blessing JA, Moore DH, et al: Cisplatin, vinblastine, and bleomycin in advanced and recurrent ovarian germ-cell tumors: a trial of the Gynecologic Oncology Group. Ann Intern Med 111:22, 1989a.

Williams SD, Blessing J, Slayton R, et al: Ovarian germ cell tumors: adjuvant trials of the Gynecologic Oncology Group (GOG). In Proceedings of the American Society of Clinical Oncology, Abstract #584, 1989b.

Yannopoulous D, Yannopoulous K, Ossowski R: Malignant struma ovarii. Pathol Annu 11:403, 1976.

Young RH, Dickersin GR, Scully RE: Juvenile granulosa cell tumor of the ovary. Am J Surg Pathol 8:575, 1984.

Young RH, Prat J, Scully RE: Ovarian Sertoli-Leydig cell tumors with heterologous elements. I. Gastrointestinal epithelium and carcinoid. Cancer 50:2448, 1982a.

Young RH, Scully RE: Ovarian sex cord-stromal tumors: recent progress. Int J Gynecol Pathol 1:101, 1982.

Young RH, Scully RE: Ovarian Sertoli cell tumors: a report of 10 cases. Int J Gynecol Pathol 2:349, 1984a.

Young RH, Scully RE: Well-differentiated ovarian Sertoli-Leydig cell tumors: a clinicopathological analysis of 23 cases. Int J Gynecol Pathol 3:277, 1984b.

Young RH, Scully RE: Ovarian Sertoli-Leydig cell tumors: a clinicopathological analysis of 207 cases. Am J Surg Pathol 9:543, 1985.

Young RH, Welch WR, Dickersin GR, Scully RE: Ovarian sex cord tumor with annular tubules. Cancer 50:1384, 1982b.

Zaloudek C, Norris HJ: Granulosa cell tumors of the ovary in young children: a clinical and pathologic study of 32 cases. Am J Surg Pathol 6:513, 1982.

Zhang J, Young RH, Arseneau J, Scully RE: Ovarian stromal tumors containing lutein or Leydig cells (luteinized thecomas and stromal Leydig cell tumors): a clinicopathological analysis of fifty cases. Int J Gynecol Pathol 1:270, 1982.

12

Tumors of the Ovary: Soft Tissue and Secondary (Metastatic) Tumors; Tumor-like Conditions

SOFT TISSUE TUMORS NOT SPECIFIC TO THE OVARY

Benign and malignant tumors may arise in the ovary from the nonspecific supporting tissues that are common to most bodily organs. Such tumors include fibromas, hemangiomas, leiomyomas, soft tissue sarcomas, lymphomas, and other rare neoplasms. The fibroma and the lymphoma are the most common and most important tumors in this category.

Fibroma

The fibroma is a benign connective tissue tumor composed of fibroblasts and collagen. It is one of the most common ovarian neoplasms and accounts for 20 percent of all solid ovarian tumors. It is not readily distinguishable from the thecoma clinically or histologically, and some authorities prefer to categorize these lesions together (see Chapter 11). The average age at diagnosis is 48 years. The fibroma is typically 6 cm in diameter; 10 percent are bilateral, and areas of calcification are common.

The fibroma is especially significant because of its role in Meigs' syndrome. In 1937, Meigs and Cass reported on the occasional coexistence of ovarian fibroma, ascites, and hydrothorax, at times complicated by cachexia. Since this clinical picture was considered diagnostic of advanced ovarian carcinoma, some women were permitted to die without therapeutic intervention. The ascites and hydrothorax are reversible after removal of the fibroma or other benign ovarian stromal neoplasm. Actually less than 5 percent of fibromas are associated with ascites

and pleural effusion, which occur almost exclusively with tumors greater than 10 cm in diameter. The hydrothorax is almost invariably on the right side and results from ascitic fluid traversing the diaphragm through congenital perforations or via lymphatics. The etiology of the ascites is unknown, but two theories have been proposed: (1) the tumor irritates the peritoneum, inducing it to produce the ascitic fluid; and (2) the tumor twists on its pedicle, obstructing lymphatic outflow from the ovary. The resultant ovarian edema leads to leakage of fluid from the tumor into the peritoneal cavity. Numerous nonmalignant gynecologic conditions have been reported to cause ascites with or without pleural fluid, including endometriosis (usually hemorrhagic), uterine fibroids, pelvic inflammatory disease, struma ovarii, massive ovarian edema, and theca-lutein cysts. Regardless of the cause, ascites and pleural effusion may be associated with a very high serum CA-125 value (Siddiqui and Toub, 1995).

Lymphoma

The genital tract in women and girls is commonly involved with generalized lymphoma or leukemia. Occasionally these diseases may present as a gynecologic problem, and in rare cases lymphoma is localized to the genital tract (Rotmensch and Woodruff, 1982; Osborne and Robboy, 1983). However, even in such cases it is disputed whether the lymphoma could originate in the ovary, since the ovary ordinarily is devoid of lymphoid structures, although variable numbers of lymphocytes are commonly present (Skodras et al, 1994). One case of a malignant lymphoma arising in a mature cystic teratoma has been reported (Seifer et al, 1986). In the paper of Chorlton et al (1974), only 19 of 9,500 cases of lymphoma had the initial manifestation in the ovary. Fox et al (1988) described 34 cases of lymphoma presenting as an ovarian tumor. The median age of the patients was 36 years; two thirds of the patients were less than 40 years of age. Fourteen of the patients presented with acute symptoms (abdominal pain, distension, vomiting). Fox and colleagues recommended utilizing the Ann Arbor staging classification of lymphomas rather than the International Federation of Gynecology and Obstetrics staging of ovarian neoplasms. Six of their 34 patients presented with disease limited to the ovary(ies) at laparotomy, but systemic disease was eventually documented in three of the six patients.

Misdiagnosis and understaging may be responsible for the generally poor prognosis of primary ovarian lymphoma. The differential diagnosis includes dysgerminoma, stromal tumors, neuroendocrine small-cell tumor, and a benign inflammatory process. Lymphoma should be suspected by the presence of bilateral solid tumors in a young patient, especially if there is lymphadenopathy. Whether or not the diagnosis of lymphoma is made by frozen section, sampling of enlarged lymph nodes is always recommended. Fresh tissue should be preserved for additional studies, including flow cytometry and cellular subtyping. Wedge biopsy of the liver and splenectomy are no longer required for staging lymphomas. Postoperatively, a computed tomography scan of the abdomen and chest, plus bone marrow biopsy, completes the staging.

Granulocytic sarcoma (chloroma) is a rare manifestation of myeloid leukemia and has been described as occurring in a wide variety of anatomic regions, including the ovary (Colle et al, 1996). The descriptive name *chloroma* refers to the greenish hue associated with these tumors.

TUMORS METASTATIC TO THE OVARY

Virchow has been quoted as saying that the organs that most frequently produce malignant neoplasms are rarely the sites of metastases. Certainly, the ovary is an exception to this dictum. From 5 to 30 percent of women dying of cancer are found to have ovarian metastases at autopsy, and one fifth of those undergoing palliative oophorectomy for metastatic breast cancer have microscopic evidence of metastases to the ovaries. At least 5 percent of patients explored for ovarian cancer have a secondary rather than a primary lesion. The most common sources of metastases to the ovary are the breast, gastrointestinal tract, and pelvic organs (Gagnon and Tetu, 1989). In 75 percent of the cases of ovarian secondaries, both ovaries are grossly involved by metastases, and, with rare exception, when metastases are present in the ovary, there is metastatic disease in other parts of the body. Occasionally, evidence of hormonal activity results from an associated reactive stromal hyperplasia.

In 1896, Krukenberg described an ovarian neoplasm that he designated as *fibrosarcoma ovarii mucocellulare* (*carcinomatodes*). He considered this to be a primary ovarian sarcoma. Schlaggenhoffer established the metastatic nature of this tumor in 1902. Although the appellation *Krukenberg tumor* has often been used to describe any secondary ovarian cancer, its application should be restricted to ovarian tumors that fit Krukenberg's original description. Grossly, these tumors are solid, kidney shaped, usually bilateral and average 10 cm in diameter. There is a tendency to retain the contour of the normal ovary. Hemorrhage and necrosis may be present, and the cut surface often displays a gelatinous consistency. Microscopically, there is a florid hyperplasia of the ovarian stroma that tends to obscure the mucus-secreting signet-ring cells. Adhesions and other intra-abdominal disease are usually absent. Virilization has been reported in association with a Krukenberg tumor in pregnancy related to abundant hyperplasia of the ovarian stroma (Silva et al, 1988).

Nearly all tumors of the ovary that fit Krukenberg's description are metastases from a primary cancer in the stomach, although other primary sites, such as the gallbladder, breast, and colon, have been reported. In about 10 percent of cases, no primary site can be identified. When gastric cancer occurs in pregnancy, it may simulate physiologic morning sickness (Cheng et al, 1994). Proposed routes of spread from the stomach to the ovary are retrograde dissemination via the aortic lymphatics, hematogenous, and transperitoneal. The occurrence of metastases to the ovary seems to be disproportionately common in premenopausal women, presumably because of the vascularity of the functioning ovary. However, the average age of women with a Krukenberg tumor is 45 to 50 years (Holtz and Hart, 1982). If a Krukenberg tumor is diagnosed intraoperatively in a patient initially thought to have an ovarian primary tumor, the focus of the operation may be changed. Unlike primary epithelial ovarian carcinoma, advanced Krukenberg tumors have a poor prognosis and are less likely to respond to chemotherapy. Indications for radical tumor-reductive surgery are therefore more restrictive.

Carcinoma of the colon metastatic to the ovary can resemble histologically primary mucinous, serous, endometrioid, or poorly differentiated adenocarcinoma of the ovary, and the clinical presentation, operative findings, and histology may be identical to a primary ovarian cancer. Serum carcinoembryonic antigen (CEA) determination and/or immunohistochemical staining of the tumor for CEA may not yield a definitive answer because both colonic and ovarian cancer are capable of producing CEA. Nuclear reactivity for estrogen receptor may assist in differentiating a primary from a secondary mucinous tumor (Darwish et al, 1988).

Because of the frequency with which carcinomas of the colon metastasize to the ovary (2 to 8 percent), some authors have recommended prophylactic oophorectomy as part of the surgical therapy for colon cancer (Morrow and Enker, 1984). However, Ballantyne et al (1985) were unable to identify a survival benefit for patients undergoing prophylactic oophorectomy. Morrow and Enker (1984) also emphasized the importance of bilateral oophorectomy at the time of palliative resection for colon cancer. Bilateral oophorectomy adds little to operative morbidity and should be done in all postmenopausal patients with colon cancer as prophylaxis against ovarian carcinoma. The procedure should also be performed on all patients with stage D colon cancer regardless of age.

TUMOR-LIKE CONDITIONS OF THE OVARY

Non-neoplastic, functional cysts and hyperplasias of the ovarian follicle and its supporting tissues are the most common, clinically detectable enlargements of the ovary occurring during the reproductive years (Table 12–1). They are of importance primarily be-

TABLE 12–1

Non-neoplastic Cysts and Hyperplasias of the Ovary

Pregnancy luteoma
Hyperthecosis
Massive edema and fibromatosis
Solitary functional cysts
   Follicle
   Corpus luteum
Polycystic ovaries
Theca-lutein cysts and multiple corpora lutea
Endometriotic cysts (endometriomas)
Germinal inclusion cysts
Simple cysts

cause they cannot be distinguished readily on clinical grounds from neoplastic enlargements.

Pregnancy Luteoma

Pregnancy luteoma is a nodular hyperplasia of ovarian lutein cells. It occurs exclusively during pregnancy, predominantly in multiparous black women. Nearly all cases have been discovered incidentally at the time of cesarean section or postpartum tubal ligation. Maternal (10 to 15 percent) and fetal (50 percent of female fetuses) virilization has been reported in association with pregnancy luteoma (Hensleigh and Woodruff, 1978). Clinical signs of maternal virilization usually appear in the second trimester of pregnancy.

Pregnancy luteomas range up to 20 cm in diameter, are frequently bilateral, and are usually multinodular. Spontaneous regression occurs postpartum, but the hyperplasia may recur with subsequent pregnancies. Scully (1979) recommends excision of uninodular lesions (with ovarian preservation) for microscopic evaluation even if the patient is virilized. If the lesion is multinodular, excision of one nodule should be done to rule out neoplasia, especially metastatic cancer.

Ovarian Hyperthecosis

Women with ovarian hyperthecosis, an androgenizing condition, have the clinical features characteristic of the polycystic ovary (PCO or Stein-Leventhal) syndrome, including familial occurrence, ovaries normal or enlarged two to three times normal, and multiple cystic follicles. In the fully manifested case, frank virilization, obesity, hypertension, and glucose intolerance are found. The characteristic microscopic ovarian lesion is a hyperplastic ovarian stroma with scattered clusters of luteinized stromal theca cells. Hyperthecosis may represent one extreme of the PCO syndrome. Women with hyperthecosis are more likely to be virilized than women with PCO, and they are less likely to ovulate in response to clomiphene citrate. Castration may be required to control the androgen excess.

Ovarian hyperthecosis is more likely than PCO to simulate clinically an ovarian or adrenal tumor, since the serum testosterone tends to be higher (150 to 200 ng/dl; a level over 300 ng/dl is strongly suspicious of tumor) than with PCO (<150 ng/dl). Although testosterone in both conditions is typically at the upper limits of normal, it may exceed 1,000 ng/dl. The onset and progression of virilization in hyperthecosis tend to be more rapid and the degree more severe, as with the virilizing tumors, in contrast to the average case of PCO.

An interesting aspect of ovarian hyperthecosis is its occasional association with *acanthosis nigricans* and the Kahn type A syndrome of hyperandrogenism (usually manifested around the time of puberty, sometimes in association with PCO, hyperthecosis, or multiple dermoid cysts) and insulin resistance, although the glucose tolerance test may be normal. Acanthosis nigricans is a cutaneous disorder characterized by symmetrical, brown, verrucous thickenings of the skin on the back of the neck, under the breasts, and in the axillae and groin (see Chapter 3). It occurs in conjunction with various endocrinopathies and malignant diseases, most often an adenocarcinoma, and it may be the only indication of insulin resistance. The type B syndrome of insulin resistance is a documented autoimmune disease with overt diabetes and acanthosis nigricans. Hyperandrogenism is not a characteristic part of the type B syndrome (Annos and Taymor, 1981; Scully et al, 1982; Barbieri and Ryan, 1983).

Massive Ovarian Edema

Massive edema of the ovary is a tumor-like condition characterized by marked enlargement of one or both ovaries as a result of an accumulation of edema fluid in the ovarian stroma. The follicles are normal, but stromal luteinization may occur, accompanied by evidence of androgen excess. Fifty-one cases of massive ovarian edema were collected from the world literature by Young and Scully

(1984). The average age of the patients was 21 years (range 6 to 33), and the most common presenting symptom was abdominal pain, at times acute and severe. Amenorrhea or menstrual irregularities were common, and about 10 percent of patients had signs of virilization. The affected ovaries averaged 11 cm in diameter, with a range from 5.5 to 35 cm. Partial or complete torsion was present in one half of the reported cases. There appears to be an association of this lesion with ovarian hyperthecosis and PCO. Ascites and hydrothorax complicating massive ovarian edema have been reported (Fukuda et al, 1984).

Grossly, the ovary resembles any edematous ovarian neoplasm, especially a fibroma or Krukenberg tumor. However, the finding of pitting edema and cystic follicles within the ovary favors the diagnosis of massive ovarian edema. The diagnosis cannot be made with certainty on the basis of operative findings, and frozen section analysis may not exclude the possibility that the lesion is an edematous neoplasm. The recommendations of Young and Scully (1984), therefore, seem to be appropriate: if the ovarian involvement is unilateral, perform an ovariectomy; if both ovaries are involved, remove the larger one for frozen section evaluation. If the diagnosis is massive ovarian edema (or fibromatosis; see later), the residual enlarged ovary should be wedged but not removed. Stabilization of the remaining ovary by reefing sutures in the ovarian ligament is recommended, since the etiology of massive ovarian edema is thought to be intermittent torsion (Thorp et al, 1990).

In their 1984 paper, Young and Scully described 14 cases of ovarian enlargement caused by pure or predominant fibromatosis (6 had areas of edema) of the ovarian stroma, with clinical features similar to those of massive ovarian edema. They suggest that fibromatosis may be the primary event leading to an increase in ovarian size and weight, with torsion and edema a secondary event. Bychkov and Kijek (1987) describe two clinical syndromes: primary ovarian edema and secondary ovarian edema.

Solitary Functional Cysts (Follicle and Corpus Luteum Cysts)

When a follicle exceeds 3 cm in diameter, it is considered to be abnormal and is designated a *follicle cyst or follicular cyst*. Such cysts are generally asymptomatic, but they may be accompanied by minor degrees of unilateral pelvic pain and occasionally dyspareunia. Some patients report menstrual irregularities. Rupture during pelvic examination is common. Spontaneous rupture can occur, accompanied by bleeding that is rarely serious unless the patient is taking anticoagulants or is thrombocytopenic. Follicular cysts infrequently undergo torsion and infarction, producing a surgical emergency. In the child, isosexual precocity can result from a persistent follicular cyst, while menometrorrhagia and anovulation may occur during the reproductive years.

Cysts of the corpus luteum are less common than follicular cysts and are more likely to be associated with symptoms related to their endocrine activity, rupture, or intracystic hemorrhage. Often the menstrual period is delayed, even in the absence of pregnancy, and vaginal spotting may occur. If pain and intra-abdominal bleeding develop and the cystic mass is palpable, the clinical picture may simulate closely an ectopic pregnancy. For those cases requiring surgery, a tissue diagnosis is recommended (Hallatt et al, 1984).

Functional cysts are characterized by their dimensions. They seldom exceed 10 cm in diameter, are unilateral, and are freely mobile. During the reproductive years, an adnexal mass of this description can be presumed to be a functional cyst rather than a true neoplasm; hormonal contraceptives do not preclude the development of benign "functional" cysts (Caillouette and Koehler, 1987; Holt et al, 1992). The rather transitory existence of functional cysts, especially the follicular variety, is of pre-eminent importance in distinguishing them from true neoplasms. Tradition and clinical experience have taught that functional cysts usually persist for only a few days or weeks, and re-examination during a different phase of the menstrual cycle has been common practice. Combination oral contraceptive pills are often prescribed to accelerate the involution of functional cysts on the presumption that these cysts are gonadotropin dependent. The inhibitory effect of the contraceptive steroids on the release of pituitary gonadotropins should therefore abbreviate the life span of these cysts, hastening their identification as functional or non-neoplastic. Failure to regress during the period of observation requires operative removal. Medicinal estrogens, however, can increase the risk of thromboembolic complications, so the routine use of oral contraceptives in the management of the patient with a suspected functional cyst may not be prudent in view of the fact that some patients will need surgery.

Spanos (1973) studied clinically unilateral functional cysts (5 to 10 cm) in 286 women. Steroid contraceptives were prescribed, and the women were re-examined in 6 weeks. In 72 percent of the women, the mass disappeared during the observation interval. Of the 81 patients whose mass persisted, none was found to have a functional cyst at laparotomy (Table 12–2). The fact that five of the removed tumors were malignant underscores the importance of avoiding delay in operative investigation. Pinotti et al (1988) reported on 499 women with adnexal cysts 3 to 8 cm in diameter (average of the two largest diameters) based on ultrasound evaluation. Most of the patients were asymptomatic and less than 50 years of age. Of those study patients without ultrasound features suggestive of malignancy, 203 were followed up to 1 year and 83.7 percent regressed spontaneously. Sixty percent of those cysts that disappeared on ultrasound follow-up did so within 3 months of diagnosis, the percentage not varying greatly with cyst diameter. Thirty-three of the monitored patients underwent surgery. Only seven had a neoplasm, none of which was malignant. Endometriomas, hydrosalpinges, simple cysts, parovarian cysts, and paratubal cysts accounted for most of the non-neoplastic persistent adnexal cystic masses.

In the reproductive period, an ovarian enlargement less than 5 cm in diameter should be investigated if it persists longer than 3 months in the absence of symptoms. Less than 5 percent of these small cysts will be

T A B L E **12–2**

Adnexal "Cysts" Persistent in 286 Women Between the Ages of 16 and 48 Years Treated With Estrogen or Combination Estrogen and Progestin for 6 Weeks*

Diagnosis	N	% of Total
Non-neoplastic cysts		
Functional	0	(0.0)
Endometriotic	28	(34.5)
Parovarian	4	(4.9)
Hydrosalpinx	3	(3.7)
Neoplasms		
Dermoid	9	(11.1)
Epithelial, benign	32	(39.5)
Epithelial, malignant	4	(4.9)
Dysgerminoma	1	(1.2)
Total	81	(100.0)

*From Spanos WJ: Preoperative hormonal therapy of cystic adnexal masses. Am J Obstet Gynecol 116:551, 1973, with permission.

neoplastic, and the risk of malignancy is less than 1 percent (Miller and Willson, 1942; see Chapter 9). Evaluation by ultrasound can be helpful if the cyst has characteristics typical of a dermoid or endometrioma, but the presence of "septa" does not exclude a reversible condition. CA-125 determination is unreliable in these reproductive-age patients and is not recommended.

Polycystic Ovaries

Bilateral ovarian enlargement may be found in young women with the PCO (Stein-Leventhal) syndrome of infertility, oligomenorrhea, and menstrual irregularities. The ovaries may be two to three times the normal size. The etiology of the ovarian enlargement usually is apparent clinically because of the characteristic history and physical features of this syndrome. Nevertheless, the nature of the ovarian enlargement needs to be documented, since PCO and ovarian neoplasia can coexist. PCO, and the related disorder ovarian hyperthecosis (see earlier), can simulate clinically ovarian and adrenal androgen-producing tumors (see Chapter 11).

Theca-Lutein Cysts and Multiple Corpora Lutea

Multiple follicle cysts with luteinization of the theca cells are referred to as *theca-lutein cysts.* They are believed to result from high levels of human chorionic gonadotropin (hCG), or an increased sensitivity of theca cells to hCG. Typically theca-lutein cysts are found in association with hydatidiform mole (in one third to one half of the cases) and choriocarcinoma, but occasionally they occur in pregnant patients with Rh sensitization, a triploid fetus, multifetal gestation, toxemia, or diabetes. Rarely does this occur in a normal singleton pregnancy. Maternal, but not fetal, virilization has been reported. Administration of gonadotropins or clomiphene to induce ovulation may produce theca-lutein cysts and multiple corpora lutea ("overstimulation syndrome"). Either of these conditions can be associated with ascites and hydrothorax. Theca-lutein cysts are characteristically bilateral and may grow to more than 25 cm in diameter. Spontaneous regression occurs as the gonadotropin level falls. Return of the ovaries to normal size, however, often lags behind the decline in gonadotropin levels. Torsion, rupture with hemorrhage, and intracystic hemorrhage are infrequent but often necessitate surgical intervention when they do occur.

Endometriotic Cysts (Endometriomas)

About 5 percent of patients with endometriosis have a clinically detectable adnexal mass. This endometriotic cyst or *endometrioma* presumably results from cyclic hemorrhage into a focus of ovarian endometriosis. Accumulation of blood within the cavity results in the classic "chocolate" cyst. These cysts are relatively thin walled, and a minor degree of leakage often occurs, producing intermittent pain and adhesions. Physical examination may reveal other findings consistent with endometriosis, including uterosacral nodularity, retroversion of the uterus, and cul-de-sac tenderness. Rupture with hemorrhage occasionally occurs, typically during the luteal or menstrual phase of the ovulatory cycle, causing acute severe abdominal pain, leukocytosis, fever, and even hypotension.

Management of the patient with an adnexal mass and suspected or proven endometriosis must be directed toward the adnexal mass. If uterosacral nodularity is present, prompt surgical evaluation is even more urgent, since the nodules may represent implants from ovarian carcinoma. The serum CA-125 value is often elevated in endometriosis and cannot be used readily to differentiate between a benign and a malignant adnexal mass (see Chapter 9). Ovarian endometriosis clearly has a malignant proclivity, and may give rise to any of the endometrial malignancies, including clear cell carcinoma, endometrioid carcinoma, stromal sarcoma, and mixed müllerian tumor (Scully et al, 1996). Epithelial atypia and adenomatous hyperplasia have also been reported (Cooper, 1978; Czernobilsky and Morris, 1979) in ovarian endometriosis. Whether endometriotic cysts of the ovary are ever true neoplasms derived from germinal inclusions in the manner of serous and mucinous tumors is disputed, but this seems to be an eminently reasonable possibility.

Germinal Inclusion Cysts

Germinal inclusion cysts are common, microscopic structures in the ovarian stroma lined by flat, cuboidal, or columnar cells that may be of the tubal, endometrial, or endocervical type. The inclusions apparently derive from the surface epithelial infoldings, which occur as a consequence of ovulation. The resultant clefts lined by germinal epithelium are pinched off by the adjacent stroma. Germinal inclusions are believed to be etiologically related to the benign and malignant epithelial neoplasms of the ovary and also the simple cysts of the ovary. Epithelial inclusions occur at all ages, even in the fetus. In the prepubertal ovary, the inclusions are lined with flat, cuboidal, or low columnar epithelium similar to mesothelial cells. In the postmenarchal female, most inclusions are lined with endotubal-type cells, suggesting that metaplasia of the multipotential celomic epithelium is induced by the changing hormonal milieu (Blaustein et al, 1982).

In a review of ovaries from 470 operated patients, Mulligan (1976) reported that 22 percent had 1 to 50 germinal inclusions lined with serous (endotubal) epithelium, 7.4 percent had 1 to 20 inclusions lined by endometrial epithelium, and 0.4 percent had 1 to 15 inclusions lined by endocervical-type epithelium. In these same patients, 63 had serous, 23 endometrioid, and 27 endocervical (mucinous) neoplasms, leading Mulligan to conclude that the mucinous inclusions had the greatest neoplastic potential.

Simple Cysts

The term *simple cyst* has been variously applied to any unilocular cyst filled with serous fluid, including functional cysts and cystadenomas. Simple cysts are defined by the World Health Organization (WHO), however, as ovarian cysts without an identifiable lining. Scully (1979) characterizes them as cysts of unknown origin in which the lining has disappeared, or has been destroyed, or consists of a thin layer of indifferent epithelial-like cells. Simple cysts are probably derived from follicular cysts, germinal inclusions, or cystadenomas; the absence or flattening of the epithelial lining reflects the effects of pressure on what has become essentially a retention cyst. Therefore, a significant feature of simple cysts is that they are not neoplastic, although they may have begun as such. If foci of serous epithelium persist, the distinction between a unilocular serous cystadenoma (or cystoma) and a simple cyst becomes fuzzy, but this is of doubtful clinical import. Regarding the clinical manifestations of simple cysts, as defined by Scully or WHO, there seems to be little information. Their size, frequency of occurrence, and associated complications are

not known. These simple cysts are encountered by the clinician, however, as an adnexal mass, an adnexal accident, or an incidental finding at surgery.

REFERENCES

Annos T, Taymor ML: Ovarian pathology associated with insulin resistance and acanthosis nigricans. Obstet Gynecol 58:662, 1981.

Ballantyne GH, Rugel MM, Wolff BG, Illstrup DM: Oophorectomy and colon cancer. Ann Surg 202:209, 1985.

Barbieri RL, Ryan KJ: Hyperandrogenism, insulin resistance, and acanthosis nigricans syndrome: a common endocrinopathy with distinct pathophysiologic features. Am J Obstet Gynecol 147:90, 1983.

Blaustein A, Kantius M, Kaganowicz A, et al: Inclusions in ovaries of females aged day 1–30 years. Int J Gynecol Pathol 1:145, 1982.

Bychkov V, Kijek M: Massive ovarian edema: four cases and some pathologic considerations. Acta Obstet Gynecol Scand 66:397, 1987.

Caillouette JC, Koehler AL: Phasic contraceptive pills and functional ovarian cysts. Am J Obstet Gynecol 156:1538, 1987.

Cheng C-Y, Chen T-Y, Lin C-K, et al: Krukenberg tumor in pregnancy with delivery of a normal baby: a case report. Chin Med J 54:424, 1994.

Chorlton I, Norris HJ, King FM: Malignant reticuloendothelial disease involving the ovary as a primary manifestation: a series of 19 lymphomas and 1 granulocytic sarcoma. Cancer 34:397, 1974.

Colle I, Lacor P, Peeters P, et al: Granulocytic sarcoma (chloroma): a report of two cases. Acta Clin Belg 51:106, 1996.

Cooper P: Mixed mesodermal tumor and clear cell carcinoma arising in ovarian endometriosis. Cancer 42:2827, 1978.

Czernobilsky B, Morris WJ: A histologic study of ovarian endometriosis with emphasis on hyperplastic and atypical changes. Obstet Gynecol 53:318, 1979.

Darwish SAE, D'Ablaing G, Taylor CR: Nuclear reactivity for estrogen, a possible diagnostic tool in differentiating colon cancer metastases in the ovary from primary mucinous ovarian tumors. Cancer 62:2203, 1988.

Fox H, Langley FA, Govan AD, et al: Malignant lymphoma presenting as an ovarian tumor: A clinicopathologic analysis of 34 cases. Br J Obstet Gynaecol 95:386, 1988.

Fukude O, Munemura M, Tohya T, et al: Massive edema of the ovary associated with hydrothorax and ascites. Gynecol Oncol 17:231, 1984.

Gagnon Y, Tetu B: Ovarian metastases of breast carcinoma: a clinicopathologic study of 59 cases. Cancer 64:892, 1989.

Hallatt JG, Steele CH Jr, Snyder M: Ruptured corpus luteum with hemoperitoneum: a study of 173 surgical cases. Am J Obstet Gynecol 149:5, 1984.

Henslight PA, Woodruff JD: Differential maternal-fetal response to androgenizing luteoma or hyperreactio luteinalis. Obstet Gynecol Surv 33:262, 1978.

Holt VL, Daling JR, McKnight B, et al: Functional ovarian cysts in relation to the use of monophasic and triphasic oral contraceptives. Obstet Gynecol 79:529, 1992.

Holtz F, Hart WR: Krukenberg tumors of the ovary: a clinicopathologic analysis of 27 cases. Cancer 50:2438, 1982.

Meigs JV, Cass JW: Fibroma of the ovary with ascites and hydrothorax with a report of 7 cases. Am J Obstet Gynecol 33:249, 1937.

Miller NF, Willson JR: Surgery of the ovary: the small ovarian cysts. NY State J Med 151:1851, 1942.

Morrow M, Enker WE: Late ovarian metastases in carcinoma of the colon and rectum. Arch Surg 119:1385, 1984.

Mulligan RM: A survey of epithelial inclusions in the ovarian cortex of 470 patients. J Surg Oncol 8:61, 1976.

Osborne BM, Robboy SJ: Lymphoma or leukemia presenting as ovarian tumors: an analysis of 42 cases. Cancer 52:1933, 1983.

Pinotti JA, de Franzin CMMO, Marussi EF, Zeferino LC: Evaluation of cystic and adnexal tumors identified by echography. Int J Gynecol Obstet 26:109, 1988.

Rotmensch J, Woodruff JD: Lymphoma of the ovary: report of twenty new cases and update of previous series. Am J Obstet Gynecol 143:870, 1982.

Scully RE: Tumors of the Ovary and Maldeveloped Gonads. Washington, DC, Armed Forces Institute of Pathology, 1979.

Scully RE, Mark EJ, McNeely BU: Case reports of Massachusetts General Hospital. N Engl J Med 306:1537, 1982.

Scully RE, Richardson GS, Barlow JF: The development of malignancy in endometriosis. Clin Obstet Gynecol 9:384, 1966.

Seifer DB, Weiss LM, Kempson RL: Malignant lymphoma arising within thyroid tissue in a mature cystic teratoma. Cancer 58:2459, 1986.

Siddiqui M, Toub DB: Cellular fibroma of the ovary with Meigs' syndrome and elevated CA 125: a case report. J Reprod Med 40:817, 1995.

Silva PD, Porto M, Moyer DL, Lobo RA: Clinical and ultrastructural findings of an androgenizing Krukenberg tumor in pregnancy. Obstet Gynecol 71:432, 1988.

Skodras G, Fields V, Kragel PJ: Ovarian lymphoma and serous carcinoma of low malignant potential arising in the same ovary: a case report with literature review of 14 primary ovarian lymphomas. Arch Pathol Lab Med 118:647, 1994.

Spanos WJ: Preoperative hormonal therapy of cystic adnexal masses. Am J Obstet Gynecol 116:551, 1973.

Thorp JM, Wells SR, Droegemueller W: Ovarian suspension in massive ovarian edema. Obstet Gynecol 76:912, 1990.

Young RH, Scully RE: Fibromatosis and massive edema of the ovary, possibly related entities: a report of 14 cases of fibromatosis and 11 cases of massive edema. Int J Gynecol Pathol 3:153, 1984.

13

Tumors of the Placental Trophoblast

The growth disturbances of the human trophoblast manifest a wide range of biologic behavior. Four distinct clinicopathologic forms are recognized: hydatidiform (hydatid) mole (from the Latin *hydatis* = watery vesicle + *moles* = a shapeless mass), invasive mole (chorioadenoma destruens), choriocarcinoma, and placental site trophoblastic tumor. The term *chorionepithelioma* was used in the past to designate both invasive mole and choriocarcinoma. Today these tumors are referred to collectively as *gestational trophoblastic neoplasia* (GTN) or *disease.* Because of the extraordinary success of chemotherapy in the management of invasive mole and choriocarcinoma, a histopathologic diagnosis has limited clinical relevance.

As a neoplastic disease, GTN is unique insofar as these tumors are derived from fetal tissue but invade almost exclusively maternal tissue. They also exhibit a number of other unusual features that make them of special interest. Both invasive mole and choriocarcinoma are capable of elaborating steroid and protein hormones. The production of large quantities of human chorionic gonadotropin (hCG) is a hallmark of these tumors. GTN is reported to undergo spontaneous regression, although such an occurrence with choriocarcinoma is rare. Of all the malignant diseases, choriocarcinoma is the greatest imitator of other pathologic conditions because of its proclivity for hematogenous spread and the production of focal hemorrhagic lesions. In addition to these traits, choriocarcinoma has the distinction of being the fist disseminated solid tumor to be cured by chemotherapy. Although a "benign" neoplasm, invasive mole is, as the name implies, locally invasive and can be deported to distant sites, a feature more characteristic of fully malignant tumors.

A review of the clinical aspects of GTN is presented in this chapter. For a more detailed exposition of the subject, the interested reader is referred to the excellent monographs by Hertig (1968), Bagshawe (1969), Park (1971), Hertz (1978) Goldstein and Berkowitz (1982), and to the symposia edited by Morrow (1984b), Patillo and Hussa (1984), Berkowitz and Goldstein (1987, 1991), and Hammond (1988), as well as to the original papers listed in the reference section.

NORMAL TROPHOBLAST

The initial mitotic cleavage of the zygote produces daughter cells of unequal size. It is believed that the larger cell gives rise to the trophoblast, while the smaller one develops into the embryonic plate. Not only the cyto- and syncytiotrophoblast but also the blood vessels and supporting tissues of the placenta originate from the multipotential, primitive trophoblastic cells. The trophoblast constitutes a major portion of the blastocyst at the time of implantation, which takes place 5 to 8 days after fertilization. It is essential to this process that the trophoblast has the capability of invading the endometrium and its blood vessels. The physicochemical means by which this is accomplished are unknown, but proteolytic enzymes do not seem to be involved. The trophoblastic tissue invades the full thickness of the decidualized endometrium within approximately 6 weeks. Some syncytiotrophoblastic cells normally penetrate the myometrium. Rarely, villi extend through the decidua basalis into the myometrium, producing the condition referred to as *placenta accreta.*

An even greater enigma of placentation is the ability of the fetal allograft, which contains both paternal and maternal haplotypes, to establish itself successfully in the material tissue without eliciting an immune response. It is known that the trophoblast is of fetal origin and that the uterus is not per se an immunologically privileged site. Immunologic

315

tolerance could be explained on the basis of antigenic immaturity of the early trophoblast, since transplantation (human leukocyte antigen [HLA]) and ABO antigens have not been conclusively demonstrated in the early human villous trophoblast (Berkowitz et al, 1984c; Sunderland et al, 1985). At the present time, the most plausible explanation for the success of this natural allograft is the presence of a nonallergenic barrier at the maternofetal (placental) interface. Electron microscopic studies suggest that every syncytiotrophoblastic cell is enveloped by a layer of mucoprotein, mainly sialomucinous in character, that prevents the fetal tissue from being recognized as foreign by the maternal lymphocytes. Maternal immunoglobulins identified on the basement membrane of trophoblastic epithelium may be protective by acting as blocking antibodies. Studies have also demonstrated that hCG has an immunosuppressive quality; however, its role in the maternal immunologic tolerance of the fetus is unknown.

The great propensity of the human trophoblast for vascular invasion is undoubtedly essential to the establishment of the hemochorial placenta. Since the epithelial coverings of the placental villi are continuously bathed by maternal blood, it is not surprising that trophoblastic cells are commonly deported to the lungs, particularly during the later weeks of pregnancy and parturition. The deportation of these cells is not known to be either beneficial or harmful to the mother.

The duration of viability of the fetal trophoblast is self-limited, but the mechanism by which this is accomplished is unknown. Hormonal and immunologic controls have been postulated. The maximum life span of the normal trophoblast under optimal conditions seems to be only slightly longer than the duration of normal gestation. This inherent limitation of survival and invasiveness of the normal trophoblast sharply distinguish it from malignant tissue.

ABNORMAL TROPHOBLAST

Hydatidiform (Hydatid) Mole

Epidemiology

The epidemiology of molar pregnancy has been reviewed by Buckley (1984), Grimes (1984), and Bracken (1987). Precise incidence figures are difficult to derive, because in most reports neither the total number of pregnancies nor the total number of hydatidiform moles (HMs) in a defined population is known. Thus the ratio of molar pregnancies to total pregnancies varies considerably more in hospital-based studies (from 1:85 to 1:1,724) than in population-based studies from (1:522 to 1:1,560; see Fig. 13–1). Furthermore, it appears that the high incidence of molar pregnancy reported from Asia is exaggerated by the currently available information, because the data are largely hospital based.

In addition to the racial implications of these geographic data, the reported incidence of HM has varied among ethnic groups. For example, in the United Sates, black women are only half as likely to have a molar pregnancy as nonblack women. Matsuura et al (1982), using the case method of investigating molar gestations in Hawaii, found that the rates per 1,000 pregnancies were as follows: Caucasians, 8.0; Filipinos, 17.5; Japanese, 16.5; and Hawaiians, 7.7. They found no differences in the rates among Asian women born and raised in Hawaii and those born in Asia. The occurrence of HM is clearly related to maternal age (Table 13–1). Women less than 20 years and over 40 years, especially the latter, have an increased risk of any gestation being an HM (Gandy et al, 1984). The outcome of prior pregnancies also correlates with the probability of molar pregnancy.

1. Once a woman has had a molar gestation, she has a 0.5 to 2.6 percent chance of another mole in subsequent gestations. After two molar pregnancies a 33 percent chance of a third mole has been observed for future gestations (Sand et al, 1984). It seems that after three molar pregnancies the prospects for a live birth are nil (Bagshawe, 1986). However, a woman having many molar pregnancies is occasionally reported (Thavarasah and Kavagalingam, 1988).
2. The risk of molar pregnancy increases with the number of previous spontaneous abortions.
3. One or more previous term pregnancies (except twins) reduces the probability of a molar pregnancy.

Other reported but unconfirmed risk factors include Rh D blood type, diet (low protein, low folate, or deficient in vitamin A), professional occupation, artificial insemina-

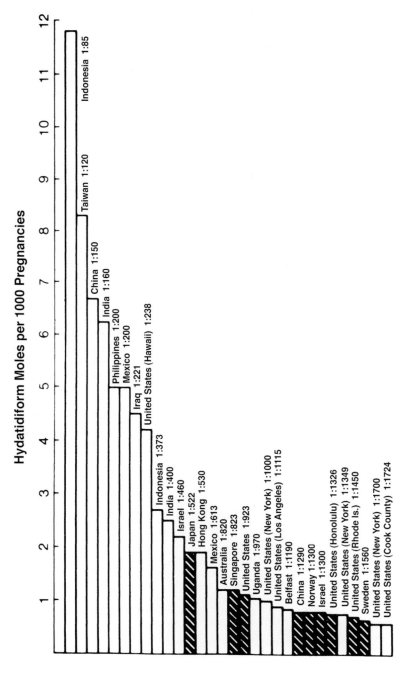

FIGURE 13-1. The reported incidence of hydatidiform mole by country. Shaded bars, the results of studies of a defined population; open bars, estimates from the records of one or more hospitals. (From Buckley JD: The epidemiology of molar pregnancy and choriocarcinoma. Clin Obstet Gynecol 27:153, 1984; reproduced with permission of Harper and Row).

TABLE **13-1**

Risk Ratios (RR) of Various Factors Reported to Correlate With Molar Pregnancy Occurrence*

Risk Factor	RR
Prior molar gestation	20–40
Maternal age	
<20 years	1.5
>40 years	5.2
Prior spontaneous abortion	1.9–3.3
Professional occupation	2.5
Vitamin A in diet above control median	0.6
Parity >1, abortions 0	0.2–0.6

*Data from Grimes (1984), Berkowitz et al (1985), Messerli et al (1985), Parazzini et al (1985), Matsuura et al (1982), and Olesnicky et al (1985).

tion, nulliparity, and consanguinity. Familial molar pregnancy has been observed (Parazzini et al, 1984).

Classification

Pregnancies characterized by the presence of hydropic villi can be classified as (1) complete moles, (2) partial moles, (3) transitional moles, or (4) one of the preceding in conjunction with a separate normal conceptus (Vassilakos et al, 1977; Szulman and Surti, 1982, 1984). Table 13–2 summarizes the clinicopathologic features of the various types of molar gestation. The *complete or classic hydatid mole* is an abnormal conceptus characterized by gross vesicular swelling involving all the placental villi (Fig. 13–2). Either no embryo, membranes, or cord ever develops or they disappear very early in the course

of development, since they are invariably absent on careful gross and microscopic examination. Microscopically, the villi are covered by various degrees of cyto- and syncytiotrophoblastic hyperplasia (Fig. 13–3). Cellular anaplasia may also be present. While microscopic confirmation is always required, the diagnosis of a complete mole based on the gross features is quite dependable. The clinical features are described in detail later.

In contrast, the *partial molar pregnancy* is invariably associated with an embryo or fetus, cord, and membranes. Although the embryo usually dies by 9 weeks' gestation, it may survive into the second or, rarely, third trimester. Hydropic swelling of the villi is haphazard, focal, and less pronounced than that in the complete mole. Consequently, it is more easily overlooked on clinical and pathologic examination. A hallmark of the partial mole is the development of functioning capillaries manifested by the presence of fetal erythrocytes. When trophoblastic hyperplasia is present, it is usually slight and limited to the syncytial trophoblastic cells.

Perhaps 80 to 90 percent of patients with partial moles present with uterine bleeding, absent fetal heart tones, and a uterus small for dates, features consistent with a diagnosis of spontaneous or missed abortion (average gestational age 17 weeks). A uterus large for dates, theca-lutein cysts, a high hCG value, and toxemia are unusual. This is consistent with the low (5 to 10 percent) frequency of malignant trophoblastic neoplasia (Czernobilsky et al, 1982; Szulman and Surti, 1982; Berkowitz et al, 1983b). The fetal component

TABLE **13-2**

Clinicopathologic Characteristics of the Various Classes of Molar Pregnancy*

Feature	Complete Mole	Partial Mole	Transitional Mole
Synonym	Classic; true	Incomplete	Blighted ovum
Villi	Pronounced swelling of all villi	Crinkled hydropic villi are focal, haphazard; many villi normal	Cystic, hydropic, and normal
Trophoblast	Cyto- and syncytial hyperplasia is variable	Mostly syncytial hyperplasia; focal, mild	No hyperplasia; may be hypoplasia
Embryo	Dies very early; no remnants found	Usually dies by 9 weeks; may survive to term	Amnion and stunted embryo
Villous capillaries	No fetal red blood cells	Many fetal red blood cells	Present
Gestational age	8–16 weeks usual	10–22 weeks	6–14 weeks
hCG value	>50,000 mlU/ml usual	75% <50,000 mlU/ml	Low
Malignant potential	15–25%	5–10%	Slight, if any
Karyotype	46,XX (95%)	Triploid (80%)	Trisomic; triploid
Size for dates			
Small	33%	65%	85%
Large	33%	10%	None

*Data from Vassilakos et al (1977) and Szulman and Surti (1984).

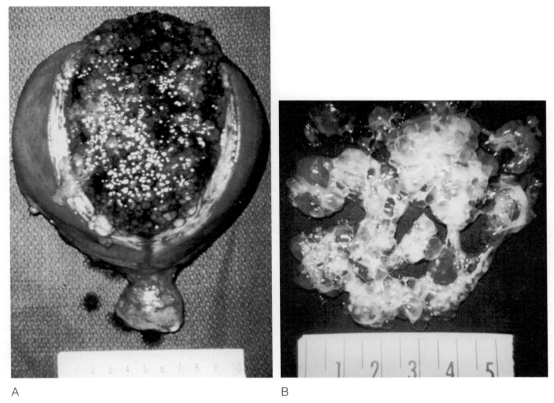

A   B

FIGURE 13–2. *A*, Specimen from an elective hysterectomy performed as primary treatment for molar gestation. The anterior myometrium was incised from the fundus to the lower segment. Note the myriad variably sized, clear vesicles. *B*, Close-up view of vesicles from the molar pregnancy in *A*.

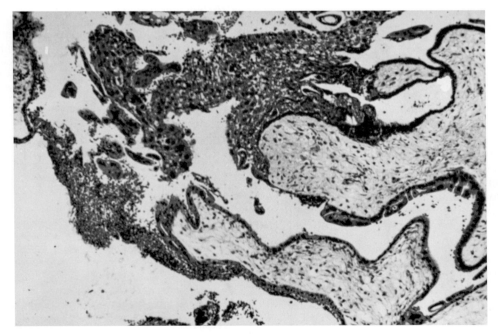

FIGURE 13–3. Photomicrograph of hydatid mole. The villi are avascular and edematous. An area of trophoblastic hyperplasia is present.

of the partial mole can be identified by ultrasound (Berkowitz et al, 1983a). This can lead to a confusing clinical picture, since a complete mole can coexist with a normal twin fetus (Szulman, 1988).

Hertig (1968) applied the term *transitional mole* to the blighted ovum with hydropic villi, because it appeared to represent a stage in the evolution of a true molar gestation. The hydropic villi are generally inconspicuous and never affect all villi. The trophoblast is normal to hypoplastic, an amnion and stunted embryo are present, and the hCG value is very low. There is no documented increased risk of trophoblastic malignancy associated with the transitional mole.

Cytogenetics

Karyotyping tissue from complete molar gestations has demonstrated that approximately 95 percent have a 46,XX composition, and the remainder are 46,XY. Of 10 documented 46,XY patients with follow-up, two developed trophoblastic malignancy (Surti et al, 1982). Thus it appears that the risk of GTN is similar for the XY and XX subsets. Genetic studies of partial moles and the associated fetuses indicate that 80 to 95 percent have a triploid genetic composition (Szulman et al, 1981). While few of these are liveborn, the deaths appear to be related more to biochemical imbalances resulting from gene-dose alterations than to anatomic anomalies. The triploid infant is rarely normal, however. According to Doshi et al (1983), the typical case is premature and growth retarded, with multiple anomalies often involving the head (hydrocephalus), the extremities (syndactyly), and the genitalia. Survival for more than a few days is unusual. However, Vejerslev et al (1986) point out that many cases of hydatid mole and fetus are the result of twinning and the fetuses have a normal diploid karyotype without anomalies.

Distinguishing between complete and partial mole, and between partial mole and hydropic degeneration, is not entirely reliable on clinical and histologic grounds. The accuracy of diagnosis is enhanced by flow cytometry determination of DNA content (Lage et al, 1992; Conran et al, 1993; Howat et al, 1993).

The startling report by Kajii and Ohama (1977) that all chromosomes in complete moles are paternal in origin has provided an important insight into their pathogenesis. The

development of an ovum under the influence of a sperm nucleus requires the absence or inactivation of the ovum nucleus ("empty egg") and a diploid sperm or duplication of the sperm haploid genome. This process, called *androgenesis*, results in a homozygous conceptus. Subsequent work has demonstrated that the 46,XX complete mole results from reduplication of a single haploid (23,X) sperm within the ovum, while the 46,XY mole originates from two separate sperm, one with 23 X and other 23 Y chromosomes (Patillo et al, 1981; Kajii et al, 1984). Kovacs et al (1991), using molecular genetic fingerprinting methods in 20 consecutive complete moles, found 12 (60 percent) to be of homozygous androgenetic origin; 4 (20 percent) were of heterozygous androgenetic origin and 4 (20 percent) were of heterozygous biparental origin. More recently, Lage et al (1992) reported that complete moles were 50 percent diploid, 43 percent tetraploid, and 3.6 percent polyploid. Thus the genetic composition of complete moles is more complicated than originally reported. The triploid partial moles, in contrast, contain two sets of paternal and one set of maternal chromosomes. An exception may be the partial moles associated with a liveborn infant. In this instance, there may be two maternal and one paternal haploid sets of chromosomes (Doshi et al, 1983).

Clinical Diagnosis

The diagnosis of HM should be suspected in any woman with bleeding in the first half of pregnancy, hyperemesis gravidarum, or toxemia before 24 weeks' gestation (Table 13–3). The suspicion may be reinforced by finding

TABLE **13–3**

Diagnosis of Hydatid Mole

Clinical data
  Bleeding in first half of pregnancy
  Lower abdominal pain
  Toxemia before 24 weeks' gestation
  Hyperemesis gravidarum
  Uterus large for dates*
  Absent fetal heart tones and fetal parts
  Evidence of hyperthyroidism
  Expulsion of vesicles

Diagnostic studies
  Ultrasound
  Chest radiograph
  Serum beta-hCG higher than normal pregnancy values

*Usually 14 to 24 weeks' size. From 50 to 60 percent of intact moles are large for dates.

TABLE 13–4

Differential Diagnosis of Hydatid Mole

Threatened or missed abortion
Normal uterine pregnancy with
   Dates wrong
   Uterine fibroid
   Ovarian neoplasm
Multifetal gestation
Hydramnios
Intrauterine fetal death
Placenta previa

on physical examination a uterus large for the estimated length of gestation and absent fetal heart tones. If the HM is intact, the uterus is almost invariably larger than 12 weeks' gestational size. Numerous clinical situations can be confused with molar pregnancy, nearly all of which can be distinguished by the use of the clinical history, physical examination, and pelvic-abdominal ultrasound (Table 13–4). In ambiguous cases, an hCG serum value in excess of the normal pregnancy range is highly supportive of the diagnosis of molar pregnancy (Romero et al, 1985).

A firm diagnosis of hydatid mole before the spontaneous expulsion of vesicles can also be made by means of transabdominal amniocentesis, but ultrasound, because it is simple and reliable, is the diagnostic method of choice. Furthermore, it is not invasive and may be performed repeatedly without apparent harm to the fetus or mother. Pelvic ultrasound should be carried out in any patient who has bleeding in the first half of preg-

nancy or a uterus larger than 12 weeks' gestational size and no fetal heart tones. This practice will facilitate the earlier diagnosis of hydatid mole. Even if the patient has expelled the pathognomonic vesicles, ultrasound is indicated if the uterine fundus remains near or above the umbilicus to rule out the presence of a fetus.

The characteristic sonographic findings of molar pregnancy are illustrated in Figure 13–4. Santos-Ramos et al (1980) scanned 318 women for molar pregnancy. There were 2 false positives, 2 false negatives, and 50 proven molar gestations. Errors are most likely in patients with a uterus less than 14 weeks in size, since the ultrasound findings are often similar to those of missed or incomplete abortion.

Prior to the availability of ultrasound, amniocentesis combined with amniography was the diagnostic test most widely used to confirm the presence of hydatid mole. If amniotic fluid is withdrawn after introducing the needle, a diagnosis of normal pregnancy is presumed and dye is not injected. A small risk to the fetus accompanies the use of amniography, and the probability of obtaining additional useful information in this circumstance is too remote to warrant its use. (Rarely, a mole may coexist with a normal fetus. This should be suspected if the patient has toxemia.) If no amniotic fluid is obtained, radiopaque dye is injected, after which roentgenograms of the abdomen are taken. The typical honeycomb appearance produced by the dispersion of the dye around the hydatid vesi-

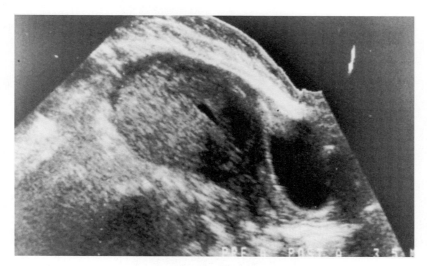

FIGURE 13–4. Ultrasound sagittal section of hydatidiform mole. Typical findings include multiple intrauterine echoes with an absent fetus and gestational sac.

cles is shown in Figure 13–5. Amniography, like sonography, is reasonably safe and accurate, but, of course, false interpretations of either study can be made.

The diagnosis of HM and coexistent normal twin fetus can be made with ultrasound or chorionic villus sampling (Hertzberg et al, 1986). Expectant management has resulted in surviving offspring delivered prematurely by cesarean section (James, 1987; Khoo et al, 1989). Neoplastic complications have not been observed following HM coexistent with a normal fetus (Thomas et al, 1987). A successful outcome in such pregnancies is unlikely, however, because spontaneous abor-

tion, severe toxemia, or fetal death usually occurs before fetal viability.

Numerous biochemical serum and urine measurements can be expected to be at variance in normal pregnancy and hydatid mole, but none has an established role in the differential diagnosis of these two conditions. Such substances include human placental lactogen, total estrogens, estradiol, estriol, estetrol, pregnanediol, progesterone, neutrophil alkaline phosphatase, leucine aminopeptidase, oxytocinase, alpha-fetoprotein, free hCG alpha- and beta-subunit, carcinoembryonic antigen, pregnancy-specific $beta_1$-globulin (SP-1), and prolactin. The mean se-

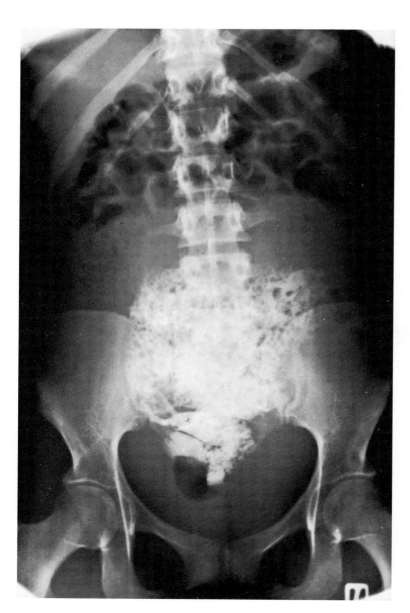

FIGURE 13–5. Classic radiologic honeycomb or moth-eaten appearance of hydatid mole obtained after intrauterine injection of water-soluble radiopaque dye.

rum hCG value for molar pregnancy at diagnosis is about 200,000 mIU/ml, compared with a peak value of 50,000 to 100,000 mIU/ml for normal pregnancy. An out-of-range hCG value in a woman with an ultrasonically normal singleton intrauterine pregnancy should alert the physician to the possibility of choriocarcinoma (gestational or germ cell), especially in a patient with an antecedent pregnancy. Evaluation should include a chest radiograph.

Non-neoplastic Complications

Although the outcome of molar pregnancy is generally uneventful, medical complications are potentially numerous and serious. Anemia from chronic blood loss, toxemia, hyperthyroidism, high-output cardiac failure, trophoblastic embolization, hemorrhage, and sepsis are constant threats that become increasingly more probable as the size of the pregnancy advances. An increased free thyroxine (T_4) index, at least in nonmolar pregnancy, is often associated with hyperemesis gravidarum (Bouillon et al, 1982). While clinical hyperthyroidism is only occasionally seen in molar pregnancy, 25 to 50 percent have total T_4 or free T_4 index values above normal pregnancy levels. These do not appear, however, to result from the high hCG levels (Amir et al, 1984), as previously believed.

A dramatic, life-threatening complication of molar pregnancy is the syndrome of *acute pulmonary insufficiency* characterized by the sudden onset of dyspnea, sometimes with cyanosis. This usually occurs within 4 hours after evacuation and affects only those patients with a uterus of 16 weeks' gestational size or larger. It rarely occurs prior to molar evacuation. The syndrome has been ascribed to massive deportation of trophoblast to the pulmonary vasculature, but some investigators suggest that the most frequent cause is pulmonary edema secondary to cardiac dysfunction and excessive fluid administration (Cotton et al, 1980; Twiggs, 1984). Aggravating factors are hyperthyroidism and dilutional anemia. Massive trophoblastic deportation does occur, as has been documented by postmortem examination of fatal cases (Llewellyn-Jones, 1967).

Management

As soon as the diagnosis of HM is confirmed, termination of the pregnancy should be carried out with no more delay than is necessary to evaluate the patient adequately and to prepare her for therapeutic intervention. If there is active bleeding, an oxytocin drip is begun until suction curettage can be initiated. Hysterotomy, pitocin induction, and prostaglandin stimulation are reserved for the patient with a fetus and a mole. Molar gestation is a contraindication to the intrauterine infusion of hypertonic solutions. HM is seldom diagnosed with the uterus less than 8 to 10 weeks' gestational size, when emptying the uterus by means of conventional curettage would be a safe procedure.

Evacuation of the uterus is carried out in the operating room under general anesthesia or paracervical block and systemic analgesia. The fragility of these patients' cardiovascular, pulmonary, and renal status must not be underestimated. Central venous or pulmonary artery and peripheral arterial lines are often helpful in managing the administration of fluid, including blood. The details of the evacuation procedure have been reviewed by Schlaerth (1984). Following suction curettage, a large, sharp curet is used to explore and gently curet the uterine cavity to ensure that evacuation has been complete.

These latter curettings have been used as a means of predicting the risk of malignancy, following the work of Hertig (1968), who devised a grading system based on the histologic and cytologic characteristics of the trophoblastic tissue. Initially, there were six groups, but he reduced these to three: apparently benign, potentially malignant, and apparently malignant. With advancing grade, there was an increased risk of developing neoplastic complications. Elston (1977) however, found no correlation between histologic appearance and clinical behavior. Although a grading system may have some predictive capacity, unless it is quite exact, the rendering of a diagnosis of "benign" mole or "malignant" mole by a pathologist has greater potential for misleading the clinician than for guiding him or her in the proper care of the patient.

Termination of molar pregnancy by primary hysterectomy is a reasonable option in the management of patients who are good surgical candidates and who desire sterilization. Parenthetically, follow-up in these patients should still include hCG testing, although the likelihood of metastatic GTN developing is remote. In 1980 Goto and colleagues demonstrated the presence of Rh D antigen on the trophoblast of invasive and noninvasive molar pregnancies. It is advisable, then, to administer RhoGam to Rh-negative women with a molar gestation and no anti–Rh D antibodies.

Enlargement of one or both ovaries by the development of multiple theca-lutein cysts complicates 25 to 50 percent of molar pregnancies (Montz et al, 1988; Fig. 13–6). The development of these cysts is attributed to the high levels of hCG, perhaps in concert with pituitary luteinizing hormone (LH), producing a form of ovarian hyperstimulation syndrome. Occasionally, ascites also develops. The ovarian enlargement may be first detected during the early follow-up period, perhaps a reflection of purely mechanical factors resulting from abdominal decompression. In extreme cases of ovarian enlargement, the abdominal distention can become more marked within a few days postevacuation than it was prior to evacuation. Involution of the theca-lutein cysts takes several weeks, reflecting the decline in the serum hCG level. If rupture, hemorrhage, or infection, of the enlarged ovary

occurs, surgery is usually necessary. Failure of the ovaries to involute in the presence of a normal hCG level suggests that the enlargement is neoplastic and surgical exploration is indicated.

The routine administration of methotrexate or actinomycin D (dactinomycin) during or immediately after the evacuation of an HM has received attention as a potential means of eliminating postmolar GTN. Because of the relatively low incidence of postmolar choriocarcinoma and invasive mole, and the almost 100 percent cure rate when adequate follow-up treatment is implemented, the use of prophylactic chemotherapy needs to be both free of significant complications and highly successful to be justifiable. Goldstein (1974) has reported the best results with this approach to the management of HM. Using actinomycin D and evacuating the mole during a 5-day treatment course reduced, but did not eliminate, the incidence of neoplastic sequelae. No serious drug effects were encountered. In view of this experience, prophylactic che-

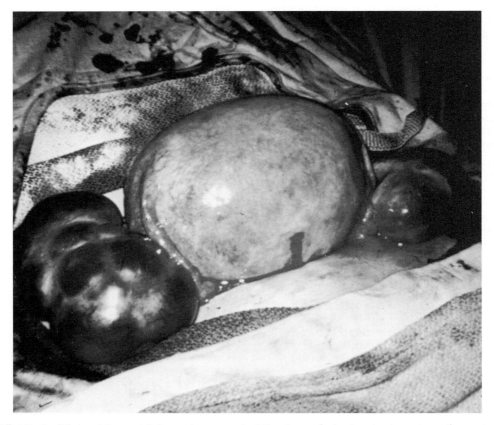

FIGURE 13–6. Bilateral theca-lutein cysts present at the time of elective hysterectomy for molar pregnancy. These cysts are characteristically thin walled and tend to rupture spontaneously. Large cysts correlate with high hCG titers and risk of trophoblastic neoplasia.

motherapy seems suitable for patients who cannot be followed after evacuation, especially those with high-risk molar pregnancies. "Covering" patients with systemic chemotherapy to prevent tumor dissemination while they undergo surgery (uterine curettage, hysterectomy) for trophoblastic disease is not recommended.

Invasive Mole

Invasion of the myometrium by molar villi produces a condition designated as invasive mole. This form of mole reportedly constitutes at least 5 to 10 percent of all molar pregnancies (Table 13–5) based on hysterectomy specimens. Although it has been suggested that the earlier surgical intervention takes place in patients with HM, the greater will be the number of invasive cases, Llewellyn-Jones (1967) found only 5 among 71 HM hysterectomy specimens.

Histologically, invasive mole is characterized by hydropic villi and proliferating trophoblastic epithelium invading the uterine muscle and blood vessels (Fig. 13–7), with associated hemorrhage and tissue necrosis. The neoplasm can penetrate the full thickness of the uterine wall (Fig. 13–8) and rupture into the broad ligament or pelvic cavity. Severe vaginal or intraperitoneal hemorrhage may occur. Invasive mole is also capable of producing "metastases," most commonly to the vagina and lung, although rare instances of secondary lesions in the brain and spinal cord have been documented. This form of GTN has all the features of a malignant tumor, with the exception that its duration of viability is self-limited. If no hemorrhagic or other serious complications occur, the tumor can be expected to involute spontaneously. Invasive mole is seldom diagnosed without excising the uterus. Even with a proven invasive mole,

however, metastases may represent choriocarcinoma. While invasive mole behaves more aggressively than noninvasive mole, it is not more likely to be complicated by choriocarcinoma.

Choriocarcinoma

Choriocarcinoma follows HM in approximately 3 to 7 percent of the cases. It is a highly malignant tumor with a predisposition to hematogenous spread. The organs most often involved by metastasis are, in decreasing order of frequency, the lung, lower genital tract (cervix, vagina, vulva), brain, liver, kidney, and gastrointestinal tract (Park, 1971). Spontaneous regression has been well documented, but this rarely occurs. Choriocarcinoma is a great imitator of other disease processes. Because of the gonadotropin excretion, amenorrhea may develop, simulating an early pregnancy. Later, vaginal bleeding occurs, and a threatened abortion or ectopic pregnancy is suggested. Some cases are manifested by intraperitoneal hemorrhage secondary to a ruptured liver, ruptured theca-lutein cyst, or bleeding ovarian metastasis. This situation can mimic ruptured ectopic pregnancy.

Patients with pulmonary spread may have cough, hemoptysis, pleuritic pain, dyspnea, "asthma," or evidence of respiratory failure. A variety of lesions are seen on the chest radiograph (Figs. 13–9 and 13–10). Gastrointestinal involvement is accompanied by chronic blood loss and melena or by massive gastrointestinal hemorrhage. Spinal and intracranial metastases are often manifested by focal neurologic signs resulting from spontaneous bleeding. The clinical picture usually suggests a brain tumor or vascular accident. A clinical syndrome with right upper quadrant pain and jaundice resembling cholecys-

TABLE **13–5**

Histologic Incidence of Invasive Mole and Choriocarcinoma
Complicating Molar Gestation

	Delfs (1959)	Brewer et al (1968)	Total	Percent
Moles	119	161	280	100.0
hCG elevated 60 days postevacuation	26	59	85	30.4
Hysterectomy	11	29	40	14.3
Invasive mole	6	16	22	7.9
Choriocarcinoma	5	13	18	6.4
Tumor deaths	2	?	2	1.7

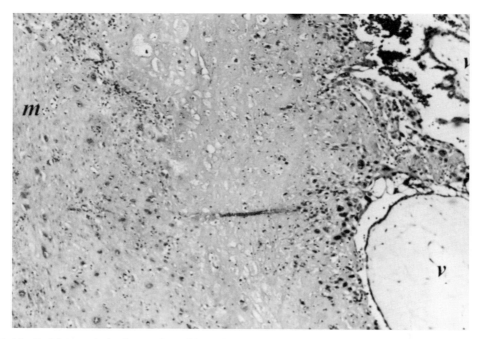

FIGURE 13–7. Histopathologic section of invasive mole (×80). At the right are hydropic villi (v) and at the left intact myometrium (m). The intervening tissue is infiltrated by trophoblastic cells and exhibits areas of necrosis.

titis is sometimes seen with extensive liver metastases. Rarely, patients have hematuria from renal involvement. Reproductive-age women presenting with any of these symptoms should be screened for choriocarcinoma by the simple expedient of pregnancy testing.

Approximately 50 percent of all cases of gestational choriocarcinoma follow HM. In the others, the antecedent pregnancies are evenly divided between abortions (including ectopic pregnancies) and normal pregnancies. Choriocarcinoma follows a term gestation about once in 40,000 cases. Considering the 3 percent risk of developing choriocarcinoma after HM, it is apparent that molar pregnancy increases the risk of choriocarcinoma at least 1,000-fold relative to normal term gestation. Trophoblastic neoplasia resulting from a normal pregnancy is always choriocarcinoma and never a benign or invasive mole.

Choriocarcinoma that follows a normal term pregnancy is sometimes manifested by delayed postpartum bleeding, a rather common complication of normal pregnancy. Because delayed postpartum bleeding is rarely due to choriocarcinoma, the diagnosis is seldom suspected. Uterine curettage is often performed for postpartum bleeding, but, even when choriocarcinoma is present, a tis-

sue diagnosis from the curettings is unusual. In the case of postpartum bleeding or, indeed, any atypical postpartum illness, it is appropriate to obtain a pregnancy test routinely in order to screen for choriocarcinoma. Unfortunately, the diagnosis is not usually made until the patient develops symptomatic metastases.

Choriocarcinoma in situ is diagnosed when a focus of choriocarcinoma is found on routine microscopic examination of a placenta. In such a rare event the baby and mother need hCG monitoring (Trask et al, 1994).

Placental Site Trophoblastic Tumor

Originally described by Kurman et al in 1976, placental site trophoblastic tumor (PSTT) was thought to be a benign relative of non-neoplastic syncytial endometritis. It was designated *trophoblastic pseudotumor.* However, according to a review article by How et al (1995), 13 of 62 patients reported in the English literature have died of metastatic disease.

Women of reproductive age are at risk, although the diagnosis is made occasionally in the sixth decade of life. The patients present at an average age of 30 years with vaginal

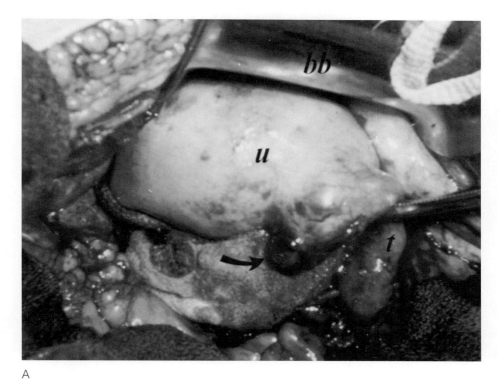

A

B

FIGURE 13–8. *A,* Operative findings in a 28-year-old woman with hemoperitoneum and a positive pregnancy test 1 year after a molar pregnancy. The bladder blade (bb), uterus (u), and right fallopian tube (t) are marked. The arrow points to the site of the uterine rupture, which proved to be invasive mole, not choriocarcinoma or a cornual pregnancy. A lap sponge is in the posterior cul-de-sac. *B,* Surgical specimen from the patient in *A.* One of the numerous hemorrhagic myometrial lesions of invasive mole is identified by the arrow. The patient also had lung metastases, which were successfully treated with chemotherapy.

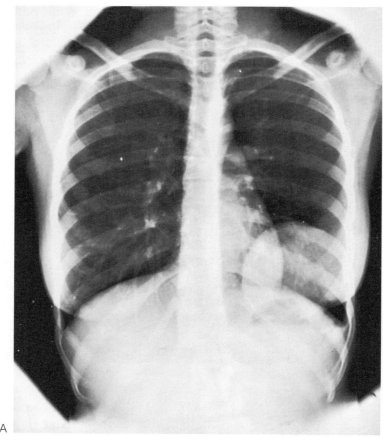

A

FIGURE 13–9. *A,* Chest posteroanterior roentgenogram demonstrating a single, large, sharply circumscribed metastasis in the left posterior lung field. *Illustration continued on opposite page*

bleeding, usually after amenorrhea of variable duration. The antecedent pregnancy may be normal, molar, or a spontaneous abortion. The uterus is usually enlarged (8 to 16 weeks), and the serum hCG level is normal to elevated but usually less than 3,000 mIU/ml. PSTT has been associated with virilization. A nephrotic syndrome with a distinctive renal lesion has been reported in a few cases. Spontaneous uterine rupture and perforation at curettage are documented complications of this disease, in addition to its malignant potential.

The tumor grows in a polyploid fashion, filling the uterine cavity or extensively infiltrating the myometrium. Microscopically, there is focal hemorrhage, moderate mitotic activity, and frequent vascular invasion by a predominantly polyhedral to round mononuclear cell population, generally considered to be intermediate trophoblastic cells. A mitotic count above 5/10 hpf seems to augur a particularly poor prognosis, although malignant behavior can be seen at lower mitotic counts (Young et al, 1988).

Most of the reported patients with PSTT are alive and well following curettage or hysterectomy. However, in at least one instance metastases appeared after an interval of 5 years. Thus longer follow-up is needed to assess the full malignant potential of this tumor. PSTT does not appear to respond well to radiation therapy or to chemotherapy, although Rustin and colleagues (1989) have reported complete remissions utilizing the EMA/CO regimen (etoposide, methotrexate, and actinomycin D alternating with cyclophosphamide and vincristine [Oncovin]).

Young et al (1988) have described a *placental site nodule,* usually an incidental finding in a hysterectomy specimen performed for leiomyomata uteri, that must be distinguished from PSTT. The clinical behavior of such nodules appears to be benign.

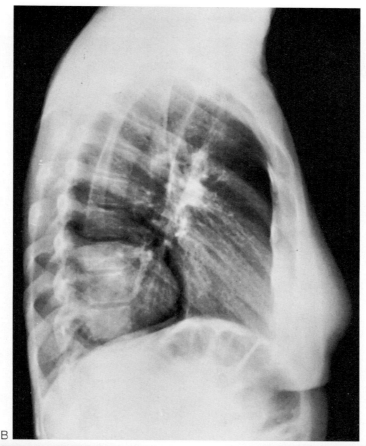

B

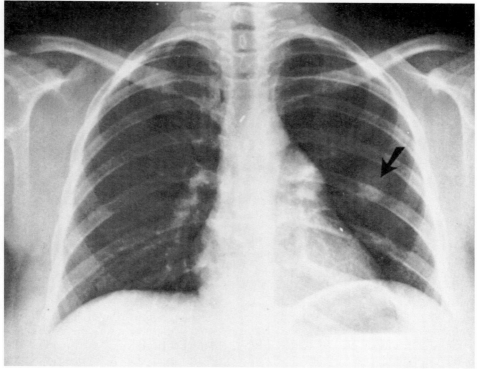

C

FIGURE 13-9. *Continued* *B*, Lateral roentgenogram of same patient as in *A*. *C*, Solitary metastasis in the left midlung field, which is smaller and less distinct than the lesion in *A*.

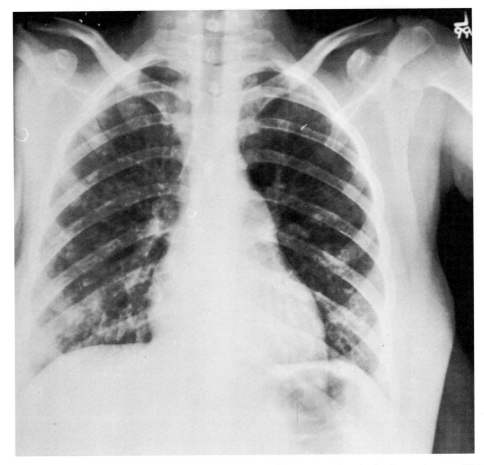

FIGURE 13–10. Bilateral diffuse pulmonary metastases from gestational choriocarcinoma. This patient also had a complete spinal cord block secondary to an extradural metastasis.

MANAGEMENT OF GESTATIONAL TROPHOBLASTIC NEOPLASIA

Human Chorionic Gonadotropin Assay

hCG is an obligate secretory product of the syncytiotrophoblast. In common with LH, follicle-stimulating hormone (FSH), and thyroid-stimulating hormone (TSH), it is a glycoprotein composed of two subunits designated alpha and beta. The molecular weight of the complete molecule is about 34,000. The smaller alpha-subunit of hCG is nearly identical to the alpha-subunits of LH, FSH, and TSH; it is the beta-subunit that gives these hormones their biologic and immunologic specificities.

The immunologic measurement of hCG in the serum and urine has been of great importance to the diagnosis and management of patients with GTN. The quantification of hCG is, however, complicated by the fact that hCG exists in several dissociated or degraded forms in addition to the whole molecule in both the serum and urine: (1) "nicked" hCG, which has a single cleavage in the β-subunit peptide; (2) nicked hCG which is missing the β-subunit C-terminal peptide; (3) free α- and β-subunits, nicked and non-nicked; and (4) β-core fragment, a terminal degradation product found principally in the urine. These products have little or no biologic activity. The proportion of the nicked subunits, free β-subunits, and β-core fragments is substantially increased in trophoblastic disease relative to pregnancy (Cole et al, 1993; Ozturk et al, 1988). Rather than the traditional polyclonal anti-β-hCG radioimmunoassay (RIA), current assays for hCG employ a two or three monoclonal antibody sandwich assay that is typically more sensitive, faster and suitable to automation. Unfortunately, there is considerable variability in the commercial monoclonal assays, some of which measure non-nicked hCG only and are clearly unsuited to monitoring patients for GTN. The best assays for this purpose measure all forms of the intact, dissociated, and degraded hCG molecule.

The interest in increasing the hCG assay sensitivity can be appreciated by considering that with current limitations probably no fewer than 10^5 syncytiotrophoblastic cells can be detected. It is believed that this lack of sensitivity explains in part the 5% relapse rate after hCG remission. Normal nonpregnant subjects, however, have serum hCG levels, most likely of pituitary origin, *which* place a practical limitation on the lower limit of detection of hCG to perhaps 1 mIU/ml.

There are many sources of error encountered in hCG testing of which the reader should be aware. One of the most common errors results from a lack of uniformity in reporting units: milli-international units per milliliter (mIU/ml, which should be the standard), IU per liter, IU per milliliter, mIU per 100 ml, nanograms per milliliter, a numerical value without units, and "negative" without a normal reference value have all been used in the past. Occasionally an error of 10 occurs so that a value of, for example, 10,000 is recorded as 1,000. The problem of discordant results from different hCG assay procedures or kits has been discussed above. Discordancy is usually manifested by a falsely negative value or a persistent low, falsely elevated value (3–8 mIU/ml) in a patient who has been or is being treated for GTN.

Postmolar Pregnancy Surveillance
(Table 13–6)

Follow-Up Routine

Flow diagrams for postmolar follow-up are presented in Figures 13–11 and 13–12. Frequent follow-up with serial hCG values is essential for every patient after molar pregnancy because of the 15 to 30 percent incidence of GTN (Table 13–7), that is, invasive mole (two thirds) and choriocarcinoma (one third). Although several clinical features of molar gestation are recognized as having a much higher than average association with GTN (Table 13–8), in general at diagnosis the

TABLE 13–6
Postmole Surveillance Program

Chest radiograph (at time of evacuation); RhoGam if Rh negative and no antibodies present

Pelvic examination at 1 week and 4 weeks*

Contraception (prefer combination oral contraceptives) for 6–12 months after hCG remission†

Quantitative serum beta-hCG determinations:
  Weekly until hCG remission†; then
  Monthly for 6 months if regression is normal, *or*
  Monthly for 12 months if regression is irregular but remission is spontaneous

*Continue examinations every 2 to 4 weeks if ovaries are enlarged (see text).
†hCG remission is defined as three consecutive weekly serum beta-hCG values less than 5.0 mIU/ml.

larger the uterus, the higher the hCG value, and the shorter the gestation, the greater the risk of GTN. However, even women having a molar gestation without these findings have a significant risk of GTN (4 percent in the series of Goldstein et al, 1979) and must be monitored. Morrow et al (1977) constructed a normal postmolar pregnancy hCG regression curve based on weekly determinations in patients undergoing spontaneous hCG remission (Fig. 13–13). This provides a reference with which random or serial values can be compared. In most instances, the postmolar hCG values exhibit a progressive decline to normal (<5.0 mIU/ml) within 14 weeks postevacuation. Once the value drops below 100 mIU/ml, an every-other-week assay of serum beta-hCG is adequate.

While serial hCG value determinations are the most important part of postmolar pregnancy surveillance, other studies are also helpful. A gynecologic examination should be done 1 week after evacuation, at which time a blood specimen is taken for the first hCG value. Observations are made about the uterine size and adnexal masses (theca-lutein cysts), and a search is made for evidence of genital tract (vulva, vagina, urethra, cervix) metastases. The examination is not repeated unless the patient develops symptoms, exhibits an hCG plateau, or has ovarian enlargement. If hCG remission occurs spontaneously and without an hCG plateau, beta-hCG is measured monthly for 6 months to complete the follow-up.

Involution of the theca-lutein cysts is documented by pelvic examination. Failure to show regression in the face of a normalizing hCG value suggests that ovarian neoplasia is present. If spontaneous hCG remission oc-

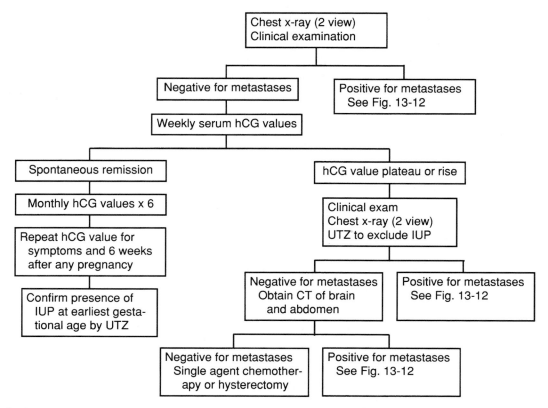

FIGURE 13–11. Algorithm for molar pregnancy follow-up after evacuation or hysterectomy (see also Fig. 13–12). Patients should be employing some means of avoiding pregnancy during postmolar follow-up and treatment. "Plateau," less than a doubling of the hCG value during a 3-week period of observation with no numerical fall in the hCG value; "Rise," a doubling or greater increase in the hCG value during a 2-week observation period. IUP = intrauterine pregnancy; UTZ = ultrasound examination; CT = computed tomography.

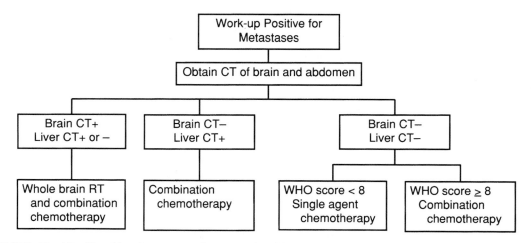

FIGURE 13–12. Algorithm for metastatic postmolar GTN (see also Fig. 13–11). CT = computed tomography; RT = radiation therapy; WHO = World Health Organization.

TABLE **13–7**

Reported Incidence Rates of Postmolar Gestational Trophoblastic Neoplasia (GTN) in the United States

Source	Total Cases	GTN (%)		
		Nonmetastatic	Metastatic	Total
Goldstein and Berkowitz (1982)	856	14.7	4.0	18.7
Lurain et al (1983)	738	16.3	3.0	19.2
Curry et al (1975)	337	16.6	3.5	20.1
Brewer et al (1968)	51	19.6	2.0	21.6
Morrow et al (1977)	121	23.1	3.3	26.4
Kohorn (1982)	127	26.0	3.1	29.1
Hatch et al (1978)	212	26.4	5.7	33.1
Total	2,442	17.6	3.6	21.2

curs but the regression curve is not normal, monthly hCG values should be obtained for 1 year rather than 6 months before the patient is released from medical supervision.

Since the hCG produced by a neoplastic trophoblast is indistinguishable biologically and immunologically from that produced during pregnancy, it is important that pregnancy be avoided during the postmole follow-up period to avoid confusion about the etiology of rising levels of hCG. An intervening pregnancy would also complicate treatment should malignant sequelae develop. Oral contraceptives (OCs) are the method of choice. Ovulation may occur within 4 weeks postevacuation, with an hCG serum level as high as 200 mIU/ml (and perhaps higher). Therefore contraception should be initiated early in the follow-up period (Ho et al, 1985). Furthermore, the OCs will suppress LH production, avoiding any interference with the hCG sensitivity.

There has been some concern that the estrogen component of OCs might enhance the risk of trophoblastic neoplasia after molar pregnancy (Brewer et al, 1979). A prospective randomized study was conducted by the Gy-

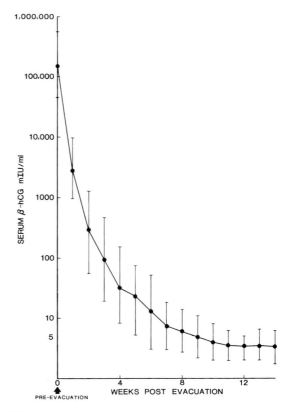

FIGURE 13–13. Normal postmolar pregnancy curve for serum beta-hCG RIA. Vertical bars indicate the 95 percent confidence limits. (From Morrow CP, Kletsky OA, DiSaia PJ, et al: Clinical and laboratory correlates of molar pregnancy and trophoblastic disease. Am J Obstet Gynecol 128:424, 1977, with permission.)

TABLE **13–8**

Relationship Between Clinical Features of Molar Pregnancy and Risk of Gestational Trophoblastic Neoplasia (GTN)*

Clinical Feature	Percent GTN
Delayed postevacuation hemorrhage	75
Theca-lutein cysts (>5 cm) plus uterus large for dates	60
Acute pulmonary insufficiency (postevacuation)	58
Theca-lutein cysts (>5 cm)	55
Uterus >20 weeks' gestational size	55
Uterus large for dates	45
Serum hCG >100,000 mIU/ml	45
Second hydatid mole	40
Uterus >16 weeks' gestational size	35
Maternal age >40 years	25

*Data from Morrow (1984a).

necologic Oncology Group comparing OCs to barrier methods in women following HM. Fewer patients had an abnormal hCG regression curve (postmolar GTN) in the OC study arm (23 vs. 33 percent). Furthermore, pregnancy complicated the postmolar follow-up twice as often in the barrier group. Thus OCs are the preferred method to prevent pregnancy after HM (Curry et al, 1989b).

Urine pregnancy tests are woefully inadequate for postmolar surveillance. Most detect concentrations of hCG no lower than 200 mIU/ml, and many are less sensitive. In addition, while the pregnancy test remains positive, it gives no indication of whether the hCG concentration is falling, has leveled off, or is rising. Today the standard of practice and the most convenient means of following patients after HM or with GTN is a quantitative serum assay for beta-hCG. The minimum acceptable sensitivity for this purpose is 5 mIU/ml.

Abnormal Serum hCG Regression

The studies of Delfs (1959), Brewer et al (1979), Bagashawe et al (1973), and others (Table 13–4) provide a basis for the interpretation of postmolar gonadotropin values relative to the diagnosis of progressive trophoblastic neoplasia and the need for therapeutic intervention. Brewer et al (1971) reported that, by 60 days after molar evacuation, approximately 70 percent of their patients achieved a normal hCG level, that is, less than 25 mIU/ml. An additional 15 percent demonstrated a continuous drop in their values, although the values were still higher than normal. In the remaining 15 percent of the group with an elevated hCG at 60 days after evacuation, the values were either level or rising. In an earlier study, Brewer et al (1968) found that nearly one half of these patients had histologic evidence of choriocarcinoma; the rest had invasive mole. It is this group of patients, those with flat or rising hCG values 60 days postevacuation, that Brewer recommended for treatment. His standard has remained the basis of all subsequent treatment plans in the United States.

Indications for Treatment

In 1983 the World Health Organization (WHO) recognized the following criteria for chemotherapy after hydatidiform mole: (1) a serum level of hCG greater than 20,000 mIU/ml or urine level greater than 30,000 mIU/ml more than 4 weeks after evacuation; (2) progressively increasing hCG values at any time after evacuation (minimum of three values in 1 month); (3) histologic evidence of choriocarcinoma; (4) central nervous system (CNS), renal, hepatic, or gastrointestinal metastases; and (5) pulmonary metastases greater than 2 cm in diameter or more than three in number. These criteria were adapted from those of Bagshawe and colleagues (1989) in the United Kingdom. In the United States a more liberal attitude toward treatment has existed because of (1) the risk of uterine hemorrhage or perforation necessitating hysterectomy; (2) the possible development of life-threatening metastases, especially to the brain, with hemorrhage and stroke; and (3) the young age of most molar pregnancy patients, which presents a significant risk, at least in some populations, of failed follow-up.

The indications for initiating therapy directed against GTN during postmolar follow-up are listed in Table 13–9. Of course, treatment should be instituted whenever there is a tissue diagnosis of choriocarcinoma (other than choriocarcinoma in situ), but histologic confirmation is unnecessary (even undesirable) since it can lead to meddlesome surgical intervention, resulting in hemorrhage, infection, and delayed therapy. The presence of metastasis is sufficient cause for initiating chemotherapy at any point in time relative to the antecedent pregnancy. Although invasive mole can be associated with pulmonary and vaginal secondary lesions, metastases may also be the result of choriocarcinoma, and delaying treatment with the expectation that the metastatic lesions may regress spontaneously is not recommended.

Usually therapy for progressive GTN after the delivery of HM is instituted because of an abnormal regression curve. A steadily falling

---

TABLE 13–9

Indications for Initiating Treatment During Postmole Follow-Up

Serum beta-hCG values rising for 2 weeks (three weekly values)*

Serum beta-hCG values on a plateau for 3 weeks or more (>500 mIU/ml)

Presence of metastasis

Significant elevation of serum beta-hCG values after reaching normal levels

Postevacuation hemorrhage not due to incomplete evacuation

*A rise in hCG is defined as a numerical doubling of the value over 2 weeks. A plateau is defined as a value that neither declines nor doubles over a 3-week period of evaluation.

hCG level portends a favorable outcome, and treatment is seldom necessary even if the value remains above normal at 14 weeks postdelivery. If there is an increase in the hCG measurement, or if it remains constant for a period of 3 weeks, treatment is recommended. The most critical period of observation is the first 4 to 6 weeks postevacuation (Fig. 13–14). Few patients whose serum hCG values follow the normal regression curve during this interval will require treatment. Occasionally, the hCG curve reaches a plateau below 500 mIU/ml. In this situation, a chest radiograph should be obtained and, if it is normal, hCG observation continued.

Repeat Uterine Curettage

Delayed bleeding which is uncommon after molar pregnancy evacuation, usually signifies the presence of invasive mole or choriocarcinoma. It is almost invariably attended by an enlarging uterus and abnormal hCG regression (rise or plateau). The enlarged uterus, on pelvic examination, may have the characteristics of an intrauterine pregnancy, and the examiner anticipates that curettage will yield much molar tissue, the result of regrowth, incomplete evacuation, or both. However, little intracavitary tissue is present in most cases. Nevertheless, the curettage is effective in stopping the bleeding. The longstanding practice of routinely recuretting patients after HM to remove residual tissue is of little value and may be harmful, at least if the initial evacuation has been accomplished by suction curettage. A gentle, sharp curettage immediately after vacuum curettage is recommended to ensure that the uterus has been completely evacuated.

Pretreatment uterine curettage has been performed at some referral centers routinely for the purpose of classifying patients into the prognostic categories of invasive mole or choriocarcinoma (Lurain et al, 1982) or into the histologic groups described by Hertig (Berkowitz et al, 1980). This information clearly correlates with the prognosis, but it has no established bearing on treatment strategy. An occasional patient will experience normalization of hCG levels from a curettage alone. This approach is not without hazard, however, because uterine perforation with hemoperitoneum has occurred, necessitating transfusion, surgery, and even hysterectomy. These complications would seem to negate any potential benefit from the curettage

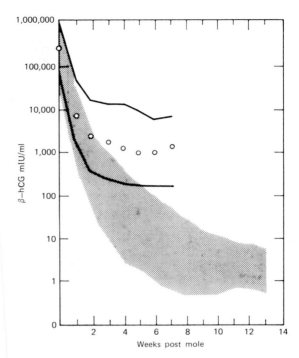

FIGURE 13–14. The 95 percent confidence corridor (stippled area) for the normal regression curve of serum beta-hCG after molar pregnancy. The circled dots and solid lines indicate the weekly mean serum beta-hCG RIA values and 95 percent confidence limits for patients with abnormal regression indicating the presence of invasive mole or choriocarcinoma. The curve stops at 7 weeks because treatment was initiated at that time for most cases. (From Schlaerth JB, Morrow CP, Kletsky OA, et al: Prognostic characteristics of serum human chorionic gonadotropin titer regression following molar pregnancy. Obstet Gynecol 58:478, 1981, with permission.)

(Schlaerth et al, 1990). Selecting patients for curettage who do not have myometrial nodules on ultrasound may be a useful strategy (Mangili et al, 1993).

Staging and Prognostic Systems

Since the first demonstration that gestational choriocarcinoma was curable with chemotherapy, there have been many attempts to devise a staging system that would allow an accurate prediction of outcome and risk for treatment failure. The initial experience of the National Institutes of Health (NIH) trophoblastic disease program indicated that successful treatment depended on the duration of disease, the rate of urinary gonadotropin excretion, and the proper administration of chemotherapeutic agents (Hertz et al, 1961; Ross et al, 1965). These criteria were refined and expanded by the Southeastern Regional Trophoblastic Disease Center (SRTDC) so that a "poor-prognosis" group of patients with metastatic disease could be identified based on duration of disease greater than 4 months, urinary hCG output greater than 100,000 IU/24 hr, or cerebral or hepatic metastases. By 1980 the poor-prognosis criteria had expanded to six features (post-term pregnancy, serum beta-hCG >40,000 mIU/ml, and failed prior chemotherapy were added), and these have become the clinical standard for managing trophoblastic disease in the United States (Hammond et al, 1980). Combination drug therapy was shown to be more effective than single-agent therapy in the poor prognosis group in the SRTDC experience (Hammond et al, 1970, 1973).

At the Charing Cross Hospital in London, Bagshawe (1976, 1989) developed a prognostic scoring system looking at 13 factors, with subsets given values from 0 to 4. This scoring system, after various revisions, was adopted by the WHO in 1983. Further analysis of the Charing Cross data has yielded yet another, more recent scoring system (Bagshawe et al, 1989).

Sung et al (1984), at the Capitol Hospital in Beijing, suggested an anatomic staging system for GTN. In 1989 The International Society for the Study of Trophoblastic Disease adopted a revised anatomic staging system based on further experience at the Capitol Hospital (Table 13–10). Three years later this system was accepted by the International Federation of Gynecology and Obstetrics (FIGO) for the reporting of treatment results in trophoblastic neoplasia (see Appendix II).

Scoring systems from the New England Trophoblastic Disease Center (Goldstein and Berkowitz, 1984) and from Hong Kong (Wong et al, 1986) are simplifications of the WHO system. Similarly, the Memorial Sloan-Kettering Cancer Center in New York City proposed a modification of the NIH/SRTDC system, the Working Group for Trophoblastic Tumors in the Netherlands has established a classification system (Dijkema et al, 1986), and another has been proposed at the John I. Brewer Trophoblastic Disease Center (Miller and Lurain, 1988).

The three most widely used prognostic/staging systems (i.e., the NIH/SRTDC classification, the prognostic scoring system of Charing Cross Hospital/WHO, and the staging system of Capital Hospital/FIGO) have been compared in several reports based on clinical analysis (Miller and Lurain, 1988; DuBeshter et al, 1991; Dubuc-Lissoir et al, 1992; Kohorn, 1995) Although there is utility in all three systems, these studies indicate that the Charing Cross Hospital/WHO system offers the greatest precision in identifying which patients will fail therapy. The FIGO system is clearly inferior (Smith et al, 1993).

Further attempts to refine the clinical understanding of trophoblastic disease have been undertaken. Most scoring or prognostic systems in use have been presented without a formal statistical basis. In 1985, Gordon et al analyzed the M.D. Anderson Hospital experience with high-risk patients using the Fisher exact test. They found that patients with only an elevated beta-hCG level did significantly better than patients with (1) liver or brain metastases ($P = 0.005$); (2) duration of disease longer than 4 months ($P = 0.005$); and (3) GTN after a full-term pregnancy ($P = 0.006$). The last group did significantly worse than those with duration of disease longer than 4 months ($P = 0.02$). All other comparisons between these factors were not significant.

Soper et al (1988) reported that patients having more than one metastatic site ($P = 0.002$), disease duration longer than 4 months ($P < 0.001$), antecedent nonmolar pregnancy ($P = 0.001$), and clinicopathologic diagnosis of choriocarcinoma ($P = 0.002$) were at significantly increased risk for treatment failure versus patients who lacked these features. Azab et al (1989) analyzed the clinical factors leading to an unfavorable outcome in a 162-patient study group. Among the 45 high-risk patients in the group, univariate and multi-

TABLE **13–10**

Staging System for Gestational Trophoblastic Neoplasms (International Society for the Study of Trophoblastic Disease)*

Stage	Description
0	Molar pregnancy: low risk or high risk[†]
I	Confined to uterine corpus
II	Metastasis to pelvis and vagina
III	Metastasis to lung
IV	Distant metastasis to liver, brain, etc.

*Data from Goldstein and Berkowitz (1984).
[†]Uterus large for dates, hCG value greater than 100,000 mIU/ml, theca-lutein cysts larger than 6 cm, maternal age over 40 years, toxemia, coagulopathy, hyperthyroidism, trophoblastic embolization, prior trophoblastic tumor.

variate analyses revealed three factors to be significant: antecedent nonmolar gestation, more than one organ involved by metastasis, and resistance to initial chemotherapy.

Nonmetastatic Gestational Trophoblastic Neoplasia

Evaluation

At the time a decision is made to initiate therapy for GTN, complete evaluation of the patient is done (Table 13–11). The majority of patients have an enlarged uterus; ovarian enlargement due to theca-lutein hyperplasia is also common. These lesions have a fairly typical appearance on ultrasound and should not be mistaken for metastases or ovarian neoplasia. Special attention is paid to the lower genital tract for evidence of metastasis, but biopsy should be avoided since major hemorrhage may ensue, particularly if the visible nodule is continuous with a pelvic metastasis. A chest radiograph is necessary but computed tomographic (CT) scanning of the brain, abdomen, and pelvis are performed in search of metastatic disease only when lung metastasis or symptoms are present (Hunter et al, 1990). For patients in whom contrast media is contraindicated, magnetic resonance imaging (MRI) should be used in place of CT scanning (Hricak et al, 1986). Baseline blood counts and renal and liver function studies are required before initiating chemotherapy. As mentioned previously, endometrial curettings have prognostic significance but are not important as a guide to treatment. Endometrial curettage therefore is unnecessary in the usual case.

Treatment

All cases of nonmetastatic GTN are considered to be curable, since no matter how extensive the uterine disease, whether it is choriocarcinoma or invasive mole, the disease can be eliminated by hysterectomy should chemotherapy fail. Hysterectomy is, of course, the treatment of choice for the healthy patient who has completed her family, but most molar pregnancy patients are quite young, with one or no children. Thus nearly all of them will choose to have the reproduction-sparing chemotherapy.

Methotrexate and actinomycin D, used singly, have demonstrated clear-cut superiority to all other cytotoxic agents in the treatment of GTN except, perhaps, etoposide. The tra-

TABLE 13–11

Staging Work-up for Gestational Trophoblastic Neoplasia

History, physical, and neurologic examinations
Chest radiograph
Pelvic sonogram to exclude intrauterine pregnancy
CT or MRI of the brain, abdomen, and pelvis*
Serum beta-hCG determination
Complete blood count, platelet count
Liver and renal function tests
Clotting screen and thyroid profile

*Selected cases only. See text.

ditional 5-day regimens for these agents are listed in Table 13–12. The therapeutic efficacy of the two drugs (90 percent primary remission rate) is apparently equivalent. Actinomycin D carries the risk of severe tissue injury if extravasation occurs. Methotrexate is contraindicated in the presence of parenchymal liver disease and impaired renal function.

Lurain and Elfstrand (1995) reported on 253 patients treated with 5-day methotrexate for nonmetastatic GTN. The primary remission rate was 89 percent and the average number of treatment cycles 4.7. A change in therapy was required in 4.7 percent of cases because of drug toxicity, usually severe stomatitis. Methotrexate resistance developed most frequently in patients with a pretreatment hCG value greater than 50,000 mIU/ml (35.7 percent) or choriocarcinoma (22.4 percent). Relapse after hCG normalization occurred in 2.4

TABLE 13–12

Traditional Single-Agent Chemotherapy for Nonmetastatic and Good-Prognosis Metastatic GTN (WHO Score <8)

Actinomycin D: 0.4–0.8 mg/m^2 IV days 1–5
OR
Methotrexate: 0.4 mg/kg or 16 mg/m^2/day IM or IV days 1–5 Repeat cycle every 2 weeks (9-day window) if granulocyte count >1,500 mm^3 and platelet count >100,000/mm^3; stomatitis and gastrointestinal toxicity recovered; liver and renal function tests normal
Continue chemotherapy 1–3 courses past normal beta-hCG value (<3.0 mIU/ml)
Beta-hCG, complete blood count, platelet count, and liver and renal function tests before each treatment cycle
After remission,* obtain monthly beta-hCG values for 12 months, then every 2 months for 12 months
Continue contraception for 1 year after remission
Seek medical care early for all subsequent pregnancies
Determine serum beta-hCG 4–6 weeks after all subsequent pregnancies

*hCG remission is defined as three weekly normal serum beta-hCG values.

percent of the study group. Altogether, five patients (0.4 percent) required hysterectomy for cure.

Each 5-day treatment cycle is repeated as soon as the normal tissues (bone marrow, gastrointestinal tract) have recovered, with a minimum 7-day rest between the last day of one course and the first day of the succeeding course. While the patients are under treatment, weekly serum hCG values and peripheral blood counts are obtained. Before each course of therapy, liver and renal function studies should also be done. Provided the hCG level continues to fall under therapy, repeat chest radiograph is not necessary. A minimum of one course of drug therapy should be given after the first normal hCG determination. On the average, about five cycles of single-drug therapy are required, but the number of treatment cycles necessary to induce remission is directly related to the magnitude of the hCG concentration at the initiation of therapy. After hCG remission has been induced and the treatment completed, hCG assays are obtained monthly for 12 months and every 2 months thereafter for the subsequent 12 months.

Numerous alternatives to the traditional 5-day methotrexate and actinomycin D single-agent regimens have been used successfully. One widely employed regimen is IM methotrexate with IM or PO folinic acid rescue (MTX-FA; Berkowitz et al, 1986; Bagshawe et al, 1989). MTX-FA has been used to treat nonmetastatic and low-risk metastatic GTN according to the schedule given in Table 13–13. In the Bagshawe et al series of 348 low-risk patients, 347 (99.7 percent) were cured. However, a treatment change was necessary in 69 (20 percent) because of drug resistance and in 23 (6 percent) because of drug-induced toxicity. The rationale of this regimen is to shorten the treatment time by giving a larger dose of methotrexate per course, simultaneously administering folinic acid (FA) to reduce the toxicity below that associated with conventional 5-day methotrexate and actinomycin D therapy.

The experience of other investigators using this regimen has not been uniformly good. For example, Smith et al (1982) reported that 27.5 percent of 29 patients with FIGO stage I GTN failed primary therapy with MTX-FA, compared with a historical failure rate of 7.7 percent among 39 stage I patients managed by the standard 5-day methotrexate regimen. In addition, Wong et al (1985) found that the MTX-FA regimen was associated with a rate of hepatic toxicity similar to that of standard 5-day methotrexate regimen. Nevertheless, the regimen is attended by less hematologic and gastrointestinal toxicity. It is interesting to note that the reduced toxicity may result from the every-other-day schedule, with almost complete interval excretion of the methotrexate, rather than from any rescue effect of the FA (Rotmensch et al, 1984). This is reassuring to those who wish to use the regimen on an outpatient basis, since it means that there may be no serious toxicity risk if the patient fails to return for the FA rescue. No one, however, has suggested omitting the FA, because serum levels of methotrexate and its excretion are somewhat unpredictable.

In an effort to increase cost-effectiveness, a study of 63 patients getting weekly IM methotrexate at a dose of 30 mg/m^2, escalating by 5 mg/m^2 every 3 weeks to 50 mg/m^2 maximum dose, was undertaken by the Gynecologic Oncology Group. This regimen proved to be minimally toxic, the total duration of therapy averaged 7 weeks, and the primary remission rate was 81 percent (Homesley et al, 1990). A follow-up study of 62 patients getting 40 mg/m^2 of IM methotrexate weekly, escalating by 5 mg/m^2 every 2 weeks to a maximum dose of 50 mg/m^2, was not more effective (Homesley et al, 1990).

Actinomycin D 1.25 mg/m^2 IV push once every 2 weeks, is another useful regimen that is especially convenient and cost-saving for the patient, since it requires only one outpatient visit every 2 weeks. In the reports of Twiggs (1983), Schlaerth et al (1984), and Petrilli et al (1987), 50 of 55 FIGO stage I patients achieved complete remission with an average of 4.5 treatment courses. There were few severe and no life-threatening toxic events. Oral etoposide, 100 mg/m^2 daily for 5 days repeated every 2 weeks, has also been used successfully (Wong et al, 1984). In a re-

---

T A B L E **13–13**

Alternative Single-Agent Chemotherapy Regimens Used to Treat Good-Prognosis GTN

5-day actinomycin D or methotrexate regimen (see Table 13–12)

Methotrexate 1.0 mg/kg or 40 mg/m^2 IM days 1, 3, 5, and 7 and FA 0.1 mg/kg IM or PO days 2, 4, 6, and 8

Actinomycin D 1.25 mg/m^2 IV push every 14 days

Methotrexate 40 mg/m^2 IM each week*

Etoposide 100 mg/m^2 daily × 5 days every 2 weeks

*The authors' recommended first-line therapy.

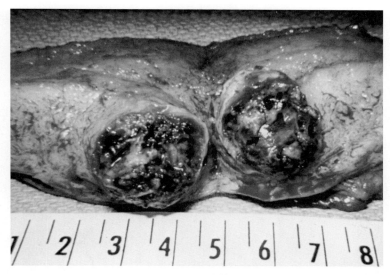

FIGURE 13–15. Hysterectomy specimen from a 24-year-old woman with gestational trophoblastic neoplasia after her second molar pregnancy. Single-agent and combination drug therapy were unsuccessful. The uterus has been opened in the frontal plane, with the endometrium facing up. The 2-cm cornual nodule has been bisected. A vesicle is visible at the arrow. The histologic diagnosis was invasive mole.

view of available therapies, Kohorn (1991) concluded that biweekly actinomycin D appears to be the protocol of choice for routine use in nonmetastatic GTN. However, many institutions, including the authors', prefer to use weekly IM methotrexate as the frontline therapy.

Ten to 20 percent of patients with nonmetastatic GTN will demonstrate resistance to single-agent therapy, invariably after an initial response. As a rule, the resistant focus is deep in the myometrium (Fig. 13–15). These patients are more likely to have high hCG levels at initiation of therapy, a longer interval since the antecedent pregnancy, and when compared to patients who do not demonstrate drug resistance. When the hCG values fail to drop significantly during two consecutive treatment courses, or if more than 8 weeks is required to induce titer remission, a change to actinomycin D or methotrexate, depending on which was the initial drug, is usually successful in eradicating the disease. If the tumor fails to respond to this change in therapy, it is reasonable to implement one of the combination chemotherapy regimens used for metastatic, high-risk GTN. If the patient does not desire further childbearing, however, hysterectomy is indicated as primary therapy for nonmetastatic GTN (Table 13–14). Hysterectomy is also indicated when the tumor manifests drug resistance. Before operation, the patient is re-evaluated for metastatic disease.

Pelvic ultrasound or angiography may be needed (Berkowitz et al, 1983a) to document the location of the neoplasm in the uterus (Fig. 13–16). The efficacy of second-line chemotherapy with hysterectomy as a backup ensures that true stage I GTN is virtually 100 percent curable.

Metastatic Gestational Trophoblastic Neoplasia

Presentation

Women with metastases from GTN, other than those diagnosed in the early months after molar pregnancy, invariably have choriocarcinoma. More often than not, the symptoms that cause them to seek medical care do not involve the reproductive system. If there is disease in the uterus and no clinical evidence of metastasis, a diagnosis of threatened abortion or ectopic pregnancy will be sug-

TABLE **13–14**

Indications for Hysterectomy in Trophoblastic Disease*

Primary management of hydatid mole—good operative candidate who requests sterilization

Primary management of nonmetastatic trophoblastic disease—good operative candidate who requests sterilization

Uterine disease resistant to chemotherapy

*Based on data in Hammond et al (1980).

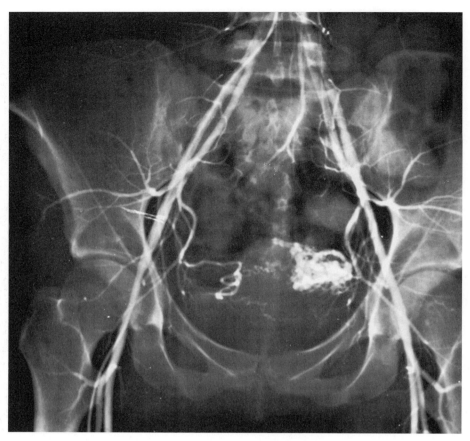

FIGURE 13–16. Pelvic arteriogram showing features characteristic of trophoblastic disease within the myometrium. The left uterine artery is enlarged and there is early filling of the ipsilateral veins as a result of arteriovenous shunting. In this case, hysterectomy was performed because of drug resistance, and a small focus of choriocarcinoma was found deep in the myometrium near the left cornu. The patient remained in remission for 5 years.

gested by the history, the physical findings, and the positive pregnancy test. Failure of the uterus to enlarge with a persistently positive pregnancy test should arouse suspicion of this lesion although the demise of a new pregnancy is by far the most frequent cause. At this juncture a chest radiograph, quantitative hCG assay, and ultrasound study of the uterus should be obtained. Among the more common manifestations of metastatic choriocarcinoma are focal neurologic signs suggestive of intracranial hemorrhage. Others include hemoperitoneum, intestinal hemorrhage, unexplained tumor metastasis, and nodular or diffuse lung disease (Table 13–15).

It is good medical practice to screen by pregnancy testing all women of reproductive age who have any of these signs. While the antecedent pregnancy usually will have terminated within 1 to 2 years prior, latency periods of several years have been documented. Rarely, metastases from choriocarcinoma appear during or immediately after the pregnancy of origin. In this case neurologic manifestations are typically interpreted as eclampsia.

TABLE 13–15

Presenting Syndromes of Patients With Gestational Choriocarcinoma

Threatened or missed abortion
Stroke—CNS tumor
Hepatitis—cholecystitis
Gastroenteritis—bleeding
Lung disease (cough, pain, dyspnea, hemoptysis)
Hemoperitoneum (ectopic pregnancy)
Unexplained metastatic cancer
Hematuria

Good-Prognosis Metastatic Disease

In 1961, Hertz et al reported a 47 percent complete remission rate among 68 women with metastatic GTN using methotrexate chemotherapy. Four years later they reported curing with actinomycin D one-half of the patients in whom methotrexate therapy had failed (Ross et al, 1965). Thus the sequential use of methotrexate and actinomycin D resulted in an overall remission rate of nearly 80 percent. As previously discussed, these investigators recognized certain characteristics of their study group that were predictive of a high probability of treatment failure. Patients with a urinary hCG output over 100,000 IU/24 hr, with disease of more than 4 months' duration, or with brain or liver metastasis remitted at a rate of only 40 percent, compared with 95 percent for patients with none of these features. The WHO/Bagshawe scoring system for assessing risk of treatment failure in patients with GTN refines this original NIH definition of high risk (Table 13–16).

Practically speaking, the great majority of patients who fail treatment have longstanding disease with liver, brain, or other visceral metastasis. Thus nearly all FIGO stage II and III cases will fall into the good-prognosis metastatic GTN category (WHO score <8). This is confirmed by the data of Goldstein and Berkowitz (1984), who reported a 100 percent cure rate in 25 stage II and 87 stage III cases compared with a 48 percent cure rate for 35 stage IV cases.

The majority of patients with good-prognosis metastatic GTN will have limited lung metastasis detected on a routine chest radiograph within 4 months of the reference pregnancy. The radiographic manifestations of lung involvement from GTN include nodular, patchy, and miliary lesions in addition to effusions and atelectasias (Figs. 13–9 and 13–10; Sung et al, 1982). Chest CT scan is helpful in clarifying the nature of lesions of uncertain significance (Mutch et al, 1986). There is a crude correlation between the serum hCG level and the extent of clinical disease that can be helpful in avoiding errors. For example, a high value in the presence of a normal uterus almost always indicates that lung metastases are present, and demonstrable metastases are distinctly unusual with an hCG value less than 200 mIU/ml.

Although it is generally recommended that all cases of metastatic GTN that fall into the good-prognosis category be treated by single-agent chemotherapy, we reserve this treatment for patients who have metastatic disease, usually in the lung, detected during the work-up for an abnormal postmolar hCG regression curve. This practice is supported by the experience of duBeshter et al (1991), who reported that single-agent therapy in low-risk metastatic GTN (prognostic score ≤4) succeeds in 86 percent of cases, whereas Roberts and Lurain (1996) had only a 67.4% primary remissions rate treating all 92 of their low risk cases with single agent chemotherapy. All other cases of good-prognosis met-

TABLE 13–16

WHO Scoring System Based on Prognostic Factors*

Prognostic Factor	Prognostic Score[†]			
	0	1	2	4
Age (years)	<39	>39		
Antecedent pregnancy	Hydatid mole	Abortion	Term	—
Interval between end of antecedent pregnancy and start of chemotherapy (months)	<4	4–6	7–12	>12
hCG (mIU/ml)	$<10^3$	$10^3–10^4$	$10^4–10^5$	$>10^5$
ABO blood groups (female × male)		O × A A × O	B AB	
Largest tumor, including uterine (cm)		3–5	>5	
Site of metastases	Lung, vagina, pelvis	Spleen, kidney	Gastrointestinal tract, liver	Brain
Number of metastases identified		1–4	4–8	>8
Prior chemotherapy			Single drug	Two or more drugs

*Data from Bagshawe (1984).
[†]The total score for a patient is obtained by adding the individual scores for each prognostic factor. Total score less than or equal to 4 = low risk; 5 to 7 = middle risk; greater than or equal to 8 = high risk.

astatic GTN are treated with methotrexate and actinomycin D, with or without cyclophosphamide combination chemotherapy. This is consistent with the advice of Bagshawe (1984), who has recommended combination chemotherapy for patients with a WHO score of 5, 6, or 7. The combined drug therapy is not so toxic that it needs to be reserved for only the most serious cases. Ishizuka and Tomoda (1990) have also employed the two-drug combination for good-prognosis metastatic GTN at a dose and schedule of methotrexate 0.4 mg/kg/day IM and actinomycin D 0.01 mg/kg/day IV for 5 days every 3 weeks.

The hCG response to therapy is more sensitive and reliable than any clinical or laboratory test. Thus failure of a lung lesion to involute completely is not sufficient evidence of persistent disease if the hCG is normal. An hCG drop of 5- to 10-fold or greater in response to the first course of chemotherapy is a good omen, while less than a 50 percent drop is very worrisome. As the hCG level falls closer to normal, however, the slope of the regression curve tends to become flatter and should not be interpreted as drug resistance. Chemotherapy is continued for two to three courses after a normal hCG value (<3 mIU/ml). If the hCG levels plateau over two consecutive courses of chemotherapy, resistance is present. Restaging with a view to changing treatment is then indicated.

Poor-Prognosis Metastatic Disease

As Table 13–17 indicates and as previously discussed, there have been a number of additions to the original NIH criteria for the poor-prognosis GTN category. All patients meeting these criteria have choriocarcinoma, usually with extensive lung, brain, or liver metastases (see also Table 13–16). Post-term pregnancy cases have been identified as having a poorer prognosis overall than post–hydatid mole or postabortal cases (65 vs. 87 percent; Olive et al, 1984). Furthermore, the post-term patients with traditional poor prognostic factors do less well than other poor-prognosis patients (47 vs. 75 percent; Miller et al, 1979). These observations can be explained partly by the higher incidence of metastases at diagnosis and the greater frequency of brain and liver metastases (Berkowitz et al, 1984a), which undoubtedly reflects the longer duration of disease, counting from the time of conception. The lion's share of poor-prognosis cases fall into the FIGO stage IV group.

However, it is the WHO scoring system that has become the standard by which therapy in the poor-prognosis group of patients is most often determined and evaluated. By this system, a score of 8 or greater identifies patients with the highest risk for treatment failure (Miller et al, 1988; DuBeshter et al, 1991). Using modifications of the WHO system, others have determined the score for high-risk GTN to be above 9 or 10 (Bagshawe, 1988; Bolis et al, 1988; Curry et al, 1989a; Surwit and Childers, 1991). It is a common practice to use the point score for high-risk metastatic GTN to determine which women should receive more intensive therapy. There are few data on outcome in individual women, however, relative to WHO scores. In one report, which used a modified WHO system, the lowest point total in a woman who died of disease was 9 (Curry et al, 1989a). Based on the unmodified WHO system, Mortakis and Braga (1990) and Dubuc-Lissoir et al (1992) reported series in which the lowest point scores in women who died of metastatic GTN were 12 and 13, respectively.

CENTRAL NERVOUS SYSTEM METASTASES

Brain metastases occur in about 10 percent of women with metastatic GTN, and death may result unnecessarily if this diagnosis is overlooked in a healthy, typically premenopausal woman who experiences focal CNS symptoms. This can be easily avoided by the simple expedient of pregnancy testing. In the series of Yordan et al (1987), 45 percent of patients with CNS metastasis died without receiving therapy and in most of these women choriocarcinoma was first diagnosed at au-

---

TABLE **13–17**

Criteria for Poor-Prognosis (High-Risk) Metastatic Gestational Trophoblastic Neoplasia

NIH criteria:
   Urinary hCG excretion >100,000 IU/24 hr
   Duration of disease longer than 4 months (interval since antecedent pregnancy)
   Brain or liver metastasis (regardless of disease duration or level of hCG)

Additional poor-prognosis features:
   Following term pregnancy*
   Serum beta-hCG >40,000 mIU/ml
   Failed prior chemotherapy
   WHO score ≥8

*Gestational choriocarcinoma metastatic to both the infant and mother has been reported.

topsy. A new aspect of the failure to diagnose CNS choriocarcinoma prior to death pertains to organ transplantation. Wallis et al (1987) and Baquero et al (1988) report three young women dying of cerebral hemorrhage whose only pregnancies were nonmolar. Their hearts, livers, and kidneys were transplanted to nine individuals, five of whom died of choriocarcinoma. Both cardiac transplant patients survived. Despite transplantation nephrectomies, three of five patients in these reports receiving cadaveric renal transplants died of choriocarcinoma, and both liver transplant patients died of choriocarcinoma.

The apparent impediment to drug therapy presented by the blood-brain barrier limits the otherwise remarkable effectiveness of systemic chemotherapy. Polar, lipid-insoluble compounds enter the CNS slowly or not at all through the capillary membranes of normal brain or cord tissue. This phenomenon is well recognized for methotrexate. In animal studies, however, the presence of tumor apparently impairs the effectiveness of the blood-brain barrier, permitting the entry of many cytotoxic drugs in therapeutic concentrations. Nevertheless, systemic chemotherapy alone has been successful in eradicating CNS disease in only 20 percent of cases (Gordon et al, 1986; Yordan et al, 1987).

Whole-brain radiation therapy in combination with systemic chemotherapy has resulted in a 50 percent survival rate of patients presenting with brain involvement in the series of 75 cases collected by Jones (1987). Evans et al (1995) reported curing 75 percent of 16 patients with whole-brain radiation therapy plus systemic chemotherapy. Two additional patients were salvaged by surgery. These results are similar to those of intrathecal methotrexate plus systemic chemotherapy reported from the United Kingdom by Rustin et al (1989). They reported that 72 percent of 25 patients presenting with CNS metastasis were cured with EMA/CO plus intrathecal methotrexate. (These patients received 1 gm/m² IV methotrexate on day 1.) Thus, while the best therapy for GTN with CNS metastasis remains somewhat controversial, either intrathecal methotrexate or whole-brain radiation therapy is needed in addition to systemic chemotherapy. Early diagnosis is also very important and is facilitated by routine head CT or MRI in patients with metastatic GTN. If the scan is negative but there is clinical evidence of CNS involvement, determining the serum-to-spinal fluid hCG ratio may be helpful. A ratio less than 60 is highly suggestive of CNS involvement (Jones, 1987). Brain metastases that appear during therapy are seldom curable.

Patients who present with CNS symptoms and elevated intracranial pressure may require surgery to evacuate a hematoma or for decompression. Otherwise, primary resection of choriocarcinoma is seldom necessary and may lead to residual neurologic deficits. In the absence of intrathecal chemotherapy or whole-brain radiotherapy, resection of a brain metastasis is potentially curative when used in conjunction with systemic chemotherapy but of little value otherwise, since nearly all cases with brain involvement have lung metastasis. Crippling or fatal spontaneous brain hemorrhage is a constant threat and must be addressed by initiating treatment as soon as possible.

The recommended whole-brain treatment course is 3,000 cGy at a rate of 1,000 cGy/week. Systemic chemotherapy may be initiated simultaneously with radiation treatments. The long-term risks of giving 3,000 cGy of whole-brain radiation over 3 weeks to adults have not been defined but are presumably quite low. Sheline et al (1980), in a review, found no reported cases of brain necrosis, a usually fatal complication, at this dose and rate. The occurrence of a secondary malignant neoplasm, glioblastoma, has been reported (Barnes et al, 1982).

LIVER METASTASES

Liver metastases from gestational choriocarcinoma are more ominous than brain metastases. From various reports, 5 to 20 percent of poor-prognosis cases have liver metastases (Surwit and Hammond, 1980; Gordon et al, 1985; Lurain and Brewer, 1985; Wong et al, 1986). With the exception of the experience of Wong et al (1986), the collected survival rate of cases with liver metastases is only 33 percent; Wong and associates reported treatment success in 12 of their 15 patients. However, 10 had lesions less than 1 cm in diameter. Without biopsy (which is not recommended), defects of this size are at the limit of diagnostic resolution.

A major issue in the management of choriocarcinoma with liver metastases has been the role of radiation therapy. Hammond and Soper (1984) recommended a dose of 2,000 cGy over 10 days in women with sizable liver lesions to diminish the risk of liver hemorrhage. Liver hemorrhage, however, has been reported in a patient undergoing radiation therapy (Lacey et al, 1983), and bleeding has been successfully dealt with by hepatic artery occlusion (Grumbine et al, 1980). Furthermore, none of the 15 patients of Wong et al treated with chemotherapy alone hemorrhaged. Since the side effects of whole-liver irradiation can be substantial, its use, in our opinion, does not have a favorable therapeutic ratio.

CHEMOTHERAPY

Because of the limited success of single-agent therapy in managing the poor-prognosis group, new approaches to treatment were investigated. Hammond et al (1973) reported 7 complete remissions among 10 patients using a modified regimen of Li's triple therapy (methotrexate, actinomycin D, and chlorambucil [MAC]) as the initial treatment. However, among seven patients who were treated with combination chemotherapy after failure with single-agent therapy, remission was achieved in only one case. The results of MAC combination chemotherapy for metastatic GTN obtained by various investigators do not necessarily reflect superiority over sequential methotrexate/actinomycin D. The differences could be explained by the composition of the treatment groups. Nevertheless, the use of MAC for high-risk metastatic GTN has become a general practice in this country, and its effectiveness is widely accepted. The treatment protocol is given in Table 13–18.

Cyclophosphamide is often substituted for chlorambucil in the MAC regimen because the latter cannot be given parenterally. The reported cure rates achieved at the major treatment centers range from 50 to 72 percent (Gordon et al, 1985; Jones and Lewis, 1985; Lurain and Brewer, 1985; DuBeshter et al,

T A B L E **13–18**

Treatment for Poor-Prognosis Metastatic GTN*

Actinomycin: 8–10 μg/kg/day IV for days 1–5
Methotrexate: 0.3 mg/kg/day IV for days 1–5
Cyclophosphamide: 3–5 mg/kg/day IV for days 1–5 (or chlorambucil: 8 mg/day PO for days 1–5)
Obtain weekly serum beta-hCG value, blood counts, liver and renal function tests
Continue for two or three courses after beta-hCG remission
After hCG remission, monitor serum beta-hCG values monthly for 1 year, then every 2 months for second year, then annually
No pregnancy for 2 years after remission
Brain metastases need emergent radiation therapy

*EMA/CO may be substituted for MAC (see Table 13–19).

1987; Soper et al, 1988; Dubuc-Lissoir et al, 1992), although higher remission rates from more recent treatment years are the rule. The variation in results from these centers probably reflects more the differences in patient tumor factors than differences in treatment protocols.

With a relatively high failure rate, it is not surprising that new, more effective regimens are being sought. Bagshawe's seven-drug CHAMOCA regimen, consisting of cyclophosphamide, hydroxyurea, actinomycin D, methotrexate, vincristine (Oncovin), citrovorum factor, and doxorubicin (Adriamycin), yielded a 75 percent success rate in his high-risk category. The CHAMOCA regimen was initially thought to be more effective and less toxic than MAC. However, a randomized study by the Gynecologic Oncology Group has shown that the standard MAC regimen appears to be at least equally effective and much less toxic than the CHAMOCA regimen (Curry et al, 1989a). A modification of MAC in which the methotrexate is given at a dose of 1.0 mg/m^2/day with FA rescue on alternate days for 8 days resulted in a 71 percent (10 of 14 cases) remission rate in poor-prognosis GTN (Berkowitz et al, 1984b).

Newlands et al (1986) have reported a 93 percent success rate by using the alternating EMA/CO combination (Table 13–19). Since then it has generally replaced MAC as the treatment of choice for high-risk disease because of greater efficacy and a lower risk of serious toxicity (Surwit, 1987; Bolis et al, 1988). An attempt has been made to improve the efficacy of EMA/CO by giving a third dose of etoposide 100 mg/m^2 and cisplatin 80 mg/m^2 on day 8 (EMA/CE); the cyclophosphamide and vincristine are deleted (Surwit and Childers, 1991). Rustin et al (1989) have used EMA/CE with high doses of cisplatin (75 mg/m^2) and etoposide (150 mg/m^2) on day 8 for patients with CNS metastases who have only partially responded to EMA/CO and intrathecal methotrexate. Renal function must be carefully monitored when using a nephrotoxic agent (cisplatin) in a patient receiving methotrexate.

A somewhat different line of developmental therapeutics has been followed by Theodore et al (1989) at the Institut Gustave Roussy. Their results with cisplatin (Platinol) plus etoposide (PE) or with PE plus actinomycin D compare favorably with all of the methotrexate-containing combinations.

Whatever combination regimen is used to treat the poor-prognosis cases, chemotherapy

T A B L E **13–19**

EMA/CO Multidrug Regimen for High-Risk Gestational Choriocarcinoma
(WHO Score >8)*

Agent	Dose	Route
Course 1		
Day 1		
Actinomycin D	0.5 mg	IV stat
Etoposide	100 mg/m^2	IV over 30 min
Methotrexate	100 mg/m^2	IV stat
Methotrexate	200 mg/m^2	IV 12-hr infusion
Day 2		
Actinomycin D	0.5 mg	IV stat
Etoposide	100 mg/m^2	IV over 30 min
Folinic acid	15 mg	PO or IM b.i.d. × 4 doses beginning 24 hr after starting methotrexate infusion
Course 2		
Day 8		
Oncovin (vincristine)	1.0 mg/m^2	IV stat
Cyclophosphamide	600 mg/m^2	IV over 30 min

Alternate courses 1 and 2 in sequence weekly as toxicity permits.

*Data from Newlands et al (1986).

should be continued three courses past the first normal hCG titer to minimize the risk of relapse. Remission for 1 year is highly indicative of a permanent cure. However, late recurrences do occasionally happen, and for that reason pregnancy should be postponed for 2 years after remission.

Salvage Chemotherapy

Cure of patients after failure on combination chemotherapy has been achieved with cisplatin, bleomycin, and vinblastine as reported by Gordon et al (1986) in 2 of 10 patients, by DuBeshter et al (1989) in 4 of 7 patients, and by Azab et al (1989) in 4 of 8 patients who failed either MAC or CHAMOCA. Surwit et al (1984) induced remission in four drug-resistant patients using cisplatin, infusion bleomycin, and etoposide (Table 13–20). The use of cisplatin-containing salvage regimens in GTN was initially based on its success in the treatment of testicular cancer. Consequently, it is of interest that the most impressive regimen developed for the treatment of resistant testicular cancer is a combination of etoposide, ifosfamide/mesna, and cisplatin (Table 13–21; Loehrer et al, 1986). In 1995 Li-Pai et al reported curing 19 of 26 patients (73 percent) with drug-resistance GTN employing a regimen of bleomycin, cisplatin, etoposide, and doxorubicin.

The feasibility of combining surgical removal with chemotherapy or radiation therapy may result in a cure not otherwise possible. This concept is particularly applicable to drug/radiation therapy–refractory metastases. As one potential application, Ishizuka and Tomoda (1990) noted in an autopsy study of 30 women who died of choriocarcinoma, all of whom had brain metastases, that most intracranial metastatic foci occur in superficial, neurosurgically accessible sites. As previously noted, Evans et al (1995) salvaged two of four patients with drug/radiation therapy–refractory brain metastases patients by surgical resection. Hysterectomy, partial pneumonectomy, and partial liver resection have also salvaged patients with drug-resistant GTN (Lehman et al, 1994).

PREGNANCY AFTER CHEMOTHERAPY FOR GESTATIONAL TROPHOBLASTIC NEOPLASIA

It is a modern marvel that gestational choriocarcinoma involving the uterus can be cured by chemotherapy, preserving intact the woman's reproductive apparatus. Once this feat is accomplished, the effect of cytotoxic drug therapy on fertility and the genetic integrity of the ova become immediate, practical concerns. Experience has clearly demonstrated that many patients who have had GTN can successfully conceive and deliver normal, healthy infants. There appears to be little, if any, increase in the risk of these drug-treated women bearing children with developmental defects (Rustin et al, 1984). This may depend

T A B L E 13–20

Salvage Regimens for Metastatic Gestational Trophoblastic Neoplasia

Drug	Surwit et al (1984)	Gordon et al (1986)	DuBeshter et al (1989)	Azab et al (1989)	Li-Pai et al (1995)
Etoposide	100 mg/m² days 1–5		9 mg/m² day 1		100 mg/m² days 1–4
Vinblastine		0.4 mg/kg day 1		0.3 mg/kg day 1	
Cisplatin	50 mg/m² day 1	100 mg/m² day 1	20 mg/m² days 1–5	100 mg/m² day 2	20 mg/m² days 1–4
Bleomycin	15 units/day as a 24-hr infusion, days 1–5	15 units/day, days 1–5	20 units/m²/day, days 1, 8, and 15	15 mg/day as a 24-hr infusion, days 1–3	10 mg/m² days 1–4
Doxorubicin					40 mg/m² day 1

Repeat cycle every 3 weeks. All drugs given intravenously.

TABLE **13-21**

Salvage Therapy for Refractory Germ Cell
Carcinoma*

Drug	Dose
Etoposide	75 mg/m^2 IV/day × 5
Ifosfamide	1.2 gm/m^2 IV/day × 5
Cisplatin	20 mg/m^2 IV/day × 5
Mesna	4 (500-mg) capsules orally q6h starting 1 hr before the first and continuing until 36 hr after the last dose of ifosfamide

*Data from Loehrer et al (1986).

partly on a 1-year period of contraception after chemotherapy to permit the wasting of damaged oocytes before pregnancy is undertaken. The use of hormonal contraception or GnRH agonists during chemotherapy may also protect the ovaries and ova from damage, reduce the likelihood of premature ovarian failure, and prevent an abnormal ovum from being fertilized (see Chapter 14).

Table 13-22 compares the reproductive performances of women after molar pregnancy and those who received chemotherapy. There is no important difference in any category (see also Berkowitz et al, 1991). Van Thiel et al (1972), however, reported a higher than expected incidence of placenta accreta. Walden and Bagshawe (1976) compared the reproductive performance of patients treated with chemotherapy for GTN with that of women having HM and with a control group. They concluded that women who develop trophoblastic tumors (including molar gestations) tend to have a poorer obstetric history that is not worsened by chemotherapy.

In the study of Rustin and colleagues (1984), only 3 percent of 217 women who tried to conceive after chemotherapy for GTN failed to do so; 86 percent had a least one live birth. The ability to conceive was not worse for women past age 30 years, but women who received polychemotherapy were less likely to have a successful pregnancy. Song et al (1988) reported on 265 patients treated with chemotherapy for GTN. There was no obvious effect on fertility, pregnancy loss or fetal anomalies of 303 live born offspring, normal growth and development was observed in all 295 who survived infancy. Peripheral lymphocyte cytogenetics were normal in all 94 tested children. It appears, then, that there is little reproductive risk for women or their offspring who are given the usual chemotherapeutic agents. Although etoposide in one study appeared to be quite gonadotoxic (Choo et al, 1985), this was based on short term follow-up. Adewole et al (1986) noted that 66 of 74 women conceived after etoposide therapy for GTN. However, women in the later years of their fertile lifetime seem to be susceptible to permanent ovarian failure from etoposide as well as polychemotherapy.

CHORIOCARCINOMA METASTATIC TO THE FETUS

Although the placenta is the site of origin of gestational choriocarcinoma, even when complicating a term pregnancy, the primary intraplacental choriocarcinoma is rarely detected (Fox and Laurini, 1988). Furthermore, transplacental metastasis to the fetus from gestational choriocarcinoma is rare (Flam et al, 1989). Some of the affected infants sustain

TABLE **13-22**

Pregnancy Outcome After Molar Gestation*

Outcome	All Molar Gestations		Chemotherapy Group†	
	No.	Percent	No.	Percent
Full term	626	67.4	154	69.1
Stillbirth	4	0.5	5	2.2
Premature	79	8.4	10	4.4
Spontaneous abortion	178	19.1	44	19.6
Induced abortion	22	2.4	6	3.0
Ectopic	7	0.8	3	1.3
Repeat mole	13	1.4	1	0.4
Congenital anomaly	32	4.5	5	3.0

*Data from Goldstein et al (1984).
†The majority of patients received either methotrexate or actinomycin D.

significant fetomaternal hemorrhage (Santa-maria et al, 1987). Symptoms of hemoptysis, melena, anemia, and gonadotropin stimulation usually develop in the infant within 6 months of birth. Liver and lung metastases are common. Most reported cases have been fatal. Early diagnosis can be facilitated by immediate hCG testing of every infant whose mother is diagnosed as having choriocarcinoma.

REFERENCES

Adewole IF, Rustin GJS, Newlands ES, et al: Fertility in patients with gestational trophoblastic tumors treated with etoposide. Eur J Cancer Clin Oncol 22:1479, 1986.

Amir SM, Osathanondh R, Berkowitz RS, Goldstein DP: Human chorionic gonadotropin and thyroid function in patients with hydatidiform mole. Am J Obstet Gynecol 150: 723, 1984.

Azab M, Droz JP, Theodore C: Cisplatin, vinblastine and bleomycin combination in the treatment of resistant high risk gestational trophoblastic tumors. Cancer 64:1829, 1989.

Azab MB, Pejovic M, Theodore C, et al: Prognostic factors in gestational trophoblastic tumors. Cancer 62:585, 1988.

Bagshawe KD: Choriocarcinoma: The Clinical Biology of the Trophoblast and Its Tumors. Baltimore, Williams & Wilkins, 1969.

Bagshawe KD: Trophoblastic tumours and teratomas. In Bagshawe KD (ed): Medical Oncology. Philadelphia, Blackwell Scientific Publications, 1975, p 453.

Bagshawe KD: Risk and prognostic factors in trophoblastic neoplasia. Cancer 38:1373, 1976.

Bagshawe KD: Treatment of high-risk choriocarcinoma. J Reprod Med 29:813, 1984.

Bagshawe KD: UK registration scheme for hydatidiform mole 1973–1983. Br J Obstet Gynecol 93:529, 1986.

Bagshawe KD: High-risk metastatic trophoblastic disease. Obstet Gynecol Clin North Am 15:531, 1988.

Bagshawe KD, Dent J, Newlands ES: The role of low-dose methotrexate and folinic acid in gestational trophoblastic tumours (GTT). Br J Obstet Gynecol 96:795, 1989.

Bagshawe KD, Wilson H, Dublon P, et al: Follow-up after hydatidiform mole: studies using radioimmunoassay for human chorionic gonadotropin (hCG). J Obstet Gynaecol Br Commonw 80:461, 1973.

Bandy LC, Clarke-Pearson DL, Hammond CB: Malignant potential of gestational trophoblastic disease at the extreme ages of reproductive life. Obstet Gynecol 64:395, 1984.

Baquero A, Bannett A, Werner DJ, Kim P: Misdiagnosis of metastatic cerebral choriocarcinoma in female cadaver donors. Transplant Proc 20:776, 1988.

Barnes AE, Liwnicz BH, Schellhas HF, et al: Case report: successful treatment of placental choriocarcinoma metastatic to brain followed by primary brain glioblastoma. Gynecol Oncol 13:108, 1982.

Berkowitz RS, Birnholz J, Goldstein DP, Bernstein MR: Pelvic ultrasonography and the management of gestational trophoblastic disease. Gynecol Oncol 15:504, 1983a.

Berkowitz RS, Cramer DW, Bernstein MR, et al: Risk factors for complete molar pregnancy from a case-control study. Am J Obstet Gynecol 152:1016, 1985.

Berkowitz RS, Desai U, Goldstein DP, et al: Pretreatment curettage: a predictor of chemotherapy response in gestational trophoblastic neoplasia. Gynecol Oncol 10:39, 1980.

Berkowitz RS, Goldstein DP (eds): Clinical update on gestational trophoblastic disease: an invitational symposium. J Reprod Med 32:621, 1987.

Berkowitz RS, Goldstein GP (eds): Advances in gestational trophoblastic disease: a symposium. J Reprod Med 36:1, 1991.

Berkowitz RS, Goldstein DP, Bernstein MR: Natural history of partial molar pregnancy. Obstet Gynecol 66:677, 1983b.

Berkowitz RS, Goldstein DP, Bernstein MR: Choriocarcinoma following term gestation. Gynecol Oncol 17:52, 1984a.

Berkowitz RS, Goldstein DP, Bernstein MR: Modified triple chemotherapy in the management of high-risk metastatic gestational trophoblastic tumors. Gynecol Oncol 19:173, 1984b.

Berkowitz RS, Goldstein DP, Bernstein MR: Ten years' experience with methotrexate and folinic acid as primary therapy for gestational trophoblastic disease. Gynecol Oncol 23:111, 1986.

Berkowitz RS, Goldstein DP, Bernstein MR: Reproductive experience after complete and partial molar pregnancy and gestational trophoblastic tumors. J Reprod Med 36:3, 1991.

Berkowitz RS, Hoch EJ, Goldstein DP, Anderson DJ: Histocompatibility antigens (HLA-A,B,C) are not detectable in molar villous fluid. Gynecol Oncol 19:74, 1984c.

Bolis G, Bonazzi C, Landoni F, et al: EMA-CO regimen in high risk gestational trophoblastic tumor. Gynecol Oncol 31:439, 1988.

Bouillon R, Naesens M, van Assche FA, et al: Thyroid function in patients with hyperemesis gravidarum. Am J Obstet Gynecol 143:922, 1982.

Bracken MB: Incidence and aetiology of hydatidiform mole: an epidemiological review. Br J Obstet Gynaecol 94:1123, 1987.

Brewer JI, Eckman TR, Dolkart RE, et al: Gestational trophoblastic disease. Am J Obstet Gynecol 109:335, 1979.

Brewer JI, Torok EE, Webster A, Dolkart RE: Hydatidiform mole: a follow-up regimen for identification of invasive mole and choriocarcinoma and for selection of patients for treatment. Am J Obstet Gynecol 101:557, 1968.

Buckley JD: The epidemiology of molar pregnancy and choriocarcinoma. Clin Obstet Gynecol 27:153, 1984.

Choo YC, Chan SYW, Wong LC, Ho K: Ovarian dysfunction in patients with gestational trophoblastic neoplasia treated with short intensive courses of etoposide (VP-16-213). Cancer 55:2348, 1985.

Cole LA, Kardana A, Parks S-Y, Braunstein GD: The deactivation of hCG by nicking and dissociation. J Clin Endocrin Metab 76:704, 1993.

Conran RM, Hitchcok CL, Popek EJ, et al: Diagnostic considerations in molar gestations. Hum Pathol 24:41, 1993.

Cotton DB, Bernstein SG, Read JA, et al: Hemodynamic observations in evacuation of molar pregnancy. Am J Obstet Gynecol 138:6, 1980.

Curry SL, Blessing JA, DiSaia PJ, et al: A prospective randomized comparison of methotrexate, dactinomycin, and chlorambucil versus methotrexate, dactinomycin, cyclophosphamide, doxorubicin, melphalan, hydroxyurea, and vincristine in "poor prognosis" metastatic gestational trophoblastic disease. Obstet Gynecol 73:357, 1989a.

Curry SL, Hammond CB, Tyrey L, et al: Hydatidiform mole: diagnosis, management, and long-term followup of 347 patients. Obstet Gynecol 45:1, 1975.

Curry SL, Schlaerth JB, Kohorn EI, et al: Hormonal contraception and trophoblastic sequelae after hydatidiform mole (a Gynecologic Oncology Group study). Am J Obstet Gynecol 160:805, 1989b.

Czernobilsky B, Barash A, Lancet M: Partial moles: a clinicopathologic study of 25 cases. Obstet Gynecol 59:75, 1982.

Delfs E: Chorionic gonadotropin determinations in patients with hydatidiform mole and choriocarcinoma. Ann N Y Acad Sci 80:125, 1959.

Dijkema HE, Aalders JG, De Bruijn HWA: Risk factors in gestational trophoblastic disease and consequences for primary treatment. Eur J Obstet Gynecol Reprod Biol 22: 145, 1986.

Doshi N, Surti U, Szulman AE: Morphologic anomalies in triploid liveborn fetuses. Hum Pathol 14:716, 1983.

DuBeshter B: High-risk factors in metastatic gestational trophoblastic neoplasia. J Reprod Med 36:9, 1991.

DuBeshter B, Berkowitz RS, Goldstein DP: Metastatic gestational trophoblastic disease—experience at the New England Trophoblastic Disease Center 1965–1985. Obstet Gynecol 69:930, 1987.

DuBeshter B, Berkowitz RS, Goldstein DP, Bernstein M: Vinblastine, cisplatin and bleomycin as salvage therapy for refractory high risk metastatic gestational trophoblastic disease. J Reprod Med 34:189, 1989.

DuBeshter B, Berkowitz RS, Goldstein DP, Bernstein M: Management of low risk metastatic gestational trophoblastic tumors. J Reprod Med 36:36, 1991.

Dubuc-Lissoir J, Zweizig S, Schlaerth JB, Morrow CP: Metastatic gestational trophoblastic disease: a comparison of prognostic classification systems. Gynecol Oncol 45:40, 1992.

Elston CW: The histopathology of trophoblastic tumours. J Clin Pathol 29(suppl):111, 1977.

Evans AC Jr, Soper JT, Clarke-Pearson DL, et al: Gestational trophoblastic disease metastatic to the central nervous system. Gynecol Oncol 59:226, 1995.

Flam F, Lundstrom V, Silfversward C: Choriocarcinoma in mother and child. Br J Obstet Gynaecol 96:241, 1989.

Fox H, Laurini RN: Intraplacental choriocarcinoma: a report of 2 cases. J Clin Pathol 41:1085, 1988.

Goldstein DP: Prevention of gestational trophoblastic disease by use of antinomycin D in molar pregnancies. Obstet Gynecol 43:475, 1974.

Goldstein DP, Berkowitz RS: Gestational Trophoblastic Neoplasms. Philadelphia, WB Saunders, 1982.

Goldstein DP, Berkowitz RS: Staging system for gestational trophoblastic tumors. J Reprod Med 29:792, 1984.

Goldstein DP, Berkowitz RS, Bernstein MR: Reproductive performance after molar pregnancy and gestational trophoblastic tumors. Clin Obstet Gynecol 27:221, 1984.

Goldstein DP, Berkowitz RS, Cohen SM: The current management of molar pregnancy. Curr Probl Obstet Gynecol 3:1, 1979.

Gordon AN, Gershenson DM, Copeland LJ, et al: High-risk metastatic gestational trophoblastic disease. Obstet Gynecol 65:550, 1985.

Gordon AN, Kavanagh JJ, Gershenson DM, et al: Cisplatin, vinblastine, and bleomycin combination chemotherapy in resistant gestational trophoblastic disease. Cancer 58: 1407, 1986.

Goto S, Nishi H, Tomada Y: Blood group Rh-D factor in human trophoblast determined by immunofluorescent method. Am J Obstet Gynecol 137:707, 1980.

Grimes DA: Epidemiology of gestational trophoblastic disease. Am J Obstet Gynecol 150:309, 1984.

Grumbine FC, Rosenshein NB, Brereton HD, Kaufman SL: Management of liver metastasis from gestational trophoblastic neoplasia. Am J Obstet Gynecol 137:595, 1980.

Hammond CB (ed): Trophoblastic disease. Obstet Gynecol Clin North Am 15(3), 1988.

Hammond CB, Borchert LG, Tyrey L, et al: Treatment of metastatic trophoblastic disease: good and poor prognosis. Am J Obstet Gynecol 115:451, 1973.

Hammond CB, Parker RT: Diagnosis and treatment of trophoblastic disease. Obstet Gynecol 35:132, 1970.

Hammond CB, Soper JT: Poor-prognosis metastatic gestational trophoblastic neoplasia. Clin Obstet Gynecol 27: 228, 1984.

Hammond CB, Weed JC, Currie JL: The role of operation in the current therapy of gestational trophoblastic disease. Am J Obstet Gynecol 136:844, 1980.

Hatch KD, Shingleton HM, Austin JM, et al: Southern Regional Trophoblastic Disease Center. South Med J 71: 1334, 1978.

Hertig AT: Human Trophoblast. Springfield, IL, Charles C Thomas, 1968.

Hertz R: Choriocarcinoma and Related Gestational Trophoblastic Tumors in Women. New York, Raven Press, 1978.

Hertz R, Lewis J Jr, Lipsett MB: Five years' experience with the chemotherapy of metastatic choriocarcinoma and related trophoblastic tumors in women. Am J Obstet Gynecol 82:631, 1961.

Hertzberg BS, Kurtz AB, Wapner RJ, et al: Gestational trophoblastic disease with coexistent normal fetus—evaluation by ultrasound guided chorionic villus sampling. J Ultrasound Med 5:467, 1986.

Ho P-C, Wong L-C, Ma H-K: Return of ovulation after evacuation of hydatidiform moles. Am J Obstet Gynecol 153: 638, 1985.

Homesley HD, Blessing JA, Schlaerth JB, et al: Rapid escalation of weekly intramuscular methotrexate for non-metastatic gestational trophoblastic disease: a Gynecologic Oncology Group study. Gynecol Oncol 39:305, 1990.

How J, Scurry J, Grant P, et al: Placental site trophoblastic tumor: report of three cases and review of the literature. Int J Gynecol Cancer 5:241, 1995.

Howat AJ, Beck S, Fox H, et al: Can histopathologists reliably diagnose molar pregnancy? J Clin Pathol 46:599, 1993.

Hricak A, Demas BE, Braga CA, et al: Gestational trophoblastic neoplasms of the uterus: MR assessment. Radiology 161:11, 1986.

Hunter V, Raymond E, Christensen C, et al: Efficacy of metastatic survey in the staging of gestational trophoblastic disease. Cancer 65:1647, 1990.

Ishizuka N, Tomoda Y: Gestational Trophoblastic Disease: Hydatidiform Mole, Invasive Mole, and Choriocarcinoma. Nagoya, Japan, The University of Nagoya Press, 1990.

James C: The conservative management of a hydatidiform mole with coexistent living fetus. Aust N Z J Obstet Gynecol 29:343, 1987.

Jones WB: Gestational trophoblastic disease: the role of radiography. In Nori D, Hilaris BS (eds): Radiation Therapy of Gynecological Cancer. New York, Alan R. Liss, 1987, p 207.

Jones WB, Lewis JL: Management of gestational trophoblastic disease—fifteen years' experience. Presented at the 16th Annual Meeting of the Society of Gynecologic Oncologists, Miami, Florida, February 3–6, 1985.

Kajii T, Kruashige H, Ohama K, Uchino F: XY and XX complete moles: clinical and morphologic correlations. Am J Obstet Gynecol 150:57, 1984.

Kajii T, Ohama K: Androgenetic origin of hydatidiform mole. Nature 268:633, 1977.

Khoo SK, Monks PL, Davies NT: Hydatidiform mole co-existing with a live fetus: a dilemma of management. Aust N Z J Obstet Gynaecol 29:356, 1989.

Kohorn EI: Hydatidiform mole and gestational trophoblastic disease in southern Connecticut. Obstet Gynecol 59:78, 1982.

Kohorn EI: Single agent chemotherapy for non-metastatic gestational trophoblastic neoplasms. J Reprod Med 36:49, 1991.

Kohorn EI: The trophoblastic tower of Babel: classification systems for metastatic gestational trophoblastic neoplasia. Gynecol Oncol 56:280, 1995.

Kovacs BW, Shahbahrami B, Tast DE, Curtin JP: Molecular genetic analysis of complete hydatidiform moles. Cancer Genet Cytogenet 54:143, 1991.

Kurman RJ, Scully RE, Norris HJ: Trophoblastic pseudotumor of the uterus: an exaggerated form of "syncytial endometritis" simulating a malignant tumor. Cancer 38:1214, 1976.

Lacey CG, Barnard D, Degefu S, et al: Irradiation of liver metastases due to gestational choriocarcinoma. Obstet Gynecol 61:71S, 1983.

Lage JM, Mark SD, Roberts DJ, et al: A flow cytometric study of 137 fresh hydropic placentas: correlation between types of hydatidiform moles and nuclear DNA ploidy. Obstet Gynecol 79:403, 1992.

Lehman E, Gershenson DM, Burke TW, et al: Salvage surgery for chemorefractory gestational trophoblastic disease. J Clin Oncol 12:2737, 1994.

Li-Pai C, Shu-Mo C, Jian-Xuan F, Zi-Ting L: PEBA regimen (cisplatin, etoposide, bleomycin, and Adriamycin) in the treatment of drug-resistant choriocarcinoma. Gynecol Oncol 56:231, 1995.

Llewellyn-Jones D: Management of benign trophoblastic tumors. Am J Obstet Gynecol 99:589, 1967.

Loehrer PJ Sr, Einhorn LH, Williams SD: VP-16 plus ifosfamide plus cisplatin as salvage therapy in refractory germ cell cancer. J Clin Oncol 4:528, 1986.

Lurain JR, Brewer JI: Treatment of high-risk gestational trophoblastic disease with methotrexate, antinomycin D, and cyclophosphamide chemotherapy. Obstet Gynecol 65:830, 1985.

Lurain JR, Brewer JI, Torok EE, Halpern B: Gestational trophoblastic disease: treatment results at the Brewer Trophoblastic Disease Center. Obstet Gynecol 60:354, 1982.

Lurain JR, Brewer JI, Torok EE, Halpern B: Natural history of hydatidiform mole after primary evacuation. Am J Obstet Gynecol 145:591, 1983.

Lurain JR, Elfstrand EP: Single-agent methotrexate chemotherapy for the treatment of nonmetastatic gestational trophoblastic tumors. Am J Obstet Gynecol 172:574, 1995.

Mangili G, Spagnolo D, Valsecchi L, Maggi R: Transvaginal ultrasonography in persistent trophoblastic tumor. Am J Obstet Gynecol 169:1218, 1993.

Matsuura J, Chiu D, Jacobs PA, Szulman AE: Complete hydatidiform mole in Hawaii: an epidemiological study. Am J Obstet Gynecol 89:258, 1982.

Messerli ML, Lilienfeld AM, Parmley T, et al: Risk factors for gestational trophoblastic neoplasia. Am J Obstet Gynecol 153:294, 1985.

Miller DS, Lurain JR: Classification and staging of gestational trophoblastic tumors. Obstet Gynecol 15:466, 1988.

Miller JM, Surwit EA, Hammond CB: Choriocarcinoma following term pregnancy. Obstet Gynecol 53:207, 1979.

Montz FJ, Schlaerth JB, Morrow CP: The natural history of theca-lutein cysts. Obstet Gynecol 72:247, 1988.

Morrow CP: Postmolar trophoblastic disease: diagnosis, management, and prognosis. Clin Obstet Gynecol 27:211, 1984a.

Morrow CP: Trophoblastic disease. Clin Obstet Gynecol 27:151, 1984b.

Morrow CP, Kletzky OA, DiSaia PJ, et al: Clinical and laboratory correlates of molar pregnancy and trophoblastic disease. Am J Obstet Gynecol 128:424, 1977.

Mortakis AE, Braga CA: "Poor prognosis" metastatic gestational trophoblastic disease: the prognostic significance of the scoring system in predicting chemotherapy failures. 76:272, 1990.

Mutch DG, Soper JT, Baker ME, et al: Role of computed axial tomography of the chest in staging patients with nonmetastatic trophoblastic disease. Obstet Gynecol 68:348, 1986.

Newlands ES, Bagshawe KD, Begent RHJ, et al: Developments in chemotherapy for medium- and high-risk patients with gestational trophoblastic tumours (1979–1984). Br J Obstet Gynaecol 93:63, 1986.

Olesnicky G, Long AR, Quinn A, et al: Hydatidiform mole in Victoria: aetiology and natural history. Aust N Z J Obstet Gynaecol 25:1, 1985.

Olive DL, Lurain JR, Brewer JI: Choriocarcinoma associated with term gestation. Am J Obstet Gynecol 148:711, 1984.

Oztruk M, Berkowitz R, Goldstein D, et al: Differential production of human chorionic gonadotropin and free subunits in gestational trophoblastic disease. Am J Obstet Gynecol 158:193, 1988.

Parazzini F, LaVecchia C, Franceschi S, Mangili G: Familial trophoblastic disease: case report. Am J Obstet Gynecol 149:382, 1984.

Parazzini F, LaVecchia C, Pampallona S, Franceschi S: Reproductive patterns and the risk of gestational trophoblastic disease. Am J Obstet Gynecol 152:866, 1985.

Park WW: Choriocarcinoma: A Study of Its Pathology. Philadelphia, FA Davis, 1971.

Patillo RA, Hussa RO: Human Trophoblast Neoplasms. New York, Plenum Press, 1984.

Patillo RA, Sasaki S, Katayama KP, Roesler M, Mattingly RF: Genesis of 46,XY hydatidiform mole. Am J Obstet Gynecol 141:104, 1981.

Petrilli ES, Twiggs LB, Blessing JA: Single-dose actinomycin-D treatment for nonmetastatic gestational trophoblastic disease: a Gynecologic Oncology Group study. Cancer 60:2173, 1987.

Roberts JP, Lurain JR: Treatment of low-risk metastatic gestational trophoblastic tumors with single-agent chemotherapy. Am J Obstet Gynecol 174:1917, 1996.

Romero R, Horgan JG, Kohorn EI: New criteria for the diagnosis of gestational trophoblastic disease. Obstet Gynecol 66:553, 1985.

Ross GT, Goldstein DP, Hertz R, et al: Sequential use of methotrexate and actinomycin D in the treatment of metastatic choriocarcinoma and related trophoblastic diseases in women. Am J Obstet Gynecol 93:223, 1965.

Rotmensch J, Rosenshein N, Donehower R, et al: Plasma methotrexate levels in patients with gestational trophoblastic neoplasia treated by two methotrexate regimens. Am J Obstet Gynecol 148:730, 1984.

Rustin GJ, Both M, Dent J, et al: Pregnancy after cytotoxic chemotherapy for gestational trophoblastic tumours. Br Med J 288:103, 1984.

Rustin GJS, Newlands ES, Begent RHJ, et al: Weekly alternating etoposide, methotrexate and actinomycin/vincristine and cyclophosphamide for the treatment of CNS metastases of choriocarcinoma. J Clin Oncol 7:900, 1989.

Sand PK, Lurain JR, Brewer JI: Repeat gestational trophoblastic disease. Obstet Gynecol 63:140, 1984.

Santamaria M, Bernirschke K, Carpenter PM, et al: Transplacental hemorrhage associated with placental neoplasms. Pediat Pathol 7:601, 1987.

Santos-Ramos R, Forney JP, Schwarz BE: Sonographic findings and clinical correlations in molar pregnancy. Obstet Gynecol 56:186, 1980.

Schlaerth JB: Methodology of molar pregnancy termination. Clin Obstet Gynecol 27:192, 1984.

Schlaerth JB, Morrow CP, Kletzky OA, et al: Prognostic characteristics of serum human chorionic gonadotropin titer regression following molar pregnancy. Obstet Gynecol 58:478, 1981.

Schlaerth JB, Morrow CP, Nalick RH, Gaddis O Jr: Single-dose actinomycin D in the treatment of postmolar trophoblastic disease. Gynecol Oncol 19:53, 1984.

Schlaerth JB, Morrow CP, Rodriguez M: Diagnostic and therapeutic curettage in gestational trophoblastic disease. Am J Obstet Gynecol 162:1465, 1990.

Sheline GE, Wara WM, Smith V: Therapeutic irradiation and brain injury. Int J Radiol Oncol Biol Phys 6:1215, 1980.

Smith DB, Newlands ES, Bagshawe KD: Correlation between clinical staging (FIGO) and prognostic groups with gestational trophoblastic disease. Br J Obstet Gynaecol 100:157, 1993.

Smith EB, Weed JC Jr, Tyrey L, Hammond CB: Treatment of nonmetastatic gestational trophoblastic disease: results of methotrexate alone versus methotrexate-folinic acid. Am J Obstet Gynecol 144:88, 1982.

Song H, Wu P, Wang Y, et al: Pregnancy outcomes after successful chemotherapy for choriocarcinoma and invasive mole: long term follow up. Am J Obstet Gynecol 158:538, 1988.

Soper JT, Clarke-Pearson D, Hammond CB: Metastatic gestational trophoblastic disease: prognostic factors in previously untreated patients. Obstet Gynecol 71:338, 1988.

Sunderland CA, Redman CWG, Stirrat GM: Characterization and localization of HLA antigens on hydatidiform mole. Am J Obstet Gynecol 151:130, 1985.

Sung HC, Wu BZ, Tang MY, et al: A staging system of gestational trophoblastic neoplasm based on the development of the disease. Chin Med J 97:857, 1984.

Sung HC, Wu P-C, Hu M-H, Su H-T: Roentgenologic manifestations of pulmonary metastases in choriocarcinoma and invasive mole. Am J Obstet Gynecol 142:89, 1982.

Surti U, Szulman AE, O'Brien S: Dispermic origin and clinical outcome of three complete hydatidiform moles with 46,XY karyotype. Am J Obstet Gynecol 144:84, 1982.

Surwit EA: Management of high-risk gestational trophoblastic disease. J Reprod Med 32:657, 1987.

Surwit EA, Alberts DS, Christian CD, Graham VE: Poor-prognosis gestational trophoblastic disease: an update. Obstet Gynecol 64:21, 1984.

Surwit EA, Childers JM: High risk gestational trophoblastic disease—a new dose intensive multiagent chemotherapeutic regimen. J Reprod Med 36:45, 1991.

Surwit EA, Hammond CB: Treatment of metastatic trophoblastic disease with poor prognosis. Obstet Gynecol 55:565, 1980.

Szulman AE: Trophoblastic disease: clinical pathology of hydatidiform moles. Obstet Gynecol Clin North Am 15:443, 1988.

Szulman AE, Philippe E, Boue JG, Boue A: Human triploidy: association with partial hydatidiform moles and nonmolar conceptuses. Hum Pathol 12:1016, 1981.

Szulman AE, Surti U: The clinicopathologic profile of the partial hydatidiform mole. Obstet Gynecol 59:597, 1982.

Szulman AE, Surti U: The syndromes and partial and complete molar gestation. Clin Obstet Gynecol 27:172, 1984.

Thavarasah AS, Kavagalingam S: Recurrent hydatidiform mole: a report of a patient with 7 consecutive moles. Aust N Z J Obstet Gynaecol 28:233, 1988.

Theodore C, Azab M, Droz JP, et al: Treatment of high-risk gestational trophoblastic disease with chemotherapy combinations containing cisplatin and etoposide. Cancer 64:1824, 1989.

Thomas EJ, Pryce WI, Maltby EL, Duncan SLB: The prospective management of a co-existent hydatidiform mole and fetus. Aust N Z J Obstet Gynaecol 27:343, 1987.

Trask C, Lage JM, Roberts DJ: A second case of "choriangiocarcinoma" presenting in a term asymptomatic twin pregnancy: choriocarcinoma in situ with associated villous vascular proliferation. Int J Gynaecol Pathol 13:87, 1994.

Twiggs LB: Pulse actinomycin D scheduling in non-metastatic gestational trophoblastic neoplasia: cost-effective chemotherapy. Gynecol Oncol 16:190, 1983.

Twiggs LB: Non-neoplastic complications of molar pregnancy. Clin Obstet Gynecol 27:199, 1984.

Van Thiel DH, Grodin JM, Ross GT, Lipsett MB: Partial placenta accreta in pregnancies following chemotherapy for gestational trophoblastic neoplasms. Am J Obstet Gynecol 112:54, 1972.

Vassilakos P, Riotton G, Kajii T: Hydatidiform mole: two entities. Am J Obstet Gynecol 127:167, 1977.

Vejerslev LO, Dueholm M, Nielsen FH: Hydatidiform mole: cytogenetic marker analysis in twin gestation. Am J Obstet Gynecol 155:614, 1986.

Walden PAM, Bagshawe KD: Reproductive performance of women successfully treated for gestational trophoblastic tumors. Am J Obstet Gynecol 125:1108, 1976.

Wallis J, Marsh JR, Esquivel CO, et al: Accidental transplantation of malignant tumor from a donor to multiple recipients. Transplantation 44:449, 1987.

Wong LC, Choo YC, Ma HK: User of oral etoposide (VP 16-213) as primary chemotherapeutic agent for gestational trophoblastic neoplasms. Am J Obstet Gynecol 150:924, 1984.

Wong LC, Choo YC, Ma HK: Methotrexate with citrovorum factor rescue in gestational trophoblastic disease. Am J Obstet Gynecol 152:59, 1985.

Wong LC, Choo YC, Ma HK: Hepatic metastases in gestational trophoblastic disease. Obstet Gynecol 67:107, 1986.

World Health Organization: Gestational Trophoblastic Diseases. Technical Report Series 692. Geneva, World Health Organization, 1983.

Yordan EL Jr, Schlaerth JB, Gaddis O Jr, Morrow CP: Radiation therapy in the management of gestational choriocarcinoma metastatic to the central nervous system. Obstet Gynecol 69:627, 1987.

Young RH, Kurman RJ, Scully RE: Proliferations and tumors of intermediate trophoblast of the placental site. Semin Diagn Pathol 5:223, 1988.

C H A P T E R

14

Cancer and Pregnancy

It is estimated that only 1 in 1,000 to 1,500 live births is complicated by a malignancy in the mother. The reports on cancer in pregnancy are often from tertiary care centers, however, where rates of occurrence may be exaggerated by referral patterns. Despite its infrequency, cancer in pregnancy has been discussed in several review articles (e.g., Antonelli et al, 1996a, 1996b). This current interest may be explained in part by the trend in delayed childbearing, increasing the concurrence of these events.

Any malignancy can occur during pregnancy, but the most common solid tumors are cervical, breast, and ovarian cancer and cutaneous melanoma. The hematologic malignancies that most frequently complicate pregnancy are the lymphomas and leukemias. Pregnancy is likely to affect the choice of treatment modality (surgery, chemotherapy, radiation therapy) for any of these cancers. Although cancer is the leading cause of death in women of reproductive age (Boring et al, 1992), it is rarely the cause of maternal mortality (Atrash et al, 1990).

The gynecologic oncologist is often consulted during the decision-making process, even when the cancer is nongynecologic in origin. With specialty knowledge in obstetrics, chemotherapy, and radiation therapy, the gynecologic oncologist can facilitate communication between the general obstetrician/gynecologist and the physician responsible for treating the cancer. The major issues to be considered are (1) the effect of pregnancy on the malignancy and its treatment, and (2) the effect of the malignancy and its treatment on the pregnancy. The effect of treatment on fertility and ovarian function are also important issues, but they are not peculiar to pregnancy.

GYNECOLOGIC CANCER

Cervical Neoplasia

Intraepithelial Neoplasia

Pregnancy provides an excellent opportunity for screening women for cervical neoplasia, and is an important component of prenatal care. Cervical dysplasia occurs with the same frequency during pregnancy as in the nonpregnant patient, but the evaluation and management are altered. Thus biopsy for diagnosis is avoided until the postpartum period unless the presence of invasive carcinoma is suspected. Furthermore, treatment of dysplasia is never undertaken during pregnancy. The rate of progression of dysplasia to invasive cancer is not accelerated during pregnancy (Madej, 1996). Coloposcopy is indicated only for a cytology consistent with a high-grade squamous intraepithelial lesion or invasive carcinoma. Follow-up cytology should be done during pregnancy for women having an abnormal smear, especially if there is no established track record of normal smears. These issues are discussed in further detail later.

Invasive Carcinoma

INCIDENCE

Estimates of the rate of invasive cervical cancer per liveborn delivery range from 1 in 1,500 to 1 in 8,000 deliveries, and are influenced by access to screening, the rate of cervical cancer in the patient population, and the methodology; for example, the inclusion of cases diagnosed postpartum increases the size of the study population but may mask any effect of pregnancy. Some reports have incorporated cases diagnosed as late as 1 year postpartum (Allen et al, 1995). In a study of patients at a large public hospital in the United States, there were only 27 cases of invasive cervical cancer diagnosed prior to delivery in 195,168 pregnant women (1 in 7,143); if the 24,944 abortions and ectopic pregnancies seen during the same time period are included, there was 1 cervical cancer per 8,333 total pregnancies (Duggan et al, 1993).

The rate at which pregnancy occurs in a population of cervical cancer patients will depend upon the incidence of cervical cancer and screening frequency in the population. In a series of over 1,000 patients with invasive cervical cancer, 40 (3.9 percent) were either pregnant at the time of diagnosis or underwent therapy in the postpartum period (Baltzer et al, 1990). The variation in rates reflects the diversity of the populations served. Cervical cancer, more than any other gynecologic tumor, is closely related to socioeconomic status. In some countries, cervical cancer is not only the leading cause of cancer death in reproductive-age women, but is also the leading cause of all deaths in women during the childbearing years.

Cervical cancer is the only malignancy for which screening is part of the routine prenatal care, a fact that may contribute to an apparently high association of both preinvasive and invasive cervical cancers during pregnancy. For many women, particularly those at risk for cervical cancer because of low socioeconomic status, pregnancy may be the only time they consult with a physician and/or midwife. After completing their childbearing, it is not uncommon for these women to not return for cervical cancer screening.

SYMPTOMS

Vaginal bleeding during the reproductive age must immediately bring to mind the two most important causes: pregnancy and cancer. When a woman is pregnant, bleeding from an already existing cervical cancer is more likely to occur and to be brought to the attention of the physician. This is especially true in the early months of pregnancy, when examination is done without hesitation. However, in one third of the cases of cervical cancer in pregnancy there is no vaginal bleeding, and the diagnosis results from the findings on physical examination or the Pap smear.

Although the symptoms of cervical cancer in pregnancy do not differ from those in the nonpregnant patient, the diagnosis may be delayed for several reasons: (1) the young age of the patient (average 32 years) may lower the physician's level of suspicion; (2) the abnormal vaginal bleeding may be attributed to pregnancy causes, especially later in pregnancy; (3) the pregnant cervix typically looks abnormal; (4) colposcopy of the pregnant cervix is often difficult to perform and evaluate; and (5) there is a greater reluctance on the part of the physician to perform a vaginal examination or cervical biopsy on the pregnant patient. Nevertheless, 85 percent of cervical cancers diagnosed in pregnancy are stage Ib or less, and two thirds are less than 4 cm in diameter. The proportion of cases found in each trimester is approximately equal (Duggan et al, 1993; Jones et al, 1996). The disproportionate number of early-stage cervical cancers diagnosed during pregnancy can be explained by the combined effect of earlier bleeding, prenatal pelvic examination, and prenatal cervical cancer screening.

DIAGNOSIS AND EVALUATION

The evaluation and diagnosis of cervical carcinoma in pregnancy is complicated by several factors vis-à-vis the nonpregnant patient, the most important and overarching factor being that there are two lives to be taken into consideration. Second, the standard diagnostic cone biopsy carries an increased risk of hemorrhage and abortion or premature labor (Table 14–1); third, endocervical curettage cannot be done because of the risk of rupturing the amniotic membrane; and fourth, diagnostic studies employing x-rays are not safe for the fetus. Therefore, the ideal situation is to be able to postpone biopsy until postpartum, or at least until the fetus is mature. Because the colposcopic findings during pregnancy are exaggerated by the increased vascularity, glandular hyperplasia, and edema of the cervix, adequate noninvasive evaluation may require the services of an expert colposcopist.

Cervical biopsy is indicated at any time during pregnancy in the presence of a lesion suspicious for cancer. In our experience and that of others (Economos et al, 1993), cervical biopsy is a reasonably safe office procedure, particularly when a small-bite instrument like the "baby" Tischler is used. Cone biopsy should be done whenever invasion is suspected on the office biopsy, or the degree of invasion cannot be determined by the office biopsy. This should be a rare event, as evi-

TABLE **14–1**

Complications and Perinatal Outcome Associated With Cone Biopsy
During Pregnancy

| | Bleeding | | | | Perinatal Deaths | |
| | Immediate | | Delayed | | | |
Source	N	(%)	N	(%)	N	(%)
Hannigan et al (1982)	10/82	(12.4)*	3/82	(3.7)[†]	3/68	(4.4)
Collected series	30/366	(8.2)	12/329	(3.6)	15/319	(4.7)
Total	40/488	(8.9)	15/411	(3.7)	18/387	(4.7)

*Estimated blood loss of more than 500 ml.
[†]Requiring hospital admission.

denced by the experience of Economos et al (1993), who performed only two cone biopsies in more than 600 pregnant patients with an abnormal Pap smear. The timing of the cone biopsy should be after 12 weeks' gestation, when the pregnancy is well established as documented by ultrasonic evaluation, but prior to the 20th week. When cone biopsy is indicated but the pregnancy has passed the 20th week of development, the cone should be postponed until after the fetus reaches maturity because of the risk of premature labor.

MANAGEMENT

A treatment algorithm for the management of the patient with invasive cervical cancer and pregnancy is presented in Figure 14–1. When cervical cancer is diagnosed at or near term,

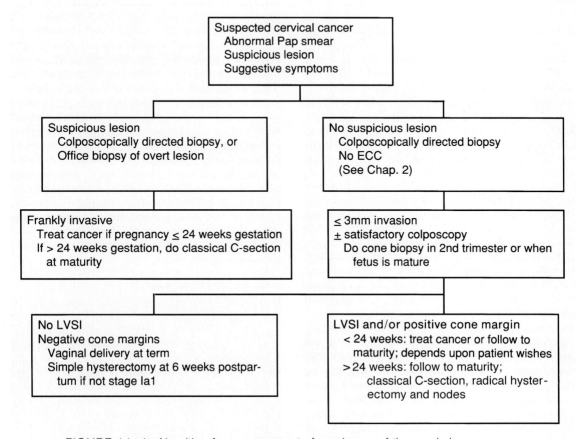

FIGURE 14–1. Algorithm for management of carcinoma of the cervix in pregnancy.

the decisions of when to deliver the infant and when to initiate therapy for the cancer are seldom problematic. Likewise, the diagnosis and treatment of an invasive cancer early in pregnancy is, for the most part, straightforward. With the exception of the lesion with 3 mm of invasion or less and no lymph–vascular space invasion, which has been removed completely by cone biopsy, invasive cervical cancer early in pregnancy is treated without regard for the outcome of the fetus. There are, however, some women who place such a high value on the pregnancy that they are willing to undertake the risk of delaying definitive treatment until after the fetus is mature. This is a very personal decision and requires the most sympathetic but informed counseling by the patient's gynecologic oncologist and obstetrician regarding the risks to the fetus and the mother.

Postponing Treatment. The time-related risk of cervical cancer progression has not been determined in either the pregnant or nonpregnant state. It is therefore impossible to accurately inform the patient of the magnitude of danger in postponing treatment. Combining the data from two reports (Duggan et al, 1993; Sorosky et al, 1995), 13 women with stage Ib cervical carcinoma up to 3 cm in diameter delayed delivery for a mean of 16 weeks (range 8 to 29) after diagnosis without evidence of progression. All patients were alive and well with a median follow-up of nearly 2 years. (In fact, progression of cervical cancer during pregnancy is rarely reported.) These data were further supported by a case-control study by Sood et al (1996). We conclude that a delay of this length is not unreasonable in terms of maternal risk, and therefore the treatment of cervical cancer, at least small stage I squamous lesions, diagnosed after 20 weeks' gestation can be postponed until fetal maturity.

Considering that some neonatal units are reporting a nearly 100 percent survival rate for infants delivered at 28 weeks' gestation, with less than 10 percent long-term morbidity, it may well be questioned whether delaying delivery until 36 weeks is necessary or desirable (Hopkins and Lavin, 1996). This is an important variable that must always be factored into the calculation of the therapeutic ratio. However, it is our view that the delivery should take place when the outcome is the same as at full term. The mother who takes the risk of postponing treatment of the cervical cancer should be given the best assurance that she will have a normal child. The risk to the fetus is almost entirely related to the degree of maturity at birth because, unlike some malignancies, cervical cancer does not metastasize to the products of conception. The final decision is, of course, ultimately the patient's.

If there is going to be a substantial delay in treatment of the cancer, additional studies such as magnetic resonance imaging may be helpful in evaluating the status of the cervical growth and retroperitoneal nodes. X-rays are contraindicated during the period of organogenesis, and exposure of the fetal gonad to gamma radiation at any time should be avoided. The frequency of follow-up evaluations must be tailored to the stage of the cancer and the risk of progression. In addition to the physical examination, cytology and colposcopy may be useful.

Delivery. Unless the lesion has been removed completely, as in the case of a microinvasive carcinoma, the recommended mode of delivery for women with invasive cervical carcinoma is cesarean section through a classical uterine incision. Although the various series in the literature have not shown that maternal survival is adversely affected by vaginal delivery, considering the different stage groups, the relatively small number of study patients, the time span, and the retrospective nature of these reviews, vaginal delivery would have to be very dangerous indeed to show an obvious adverse effect. It is simply not logical to believe that the trauma of labor and dilation does not carry some risk of local or distant tumor dissemination. If the tumor is large, there is also undoubtedly some risk for hemorrhage. Albeit uncommon, several instances of carcinoma of the cervix implanting at the episiotomy site have been well documented (Cliby et al, 1994), another reason for abdominal delivery.

Surgical Treatment. If the patient has a technically operable lesion, and she is medically operable, then a radical hysterectomy and pelvic lymphadenectomy are performed according to the usual clinicopathologic criteria, either with the fetus in situ or at the time of cesarean section, depending upon the stage of gestation. A classical cesarean section incision should be performed, staying away from the lower uterine segment and the cervical cancer. When the radical hysterectomy is done prior to fetal maturity (i.e., if the fetus is going to be sacrificed), it is not necessary to perform a hysterotomy, which may significantly increase the blood loss.

Because radical cesarean hysterectomy is associated with an increase in blood loss and other complications relative to radical hysterectomy in the nonpregnant patient, consideration should be given to performing the surgery 4 to 6 weeks postpartum, particularly when the conditions for surgery are not optimal. Surgical staging can be done at the time of operative delivery in those patients to be treated with radiation therapy.

Radiation Therapy. The use of radiation to treat cervical cancer in pregnancy is generally reserved for patients who are not good candidates for surgery (i.e., those with disease more advanced than stage IIa, those with lesions >4 cm, and those who are poor candidates for radical surgery on medical or technical grounds). When treatment is indicated before fetal viability, the radiation is given with the fetus in situ, in keeping with the thesis that cervical trauma has the potential to disseminate the cancer. Spontaneous abortion typically occurs before completion of the external beam therapy, or the uterus is evacuated at the time of intracavitary therapy. If hysterotomy is required, surgical staging can be performed at the same time.

OUTCOME

The overall survival for the patient with cervical cancer diagnosed during pregnancy does not appear to differ from that of the nonpregnant patient when prognostic factors such as age, stage, lymph node metastases, and histology are controlled for. The prognosis for patients with cervical cancer complicating pregnancy is not different stage for stage than that for cervical cancer in the nonpregnant population (van der Vange et al, 1995). Nevertheless, the incidences of capillary space involvement and lymph node metastasis have been reported to be higher in early invasive cervix cancer that is associated with pregnancy (Zemlickis et al, 1991; Hopkins and Morley, 1992; Monk and Montz, 1992; Duggan et al, 1993; Sivanesaratnam et al, 1993; Nevin et al, 1995).

Ovarian Neoplasia

The incidence of ovarian tumors is approximately 1 in 500 pregnancies; however, only 30 to 50 percent of these tumors are true neoplasms, and only 2 to 5 percent are malig-

TABLE **14–2**

Relative Frequency of Ovarian Neoplasms Diagnosed During Pregnancy*

	N	% Total
Non-Neoplastic Cysts		
Corpus luteum; follicular	73	32
Neoplastic—Benign		36.4
Dermoid cyst	83	17.5
Serous cystadenoma	40	7.5
Mucinous cystadenoma	17	1
Brenner tumor	2	1
Fibroma/thecoma	2	
Total	144	63
Neoplastic—Malignant		
Low malignant potential	7	3
Adenocarcinoma	2	1
Germ cell/stromal	2	1
Total	11	5

*Data from Ballard (1984), Hess et al (1988), and Thornton and Wells (1987).

nant (Table 14–2). The nearly universal application of ultrasound during pregnancy has lately been responsible for an increase in the detection of ovarian tumors. Of the benign ovarian neoplasms that occur during pregnancy, the dermoid cyst and the serous cystadenoma account for 85 percent in collected series. When considered under the classification of adnexal masses, the second most common diagnosis after benign neoplasms is non-neoplastic or tumor-like conditions of the ovary (i.e., corpus luteum, follicular cyst, endometrioma) and uterine fibroids (Hess et al, 1988). Consistent with the young age of the pregnant population, the malignant ovarian tumors in pregnancy are disproportionately tumors of low malignant potential and germ cell tumors, as compared with malignant ovarian neoplasms in the general population.

Symptoms of ovarian tumors diagnosed during pregnancy include pain, increased abdominal girth, and shock caused by intraabdominal hemorrhage. Hess et al (1988) reported that 15 of 54 patients (28 percent) with an adnexal mass during pregnancy underwent emergency laparotomy because of acute symptoms related to the ovarian neoplasm. Others have reported a similar experience (El Yahia et al, 1991). Asymptomatic ovarian tumors are discovered during pregnancy on the basis of ultrasound examination, at cesarean section, and occasionally on routine physical examination.

Ovarian masses that are more than 6 cm in diameter, increase in size during serial ultra-

sound evaluation, have features of malignancy, or are symptomatic require laparotomy during pregnancy. The importance of
patient selection is demonstrated by the experience of Platek et al (1995). None of 31
women with an ultrasonically persistent ovarian cyst larger than 6 cm removed during
pregnancy had a malignancy, and nine of the
cysts were functional. Furthermore, after surgery one patient aborted and another had
premature rupture of the membranes. To
minimize the risk for abortion or premature
labor, the surgery should be performed at 12
to 16 weeks' gestation. If the tumor is discovered during the third trimester, therapy is delayed until postpartum. Unless the tumor is
obstructing the pelvic outlet, the patient is delivered vaginally or abdominally according to
conventional obstetric indications. When the
patient requires an elective or emergency cesarean section, the ovarian tumor can be
removed at that time. Predelivery serum CA-
125 and alpha-fetoprotein levels may be misleading because pregnancy itself may cause
an increase in these values.

Treatment of ovarian malignancy in the
pregnant patient is similar to that in the nonpregnant patient. Hysterectomy with the fetus
in situ is not necessary in carcinoma of the
ovary unless the tumor involves the uterus.
The contralateral uninvolved ovary can be
preserved. In more advanced stages, the extent of surgery, including tumor debulking,
will depend upon the maturity of the fetus
and the patient's wishes with regard to the
pregnancy (Altaras et al, 1989). If removal of
the uterus does not contribute significantly to
tumor reduction, it will also not contribute to
curing the patient. With more advanced disease, the patient should be informed that chemotherapy may be a very effective interim
treatment for the cancer in lieu of immediate
surgical cytoreduction (neoadjuvant chemotherapy) if she desires to have the child. In
this case the surgical therapy can be completed at the time of cesarean section. Several
reports have documented successful chemotherapy for the management of germ cell and
the common epithelial ovarian malignancies
in pregnancy in the adjuvant and nonadjuvant
setting (Malone et al, 1986; King et al, 1990;
Malfetano and Goldkrand, 1990; van der Zee
et al, 1991).

Because ovarian cancer complicating pregnancy is more frequently diagnosed at an earlier stage than in the nonpregnant patient, the
overall prognosis is better (Antonelli et al,

1996a). For example, Dgani et al (1989) reported on 23 cases of an ovarian malignancy
in pregnancy from the Israel Cancer Registry.
Fifteen of the 23 cases were epithelial neoplasms; over one half were low-malignant-
potential tumors. Seven of the 23 cases were
either germ cell tumors (dysgerminoma) or
stromal tumors. Seventeen of the 23 patients
had stage I ovarian tumors. Survival was related to stage of disease; it was 91 percent for
patients with stage I cancer. There were no
survivors among the six patients with more
advanced disease, in spite of aggressive
therapy.

Other Gynecologic Tumors

Endometrial/Uterine

Only 5 to 10 percent of endometrial cancers
occur in women under age 40, and many of
these women have an endocrinologic disorder (i.e., obesity, polycystic ovarian syndrome) associated with infertility. Furthermore, neoplasms of the endometrium may
present an environment hostile to embryo
implantation. Thus it is not surprising that
adenocarcinoma of the endometrium associated with pregnancy is very rare. Of the
dozen or so patients reported in the literature,
most were diagnosed at the time of uterine
curettage for spontaneous or elective termination of pregnancy, but two delivered live
term infants. The patients' ages ranged from
21 to 43 years, and some were multiparous.
Two patients had concomitant, histologically
similar ovarian carcinomas (one papillary serous, one endometrioid). The only reported
recurrence was in a patient with a stage II
lesion. Hysterectomy was not performed on
two patients (ages 26 and 28), one of whom
was well 10 years later (Hoffman et al, 1989;
Schneller and Nicastri, 1994; Kodama et al,
1997). Several cases of endometrial carcinoma diagnosed within 10 months after the
last pregnancy have been reported. All presented with vaginal bleeding. One tumor was
poorly differentiated with nodal metastases
(Kodama et al, 1997). Carcinosarcoma and
leiomyosarcoma have also been reported to
occur concomitantly with an intrauterine
pregnancy.

Vulva

In the event vulvar dysplasia occurs coincident with pregnancy, invasion must be ruled
out but treatment should be postponed until

after the pregnancy has resolved. Some vulvar intraepithelial neoplasia lesions, presumably as a result the immune suppression of pregnancy, appear during pregnancy and involute spontaneously afterward (see Chapter 2).

Gitsch et al (1995) reported two cases of invasive vulvar carcinoma, one stage II and one stage III, treated surgically during pregnancy in women who were ultimately delivered by cesarean section. In their literature review of an additional 16 patients, most had had definitive surgery during pregnancy. Two patients whose treatment was delayed for several months progressed. As expected, squamous cancers predominate over the less common adenocarcinomas. Treatment of vulvar carcinoma should be the same in the pregnant and the nonpregnant patient (see Chapter 3). The surgery poses little risk to the fetus. We do not believe therapy should be delayed more than 4 weeks to await delivery or to allow the pregnancy to reach the second trimester. If delivery is to precede surgical therapy, it is advisable to perform a cesarean section unless the lesion is anterior and will not be traumatized or lacerated by vaginal delivery. Treatment prior to delivery may result in scarring or weaking of the pelvic floor, or require reconstructive surgery such that vaginal delivery is undesirable. If adjuvant radiation is indicated, it must be applied postpartum (Gitsch et al, 1995).

Vulvar leiomyosarcoma has been reported to complicate pregnancy (Kuller et al, 1990). As is true of other soft tissue neoplasms, the histologic diagnosis of smooth muscle tumors in pregnancy may be more difficult because of the local effect of increased maternal hormone levels; the cellular changes may include increased mitotic activity, hyperchromatic nuclei, and/or atypia, all of which are criteria for predicting the natural history and biologic potential of soft tissue tumors.

NONGYNECOLOGIC CANCERS

Solid Tumors

Melanoma

The incidence of malignant melanoma is increasing at a rapid rate, primarily related to increased sun exposure, particularly during childhood and adolescence. Cutaneous melanoma is diagnosed in women at a median age of 45 years. Women are afflicted more frequently than men, and their overall survival is better (Friedman et al, 1991; Koh, 1991). While its incidence has increased dramatically, melanoma is now more commonly diagnosed at an earlier stage. There is no evidence that the risk for cutaneous melanoma is increased by pregnancy (Dillman et al, 1996).

The incidence of malignant melanoma in pregnancy is difficult to estimate. However, reports from large referral centers do provide some indication of the population at risk. Wong et al (1989) reported that, of 1,851 women with malignant melanoma identified in a 15-year review, 887 (48 percent) were of childbearing age (15 to 40 years old) at diagnosis. Of these 887 women, 77 were pregnant (8.7 percent) at the time of diagnosis.

The majority of patients with cutaneous melanoma who are pregnant have stage I disease, that is, there is no evidence of lymphatic and/or distant metastasis (Table 14–3). The most common presenting complaint is an increase in the size (88 percent) or a change in color (44 percent) of a pre-existing mole, or both. The most common site for melanoma in pregnant women is the extremities (Wong et al, 1989; MacKie et al, 1991). This tendency is similar for nonpregnant women.

For patients with stage I malignant melanoma, prognosis is related primarily to the thickness of the lesion, as determined by the

T A B L E **14–3**

Melanoma Associated With Pregnancy

Source	Total N	Stage	Outcome
Wong et al (1989)	66	I	No difference in survival
McManamny et al (1989)	23	I	No difference in survival
Slingluff et al (1990)	88	I	No difference in survival
	10	II	Significant decrease in
	2	III	survival
MacKie et al (1991)	92	I	Pregnant patients more likely to have thicker lesions

microstaging methods of Clark, Breslow, or both. Two series, reporting a combined 154 patients, found no significant difference in median tumor thickness when pregnant patients with melanoma were compared to nonpregnant patients (Wong et al, 1989; Slingluff et al, 1990). Conversely, MacKie et al (1991), reporting on the results of the World Health Organization (WHO) study of melanoma in pregnancy, found that the mean tumor thickness was significantly greater (2.38 mm) for pregnant women compared to three other cohorts of women with melanoma (range 1.48 to 1.96 mm). Travers et al (1995) also found that pregnant women had thicker lesions, while there was no difference in histologic type or location.

In an analysis of the survival data, pregnant patients with melanoma do not appear to have a poorer outcome than nonpregnant melanoma patients when controlling for stage, lesion characteristics, site, and patient age (Table 14–3). After reviewing the literature, Grin et al (1996) concluded, on the basis of the reported controlled trials, that pregnancy before, after, or during the time of diagnosis of stage I cutaneous melanoma did not appear to affect survival. Some authors report that pregnant patients are more likely to develop nodal metastases (stage II disease), which are often amenable to surgical treatment (Slingluff et al, 1990; Dillman et al, 1996). Thus pregnant patients may be candidates for elective lymph node dissection, although its value is otherwise debated (Balch, 1988).

After therapy for stage I melanoma, it is recommended by many authors that the patient wait 2 to 3 years before attempting pregnancy because of the concern that a pregnancy may increase the risk for tumor relapse. The literature on the subject unfortunately gives conflicting results. The largest series, a WHO cooperative study, identified 85 women who were treated for malignant melanoma and became pregnant at a later date. Their disease-free survival was not different from that of women whose melanoma was treated after they had completed childbearing (MacKie et al, 1991). Grin et al (1996), after reviewing the literature, came to the same conclusion. A better rationale for postponing childbearing after treatment of melanoma relates to the natural history of the malignancy. Seventy-five to 80 percent of recurrences will develop in the first 2 to 3 years after diagnosis (McManamny et al, 1989;

Wong et al, 1989; Slingluff et al, 1990; MacKie et al, 1991). Therefore, the woman who undertakes a pregnancy during this time, especially when the risk of recurrence is high, must consider the possibility of dying, leaving a young child motherless.

Another consideration in the pregnant patient with melanoma is the significant potential for metastasis to the placenta and fetus. In a literature review, Eltorky et al (1995) found 54 cases of maternal cancers metastatic to the placenta, over half of which were melanomas. Fourteen of the 54 cases also metastasized to the fetus. Although pregnancy termination has no therapeutic benefit (Dillman et al, 1996), in view of the small risk to the fetus, early delivery may be warranted in patients with advanced melanoma.

The occurrence and progression of melanoma has long been thought to be adversely influenced by female sex hormones associated with pregnancy and puberty. It is of interest, therefore, that sophisticated immunohistochemical staining of melanoma tissue has demonstrated a complete lack of nuclear estrogen and progesterone receptors (Duncan et al, 1994). In view of this fact and the rather large body of evidence that pregnancy does not have an adverse influence on survival with melanoma, there seems to be no valid reason to withhold oral contraceptives (OCs) from these patients.

Breast Cancer

INCIDENCE

In the United States breast cancer is the most common malignancy in women. With approximately 180,000 new cases diagnosed annually (Parker et al, 1997), breast cancer accounts for one fourth of all cancers in women and one sixth of all cancer deaths in women. The peak age of occurrence is 53 years, but 20 percent of patients are less than 45 years old at diagnosis. Approximately one in seven women age 35 years or less with breast cancer is pregnant at the time of diagnosis, and 2 to 5 percent of women are pregnant when diagnosed with breast cancer (Treves and Holleb, 1958; Doll et al, 1988). The estimated incidence of breast cancer in pregnant women is 1 per every 3,000 live births.

DETECTION AND DIAGNOSIS

Physiologic changes in the breast that are related to pregnancy and lactation not only increase the frequency and range of breast problems, but make the detection of breast cancer more difficult. For example, lactating adenomas, galatoceles, and milk-filled cysts may appear, and fibroadenomas may enlarge during pregnancy or lactation (Collins et al, 1995; Scott-Conner and Schorr, 1995). Furthermore, when a mass is noted during pregnancy, the patient and her physician may be reluctant to proceed with an appropriate diagnostic work-up. Estimates of the average delay range from 6 weeks to 6 months (Barnavon and Wallach, 1990). In a series of 44 women whose breast cancer was diagnosed within 1 year of pregnancy, 50 percent had a mass that was documented but not evaluated during pregnancy (Petrek et al, 1991).

The obstetrician who examines the pregnant patient may be the only physician that the patient consults. In addition to a careful breast examination, a family history should be obtained to identify the risk for early-onset breast cancer. Although the sensitivity of mammography is diminished by the breast changes in pregnancy, the study should still be recommended for screening high-risk patients, and for those women with an inconclusive breast examination. With appropriate shielding during low-dose mammography, fetal exposure is negligible (Parente et al, 1988). Nevertheless, the procedure should be avoided during the first trimester.

Approximately one half of breast cancer occurrences in pregnancy are first discovered by the patient (Greene, 1988; Parente et al, 1988). Most of the remaining tumors are detected at physical examination. When a breast mass is discovered, evaluation should be carried out in a manner similar to that for the nonpregnant patient (see Chapter 15). The majority of pregnant patients are in their third trimester at the time of diagnosis. The stage of breast cancer tends to be more advanced when diagnosis is made during pregnancy, but disseminated cancer is rarely present.

MANAGEMENT

Appropriate counseling regarding therapy is important for all patients with breast cancer. Most literature series report that the standard curative surgical procedure during pregnancy is the modified radical or radical mastectomy, which avoids the need for adjuvant radiation therapy (Greene 1988; Parente et al, 1988; Barnavon and Wallach, 1990; Petrek et al, 1991). Thus breast-conserving surgery, which must be combined with adjuvant radiotherapy, is not feasible unless the surgery or the

radiation can be postponed until after delivery. Although it is supradiaphragmatic, radiotherapy for breast cancer will result in significant scatter to the pelvis and fetus, much of which is internal and cannot be blocked by abdominal shielding. Localized radiation to the axilla and/or chest wall may be safe for the fetus after the first trimester. If the breast-conserving segmental mastectomy plus axillary lymph node dissection is the selected surgical procedure, adjunctive radiation therapy should begin within 8 weeks of surgery (Barnavon and Wallach, 1990).

Adjuvant chemotherapy is often recommended for premenopausal women with breast cancer. The most commonly prescribed regimen is cyclophosphamide, methotrexate, and 5-fluorouracil (5-FU) (CMF). Because of the association of methotrexate with congenital abnormalities, this regimen is not recommended during pregnancy (Doll et al, 1988). An alternative to CMF chemotherapy is the combination of cyclophosphamide, doxorubicin, and 5-FU. When these agents are given during the second and third trimesters, the data in the literature indicate that there is no increase in the risk for congenital malformations. There is, however, an increased incidence of intrauterine growth retardation and prematurity (Willemse et al, 1990; Petrek, 1994).

There is no contraindication to breast feeding after completion of treatment for breast cancer, but it should not be done during chemotherapy, tamoxifen therapy, or radiation therapy. It must be recognized that the sensitivity of mammography is substantially reduced during lactation and, therefore, the period of lactation should be restricted to allow proper follow-up after breast cancer treatment. There is no contraindication to the use of hormonal contraceptives or to undertaking a subsequent pregnancy. The patient may be well advised to postpone pregnancy until after the period of greatest risk for recurrence (DiFronzo and O'Connell, 1996). It would be helpful to get a mammogram just prior to pregnancy because of the loss of sensitivity of this screening test as a result of the changes of pregnancy. As previously mentioned, the issue of pregnancy after cancer therapy is largely a social issue related to the risk of leaving an infant or child motherless. Pregnancy does not increase the risk for recurrence or death from breast cancer, and breast cancer treatment does not affect the health or development of the subsequent offspring. Furthermore, quality-of-life studies indicate no adverse effect of childbearing after breast cancer (Dow et al, 1994; Malamos et al, 1996).

OUTCOME

Breast cancer is well known to be a hormonally dependent tumor, and the potential adverse effects of the high serum level of maternal estrogen on breast cancer have been a cause for concern. In the past, many physicians assumed that breast cancer in pregnancy would have a worse prognosis than for nonpregnant women and that termination of the pregnancy would improve survival. This assumption has not been validated by clinical or laboratory data, however (Isaacs, 1995; Merkel, 1996). Women with breast cancer in pregnancy have estrogen receptor–negative tumors, and the survival of pregnant breast cancer patients does not appear to differ from that of nonpregnant patients with breast cancer when the results are controlled for stage, lymph node status, and age (Greene, 1988; Parente et al, 1988; Petrek et al, 1991) (Table 14–4). Zemlickis and colleagues (1992) reviewed the maternal and fetal outcome in 118 patients having breast cancer associated with pregnancy, as compared to 269 matched, non-pregnancy-associated breast cancer patients. Survival did not differ statistically between the women with pregnancy-associated breast cancer and the control group (Fig. 14–2). The pregnancy-associated breast cancer patients were, however, 2.5 times more likely to have metastatic disease; conversely, they were less likely to have stage I disease at diagnosis. The difference in survival is probably due to a delay in diagnosis, as discussed previously.

In their review, Zemlickis et al (1992) also reported that the infants born to women with breast cancer were small for gestational age, possibly related to the disease or treatment. Preterm delivery was more common, but this was often the result of performing an elective, preterm cesarean section to allow for earlier initiation of cancer therapy.

Other Solid Tumors

Single case reports of various solid tumors associated with pregnancy abound in the literature. Literature reviews of primary brain and spinal tumors (Roelvink et al, 1987; Antonelli et al, 1996a) as well as thyroid cancer (Hod et al, 1989; Antonelli et al, 1996a) in pregnancy are comprised of reports of one to four patients. About 90 percent of central nervous system (CNS) tumors arise in the brain. One third are gliomas and one third meningiomas. The rest are acoustic neuromas and other rarer tumors such as pituitary adenomas. The most common spinal tumors are hemangiomas and meningiomas. CNS tumors often enlarge during pregnancy, especially meningiomas, which typically are progestin receptor positive. Symptoms may be exacerbated in the third trimester or during labor, only to disappear after delivery. In one review of cancer-related maternal mortality, CNS tumors were the leading cause of cancer deaths in pregnant women (Sachs et al, 1990).

Thyroid nodules discovered during pregnancy are evaluated the same as in the nonpregnant female. When carcinoma is diagnosed, thyroidectomy should be performed during the second trimester, while benign neoplasms can be treated postpartum. Pregnancy has no deleterious effect on thyroid cancer, and the cancer is not inimical to the fetus (Tan et al, 1966). Gastrointestinal tumors complicating pregnancy are rare and may have a poorer prognosis. Two thirds of the colon cancers are rectal in origin (Parry et al, 1994; Antonelli et al, 1996a). Attributing rectal bleeding to hemorrhoids is especially prone to occur, leading to delay in diagnosis. Gastric cancer complicating pregnancy can mimic the symptoms of morning sickness, and it is more

TABLE **14–4**

Breast Cancer in Pregnancy and Lactation

Source	Pregnant N	Lactating N	Outcome
Petrek et al (1991)	2	44	No difference in survival for pregnant vs. nonpregnant
Greene (1988)	8	—	
Parente et al (1988)	8	—	
Tretli et al (1988)	20	15	17/20 pregnant breast cancer patients died within 4 years; significant decrease in survival

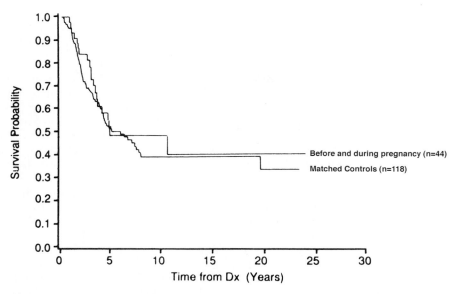

FIGURE 14-2. Survival curve for breast cancer comparing pregnant woman with nonpregnant matched controls. (From Zemlickis D, Lishner M, Degendorfer P, et al: Maternal and fetal outcome after breast cancer in pregnancy. Am J Obstet Gynecol 166:781, 1992, with permission.)

likely to produce ovarian metastases than in the nonpregnant state (Maeta et al, 1995).

Antonelli et al (1996a) reviewed the literature on pheochromocytoma complicating pregnancy. More than 200 cases have been reported but only 4 were malignant. Clinically, pheochromocytoma in pregnancy is commonly mistaken for pregnancy-induced hypertension with or without convulsions, and failure to make the diagnosis may have serious consequences related to the onset of a hypertensive crisis during labor, anesthesia, and vaginal delivery. Currently there has been a reported 15 percent fetal loss (intrauterine growth retardation, spontaneous abortion) and a similar high level of maternal mortality. When the diagnosis is made during pregnancy, medical therapy with beta-blockers and delivery by cesarean section seem to be the preferred management.

Hematologic Malignancies

Among the most common malignancies in women of reproductive age are the lymphomas and leukemias. The great majority of leukemias are acute, either myeloid or lymphoblastic. Unlike many of the solid tumors, the acute leukemias require immediate chemotherapy, so postponing treatment for fetal maturity is not feasible. The high complete remission rate (70 to 90 percent) and long-term disease free survival (30 to 40 percent) of

these malignancies do not seem to be affected by pregnancy. There are, however, numerous subcategories of the hematologic cancers and many prognostic factors, resulting in a rather wide variation in outcome.

With regard to the effect of leukemia and lymphoma on pregnancy outcome, data from the literature are limited, and it is difficult to distinguish between the direct effect of the leukemia and the effects of chemotherapy. Approximately half the patients receiving chemotherapy give birth prematurely regardless of the trimester of diagnosis (Reynoso et al, 1987; Caligiuri and Mayer, 1989). Several cases of placental involvement by leukemia have been reported, and the children of patients with acute leukemia should be examined and followed for vertical transmission of leukemia. Of the 300 reported pregnancies complicated by maternal leukemia, there have been 3 instances of vertical transmission of the leukemia to the child. In one case, the interval from delivery of the infant to the diagnosis of leukemia was 20 months (Osada et al, 1990).

The generally good prognosis for patients with Hodgkin's lymphoma, which accounts for most lymphomas diagnosed during pregnancy, evidently is not altered by pregnancy (Lishner et al, 1992). In the Stanford experience the diagnosis is made at an average gestation of 22 weeks. Most patients have stage II and III disease and defer treatment until after delivery, with excellent results (Gelb et al, 1996). The overall prognosis for pregnant women with non-Hodgkins lymphoma is reported to be poorer than for those with Hodgkin's disease. These patients more often have disseminated disease at diagnosis, and the outcome, therefore, is thought to be independent of the pregnancy (Gelb et al, 1996), although the immune suppression of pregnancy could be invoked as a contributing factor. Treatment with chemotherapy after the first trimester would be expected to have little effect on fetal outcome; however, the administration of radiation therapy, even supradiaphragmatic, is potentially harmful to the fetus (see later). Lymphoma metastatic to the placenta and also to the fetus has been rarely reported (Dildy et al, 1989).

FETAL EFFECTS OF RADIATION THERAPY AND CHEMOTHERAPY

Of great importance in managing the pregnant woman with cancer is the effect of treatment on the fetus. Surgical therapy may, of course, necessitate hysterectomy, or result in pregnancy loss because of spontaneous abortion or premature labor, but it is the administration of chemotherapy and radiation therapy that raises the greatest concern with regard to the fetus because of their potential for genetic damage and carcinogenesis. Most of the scant data available come from observations on patients treated for a hematologic malignancy or breast cancer. Congenital anomalies have been reported, particularly after cytotoxic therapy administered during the first trimester of pregnancy, but most of these reports derive from small series and the outcomes are not consistent. For example,

one woman treated with multiagent chemotherapy during the first trimester of pregnancy gave birth to twins. The male infant was later noted to have a congenital malformation while his twin sister was normal (Reynoso et al, 1987). Reichman and Green (1994), after a literature review of the reproductive effects of chemotherapy in breast cancer patients, concluded that there was no evidence for an increased risk of teratogenesis in the fetus if drug exposure occurred after the first trimester.

The most extensive study, which provides thorough, long-term follow-up of infants exposed to chemotherapy in utero, was reported by Aviles et al (1991). A total of 43 children were born to women who were treated during pregnancy (many during the first trimester) for leukemia or lymphoma: 18 non-Hodgkin's lymphoma, 14 Hodgkin's lymphoma, 7 acute leukemia, and 4 chronic granulocytic leukemia patients. The physical, neurologic, psychological, and hematologic evaluation and cytogenetics analysis of bone marrow aspirates for the 43 children were normal (Table 14–5). At follow-up of 3 to 19 years, all of the children had normal intelligence scores. Sexual development was normal in the subgroup of adolescents. Although all 43 children were alive and well, the grave nature of these hematologic malignancies is underscored by the fact that 17 of the mothers died of their disease.

As mentioned previously in this chapter, the potential deleterious effects of fetal radiation exposure, especially during the first trimester, are well known. Cancerocidal doses of radiation cannot be administered for gynecologic or other pelvic malignancies with pregnancy preservation, but radiation therapy to areas remote to the pregnancy is often required for other cancers, such as breast and

TABLE **14–5**

Pregnancy and Hematologic Malignancy — Outcome Related to Chemotherapy Exposure by Gestational Age

Source	Total Pregnancies	Anomalies/Births by Trimester			Total Live Births
		1st	2nd	3rd	
Reynoso et al (1987)	7	1/2	0/3	0/3	1/8*
Review of literature	51	0/10	0/12	0/20	0/42
Zuazu et al (1990)	22	0/7	0/4	0/2	0/13
Aviles et al (1991)	47	0/20	0/16	0/7	0/43
Total	127	1/39	0/35	0/32	1/106†

*One twin gestation; one twin exposed during first trimester had major congenital anomalies.
†Twenty-one patients had either a spontaneous or elective abortion.

lymphoma. Nevertheless, because of scatter, even supradiaphragmatic radiation therapy can result in doses above 200 cGy to the closest fetal part, depending upon the stage of gestation. Because some of the scatter is internal, it is not possible to completely shield the pregnancy. Stovall et al (1995) report that, with proper shielding, the fetal dose can be reduced 50 percent. While a high level of fetal wastage has been reported to attend radiation exposure (Mulvihill et al, 1987), the collective evidence in the literature indicates that indirect (e.g., supradiaphragmatic) radiation to the fetus even during the first trimester of pregnancy is attended by a low risk to the fetus (Woo et al, 1992; Friedman and Jones, 1993).

OVARIAN FUNCTION AND REPRODUCTION AFTER CANCER THERAPY

Sterilization is frequently an unavoidable side-effect of cancer therapy, especially when the primary tumor involves the pelvic organs. Although the importance of reproductive integrity in the physical and emotional development of the child or young woman cannot be lightly regarded, conservatism is often not the best course. Any disease that threatens both the life of a patient and her sexual or reproductive faculties invariably produces an intensely emotional atmosphere. Under these circumstances, assessment of the risks and benefits becomes more difficult. Nevertheless, there should be no hesitation to recommend removal or irradiation of the reproductive organs, or administration of gonadotoxic chemotherapy in the course of cancer treatment, if there is a reasonable expectation that doing so will contribute to a remission or cure. In the face of disease that can only be palliated, the deleterious effects on the reproductive tract cannot be considered a major impediment to therapy, unless the patient is pregnant.

Gonadal Function

Stillman and associates (1982) reviewed the effects of radiation therapy and chemotherapy on gonadal function. When the ovaries were outside the radiation treatment field, no cases of ovarian failure were observed (average gonadal dose 54 rad); one fourth of the patients with the gonads at the edge of the field developed ovarian failure (average gonadal dose 290 rad); and two thirds of the patients with the ovaries in the field of radiation developed ovarian failure (average gonadal dose 3,200 rad). Moving the ovaries to the midline or to the iliac fossae (oophoropexy) can avoid ovarian destruction in many cases.

It is clear that some chemotherapeutic agents, especially of the alkylating class, when administered to the postmenarchal female, cause amenorrhea, oocyte depletion, and ovarian failure. The longer the treatment, the higher the dose, and the older the patient, the greater the risk of immediate or delayed premature gonadal failure (Reichman and Green, 1994). Ovarian damage is most pronounced in women over age 35 years. Up to 50 percent of women under age 35 will continue to menstruate after combination chemotherapy (Hortobagyi et al, 1986). Regarding the effect of chemotherapy on the prepubertal ovary, Stillman et al (1982) found a 15 percent incidence of premature ovarian failure among 79 females who were long-term survivors of childhood cancer treated with alkylating chemotherapy.

More recently, Byrne et al (1992) reviewed menstrual outcome in a cohort of long-term cancer survivors whose initial treatment was administered at ages 13 through 19 years. The menstrual rate for patients treated by surgery alone was not significantly different from that in control patients. The highest risk for early menopause was in the group of patients who received radiotherapy below the diaphragm along with alkylating agent chemotherapy; 42 percent of these women were menopausal at age 31 (Fig. 14–3).

Complete suppression of ovarian function with gonadotropin-releasing hormone (GnRH) agonists has been reported to provide protection to the ovary against chemotherapy (Blumenfeld et al, 1996) (see Chapter 11). OCs have been prescribed during chemotherapy primarily to prevent pregnancy but also to minimize ovarian damage. However, it is less probable that OCs will protect the ovaries, because, while OCs do prevent ovulation, unlike the GnRH agonists, they do not shut down ovarian follicular activity.

Pregnancy Outcome

Low-dose radiation to the gonads involves a theoretical risk of genetic damage to the oocytes, which might not be manifested until

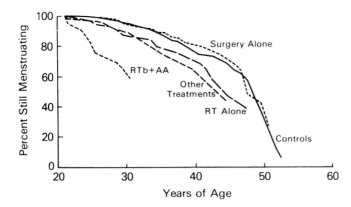

FIGURE 14-3. Percentage of woman menstruating, grouped by therapy, after cancer treatment compared with control patients. RT = radiation therapy; RTb = radiation therapy below the diaphragm; AA = alkylating agent chemotherapy. (From Byrne J, Fears TR, Gail MH, et al: Early menopause in long-term survivors of cancer during adolescence. Am J Obstet Gynecol 166:788, 1992, with permission.)

later generations, and there is also a theoretically increased risk for ovarian cancer. However, from the study of Japanese children born to survivors of the atomic bomb, and/or the progeny of men and women receiving irradiation for cancer treatment, there is no evidence that low-dose gonadal irradiation has produced an increase in mutations, congenital anomalies, or other fetal disorders (Stillman et al, 1982).

Patients treated for pediatric tumors retain ovarian function and fertility potential. In a survey of a large cooperative study group involved in the treatment of lymphoma and leukemia patients, 58 pregnancies occurred in 40 women after therapy for malignancy. Although there was an increased number of abnormal pregnancy outcomes in this group of patients (40 percent of pregnancies), the abnormalities were low birth weight and prematurity rather than congenital anomalies (Mulvihill et al, 1987). The authors theorized that many of the abnormal outcomes occurred because the pregnancies began during the first 12 months after completion of therapy. In the same article, Mulvihill et al reviewed the literature on pregnancy in the survivors of cancer therapy. They found a total of 993 pregnancies, with 747 liveborn children (75 percent). Thirty-two of the liveborn children (4 percent) were reported to have major anomalies, an incidence similar to the frequency of anomalies in the general population. In a review of premenopausal breast cancer patients, 25 of 227 patients (10 percent) who had received adjuvant chemotherapy became pregnant. Ten of the 33 total pregnancies were electively terminated, 2 spontaneously aborted, and 19 pregnancies resulted in normal, full-term infants. There were no congenital anomalies among the term pregnancies (Sutton et al, 1990).

Among gynecologic cancers, the largest group of patients that has been studied for adverse reproductive effects of chemotherapy was treated for gestational trophoblastic tumors, either with single-agent or combination chemotherapy. Follow-up of subsequent pregnancies in the gestational trophoblastic neoplasia group demonstrates no increase in the incidence of congenital anomalies (Ross, 1976; Rustin et al, 1984). Green et al (1991) calculated the frequency of congenital anomalies in the children of both male and female cancer patients. The frequency of major anomalies, 8.1 percent among children delivered of female cancer patients and 7.9 percent among children whose fathers had been treated for cancer, was not statistically different from that in the general population. It is possible for women to have normal pregnancies after recovery from successful bone marrow transplantation, either pre- or postpubertal, according to Sanders et al (1996). In their study of 708 postpubertal women undergoing high-dose chemotherapy with bone marrow transplantation, these authors found that 110 recovered normal ovarian function and 32 subsequently became pregnant. There was no increased risk for congenital anomalies, but a higher rate of preterm labor and low-birth-weight infants was observed. Those women who received total-body irradiation in addition to the chemotherapy had more spontaneous abortions.

REFERENCES

Allen DG, Planner RS, Tang PT, et al: Invasive cervical cancer in pregnancy. Aust N Z J Obstet Gynaecol 35:408, 1995.

Altaras M, Rosen D, Shapiro J, et al: Advanced primary ovarian carcinoma in pregnancy. Am J Obstet Gynecol 160:5, 1989.

Antonelli NM, Dotters DJ, Katz VL, Kuller JA: Cancer in pregnancy: a review of the literature. Part I. Obstet Gynecol Surv 51:125, 1996a.

Antonelli NM, Dotters DJ, Katz VL, Kuller JA: Cancer in pregnancy: a review of the literature. Part II. Obstet Gynecol Surv 51:135, 1996b.

Atrash HK, Koonin LM, Lawson HW, et al: Maternal mortality in the United States, 1979–1986. Obstet Gynecol 76:1055, 1990.

Aviles A, Diaz-Maqueo JC, Talavera A, et al: Growth and development of children of mothers treated with chemotherapy during pregnancy: current status of 43 children. Am J Hematol 36:243, 1991.

Balch CM: The role of elective lymph node dissection in melanoma: rationale, results, and controversies. J Clin Oncol 6:163, 1988.

Ballard C: Ovarian tumors associated with pregnancy termination patients. Am J Obstet Gynecol 149:4, 1984.

Baltzer J, Regenbrecht ME, Kopcke W, Zander J: Carcinoma of the cervix and pregnancy. Int J Gynecol Obstet 31:317, 1990.

Barnavon Y, Wallach MK: Management of the pregnant patient with carcinoma of the breast. Gynecol Obstet 171:347, 1990.

Blumenfeld Z, Avivi I, Linn S, et al: Prevention of irreversible chemotherapy induced ovarian damage in young women with lymphoma by a gonadotrophin releasing hormone agonist in parallel to chemotherapy. Hum Reprod 11:1620, 1996.

Boring CC, Squires TS, Tong T: Cancer statistics, 1992. CA Cancer J Clin 42:19, 1992.

Byrne J, Fears TR, Gail MH, et al: Early menopause in long-term survivors of cancer during adolescence. Am J Obstet Gynecol 166:788, 1992.

Caligiuri SG, Mayer RJ: Pregnancy and leukemia. Semin Oncol 16:338, 1989.

Cliby WA, Dodson MK, Podratz KZ: Cervical cancer complicated by pregnancy: episiotomy site recurrences following vaginal delivery. Obstet Gynecol 84:179, 1994.

Collins JC, Liao S, Wile AG: Surgical management of breast masses in pregnant women. J Reprod Med 40:785, 1995.

Dgani R, Shoham Z, Atar E, et al: Ovarian carcinoma during pregnancy: a study of 23 cases in Israel between the years 1960 and 1984. Gynecol Oncol 33:326, 1989.

DiFronzo LA, O'Connell TX: Breast cancer in pregnancy and lactation. Surg Clin North Am 76:267, 1996.

Dildy GA, Moise KJ Jr, Carpenter RJ Jr, Klima T: Maternal malignancy metastatic to the products of conception: a review. Obstet Gynecol Surv 44:7, 1989.

Dillman RO, Vandermolen LA, Barth NM, Bransford KJ: Malignant melanoma and pregnancy: 10 questions. West J Med 164:156, 1996.

Doll DC, Ringenberg QS, Yarbro JW: Management of cancer during pregnancy. Arch Intern Med 148:2058, 1988.

Dow DH, Harris JR, Roy C: Pregnancy after breast-conserving surgery and radiation therapy for breast cancer. Monogr Natl Cancer Inst 16:131, 1994.

Duggan B, Muderspach LI, Roman LD, et al: Cervical cancer in pregnancy: reporting on planned delay in therapy. Obstet Gynecol 82:598, 1993.

Duncan LM, Travers RL, Koerner FC, et al: Estrogen and progesterone receptor analysis in pregnancy-associated melanoma: absence of immuno-histochemically detectable hormone receptors. Hum Pathol 25:36, 1994.

Economos K, Veridiano NP, Delke I, et al: Abnormal cervical cytology in pregnancy: a 17 year experience. Obstet Gynecol 81:915, 1993.

Eltorky M, Khare VK, Osborne P, Shanklin DR: Placental metastasis from maternal carcinoma: a report of 3 cases. J Reprod Med 40:399, 1995.

El Yahia AR, Rahman J, Rahman MS, et al: Ovarian tumors in pregnancy. Aust N Z J Obstet Gynaecol 31:327, 1991.

Friedman E, Jones GW: Fetal outcome after maternal radiation treatment of supradiaphragmatic Hodgkin's disease. Can Med Assoc J 149:1281, 1993.

Friedman RJ, Rigel DS, Silverman MK, et al: Malignant melanoma in the 1990's: the continued importance of early detection and the role of physician examination and self-examination of the skin. CA Cancer J Clin 41:4, 1991.

Gelb AB, van de Rijn M, Warnke RA, Kamel OW: Pregnancy associated lymphomas: a clinicopathologic study. Cancer 78:304, 1996.

Gitsch G, van Eijkeren M, Hacker N: Surgical therapy of vulvar cancer in pregnancy. Gynecol Oncol 56:312, 1995.

Green DM, Zevon MA, Lowrie G, et al: Congenital anomalies in children of patients who received chemotherapy for cancer in childhood and adolescence. N Engl J Med 325:3, 1991.

Greene FL: Gestational breast cancer: a ten-year experience. South Med J 81:12, 1988.

Grin CM, Driscoll MS, Grant-Kelo JM: Pregnancy and prognosis of malignant melanoma. Semin Oncol 23:734, 1996.

Hannigan EV, Whitehouse HH, Atkinson WD, Becker SN: Cone biopsy during pregnancy. Obstet Gynecol 60:450, 1982.

Hess LW, Peaceman A, O'Brien WF, et al: Adnexal mass occurring with intrauterine pregnancy: report of fifty-four patients requiring laparotomy for definitive management. Am J Obstet Gynecol 158:5, 1988.

Hod M, Sharony R, Friedman S, Ovadia J: Pregnancy and thyroid carcinoma: a review of incidence, course, and prognosis. Obstet Gynecol Surv 44:11, 1989.

Hoffman MS, Cavanagh D, Walter TS, et al: Adenocarcinoma of the endometrium and endometrioid carcinoma of the ovary associated with pregnancy. Gynecol Oncol 32:82, 1989.

Hopkins MP, Lavin JP: Cervical cancer in pregnancy [editorial]. Gynecol Oncol 63:293, 1996.

Hopkins MP, Morley GW: The prognosis and management of cervical cancer associated with pregnancy. Obstet Gynecol 80:9, 1992.

Hortobagyi GN, Buzdar AU, Marcus CE, Smith TL: Immediate and long-term toxicity of adjuvant chemotherapy regimens containing doxorubicin in trials at M.D. Anderson Hospital and Tumor Institute. NCI Monogr 1:105, 1986.

Isaacs JH: Cancer of the breast in pregnancy. Surg Clin North Am 75:47, 1995.

Jones WB, Shingleton HM, Russell A, et al: Cervical carcinoma and pregnancy: a National Patterns of Care study of the American College of Surgeons. Cancer 77:1479, 1996.

King LA, Nevin PC, Williams PP, Carson LF: Case report: treatment of advanced epithelial ovarian carcinoma in pregnancy with cisplatin-based chemotherapy. Gynecol Oncol 41:78, 1990.

Kodama J, Yoshinouchi M, Miyagi Y, et al: Advanced endometrial cancer detected at 7 months after childbirth. Gynecol Oncol 64:501, 1997.

Koh HK: Cutaneous melanoma. N Engl J Med 325:3, 1991.

Kuller JA, Zucker PK, Peng CC: Vulvar leiomyosarcoma in pregnancy. Am J Obstet Gynecol 162:164, 1990.

Lishner M, Zemlickis D, Degendorfer P, et al: Maternal and fetal outcome following Hodgkin's disease in pregnancy. Br J Cancer 65:114, 1992.

MacKie RM, Bufalino R, Morabito A, et al: Lack of effect of pregnancy on outcome of melanoma. Lancet 337:653, 1991.

Madej JG Jr: Colposcopy monitoring in pregnancy complicated by CIN and early cervical cancer. Eur J Gynaecol Oncol 17:59, 1996.

Maeta M, Yamashiro H, Oka A, et al: Gastric cancer in the young, with special reference to 14 pregnancy-associated cases: analysis based on 2,325 consecutive cases of gastric cancer. J Surg Oncol 58:191, 1995.

Malamos NA, Stathopoulos GP, Keramopoulos A, et al: Pregnancy and offspring after the appearance of breast cancer. Oncology 53:471, 1996.

Malfetano JH, Goldkrand JW: Cis-platinum combination chemotherapy during pregnancy for advanced epithelial ovarian carcinoma. Obstet Gynecol 75:3, 1990.

Malone JM, Gershenson DM, Creasy RK, et al: Endodermal sinus tumor of the ovary associated with pregnancy. Obstet Gynecol 68(suppl):88, 1986.

McManamny DS, Moss ALH, Pocock PV, Briggs JC: Melanoma and pregnancy: a long-term follow-up. Br J Obstet Gynaecol 96:1419, 1989.

Merkel DE: Pregnancy and breast cancer. Semin Surg Oncol 12:370, 1996.

Monk BJ, Montz FJ: Invasive cervical cancer complicating intrauterine pregnancy: treatment with radical hysterectomy. Obstet Gynecol 80:199, 1992.

Mulvihill JJ, McKeen EA, Rosner F, Zarrabi MH: Pregnancy outcome in cancer patients: experience in a large cooperative group. Cancer 60:1143, 1987.

Nevin J, Soeters R, Dehaeck K, et al: Cervical carcinoma associated with pregnancy. Obstet Gynecol Surv 50:228, 1995.

Osada S, Horibe K, Oiwa K, et al: A case of infantile acute monocytic leukemia caused by vertical transmission of the mother's leukemic cells. Cancer 65:5, 1990.

Parente JT, Amsel M, Lerner R, Chinea F: Breast cancer associated with pregnancy. Obstet Gynecol 71:6, 1988.

Parker SL, Tong T, Bolden S, Wingo PA: Cancer statistics, 1997. CA Cancer J Clin 47:5, 1977.

Parry BR, Tan BK, Chan WB, Goh HS: Rectal carcinoma during pregnancy. Aust N Z J Surg 64:618, 1994.

Petrek JA: Pregnancy safety after breast cancer. Cancer 74:528, 1994.

Petrek JA, Dukoff BA, Rogatko A: Prognosis of pregnancy-associated breast cancer. Cancer 67:869, 1991.

Platek DN, Henderson CE, Goldberg GL: The management of a persistent adnexal mass in pregnancy. Am J Obstet Gynecol 173:1236, 1995.

Reichman BS, Green KB: Breast cancer in young women: effect of chemotherapy on ovarian function, fertility, and birth defects. Monogr Natl Cancer Inst 16:125, 1994.

Reynoso EE, Shepherd FA, Messner HA, et al: Acute leukemia during pregnancy: the Toronto Leukemia Study Group experience with long-term follow-up of children exposed in utero to chemotherapeutic agents. J Clin Oncol 5:7, 1987.

Roelvink NCA, Kamphorst W, van Alphen HAM, Rao BR: Pregnancy-related primary brain and spinal tumors. Arch Neurol 44:209, 1987.

Ross GT: Congenital anomalies among children born of mothers receiving chemotherapy for gestational trophoblastic neoplasms. Cancer 37(suppl 2):1043, 1976.

Rustin GJS, Booth M, Dent J, et al: Pregnancy after cytotoxic chemotherapy for gestational trophoblastic tumours. Br Med J 288:103, 1984.

Sachs BP, Penzias AS, Brown AJ, et al: Cancer-related maternal mortality in Massachusetts 1954–1985. Gynecol Oncol 36:395, 1990.

Sanders JE, Hawley J, Levy W, et al: Pregnancies following high-dose cyclophosphamide with or without high dose busulfan or total body irradiation and bone marrow transplantation. Blood 87:3045, 1996.

Schneller JA, Nicastri AD: Intrauterine pregnancy coincident with endometrial carcinoma: a case study and review of the literature. Gynecol Oncol 54:87, 1994.

Scott-Conner CE, Schorr SJ: The diagnosis and management of breast problems during pregnancy and lactation. Am J Surg 170:404, 1995.

Sivanesaratnam V, Jayalakshmi P, Loo C: Surgical management of early invasive cancer of the cervix associated with pregnancy. Gynecol Oncol 48:68, 1993.

Slingluff CL, Reintgen DS, Vollmer RT, Seigler HF: Malignant melanoma arising during pregnancy: a study of 100 patients. Ann Surg 211:5, 1990.

Sood AK, Sorosky JI, Krogman S, et al: Surgical management of cervical cancer complicating pregnancy: a case control study. Gynecol Oncol 63:294, 1996.

Sorosky JI, Squatrito R, Ndubisi BU, et al: Stage I squamous cell cervical carcinoma in pregnancy: planned delay in therapy awaiting fetal maturity. Gynecol Oncol 59:207, 1995.

Stillman RJ, Schiff I, Scheinfeld J: Reproductive and gonadal function in the female after therapy for childhood malignancy. Obstet Gynecol Surv 37:385, 1982.

Stovall M, Blackwell CR, Cundiff J, et al: Fetal dose from radiotherapy with photon beams: report of AAPM Radiation Therapy Committee Task Group no. 36. Med Phys 22:1353, 1995.

Sutton R, Buzdar AU, Hortobagyi GN: Pregnancy and offspring after adjuvant chemotherapy in breast cancer patients. Cancer 65:847, 1990.

Tan GH, Gharib H, Goellner JR, et al: Management of thyroid nodules in pregnancy. Arch Intern Med 156:2317, 1996.

Thornton JG, Wells M: Ovarian cysts in pregnancy: does ultrasound make traditional management inappropriate? Obstet Gynecol 69:5, 1987.

Travers RL, Sober AJ, Berwick M, et al: Increased thickness of pregnancy associated melanoma. Br J Dermatol 132:876, 1995.

Tretli S, Kvalheim G, Thoresen S, Host H: Survival of breast cancer patients diagnosed during pregnancy or lactation. Br J Cancer 58:382, 1988.

Treves N, Holleb AI: A report of 549 cases of breast cancer in women 35 years of age and younger. Surg Gynecol Obstet 107:271, 1958.

van der Vange N, Weverling GJ, Ketting BW, et al: The prognosis of cervical cancer associated with pregnancy: a matched cohort study. Obstet Gynecol 85:1022, 1995.

van der Zee AGJ, de Bruijn HWA, Bouma J, et al: Endodermal sinus tumor of the ovary during pregnancy: a case report. Am J Obstet Gynecol 164:2, 1991.

Willemse PHB, van der Sijde R, Sleijfer DT: Combination chemotherapy and radiation for stage IV breast cancer during pregnancy. Gynecol Oncol 36:281, 1990.

Wong JH, Sterns EE, Kopald KH, et al: Prognostic significance of pregnancy in stage I melanoma. Arch Surg 124:1227, 1989.

Woo SY, Fuller LM, Cundiff JH, et al: Radiotherapy during pregnancy for clinical stages IA and IIA Hodgkin's disease. Int J Radiat Oncol Biol Phys 22:407, 1992.

Zemlickis D, Lishner M, Degendorfer P, et al: Maternal and fetal outcome after invasive cervical cancer in pregnancy. J Clin Oncol 9:1956, 1991.

Zemlickis D, Lishner M, Degendorfer P, et al: Maternal and fetal outcome after breast cancer in pregnancy. Am J Obstet Gynecol 166:781, 1992.

Zuazu J, Julia A, Sierra J, et al: Pregnancy outcome in hematologic malignancies. Cancer 67:703, 1990.

C H A P T E R

15

Breast Disease

■

William H. Hindle

The female breasts are an integral part of the female reproductive tract. Gynecologists, in their role as primary health care providers to women, are responsible for routine breast examinations, evaluating breast symptoms and findings, and ordering screening mammography for their patients. Every annual examination should include bilateral breast examination, instruction in breast self-examination, and screening mammography following the American College of Obstetricians and Gynecologists (ACOG, 1989a,b, 1993) guidelines listed in Table 15–1. Documentation of these essential preventative medicine procedures, including specific recommendations for follow-up, should be recorded in the medical record.

CANCER INCIDENCE AND MORTALITY

The incidence of breast cancer continues to increase every year in the United States. Despite improvements in surgical technique, chemotherapy, hormone therapy, and radiation therapy, the breast cancer mortality rate has remained unchanged for more than 60 years. The overall 5-year survival for women diagnosed with invasive breast cancer remains about 50 percent. Only routine population-based screening mammography, with its increased detection of small cancers, has been demonstrated to alter this prognosis significantly (Andersson et al, 1988). Ten-year follow-up figures have shown a 40 percent decrease in the mortality from breast cancer for women offered screening mammography compared with a control group who did not have mammography (Feig, 1988). Furthermore, small cancers detected by mammography are usually amenable to breast-

conserving surgery with the same 10-year disease-free survival rates as similar cancers treated with the traditional modified radical mastectomy.

For 1996, the American Cancer Society estimated that in the United there were 184,300 new cases of invasive breast cancer diagnosed and that 44,300 women died of breast cancer (Parker et al, 1996). This represents 31 percent of the total cancer incidence and 17 percent of all cancer deaths in women. The lifetime risk of breast cancer for a white woman born in the United States in 1996 is now 1 in 9 for the mean life expectancy.

The incidence (Fig. 15–1) and mortality of female breast cancer is more than twice the total incidence and mortality of all the gynecologic pelvic malignancies combined. The routine application of screening mammography for all women following ACOG guidelines should reduce the mortality from breast cancer similarly to that achieved for cervical cancer by the routine application of annual Pap smears.

ANATOMY

The Breast

The anatomy of the breast is shown in Figure 15–2. Most of the breast is composed of fat. The glandular tissue spreads out from the nipple within the fat. Beginning at about age 20 years there is progressive fatty replacement of the glandular tissue. Each lobe of the breast is anatomically distinct, not connected to any other, and drains through a single duct opening of the nipple. Thus, intrinsic breast pathology within a lobe will present with nipple discharge from a single nipple duct opening. Cooper's ligaments are thin, fibrous, in-

ACOG Guidelines for Breast Self-Examination,
Clinical Breast Examination, and
Screening Mammography

Breast self-examination
  Monthly beginning at age 18 years
Clinical breast examination
  Annually beginning at age 18 years
Screening mammography
  Baseline between ages 35 and 40 years
  Every 1 to 2 years ages 40 to 50 years
  Annually after age 50 years

terwoven bands between the lobes. When invaded by carcinoma, the ligaments contract and can produce nipple retraction, skin dimpling, and the characteristic peau d'orange of the overlying skin. Figure 15–3 is an anatomic diagram of a single breast lobe and the terminal duct lobular unit (TDLU). The TDLU is the site of the physiologic function of the breast, lactation. At all times other than during lactation, the breast epithelium is in a resting state, although changes do occur correlated with the hormonal sequence of the menstrual cycle.

The exact initiation and promotion of human breast cancer is not known. The current theory is that there is a genetic susceptibility to environmental carcinogens that can lead to malignant transformation of breast ductal epithelium. This is probably a continuous spectrum of change that is reversible until cytologic malignancy occurs. However, it is possible that, if women lived long enough, all the preinvasive malignant lesions might become invasive. Once malignant, a typical ductal carcinoma cell's doubling time is about 100 days. However, the range is probably 30 to 300 days, and serial mammography has shown that some cancers do not double in size at a constant rate.

The Lymph Nodes

The axillary lymph nodes perform the major lymphatic draining of the breast and are important in estimating prognosis and in making decisions about adjuvant therapy for breast cancer. The level I axillary lymph nodes are located lateral to the insertion of the pectoralis minor muscle, the level II axillary lymph nodes are under the insertion of the pectoralis minor muscle, and the level III axillary lymph nodes are medial and superior to the pectoralis minor muscle. Axillary lymph node dissection includes the level I and II nodes, which number about 35. Adverse prognosis correlates with the number of axillary lymph nodes containing metastatic cancer.

ENDOCRINOLOGY

The endocrinology of the development and function of the human female breast is species specific and not analogous to other reproductive endocrine end-organs. Adrenal corticosteroids, estrogen, growth hormone, insulin, progesterone, and prolactin are required for the functional development of the female breast. Additionally, placental lactogen and chorionic gonadotropin are necessary for lactation. Throughout the glandular

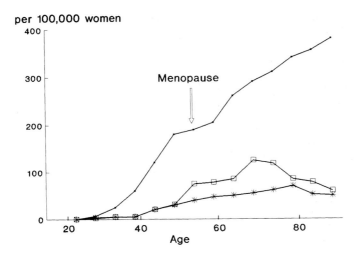

FIGURE 15–1. Incidence rate versus age for breast (·—·), cervical (*—*), and endometrial (□—□) carcinoma. (Redrawn from Gambrell RD Jr: Breast disease in the postmenopausal years. Semin Reprod Endocrinol 1:27, 1983, with permission.)

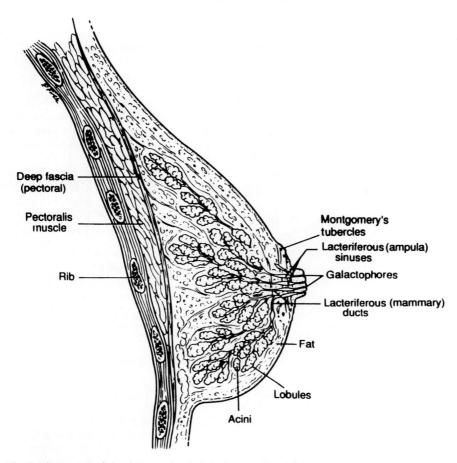

FIGURE 15-2. Anatomy of the breast depicting the separate lobes in the surrounding adipose tissue.

tissue there is a heterogeneous response to the concerted action of these hormones. This hormonal interaction is complex and poorly understood (Vogel et al, 1981). There are few clinical data available on the endocrinology of the human female breast.

It is clear that the breast ductal epithelium is not analogous to the endometrium in its response to estrogen and progesterone (Longacre and Bartow, 1986). Studies of mitotic/DNA activity in the human female ductal epithelium reveal elevated levels in the luteal phase of the menstrual cycle, in contrast to the known increased mitotic/DNA activity that occurs in the follicular phase of the endometrium (Ferguson and Anderson, 1981). Human female breast ductal epithelium follows a cyclic pattern of cellular proliferation and regression during the menstrual cycle (Fig. 15–4) (Anderson et al, 1982; Going et al, 1988).

DIAGNOSIS

History

The patient's age, last menstrual period, previous breast cancer and breast surgery history, age at diagnosis of first-degree relatives (mother, sisters, or daughters) with breast cancer, and current or past hormone therapy are clinically significant.

Symptoms

Presenting breast symptoms are pain, mass, and nipple discharge. Most women presenting with breast symptoms have a profound underlying fear of breast cancer. They fear death, disfigurement, defeminization, chemotherapy, domestic stress, and sexual rejection. At the time of diagnosis and with treat-

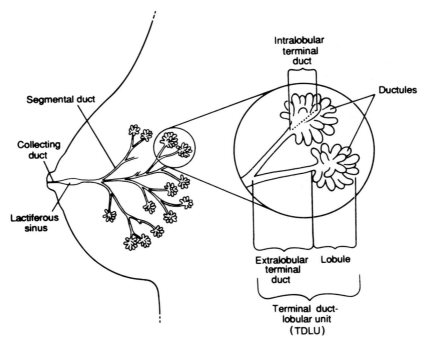

FIGURE 15-3. A single breast lobe and the terminal duct lobular unit.

ment, a woman with breast cancer often manifests the sequential grieving/loss emotions characterized by (1) denial, (2) bartering, (3) anger, (4) guilt, (5) depression, and, finally, (6) grief (Kubler-Ross, 1969). The physician should be empathetic and sensitive to

the anxieties, fears, and concerns of women who present with breast symptoms. No matter how trivial the symptoms and physical findings may seem to the physician, all breast complaints should be taken seriously and thoroughly evaluated. Only after complete, exact evaluation can the patient be reassured. As long as she remains anxious, continuing follow-up is indicated.

Breast Self-Examination

Breast self-examination (BSE) is useful for women in familiarizing themselves with their breasts and axillae. The teaching of BSE should be done by one-on-one demonstration and then having the patient demonstrate the technique she has learned. This BSE teaching process should be repeated at each annual examination. The ACOG (1989a,b) recommends beginning monthly BSE at age 18 years. The optimum time for BSE is a few days after menstruation ceases or on a scheduled calendar basis for women who are not having regular periods. Although helpful, pamphlets and video instructions have not resulted in high levels of compliance or effective BSE. Traditionally most breast masses are found by chance by the patient herself and are usually 2 to 3 cm when discovered. Although it seems logical that finding smaller

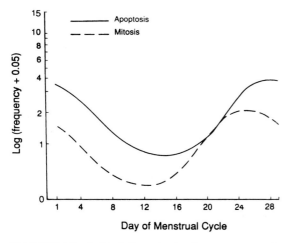

FIGURE 15-4. Variation of mitosis and apoptosis measured in human female breast epithelium versus the day of the menstrual cycle. (Adapted from Ferguson DJ, Anderson TJ: Morphological evaluation of cell turnover in relation to menstrual cycle in the "resting" human breast. Br J Cancer 44:177, 1981, with permission.)

masses earlier by BSE would result in improved prognosis, a significant change in overall survival has not been documented. There are some reports that the clinical stage of breast cancers found by BSE are somewhat "earlier" than breast cancers found by chance (Hill et al, 1988).

Screening Mammography

Screening mammography is the only proven technique for decreasing the mortality rate from breast cancer (Verbeek et al, 1984; NCI Breast Cancer Screening Consortium, 1990). First demonstrated to be effective in diagnosing small lesions in asymptomatic women by the Health Insurance Plan (HIP) study in New York (Shapiro et al, 1971, 1982; Chu et al, 1988), screening mammography has been shown by numerous studies to be effective in detecting nonpalpable breast cancers, which have an excellent prognosis with current methods of treatment. The HIP screening mammography study demonstrated a significant downgrading of the expected stage of cancer at the time of diagnosis from inoperable stages III and IV to operable stages I and II. The Breast Cancer Detection Demonstration Project found six cancers per 1,000 initial mammographic screens and three cancers per 1,000 on interval follow-up screening mammograms (Baker, 1982; Seidman et al, 1987). The Swedish population-based study, which was conducted with less than optimum screening intervals and only a single-view mammogram, showed a 40 percent reduction of the breast cancer mortality rate 10 years after the study was begun (Tabar et al, 1985, 1989). The study includes all the women who were offered screening mammography, had a screening interval of about 2 years, and utilized only a mediolateral oblique view mammogram. The recall rate for mammographic evaluation was about 5 percent. For optimum results, screening mammography requires skilled, compassionate mammographic technicians, dedicated mammography machines, extended processing of the films, and a perceptive and experienced mammographer.

Mammography can detect a mass as small as 1 mm in diameter. Given the doubling time of 100 days, mammography has the potential to detect a cancer 3 to 4 years before it has grown large enough to palpate. However, 10 percent of palpable breast cancers are not detected by mammography (Edeiken, 1989). Clinical breast examination should always supplement mammographic evaluation.

THE DIAGNOSTIC TRIAD FOR A PALPABLE MASS

The evaluation of breast lesions (see Table 15–2) includes the diagnostic triad for a palpable dominant breast mass of (1) clinical breast examination (CBE), (2) fine-needle aspiration (FNA), and (3) diagnostic mammography (Hindle, 1990).

Clinical Breast Examination

Bilateral CBE should include the entire anterior chest wall, including both axillae and both supraclavicular areas. Visual inspection should take place with the patient (1) sitting up, (2) raising her arms over her head, (3) pressing her hands on her hips, and (4) leaning forward. With the patient lying flat, palpation should be with the pads of the second, third, and fourth fingers in a dime-sized circular motion with varying degrees of pressure (superficial, medium, and deep). The vertical strip method is the most effective search pattern (Saunders et al, 1986). Careful attention should be paid to the nipple/areolar area, because 15 percent of cancers are located under the areola. This area is very sensitive to the patient. It feels irregular to palpation because of the underlying collecting ducts. A prominent lateral ridge is often felt in this area where the lobes fan out into the adipose tissue of the remainder of the breast. Particular attention should be paid also to any area where the patient thinks she has felt a mass. Studies have shown that the effectiveness of CBE is directly related to the time spent palpating the breast. Any breast mass larger than 1 cm in diameter should be detected by palpation. With special training and enough time to palpate the breast thoroughly and systematically, it is possible to detect a mass as small as 0.5 cm in diameter. All palpable, dominant, three-dimensional persistent masses should be diagnosed. The written documentation in the patient's medical record should state at

TABLE **15–2**

Evaluation of Breast Lesions

History
Clinical breast examination
Mammography
Fine-needle aspiration of palpable masses
  Aspiration of cyst fluid
  Aspiration cytology of solid masses

least that "bilateral breast and axillary examination was performed and no dominant masses were felt."

Fine-Needle Aspiration

Technique

FNA (Fig. 15–5) is readily learned, accurate, efficient, and cost effective (Zajicek et al, 1967; Zajdela et al, 1975; Hindle, 1990). FNA is no more painful than a venipuncture and takes only a little more time. Local anesthesia is not necessary. The essential equipment is already available in most physicians' offices: a 22-gauge 1.5-inch needle with transparent plastic hub, a 10-ml syringe, an alcohol or equivalent skin wipe, and a 4 × 4-inch sterile gauze pad (Bell et al, 1983; Hindle and Navin, 1983). The slides must be prepared quickly to avoid drying and then are processed in a manner similar to Pap smears. The most difficult part of FNA is to stabilize the mass completely, preferably over a rib, which can be done by downward and outward pressure of the index and third fingers of the nonaspirating hand (Fig. 15–6). Once the mass is stabilized between the fingers, the skin over the mass is cleaned with antiseptic. Then the needle, with the syringe attached, is inserted directly into the center of the mass (Fig. 15–7). It is important to visualize the mass mentally at all times during FNA, particularly as to its depth below the skin, because the compression provided by the fingers stabilizing the mass usually brings the mass closer to the skin surface. The cytology obtained will accurately reflect the tissue exactly where the needle tip was during the FNA.

Tactile information is obtained upon the needle's entering the mass: normal breast tissue is soft and offers little resistance; a cyst tends to "pop" when entered; fibroadenomas

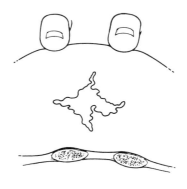
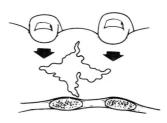

FIGURE 15–6. Technique of immobilizing a palpable dominant breast mass for fine-needle aspiration.

feel dense and rubbery; and most cancers are gritty and resistive to FNA. Once the needle is within the mass, it is moved back and forward in "jackhammer" fashion, the tip remaining inside the mass at all times. The back-and-forth action uses about a 1- to 2-cm

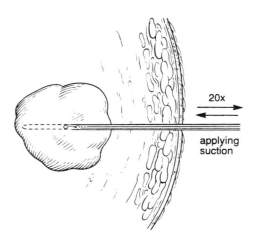

FIGURE 15–7. The back-and-forth motion of the needle tip within the mass during fine needle aspiration for cytology.

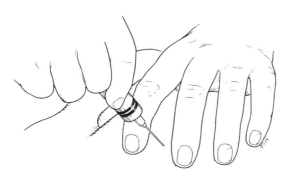

FIGURE 15–5. Fine-needle aspiration of a palpable solid breast mass.

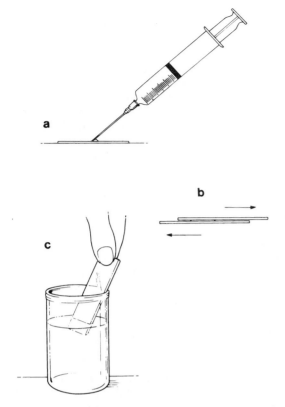

FIGURE 15–8. Technique for preparing fixed slides before staining.

without a syringe and negative pressure, the cellular harvest is less (Zajdela et al, 1987).

The negative pressure is released *before* the needle is removed from the mass and the skin. The needle is then detached, air drawn up into the syringe, the needle reattached, and air forcefully ejected down the needle tip, touching a glass slide at about a 45-degree angle. The drop of tissue fluid is then quickly smeared similarly to preparing a hematology smear and the slide is placed in a Pap smear bottle of fixative (Fig. 15–8). Alternately, spray fixative can be used. After fixation, the slides can be stained at any time. Particularly when first learning the technique of FNA, it is helpful to apply a rapid stain such as Diff-Quik (Harleco, Division of American Hospital Supply Corp., Gibbstown, NJ) so that the aspirator can confirm that there is an adequate cell sample preserved on the slide.

Cytology

Each benign and malignant neoplasm of the breast has characteristic cytologic findings. A specific cytologic diagnosis can be made if there is a well-preserved, adequate cell sample on the slide. Typical FNA cytology (FNAC) patterns of normal breast tissue, fibroadenoma, and carcinoma are drawn in Figure 15–9. Unlike Pap smears, in which one must search for a few scattered malignant cells in a sea of benign cells, with FNAC almost all the cells on the smear are from the neoplasm (if the aspirator kept the needle tip within the mass). The differentiation between normal breast tissue and neoplasm, benign and malignant, is usually clear under the microscope.

stroke and should be repeated about 20 times (Fig. 15–7). During this time, negative pressure in the syringe helps to draw more tissue fluid and cells into the barrel of the needle. Various pistol syringe holders are available to maintain the negative pressure during the FNA, but they are not necessary. While capillary action alone is sufficient to draw cells and tissue fluid into the barrel of the needle

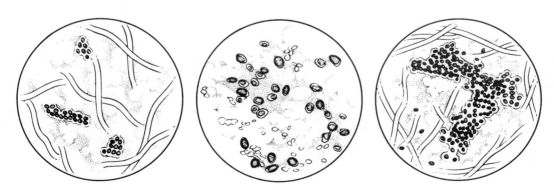

FIGURE 15–9. Microscopic appearance of fine-needle aspiration cytology of normal breast tissue, invasive ductal carcinoma, and fibroadenoma.

At the Los Angeles County–University of Southern California Medical Center and several other institutions (Wanebo et al, 1984; Gelabert et al, 1990), the surgeons accept the cytologic FNA diagnosis of adenocarcinoma and will perform a modified radical mastectomy without requiring histologic verification.

Complications and Contraindications

There is no evidence that any risk exists for spreading cancer or adversely affecting the prognosis of women who have breast cancer diagnosed by FNA (Robbins et al, 1954; Berg and Robbins, 1962; Engzell et al, 1971). The indication for FNA is a persistent dominant breast mass; there are no contraindications. The risk for hematoma formation can be minimized if a folded 4 × 4-inch gauze pad is pressed over the area of the aspiration for 2 minutes immediately after the FNA. Pneumothorax has been reported but should be readily avoided if the mass is stabilized over a rib and the aspirator mentally visualizes exactly were the needle tip is at all times during the FNA.

Mammography

Timing of FNA and Mammography

FNA has been reported to produce bleeding into the breast tissue, which can be mistaken for a "suspicious" lesion on mammography. Thus mammograms should be scheduled before or 2 weeks after FNA to avoid this possible mammographic confusion (Klein and Sickles, 1982; Sickles et al, 1983).

Diagnostic Mammography

Diagnostic mammography is essential to the evaluation of the breast containing the mass and the contralateral breast. In addition, clinically useful information about the mass itself often will be obtained by mammography. However, the clinical opinion given by the mammographer is at best a tentative diagnosis and must be confirmed by either FNA or open surgical biopsy if there is a question of malignancy either on CBE or mammography.

Young women often have mammographically dense breast tissue, which markedly decreases the accuracy of mammographic interpretation. However, as there is progressive fatty replacement of the glandular breast with advancing age, the accuracy of mammographic interpretation increases with age (Edeiken, 1989), as does the incidence of breast cancer.

Significant Findings. Stellate lesions, circumscribed lesions, microcalcifications, asymmetric densities, and skin changes are clinically significant mammographic findings that should be specifically reported. In addition, the report should state if the findings are mammographically normal, benign, suspicious, or malignant. If the mammographic impression is of a suspicious or malignant lesion, an appropriate recommendation (e.g., biopsy) should be in the mammography report. Furthermore, a "negative" mammogram does not rule out cancer. Such a report only indicates that no abnormalities were noted.

Cysts and Ultrasound. Mammography detects nonpalpable breast masses but cannot reliably distinguish cysts from solid masses. Ultrasound can usually differentiate nonpalpable cysts from solid masses and is a useful adjunct to mammography. Ultrasound is not useful is delineating microcalcifications.

Microcalcifications. The most common suspicious, nonpalpable lesions are clustered, irregular, dense, often branching, microcalcifications. These are best seen on magnification views, with the aid of a magnifying glass.

When suspicious clustered microcalcifications are excised, associated ductal carcinoma is found in about 25 percent. This may be either ductal carcinoma in situ (DCIS) or invasive carcinoma. Typically, these suspicious microcalcifications occur as the cancer outgrows its blood supply, with resultant intraductal tumor necrosis and subsequent intraductal calcification of the necrotic debris.

Needle Localization Biopsy. Mammographically suspicious, nonpalpable breast lesions are excised utilizing preoperative mammographic needle localization techniques so that the surgeon can excise the entire area of the suspicious lesion (Meyer et al, 1990; Thompson et al, 1991). Such lesions are usually not visible or palpable even at surgery. A specimen radiograph, obtained before completion of the operation, is essential to confirm that the mammographic lesion has been excised. If the lesion has not been totally excised, or if there is a question about the margins, further breast tissue should be excised and similarly radiographically evaluated.

Stereotactic FNA and Needle Biopsy. Mammographically guided stereotactic techniques are available for FNAC of nonpalpable breast lesions. Careful technique, usually with multiple passes of the needle, is required to avoid sampling error and the possibility of missing the lesion. Biopsy gun technique, with a 14-gauge needle and local anesthesia, which removes a needle core of tissue for histologic diagnosis, can also be used (Parker et al, 1991). If a definitive diagnosis is not obtained by either technique, mammographic needle localization biopsy should be performed to excise the entire suspicious area and obtain a definitive histologic diagnosis. Ultrasound also is being used for FNA and needle gun biopsy of nonpalpable lesions utilizing a 7.5- or 10-mHz linear array, hand-held transducer. With solid masses, the accuracy is similar to that of stereotactic mammography.

Clinical Correlations

Although a high degree of clinical correlation is possible, CBE and mammography yield only presumptive diagnoses. A definitive diagnosis is established by FNAC (with an adequate cell sample) or open surgical biopsy histology. A clinical algorithm for the evaluation of a persistent palpable dominant breast mass is presented in Figure 15–10.

The Diagnostic Team

Optimum diagnostic evaluation of breast lesions requires the close cooperation and direct communication of a dedicated multispecialty team composed of the patient's physician, a cytopathologist, a mammographer, an oncologic surgeon, and a pathologist. Each of these specialists should have had training in breast disease, have a clinical orientation and patient sensitivity, see an adequate volume of breast cases, and have a continuing keen interest in breast disease.

BENIGN BREAST DISEASE

Mastalgia

Mastalgia is a common breast symptom, particularly in the early reproductive years. Mastalgia is usually cyclic but can be noncyclic. The pain is usually diffuse and often bilateral. After complete evaluation, most patients with mastalgia can be appropriately treated by reassurance and explanation. Almost all patients with breast pain have an underlying fear of breast cancer. When specific treatment is required for mastalgia, it should be prescribed in a stepwise fashion beginning with simple nonpharmacologic recommendations (Goodwin et al, 1988), as listed in Table 15–3. Danazol is the only prescription medicine approved by the Food and Drug Administration for the treatment of mastalgia. Although it is effective in 80 percent of the cases, danazol is rarely used because of the masculinizing side effects of long-term treatment. Also, as many as 50 percent of the women treated with danazol for mastalgia experience a recurrence of their breast pain within 6 months of completing therapy. However, those women who require danazol therapy for mastalgia can often be maintained on a reduced dosage after the symptoms have been controlled on the initial standard dosage.

Response to any therapy is significantly greater for cyclic mastalgia compared with noncyclic mastalgia. Careful evaluation should confirm that the breast pain is mastalgia and not nonbreast pain referred to the anterior chest area, such as achalasia, angina, cervical rib, cervical spondylosis, cholelithiasis, costochondritis, hiatus hernia, myalgia, neuralgia, or pleurisy.

Nipple Discharge

Nipple discharge can be elicited from the breasts of more than 75 percent of women by repeated compression or gentle suction (Devitt, 1985). Pathologic nipple discharge is spontaneous, is often unilateral, and, except for galactorrhea, presents from a single duct opening in the nipple (Leis et al, 1985; Leis, 1989). Milky discharge is physiologic and does not represent intrinsic breast pathology. Greenish nipple discharge is usually from mammary duct ectasia (periductal mastitis). Bloody nipple discharge can be from underlying carcinoma, as can watery, serous, and serosanguineous nipple discharge. Blood can be identified in nipple discharge by the use of a Hemostix or similar dipstick test. Intraductal papilloma is the etiology of most cases of spontaneous single-duct nipple discharge. A ductogram can specifically localize the lesions but cannot reliably differentiate benign from malignant papillomas, so all such lesions must be surgically excised (Katz et al, 1982; Tabar et al, 1983). The incidence of underlying carcinoma as the etiology of nipple discharge is about 6 percent for watery/serous discharge and 13 percent for grossly

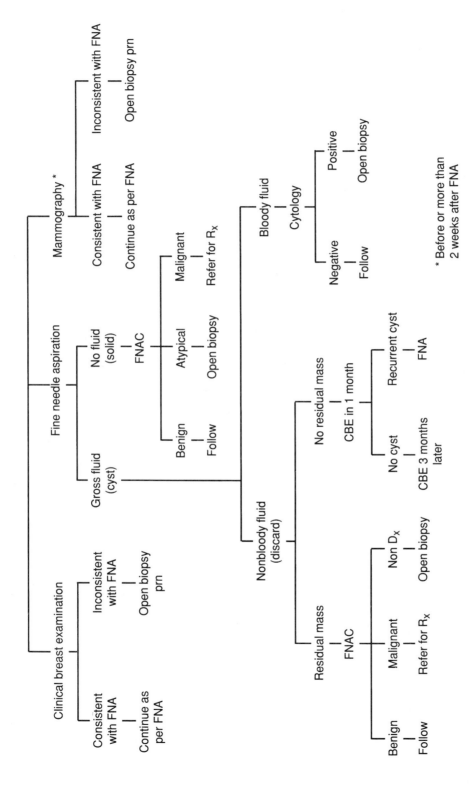

FIGURE 15–10. Clinical algorithm for the evaluation of a persistent palpable dominant breast mass. FNA, fine needle aspiration; FNAC, fine needle aspiration cytology; CBE, clinical breast examination; D$_x$, diagnostic; R$_x$, treatment; prn, as indicated.

TABLE 15–3
Treatment of Mastalgia
Reassurance
Fitted supportive brassiere
Salt restriction before menstruation
Nonsteroidal analgesia
Low-estrogen oral contraceptives
Danazol

bloody discharge (Tabar et al, 1983). Cytology of nipple discharge is rarely of clinical value because the cellular yield is low. A definitive histologic diagnosis can only be made on permanent sections of the surgically excised specimen.

Mastitis

Mastitis demands immediate antibiotic treatment and careful, frequent follow-up. Acute mastitis is usually caused by *Staphylococcus aureus* (Edmiston et al, 1990). Empirical antibiotic therapy, such as dicloxacillin for puerperal mastitis and amoxicillin/clavulanate for nonpuerperal mastitis should be given as soon as a breast infection is clinically suspected. If there is evidence of abscess formation, the abscess should be drained. This can be done with an 18-gauge needle using local anesthesia if the abscess is small (Dixon, 1988). Large abscesses require surgical incision and drainage, usually performed under general anesthesia, to ensure that all the loculi (Cooper's ligaments) are broken up within the abscess cavity. The patient should be seen in 3 days to confirm that the infection is responding and then seen again every 3 days until all clinical evidence of the infection clears. Abscess formation should be aggressively treated whenever it occurs. Antibiotics should be changed if the infection is not responding to treatment. Lactating mothers should continue breast-feeding or pump the infected breast. Cultures and antibiotic sensitivity studies are of limited value except in chronic infections or acute infections that are not responding to treatment. Blood cultures are not indicated. Chronic and recurrent mastitis are usually caused by mixed aerobic and anaerobic bacteria and should be treated with combined antibiotics such as dicloxacillin and metronidazole. Chronic, recurrent subareolar fistulas usually require surgical excision.

Fibrocystic Changes

A multitude of histologic diagnoses used to be collectively referred to by the wastebasket term *fibrocystic disease.* This is not a proper medical term and does not denote a specific histologic diagnosis. Furthermore, the term *fibrocystic disease* has inappropriately acquired a premalignant connotation that causes patient anxiety and has influenced insurance companies to change life and health insurance rates adversely for women thus labeled. The use of the term is equally inappropriate clinically. As many as 75 percent of women have histologic breast changes that previously could have been called fibrocystic disease (Frantz et al, 1951). Within the heterogeneous histologic variability of the human female breast, many of these changes are normal (Love et al, 1983; Carter et al, 1988). In 1985, the College of American Pathologists (1986) formally abandoned the term. Clinically, many women have nodular, lumpy breasts by examination. Specific physical findings should be described exactly as they are, with terms such as *diffuse fullness*, *lumpiness*, *nodularity*, or *thickening*.

Methylxanthines

After initial published suggestions that the methylxanthines found in caffeine, chocolate, coffee, cola, peanuts, and tea are an etiologic factor in mastalgia and breast nodularity, several double-blind crossover studies demonstrated no correlation between methylxanthine intake and the symptoms of breast pain and findings of diffuse breast nodularity (Ernster et al, 1982; Marshall et al, 1982; Lubin et al, 1985; Schairer et al, 1986). However, individual patients with such symptoms do occasionally seem to respond to restriction of methylxanthines. Although it is a simple "therapeutic" approach, it is not based on scientific data (Rohan et al, 1989). No correlation with, or increased relative risk of breast cancer has been documented to be associated with methylxanthine intake (Allen and Froberg, 1986).

Cysts

Microcysts of the breast are common during the reproductive years and can be associated with diffuse tender nodularity by palpation. Although estrogen is thought to stimulate breast cysts, the breast is typically most tender before the onset of menstruation.

TABLE 15-4

Evaluation and Follow-Up of a Breast Cyst

Diagnosis by fine-needle aspiration
Aspirate all cyst fluid
No residual mass by palpation
Nonbloody fluid
   (rule out intracystic carcinoma if fluid is bloody)
No recurrence within 3 months
   (re-examine 1 month and 3 months after aspiration)

Cysts are usually multiple, bilateral, and not premalignant. Ultrasound can differentiate a cyst from a solid mass. Macrocysts are often symptomatic and should be evaluated as described in Table 15–4. FNA can readily diagnose a palpable cyst and is usually therapeutic if there is no residual mass after complete aspiration of all cyst fluid (Rosemond, 1963; Rosemond et al, 1969; Tabar et al, 1981). Intracystic carcinomas are rare (less than 1:1,000) (Rosemond et al, 1955; Abramson, 1974) and will be clinically manifested by a residual solid mass after aspiration, grossly bloody cyst fluid, or persistent recurrence of the cyst. Careful follow-up is essential, with repeat examination in 1 month (with re-aspiration if the cyst recurs) and then again 2 months after that. If there is no evidence of a recurrent cyst or mass within 3 months, the patient can be followed in the same routine manner as women without cysts. Cytology of cyst fluid is able to identify malignant cells, but this is likely only with grossly bloody fluid. Clear and straw-colored fluids are usually acellular, and cytologic examination is not recommended. Mammography does not reliably differentiate solid from cystic masses. A palpable mass should be aspirated to determine if it is cystic and a nonpalpable mass detected by mammography should be evaluated by ultrasound.

Fibroadenomas

Fibroadenomas are the most common benign neoplasms of the breast. They are initially palpable most commonly during the early reproductive years. Fibroadenomas do not transform into carcinomas. However, carcinomas have been reported within fibroadenomas (Yoshida et al, 1985). Most of the reported malignancies were lobular carcinoma in situ (LCIS), with the others evenly divided between DCIS and invasive ductal carcinoma. Few metastatic malignancies have been reported. However, fibroadenomas, particularly

if progressing in size, must be differentiated from phyllodes tumors, especially malignant ones. Because of the overlapping ranges, neither the patient's age nor the size of the tumor reliably differentiates fibroadenomas from phyllodes tumors (Hindle and Alonzo, 1991; Hindle and Pan, 1991). Phyllodes tumors, particularly the malignant variety, have been described as growing rapidly. Palpation and mammography do not reliably differentiate fibroadenomas from phyllodes tumors. With an adequate cell sample, FNA can identify malignant cells.

Fibroadenomas can be cytologically diagnosed with a well-preserved, abundant cell sample by the characteristic trial of numerous bipolar naked nuclei (without cytoplasm), normal stroma without increased cellularity or overgrowth, and numerous monolayer sheets of benign ductal epithelial cells. If there is doubt about the specific cytologic diagnosis, particularly if there is any question of a phyllodes tumor or malignancy, surgical excision biopsy should be performed, with definite histologic diagnosis based on multiple permanent sections. In any case, a fibroadenoma can be surgically excised upon the patient's request (Dent and Cant, 1989; Wilkinson et al, 1989).

Other Benign Lesions

The common benign breast diseases are listed in Table 15–5. An adenolipoma can present as a palpable mass or be seen on a mammogram. Cysts can be micro (nonpalpable) or macro (palpable). Ductal epithelial hyperplasia is a specific histologic diagnosis with no manifestations by physical examination. Fat necrosis is usually associated with a history of trauma, is self-limited, and re-

TABLE 15-5

Benign Breast Diseases

Adenolipoma (hamartoma)
Cysts
Ductal epithelial hyperplasia
Fat necrosis
Fibroadenoma
Fibrocystic changes
Galactocele
Intraductal papilloma
Lipoma
Lobular epithelial hyperplasia
Mammary duct ectasia (periductal mastitis)
Mastitis
Mondor's disease (superficial venous thrombosis)

sponds without specific treatment. Galactoceles are usually associated with pregnancy and lactation and are readily diagnosed by FNA. Lipomas can present as distinct palpable masses and have consistent findings by mammography and FNA. Lobular epithelial hyperplasia is a histologic diagnosis with no clinical manifestations. Mammary duct ectasia (periductal mastitis) is often associated with dark green nipple discharge and usually occurs in perimenopausal women. Mondor's disease is clotting of the superficial veins of the breast and can be mistaken for carcinoma, but regresses spontaneously.

PREMALIGNANT LESIONS OF THE BREAST

Long-term follow-up study of more than 10,000 consecutive benign breast biopsies revealed that atypical proliferative changes of the ductal and lobular epithelium have a five-fold increased risk of invasive breast cancer (Dupont and Page, 1985). This risk was increased to 11-fold if there was also a first-degree relative with breast cancer. Hyperplasia (moderate or florid, solid or papillary) and papilloma with a fibrovascular core were associated with a 1.5- to 2.0-fold increased relative risk of invasive breast cancer.

Ductal Carcinoma In Situ

DCIS is the preinvasive lesion for invasive ductal carcinoma, although clinically not all DCIS progresses to invasion (Lagios et al, 1982; Page and DuPont, 1982; Fisher et al, 1986; Silverstein et al, 1990). This may be because the patient does not live long enough for invasion to occur. Comedo carcinoma (large-cell carcinoma in situ with high nuclear grade and solid cell proliferation) is a particular presentation of DCIS that has a typical mammographic appearance, is multifocal and even multicentric, and tends to cover a large area of the breast, with involvement extending up the duct system toward the nipple. An extensive intraductal component associated with invasive ductal carcinoma typically involves a large area of the breast (multiple quadrants) and has a poor prognosis in spite of therapy (Holland et al, 1990a,b).

Lobular Carcinoma In Situ

The biologic behavior and significance of LCIS are controversial, as is the recommended treatment (Rosen et al, 1987; Beute et al, 1991). Some authors prefer the term *lobular neoplasia* and the concept of LCIS as a tumor marker and not a preinvasive lesion per se (Haagensen et al, 1978). Patients with LCIS have a 1 percent/year chance of developing invasive carcinoma, which most often will be invasive ductal carcinoma (not invasive lobular carcinoma) and will occur with equal frequency in either breast.

INTRADUCTAL PAPILLOMAS

Intraductal papillomas, like phyllodes tumors, can be benign or malignant. Neither of these neoplasms has established criteria with which to separate the benign from the malignant form by history, CBE, FNAC, or mammography. Intraductal papillomas usually present with spontaneous, single duct, nonmilky nipple discharge. Ductograms (galactography) can demonstrate the intraductal lesions and assist the surgeon in locating the exact duct system to be excised (Tabar et al, 1983). Benign intraductal papillomas are usually single, whereas the papillary carcinomas are usually multiple intraductal lesions. However, both forms must be excised for definitive histologic diagnosis. Sometimes large papillomas are palpable as soft subareolar masses, but often there are no palpable changes. If a ductogram is not available, the surgeon can localize the involved duct by passing a fine probe down the duct and excise that single lobular collecting duct system.

PHYLLODES TUMORS

Phyllodes tumors usually present in the same fashion as fibroadenomas. Some phyllodes tumors increase rapidly in size. The range of patient age and size of the tumor at the time of excision widely overlap and do not allow clinical differentiation on that basis. FNAC can detect malignant cells in phyllodes tumors but is not reliable in differentiating benign fibroadenomas from benign phyllodes tumors even with adequate cell samples. When there is a possibility of a phyllodes tumor by any diagnostic modality, the mass should be excised, with clear surgical margins, for specific permanent section histologic diagnosis.

MALIGNANT BREAST DISEASE

Epidemiologic Risk Factors

Female gender and advancing age are the two most significant risk factors for the development of breast cancer. Clinically increased risk occurs in the contralateral breast of women who have had breast cancer and in first-degree relatives (mother, sister, daughter) of women with breast cancer. This familial risk is markedly increased if the breast cancer was premenopausal in onset and especially if it occurred bilaterally.

Numerous epidemiologic risk factors for increased incidence of breast cancer have been reported (see Table 15–6), but these variables do not exist in the clinical evaluation and management of individual patients. Augmentation mammoplasty with a prosthesis does not increase the relative risk for breast cancer (Silverstein et al, 1988) but, even with optimum positioning techniques, does decrease the amount of breast tissue that can be seen by mammography.

Viewed collectively, studies of women who have taken or are taking oral contraceptives (OCs) demonstrate no meaningful increased risk of breast cancer (Brinton et al, 1982; Centers for Disease Control, 1983; Vessey, 1987; Rohan and McMichael, 1988; Mishell, 1989; Stanford et al, 1989; Paul et al, 1990; UK National Case-Control Study Group, 1990; Clavel et al, 1991; Harlap, 1991; Wingo et al, 1991). A review of 54 prospective and case-control studies calculated an overall 1.07 relative risk of breast cancer for ever-users of OCs and a 1.24 relative risk for current users (Collaborative Group on Hormonal Factors in Breast Cancer, 1996). This epidemiologically increased relative risk diminished with years after OC use was stopped, with no effect seen after 10 years. Clinically meaningful increased relative risk was not demonstrated in this review. Furthermore, there was no evidence of dose or duration effect, which would have implied causality. Reviews of the published data on the influence of estrogen replacement therapy (ERT) on breast cancer risk demonstrate a mean epidemiologic increased risk of about 1.2 times (Hulka, 1987; Barrett-Connor, 1989; Dupont et al, 1989; Dupont and Page, 1991, Steinberg et al, 1991). This compares with the 5-fold increased risk of endometrial cancer in women taking unopposed estrogen and the 10-fold increased risk of invasive breast cancer in women with diagnosed DCIS. Caffeine is not a risk factor for breast cancer.

TABLE 15–6

Factors Reported to be Epidemiologically Associated With an Increased Relative Risk of Breast Cancer

Affluent economic status
Birth of first child after age 30 years
Caucasian race
Chronic psychological stress
Cold climate
Diabetes
Diethylstilbestrol therapy during pregnancy
Endometrial carcinoma
Ethnic background
Geography
High-fat diet
History of benign breast disease
History of breast biopsy
Hypertension
Irradiation
Jewish background
Living in the western hemisphere
Menarche before age 12 years
Menopause after age 55 years
Menstruation for more than 30 years
Nonatypical ductal/lobular epithelial hyperplasia
Nulliparity
Number of mentrual cycles before first term pregnancy
Oral contraceptives taken for 10 years prior to first pregnancy
Ovarian carcinoma
Overnutrition
Polygenetic predisposition
Postmenopausal obesity
Second-degree relative (aunt or grandmother) with breast cancer

Genetic Advances

The *BRCA-1* gene has been sequenced (Miki et al, 1994) in the long arm of chromosome 17 (17q21). More than 100 breast cancer–associated mutations subsequently were identified within the *BRCA-1* gene (Shattuck-Eidens et al, 1995). *BRCA-1* is an autosomal dominant gene that carries an 80 percent lifetime risk of breast cancer and a 60 percent lifetime risk of ovarian cancer. The incidence of *BRCA-1* is estimated to be 1:800 in women in the United States and 1:100 in women of Ashkenazi Jewish ancestry. *BRCA-2*, on chromosome 13q12-13, has been sequenced and appears to be associated with early-onset breast cancer. Commercial genetic testing is available and is suggested for women who have a family history of breast cancer with an autosomal dominant pattern, usually over three generations (Hoskins et al, 1995). If such a patient is found to carry *BRCA-1*, then testing of immediate relatives may be indicated (Lerman et al, 1996). There is no consensus as to recommendations for women who carry *BRCA-1* or *-2*.

Oncologic Work-up

At the time of initial malignant diagnosis, the oncologic work-up includes complete physical examination, bilateral diagnostic mammography, complete blood count, alkaline phosphatase level (and complete liver profile if this value is elevated), and chest radiograph. Many oncologists routinely order bone and liver scans as a baseline measure, but cost-effectiveness analyses indicate no proven outcome advantage over waiting for clinical evidence of metastasis before ordering such special studies.

Types of Invasive Cancer

The breast is the site of a heterogeneous group of malignancies with variable biologic behavior. The World Health Organization classification and approximate percentage incidences are listed in Table 15–7. In addition, there are code classifications for invasive ductal carcinoma with a predominant intraductal component and for rare carcinomas with metaplasia of squamous, spindle cell, cartilaginous, and osseous types. Most breast cancers are invasive ductal carcinomas or mixed malignancies with ductal carcinoma and respond biologically the same as pure invasive ductal carcinoma. Generally, the nonductal carcinomas have a slower growth pattern and better prognosis than invasive ductal carcinoma. Paget's disease of the nipple is associated with underlying in situ or invasive ductal carcinoma (Lagios et al, 1984; Dixon et al, 1991). Inflammatory carcinoma is a particular clinical manifestation of invasive ductal carcinoma with extensive involvement of the dermal lymphatics (Moore et al, 1991).

Treatment Planning Conference

A treatment planning conference with a consensus opinion of a multispecialty team offers the optimum therapeutic recommendation for women with breast cancer. The ideal would be a coordinated, dedicated multidisciplinary team consisting of the woman's primary care physician and one or more surgical oncologists, medical oncologists, radiation oncologists, plastic surgeons, mammographers, cytopathologists, pathologists, and ancillary medical support personnel such as psychologists, social workers, rehabilitation specialists, oncologic nurses, and treated breast cancer patients. The team should meet together, review all the pertinent medical data, including the patient's history and physical examination findings, the cytology slides, the histology slides, the mammograms, and the operative reports, and then, after full discussion with each other and the patient, render a consensus recommendation for that patient. It is essential that the patient's primary support person, usually her spouse, and her immediate family be counseled and appropriately informed.

Second Opinions

With the complexity and uncertainty of optimum treatment for breast cancer, patients often seek a second opinion. This has become accepted practice and in fact is encouraged by most breast centers. There is no agreed upon "best treatment" of breast cancer. Each case must be individualized and requires in-depth counseling of the patient and her primary support person prior to the patient's final decision.

Staging and Survival

TNM staging (Table 15–8) tabulates the size of the tumor at diagnosis and the involvement of surrounding structures, axillary lymph

TABLE **15–7**

Histologic Type and Incidence of Invasive Breast Cancer*

Type	Incidence (%)
Ductal carcinoma	53
Mixed ductal carcinoma	28
Medullary carcinoma	6
Lobular carcinoma	5
Mixed nonductal carcinoma	2
Mucinous carcinoma	2
Paget's disease	2
Tubular carcinoma	1
Adenoid cystic carcinoma	<1
Apocrine carcinoma	<1
Papillary carcinoma	<1
Secretory (juvenile) carcinoma	<1
Carcinosarcoma	<1

*Data from World Health Organization. In Histologic Typing of Breast Tumours, 2nd ed. Geneva, World Health Organization, 1981, p 15; and DeVita VT Jr, Hellman S, Rosenberg SA, et al: Cancer: Principles and Practice of Oncology, 3rd ed., Vol. 1. Philadelphia, JB Lippincott, 1989, p 1205.

TABLE 15–8

T A B L E **15–8**

Definition of Tumor, Node, Metastasis (TNM) Staging System*

Stage	Definition	Stage	Definition
Primary tumor (T)		Distant metastasis (M)	
TX	Primary tumor cannot be assessed	MX	Presence of distant metastasis cannot be assessed
T0	No evidence of primary tumor	M0	No distant metastasis
Tis	Carcinoma in situ: intraductal carcinoma, lobular carcinoma in situ, or Paget's disease of the nipple with no tumor	M1	Distant metastasis (includes metastasis to ipsilateral supraclavicular lymph node[s])
		Grouping	
T1	Tumor 2 cm or less in greatest dimension	0	Tis, N0, M0
T1a	0.5 cm or less in greatest dimension	I	T1, N0, M0
T1b	More than 0.5 cm but not more than 1 cm in greatest dimension	IIa	T0, N1, M0
			T1, N1, M0
			T2, N0, M0
T1c	More than 1 cm but not more than 2 cm in greatest dimension	IIb	T2, N1, M0
			T3, N0, M0
T2	Tumor more than 2 cm but not more than 5 cm in greatest dimension	IIIa	T0, N2, M0
			T1, N2, M0
			T2, N2, M0
			T3; N1, N2; M0
T3	Tumore more than 5 cm in greatest dimension	IIIb	T4, any N, M0
			Any T, N3, M0
T4	Tumor of any size with direct extension to chest wall or skin	IV	Any T, any N, M1
T4a	Extension to chest wall		
T4b	Edema (including peau d'orange) or ulceration of the skin of the breast or satellite skin nodules confined to the same breast		
T4c	Both T4a and T4b		
T4d	Inflammatory carcinoma		
Regional lymph nodes (N)			
NX	Regional lymph nodes cannot be assessed (e.g., previously removed)		
N0	No regional lymph node metastasis		
N1	Metastasis to movable ipsilateral axillary lymph node(s)		
N2	Metastasis to ipsilateral axillary lymph node(s) fixed to one another or to other structures		
N3	Metastasis to ipsilateral internal mammary lymph node(s)		

*From American Joint Committee on Cancer: Manual for Staging of Cancer, 3rd ed. Philadelphia, JB Lippincott, 1988, with permission.

nodes, and distant metastases. Even today, most breast cancers are found by the patients themselves and are usually 2.5 cm in diameter or larger, with 50 percent showing involvement of the axillary lymph nodes. Of such patients, 50 percent will die from their breast cancer, in spite of all the improvements and innovations in treatment. Conversely, 10-year follow-up data demonstrate that, with current methods of treatment, up to 90 percent of women diagnosed with invasive cancers less than 1 cm in diameter will have a disease-free survival (Rosen et al, 1989). With the patient's informed consent and choice, most invasive cancers of this small size can be treated by breast-conserving therapy.

Impact of Screening Mammography

The widespread application of screening mammography shifts the incidence of invasive carcinoma to smaller lesions, earlier stages, and less axillary lymph node involvement. Potentially, with current methods of treatment, patients with preclinical, mammographically diagnosed carcinomas have a significantly improved long-term disease-free survival rate, and may have increased overall survival. Unfortunately breast cancer can recur, and metastases can become clinically apparent 10 to 30 years after the initial diagnosis and treatment. Thus long-term (e.g., 20-year) follow-up studies are required for definitive analysis and validation of ultimate outcome.

Pregnancy and Lactation

During pregnancy and lactation, a dominant breast mass should be evaluated in the same manner as for nonpregnant women. Screening mammography should be deferred because there may be some risk to the fetus and congested breasts are difficult to evaluate mammographically. However, if cancer is the probable clinical diagnosis, lead shielding will largely protect the fetus and diagnostic mammography can be done. The treatment for breast cancer is the same for pregnant and lactating women as it is for other women (Bunker and Peters, 1963; Peters, 1968; Donnegan, 1979; Harvey et al, 1981; Murray et al, 1984; Greene, 1988). Although some breast cancers have been anecdotally reported to progress rapidly during pregnancy, review of the available published data does not demonstrate an adverse outcome of breast cancer diagnosed during pregnancy or lactation when compared stage for stage with nonpregnant patients of the same age (Petrek et al, 1991) (see Chapter 14). Thus there is no proven medical indication for the termination of pregnancy when breast cancer is diagnosed, although the woman herself may elect to do so. After treatment for breast cancer, there is no contraindication to pregnancy for the patient who is clinically in remission, because there are no published data to indicate any adverse effect of pregnancy after breast cancer treatment (Mignot, 1986; Sutton et al, 1990). Traditionally, however, many oncologists have advised waiting for at least a 2-year disease-free interval before attempting pregnancy, because the majority of recurrences will be clinically manifested within 2 years of initial treatment.

Treatment

NIH Consensus Conference Treatment Recommendations

The list in Table 15–9 summarizes the recommendations of the NIH Consensus Conference (1991) on the treatment of early-stage breast cancer. Breast-conserving treatment (lumpectomy, axillary lymph node dissection, and postoperative radiation therapy) is recommended as the preferred treatment of stages I and II invasive breast cancer. Since the 10-year disease-free survival for patients

TABLE **15–9**

NIH Consensus Conference Recommendations on the Treatment of Early-Stage Breast Cancer

Breast-conserving treatment is the preferred treatment of most stage I and II breast cancers

Breast-conserving treatment should be local excision with clear margins, dissection of levels I and II axillary lymph nodes, and radiation up to 50 cGy to the affected breast

Patients with node-negative breast cancer should be urged to enroll in adjuvant therapy clinical trials

Most women with node-negative breast cancer are cured by primary surgical treatment

Adjuvant combination cytotoxic chemotherapy and adjuvant tamoxifen reduce the rate of local and distant recurrence

Women with cancers less than 1 cm in diameter do not require adjuvant systemic therapy

with invasive cancers of 1 cm or less is 90 percent, systemic adjuvant therapy is not recommended for these women. Adjuvant combination cytotoxic chemotherapy (generally for premenopausal women) or adjuvant tamoxifen therapy (generally for postmenopausal women) should be offered to all other patients with invasive carcinoma (Gelber et al, 1991). Modified radical mastectomy with preservation of the pectoralis muscle and concomitant axillary lymph node dissection is an equal alternative to breast-conserving surgery (Fisher et al, 1985, 1989) and has been the standard surgical treatment for about 20 years. Before that, beginning at the turn of the century, the Halsted radical mastectomy, which included removing the pectoralis muscle, was the standard surgical treatment. Lymphedema of the arm, limitation of motion of the arm, slough of the skin over the rib cage, and gross disfigurement of the anterior chest wall were significant complications after the Halsted radical mastectomy. In all cases, the patient's fully informed consent should be obtained following complete explanation of treatment options and consequences, including quality-of-life issues.

Axillary Lymph Node Dissection

Axillary lymph node dissection is not therapeutic but provides a general statistical prognosis and can be useful in the decision about adjuvant therapy: chemotherapy, hormone manipulation, or both (Siegel et al, 1990). There is an inverse correlation between the number of lymph nodes involved and a statistically favorable prognosis. However, the biologic behavior of a specific invasive cancer in an individual may or may not follow this statistical correlation.

Prognostic Indications

The continuing search for clinically useful prognostic indicators is promulgated by the need for accurate prognostic information for individual patients and to aid in making recommendations for systemic therapy. Axillary lymph node involvement and tumor size (greatest measured diameter) are the most reliable prognostic factors. Estrogen and progesterone receptor status are generally useful in predicting risk of recurrent cancer and response to adjuvant therapy. The correlations with estrogen and progesterone receptor levels are general and do not necessarily apply to a given individual. Generally, patients whose cancers have high estrogen receptor levels respond better to hormonal manipulation and have a more favorable prognosis. Tumor grade; nuclear grade; DNA synthesis (ploidy and S phase); carcinoembryonic antigen; CA-15-3; the HER-2/*neu* and p53 oncogenes; epidermal growth factor receptors; transforming growth factor-alpha; and cathepsin D are under clinical investigation as prognostic indicators.

Chemotherapy

A multitude of combinations and dosages of systemic cytotoxic therapy are under clinical investigation (Early Breast Cancer Trialist Collaborative Group, 1988). Cyclophosphamide, methotrexate, and 5-fluorouracil (5-FU), and 5-FU, doxorubicin, and cyclophosphamide, are the most commonly used multidrug chemotherapies. Chemotherapy is usually given in sequential courses over a 6-month period. The overall response rate is about 70 percent. Malaise, nausea, leukopenia, hair loss, amenorrhea, and sterility are common side effects of these chemotherapy regimens.

Hormone Manipulation

Hormone therapy is usually given in the form of tamoxifen 10 to 20 mg orally twice a day for at least 5 years and probably lifelong if there is not evidence of recurrent cancer (Early Breast Cancer Trialist Collaborative Group, 1988; Love, 1989). Some patients experience hot flashes with tamoxifen, but the drug is otherwise well tolerated. Megesterol acetate is also used in the treatment of advanced breast cancer.

Reconstructive Surgery

After full informed consent, if the patient elects to have a modified radical mastectomy, she should be offered immediate or delayed reconstruction of the breast. Immediate reconstruction requires close coordination between the oncologic surgeon and the plastic surgeon. The combined operation is usually long but offers the patient the psychological value of recovering from her surgery with a "breast" in place. Nipple reconstruction is usually done at a later date as an office or outpatient procedure and can require several operations for optimum cosmesis. Traditionally, oncologists have often recommended delaying breast reconstruction until 2 years after initial surgery. This was largely based on the incidence of recurrence during that time (as many as 70 percent of the recurrences are clinically apparent within 2 years). Reconstruction is accomplished with a prosthesis or autologous flaps. The most commonly used flaps are the transverse rectus abdominus myocutaneous flap and the latissimus dorsi myocutaneous flap.

Rehabilitation and Post-treatment Follow-up

Counseling and Support

Psychological support of the patient and her family is essential to the complete recovery of a woman with breast cancer. A positive self-image and return to normal activities should be encouraged. Formal and informal counseling should be available and usually includes the participation of the patient's primary support person (frequently her spouse). It should provide emotional ventilation, information giving, and sexual counseling. Hospitals often have volunteer support groups composed of recovered cancer patients. The American Cancer Society "Reach to Recovery" and the Y-ME (National Association for Breast Cancer Information and Support, Inc.) programs are available in most urban areas. Physical therapy may be beneficial for some post–modified radical mastectomy patients. The goal is to have the breast cancer patient return to the quality of life and activities that were natural for her prior to her diagnosis.

Follow-up Schedule

A common follow-up plan is examination every 3 months for 1 year, then every 6 months for 5 years, and annually for the remainder of the patient's life. An annual mammogram, chest film, and alkaline phosphatase level, with full liver function testing if elevated, should be performed. Physical examination should focus on possible local recurrence and on the remaining breast (Loomer et al, 1991). Common sites of relapse are the lymph nodes, lung, liver, bone, adrenal gland, and ovary.

Oral Contraceptive Use

OCs have not been demonstrated to adversely affect outcome when given to disease-free patients after treatment for breast cancer. However, reliable nonhormonal methods of contraception are readily available and should be recommended (ACOG, 1991).

Estrogen Replacement Therapy

ERT after treatment of breast cancer continues to be controversial (Ross et al, 1980). There are no randomized clinical trials or statistically significant data reported in the literature on this subject. Anecdotal cases of progression of breast cancer in patients on ERT are mentioned in surgical textbooks. Paradoxically, estrogens have proven useful in the treatment of certain subsets of patients with advanced or recurrent breast cancer.

Considering the significant reduction in cardiovascular disease, coronary artery disease, and osteoporosis that has been achieved by ERT for women with estrogen deficiency (Ernster et al, 1989; Barrett-Connor and Bush, 1991), there is a growing clinical opinion that ERT may be recommended to women who have been treated for breast cancer, are clinically disease free, and have diagnosed estrogen deficiency (ACOG, 1991; Creasman, 1991; Cobleigh, 1994; DiSaia et al, 1996).

Recurrent and Metastatic Breast Cancer

The treatment of recurrent carcinoma should be individualized in each specific situation. Cytoreductive surgery, resection of local cancer, sequential chemotherapy, various hormone manipulations, radiation therapy, and bone marrow transplant are used. None of these modalities of therapy cures recurrent breast cancer. However, significant prolongation of life (e.g., 2 years) and improved patient comfort can be achieved.

TABLE **15–10**

Recommendations for Avoiding Breast Cancer Lawsuits

1. Follow ACOG guidelines for screening mammography, clinical breast examinations, and breast self-examinations
2. Take the patient's complaint seriously
3. Discuss the family history relative risk
4. Carefully evaluate young patients
5. Definitively diagnose a persistent dominant mass
6. Perform a complete evaluation in spite of a "negative" mammogram report
7. Explain the probable diagnosis
8. Explain your action plan each visit
9. Explain that "negative" results are not a guarantee
10. If you or the patient have diagnostic doubts, obtain a consultation
11. Communicate directly with your consultants
12. Schedule the follow-up visit
13. Follow up on the patient's compliance
14. Record all of the above in the patient's medical record
15. Record phone calls to and from the patient

LEGAL CONCERNS

Failure to diagnose breast cancer is a leading cause of lawsuits against primary care providers for women. Most of the closed legal cases were brought by women under the age of 40 years who often had developed recurrent disease. The initial mass found by the patient was ignored or thought by the physician to be unimpressive. The mammogram, if performed, was often interpreted as "negative." Beware! A mammogram cannot rule out cancer. Abnormal mammographic findings are significant, but serious lesions are not always apparent with mammography. The medical record with documentation of the patient's complaint, physical and other findings, and specific recommendations is the best legal defense. Steps to avoid breast cancer lawsuits are listed in Table 15–10.

REFERENCES

Abramson DJ: A clinical evaluation of aspiration of cysts of the breast. Surg Gynecol Obstet 139:531, 1974.

Allen SS, Froberg DC: The effects of decreased caffeine consumption on benign proliferative breast disease: a randomized clinical trial. Surgery 101:720, 1986.

American College of Obstetricians and Gynecologists: Report of Task Force on Routine Cancer Screening. ACOG Committee Opinion 68. Washington, DC: American College of Obstetricians and Gynecologists, 1989a.

American College of Obstetricians and Gynecologists: Standards for Obstetric-Gynecologic Services, 7th ed. Washington, DC, American College of Obstetricians and Gynecologists, 1989b.

American College of Obstetricians and Gynecologists: Carcinoma of the Breast. Technical Bulletin No. 158. Washington, DC, American College of Obstetricians and Gynecologists, 1991.

American College of Obstetricians and Gynecologists: Routine Cancer Screening. Committee on Gynecologic Practice Committee Opinion No. 128. Washington, DC, American College of Obstetricians and Gynecologists, 1993.

American Joint Committee on Cancer: Manual for Staging of Cancer, 3rd ed. Philadelphia, JB Lippincott, 1988.

Anderson TJ, Ferguson DJ, Rabb GM: Cell turnover in the "resting" human breast: influence of parity, contraceptive pill, age and laterality, Br J Cancer 46:376, 1982.

Andersson I, Aspergren K, Janzon L, et al: Mammographic screening and mortality from breast cancer: the Malmo mammographic screening trial. Br Med J 297:943, 1988.

Baker LH: Breast Cancer Detection Demonstration Project: five-year summary report. Cancer 32:194, 1982.

Barrett-Connor E: Postmenopausal estrogen replacement and breast cancer. N Engl J Med 321:319, 1989.

Barrett-Connor E, Bush TL: Estrogen and coronary heart disease in women. JAMA 265:1861, 1991.

Bell DA, Hajdu SI, Urban UA, Gaston JP: Role of aspiration cytology in the diagnosis and management of mammary lesions in office practice. Cancer 51:1182, 1983.

Berg JW, Robbins GF: A late look at the safety of aspiration biopsy. Cancer 15:826, 1962.

Beute BJ, Kalisher L, Hutter RV: Lobular carcinoma in situ of the breast: clinical, pathological, and mammographic features. AJR Am J Roentgenol 57:21, 1991.

Brinton LA, Hoover R, Szklo M, Fraumeni JF Jr: Oral contraceptives and breast cancer. Int J Epidemiol 11:316, 1982.

Bunker ML, Peters MV: Breast cancer associated with pregnancy and lactation. Am J Obstet Gynecol 85:312, 1963.

Carter CL, Corle DK, Micozzi MS, et al: A prospective study of the development of breast cancer in 16,692 women with benign breast disease. Am J Epidemiol 128:467, 1988.

Centers for Disease Control: Centers for Disease Control Cancer and Steroid Hormone Study: long-term oral contraceptive use and the risk of breast cancer. JAMA 249:1591, 1983.

Chu KC, Smart CR, Tarone RE: Analysis of breast cancer mortality and stage distribution by age for the Health Insurance Plan clinical trial. J Natl Cancer Inst 14:1195, 1988.

Clavel F, Andrieu N, Gairard B, et al: Oral contraceptives and breast cancer: a French case-control study. Int J Epidemiol 20:32, 1991.

Cobleigh MA, for the Breast Cancer Committee of the Eastern Cooperative Oncology Group: Estrogen replacement therapy in breast cancer survivors: time for change. JAMA 272:540, 1994.

Collaborative Group on Hormonal Factors in Breast Cancer: Breast cancer and hormonal contraceptives: collaborative reanalysis of individual data on 53,297 women with breast cancer and 100,239 women without breast cancer from 54 epidemiological studies. Lancet 347:1713, 1996.

College of American Pathologists: Is "fibrocystic disease" of the breast precancerous? Arch Pathol Lab Med 110:171, 1986.

Creaseman WE: Estrogen replacement therapy: is previously treated cancer a contraindication? Obstet Gynecol 707:308, 1991.

Dent DM, Cant PJ: Fibroadenoma. World J Surg 13:706, 1989.

DeVita VT Jr, Hellman S, Rosenberg SA, et al: Cancer: Principles and Practice of Oncology, 3rd ed, Vol. 1. Philadelphia, JB Lippincott, 1989, p 1205.

Devitt JE: Management of nipple discharge by clinical findings. Am J Surg 149:789, 1985.

DiSaia PJ, Grosen EA, Kurosaki T, et al: Hormone replacement therapy in breast cancer survivors: a cohort study. Am J Obstet Gynecol 174:1494, 1996.

Dixon AR, Galea MH, Ellis IO, et al: Paget's disease of the nipple. Br J Surg 78:722, 1991.

Dixon JM: Repeated aspiration of breast abscesses in lactating women. Br Med J 297:1517, 1988.

Donnegan WL: Mammary carcinoma and pregnancy. Major Prob Clin Surg 5:448, 1979.

Dupont WD, Page DL: Risk factors for breast cancer in women with proliferative disease. N Engl J Med 312:146, 1985.

Dupont WD, Page DL: Menopausal estrogen replacement therapy and breast cancer. Arch Intern Med 151:67, 1991.

Dupont WD, Page DL, Rogers LW, Pearl FF: Influence of exogenous estrogens, proliferative breast disease, and other variables on breast cancer risk. Cancer 63:948, 1989.

Early Breast Cancer Trialist Collaborative Group: Effects of adjuvant tamoxifen and of cytotoxic therapy on mortality in early breast cancer: an overview of 61 randomized trials among 28,896 women. N Engl J Med 319:1681, 1988.

Edeiken S: Mammography in the symptomatic woman. Cancer 63:1412, 1989.

Edmiston CE Jr, Walker AP, Krepel CJ, Gohr C: The nonpuerperal breast infection: aerobic and anaerobic microbial recovery from acute and chronic disease. J Infect Dis 162:695, 1990.

Engzell U, Esposti Rubio C, et al: Investigation of tumour spread in connection with aspiration biopsy. Acta Radiol Ther Phys Biol 10:385, 1971.

Ernster VL, Bush TL, Huggins GR, et al: Benefits and risks of menopausal estrogen and/or progestin hormone use. Prev Med 17:201, 1988.

Ernster VL, Mason L, Goodson WH III, et al: Effects of caffeine free diet on benign breast disease: a randomized trial. Surgery 91:263, 1982.

Feig SA: Decreased breast cancer mortality through mammographic screening: results of clinical trials. Radiology 167:659, 1988.

Ferguson DJ, Anderson TJ: Morphological evaluation of cell turnover in relation to menstrual cycle in the "resting" human breast. Br J Cancer 44:177, 1981.

Fisher B, Bauer M, Margolese R, et al: Five-year results of a randomized clinical trial comparing total mastectomy and segmental mastectomy with or without radiation in the treatment of breast cancer. N Engl J Med 312:665, 1985.

Fisher B, Redmond C, Poisson R, et al: Eight-year results of a randomized clinical trial comparing total mastectomy and lumpectomy with or without irradiation in the treatment of breast cancer. N Engl J Med 320:822, 1989.

Fisher ER, Sass R, Fisher B, et al: Pathologic findings from the National Surgical Adjuvant Breast Project (Protocol 6). 1. Intraductal Carcinoma (DCIS). Cancer 57:197, 1986.

Frantz VK, Pickren JW, Melcher FW: Incidence of chronic cystic disease in so-called "normal breast": a study based on 225 postmortem examinations. Cancer 4:762, 1951.

Gambrell RD Jr: Breast disease in the postmenopausal years. Semin Reprod Endocrinol 1:27, 1983.

Gelabert HA, Hsiu JG, Mullen JT, et al: Prospective evaluation of the role of fine-needle aspiration biopsy in the diagnosis and management of patients with palpable solid breast lesions. Am Surg 56:263, 1990.

Gelber RD, Goldhirsch A, Cavalli F: Quality-of-life adjusted evaluation of adjuvant therapies for operable breast cancer. Ann Intern Med 114:621, 1991.

Going JJ, Anderson TJ, Battersby S, MacIntyre CC: Proliferative and secretory activity in human breast during natural and artificial menstrual cycles. Am J Pathol 130:193, 1988.

Goodwin PJ, Neelam M, Boyd NF: Cyclical mastopathy: a critical review of therapy. Br J Surg 75:83, 1988.

Greene FL: Gestational breast cancer: a ten-year experience. South Med J 81:1509, 1988.

Haagensen CD, Lane N, Lattes R, Bodian C: Lobular neoplasia (so-called lobular carcinoma in situ) of the breast. Cancer 42:737, 1978.

Harlap S: Oral contraceptives and breast cancer: cause and effect? J Reprod Med 36:374, 1991.

Harvey JC, Rosen PT, Ashikari R, et al: The effect of pregnancy on the prognosis of carcinoma of the breast following radical mastectomy. Surg Gynecol Obstet 153:723, 1981.

Hill D, White V, Jolley D, Mapperson K: Self-examination of the breast: is it beneficial? Meta-analysis of studies investigating breast self-examination and extent of disease in patients with breast cancer. Br Med J 297:271, 1988.

Hindle WH: Breast masses: in-office evaluation with diagnostic triad. Postgrad Med 88:85, 1990.

Hindle WH, Alonzo LJ: Conservative management of breast fibroadenomas. Am J Obstet Gynecol 164:1647, 1991.

Hindle WH, Navin J: Breast aspiration cytology: a neglected gynecologic procedure. Am J Obstet Gynecol 146:482, 1983.

Hindle WH, Pan EY: Phyllodes tumors—diagnosis & treatment—a double dilemma. Trans Pacific Coast Obstet Gynecol Soc 59:189, 1991.

Holland R, Connolly JL, Gelman R, et al: The presence of an extensive intraductal component following a limited excision correlates with prominent residual disease in the remainder of the breast. J Clin Oncol 8:113, 1990a.

Holland R, Hendriks JH, Verbeek AL, et al: Extent, distribution, and mammographic/histological correlations of breast ductal carcinoma in situ. Lancet 335:519, 1990b.

Hoskins KF, Stopfer JE, Calzone KA, et al: Assessment and counseling for women with a family history of breast cancer: a guide for clinicians. JAMA 273:577, 1995.

Hulka BS: Replacement estrogens and risk of gynecologic cancers and breast cancer. Cancer 60:1960, 1987.

Katz R, Lerner MA, Feller N: Galactography in nipple discharge: a statistical analysis and comparison with mammography. Breast 8:18, 1982.

Klein DL, Sickles EA: Effects of needle aspiration on the mammographic appearance of the breast: a guide to the proper timing of the mammography examination. Radiology 145:44, 1982.

Kubler-Ross E (ed): On Death and Dying. New York, Macmillan, 1969.

Lagios MD, Westdahl PR, Margolin FR, Rose MR: Duct carcinoma in situ: relationship of extent of noninvasive disease to the frequency of occult invasion, multicentricity, lymph node metastases, and short-term treatment failures. Cancer 50:1309, 1982.

Lagios MD, Westdahl PR, Rose MR, Concannon S: Paget's disease of the nipple: alternative management in cases without or with minimal extent of underlying breast carcinoma. Cancer 54:545, 1984.

Leis HP Jr: Management of nipple discharge. World J Surg 13:736, 1989.

Leis HP Jr, Cammarata A, LaRaja RD: Nipple discharge: significance and treatment. Breast 11:6, 1985.

Lerman C, Narod S, Schulman K, et al: BRCA1 testing in families with hereditary breast-ovarian cancer. JAMA 275:1885, 1996.

Longacre TA, Bartow SA: A correlative morphologic study of human breast and endometrium in the menstrual cycle. Am J Surg Pathol 10:382, 1986.

Loomer L, Brockschmidt JK, Muss HB, Saylor G: Postoperative follow-up of patients with early breast cancer: patterns of care among clinical oncologists and a review of the literature. Cancer 67:55, 1991.

Love RR: Tamoxifen therapy in primary breast cancer: biology, efficacy and side effects. J Clin Oncol 7:803, 1989.

Love SM, Gelman SR, Silem W: Fibrocystic "disease" of the breast—a nondisease. N Engl J Med 307–1010, 1983.

Lubin F, Ron E, Wax Y, et al: A case-control study of caffeine and methylxanthines in benign breast disease. JAMA 253:2388, 1985.

Marshall J, Graham S, Swanson M: Caffeine consumption and benign breast disease: a case-control comparison. Am J Public Health 72:610, 1982.

Meyer JE, Eberlein TJ, Stomper PC, Sonnenfeld MR: Biopsy of occult breast lesions: analysis of 1,261 abnormalities. JAMA 263:2341, 1990.

Mignot L: Breast cancer and subsequent pregnancy. Am Soc Clin Oncol Proc 5:57, 1986.

Miki Y, Swensen J, Shattuck-Eidens D, et al: A strong candidate for the breast and ovarian cancer susceptibility gene BRCA1. Science 266:66, 1994.

Mishell DR Jr: Contraception. N Engl J Med 320:777, 1989.

Moore MP, Ihde JK, Crowe JP Jr, et al: Inflammatory breast cancer. Arch Surg 126:304, 1991.

Murray CL, Reichert AA, Anderson J, Twiggs L: Multimodal cancer therapy for breast cancer in the first trimester of pregnancy. JAMA 252:2607, 1984.

NCI Breast Cancer Screening Consortium: Screening mammography: a missed clinical opportunity? Results of the NCI Breast Cancer Screening Consortium and National Health Interviews Survey studies. JAMA 264:54, 1990.

NIH Consensus Conference: Treatment of early-stage breast cancer. JAMA 265:391, 1991.

Page DL, Dupont WD: Intraductal carcinoma of the breast. Cancer 49:751, 1982.

Parker SH, Lovin JD, Jobe WE, et al: Nonpalpable breast lesions: stereotactic automated large-core biopsies. Radiology 180:403, 1991.

Parker SL, Tong T, Boldon S, Wingo PA: Cancer statistics, 1996. CA Cancer J Clin 65:5, 1996.

Paul C, Skegg DC, Spears GF: Oral contraceptives and risk of breast cancer. Int J Cancer 46:366, 1990.

Peters M: The effect of pregnancy in breast cancer. In Prognostic Factors in Breast Cancer. Proceedings of the first Tenovus Symposium, Cardiff. Forest APM, Kunkler PB (eds). Baltimore, Williams & Wilkins, 1968, p 115.

Petrek JA, Dukoff R, Rogatko A: Prognosis of pregnancy associated breast cancer. Cancer 67:869, 1991.

Robbins GF, Brothers UH III, Eberhart WF, Quan S: Is aspiration biopsy of breast cancer dangerous to the patient? Cancer 7:774, 1954.

Rohan TE, Cook MG, McMichael AJ: Methylxanthines and benign proliferative epithelial disorders of the breast in women. Int J Epidemiol 18:626, 1989.

Rohan TE, McMichael AJ: Oral contraceptive agents and breast cancer: a population-based case-control study. Med J Aust 149:520, 1988.

Rosemond GP: Differentiation between the cystic and solid breast mass by needle aspiration. Surg Clin North Am 43:1433, 1963.

Rosemond GP, Burnett WE, Caswell HT: Aspiration of breast cysts as a diagnostic and therapeutic measure. Arch Surg 71:223, 1955.

Rosemond GP, Maier WP, Brobyn TJ: Needle aspiration of breast cysts. Surg Gynecol Obstet 128:351, 1969.

Rosen PP, Groshen S, Saigo PE, et al: A long-term follow-up study of survival in stage I (T1N0M0) and stage II (T1N1M0) breast carcinoma. J Clin Oncol 7:355, 1989.

Rosen PP, Lieberman PH, Braun DW: Lobular carcinoma of the breast. Am J Surg Pathol 2:225, 1987.

Ross RK, Paganini-Hill A, Gerkins VR, et al: A case-control study of menopausal estrogen therapy and breast cancer. JAMA 243:1635, 1980.

Saunders KJ, Pilgrim CA, Pennypaker HS: Increased proficiency of search in breast self-examination. Cancer 58:2531, 1986.

Schaire C, Brinton LA, Hoover RN: Methylxanthines and benign breast disease. Am J Epidemiol 124:603, 1986.

Seidman H, Gelb SK, Silverberg E, et al: Survival experience in the Breast Cancer Detection Demonstration Project. CA Cancer J Clin 37:258, 1987.

Shapiro S, Strax P, Venet L: Periodic breast screening in reducing mortality in breast cancer. JAMA 215:1777, 1971.

Shapiro S, Venet W, Strax P, et al: Ten- to fourteen-year effects of screening on breast cancer mortality. J Natl Cancer Inst 69:349, 1982.

Shattuck-Eidens D, McClure M, Simard J, et al: A collaborative survey of 80 mutations in the BRCA1 breast and ovarian cancer susceptibility gene: implications for presymptomatic testing and screening. JAMA 273:535, 1995.

Sickles EA, Klein DL, Goodson WH III, Hunt TK: Mammography after fine needle aspiration of palpable breast masses. Am J Surg 145:395, 1983.

Siegel BM, Mayzel KA, Love SM: Level I and II axillary dissection in the treatment of early-stage breast cancer: an analysis of 259 consecutive patients. Arch Surg 135:1144, 1990.

Silverstein MJ, Handel N, Gamagami P, et al: Breast cancer in women after augmentation mammoplasty. Arch Surg 123:681, 1988.

Silverstein MJ, Waisman JR, Gamagami P, et al: Intraductal carcinoma of the breast (208 cases). Cancer 66:102, 1990.

Stanford JL, Brinton LA, Hoover RN: Oral contraceptives and breast cancer: results from an expanded case-control study. Br J Cancer 60:375, 1989.

Steinberg KK, Thacker SB, Smith SJ, et al: A meta-analysis of the effect of estrogen replacement therapy on the risk of breast cancer. JAMA 265:1985, 1991.

Sutton R, Buzdar AU, Hortobagyi GN: Pregnancy and offspring after adjuvant chemotherapy in breast cancer patients. Cancer 65:847, 1990.

Tabar L, Dean PB, Pentek Z: Galactography: the diagnostic procedure of choice for nipple discharge. Radiology 149:31, 1983.

Tabar L, Fagerberg G, Duffy SW, Day NE: The Swedish two county trial of mammographic screening for breast cancer: recent result and calculation of benefit. J Epidemiol Community Health 43:107, 1989.

Tabar L, Fagerberg CJ, Gad A, et al: Reduction in mortality from breast cancer after mass screening with mammography randomized trial from the Breath Cancer Screening Working Group of the Swedish National Board of Health and Welfare. Lancet 1:829, 1985.

Tabar L, Pentek Z, Dean PB: The diagnostic and therapeutic value of breast cyst puncture and pneumocystography. Radiology 14:1659, 1981.

Thompson WR, Bowen R, Dorman BA, et al: Mammographic localization and biopsy of nonpalpable breast lesions: a 5-year study. Arch Surg 126:730, 1991.

UK National Case-Control Study Group: Oral contraceptive use and breast cancer risk in young women: subgroup analyses. Lancet 335:1507, 1990.

Verbeek AL, Hendriks JH, Holland R, et al: Reduction in breast cancer mortality through mass screening with modern mammography: first results of Nijmegen Project 1975–1981. Lancet 1:1222, 1984.

Vessey MP: Oral contraceptives and breast cancer. ITTF Med Bull 21:1, 1987.

Vogel PM, Georgiade NG, Fetter BF, et al: The correlation of histologic changes in the human breast with the menstrual cycle. Am J Pathol 104:23, 1981.

Wanebo HJ, Feldman PS, Wilhelm MC, et al: Find needle aspiration cytology in lieu of open biopsy in management of primary breast cancer. Ann Surg 199:569, 1984.

Wilkinson S, Anderson TJ, Rifkind E, et al: Fibroadenoma of the breast: a follow-up of conservative management. Br J Surg 76:390, 1989.

Wingo PA, Lee NC, Ory HW, et al: Age-specific differences in the relationship between oral contraceptive use and breast cancer. Obstet Gynecol 78:161, 1991.

World Health Organization. In Histologic Typing of Breast Tumors. 2nd ed. Geneva, World Health Organization, 1981, p 15.

Yoshida Y, Takaoka M, Fukumoto M: Carcinoma arising in fibroadenoma: case report and review of the world literature. J Surg Oncol 29:132, 1985.

Zajdela A, Ghossen NA, Pilleron JP, Ennuyer A: The value of aspiration cytology in the diagnosis of breast cancer: experience at the Foundation Curie. Cancer 35:499, 1975.

Zajdela A, Zillhardt P, Voillemot N: Cytological diagnosis by fine needle sampling without aspiration. Cancer 59:1201, 1987.

Zajicek J, Franzen S, Jakobsson P, et al: Aspiration biopsy of mammary tumors in diagnosis and research—a critical review of 2,200 cases. Acta Cytol 11:169, 1967.

C H A P T E R

16

Principles of Chemotherapy

Augustin A. Garcia
J. Tate Thigpen

GENERAL PRINCIPLES

Principles of Pharmacology

Chemotherapeutic agents act on macromolecules (DNA, RNA, protein) in target cells. However, in order to produce their effect on the target molecules, drugs must be present at an appropriate concentration within the cell. The concentration is determined primarily by the amount of drug administered and the time of administration. Nonetheless, several other factors have a major influence on the final concentration at the target site. These factors are absorption, distribution, biotransformation, cellular penetration, and excretion of the drug.

Absorption is the process by which a drug leaves the site of administration. In oncology most drugs are administered parenterally, a method that assures a rapid and predictable effect. Parenteral routes include intravenous, intra-arterial, intrathecal, and intraperitoneal. A few drugs are administered orally. The advantages of the oral route are convenience and lower cost. The disadvantages which apply to some but not all drugs, include irregularities in absorption, limitation of absorption as a result of their chemical characteristics, and inactivation by digestive enzymes or pH. Furthermore, before reaching the systemic circulation, many drugs are metabolized in the liver. Among the cytotoxic drugs that can be administered orally are the nitrosureas, etoposide, melphalan, and cyclophosphamide.

After a drug is absorbed into the bloodstream, it is distributed into the interstitial and cellular fluids. Regional blood flow, protein binding, and liposolubility will determine the concentrations reached at different sites. Some organs are considered "drug sanctuaries" (e.g., the central nervous system and the testicle) because of the lower level of drug achieved in them.

The biotransformation of drugs refers to the metabolic changes to which the drug is subjected. The metabolic pathways can increase, decrease, or have no significant effect on the activity of the parent drug. Drug metabolism occurs mainly in the liver, but other organs that may also play a significant role are the kidneys, gastrointestinal tract, lungs, and skin.

Cellular penetration is the ultimate and most important step that anticancer drugs must undergo before producing their effect. Drugs penetrate cells by different mechanisms. *Passive diffusion* is a process by which drugs cross cell membranes by diffusion along a concentration gradient. The rate of transfer depends upon the magnitude of the gradient and the liposolubility of the drug. Passive diffusion is a nonsaturable process, meaning that diffusion into the cell will continue until the concentration of the drug is the same on both sides of the cell membrane. Some drugs penetrate into the cells by *facilitated diffusion*, in which a carrier-mediated transport system facilitates the process. Selectivity and saturability characterize facilitated diffusion. *Carrier-mediated active transport* shares characteristics with facilitated diffusion. However, it differs in that this method requires energy, usually in the form of ATP, and can occur against an electrochemical gradient.

Drugs can be excreted in their parent form, but most drugs are excreted as inactive metabolites. The kidneys, liver, and gastrointestinal tract are the major routes of drug excretion.

Mechanisms of Cytotoxicity

The mechanism by which virtually all available effective chemotherapeutic agents act is an attack on either the function or the synthesis of macromolecules (DNA, RNA, protein) in target cells. The attack may focus on any step in the process, from purine or pyrimidine synthesis to the function of end products such as enzymes or the microtubules of the mitotic spindle. The specific way in which interference with these aspects of cellular function is consummated depends on the particular drug employed.

Regardless of the specific site of the drug-induced metabolic lesion, cytotoxic effects are usually manifested only after the cell attempts to divide. The consequences of drug exposure thus are intimately related to the cell cycle (Fig. 16–1). This cycle is divided into four unequal phases: G_1, the intermitotic phase, in which a number of events prepare the cell for subsequent steps in the cycle; S, the phase of DNA synthesis; G_2, the premitotic phase, in which specific preparation for cell division, such as the synthesis of spindle proteins, takes place; and M, mitosis, a four-step phase leading to actual cell division. G_1 has the greatest variation in length and is generally the longest phase, while mitosis is the shortest.

Certain drugs act in only one of these four phases (e.g., 5-fluorouracil [5-FU] interferes with pyrimidine synthesis specifically in S phase) and are *cell cycle specific*. Most such drugs act in S phase to interfere with DNA synthesis. A few, such as the vinca alkaloids, interfere with the synthesis of the protein macromolecules of the mitotic spindle.

Other drugs attack existing macromolecules and interfere with either their function or their replication: for example, the alkylating agents crosslink strands of DNA to inter-

fere with the subsequent function of these macromolecules. These drugs are referred to as *cell cycle nonspecific* in the sense that the cell is not required to be in one specific phase of the cell cycle for a drug effect to be exerted. However, cytotoxicity usually results only if the cell attempts to divide before repair takes place. For the most part, the target molecule of these agents is DNA.

Assuming a homogeneous population of sensitive, actively cycling cells, the cytocidal effect of anticancer drugs follows first-order kinetics (Skipper et al, 1964). This means that a given dose of a drug will kill a constant percentage of the remaining cells rather than an absolute number of cells. This is usually expressed as the log of cell kill. Thus a 90 percent cell kill would be a one-log kill, a 99.99 percent kill a four-log kill, and so forth.

Factors Influencing Response

Considerations thus far have assumed a uniform cell population sensitive to the effects of available drugs. Unfortunately, such an ideal situation is not characteristic of human neoplasia. Human tumors exhibit a number of features that necessitate modification of the principles discussed thus far.

Growth Fraction

Under ideal circumstances, the rate of change in the size of a neoplastic mass is a reflection of the length of the cell cycle. The situation in actuality is a great deal more complex. Two major factors in addition to the length of the cell cycle influence the rate of change of mass size: the growth fraction, or percentage of cells actively in the cell cycle, and the rate of cell death and lysis.

Of these factors, by far the more important in terms of treatment implications is the growth fraction. Unlike the ideal tumor mass, human neoplasms have a significant proportion of cells that are in a resting state (G_0). These cells are capable of re-entering the cell cycle at any time, contributing to further growth of the neoplasm, but the resting state renders them relatively impervious to the effects of most drugs. The growth fraction of a mass decreases as the mass increases in size; hence the proportion of cells relatively resistant to drug effects will increase as the mass increases in size.

This fact has obvious implications for therapy. The optimal time to initiate therapy in terms of the first-order kinetics of cell kill is

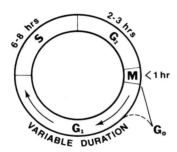

FIGURE 16–1. The cell cycle. G_1, intermitotic phase; G_2, premitotic phase; M, mitosis; S, DNA synthesis.

when the tumor is small, because there will be proportionately fewer cells in the relatively resistant resting state. Variation in the growth fraction is also thought to account for differences in the sensitivity of neoplastic and normal tissue to the effects of chemotherapy. Observations suggest that neoplastic tissue is more sensitive to cytotoxic drugs primarily because of a higher growth fraction, a difference that is even greater when the neoplastic mass is small.

Tissue Exposure to Drug

The sensitivity of neoplastic tissue to cytotoxic drugs depends not only on those cellular factors already discussed but also on adequate exposure of the tissue to drug. It must be possible to expose cells to an adequate concentration (C) of drug for an adequate period of time (t) in order to achieve a significant cell kill ($C \times t$). Along with the principles of pharmacology discussed earlier, a number of factors can act to prevent an adequate exposure: large tumor mass, altered blood supply to the tumor (e.g., tumor in a previously irradiated field), tumor cells in a sanctuary site (e.g., the central nervous system), poor normal tissue tolerance of drug effects, physician reluctance to employ aggressive therapy, and so on.

In addition to the drug dose, the rate of drug exposure (i.e. the rate at which a drug is administered) appears to be important. This aspect of chemotherapy deals not only with the dose of drug given with each course but also with the interval between courses. This concept of the importance of drug dose and interval is known as *dose intensity* and is expressed usually as milligrams of drug per square meter of body surface area per unit of time (e.g., mg/m^2/wk). Preclinical models, such as the classical experiments of Skipper et al (1964), using an osteosarcoma tumor model, showed that a reduction in the average dose intensity of two drugs produced a significant decrease in the cure rate before a significant reduction in the complete response rate occurred. Early trials of adjuvant chemotherapy with cyclophosphamide, methotrexate, and 5-FU (CMF) in patients with breast cancer also support the importance of dose intensity (Bonadonna and Valagussa, 1981). In these studies the doses of CMF were reduced based on age and toxicity. When the effect of these reductions was related to relapse-free survival, there was a sug-

gestion of a negative effect. Additional support is found in meta-analyses of numerous studies involving patients with ovarian carcinoma (Levin and Hryniuk, 1987). These authors demonstrated from pooled data that increasing the dose intensity of a platinum compound increased the frequency of response, which in turn correlated with enhanced survival. There is considerable evidence, however, that dose intensity within the limitations imposed by drug toxicity is not a major factor in clinical outcome (vide infra).

Mechanisms of Resistance

Data from murine models and dose intensity studies imply that cure of the patient with cancer is a simple matter of achieving sufficient dose intensity of active cytotoxic agents to kill the entire neoplastic cell population. This would, of course, necessitate developing methods to prevent or ameliorate adverse effects that limit the amount of drug that can be given safely. The matter is not so simple, however, as evidenced by one study that showed no advantage to a doubling of the dose intensity of a cisplatin-cyclophosphamide combination in patients with advanced ovarian carcinoma (McGuire et al, 1992).

Failure of neoplasms to respond to chemotherapy can be explained by factors already discussed, such as low growth fraction, drug sanctuaries, and inadequate drug delivery. The most significant reason for failure to respond, nevertheless, is cellular resistance to drug. Such resistance may be a de novo characteristic of some cells or, more commonly, may develop as a result of exposure to drug.

Goldie and Coldman (1979) used a bacterial model to study cellular resistance to anticancer drugs and provided further evidence for the observed relationship between increasing tumor size and decreasing curability. They formulated a hypothesis stating that mutation toward resistance occurs spontaneously at a rate of one mutation per 10^6 cell divisions or higher. As the number of cells in a mass increases, the likelihood of spontaneous mutation resulting in a resistant clone increases. Although these mutations occur independently of drug exposure, exposure selects for the resistant clone. This selection process explains recurrence in patients who develop a complete response to a drug regimen and then relapse despite continued drug therapy.

It is now evident that neoplastic cells can become resistant to cytotoxic agents by diverse mechanisms. Several mechanisms have been studied, including

1. Multidrug resistance (MDR) mediated by overexpression of the *MDR* gene. The gene product, P-glycoprotein, acts as an efflux cellular pump, resulting in decreased intracellular concentration of antineoplastic agents. This mechanism protects cells against damage from anthracyclines, plant alkaloids, epipodophyllotoxins, and taxanes.
2. Increased intracellular levels of gluthathione transferase. This enzyme protects cells from damage produced by free radicals, leading to resistance to alkylating agents, platinum compounds, and anthracyclines.
3. Alterations in tubulin, which produces resistance to taxanes and plant alkaloids.
4. Modification of target enzymes (thymidylate synthatase, dihydrofolate reductase), which produces resistance to antimetabolites (5-fluorouracil, methotrexate).

The overexpression of *MDR* is the most studied mechanism. Several trials have been conducted to evaluate drugs than can inhibit P-glycoprotein, including verapamil, quinine, tamoxifen, and cyclosporin. In general these efforts have not demonstrated an advantage in outcome.

CURRENT PRACTICE

The principles discussed thus far form the basis for clinical chemotherapy and may be summarized as follows: (1) chemotherapy exerts its effects on macromolecular synthesis or function within the cell; (2) these effects are usually manifested as a result of attempted cell division; (3) relative resistance to drug effects is characteristic of cells in the resting state and results from repair of drug-induced damage; (4) the percentage of resting cells increases (growth fraction decreases) as a neoplastic mass enlarges; (5) the drug effect depends upon adequate exposure of cells to the drug: an adequate dose for an adequate period of time (dose intensity); and (6) development of cellular resistance is a result of spontaneous mutation together with drug-pressured selection of resistant clones. Dose intense chemotherapy not only increases the response rate but reduces the likelihood of drug resistance developing (Coldman and Goldie, 1987). Attention is now focused on

the manner in which these concepts are applied to clinical practice.

Combination Chemotherapy

The first natural outgrowth of this insight into drug resistance was the use of combinations of drugs as opposed to single agents. A properly designed combination should offer significant advantages over single agents. First, combining drugs that act on different parts of the cell's metabolic machinery should provide broader coverage of de novo resistant cells and prevent or slow the development of newly resistant cell lines. Second, selecting drugs with differing toxicities should permit the use of each agent in its optimal dose and schedule (greater dose intensity), and thus result in greater cell kill than could be achieved with any of the agents alone (DeVita, 1981).

That properly designed combination chemotherapy does in fact lead to a greater frequency and durability of response has been demonstrated in those neoplasms for which a variety of effective drugs are available: acute leukemia, Hodgkin's disease, high-grade lymphomas, diffuse histiocytic lymphoma, testicular carcinoma, breast carcinoma, and ovarian carcinoma. This approach is unfortunately limited for most cancers because there are an insufficient number of effective drugs to formulate a combination with different mechanisms of action and different toxicities that would permit the use of each drug at its optimal dose and schedule. Only under such circumstances can the combination be expected to provide a major therapeutic advantage. Not only are there too few active drugs available for most common neoplasms, but there is also a reluctance on the part of physicians and their patients to accept the greater variety of toxicities that invariably result from a properly selected combination.

Drug Dose and Schedule

On the basis of the principles that have been outlined, at least three aspects of drug dose and scheduling are important. First, the schedule for each drug on any given course of therapy should be governed by the drug's interrelationship with the cell cycle. Drugs that act in a specific phase of the cell cycle (cell cycle–specific agents) must be administered longer or at more frequent intervals to ensure that the cells are exposed to the drugs during the appropriate phase of the cycle.

Second, the greater sensitivity of neoplastic tissue to the cytocidal effects of chemotherapy and the greater rapidity with which normal tissue recovers from drug-induced suppression suggest that high-dose, intermittent or cyclic schedules will be more effective than continuous or low-dose maintenance schedules. A corollary to this reasoning is that the interval between drug courses is crucial to the success of treatment. The interval should be geared to coincide with the recovery of normal tissue in order to minimize the recovery of the malignant tissue. Unnecessary delay defeats the purpose of cyclic therapy. A further corollary is that the optimal drug therapy should be continued for a maximum period of time and not replaced with a less toxic, lower dose maintenance schedule.

Finally, the doses of the drugs that make up the combination should provide adequate dose intensity. Successful application of this concept offers the greatest challenge. Three possible relationships between dose intensity and response to therapy are depicted in graph A in Figure 16–2. The simplest relationship is depicted by line 1, a relationship in which response rate continues to increase as dose intensity increases. A second possible relationship is demonstrated by line 2. In this setting, escalation of dose intensity results in a higher response rate until a specific level of dose intensity is reached (presumably the point at which all sensitive cells have been eradicated); beyond this point, further increases in dose intensity yield no additional

benefit. A third possible relationship is presented by line 3. This scenario postulates a gradual increase in response rate with escalation of dose intensity over a low dose range until the intensity reaches a threshold beyond which response rate rises more rapidly.

Available data suggest that, over a lower range of drug doses (Levin and Hryniuk, 1987), response rates and survival improve as drug dose intensity escalates. Other data suggest that, beyond this lower range, escalation of dose intensity is not rewarded with enhanced therapeutic benefit (McGuire et al, 1992). These data fit best with the relationship postulated by line 2 on Graph A. One possible interpretation of these results is that sufficient dose intensity is required to eradicate all cells sensitive to the drugs employed, but that further escalation beyond this point does not yield further benefit because dose intensity cannot overcome cellular resistance.

Line 4 (graph B) in Figure 16–2 depicts a fourth possible relationship between dose intensity and response to therapy. The initial part of this graph is identical to line 2 of graph A, but a second threshold is proposed, a threshold that would theoretically correspond to the achievement of a dose intensity that successfully overcomes cellular resistance. To date, there are no clinical data that support the existence of such a threshold.

Based on these considerations, the challenges that confront us are three in number. First, assuming that the data supporting line 2 are correct, what is the dose intensity level

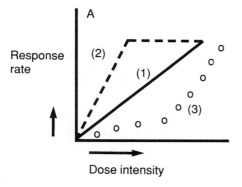
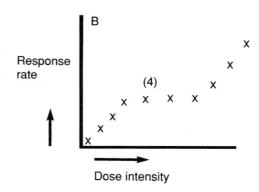

FIGURE 16–2. *A,* Three possible relationships between dose intensity and response rate. *1* (solid line): As dose intensity escalates, response rate continues to increase. *2* (dashed line): As dose intensity escalates, the response rate increases until all sensitive cells have been eradicated; further escalation yields no additional benefit. *3* (open circles): As dose intensity escalates, the response rate rises slowly until a threshold is reached; beyond this point, response increases at a much more rapid rate. *B,* A fourth possible interpretation (crosses): As dose intensity escalates, the response rate rises until a plateau is reached at which point presumably all sensitive cells have been eradicated. Further dose escalation yields no increase in response until cellular resistance is overcome, with a resultant further increase in the response rate.

beyond which no further therapeutic benefit is seen for each individual tumor and regimen? Second, is there a second threshold as postulated by line 4? Third, if a second threshold is proven, what is that threshold for each tumor and regimen?

Further complicating this issue is evidence that points to the importance of tumor volume at the time of initiation of chemotherapy and total drug dose (Kaye et al, 1992; Levin and Hryniuk, 1987). The relative importance of total dose as opposed to dose intensity is discussed at length in the section "Chemotherapy of Ovarian Cancer," but the data suggest that the increase in dose intensity of platinum compounds that can be safely achieved in clinical practice (approximately twofold) does not produce a major improvement in survival. Thus the ultimate role of high-dose and dose-intense regimens in patient management is not clear at the present time. Further studies evaluating total dose and larger differences in dose intensity in small-volume and large-volume disease will be required.

The current utility of hematopoietic growth factors, in particular granulocyte colony-stimulating factor and granulocyte-macrophage colony-stimulating factor, must be evaluated in light of the foregoing discussion on dose intensity. These two growth factors act primarily to support the number of available segmented neutrophils. Initial research raised the hope that these agents would lead to clinically tolerable higher dose intensity of drug therapy and thereby improve treatment re-sults. Current use, however, is better confined to support those patients who could not otherwise tolerate standard-dose therapy because of neutropenia (Demetri and Griffin, 1990).

Adjuvant Chemotherapy

The term *adjuvant chemotherapy* refers to the use of drugs in patients who have been rendered clinically disease free by surgical therapy but are known to be at high risk for the presence of micrometastases, and therefore recurrence, because of adverse tumor characteristics. The rationale for adjuvant chemotherapy is based in part on the principles that smaller masses have a higher growth fraction than larger masses and that a higher growth fraction is associated with greater sensitivity to drug therapy. The best application of these principles requires that treatment be given before the tumor achieves a clinically detectable size, because clinically detectable masses already have a declining growth rate reflective of a declining growth fraction (Fig. 16–3).

An additional scientific basis for adjuvant chemotherapy is the Goldie-Coldman hypothesis: As a neoplastic mass enlarges, the likelihood of spontaneous mutations, which result in resistant clones, increases. This suggests that the earlier chemotherapy is given, the greater the chance that all cells in the mass will be sensitive to the cytotoxic effects of the drugs and hence the greater the like-

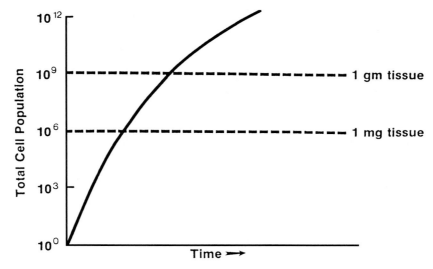

FIGURE 16–3. Growth of cancer follows a Gompertzian pattern. Early growth is exponential, but the growth rate slows as the mass enlarges, reflecting a declining growth fraction. This decline in growth rate occurs prior to the level of clinical detectability.

lihood that the entire neoplastic cell population will be eradicated. The most publicized example of the successful use of adjuvant chemotherapy is in the management of early breast cancer. This example also illustrates several other principles discussed here.

Special Cases

Every principle discussed thus far points to the importance of using effective drugs and achieving optimal cell exposure to the drugs. The crucial nature of these two aspects of chemotherapy has led to alternative approaches in an attempt to maximize both tumor sensitivity and exposure to drugs. None of these approaches can be considered a part of standard treatment at present, but each represents a current experimental approach with a certain amount of promise.

Drug Sensitivity Testing

Although numerous attempts to assess the sensitivity of specific neoplasms to drugs in vitro have been made since the early 1970s, the report from Salmon and colleagues in 1978 stimulated renewed interest in such an approach to the development of effective chemotherapy. This human tumor stem cell or clonogenic assay has yielded successful in vitro growth in about 50 percent of cases, with a predictive accuracy of 83 to 100 percent for drug resistance and 60 to 90 percent for drug sensitivity. Improved survival for patients with relapsed ovarian carcinoma treated on the basis of assay results as opposed to the basis of the physician's judgment has been reported in one series (Alberts et al, 1981). Despite some apparent successes, however, the relatively low colony-forming efficiency, the 2-week time period required to culture the cells, and the small pool of effective drugs for most tumors currently limit the clinical usefulness of the assay.

At least five other techniques have been reported (Kochli et al, 1994). These include a dye exclusion assay (Weisenthal et al, 1983) and a subrenal capsule assay (Griffin et al, 1983). The former is based on differential uptake of certain vital dyes to identify surviving cells after drug exposure, while the latter utilizes human tumor xenografts implanted under the renal capsule of athymic mice. Each of these techniques has disadvantages that have hampered their clinical utility. Furthermore, clinical trials with some of these assay techniques have been unable to demonstrate any association between the results of the assay and clinical response or survival (Federico et al, 1994; von Hoff et al, 1990; Maenpaa et al, 1995).

A somewhat different approach has been the development of chemoresistance assays such as that of Kern et al (1991). In their assay, human tumor cells are cultured in soft agar and exposed to suprapharmacologic concentrations of cytotoxic drugs. The tumor cells that survive this unusual drug exposure are considered to demonstrate "extreme drug resistance." The authors have shown that this assay has a negative predictive value of greater than 99 percent. The ability of this assay to accurately identify inactive chemotherapeutic agents helps the treating physician avoid ineffective therapy and unnecessary toxicity. The major clinical limitation of this assay is that the identification of chemoresistance to one or more drugs does not imply that other drugs will be effective.

At present, none of these assays should be used to select primary therapy in cases where an effective standard regimen exists. Whether they are of use in selection of therapy in relapsed cases of, for example, ovarian carcinoma is debatable.

Directed Chemotherapy

The term *directed chemotherapy* refers to the delivery of chemotherapeutic agents to specific areas that contain either all or the bulk of the tumor burden. This may take one of several forms: intracavitary therapy, intra-arterial infusion, or attaching the drug to vehicles such as monoclonal antibodies or liposomes, which concentrate in the area of the neoplasm. The first of these approaches is the most important in gynecologic oncology today and consists for the most part in the use of intraperitoneal (IP) chemotherapy to treat ovarian carcinoma.

The rationale for *IP chemotherapy* in ovarian carcinoma begins with the observations that the principal route of spread of the tumor is via direct peritoneal seeding, and that the bulk of the tumor remains confined to the peritoneal cavity in a significant proportion of patients. Solutions have been developed to several of the problems that plagued early attempts to take advantage of these observations. First, the problem of access to the abdominal cavity for repeated drug administration has essentially been solved by the use of catheters developed for peritoneal dialysis and central venous access. Second, the problem of achieving an even distribution of drug in patients who previously had undergone laparotomy was at least partly overcome by administering a relatively large volume of fluid with the drug. Finally, studies on the pharmacokinetics of drugs put into the peritoneal cavity indicate a distinct regional advantage for several drugs as measured by the peak peritoneal concentration over the peak serum level: from a 7- to more than 7,000-fold greater concentration in the peritoneal cavity.

This information has been brought to bear on the treatment of patients with recurrent ovarian carcinoma confined to the abdominal cavity. No fewer than nine drugs have been employed as single agents in human IP studies with acceptable adverse effects: melphalan, mitomycin C, 5-FU, 5-fluorodeoxy-uridine (floxuridine; FUDR), methotrexate, doxorubicin, mitoxantrone, cisplatin, carboplatin, and cytosine arabinoside (Markman and Muggia, 1985; Myers, 1984). In addition, combinations of cisplatin with other agents (5-FU, cytarabine, etoposide, melphalan, cytarabine and doxorubicin, cytarabine and bleomycin, and recombinant alpha-interferon) have been tested with demonstration of responses and safety (Markman, 1991). The largest series of patients with ovarian carcinoma reports significant responses, including complete responses to the combination of cisplatin and cytosine arabinoside, in patients with small-volume disease who had prior cisplatin-based intravenous (IV) chemotherapy (Markman et al, 1985, 1991a). Patients with large-volume (>2 cm largest diameter) disease did not demonstrate significant response to IP therapy. A more critical analysis of results with IP cisplatin plus cytarabine (Markman et al, 1991b), however, reveals that essentially all of the responses of small-volume disease occur in patients who initially responded to an IV platinum-based regimen and later relapsed, not in those patients who progressed while receiving the prior platinum-based regimen.

Although no major randomized study of second-line IP chemotherapy has been conducted, some drugs show promising results in uncontrolled clinical trials. Two of these drugs are mitoxantrone and FUDR. On the basis of the results of a randomized Phase II study of these two drugs, FUDR, which showed a longer progression-free survival

and higher median overall survival, was recommended by the authors for further investigation (Markman et al, 1990; Muggia et al, 1996).

The major objective for IP therapy in ovarian carcinoma is to achieve greater drug exposure of a cancer that characteristically is limited to the peritoneal space for much of its natural history. The greater local dose intensity thus attained should result in more frequent responses and response in some patients whose disease would be resistant to the lower concentration of drug achievable by IV administration. The data cited previously suggest, however, that in fact those patients who do respond to IP therapy are the same patients who also respond to retreatment with IV platinum-based therapy (Markman et al, 1991b). This raises serious questions about the value of IP therapy, which is attended by additional significant toxicity, including infection, hemorrhage, bowel perforation or obstruction, and abdominal pain (Kaplan et al, 1985; Markman, 1991; Runowicz et al, 1986).

The results of an intergroup trial comparing the IP approach to standard IV therapy in previously untreated patients were reported by Alberts et al (1996). In this trial patients with small-volume advanced-stage ovarian cancer were randomized to treatment with IV cyclophosphamide (Cytoxan) plus IV or IP cisplatin. This study demonstrated a 20 percent improvement in median survival and a 24 percent reduction of death. However, it is unclear how the results of IP therapy relate to regimens where taxol is employed, because it was shown that the combination of IV taxol and IV cisplatin is superior to IV Cytoxan and IV cisplatin (McGuire et al, 1996).

In short, it is currently controversial whether IP chemotherapy should have any role in the treatment of advanced or recurrent ovarian carcinoma in either the first- or second-line setting. It is the authors' opinion that its use should for the time being remain confined to the investigational setting.

Summary

The principles and applications that have been discussed may be summarized in the simple tenet that success in the use of chemotherapy requires aggressive management combined with measures to minimize both resistance and adverse effects. Aggressive intermittent combination chemotherapy with active drugs given at the shortest interval consistent with reasonable normal tissue recovery should be administered, if at all possible, when the tumor burden is minimal so as to achieve maximum drug exposure to neoplastic tissue while it has a high growth fraction and the minimum chance of containing resistant clones. Such therapy should be continued for an extended period of time and should not be replaced with low-dose maintenance chemotherapy in the interest of decreasing toxicity. This requires a willingness to accept significant toxicity as the price of optimum neoplastic cell kill.

DRUG DEVELOPMENT: CLINICAL TRIALS

Clinical Trials

Potential anticancer drugs that reach clinical trials are evaluated in a series of four phases designed to determine their toxicity, their spectrum of activity, and ultimately their place in the therapeutic armamentarium for specific human tumors.

Evaluation Parameters

The efficacy of chemotherapy is typically evaluated by three parameters: objective response, interval to progression of disease (progression-free interval, or PFI), and overall survival. Objective response is assessed in terms of the size of lesions measurable in at least two dimensions (Table 16–1). The definitions of the various response categories, with minor variations, are essentially the same among all major clinical trial groups in the United States. This parameter is an attempt to determine, albeit crudely, the ability of a drug or treatment regimen to induce a significant cell kill. It is usually reported in terms of overall (complete plus partial) and complete response rates. The PFI is a reflec-

tion of the durability and hence the usefulness of a response. Survival would seem to be the ultimate test of the efficacy of a drug or regimen, but the value of the parameter is confounded to some extent by the variety of management approaches used once the patient progresses and is taken off the study.

Both the type and the severity of toxicity are recorded. A reasonably standard set of criteria for grading the severity of each type of adverse effect has evolved in the United States. Such effects are classified as mild (grade 1), moderate (grade 2), or severe (grade 3). For certain types of toxicity, such as myelosuppression, a fourth grade for exceptionally severe or life-threatening toxicity is added. This grading system, although imprecise, does provide a reasonable estimate of the adverse effects to be expected with a given drug or regimen and is equally important to parameters measuring therapeutic efficacy.

It has been emphasized that a measurement of the quality of life of cancer patients undergoing chemotherapy is also of great importance. Efforts have been directed to develop instruments to measure quality of life. Several techniques are currently in use in Phase II and III clinical trials: the Functional Assessment of Cancer Therapy, the Memorial Symptom Assessment Scale, and the European Organization for Research and Treatment of Cancer (EORTC) Quality of Life Questionnaire. These scales measure physical, functional, emotional, and social well-being characteristics of patients with cancer as well as the impact of chemotherapy on these same parameters.

Evaluation Phases

The initial step in the clinical evaluation of a new drug is the determination of the maximum tolerable dose, optimal schedule, and dose-limiting toxicity of the agent. This type

TABLE **16–1**

Definitions of the Objective Response Employed by the Gynecologic Oncology Group

Response	Definition
Complete response (CR)	Complete disappearance of all evidence of disease for at least 1 month
Partial response (PR)	Reduction of the product of the greatest diameter of a lesion and its perpendicular by at least 50% for at least 1 month; these criteria must be exhibited by each measureable lesion
Stable disease (SD)	Maintenance for each lesion of criteria less than those required for either a partial response or increasing disease
Increasing disease (ID)	Increase of the product of the greatest diameter of a lesion and its perpendicular by at least 50% or the appearance of a new lesion within 1 month

of study, the *Phase I trial*, is conducted in a population of 15 to 30 patients with no other reasonable therapeutic options. The dose begins at a low level (usually 10 percent of the 10 percent lethal dose) and is escalated after three patients have been treated safely at each dose level. The scheme for dose escalation follows a set pattern, usually a modified Fibonacci system (Muggia et al, 1979), in which the dose is initially doubled and then increased by 66, then 50, and then 33 percent, and so on, for each succeeding group of three patients until toxicity is noted. Patients treated at one dose level are not used for testing subsequent dose levels in order to avoid the confounding effects of delayed and cumulative toxicity.

Those drugs with acceptable toxicity in Phase I testing proceed to a *Phase II trial*, which seeks to study each drug in a panel of human tumors that includes at a minimum breast carcinoma, colon carcinoma, lung carcinoma, melanoma, acute leukemia, and lymphoma. Multiple doses and schedules are usually tested, and each requires sufficient patients per tumor type to obtain an estimate of the response rate. Multiple statistical and sample size methods have been developed for Phase II studies. One of the most commonly used methods is the optimal two-stage design (Simon et al, 1989). In this method a number of evaluable patients are entered into the first stage of the trial. If there were fewer than a specified number of responses, the accrual is terminated and the drug is considered to have minimal activity. Otherwise accrual continues until a predetermined total number of evaluable patients is achieved. Under this method the researchers specify a target activity for the drug, typically a 20 percent response rate, although the occurrence of durable complete responses is also of interest. Using this method, the number of patients required to evaluate the drug activity against each type of tumor can be strictly limited. Even so, the Phase II evaluation of each drug will require several hundred patients. Those drugs that meet the target criteria are selected for further study if the observed toxicity is acceptable.

Drugs with activity in Phase II trials are evaluated next in randomized *Phase III trials*, either alone or as a part of a combination with other active agents. In this setting the new agents are most often compared to the standard treatment for the tumor type in question. Where effective standard therapy is not available, all study regimens might be investigational. The purpose of this type of trial is to establish the place of the new drug(s) in the chemotherapeutic armamentarium for each tumor type.

Especially promising drugs or regimens are finally evaluated as part of an integrated, multimodality treatment program that includes surgery and/or radiotherapy. These *Phase IV trials* are also randomized, with the control group representing either standard therapy or another experimental regimen.

CLASSIFICATION AND CHARACTERISTICS OF SPECIFIC DRUGS

Current cytotoxic agents used in the systemic treatment of cancer have three properties in common. First, their cytotoxic capability was demonstrated as a part of the drug development process prior to using the agent to treat human neoplasms. Second, their toxicity is controllable and tolerable. Third, their efficacy in the treatment of human cancer must have been demonstrated in clinical trials.

Available anticancer drugs that meet these criteria fall into three broad categories according to their mechanism of action: the alkylating agents, the antimetabolites, and the plant alkaloids. In this section the mechanisms of action are discussed for the general categories. In addition, the individual drug's place in the therapeutic armamentarium and its important peculiarities are discussed. This section does not attempt to replace those sources that provide extensive, detailed discussion of individual drugs. For a complete description of the pharmacology, adverse effects, indications, and other facts relative to chemotherapeutic agents, the reader should consult reference works (e.g., Perry, 1996).

Alkylating Agents

The alkylating agents comprise a class of drugs that interact with macromolecules, particularly DNA, in such a way as to interfere with their function, typically by suppressing their role in the synthesis of one or more macromolecules essential to cell replication. Alkylating agents are therefore cell cycle nonspecific, although usually their lethal effect is dependent on subsequent cell division. There are four distinct groups of compounds that act as alkylating agents: the classic alkylating agents, the nitrosoureas, the antitumor antibiotics, and a group of miscellaneous drugs with alkylating properties.

Classic Alkylating Agents

The classic alkylating agents have the ability to form highly reactive carbonium ions that attack nucleophilic or electron-rich sites on macromolecules within the target cell to form covalent bonds. Although RNA and protein molecules as well as DNA can be alkylated, the principal target is DNA. Certain compounds can form two or more such groups per molecule and hence can alkylate more than one DNA site either on the same or on different strands. The favored site for alkylation appears to be the N7 position of guanine. Such interaction may produce one of several effects on DNA: (1) miscoding with thymidine to produce abnormal base pairs, (2) destruction of the imidazole ring of guanine, (3) crosslinking of two strands of DNA by covalent bonds, and (4) actual breaking of DNA strands by depurination. The net result is cell death unless the cell has sufficient time to effect repair prior to entering the S phase of the cell cycle. For this reason, these agents are far more effective against cycling cells than against resting cells.

The prototype for this class of alkylating agents is mechlorethamine, or nitrogen mustard. Spurred by evidence for activity of this drug in lymphomas, investigations over three decades have led to the development of a number of currently employed drugs that fall into three chemical groups: the bis(chloroethyl) amines, the ethyleneimines, and the alkyl sulfonates.

BIS(CHLOROETHYL) AMINES

Bis(chloroethyl) amines, the most commonly used alkylating agents in gynecologic cancer therapy, are derivatives of mechlorethamine. The common adverse effects seen with all members of this class are myelosuppression and second malignancies such as acute leukemia. Uncommonly, interstitial pneumonitis and pulmonary fibrosis occur. Additional more common adverse effects are seen with individual agents. Four of these drugs are used frequently enough in gynecologic malignancies to warrant further discussion.

Cyclophosphamide (Cytoxan; CTX). This agent is a cyclic phosphamide ester of mechlorethamine (Fig. 16–4) designed in an unsuccessful attempt to improve the selectivity

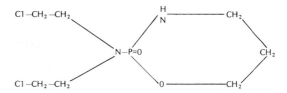

2—[Bis(β—chloroethyl)amino]—2H—1,3,2—oxazaphosphorinane 2—oxide

FIGURE 16–4. Cyclophosphamide (Cytoxan, Endoxan).

of mechlorethamine. However, the compound has proved to have a wide spectrum of activity and is currently the most commonly used alkylating agent. It does require activation by hepatic microsomal enzymes and hence is not useful for directed chemotherapy, such as intracavitary administration. The dose-limiting toxicity for CTX, as for virtually all of the alkylating agents, is myelosuppression characterized by a greater effect on leukocytes than on platelets. The nadir cell counts can be expected between day 7 and day 14 after administration of CTX, with recovery usually by day 21.

Several unique aspects of CTX deserve mention. First, drugs such as allopurinol and barbiturates, which induce hepatic microsomal enzymes, may enhance the conversion of CTX to its active metabolites and thus increase toxicity. Corticosteroids, in contrast, may inhibit microsomal enzymes and reduce the effect of CTX. These drugs should either be avoided or, in the case of steroids, given at a consistent dosage to prevent sudden changes in the effects of the drug. Second, CTX, if allowed to concentrate in the bladder, can produce hemorrhagic cystitis from one to several days after administration. This effect can be prevented by adequate fluid intake (3 liters/day) before, during, and after drug administration. Caution with hydration is warranted, however, because CTX can induce water retention mediated by its effect on the renal tubule. Successful management of severe hemorrhagic cystitis has been reported by irrigating the bladder with thiol compounds, and by systemic administration of acetylcysteine or sodium-2-mercaptoethane sulfonate (mesna) (Brock et al, 1981). If the problem persists despite adequate hydration, cessation of therapy with CTX is indicated to prevent the development of a small, fibrotic bladder.

Ifosfamide. Chemically similar to CTX, ifosfamide has an oxazaphosphorine ring structire and requires activation by hepatic microsomes. Hemorrhagic cystitis, which prevented the clinical use of ifosfamide for many years, can be prevented now by the concomitant administration of mesna. Other adverse effects include myelosuppression and central nervous system toxicity manifested as varying degrees of confusion, aphasia, hallucinations, and coma. The frequency of central nervous system toxicity correlates with drug dose and schedule (e.g., high-dose single-day regimen), renal function, and serum albumin level (Antman et al, 1989; Cerny and Kupfer, 1989; Curtin et al, 1991).

Ifosfamide has a broad spectrum of activity among gynecologic malignancies, with evidence of efficacy in ovarian cracinoma, carcinoma of the cervix, uterine sarcomas, and germ cell neoplasms of the ovary (Thigpen et al, 1990). Perhaps more importantly, there is evidence of drug activity in the face of platinum resistance in ovarian carcinoma (Markman et al, 1992).

Melphalan (Alkeran; L-Phenylalanine Mustard [L-PAM]). Melphalan, a phenylalanine derivative of mechlorethamine, was, along with chlorambucil, the treatment of choice for ovarian carcinoma in the 1960s. It is available only for oral administration because it is highly insoluble. Absorption from the gastrointestinal tract appears to be quite variable, with a fourfold difference among patients. Evidence supports the requirement for a carrier-mediated active transport mechanism for the drug to enter cells. The dose-limiting toxicity is myelosuppression with a delayed nadir of 14 to 21 days, but occasionally as long as 6 weeks, after drug administration. The drug is more toxic to the platelet series than it is to the white cells. Of particular note is the association of this drug with prolonged bone marrow suppression and an increased incidence of acute leukemia (Kaldor et al, 1990).

Chlorambucil (Leukeran). This is another derivative of mechlorethamine that is available only for oral use, but, unlike melphalan, it apparently has excellent absorption from the gastrointestinal tract. It was often used in the past as a substitute for CTX in those patients with hemorrhagic cystitis not correctable by adequate hydration. The dose-limiting toxicity is myelosuppression.

ETHYLENEIMINES

The ethyleneimines are polyfunctional alkylating agents pharmacologically similar to the bis(chloroethyl) amines. The active alkylating moieties are the ethyleneimine radicals. The only member of this group available for clinical use is triethylene thiophosphoramide (*thio-TEPA*), which was commonly used to treat malignant effusions by intracavitary instillation. This compound is relatively nonpolar and hence lipid soluble; as a result, it can enter the central nervous system. The dose-limiting adverse effect is myelosuppression, which may be seen after intracavitary as well as IV administration. Other forms of toxicity are unusual.

Nitrosoureas

The nitrosoureas are characterized by their lipid solubility. They have a theoretical advantage over the classic alkylating agents because their decomposition yields isocyanates, the carbamoylate amine groups of which inhibit DNA repair and alter maturation of RNA. Despite this theoretical advantage, alkylation appears to be their major modus operandi. There are five drugs that belong to the nitrosourea group: carmustine (BCNU), lomustine (CCNU), methyl CCNU, streptozotocin, and chlorozotocin. None of the nitrosoureas is currently used to treat gynecologic malignancy.

Antitumor Antibiotics

This group of drugs is composed of microbial fermentation products that possess cytotoxic properties. Included are the anthracyclines, the chromomycins, mitomycin, and the bleomycins. The diverse characteristics of the individual drugs and families that make up this group are discussed in the following paragraphs.

ANTHRACYCLINES

The anthracyclines are a family of drugs that includes daunorubicin and doxorubicin (Adriamycin [ADR]), as well as a group of analogs and related compounds such as rubidazole, aclacinomycin a, carminomycin, demethoxydaunorubicin (idarubicin), deoxydoxorubicin, 4'-epi-doxorubicin (epirubicin), dihydroxyanthracenedione (mitoxantrone; DHAD), and anthracene dicarboxaldehyde (bisantrene). Although there are advantages to the various newer anthracyclines, no study to date has confirmed their clinical value in gynecologic oncology. Attention is therefore directed to the two primary agents and in particular to ADR, the most commonly used anthracycline.

The anthracyclines act primarily to interfere with nucleic acid synthesis by intercalating adjoining DNA nucleotide pairs and thereby creating a block of DNA-directed RNA and DNA transcription. This process attacks pre-existing macromolecules and is cell cycle nonspecific. Other effects that may be important in the antitumor activity of these compounds include the chelation of divalent cations, interaction with cell membranes to alter membrane function, and participation in oxidation-reduction reactions. These drugs are metabolized by the liver and excreted through the biliary tract; hence dose adjustment is indicated in patients with evidence of impairment of hepatic excretory function.

There are a number of adverse effects shared by the members of the anthracycline family. The dose-limiting toxicity of anthracyclines is myelosuppression. Leukopenia is far more common than thrombocytopenia or anemia. The nadir cell counts occur at 10 to 14 days and recovery by 21 days after drug administration. Extravasation of the anthracyclines can produce severe local skin and soft tissue necrosis. Although surgical debridement and skin grafting may be required for severe injuries, immediate infiltration of the area with sodium bicarbonate and corticosteroids followed by application of ice can prevent much of the tissue damage. Other skin effects include alopecia, hyperpigmentation, reactivation of radiation skin reactions (recall phenomenon), and inflammation of the veins used for administration. Also common to some degree with all anthracyclines are stomatitis, nausea, vomiting, and diarrhea.

The most important and a unique adverse effect seen with the anthracyclines is cardiotoxicity. This includes the acute toxicities of pericarditis, myocarditis, and electrophysiologic aberrations, as well as a cardiomyopathy that is cumulative. The former effects appear to be reversible and do not contraindicate further therapy. The cardiomyopathy, conversely, presents as classic congestive heart failure, which may be refractory to the usual measures and is irreversible. The mechanism by which anthracyclines induce cardiomyopathy is not well understood, but it appears to be mediated by the development of oxidizing agents through an iron-dependent process. The pathology associated with this complication is that of fragmentation and dropout of myofibrils. There appears to be a close relationship between the incidence of cardiomyopathy and several factors: total dose of anthracycline received, age of the patient, and schedule of the drug. Older patients and those who received higher individual doses appear to be at greater risk. No method to monitor for early signs of cardiomyopathy has been totally successful. Serial echocardiography and endomyocardial biopsy appear to be the best predictors of cardiomyopathy, but limitation of the total dose is still the standard means employed to avoid this complication.

Adriamycin (doxorubicin) is a hydroxylated congener of daunorubicin (Fig. 16–5). Current evidence suggests a mechanism of action and a spectrum of adverse effects similar to those of daunorubicin. The incidence of cardiomyopathy is less than 1 percent at total doses below 500 mg/m^2, rises to 11 percent between 501 and 600 mg/m^2, and ex-

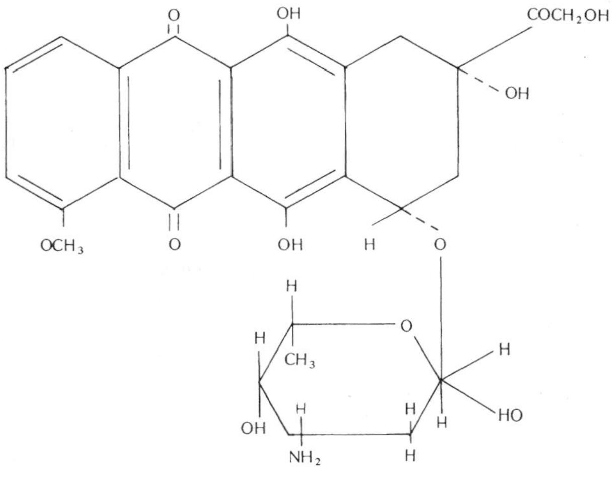

FIGURE 16–5. Doxorubicin (Adriamycin).

ceeds 30 percent at doses beyond 600 mg/m^2 (Minow et al, 1975). A number of measures to decrease the incidence of ADR cardiomyopathy have been investigated: smaller weekly doses, continuous IV infusion, digitalis, and the administration of alpha-tocopherol, among others. A low weekly dose schedule of ADR does permit the safe administration of a higher cumulative dose, but the therapeutic value of this additional 160 mg/m^2 is not clear (Lum et al, 1985).

Current practice includes several measures to deal with the cardiotoxicity of ADR (Allen, 1992). The foremost is to limit the cumulative dose of ADR to 550 mg/m^2 maximum. The maximum dose should be reduced to 450 mg/m^2 in the presence of any factor that might enhance the cardiotoxicity of ADR: mediastinal radiation therapy, pre-existing cardiotoxicity, the extremes of age, poor nutritional status, and possibly concomitant use of CTX, etoposide, actinomycin D, mitomycin C, melphalan, vincristine, or bleomycin. Monitoring cardiac function is of uncertain value, but clinical practice generally includes serial multiple gated acquisition scans (MUGA), the interval depending upon the patient risk factors and expected total dose. A persistent decline in the ejection fraction, or a drop below 50 percent, should prompt consideration of discontinuing ADR therapy.

Dexrazoxane (ICPF-187), an analog of ethylene diamine-tetraacetic acid, has been approved as an ADR cardioprotective agent. Its mechanism of action is mediated by iron chelation, thereby reducing the amount of available iron and preventing the formation of oxygen radicals. Several clinical trials have confirmed the ability of dexrazoxane to produce smaller decreases in left ventricular ejection fraction, a lower incidence of congestive heart failure, and to allow the administration of a higher cumulative dose of ADR (Speyer et al, 1988).

Adriamycin has enjoyed by far the greatest utilization of any of the anthracyclines in gynecologic cancer. These data are discussed in detail later under each specific gynecologic neoplasm. Although not available in the United States, *epirubicin* is a widely studied analog of ADR (Plosker and Faulds, 1993). Its clinical efficacy in several tumors is equivalent to ADR, but it appears to have lower hematologic and cardiac toxicity. Data suggest it may have a role in recurrent ovarian cancer (Havsteen et al, 1996; Vermorken et al, 1995).

Doxil is a preparation of ADR in a liposome (Vaage et al, 1992). Preclinical studies indicate a superior activity compared to free doxorubicin. It appears to be devoid of cardiotoxicity, and hematological toxicity is minimal. The dose-limiting toxicities of this drug are mucosal and cutaneous (Uziely et al, 1995). Some studies suggest it may also play a role in refractory ovarian cancer (Muggia et al, 1997b).

Mitoxantrone, an anthracenedione, possesses many similarities to ADR. Two significant differences suggest a potential role for this agent in gynecologic cancers. First, the mechanism by which drug resistance develops appears to be different (Harker et al, 1989). Second, the potential for producing cardiotoxicity appears to be less than that for ADR (Mather et al, 1987). No evidence to date, however, defines a clear-cut role for mitoxantrone in treating any gynecologic cancer.

CHROMOMYCINS

The chromomycin family of antitumor antibiotics includes at least two clinically useful drugs: actinomycin D (dactinomycin; ACT-D) and mithramycin. These agents act to block DNA-directed RNA synthesis and, to a lesser extent, DNA synthesis, by intercalating adjoining DNA nucleotide pairs. This action is cell cycle nonspecific. The other characteristics of the two drugs are sufficiently different to warrant separate discussion.

Actinomycin D, a product of *Streptomyces v. parvullus*, has been in clinical use for over 25 years. The dose-limiting toxicity of ACT-D is usually myelosuppression manifested as both leukopenia and thrombocytopenia, with a nadir at 7 to 10 days and recovery 21 days after drug administration. Equally important, however, are adverse effects such as mucositis, nausea, vomiting, and diarrhea. These may also be dose limiting on occasion. Other significant toxicities include immunosuppression, alopecia, maculopapular rash, radiation recall reaction, and skin and soft tissue necrosis upon extravasation. Excretion of ACT-D involves both the liver and the kidney; hence dose reduction is called for in the face of impairment of either organ system.

Mithramycin, a product of *Streptomyces tanashiensis*, is an intercalating agent similar to ACT-D and the anthracyclines. Its principal use in clinical medicine relates to its ability to lower serum calcium by inhibiting osteoclasts and blocking parathormone. Although it has a potent effect on germ cell neoplasms, its use is limited by severe and unpredictable toxicity manifested primarily as a hemorrhagic diathesis independent of measurable platelet and coagulation deficiencies. Other significant adverse effects include hepatic and renal toxicity; acute gastrointestinal toxicity, such as nausea, vomiting, and diarrhea; and acute central nervous system effects manifested by headache and irritability progressing to lethargy.

MITOMYCIN

Mitomycin, a product of *Streptomyces caespitosus*, has three potentially active groups: quinone, urethane, and aziridine moieties. The major mechanism of action appears to result from reduction of the quinones to yield a bifunctional or possibly trifunctional alkylating agent capable of producing DNA crosslinks. As in the case of the other alkylating agents, this action is cell cycle nonspecific.

The dose-limiting adverse effect is myelosuppression characterized by a delayed nadir between 3 and 8 weeks after drug administration; the effect is cumulative with repeated doses. All three formed elements of the blood are affected. Nausea and vomiting are also seen. Other significant but less common side effects include nephrotoxicity, interstitial pneumonitis, pulmonary fibrosis and tissue necrosis with extravasation. This complication is handled in the same fashion as anthracycline extravasation.

BLEOMYCINS

The bleomycins are a group of 13 glycopeptide fractions, the main component of which has been designated bleomycin A2. These substances are fermentation products of *Streptomyces verticillus*. Convention now designates 1 mg as equal to 1 unit of activity even though the potency varies between 1.2 and 1.7 units/mg. The drug binds to DNA, causing strand breaks and inhibition of DNA polymerase. This action is cell cycle specific, with the major effect falling in the G_2 and M phases; as a result, this antibiotic tends to be administered at more frequent intervals or by prolonged infusion.

The bleomycins, unlike other antitumor antibiotics and most alkylating agents, do not produce significant myelosuppression. Acute toxicities of note include anaphylactoid reactions and fever associated with sweating, dehydration, and hypotension within the first 24 hours after drug administration. The fever results from the liberation of endogenous pyrogen from leukocytes. Dermatologic toxicity, the most common adverse effect seen with bleomycin, is characterized by blistering, hyperpigmentation, and alopecia.

The most significant adverse effect observed with the bleomycins, however, is delayed pulmonary toxicity. Presenting symptoms include dry cough and shortness of breath; the chest radiograph shows infiltrates, a reflection of pneumonitis that can progress to fibrosis. This toxicity is dose related, with an incidence as high as 55 percent in patients who receive a cumulative drug dose in excess of 283 mg/m² (Sostman et al, 1977). Reversible impairment of pulmonary function and a hypersensitivity pneumonitis responsive to steroids can be seen in association with a much lower total dose of bleomycin. The overall incidence of this complication is 11 percent, with a 0 to 6 percent mortality in various series. The appearance of signs and symptoms suggestive of the problem should therefore prompt cessation of further bleomycin therapy.

Although changes in pulmonary function tests are seen with bleomycin pulmonary toxicity, no single test provides a specific means of monitoring for the appearance of a premonitory change. Serial measurement of carbon monoxide diffusion capacity (D_{CO}) has been recommended, but its value is disputed, and Piotti et al (1984) reported that there is little correlation between D_{CO} and bleomycin-induced pulmonary toxicity. Cognizance of high-risk factors can affect clinical decisions, however. The known risk factors include age greater than 70 years, cumulative dose greater than 400 units, radiotherapy to the chest, renal dysfunction, and bolus administration. In addition, patients who receive a high cumulative dose of bleomycin have an increased risk of serious pulmonary toxicity when exposed to a high forced inspiratory oxygen concentration (FiO_2). When such a patient undergoes general anesthesia, the FiO_2 should be maintained below 35 percent.

Other Alkylating Agents

There are several additional agents with alkylator-like activity that merit consideration: the metal coordination complexes and hexamethylmelamine. The metal coordination complexes contain platinum or another heavy metal as the base molecule, and represent a relatively new class of antineoplastic drugs. The only commercially available members of this class are cisplatin and carboplatin.

PLATINUM COMPOUNDS

Cisplatin (*cis*-diamminedichloroplatinum II; Fig. 16–6) has significant activity against a broad spectrum of tumors. Several mechanisms of action are proposed: inhibition of DNA precursors, intrastrand crosslinking of DNA, and unmasking of antigenic sites on the cell membrane. Regardless, the effect is cell cycle nonspecific.

The drug has significant multiple adverse effects. At the time of the initial trials, the major and dose-limiting toxicity was manifested by renal tubular damage with a consequent rise in blood urea nitrogen and creatinine and, occasionally, severe depletion of potassium, magnesium, and calcium. This effect is usually reversible and may be prevented by the use of vigorous diuresis, with or without mannitol, before, during, and after the administration of the drug. Use of other nephrotoxic agents, such as the aminoglycoside antibiotics, concomitantly with cisplatin can worsen the nephrotoxicity and should be avoided or approached with caution.

The development of reasonably effective preventive measures for the nephrotoxicity of cisplatin has turned attention to certain other adverse effects of the drug. Cumulative, dose-related neurotoxicity manifested by paresthesias, ototoxicity initially involving high-frequency hearing loss, and seizures have assumed increasing importance as long-term, dose-limiting effects. The neurotoxicity is enhanced when other neurotoxic agents such as the vinca alkaloids are used with cisplatin.

Acute toxicities seen with cisplatin include transient myelosuppression, severe nausea and vomiting, and allergic phenomena, including anaphylactic reactions. The myelosuppression is usually not severe and exhibits nadir leukocyte and platelet counts at 2 weeks after drug administration, with recovery by 3 weeks. The emesis is severe, immediate, and usually short in duration. This may be ameliorated by high-dose metoclopramide and/or steroids given prior to and following cisplatin administration. The antiemetics ondansetron and granisetron are even more effective than metoclopromide in preventing the nausea and vomiting associated with cisplatin administration, especially in combination with dexamethasone (Roila et al, 1991).

The plethora and severity of adverse effects seen with cisplatin generated interest in certain analogs that appeared to have less toxicity in early clinical studies. One of these, the platinum II compound *carboplatin* (1,1-cyclobutane-dicarboxylatodiammine-platinum II; JM-8; CBDCA) (Fig. 16–6), was initially released for use as second-line chemotherapy for ovarian carcinoma. Carboplatin is associated with less nephrotoxicity, nausea and vomiting, and neurotoxicity but greater myelotoxicity than cisplatin. The current role of carboplatin in the treatment of gynecologic cancer is quite extensive and is discussed in detail later.

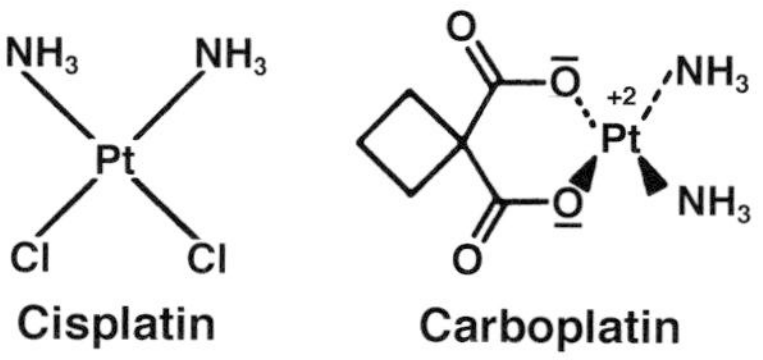

HEXAMETHYLMELAMINE

Hexamethylmelamine (altretamine; Hexalen; HMM) is a derivative of cyanuric chloride. Although the precise mechanism of action is not known, it is believed that alkylation is an important part of its cytotoxicity based on its similarity to a known alkylating agent, triethylenemelamine. The dose-limiting toxicity is gastrointestinal: anorexia, nausea, vomiting, diarrhea, and abdominal cramps. Neurotoxicity may also occur in the form of peripheral neuropathy and central nervous system effects such as confusion, hallucinations, depression, and Parkinson-like symptoms. Myelotoxicity is usually mild (Foster et al, 1986). Hexamethylmelamine has been put on the market for use as a second-line agent in ovarian carcinoma.

Antimetabolites

Unlike the alkylating agents, the antimetabolites are all cell cycle specific and exert their effect in S phase by interference with the process of DNA synthesis. This fact indicates that only those cells actively participating in the cell cycle at the time of drug administration will be affected, and argues for a more prolonged or frequent period of administration for these drugs as compared to the cycle-nonspecific alkylating agents. Four broad groups of compounds fit into this class: the

FIGURE 16–6. The currently available platinum compounds. Both are very useful, active agents in gynecologic oncology.

folate antagonists, the purine antagonists, the pyrimidine antagonists, and the ribonucleotide reductase inhibitors.

Folate Antagonists

METHOTREXATE

Methotrexate (MTX), a 4-amino-10-methyl analog of folic acid (Fig. 16–7), is the only commercially available folic acid antagonist currently in use in the treatment of gynecologic neoplasms. The drug acts by binding reversibly to dihydrofolate reductase, preventing the reduction of folic acid to tetrahydrofolate, which is essential to the production of thymidine and purine bases. The drug inhibits the synthesis of DNA, RNA, and protein, but its effects quickly abate when the drug leaves the cell. Methotrexate requires active transport into the cell. Resistance results when either the intracellular quantity of dihydrofolate reductase rises to levels greater than can be successfully bound by the available MTX, or the transport mechanism is no longer available in the target cells. The latter mechanism is probably the more important. Very high doses of MTX have been employed to overcome tumor resistance (see later).

The dose-limiting toxicity for conventional therapy with methotrexate is myelosuppression manifested by leukopenia, thrombocytopenia, and anemia. Nausea and vomiting may also be seen, as well as mucositis, which, if severe, causes diarrhea, hemorrhage, and even intestinal perforation. Thus significant gastrointestinal adverse affects are an indication for cessation of therapy until recovery occurs; a dose reduction is required upon resumption of therapy. A variety of dermatologic adverse effects also may be seen, including rashes, alterations in pigmentation, photosensitivity, and alopecia.

Hepatic, renal, and central nervous system toxicity occur on occasion. Of particular note is the association between long-term MTX therapy and hepatic fibrosis or cirrhosis, which can lead to death (Perry, 1996). Renal failure, which is more prone to develop in association with the high-dose schedule, may be prevented by alkalinization of the urine and hydration. Adverse effects on the central nervous system, seen with intrathecal administration, may assume the form of an encephalopathy or dizziness and blurred vision.

High-dose MTX followed by administration of leucovorin (folinic acid) exploits the facts that both MTX and leucovorin require the same active transport system, and that neoplastic cells, but not normal cells, can apparently delete this transport mechanism. High-dose MTX presumably achieves cell entry independent of active transport. The follow-up doses of leucovorin bypass the block of dihydrofolate reductase, "rescuing" the normal tissues that retain this transport mechanism. The neoplastic tissues, which do not retain the transport mechanism, are not rescued. However, it has been difficult to prove clinically that such an approach offers a significant therapeutic advantage over conventional doses; hence it cannot be recommended for routine clinical use, especially in view of the marked increase in cost as compared to conventional doses. Nevertheless, higher than standard doses of MTX are still employed in some popular trophoblastic disease treatment protocols.

OTHER ANTIFOLATES

Over the last few years several new antifolates have been developed with the intent of avoiding some of the mechanisms of resistance to MTX. Trimetrexate (Neutrexin) and tomudex (ZD1694) are among the more promising agents. Trimetrexate is characterized by a greater liposolubility than MTX, not requiring a carrier system for cellular transport, and by an absent potential for polyglutamation. The main toxicity seen with this drug is myelosuppression. Other side effects are skin toxicity, mucositis, fever, nausea, and vomiting (Lin and Bertino, 1991). Tomudex is a quinazoline antifolate that is also a potent inhibitor of thymidylate synthetase. Like MTX,

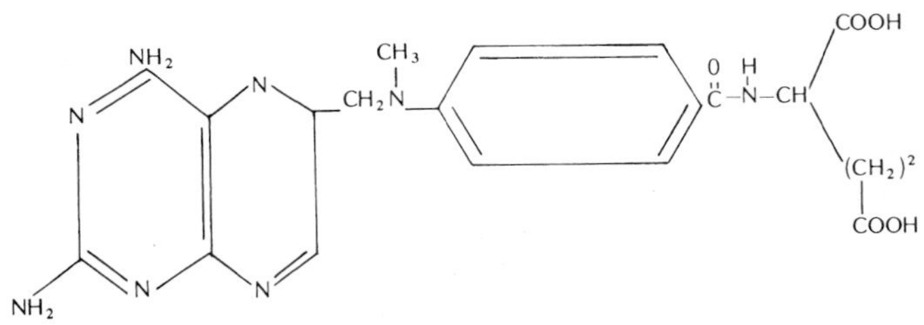

FIGURE 16–7. Methotrexate (Amethopterin).

it requires a folate carrier to enter cells. Its principal mechanism of action is by inhibition of thymidylate synthetase, producing a depletion of deoxythymidine triphosphate (dTTP), which is required for repair and synthesis of DNA. The major toxicities are anorexia, fatigue, diarrhea, myelosuppression, and reversible transaminasemia (Clark et al, 1994). Neither of these compounds has shown significant activity in gynecologic tumors.

Purine Antagonists

Purine antagonists inhibit DNA synthesis by acting as false metabolites as a result of their similarities to natural purines. The two members of this group currently in use as antineoplastic agents, 6-mercaptopurine (6-MP) and 6-thioguanine, are rarely indicated for treatment of gynecologic cancers. The first is an analog of hypoxanthine and hence interferes with the proper incorporation of adenine into DNA. The second is an analog of guanine and exerts its influence in relation to that moiety. The actions of both agents are specific for the S phase and primarily interfere with DNA synthesis. For both drugs, the dose-limiting toxicity is myelosuppression. Gastrointestinal toxicity and intrahepatic cholestasis are occasionally seen. The use of allopurinol with 6-MP should be avoided because 6-MP is metabolized by xanthine oxidase, the target enzyme for allopurinol.

Pyrimidine Antagonists

The pyrimidine antagonists are similar to the pyrimidine bases that make up DNA and RNA. The principal effect of the drugs is on DNA synthesis, however. Thus they are cell cycle specific for the S phase. The drugs that make up this group can be divided into two subgroups, the fluoropyrimidines and the cytidine analogs.

FLUOROPYRIMIDINES

The fluoropyrimidines include three agents: 5-FU, FUDR, and ftorafur. The most commonly used fluoropyrimidine is 5-FU, which achieves its cytotoxic effect by acting as a false pyrimidine to compete successfully for the enzyme thymidylate synthetase. This interferes with the production of thymidine and ultimately with the synthesis of DNA. 5-Fluorouracil is not only an active chemotherapeutic agent but is also an effective radiation sensitizer. The adverse effects seen with 5-FU include gastrointestinal toxicity, myelosuppression, and dermatologic problems. The gastrointestinal toxicity is often dose limiting and is manifested as nausea, vomiting, diarrhea, and stomatitis. The last is the most important because its appearance portends extensive ulceration of the mucosal surface of the gastrointestinal tract. The myelosuppression affects both leukocytes and platelets, with a nadir at 7 to 14 days. The dermatologic adverse effects consist of alopecia, hyperpigmentation, photosensitivity, and occasionally a maculopapular rash, which rarely progresses to become a severe problem. The other two fluoropyrimidines, *FUDR* and *ftorafur*, are similar to 5-FU in their spectrum of activity and their adverse effects. FUDR has been advocated for arterial and intraperitoneal infusion. 5-Fluorouracil is employed topically to treat vaginal and vulvar intraepithelial squamous lesions. Neither 5-FU (except as a radiation sensitizer; see Chapter 17) nor FUDR has a major role in gynecologic cancer therapy.

CYTIDINE ANALOGS

The cytidine analogs include cytosine arabinoside, azacytidine, and gemcitabine. *Cytosine arabinoside* is metabolized by deoxycytidine kinase to its triphosphorylated derivative, which in turn acts as a competitive inhibitor of DNA polymerase to block DNA synthesis. This action is cell cycle specific for the S phase. The dose-limiting and only major toxicity of the drug is myelosuppression manifested as leukopenia and thrombocytopenia. Nausea, vomiting, and stomatitis are occasionally seen, and a flu-like syndrome with fever, arthralgias, and rash is also reported.

Gemcitabine is an analogue of deoxycytidine that resembles cytosine arabinoside in structure and metabolism (Plunkett et al, 1996). It reduces deoxynucleotide pools by inhibiting ribonucleotide reductase. It is also incorporated into DNA, blocking further elongation of the DNA chain. Gemcitabine has a low incidence of side effects. Myelosuppression is mild, and serious complications are rare. Proteinuria, hematuria, elevation of liver transaminases, nausea, vomiting, flu-like symptoms, and peripheral edema have been reported (Green et al, 1996).

Ribonucleotide Reductase Inhibitors

The single ribonucleotide reductase inhibitor currently in use in gynecologic cancer therapy is *hydroxyurea* (HU). The conversion of ribonucleotides to deoxyribonucleotides is one pathway by which the components of DNA can be generated in cells. This step, catalyzed by the enzyme ribonucleotide reductase, is blocked by HU, which results in the inhibition of DNA synthesis. Hydroxyurea is thus specific for the S phase. Whether there are other effects of this drug is not known. The major and dose-limiting toxicity is myelosuppression manifested primarily as leukopenia. Nausea, vomiting, and diarrhea are also commonly seen at high doses. Less commonly, rashes and impairment of renal tubular function may be seen. Hydroxyurea is employed primarily as a radiation sensitizer in the treatment of cervical carcinoma.

Plant Alkaloids

The plant alkaloids are naturally occurring compounds derived from certain species of plant life. Despite the fact that the plant of origin varies, the mechanism of action for each of the six agents in clinical use is similar. They produce an arrest of the cell's progression through mitosis in metaphase; hence these drugs are cell cycle specific for M phase. The drugs in this class fit into three groups according to their source: the vinca alkaloids, the podophyllotoxins, and the taxanes.

Vinca Alkaloids

Vinca alkaloids are derived from the periwinkle plant. Three members of this group are in current clinical use: vincristine, vinblastine, and vinorelbine. They are similar in chemical structure and mechanism of action, yet their spectrum of antitumor activity and adverse effects are surprisingly different. Only vicristine and vinblastine are used frequently in the treatment of gynecologic cancers, but vinorelbine has prospects for ovarian cancer therapy.

VINCRISTINE

Vincristine, like the other vinca alkaloids, binds to the microtubular protein of the mitotic spindle, causing tubule polymerization. Not all cells are irreversibly damaged; a certain proportion can escape and proceed with cell division. Other effects that might explain the cytotoxicity of the drug appear only at concentrations higher than those normally achieved in the cell.

Vincristine exhibits neurotoxicity as its dose-limiting side effect. This adverse effect is secondary to interference with the function of microtubules in axons. Peripheral neuropathies manifested by a loss of deep tendon reflexes, weakness, and paresthesias are the earliest clinical signs to appear, but autonomic neuropathies, severe jaw pain (probably secondary to a trigeminal neuralgia), and central nervous system toxicity, including coma, may appear later. These effects are usually reversible but may take months to disappear. Although neurotoxicity is seen with the other vinca alkaloids, the degree and frequency are much greater with vincristine, probably because of its greater polarity and binding affinity for tubulin.

Other adverse effects are relatively less important. The drug appears to be minimally myelosuppressive and capable of producing a syndrome of inappropriate secretion of antidiuretic hormone. Alopecia is usually total and consistent, and the drug can produce significant tissue irritation at sites of extravasation.

VINBLASTINE

Vinblastine differs from vincristine only in the replacement of a formyl side chain with a methyl group on one portion of the molecule. Despite this relatively minor difference and an apparently identical mechanism of action, vinblastine neurotoxicity is infrequent. Its dose-limiting toxicity is myelosuppression manifested primarily as leukopenia, although thrombocytopenia can be seen. Other adverse effects include nausea, vomiting, skin rash, photosensitivity, and stomatitis, all typically mild and reversible. Alopecia is consistent and total, as with vincristine, and the drug causes severe irritation and tissue necrosis at sites of extravasation.

VINORELBINE

Vinorelbine differs from other vinca alkaloids in that the catharantine nucleus contains an eight-member ring that replaces the traditional nine-member ring (Potier et al, 1989). The dose-limiting toxicity is neutropenia; severe anemia and thrombocytopenia are uncommon. Mild peripheral neuropathy occurs frequently. Reversible, asymptomatic elevations of alkaline phosphatase can appear. Phlebitis is frequently encountered. In preclinical models vinorelbine is more active than vinblastine or vincristine (Burris and Fields, 1994).

Epipodophyllotoxins

The podophyllotoxins are derived from the root of the May-apple plant (*Podophyllum peltatum*). Two semisynthetic derivatives are used in clinical oncology: etoposide and teniposide. Although the mechanism of action for the natural podophyllotoxin is similar to that of the vinca alkaloids, these derivatives induce cytotoxicity by a different mechanism. Both etoposide and teniposide bind to topoisomerase-11, inhibiting regulation of DNA and inducing breaks in DNA.

Etoposide is the only podophyllotoxin with activity in gynecologic tumors. In addition to the observed metaphase arrest, the drug causes an inhibition of cell entry into mitosis and suppression of DNA synthesis. These observations suggest that etoposide is cell cycle specific not only for M phase but also, to some extent, for G_2 and S phases. The dose-limiting toxicity for etoposide is to the bone marrow, manifested as leukopenia and thrombocytopenia, with a nadir at 2 weeks and recovery by 3 weeks. Nausea and vomiting are not uncommon, and severe hypotension can be seen, especially with too-rapid infusion of the drug. Bronchospasm responsive to antihistamines has also been noted, and alopecia does occur.

Because etoposide is phase specific and preclinical data suggest schedule dependency, its administration as a daily oral regimen has been evaluated. Oral etoposide has an average bioavailability of approximately 50 percent, but there is marked inter- and intrapatient variability. As with the standard IV administration, myelosuppression is the dose-limiting toxicity of the oral route.

Taxanes

The taxanes are complex esters consisting of a 15-member taxane ring linked to a 4-member oxetane ring. Two taxanes are commercially available and show activity in gynecologic neoplasms: taxol (paclitaxel) and taxotere (docetaxel). Both drugs share a unique mechanism of action, the enhancement of tubulin polymerization and microtubule stability, to produce microtubule bundling throughout the cell (Rowinsky et al, 1988). This inhibits the dynamic reorganization of the microtubular structure of the cell before cell division. This unique mechanism of action probably accounts for the apparent lack of cross-resistance between these drugs and the platinum analogs.

TAXOL

Taxol was isolated from the bark of the Western yew tree (*Taxus brevifolia*) (Fig. 16–8). Early on, the drug was in short supply because of environmental concerns and the limited number of Western yew trees. Currently the supply of taxol is not a problem because the drug is produced semisynthetically. Taxol is characterized by its insolubility, which requires the use of a vehicle (Cremaphor) for administration. In early trials Cremaphor hypersensitivity was the dose-limiting toxicity, but this has been largely overcome by administration of the drug after premedication with steroids as well as histamine-1 and -2 blockers, which prevents nearly all hypersensitivity reactions.

Adverse effects, in addition to hypersensitivity, include myelosuppression, neuropathy, cardiotoxicity, alopecia, and gastrointestinal toxicity manifested as mucositis, diarrhea, nausea, and vomiting (Donehower et al, 1987; Grem et al, 1987; Ohnuma et al, 1985; Wiernik et al, 1987). Noteworthy in early trials was the cardiotoxicity, manifested by bradycardia, atrioventricular conduction block, left bundle-branch block, ventricular tachycardia, and evidence of cardiac ischemia. The more serious arrhythmias were observed in 5 percent of patients (Rowinsky et al, 1991b).

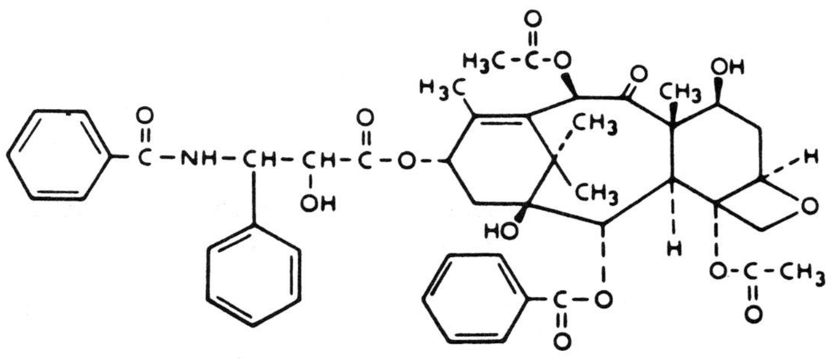

FIGURE 16–8. Paclitaxel (Taxol) is a diterpenoid derived from the Western yew tree. It is an active agent in the treatment of many gynecologic malignancies, especially ovarian carcinoma.

Because of these cardiac effects, a continuous infusion for up to 24 hours and cardiac monitoring were initially recommended. Myelosuppression is the most common dose-limiting toxicity, with a majority of patients experiencing severe leukopenia and/or thrombocytopenia at an initial dose of 175 mg/m^2 over 24 hours every 3 weeks. The period of myelosuppression, however, tends to be of brief duration.

It has become evident that taxol is schedule dependent. Preclinical data suggest an increase in cytotoxicity with prolonged exposure to the drug. Clinical trials have compared the effects of administering the drug as either a 3-hour or 24-hour infusion (Eisenhauer et al, 1994). These studies demonstrated that the drug could be safely administered as a 3-hour infusion. Current studies are evaluating a 1-hour infusion schedule. The toxicity profile of taxol is modified with the duration of administration. Prolonged infusions produce more severe mucositis, diarrhea, and hematologic toxicity; shorter infusions produce more peripheral neuropathy, arthralgias, and myalgias. Taxol has a broad spectrum of activity and has become one of the most important agents in the treatment of gynecologic cancers, particularly ovarian carcinoma. The optimal dose and schedule of administration are still under investigation.

TAXOTERE

Taxotere is a semisynthetic analog of taxol, initially extracted from the European yew tree (*Taxus baccata*). It shares its mechanism of action with taxol, but preclinical data show it to be more active. The drug is administered as a 1-hour infusion. The dose-limiting toxicity is to the bone marrow: neutropenia, anemia, and thrombocytopenia are common. Other side effects are hypersensitivity cutaneous reactions and alopecia. Taxotere has shown an activity profile similar to that of taxol (Cortes and Pazdur, 1995).

Other Useful Agents

Not included in those classes of drugs already discussed are two compounds that deserve consideration because of their potential or demonstrated clinical utility in gynecologic cancer. These are topotecan and dimethyl-triazeno-imidazole carboxamide (DTIC).

Topotecan is a semisynthetic analog of camptothecin, whose mechanism of action is to inhibit topoisomerase-1. Topotecan is administered as a 5-day intravenous infusion. The dose-limiting toxicity is severe myelosuppression, particularly neutropenia. The neutropenia is of short duration, however. Gastrointestinal toxicity is mild. No significant fluid retention, fever, or neurologic, cardiac, or renal toxicities are seen. Topotecan has proven activity against platinum-resistant ovarian carcinoma.

DTIC (dacarbazine) is an analog of a purine intermediate. It probably acts as an alkylating agent, but other possible mechanisms of action include inhibition of DNA synthesis as a purine precursor and interaction with protein sulfhydryl groups. Whatever the mechanism, the drug does not appear to be cell cycle specific. The dose-limiting toxicity is myelosuppression affecting both leukocytes and platelets, with a nadir 3 weeks after drug administration. Other adverse effects include severe, frequent nausea and vomiting and a flu-like syndrome of fever and myalgias.

CHEMOTHERAPY OF OVARIAN CANCER

Ovarian cancer is a heterogeneous group of neoplasms that contains four broad categories: celomic epithelial, germ cell, stromal, and miscellaneous. The role of chemotherapy in each of the first three of these categories is considered in detail in this section.

Epithelial Carcinoma

The malignant lesions of epithelial origin comprise 85 to 90 percent of ovarian cancers. Chemotherapy is an essential part of the treatment of the majority of patients with epithelial carcinoma of the ovary, both because these patients tend to present with advanced disease and because these lesions are very sensitive to cytotoxic drugs. The principal factor influencing the selection of therapy is the extent of disease at the time of diagnosis. Because these tumors spread principally by the intraperitoneal route, evaluation necessarily focuses on the abdominal cavity and includes a detailed staging laparotomy. The results of such an evaluation allow the division of patients into two groups: those with advanced (stages III and IV) disease and those with early (stages I and II) disease (see Chapter 10). The management of only the advanced stages is discussed in this chapter.

There are three basic clinical situations that confront the physician with therapeutic decisions in regard to patients with advanced ovarian carcinoma: surgical decisions at the time of initial patient presentation, decisions regarding the choice of chemotherapy following primary surgery, and selection of appropriate salvage therapy at the time of disease recurrence.

Initial Surgical Decisions — Cytoreductive Surgery

There is a general consensus that advanced epithelial carcinoma of the ovary requires as the initial step in management a detailed exploratory laparotomy for diagnosis, to assess extent of disease, and to attempt maximal surgical reduction of disease. Patients who have only small-volume disease after such an effort have an improved frequency of response to chemotherapy and a significantly improved survival (Omura et al, 1991). The definition of small-volume (optimal) residual disease has varied from no gross residual to nodules no larger than 3 cm in maximum diameter. Regardless of the definition, these data suggest that the survival of patients with "small-volume" disease is better than the survival of those with large-volume disease, that surgical tumor reduction should be attempted, and that clinical trials of advanced ovarian carcinoma must take tumor volume into account in order to yield a valid assessment of differences between treatments.

Criticism of these conclusions has focused on the fact that a significant proportion of patients present with small-volume disease (and thus require no surgical cytoreduction to achieve small-volume status), and that these patients could account for the entire improvement in survival simply as a reflection of the innate biologic characteristics of their neoplasms. Implicit in this line of reasoning is the hypothesis that surgical cytoreduction has no impact on outcome. An analysis of a large population of patients with postsurgical small-volume residual disease confirms that patients who achieved small-volume status as a result of surgical cytoreduction had a significantly greater likelihood of shorter PFI and survival than those who did not require surgical cytoreduction to achieve small-volume status (Hoskins et al, 1992). The group that was cytoreduced to the small-volume category, however, did appear to do better than those patients who were left with

large-volume disease. Although this neither proves nor disproves the value of surgical cytoreduction, the most probable interpretation is that the advanced disease population consists of three groups: those with small-volume disease at the time the abdomen is opened (the "best" group), those who achieve small-volume disease a a result of surgical cytoreduction (the "intermediate" group), and those left with large-volume disease (the "worst" group).

Additional support for the role of cytoreductive surgery came from a randomized trial of the EORTC (van der Burg et al, 1995). This study demonstrated that interval surgical cytoreduction results in a superior progression-free and overall survival as compared to chemotherapy alone. The results of this trial conclusively prove that there is a survival benefit from cytoreductive surgery. This topic is discussed in more detail in Chapter 10.

First-Line Chemotherapy

After evaluation and initial surgical tumor reduction, systemic chemotherapy is the treatment of choice. Selection of appropriate first-line chemotherapy requires that six issues be addressed:

1. Should the patient receive combination chemotherapy or a single agent?
2. Is a platinum compound an essential part of therapy?
3. If a platinum compound is essential, which one is the optimal agent?
4. What is the optimal platinum-based combination of drugs?
5. What is the role of paclitaxel (taxol)?
6. What dose, schedule, and route of administration should be chosen?

COMBINATION VERSUS
SINGLE-AGENT THERAPY

In regard to combination as opposed to single-agent chemotherapy, a number of systemic agents (Table 16–2) have demonstrated activity against ovarian carcinoma. Prior to 1976, standard therapy consisted of a single alkylating agent, usually melphalan or leukeran. The response rate as demonstrated by the Gynecologic Oncology Group (GOG) in the melphalan control arm of three different studies of suboptimal ovarian cancer (dose = 0.2 mg/kg/day for 5 days every 4 to 6 weeks), was 33 percent, with half of the responses being clinically complete. The median dura-

Single-Agent Activity in Celomic Epithelial Carcinoma of the Ovary*

Drug	Patients	Response Rate (%)
Alkylating agents	1,371	33
Ifosfamide	37	22
Cisplatin	190	32
Carboplatin	82	24
Doxorubicin	102	33
5-Fluorouracil	126	29
Methotrexate	34	18
Mitomycin	49	16
Hexamethylmelamine	215	24
Paclitaxel	155	35
Oral etoposide	41	27[†]
Topotecan	67	13[†]
Gemcitabine	27	22
Doxil	34	29
Navelbine	24	21
Progestins	176	12
Antiestrogens	42	19
Alpha-interferon	21	19
Gamma-interferon	14	29

*Modified from Thigpen JT: Chemotherapy of gynecologic cancer. In Perry MC (ed): The Chemotherapy Source Book, 2nd ed. Baltimore, Williams & Wilkins, 1996, p 1253, with permission.
[†]Platinum/paclitaxel-resistant patients only.

tion of the response for these suboptimal cases was 7 months, and the median survival was 12 months. A randomized trial in patients with large-volume disease (Omura et al, 1983b, 1991) demonstrated that ADR plus CTX produced a superior frequency of clinically complete responses (but similar survival) to melphalan alone.

NEED FOR A PLATINUM COMPOUND

The GOG then compared ADR plus CTX to ADR plus CTX plus cisplatin (PAC) (Table 16–3). The platinum-based combination (PAC) yielded results significantly superior to those of the two-drug combination in regard to the clinically complete response rate, overall response rate, and duration of remission. For those patients with measurable disease, overall survival was also significantly better with the cisplatin combination. Although there were too few patients with second-look laparotomy to determine whether the pathologically complete response rate was significantly better with the three-drug regimen, the trend was definitely in that direction. These results suggested that platinum-based combination chemotherapy is superior to therapy with a single alkylating agent and also to CTX + ADR in patients with large-volume residual disease. The addition of the platinum compound to the combination, however, added significantly to the toxicity of the regimen.

In addition to the evidence already cited, long-term follow-up of a study of The Netherlands Joint Study Group for Ovarian Cancer comparing a non-platinum-containing regimen (HMM plus CTX plus MTX plus 5-FU; Hexa-CAF) to a platinum-based combination (CTX plus HMM plus ADR plus cisplatin; CHAP-5) provides further support for the central role of the platinum compound in optimal therapy (Neijt et al, 1984, 1991). At a median follow-up of 9.5 years, 9 percent of the Hexa-CAF patients and 21 percent of the CHAP-5 patients were alive. This points to the superiority of the platinum-based regimen. Even more significantly, half of the surviving Hexa-CAF patients had relapsed but were alive at 9.5 years as a result of response to salvage platinum-based therapy.

CARBOPLATIN VERSUS CISPLATIN AS THE OPTIMAL AGENT

The introduction of a second platinum compound, carboplatin, raised the question of which platinum compound should be a part of first-line therapy. Three randomized trials comparing cisplatin 100 mg/m² every 4 weeks to carboplatin 400 mg/m² every 4 weeks (Adams et al, 1989; Pecorelli et al, 1988; Wiltshaw, 1985) have been completed. A meta-analysis of these three studies (Table 16–4) demonstrates similar response rates, PFI, and survival for the two drugs (Rosencweig et al, 1990). Expected differences in the adverse effects include a greater frequency of neutropenia and thrombocytopenia with carboplatin and a greater frequency of neurotoxicity with cisplatin. Very little nephrotoxicity was seen with either drug. Although these trials were not designed as equivalency studies, the meta-analysis certainly suggests that the drugs have equal efficacy.

An additional four randomized trials evaluated the relative efficacy of cisplatin-based combination chemotherapy versus the same combination based on carboplatin (Table 16–5). These trials were designed to look for a stated difference in either response rate or survival between the two regimens. The only trial to demonstrate any statistically significant difference was the Edmondson et al (1989) study of CTX plus either cisplatin or carboplatin, in which the cisplatin regimen produced superior survival. This study was

T A B L E **16–3**

GOG Trials of Combination Chemotherapy in Advanced
Ovarian Carcinoma*,†

Parameter	Protocol 22 (L-PAM vs. AC)		Protocol 47 (AC vs. PAC)	
Patients	64	72	120	107
Complete response (CR) (%)	20	32	26	51
Total response (CR + PR) (%)	37	49	48	76
Pathologic CR	4/23	13/39		
PCR/total (%)	3	12		
Duration (mo)	8	10	9	15
Median survival (mo)	12	14	16	20

*Data from Omura et al. (1986a, 1989).
†L-PAM = melphalan 0.2 mg/kg/day orally for 5 days every 4–6 weeks for 10 courses; AC = Adriamycin 50 mg/m² plus Cytoxan 500 mg/m² both IV every 3 weeks for eight courses; PAC = Cisplatin 50 mg/m² plus Adriamycin and Cytoxan as in AC given IV every 3 weeks for eight courses; PR = partial response; CR = complete response; PCR = pathologic complete response.

potentially flawed by a difference in the dose intensity of the platinum compound between the two regimens (the carboplatin dose was only 150 mg/m², significantly less dose intense than the cisplatin dose of 60 mg/m²). This difference in dose intensity could well explain the observed difference in survival. [An alternative explanation could be that all of the regimens had 4-week cycles, but the cisplatin was administered at doses employed for a 3-week cycle. —Editors]

The weight of evidence favors the conclusion that cisplatin and carboplatin are therapeutically equivalent. The choice of a platinum compound thus rests on the differing spectrum of adverse effects, a choice that fa-

vors carboplatin. Furthermore, under ordinary circumstances, ease of administration on an ambulatory basis and cost also favor carboplatin.

The Advanced Ovarian Cancer Trialists Group (1991) addressed each of these first three issues in a meta-analysis. The study involved 8,139 patients from 45 different trials. Five separate comparisons were conducted. The first three comparisons looked at (1) single nonplatinum agents versus non-platinum-based combinations, (2) single nonplatinum agents versus platinum-based combinations, and (3) combination regimens with or without a platinum compound. None of these comparisons showed a significant difference,

T A B L E **16–4**

Meta-Analysis Comparing Cisplatin to Carboplatin as Single
Agents in Ovarian Carcinoma*

Parameter	Cisplatin	Carboplatin
Patients	195	190
Response	71/120 (59%)	80/142 (56%)
Complete	31/120 (26%)	36/142 (25%)
Partial	40/120 (33%)	44/142 (31%)
Survival (median, mo)	23	22
Adverse effects†		
Leukopenia	30/171 (18%)	57/187 (30%)
Thrombocytopenia	2/171 (1%)	40/187 (22%)
Emesis	120/173 (69%)	100/187 (53%)
Neuropathy	30/173 (17%)	1/187 (1%)
Ototoxicity	22/173 (13%)	4/187 (2%)
Azotemia	2/161 (1%)	1/178 (1%)
Hypomagnesemia	15/39 (38%)	11/32 (34%)

*From Rozencweig M, Martin A, Beltangady M, et al: Randomized trials of carboplatin versus cisplatin in advanced ovarian cancer. In Bunn P, Canetta R, Ozols R, Rozencweig M (eds): Carboplatin (JM-8): Current Perspectives and Future Directions. Philadelphia, WB Saunders, 1990, p. 175, with permission.
†World Health Organization grade 2 or higher.

TABLE 16–5

TABLE 16–5

Randomized Trials Comparing Cisplatin-Based to Carboplatin-Based
Combination Chemotherapy for Ovarian Carcinoma

Study and Regimen	Response*	Survival
Alberts et al. (1992) (N = 342)		
Carboplatin 300 mg/m² q4wk	cCR = 34%	20 mo
Cytoxan 600 mg/m² q4 wk	pCR = 12%	
vs.		
Cisplatin 100 mg/m² q4 wk	cCR = 27%	16.8 mo
Cytoxan 600 mg/m² q4 wk	pCR = 7%	
ten Bokkel Huininks et al. (1988) (N = 339)		
Cytoxan 100 mg/m² po d14–28	cCR = 24%	24.8 mo
HMM 150 mg/m² po d14–28		
Adriamycin 35 mg/m² IV d1		
Carboplatin 350 mg/m² IV d1		
vs.		
Cytoxan 100 mg/m² po d14–28	cCR = 23%	25 mo
HMM 150 mg/m² po d14–28		
Adriamycin 35 mg/m² IV d1		
Cisplatin 20 mg/m² IV d1–5		
Swenerton et al. (1992) (N = 447)		
Carboplatin 300 mg/m² q4 wk	pCR = 13%	24 mo
Cytoxan 600 mg/m² q4wk		
vs.		
Cisplatin 75 mg/m² q4 wk	pCR = 18%	23 mo
Cytoxan 600 mg/m² q4wk		
Edmondson et al. (1989) (N = 103)		
Carboplatin 150 mg/m² q4 wk		20 mo
Cytoxan 1000 mg/m² q4 wk		
vs.		
Cisplatin 60 mg/m² q4wk		27 mo
Cytoxan 1000 mg/m² q4 wk		

*p = pathologic; c = clinical; CR = complete response.

an observation that probably results from the fact that all but one study included in the analysis permitted the administration of a platinum-based regimen to those patients who failed non-platinum-based chemotherapy. *In essence, these comparisons evaluated immediate versus delayed platinum-based therapy.*

The fourth comparison looked at six studies that compared a platinum compound alone versus a platinum-based combination regimen. An analysis involving all six studies shows no significant difference. One of the six studies, however, compared cisplatin 100 mg/m² alone to a combination of cisplatin 20 mg/m² and chlorambucil—a fivefold difference in the platinum dose intensity between the single agent and combination arms (Wiltshaw et al, 1986). Exclusion of this trial results in a significant difference favoring platinum-based combination therapy, which yielded a 15 percent reduced risk of recurrence and death as compared to platinum alone. The fifth comparison analyzed pooled data from trials comparing carboplatin regi-

mens to cisplatin regimens. No significant differences were noted.

The meta-analysis thus supports the conclusions drawn thus far: (1) platinum-based combination chemotherapy is superior, and should be the standard of care for patients with advanced disease after initial surgery; (2) a platinum compound is the most essential element of first-line chemotherapy; and (3) cisplatin and carboplatin are equally effective but differ in their spectrum of adverse effects, ease of administration, and cost.

OPTIMAL COMBINATION THERAPY

Another critical issue is the optimum composition of the combination regimen. Although the specific drugs included in regimens vary from study to study, most combinations include at least a platinum compound plus an alkylating agent. Investigations have focused on whether ADR and, in some instances, HMM should be added to the combination. Two well-conducted randomized trials address this issue. The first was conducted by the GOG in a population of patients with small-volume advanced disease randomized to cisplatin plus CTX or cisplatin plus ADR plus CTX (Table 16–6). One critical feature of this trial is the higher dose of CTX in the two-drug arm, a feature that makes the relative dose intensity of the two regimens roughly the same (i.e., equitoxic). There was no difference in the frequency of pathologic complete response, PFI, or survival (Omura et al, 1989).

The second trial (Neijt et al, 1987), which involved both small- and large-volume disease categories, compared a combination of cisplatin and CTX every 3 weeks to cisplatin days 1 to 5 plus ADR day 1, oral CTX days 15 to 28, and oral HMM days 15 to 28. The four-drug combination was administered every 5 weeks. As in the case of the GOG trial, the two regimens in this study called for similar dose intensities in the two arms. There were no differences observed between the two arms in regard to response rate, PFI, and survival.

These two trials indicate that there is no need to include either ADR or HMM as a part of first-line chemotherapy so long as dose intensity is maintained. Nevertheless, certain studies are not in agreement, which leaves the issue open to question. Four studies (Bertelsen et al, 1987; Conte et al, 1986; Gruppo Interegionale Cooperativo Oncologico Ginecologia [GICOG], 1987; Ovarian Cancer Meta-Analysis Project, 1991) concluded that a combination including ADR was superior, but the regimens in these studies were not equitoxic, favoring the ADR arm. Thus dose intensity could explain the differences in outcome. Edmondson et al (1990),

Bruckner et al (1989), and Hainsworth et al (1990) reported that the addition of HMM improved long-term survival, but these trials have not been confirmed.

ROLE OF PACLITAXEL

The introduction of the platinum compounds into the therapeutic armamentarium for ovarian carcinoma reduced morbidity and mortality by 31 percent for patients with advanced disease and established platinum-based chemotherapy as the standard of care by the end of the 1980s (Omura et al, 1986a). Paclitaxel represents a second major addition to the therapeutic armamentarium. Interest in paclitaxel in ovarian carcinoma stemmed from the observation of responses in patients with drug-resistant ovarian carcinoma included in early Phase I trials (McGuire et al, 1989b). Subsequent Phase II trials produced an overall 35 percent response rate among 155 patients and, more importantly, a 27 percent response rate in the 52 patients deemed to be clinically resistant to initial platinum-based chemotherapy (Rowinsky et al, 1996). These Phase II results not only established paclitaxel as an active drug in ovarian carcinoma but also suggested that the drug was clinically non-cross-resistant with the platinum compounds and the alkylating agents.

In regard to the identification of an appropriate dose and schedule for a paclitaxel plus cisplatin combination, a Phase I trial yielded two important observations (Rowinsky et al, 1991a). First, paclitaxel given before cisplatin produced greater cytotoxicity with fewer side effects. Second, paclitaxel 135 mg/m^2 over 24 hours followed by cisplatin 75 mg/m^2 every 3 weeks proved to be a feasible regimen. This combination then became the first paclitaxel-based regimen to be studied in first-line therapy (GOG Protocol 111). Three randomized Phase III studies of paclitaxel-based chemotherapy have been reported.

GOG Protocol 111 (Table 16–7). The GOG randomized 386 newly diagnosed patients with large-volume advanced ovarian carcinoma to six cycles of cisplatin plus either CTX or paclitaxel preceding the cisplatin (McGuire et al, 1996). The paclitaxel-based regimen proved superior in regard to overall response rate, clinical complete response rate, percentage grossly disease free at second-look laparotomy, progression-free survival, and overall survival. Analysis of comparative risk demonstrated a 33 percent reduction in mor-

---

TABLE **16–6**

Platinum-Based Combination Chemotherapy with and without Adriamycin in Stage III Small-Volume Ovarian Carcinoma*,†

Parameter	PAC	PC
Patients	173	176
Early recurrence	19	30
Refused second look	36	37
Residual disease	73	67
Pathologic complete response	45 (26%)	42 (24%)

*From Omura G, Bundy B, Berek J, et al: Randomization of cyclophosphamide plus cisplatin with or without doxorubicin in ovarian carcinoma: a Gynecologic Oncology Group Study. J Clin Oncol 7:457, 1989, with permission.
†PC = cisplatin 50 mg/m^2 plus Cytoxan 1,000 mg/m^2 IV q3wk for eight cycles; PAC = cisplatin 50 mg/m^2 plus Adriamycin 50 mg/m^2 plus Cytoxan 500 mg/m^2 IV q3wk for eight cycles.

TABLE **16-7**

Results of GOG Protocol 111, a Randomized Phase III Trial of Cisplatin plus Cytoxan
or Paclitaxel in 386 Patients with Suboptimal Ovarian Cancer*,†

Parameter	Paclitaxel/Cisplatin	Cytoxan/Cisplatin	p Value
Clinical response rate	73%	60%	.01
Clinical complete response rate	51%	31%	.01
Grossly disease free at second look	40%	24%	.001
Pathologic complete response	26%	20%	.08
Progression-free survival	18 months	13 months	.001
Overall survival	38 months	24 months	.001

*From McGuire WP, Hoskins WJ, Brady NW, et al: Cyclophosphamide and cisplatin compared with paclitaxel and
cisplatin in patients with stage III and stage IV ovarian cancer. N Engl J Med 334:1, 1996, with permission.
†Dosages: paclitaxel = 135 mg/m² over 24 hours; cisplatin = 75 mg/m²; Cytoxan = 750 mg/m².

tality with the addition of paclitaxel to first-line chemotherapy. Although there were increased myelosuppression, cardiac problems, and alopecia with the paclitaxel-based regimen, there were no major clinical consequences. In particular, the frequency of grade 3 or 4 neurotoxicity was the same with the two regimens. The conclusion of the GOG is that paclitaxel plus cisplatn should be the standard chemotherapy for women with advanced ovarian carcinoma.

GOG Protocol 132. In this trial, 613 newly diagnosed patients with large-volume residual ovarian cancer were randomized postoperatively to six cycles at 3-week intervals of cisplatin (100 mg/m²), or paclitaxel (200 mg/m² over 24 hours), or paclitaxel plus cisplatin dosed as in GOG Protocol 111 (Muggia et al, 1997a). No differences were observed among the three arms with respect to overall survival (26.0 vs. 30.2 vs. 26.6 months, respectively), but the paclitaxel regimen arm was inferior with respect to response (46 vs. 74 vs. 72 percent, respectively) and progression-free survival (11.4 vs. 16.4 vs. 14.1 months, respectively). This trial cannot confirm the results of GOG Protocol 111, however, because less than half of the patients on the nonpaclitaxel regimen in GOG Protocol 111 received paclitaxel at the time of first relapse, whereas the vast majority of patients on the single-agent regimens of GOG Protocol 132 received the other drug prior to progression of disease. The combination is considered the regimen of choice because it is less toxic while yielding similar results to cisplatin alone, and it is superior to taxol alone in regard to response and progression-free survival.

Protocol OV-10. A Canadian-European consortium randomized patients with advanced ovarian cancer to cisplatin (75 mg/m²) plus either CTX (750 mg/m²) or 3-hour paclitaxel (175 mg/m²), each regimen given every 3 weeks for 6 cycles (Piccart et al, 1997). This trial shows superiority for the paclitaxel plus cisplatin regimen with regard to response (66 vs. 77 percent), clinical complete response (36 vs. 50 percent), and progression-free survival (12 vs. 16.6 months). The data are insufficiently mature for overall survival analysis at the present time. This study confirms GOG Protocol 111 and conclusively establishes paclitaxel plus a platinum compound as the current standard for treating advanced epithelial carcinoma of the ovary. The 24 percent rate of grade 3 neurotoxicity with the shorter paclitaxel infusion compared to 4 percent in GOG Protocol 111 indicates that carboplatin should be substituted for cisplatin if a short infusion of paclitaxel is to be used. This observation is supported by similar results in at least one other trial (Markman et al, 1996a).

DOSE, SCHEDULE, AND ROUTE
OF ADMINISTRATION

Although paclitaxel plus a platinum compound is now the accepted standard of care in the United States, efforts continue to identify the optimal dose, schedule, and route of administration. The question that has received the greatest attention is the optimal dose and schedule of the agents.

Platinum Dose Intensity.

Intravenous Dose Intensity. Because the platinum compounds are the most active agents in ovarian carcinoma, the determination of the optimal dose and schedule is the subject of much ongoing clinical investigation. In vitro data suggest a steep dose-response relationship for cisplatin (Frei and Canellos,

1980). In 1987, Levin and Hryniuk published a meta-analysis of over 60 randomized trials in ovarian carcinoma. The key observation was the correlation between response to chemotherapy and the dose intensity of cisplatin over a range of 6 to 12 mg/m²/wk (18 to 36 mg/m² every 3 weeks), a range below the lowest commonly used dose of 50 mg/m².

An extended meta-analysis by the same investigators (Levin et al, 1993) included more studies in the higher dose range. This study noted a correlation between response and cisplatin dose up to a level of 25 mg/m²/wk (75 mg/m²/every 3 weeks). Neither meta-analysis, therefore, offered any evidence supporting the importance of dose intensity (or total dose) for cisplatin beyond the standard doses used in clinical practice. Evidence for the value of greater dose intensity, if it is to be credible, must ultimately come from randomized trials. To establish the importance of dose intensity over a clinically relevant range, eight randomized trials have been conducted (Table 16–8). Six of these showed no advantage for the higher dose schedule.

In the GOG (McGuire et al, 1995) and GICOG (Colombo et al, 1993) trials, each regimen gave the same total dose of drugs with a twofold difference in dose intensity. Some investigators have suggested that the failure to observe improved efficacy with the higher

but more toxic dose related to the failure to give a greater total dose. The Gruppo Oncologico Nord-Ovest (GONO) (Conte et al, 1996), London GOG (Gore et al, 1996), and Danish (Jakobsen et al, 1997) trials increased not only the dose intensity but also the total dose of at least the platinum compound. No significant differences were observed in response or survival in any of these studies. In all three trials, a doubling of dose intensity and an increase in total dose yielded only increased toxicity.

The Austrian trial increased the dose intensity of the platinum compounds by combining cisplatin and carboplatin in the same regimen (Dittrich et al, 1996). This increase in total dose and 1.6-fold increase in dose intensity of the platinum compounds, as in the other studies, led to increased toxicity with no increase in response, progression-free survival, or overall survival.

In contrast, the Scottish trial (Kaye et al, 1996) and the Hong Kong trial (Ngan et al, 1989) showed an advantage for increasing dose intensity. In the Scottish trial the response rate was superior with the high-dose regimen and there was a 5 percent improvement in survival at 4 years. Despite the fact that one third of the patients in the trial had stage IC disease, the high-dose regimen yielded results no better than those reported

---

T A B L E **16–8**

Eight Randomized Trials of Platinum Dose Intensity in Advanced Ovarian Carcinoma

Trial	Platinum Dose Intensity (Prescribed Dose)	Response Rate (%)	Survival (Median)
Trials Showing No Difference			
GOG (McGuire et al., 1995)	Cisplatin 16.7 mg/m²/wk	65%	21 mo
	Cisplatin 33.3 mg/m²/wk	59%	24 mo
GICOG (Colombo et al., 1993)	Cisplatin 25 mg/m²/wk	61%	33 mo
	Cisplatin 50 mg/m²/wk	66%	36 mo
GONO (Conte et al., 1996)	Cisplatin 12.5 mg/m²/wk	61%	24 mo
	Cisplatin 25 mg/m²/wk	58%	29 mo
London GOG (Gore et al., 1996)	Carboplatin AUC* 6/4 wk	57%	(Hazard ratio
	Carboplatin AUC 12/4 wk	63%	= 0.91)
Danish (Jakobsen et al., 1997)	Carboplatin 4/4 wk	32%	19 mo
	Carboplatin 8/4 wk	30%	19 mo
Austrian† (Dittrich et al., 1996)	Cisplatin 25 mg/m²/wk	42%	38 mo
	Cisplatin + carboplatin‡	39%	42 mo
Trials Showing a Difference			
Scottish (Kaye et al., 1997)	Cisplatin 16.7 mg/m²/wk	34%	27% at 4 yr
	Cisplatin 33.3 mg/m²/wk	61%	32% at 4 yr
Hong Kong (Ngan et al., 1989)	Cisplatin 15–20 mg/m²/wk	30%	30% at 3 yr
	Cisplatin 30–40 mg/m²/wk	55%	60% at 3 yr

*AUC = area under curve.
†Platinum dose intensity advantage for the cisplatin/carboplatin regimen, 1.6.
‡Cisplatin 25 mg/m²/wk; carboplatin 75 mg/m²/wk.

by the GOG with a lower dose intensity of CTX and cisplatin in patients with large-volume advanced disease. The Hong Kong trial reported a superior response rate and 3-year survival for the high-dose arm, but the small size of this trial (50 patients total) and poor characterization of the patient population make these results uninterpretable.

Intraperitoneal (IP) Dose Intensity. The rationale for IP therapy is based on the observation that ovarian carcinoma spreads primarily by IP seeding. Because the disease remains at least grossly confined to the peritoneal cavity for a significant portion of its course, the administration of chemotherapy via the IP route is logical. Furthermore, when given IP, a number of cytotoxic drugs achieve peak peritoneal-to-plasma concentration ratios of 18 to over 1,000 (Markman, 1993). Included among these are cisplatin and carboplatin. The obvious limitation of intraperitoneal therapy is the depth of penetration of drug, which dictates that only patients with small-volume disease (the smaller the better) be considered.

Uncontrolled Phase II trials of IP platinum therapy in small-volume persistent or recurrent ovarian cancer have shown that 25 to 35 percent of patients achieve a pathologic complete response (Hacker et al, 1987; Markman et al, 1991a; Piver et al, 1988; Reichman et al, 1989). Subsequent results of Phase II trials in persistent or recurrent disease, however, indicate that the case for IP therapy is not straightforward (Markman et al, 1991b). Patients with platinum-sensitive disease (relapse interval greater than 6 months) had response rates to IP therapy of 40 to 60 percent, rates that were in fact similar to those reported with the same therapy given IV. Those patients whose disease was platinum resistant responded less than 10 percent of the time. At least in the salvage setting, therefore, no advantage for the IP approach was observed.

Only one randomized trial of IP therapy has been completed to date (Alberts et al, 1996). This trial involved 654 newly diagnosed stage III ovarian cancer patients with residual nodules 2 cm or less in diameter randomized to CTX 600 mg/m^2 IV plus cisplatin 100 mg/m^2 either IV or IP every 3 weeks for six cycles. The final analysis showed no statistically significant difference in surgically determined complete responses but a significant difference in overall survival ($p = .02$) favoring the IP regimen (hazard ratio 0.77). This would seem to establish the case for front-line IP therapy for small-volume ovarian carcinoma. Unfortunately, certain design aspects of the randomized trial cast doubt on the conclusions. The study did not reach its original goal of a hazard ratio of 0.67 despite extension of accrual to include larger numbers of the most favorable group. This leaves serious questions about the conclusions of the trial. Hopefully another ongoing trial will finally resolve this important issue.

Stem Cell–Supported Dose Intensity. Regarding another controversial approach to high-dose therapy, reviews of available Phase I and II trials of stem cell–supported high-dose chemotherapy (Fennelly and Schneider, 1995; Kotz and Schilder, 1995) demonstrate the feasibility of administering active regimens in very high doses (8- to 10-fold increase in dose intensity) together with stem cell support. Although response rates are high, the patient populations are poorly characterized as to whether the disease is platinum sensitive or platinum resistant, and the response durations are brief. These results are achieved at the cost of significant toxicity and expense, and do not support the use of this approach outside of clinical trials. A randomized trial as a national effort is underway that should establish the role for stem cell–supported drug dose enhancement.

Paclitaxel Dose Intensity. Two studies provide information on the efficacy of paclitaxel dose intensity. The first is a meta-analysis of Phase II data from studies of previously treated ovarian carcinoma patients (Rowinsky et al, 1996). Of 157 patients who initially had stage III or IV ovarian carcinoma for whom platinum sensitivity could be assessed, 121 (77 percent) were judged to be platinum resistant. Paclitaxel dosing ranged from 110 to 312 mg/m^2, with a mean dose of 195 mg/m^2 and a mean dose intensity of 61 mg/m^2/wk. The overall response rate was 27 percent. Neither dose nor dose intensity correlated with response. These data provide no support whatsoever for escalating the dose of paclitaxel above the range of 135 to 175 mg/m^2 every 3 weeks.

The second study randomized 338 patients previously treated with first-line platinum-based combination chemotherapy to either 175 or 250 mg/m^2 of paclitaxel over 24 hours every 3 weeks. The latter group got granulocyte colony-stimulating factor support (Omura et al, 1996). The higher dose produced a higher response rate (36 versus 28 percent), but no difference in progression-free survival (5.3 vs. 4.8 months median) or overall survival (11.9 months vs. 12.5 months median) was observed. The higher dose caused significantly more anemia, thrombocytopenia, gastrointestinal toxicity, neurotoxicity, and myalgias.

Data on Dose Intensity for Other Drugs. Many of the agents other than the platinums and taxanes that have activity in ovarian carcinoma have been examined in meta-analyses with little or no evidence of a dose-response relationship (Levin and Hryniuk, 1987; Levin et al, 1993). Formal studies of dose intensity for alkylating agents provide no support for the use of doses higher than the standard ranges.

Summary of Dose Intensity Data. Clinical studies indicate that the frequency of response to drugs can be enhanced over a low dose range by escalating the dose intensity. Beyond a threshold dose, however, no further therapeutic benefit is observed by increasing the dose. For cisplatin, the threshold appears to fall in the range from 15 to 25 mg/m^2/wk (45 to 75 mg/m^2 every 3 weeks). Hints of a second threshold at very high dose intensities come from studies of IP therapy and regimens supported by stem cells. For carboplatin, the threshold falls at an area under the curve of 4 to 5 every 4 weeks, and for paclitaxel at a dose of 175 mg/m^2 every 3 weeks.

With regard to schedule, clinical trials have focused primarily on paclitaxel. Ongoing studies are evaluating 3-hour, 24-hour, and 96-hour infusions as well as 1-hour weekly infusions. Based on the weight of evidence in the current literature, either a 24-hour or a 3-hour schedule is acceptable. The 3-hour schedule is more suited to outpatient therapy but should not be used in combination with cisplatin because of unacceptable neurotoxicity.

Second-Line (Salvage) Chemotherapy

The characteristic that best reflects the potential for response to salvage chemotherapy is the response to front-line platinum-based chemotherapy. Patients who respond to platinum-based therapy and demonstrate a significant relapse-free interval have a high probability of responding again to platinum-based treatment (Markman et al, 1991a,b; Ozols et al, 1985, 1987; van der Burg et al, 1991; Weiss et al, 1991; Zanaboni et al,

TABLE 16–9

Definition of Platinum Sensitivity and Platinum Resistance

Clinical sensitivity	Initial response to platinum *and* Platinum-free interval >6 months
Clinical resistance	Progression on platinum therapy *or* Best response stable disease *or* Relapse <6 months after platinum

1991). Conversely, patients who progress during or shortly after completion of platinum-based therapy are unlikely to respond to further treatment with a platinum compound and should receive therapy with non-cross-resistant agents. This division of patients into platinum "sensitive" and "resistant" populations will govern the choice of salvage therapy (Table 16–9). The definition of what constitutes a "significant platinum-free interval" is not clear, although the data suggest that the longer the interval, the more likely it is that there will be a tumor response on retreatment with a platinum compound.

SALVAGE AFTER
PLATINUM-BASED CHEMOTHERAPY

Platinum-Sensitive Tumors. The role of IV cisplatin-based therapy as salvage treatment was evaluated retrospectively in a series of 72 measurable-disease patients (Markman et al, 1991c) who had received at least two cisplatin or carboplatin-based regimens, and who had demonstrated a platinum-free interval of at least 4 months between the completion of the first regimen and the initiation of the second (Table 16–10). This "platinum-sensitive"

TABLE 16–10

Results of Salvage Platinum-Based Therapy for Ovarian Carcinoma as a Function of the Time from Completion of the Previous Treatment to Relapse*

Cisplatin-Free Interval (mo)	Clinical Response (%)	pCR[†] (%)
>4 (all cases)	31/72 (43)	10/72 (14)
5–12	(27)	(5)
13–24	(33)	(11)
<24	(59)	(22)

*From Markman M, Rothman R, Hakes T, et al: Second-line platinum therapy in patients with ovarian cancer previously treated with cisplatin. J Clin Oncol 9:389, 1991, with permission.
[†]pCR = pathologic complete response.

population demonstrated an overall response rate of 43 percent, with an increasing frequency of response as the platinum-free interval increased.

Similar results were reported with salvage regimens of weekly cisplatin combined with either epirubicin or etoposide (Zanaboni et al, 1991), carboplatin and CTX (van der Burg et al, 1991), and the platinum analog iproplatin (Weiss et al, 1991). In each instance, "platinum-sensitive" patients experienced a higher response rate than "platinum-resistant" patients.

Platinum-Resistant Tumors. The management of patients with platinum-resistant tumors has focused on two approaches: more dose-intense platinum-based regimens and non-cross-resistant drugs. Regarding the dose-intense approach, there are two reports that provide information on prior response of the study group to platinum-based treatment. Ozols et al (1985, 1987) administered carboplatin 800 mg/m^2 to 30 patients previously treated with cisplatin. None of the eight objective responses (27 percent) was observed in a patient who had progressive disease during initial cisplatin therapy. Markman et al (1991b) examined retrospectively two Phase II trials of cisplatin-based IP therapy in patients with persistence or recurrence after initial platinum-based chemotherapy (Table 16–11). Among the 52 patients with a platinum-sensitive tumor, 29 (56 percent) exhibited an objective response, 17 of which were pathologic complete responses. Only 11 percent of the 37 platinum-resistant tumors responded, all partially.

These two reports suggest that the increase in dose intensity achievable by IV dose escalation or IP administration of drug cannot overcome true platinum resistance. Successful management of these patients depends on the identification of active agents that are non-cross-resistant with the platinum compounds. Three cytotoxic agents have been shown to produce objective responses in patients whose tumors have proven to be resistant to platinum-based initial therapy: paclitaxel (taxol), ifosfamide, and HMM.

Three Phases II studies of *paclitaxel* in patients who previously received platinum-based therapy have confirmed major activity of this drug in ovarian carcinoma (Einzig et al, 1990; McGuire et al, 1989b; Thigpen et al, 1992a). Of greatest significance in the Phase II trials was the observation of a relatively high response rate (24 to 30 percent) in

platinum-resistant patients. In the GOG trial (Thigpen et al, 1992a), a response rate of 25 percent was observed even in the patients who actually progressed during platinum therapy. Paclitaxel is the most active agent yet tested in patients with a platinum-resistant tumor. However, its use as salvage therapy is very limited by the fact that it has become a standard part of front-line therapy.

Ifosfamide is chemically similar to CTX. In Phase II trials, ifosfamide has produced objective responses in patients whose tumor has demonstrated resistance to platinum plus CTX combinations (Markman et al, 1992; Thigpen et al, 1992b). The best data come from a report of 52 patients who received ifosfamide 1.0 to 1.2 gm/m^2 IV daily for 5 days every 4 weeks plus mesna (60 percent of the ifosfamide dose). Among 41 patients with a platinum-resistant tumor, there were five responses (one complete). Among the 11 platinum-sensitive patients, there were two responses (one complete) (Markman et al, 1992). Ifosfamide thus does have sufficient activity against platinum-resistant ovarian carcinoma to give it a place in salvage therapy.

Hexamethylmelamine's role in salvage therapy for platinum-resistant disease is less clear. Three Phase II trials in patients who had received prior chemotherapy document clear activity for the drug in the salvage setting (Manetta et al, 1990; Moore et al, 1991; Rosen et al, 1987). None of these reports, however, provides a detailed breakdown of the patients into platinum-sensitive and resistant categories; hence the value of the drug as a salvage therapy for patients with resistant disease cannot be determined based on currently published data.

SALVAGE AFTER PLATINUM-PACLITAXEL–BASED CHEMOTHERAPY

More recently, with the advent of widespread use of paclitaxel plus platinum as the standard front-line chemotherapy, efforts have been directed to identify agents that can induce responses in patients resistant to both paclitaxel and a platinum compound. Eight trials focus on treatment of this group of patients (Table 16–12).

Paclitaxel. The first of these trials evaluated the use of paclitaxel at variable doses and schedules after prior taxane treatment (Aghajanian et al, 1996). The response rate was 25 percent among patients with a treatment-free interval exceeding 6 months, and 6 percent if the interval was less than 4 months. These

TABLE **16–11**

Results of Salvage Intraperitoneal Cisplatin by Prior Response to Platinum-Based Therapy*

Tumor Size	Prior Response (N = 52)		No Prior Response (N = 37)	
	Response (%)	CR (%)	Response (%)	CR (%)
Microscopic only	6/13 (46)	6/13 (46)	1/4 (25)	0/4 (0)
<0.5 cm	12/17 (71)	7/17 (41)	0/7 (0)	0/7 (0)
0.5–1.0 cm	3/6 (50)	2/6 (33)	0/3 (0)	0/3 (0)
>1.0 cm	8/16 (50)	2/16 (13)	3/23 (13)	0/23 (0)

*From Markman M, Reichman B, Hakes T, et al: Responses to second-line cisplatin-based intraperitoneal therapy in ovarian cancer: influence of a prior response to intravenous cisplatin. J Clin Oncol 9:1801, 1991, with permission.

data indicate that paclitaxel may be of value if the patient's tumor is taxane sensitive but is inappropriate in taxane-resistant cases.

Etoposide. A second trial gave previously treated patients oral etoposide 50 mg/m^2/day for 21 days every 4 weeks (Rose et al, 1996). Among 41 patients resistant to first-line therapy, which for the most part consisted of paclitaxel plus cisplatin, a 27 percent response rate (percent complete) was observed. Among 29 patients sensitive to first-line therapy, a 34 percent response rate (17 percent complete) resulted. The response rate among those patients with resistant disease is impressive, and establishes oral etoposide as a reasonable treatment option for resistant tumors and also a potential third drug to add to first-line chemotherapy.

Topotecan. Two trials evaluated topotecan 1.5 mg/m^2/day for 5 days every 3 weeks in previously treated ovarian cancer patients (Carmichael et al, 1996; Gordon et al, 1996). In those tumors resistant to platinum but not the taxanes, a response rate of 23 percent was observed, whereas of those resistant to both

the taxanes and platinum, only 13 percent responded. Topotecan is clearly an active agent in the salvage setting.

Tamoxifen. The GOG evaluated tamoxifen in patients with prior treatment with a platinum and a taxane (Markman et al, 1996b). Of the 77 patients with resistant disease, 13 percent responded at a dose of 20 mg orally twice daily. Of those 20 patients with sensitive disease, 15 percent responded.

Navelbine. One study evaluated the activity of navelbine in patients with ovarian carcinoma resistant to both platinums and taxanes (Gershenson et al, 1996). Among 20 evaluable patients receiving 25 mg/m^2/day for 3 days every 3 weeks, 15 percent responded (two completely).

Gemcitabine and Doxil. Studies suggest that gemcitabine (Shapiro et al, 1996) and Doxil (Muggia et al, 1997b) may have activity against platinum-resistant tumors. Two of 13 patients (15 percent) with resistant disease and 2 of 14 (14 percent) with sensitive tumors responded to gemcitabine, and 9 of 34 pa-

TABLE **16–12**

Results of Salvage Therapy in Ovarian Cancer Patients Previously Treated with Platinum and/or Paclitaxel

Regimen	Study	Sensitive	Resistant
Paclitaxel	Aghajanian et al (1996)	15/60 (25%)	1/16 (6%)
Etoposide (oral)*	Rose et al (1996)	10/29 (34%)	11/41 (27%)
Topotecan	Gordon et al (1996)	22/96 (23%)	9/67 (13%)
	Carmichael et al (1996)		
Tamoxifen	Markman et al (1996b)	3/20 (15%)	10/77 (13%)
Navelbine	Gershenson et al (1996)	3/20 (15%)	
Gemcitabine	Shapiro et al (1996)	2/14 (14%)	2/13 (15%)
Doxil	Muggia et al (1997b)	9/34 (29%)†	

*5.0 mg/m^2/day on days 1–21.
†Status of resistance not entirely clear.

tients (26 percent) with platinum/taxane resistance had a clinical response to Doxil.

Summary. Treatment of patients who have received prior chemotherapy should be based on their response to initial therapy. Those deemed to be clinically sensitive to initial therapy should receive retreatment with the same drugs with the expectation of a high response rate. Those resistant to either a platinum compound or paclitaxel but not both should be treated with the class of drug to which they have not been exposed. Those resistant to a combination of the two classes of agents should be treated with a drug that is clinically non-cross-resistant. Among these agents, oral etoposide has the highest reported response rate.

Germ Cell Neoplasms

Approximately 5 percent of ovarian cancers are of germ cell origin. These neoplasms are classified into two broad groups: dysgerminomas and nondysgerminomatous tumors. The management of these patients begins with exploratory laparotomy to determine the extent of disease and to carry out surgical resection. Subsequent therapy depends on the histology and the findings at laparotomy, on the basis of which patients can be divided into two groups: those with completely resected stages I through III disease and those with incompletely resected stages III and IV disease. Unlike the epithelial carcinomas, however, the relative efficacy of new therapeutic regimens must be based on comparisons to historical controls because these lesions are not sufficiently common to make randomized trials feasible.

Patients with completely resected stage I, II, or III endodermal sinus tumor, mixed cell tumors, embryonal carcinomas, choriocarcinomas, and most immature teratomas have a sufficiently high recurrence rate that adjuvant therapy is warranted (see Chapter 11). The largest experience with adjuvant chemotherapy is that of the GOG, which evaluated regimens of vincristine, ACT-D, and CTX (VAC) and bleomycin, etoposide, and cisplatin (BEP) (Table 16–13).

Assessment of the relative value of these regimens is best accomplished by comparison with historical data on patients who received no adjuvant therapy. These data show a steady increase in the percentage of patients remaining disease free at 16 months of follow-up as one goes from no adjuvant

TABLE 16–13

GOG Trials of Adjuvant Chemotherapy in Ovarian Germ Cell Cancer[*,†]

Adjuvant Therapy	EST and Mixed Tumors NED (%)[‡]	Immature Teratoma NED (%)[‡]
None	34/165 (21)	36/56 (64)
VAC	53/82 (65)	59/70 (84)
BEP	30/31 (97)	18/19 (95)

[*]Data from Slayton et al (1985) and Williams et al (1989b).
[†]EST = endodermal sinus tumor; VAC = vincristine 1.5 mg/m² IV (max 2 mg) q2wk × 12 plus actinomycin-D 350 μg/m² IV daily × 5 days q4wk × 6 plus Cytoxan 150 mg/m² IV daily × 5 days q4wk × 6; BEP = bleomycin 20 units/m² IV (max 30 units) q1wk × 9 plus etoposide 100 mg/m² IV daily × 5 q3wk × 3 plus cisplatin 20 mg/m² IV daily × 5 q3wk × 3.
[‡]Percentage of patients with no evidence of disease (NED) at a median of 16 months following completion of therapy.

through VAC to BEP. These data also indicate that BEP is the treatment of choice in the adjuvant setting for immature teratomas of grades 2 and 3, endodermal sinus tumors, mixed germ cell tumors, and probably also embryonal carcinoma and choriocarcinoma. For other histologies, insufficient data exist to permit a definite recommendation.

For patients with stage III incompletely resected or stage IV disease, at least two chemotherapy regimens have been shown by the GOG to be active: VAC and vinblastine, bleomycin, and platinum (Table 16–14). However, the cisplatin-based combination yields a higher response rate and a greater percentage of durable complete responses or cures. Currently the GOG is studying BEP in this patient population.

Stromal Cell Malignancies

Malignant tumors arising from the ovarian stroma account for less than 3 percent of malignant ovarian neoplasms and include principally granulosa cell tumors and androblastomas (Sertoli-Leydig cell tumors). The chemotherapy experience in these neoplasms is purely anecdotal (Slayton et al, 1985). Drugs that have been reported to produce one or more responses include CTX, vincristine, ACT-D, 5-FU, ADR, bleomycin, and cisplatin. None has been evaluated in a sufficient number of patients to determine a reasonable level of activity. Combinations that have produced responses include PAC, VAC, BEP, and ACT-D plus 5-FU and CTX.

A recommendation for an optimal chemotherapy regimen in these neoplasms is im-

T A B L E **16–14**

GOG Trial of Incompletely Resected Stages II, III, IV and Recurrent Germ Cell Cancers of the Ovary[*,†,‡]

Histology	Total Cases	Measurable	CR	PR	NED (%)
Dysgerminoma	8	4	3	1	(88)
Immature Teratoma	24	9	2	2	(54)
Endodermal Sinus Tumor	28	12	7	4	(55)
Mixed Cell Tumor	27	9	5	4	(52)
Embryonal Carcinoma	3	2	1	0	(33)
Choriocarcinoma	3	3	2	1	(67)

*From Williams SD, Blessing JA, Moore DH, et al: Cisplatin, vinblastine, and bleomycin in advanced and recurrent ovarian germ cell tumors: a trial of the Gynecologic Oncology Group. Ann Intern Med 111:22, 1989, with permission. (Some of these data not published)
[†]37% of non-dysgerminoma patients had prior chemotherapy.
[‡]Five of 12 IT and EST patients were salvaged with VAC chemotherapy.
VBP = Vinblastine 12 mg/m^2 IV q3wk × 3–4; Bleomycin 20 units/m^2 IV (maximum 30 units) q1wk × 12; Cisplatin 20 mg/m^2 IV daily × 5 q3wk × 3–4.

possible on the basis of available data. It seems clear that some form of systemic therapy should be employed in patients with advanced or recurrent disease. Readers may refer to Chapter 11 for additional information regarding therapy of specific tumors.

CHEMOTHERAPY OF CERVICAL CANCER

Squamous Cell Carcinoma

Chemotherapy for squamous carcinoma of the female genital tract has for the most part been reserved for those patients with advanced (stage IVb) or recurrent cervical cancer, although neoadjuvant chemotherapy is currently under study (see Chapters 5 and 17). Evaluation of chemotherapy in such a patient population is difficult for two reasons. First, most of the patients have had prior therapy with radiation, which not only impairs bone marrow reserve but also interferes with the vascular supply to the tumor and delivery of the drug. Second, many of these patients have ureteral obstruction with impaired excretion of many drugs, thus limiting the tolerance to these agents. Despite these problems, there is considerable information regarding the role of systemic therapy in cervical carcinoma, a relatively common malignancy. Attention is directed first to the management of advanced and recurrent squamous cell carcinoma of the cervix with single and combination chemotherapy regimens, and then to other possible uses of systemic therapy in patients with this neoplasm.

Advanced and Recurrent Squamous Carcinoma

SINGLE-AGENT THERAPY

Platinum. Advanced and recurrent squamous cell carcinoma of the cervix no longer amenable to control with surgery and/or radiotherapy has been managed with a variety of chemotherapeutic agents (Table 16–15). Although certain of these agents have moderate activity, most attention has been directed to the platinum compounds. Platinum, which has been studied extensively in a variety of dosages and schedules, yields an objective response rate of 20 to 25 percent as first-line chemotherapy. Response of tumor outside the field of radiation is more frequent than in-field tumor response. There is marginal evidence that the 100-mg/m^2 regimen may be better (response rate 31 vs. 21 percent; p = .05) than 50 mg/m^2 (Bonomi et al, 1985). Results with carboplatin suggest a lower level of efficacy but a decrease in adverse effects, most notably nephrotoxicity and neurotoxicity (Arseneau et al, 1985; McGuire et al, 1989a).

Ifosfamide. In Phase II trials from Europe, ifosfamide produced a 29 percent response rate among 84 patients (Thigpen et al, 1990), but the GOG reported only a 14 percent response rate among 73 patients (Sutton et al, 1989a,b).

Dibromodulcitol (mitolactol). This halogenated sugar, was reported to have significant activity in squamous cell carcinoma of the cervix by Lira-Puerto et al (1985). This report prompted a GOG study that observed a 29

TABLE 16–15

Single-Agent Activity in Squamous Cell Carcinoma of the Cervix*

Drug	Prior Treatment	Clinical Response (%)[†]
Alkylating agents		
Cytoxan	Mixed	38/351 (15)
Chlorambucil	Mixed	11/44 (25)
Melphalan	Mixed	4/20 (20)
Ifosfamide	No	7/46 (15)
	Yes	3/27 (11)
	Mixed	25/84 (29)
Dibromodulcitol	No	16/55 (29)
Galactitol	No	7/47 (15)
	Mixed	7/36 (19)
Heavy metal complexes		
Cisplatin	No	182/785 (23)
	Yes	8/30 (27)
Carboplatin	No	27/175 (15)
Iproplatin	No	19/177 (11)
Antibiotics		
Adriamycin	No	12/61 (20)
	Mixed	33/205 (16)
Mitomycin C	No	6/52 (12)
Piperazinedione	No	5/38 (13)
Porfiromycin	No	17/78 (22)
Antimetabolites		
5-Fluorouracil	Mixed	29/142 (20)
Methotrexate	Mixed	17/96 (18)
Baker's Antifol	Mixed	5/32 (16)
Plant alkaloids		
VM-26	Yes	3/22 (14)
Vincristine	Mixed	10/55 (18)
Vinblastine	Mixed	2/20 (10)
Vindesine	Mixed	5/21 (24)
Other agents		
Paclitaxel	Yes	9/52 (18)
ICRF-159	Mixed	5/28 (18)
Hexamethylmelamine	No	12/64 (19)

*From Thigpen JT: Chemotherapy of gynecologic cancer. In Perry MC (ed): The Chemotherapy Source Book, 2nd ed. Baltimore, Williams & Wilkins, 1996, p. 1253, with permission.
[†]Aminothiodiazole, amsacrine, CCNU, diaziquone, dichloromethotrexate, echinomycin, esorubicin, etoposide, hydroxyurea, maytansine, methyl CCNU, mitoxantrone, 6-MP, N-methylformamide, PALA, spirogermanium, and Yoshi 864 have produced a less than 10 percent response rate.

percent response rate among 55 evaluable patients (Stehman et al, 1989). These results suggest that the drug should be investigated further as part of a combination regimen.

COMBINATION DRUG THERAPY

Numerous drug combinations have been tried in patients with advanced or recurrent squamous cell carcinoma of the cervix (Bonomi and Yordan, 1984). Most attention has been directed to cisplatin-containing combinations and, in particular, the combination of mitomycin C, vincristine, and bleomycin with cisplatin. Initial reports suggested a response rate exceeding 50 percent, with a complete response rate of 25 percent and long-lasting complete responses. However, a randomized trial conducted by the Southwest Oncology Group (Baker et al, 1985) revealed no advantage for the combination over single-agent cisplatin. In a similar vein, no other data exist in the form of a controlled trial to support the use of any combination of chemotherapeutic agents over cisplatin alone in terms of overall survival (see below).

The greatest interest focuses on attempts to study combinations of ifosfamide with other presumably active agents. Nishida et al (1989) reported six responses (three complete) among nine patients receiving the combination of ifosfamide plus cisplatin 50 mg/m^2 and ADR 50 mg/m^2 plus bleomycin 30 mg over 24 hours, all on day 1, and ifosfamide 1 gm/m^2 (plus mesna 1 gm/m^2) on days 1 through 5, repeated every 4 weeks. All patients had advanced or recurrent cervical carcinoma previously irradiated but not previously exposed to chemotherapy. Buxton et al (1989) investigated the combination of bleomycin 30 mg over 24 hours on day 1 followed by cisplatin 50 mg/m^2 and then ifosfamide 5 gm/m^2 over 24 hours (plus mesna 6 gm/m^2 over 36 hours) repeated every 3 weeks. Among 49 patients, most of whom had received prior radiotherapy and none of whom had received prior chemotherapy, 10 complete and 24 partial responses were observed (69 percent).

A third study (Lara et al, 1990) of combination chemotherapy utilized cisplatin 20 mg/m^2/day for 5 days plus ifosfamide 1.5 gm/m^2/day and mesna 900 mg/m^2/day each for 5 days repeated every 4 weeks. Twenty-four patients with measurable disease were included in the study, of whom 62 percent exhibited a partial response. None had received prior radiotherapy or chemotherapy. Kuhnle et al (1990) employed carboplatin 300 mg/m^2 on day 1 followed by ifosfamide 5 gm/m^2 over 24 hours and mesna 9.2 gm over 36 hours, repeated every 4 weeks. Of 32 patients treated in the study, 59 percent responded (three completely). None had received either chemotherapy or radiotherapy previously.

The GOG completed a randomized Phase III trial of cisplatin alone or combined with either ifosfamide or mitolactol (Omura et al, 1997). The combination of ifosfamide plus cisplatin produced a superior total complete response rate and progression-free survival with no change in overall survival (Table

16–16). Two follow-up randomized Phase III trials of ifosfamide plus cisplatin with or without bleomycin and cisplatin with or without paclitaxel are either ongoing or completed with no results.

SUMMARY

Numerous drugs have shown activity in squamous carcinoma of the cervix. At least three of these are currently under study as part of potentially interesting combination regimens. For now, there is no treatment of choice for these neoplasms when radiation and/or surgery are not applicable. Reasonable options include single-agent therapy with one of the three promising drugs (cisplatin, ifosfamide, and dibromodulcitol) or a combination of ifosfamide plus cisplatin. It should be noted that one common combination, cisplatin plus 5-FU, yielded only a 22 percent response rate among 55 patients in a GOG Phase II trial, a rate similar to that with cisplatin alone (Bonomi et al, 1989).

Locally Advanced Carcinoma

Another role for chemotherapy is in combination with radiotherapy in patients with locally advanced disease to improve on results achievable with radiotherapy. The literature is replete with nonrandomized trials evaluating concomitant single-agent or combination chemotherapy, neoadjuvant chemotherapy, intra-arterial chemotherapy, and postradiation adjuvant chemotherapy, but only randomized trials are cited here to form a basis for current practice.

Hydroxyurea, given orally during radiation therapy, has been shown to improve outcome compared to radiation alone in a ran-

domized GOG study involving 190 patients with locally advanced cervical carcinoma. Complete response (68 vs. 32 percent), progression-free survival (14 vs. 8 months), and total survival (20 vs. 11 months) were all superior in the HU treatment arm (Hreshchyshyn et al, 1979). An independent study also favored the use of HU (Piver et al, 1987). The results of these studies have been challenged, however, because the patients were not surgically staged prior to study entry, and in the GOG study half of the patients entered were inevaluable. Subsequently the GOG conducted a Phase III study on surgically staged patients, excluding those with aortic nodes metastases (Stehman et al, 1988). There were 296 patients with clinical stages IIb through IVa disease randomized to radiation plus HU or misonidazole, another radiation sensitizer. The preliminary analysis shows a marginal advantage for the HU arm.

The results of these randomized Phase III trials support the use of concomitant HU and radiation in the management of locally advanced carcinoma of the cervix. Alternative approaches are under investigation, including Phase III GOG trial randomizing patients with stage IIb through IVa cervical carcinoma to radiation plus either HU or cisplatin plus 5-FU. Uncontrolled trials seek to determine feasibility for such approaches as hyperfractionated radiation plus radiosensitizer, neoadjuvant chemotherapy (see Chapters 5 and 17), adjuvant chemotherapy, and intra-arterial chemotherapy.

Nonsquamous Carcinoma

Data on the use of chemotherapy in nonsquamous carcinomas of the cervix come pri-

TABLE **16–16**

Results of GOG Protocol 110, a Randomized Phase III Trial of Patients with Advanced or Recurrent Squamous Cell Carcinoma of the Cervix*

Regimen[†]	N	Response[§]	Rate (%)
Cisplatin 50 mg/m² IV	137	9 CR, 16 PR	19
Cisplatin 50 mg/m² IV + Ifosfamide 5 gm/m² IV 24 hours	140	19 CR, 28 PR	33
Cisplatin 50 mg/m² IV + Mitolactol 180 mg/m² po days 2–6	141	14 CR, 17 PR	22

*From Omura G, Blessing J, Vacarello L, et al: Ramdomized trial of cisplatin plus mitolactol versus cisplatin plus ifosfamide in advanced squamous cell carcinoma of the cervix: a Gynecologic Oncology Group Study. J Clin Oncol 15:165, 1997, with permission.
†Cisplatin infused at 1 mg/minute; ifosfamide infused over 24 hours with mesna. All regimens repeated every 3 weeks.
‡Author's comment: Progression-free survival (4–5 months) and overall survival (8 months) was not significantly different among the regimens.
§CR = complete response; PR = partial response.

marily from studies of the GOG (Table 16–17). These are all single-agent trials involving mostly patients with an adenocarcinoma or adenosquamous carcinoma who had received prior radiotherapy and, in some instances, prior chemotherapy. Of the 10 agents studied, 3 demonstrated moderate activity: cisplatin (20 percent of 20 patients), piperazinedione (14 percent of 14 patients), and ifosfamide (12 percent of 24 patients). There are no reported studies of combination chemotherapy in this patient population.

CHEMOTHERAPY OF ENDOMETRIAL CANCER

Endometrial carcinoma, the most common invasive malignancy of the female genital tract, tends to present at an early stage of development. The cure rate for patients with such early lesions is high; hence the development of adequate systemic therapy for the patients who have advanced or recurrent disease has been slow. This section focuses on the use of systemic therapy in patients with advanced (stage III or IV) and recurrent disease.

Patients who have disease beyond the uterus clinically can be divided into two groups: those with loco-regional disease only, and those with disseminated disease with or without loco-regional involvement. Those with loco-regional involvement only may be candidates for surgery and/or radiotherapy to control their disease. Most other patients in this category will be candidates for systemic therapy, either hormonal therapy or chemotherapy.

Hormonal Therapy

The older literature reports objective regression of metastatic endometrial carcinoma in 33 percent of patients treated with progestational agents. Responses correlate with histologic grade and receptor status. Well-differentiated lesions are more likely to respond, and as expected are more likely to be positive for estrogen and progesterone receptors (Table 16–18). Most of the clinical trials of hormonal therapy have been conducted with parenteral progestins.

The GOG conducted a Phase II study of oral medroxyprogesterone acetate (MPA) 150 mg/day in patients with advanced or recurrent endometrial carcinoma not previously treated with systemic therapy. Among 331 pa-

TABLE 16–17
Single-Agent Activity in Nonsquamous Carcinoma of the Cervix*

Prior Drug	Treatment	Response (%)
Cisplatin	None	4/20 (20)
Piperazinedione	Mixed	2/14 (14)
VP-16	Mixed	1/19 (5)
Galactitol	Mixed	2/27 (7)
ICRF-159	Mixed	1/25 (4)
Mitoxantrone	Mixed	2/25 (8)
Diaziquone	Mixed	2/26 (8)
Aminothiadiazole	Mixed	2/26 (8)
VM-26	Mixed	1/23 (4)
Ifosfamide	Mixed	3/24 (12)

*From Thigpen JT: Chemotherapy of gynecologic cancer. In Perry MC (ed): The Chemotherapy Source Book, 2nd ed. Baltimore, Williams & Wilkins, 1996, p. 1253, with permission.

tients with measurable disease, there were 32 complete (10 percent) and 26 partial (8 percent) responses (Table 16–19). The median PFI was 4 months and median survival was 10.5 months. Only 51 patients had receptor data, but response, PFI, and survival were superior in patients with tumors positive for both estrogen and progesterone receptors. These results indicate that the actual activity of progestins in advanced or recurrent endometrial carcinoma is somewhat less than previously reported.

A follow-up GOG study (Thigpen et al, 1991b) randomized patients to receive either 200 or 1,000 mg/day of MPA, and required that blood levels of progestin be assessed to confirm patient compliance. Surprisingly, the lower dose of MPA offered a marginal advantage in terms of PFI with a similar response rate (16.7 vs. 10.0 percent complete response; 9.4 vs. 7.9 percent partial response).

These two trials support the longstanding practice of using hormonal therapy in selected patients with advanced or recurrent

TABLE 16–18
Receptor Status and Response to Progestin Therapy in Endometrial Carcinoma*

Study	ER+ PR+ Response	(%)	ER− PR− Response	(%)
Creasman et al (1980)	3/5	(60)	1/8	(12)
Ehrlich et al (1981)	7/8	(80)	1/16	(7)
Benraad et al (1980)	5/6	(83)	0/5	(0)
Martin et al (1979)	13/13	(100)	1/7	(14)
McCarty et al (1979)	4/5	(80)	0/8	(0)
Total	32/37	(86)	3/44	(7)

*ER = estrogen receptor; PR = progesterone receptor.

TABLE 16–19

Phase II Trial of MPA 150 mg/day Orally in Advanced and Recurrent Endometrial Carcinoma*

Patients	Response (%)	PFI (mo)	Survival (mo)
Known receptor status[†]			
ER⁺PgR⁺	4/10 (40)	8.5	13.5
ER⁺PgR⁻	2/16 (12)	4.5	9.0
ER⁻PgR⁻	3/25 (12)	2.5	9.5
Overall	58/331 (18)	4.0	10.5

*From Thigpen T, Blessing J, DiSaia P, Ehrlich C: Oral medroxyprogesterone acetate in advanced or recurrent endometrial carcinoma: results of therapy and correlation with estrogen and progesterone receptor levels. In Baulier E, Iacobelli S, McGuire W (eds): Endocrinology and Malignancy. 1986, p. 446, with permission.
[†]ER = estrogen receptor; PgR = progesterone receptor.

endometrial cancer. Such therapy is particularly suitable for those patients with known receptor positivity or a well-differentiated neoplasm. The hormones of choice are progestational agents (see Chapter 6).

Chemotherapy

Single-Agent Therapy

A summation of the reported activity of cytotoxic agents in treating endometrial carcinoma is presented in Tables 16–20 and 16–21. The clinically useful drugs are discussed in detail in the following paragraphs.

Adriamycin is the most extensively studied chemotherapeutic agent in endometrial carcinoma. A Phase II GOG trial of ADR 60 mg/m^2 every 3 weeks produced a response rate of 38 percent (Thigpen et al, 1979). The same dose and schedule were employed as a control arm in two subsequent randomized GOG trials (Thigpen et al, 1985, 1993) with response rates of 24 and 28 percent, respectively. This combined experience in over 250 patients confirms the modest activity of ADR.

Platinum compounds also appear to be active. Cisplatin at doses varying from 50 to 100 mg/m^2 has yielded response rates ranging from 20 to 42 percent, and carboplatin at doses of 300 to 400 mg/m^2 has yielded response rates of 28 to 33 percent (Thigpen et al, 1995).

Although most attention has focused on ADR and the platinum compounds, a GOG report on *paclitaxel* has generated considerable interest (Thigpen et al, 1995). In a Phase II study involving 28 evaluable patients, four complete and six partial responses (35 percent) were observed with a paclitaxel regimen of 250 mg/m^2 over 24 hours every 3 weeks. In light of this significant level of activity, and taking into consideration observations in other solid tumors (ovary, breast) paclitaxel exhibits clinical non-cross-resistance with the platinum compounds, it must be concluded that paclitaxel has great potential for first-line combination chemotherapy in endometrial cancer patients.

In terms of progression-free and overall survival, none of the single agents yields results that differ significantly from those seen with hormonal therapy. Median progression-free survival is in the range of 4 to 6 months and overall survival 9 to 12 months, with responders living longer than nonresponders. It should be noted, however, that chemother-

TABLE 16–20

Single-Agent Activity in Endometrial Carcinoma with No Prior Chemotherapy*

Drug	Schedule	Response (%)
Adriamycin	60 mg/m^2/3 wk	16/43 (38)
	50 mg/m^2/3 wk	4/21 (19)
Cisplatin	50 mg/m^2/3 wk	10/49 (20)
	50 mg/m^2/3 wk	4/11 (36)
	50–100 mg/m^2/3 wk	11/26 (42)
Carboplatin	400 mg/m^2/4 wk	7/25 (28)
	400 mg/m^2/4 wk	9/27 (33)
Hexamethylmelamine	280 mg/m^2 × 14 days/4 wk	3/34 (9)
	8 mg/kg/day	6/20 (30)
Methotrexate	40 mg/m^2/wk	2/33 (6)
Cytoxan	666 mg/m^2/3 wks	0/19 (0)
Ifosfamide	1.2 gm/m^2/day × 5 days/4 wk	2/16 (13)
Paclitaxel	250 mg/m^2/24 hr/3 wk	10/28 (35)

*From Thigpen JT: Chemotherapy of gynecologic cancer. In Perry MC (ed): The Chemotherapy Source Book, 2nd ed. Baltimore, Williams & Wilkins, 1996, p. 1253, with permission.

T A B L E **16–21**

Single-Agent Activity in Endometrial Carcinoma with Prior Chemotherapy*

Drug	Schedule	Response (%)
Piperazinedione	9 mg/m^2/3 wk	1/22 (5)
Cisplatin	50 mg/m^2/3 wk	1/25 (4)
	3 mg/kg/3 wk	4/13 (31)
Aminothiadiazole	125 mg/m^2/wk	0/21 (0)
Teniposide	100 mg/m^2/wk	2/22 (9)
Diaziquone	22.5 mg/m^2/3 wk	2/26 (8)
Mitoxantrone	12 mg/m^2/3 wk	1/19 (5)
Razoxane	1.5 gm/m^2/wk	0/24 (0)
Etoposide	100 mg/m^2 × 3 days/4 wk	1/29 (3)
Galactitol	60 mg/m^2/wk	1/17 (6)
Vinblastine	1.5 mg/m^2/day × 5 days/3 wk	4/34 (12)
MGBG	500 mg/m^2/day/wk	3/21 (14)
Amsacrine	—	1/19 (5)

*From Thigpen JT: Chemotherapy of gynecologic cancer. In Perry MC (ed): The Chemotherapy Source Book, 2nd ed. Baltimore, Williams & Wilkins, 1996, p. 1253, with permission.

apy is not recommended for patients with potentially hormone-sensitive tumors.

Combination Chemotherapy

Although a number of combination regimens have been studied in uncontrolled trials of endometrial cancer patients, only a small number of randomized trials have been conducted. Two GOG trials compared single-agent ADR with ADR-based combinations. The first randomized patients with advanced or recurrent uterine cancer to ADR 60 mg/m^2 with or without CTX 500 mg/m^2 every 3 weeks (Thigpen et al, 1985). No significant differences were observed between the two arms. The second randomized patients with advanced or recurrent disease to ADR with or without cisplatin 50 mg/m^2 every 3 weeks (Table 16–22) (Thigpen et al, 1993). The combination regimen yielded a statistically significantly superior response rate (44 vs. 28 percent). Progression-free survival was also significantly superior for the combination regimen, but overall survival was not. These data indicate that a combination of doxorubicin 60 mg/m^2 plus cisplatin 50 mg/m^2 every 3 weeks should be considered the standard front-line chemotherapy regimen for patients with advanced or recurrent endometrial carcinoma.

CHEMOTHERAPY OF UTERINE SARCOMAS

Uterine sarcomas, far less common than endometrial carcinoma, are further distinguished by a relapse rate of at least 50 per-

cent in stage I disease. This fact, plus their propensity to recur at distant sites, makes the use of chemotherapy a prime therapeutic option for uterine sarcomas. The relative infrequency of these lesions, however, has limited the amount of meaningful information available on the use of chemotherapy.

Several general considerations are important to the choice of systemic therapy. Uterine sarcomas are a heterogeneous group of neoplasms that include malignant mixed mesodermal tumors (MMMTs), leiomyosarcomas (LMSs), endometrial stromal sarcomas, and certain rare histologic types. The first two of these, the MMMTs and the LMSs, constitute 90 percent of the cases and are the only two types for which meaningful data are avail-

T A B L E **16–22**

Gynecologic Oncology Group Protocol 107, a Randomized Trial of Adriamycin with or without Cisplatin in Women with Advanced or Recurrent Endometrial Carcinoma*[*,†]

Response Status	Adriamycin	Adriamycin + Cisplatin[‡]
Complete response	10 (8%)	23 (21%)
Partial response	25 (20%)	25 (23%)
Stable disease	60 (47%)	46 (42%)
Increasing disease	32 (25%)	16 (15%)
Total	127 (100%)	110 (100%)

*From Thigpen T, Blessing J, Homesley H, et al: Phase III trial of doxorubicin ± cisplatin in advanced or recurrent endometrial carcinoma: a Gynecologic Oncology Group Study. Proc Am Soc Clin Oncol 12: 261, 1993, with permission.
†Dosages: Adriamycin = 60 mg/m^2; cisplatin = 50 mg/m^2.

able. Because these two histologic types appear to respond differently to chemotherapy, they should be studied as separate patient populations. Within each population, there are two clinical situations in which chemotherapy has been studied: management of patients with advanced or recurrent disease, and adjuvant treatment of patients with stage I disease following complete surgical resection.

Advanced and Recurrent Sarcoma

Malignant Mixed Mesodermal Sarcoma

Among patients with MMMTs, two drugs appear to be active: ifosfamide and cisplatin (Table 16–23). *Ifosfamide* in a 5-day schedule at a dose of 1.5 mg/m^2/day for 5 days every 4 weeks produced five complete and four partial responses among 28 patients with no prior chemotherapy (Sutton et al, 1989c). This agent appears to be the most active drug studied to date.

Cisplatin was tested in patients with prior chemotherapy and achieved an 18 percent response rate in 28 patients (Thigpen et al, 1986d). A repeat trial in patients with no prior chemotherapy produced a 19 percent response rate among 63 patients (Thigpen et al, 1991a). Both of these trials employed a relatively low dose of cisplatin (50 mg/m^2 every 3 weeks). Investigators at M.D. Anderson Hospital used cisplatin in doses ranging from 75 to 100 mg/m^2 every 3 weeks (Gershenson et al, 1987a). Only 12 patients with measurable disease were entered into the study, but one complete and four partial responses were observed (42 percent). Because of the small number of cases and the lack of a randomized control group, no conclusions can be made about the merits of the higher dose.

Surprisingly, *ADR* demonstrated little activity in two trials of patients with uterine MMMT. The first, conducted as one arm of a Phase III trial, produced only four responses among 41 patients at a dose of 60 mg/m^2 every 3 weeks (Omura et al, 1983a). The second used doses from 50 to 90 mg/m^2 every 3 weeks, with most of the patients receiving either 75 or 90 mg/m^2 (Gershenson et al, 1987b). No responses were seen among the nine patients with measurable disease.

Leiomyosarcoma

SINGLE-AGENT THERAPY

The most active single agent for chemotherapy of LMS appears to be ADR (Table 16–24). Seven responses were observed among 28 patients treated with a 60-mg/m^2 dose every 3 weeks. Ifosfamide (four partial responses in 28 patients) and etoposide (one complete and two partial responses in 28 patients) demonstrated moderate activity.

COMBINATION CHEMOTHERAPY

Adequate evaluation of combination chemotherapy requires randomized Phase III trials, which have been completed in only two instances. The first randomized trial compared ADR alone to ADR plus DTIC (Table 16–25). No significant differences between the two regimens were noted (Omura et al, 1983a). The study was designed, however, before the

TABLE **16–23**

Single-Agent Activity in Malignant Mixed Mesodermal Tumor of the Uterus*

Drug	Prior Treatment	Schedule	N	Response† (%)
Ifosfamide	Yes	1.5 gm/m^2/day plus mesna 0.3 gm/m^2/day for 5 days q4wk	28	5 CR, 4 PR (32)
Cisplatin	No	50 mg/m^2 q3wk	63	5 CR, 7 PR (19)
	Yes	50 mg/m^2 q3wk	28	2 CR, 3 PR (18)
	No	75–100 mg/m^2 q3wk	12	1 CR, 4 PR (42)
Adriamycin	No	60 mg/m^2 q3wk	41	4 (10)
	No	50–90 mg/m^2 q3wk	9	0 (0)
Etoposide	Yes	100 mg/m^2/day for 3 days q4wk	31	0 CR, 2 PR (6)
Mitoxantrone	Yes	12 mg/m^2 q3wk	17	0 (0)
Piperazinedione	Yes	9 mg/m^2 q3wk	6	0 (0)

*From Thigpen JT: Chemotherapy of gynecologic cancer. In Perry MC (ed): The Chemotherapy Source Book, 2nd ed. Baltimore, Williams & Wilkins, 1996, p. 1253, with permission.
†CR = complete response; PR = partial response.

TABLE 16–24

Single-Agent Activity in Leiomyosarcoma of the Uterus*

Drug	Prior Treatment	Schedule	N	Response[†] (%)
Adriamycin	No	60 mg/m² q3wk	28	7[‡] (25)
Ifosfamide	No	1.5 gm/m²/day plus mesna 0.3 gm/m²/day for 5 days q4wk	28	4 PR (14)
Cisplatin	No	50 mg/m² q3wk	33	1 PR (3)
	Yes	50 mg/m² q3wk	17	1 PR (5)
Etoposide	Yes	100 mg/m²/day for 3 days q4wk	28	1 CR, 2 PR (11)
Mitoxantrone	Yes	12 mg/m² q3wk	12	0 (0)
Piperazinedione	Yes	9 mg/m² q3wk	11	1[‡] (9)

*From Thigpen JT: Chemotherapy of gynecologic cancer. In Perry MC (ed): The Chemotherapy Source Book, 2nd ed. Baltimore, Williams & Wilkins, 1996, p. 1253, with permission.
[†]CR = complete response; PR = partial response.
[‡]Responses not characterized.

differences in response to chemotherapy for LMS and MMMT were observed. As a consequence, there are insufficient numbers of each histologic type in this study to permit subset analysis. The second randomized trial of combination chemotherapy in uterine sarcomas randomized patients to ADR with or without CTX (Muss et al, 1985). The study was closed early because the likelihood of identifying differences was extremely small. The overall response rate for the combined data was similar to that seen in the first randomized trial.

SUMMARY

With recognition of the difference in response between LMS and MMMT, future randomized trials must regard each of the two major histologic types as a separate patient population. An ongoing Phase III GOG trial studying only MMMT patients is comparing ifosfamide therapy with or without cisplatin. The study is too early in accrual to permit any conclusions. Patients with LMS are entered into single-agent trials in an attempt to identify a second active agent.

Early-Stage Sarcoma

There is no defined role for adjuvant chemotherapy for stage I uterine sarcoma after complete surgical resection. The one meaningful study randomized patients to receive either ADR 60 mg/m² every 3 weeks for eight cycles or no further therapy (Table 16–26). No significant differences in recurrence rate, PFI, or survival were observed, although in each subset a 12 percent or greater difference in recurrence rate was noted favoring the ADR treatment arm. In the overall population, the median survival was 73.7 months for the ADR patients and 55.0 months for the patients getting no ADR (Omura et al, 1986b). It must be concluded that there is no convincing evidence that adjuvant chemotherapy is of any value in the management of patients with high-risk uterine sarcoma.

TABLE 16–25

Randomized Trial of Adriamycin with or without DTIC in Advanced and Recurrent Uterine Sarcoma*

Histologic Type	Adriamycin Response (%)	Adriamycin + DTIC Response (%)
Leiomyosarcoma	7/28 (25)	6/20 (30)
Malignant mixed mesodermal tumor	4/41 (10)	7/31 (23)
Other sarcomas	2/11 (18)	3/15 (20)

*From Omura GA, Major F, Blessing JA: A randomized study of Adriamycin with and without dimethyl-triazenoimidazole carboxamide in advanced uterine sarcomas. Cancer 52:626, 1983, with permission.

TABLE **16–26**

GOG Randomized Trial of Adriamycin Versus No Further Therapy in Completely Resected Stage I and II Uterine Sarcomas***

Cell Type	Adriamycin Relapse (%)	No Therapy Relapse (%)	Total (%)
Leiomyosarcoma	11/25 (44)	14/23 (61)	25/48 (52)
Malignant mixed mesodermal tumor	17/44 (39)	25/49 (51)	42/93 (45)
Other sarcoma	3/6 (50)	4/9 (44)	7/15 (47)
Total	31/75 (41)	43/81 (53)	74/156 (47)

*From Omura GA, Blessing JA, Major F, et al: A randomized clinical trial of adjuvant adriamycin in uterine sarcomas: a Gynecologic Oncology Group Study. J Clin Oncol 3:1240, 1986, with permission.

CHEMOTHERAPY OF OTHER GYNECOLOGIC MALIGNANCIES

In regard to squamous cell carcinoma of the *vulva*, only four agents have been used in a sufficient number of patients to make conclusions regarding activity. A review by Yordan et al (1984) drew from 12 different series to note 27 responses (59 percent) among 46 patients treated with bleomycin. With the variety of response definitions in the diverse sources, however, the true level of bleomycin activity is certainly in question. Cytembena was noted to have induced four responses among 26 patients (15 percent) in one series. Piperazinedione and cisplatin appear to be inactive (Thigpen et al, 1986c). Other single-agent data and all combination chemotherapy data are purely anecdotal.

For *vaginal* squamous carcinoma, only cisplatin has been evaluated in a sufficient number of patients, and it appears to be inactive (one response in 16 patients) (Thigpen et al, 1986c). All other data for vulvar or vaginal carcinoma of any cell type are anecdotal.

REFERENCES

Adams M, Kerby IJ, Unger L, et al: A comparison of first- and second-line efficacy of cisplatin and carboplatin in advanced ovarian cancer. In Proceedings of the Sixth NCI-EORTC Symposium on New Drugs in Cancer Therapy, 1989 (abstr 315).

Advanced Ovarian Cancer Trialists Group: Chemotherapy in advanced ovarian cancer: an overview of randomized clinical trials. BMJ 303:884, 1991.

Aghajanian C, Gogas H, Kennelly D, et al: Second-line paclitaxel therapy in patients with ovarian cancer previously treated with a taxane. Proc Am Soc Clin Oncol 15:286, 1996.

Alberts DS, Chen H, Young L, et al: Improved survival for relapsing ovarian cancer patients using the human tumor stem cell assay to select chemotherapy. Proc Am Soc Clin Oncol 22:462, 1981.

Alberts DS, Green SJ, Hannigan EV, et al: Improved efficacy of carboplatin plus cyclophosphamide versus cisplatin plus cyclophosphamide: preliminary report by the Southwest Oncology Group of a Phase III randomized trial in stages III and IV suboptimal ovarian cancer. J Clin Oncol 10:706, 1992.

Alberts D, Liu P, Hannigan E, et al: Intraperitoneal cisplatin plus intravenous cyclophosphamide versus intravenous cisplatin plus intravenous cyclophosphamide for stage III ovarian cancer. N Engl J Med 335:1950, 1996.

Allen A: The cardiotoxicity of chemotherapeutic drugs. In Perry MC (ed): The Chemotherapy Source Book. Baltimore, Williams & Wilkins, 1992, p 582.

Antman KH, Ryan L, Elias A, et al: Response to ifosfamide and mesna: 124 previously treated patients with metastatic or unresectable sarcoma. J Clin Oncol 7:126, 1989.

Arseneau JC, Hatch K, Stehman FB, Blessing JA: Phase II study of carboplatin in advanced squamous cell carcinoma of cervix. Proc Am Soc Clin Oncol 4:120, 1985.

Baker L, Boutselis J, Alberts D, et al: Combination chemotherapy for patients with disseminated carcinoma of the uterine cervix. Proc Am Soc Clin Oncol 4:120, 1985.

Benraad TJ, Friberg LG, Koenders AJ, Kullander S: Do estrogen and progesterone receptors in metastasizing endometrial cancers predict the response to gestagen therapy? Acta Obstet Gynecol Scand 59:155, 1980.

Bertelsen K, Jakobsen A, Andersen JE, et al: A randomized study of cyclophosphamide and cisplatin with or without doxorubicin in advanced ovarian carcinoma. Gynecol Oncol 28:161, 1987.

Bonadonna G, Valagussa P: Dose-response of adjuvant chemotherapy in breast cancer. N Engl J Med 304:10, 1981.

Bonomi P, Blessing J, Ball H, et al: A phase II evaluation of cisplatin and 5-fluorouracil in patients with advanced squamous cell carcinoma of the cervix: a Gynecologic Oncology Group study. Gynecol Oncol 34:357, 1989.

Bonomi P, Blessing JA, Stehman FB, et al: Randomized trial of three cisplatin dose schedules in squamous-cell carcinoma of the cervix: a Gynecologic Oncology Group study. J Clin Oncol 3:1079, 1985.

Bonomi P, Yordan E: Chemotherapy of cervical carcinoma. In Deppe G (ed): Chemotherapy of Gynecologic Cancer. New York, Alan R. Liss, 1984, p 103. Brock et al: 1981.

Brock N, Pohl J, Stekar J: Detoxification of urotoxic oxazaphosphorines by sulfhydryl compounds. J Cancer Res Clin Oncol 100:311, 1981.

Bruckner HW, Cohen CJ, Feuer E, Holland JF: Modulation and intensification of a cyclophosphamide, hexamethylmelamine, doxorubicin, and cisplatin ovarian cancer regimen. Obstet Gynecol 73:349, 1989.

Burris HA, Fields S: Summary of data from in vitro and phase I vinorelbine (Navelbine) studies. Semin Oncol 21: 14, 1994.

Buxton EJ, Meanwell CA, Hilton C, et al: Combination bleomycin, ifosfamide, and cisplatin chemotherapy in cervical cancer. J Natl Cancer Inst 81:359, 1989.

Carmichael J, Gordon A, Malfetano J, et al: Topotecan, a new active drug, vs. paclitaxel in advanced epithelial ovarian carcinoma: International Topotecan Study Group trial. Proc Am Soc Clin Oncol 15:283, 1996.

Cerny T, Kupfer A: Stabilization and quantitative determination of the neurotoxic metabolite chloracetaldehyde in the plasma of ifosfamide treated patients. Proc ECCO 5: 147, 1989.

Clarke SJ, Ward J, de Boer M, et al: Phase I study of the new thymidylate synthetase inhibitor Tomudex (ZD 1694). Ann Oncol 5:241, 1994.

Coldman A, Goldie J: Impact of dose-intense chemotherapy on the development of permanent drug resistance. Semin Oncol 14:29, 1987.

Colombo N, Pittelli M, Parma G, et al: Cisplatin dose intensity in advanced ovarian cancer: a randomized study of conventional dose versus dose-intense cisplatin monochemotherapy. Proc Am Soc Clin Oncol 12:255, 1993.

Conte P, Bruzzone M, Carnino F, et al: High-dose versus low-dose cisplatin in combination with cyclophosphamide and epidoxorubicin in suboptimal ovarian cancer: a randomized study of the Gruppo Oncologico Nord-Ovest. J Clin Oncol 14:351, 1996.

Conte PF, Bruzzone M, Chiara S, et al: A randomized trial comparing cisplatin plus cyclophosphamide versus cisplatin, doxorubicin, and cyclophosphamide in advanced ovarian cancer. J Clin Oncol 4:965, 1986.

Cortes JE, Pazdur R: Docetaxel. J Clin Oncol 13:2643, 1995.

Creasman WT, McCarty KS Sr, Barton TK, McCarty KS Jr: Clinical correlates of estrogen and progesterone binding proteins in human endometrial adenocarcinoma. Obstet Gynecol 55:363, 1980.

Curtin JP, Koonings PP, Gutierrez M, et al: Ifosfamide-induced neurotoxicity. Gynecol Oncol 42:193, 1991.

Demetri GD, Griffin JD: Hematopoietic growth factors and high dose chemotherapy: will grams succeed where milligrams fail? J Clin Oncol 8:761, 1990.

DeVita VT Jr: The consequences of the chemotherapy of Hodgkin's disease: the 10th annual David A. Karnofsky lecture. Cancer 47:1, 1981.

Dittrich C, Obermair A, Kurz C, et al: Prospective randomized trial of cisplatin/carboplatin versus conventional cisplatin/cyclophosphamide in epithelial ovarian cancer: first results of the impact of platinum dose intensity on patient outcome. Proc Am Soc Clin Oncol 15:279, 1996.

Donehower RC, Rowinsky EK, Grochow LB, et al: Phase I trial of taxol in patients with advanced cancer. Cancer Treat Rep 71:1171, 1987.

Edmondson JH, McCormack GW, Wieand HS: Late emerging survival differences in a comparative study of HCAP vs CP in stage III–IV ovarian carcinoma. In Salmon S (ed): Adjuvant Therapy VI. New York, Grune & Stratton, 1990, p 512.

Edmondson JH, McCormack GM, Wieand HS, et al: Cyclophosphamide-cisplatin versus cyclophosphamide-carboplatin in stage III–IV ovarian carcinoma: a comparison of equally myelosuppressive regimens. J Natl Cancer Inst 81:1500, 1989.

Ehrlich C, Young P, Cleary R: Cytoplasmic progesterone and estradiol receptors in normal, hyperplastic, and carcinomatous endometria: therapeutic implications. Am J Obstet Gynecol 141:539, 1981.

Einzig AI, Wiernik PH, Sasloff J, et al: Phase II study of taxol in patients with advanced ovarian cancer. Proc Am Assoc Cancer Res 31:187, 1990.

Eisenhauer EA, ten Bokkel Huinink WW, Swenerton KD, et al: European-Canadian randomized trial of paclitaxel in relapsed ovarian cancer: high-dose versus low-dose and long versus short infusion. J Clin Oncol 12:2654, 1994.

Fennelly D, Schneider J: Role of chemotherapy dose intensification in the treatment of advanced ovarian cancer. Oncology 9:911, 1995.

Fojo A, Hamilton T, Young RC, et al: Multidrug resistance in ovarian cancer. Cancer 60:2075, 1987.

Foster BJ, Clagett-Carr K, Marsoni S, et al: Role of hexamethylmelamine in the treatment of ovarian cancer: where is the needle in the haystack? Cancer Treat Rep 70: 1003, 1986.

Federico M, Alberts DS, Garcia DJ, et al: In vitro drug testing of ovarian cancer using the human tumor colony-forming assay: comparison of in vitro response and clinical outcome. Gynecol Oncol 55:S156, 1994.

Frei E, Canellos G: Dose: a critical factor in cancer chemotherapy. Am J Med 69:585, 1980.

Gershenson D, Burke T, Levenback B, et al: A phase I study of a daily x3 schedule of intravenous navelbine for refractory epithelial ovarian cancer. Proc Am Soc Clin Oncol 15:811, 1996.

Gershenson DM, Kavanagh JJ, Copeland LJ, et al: Cisplatin therapy for disseminated mixed mesodermal sarcoma of the uterus. J Clin Oncol 5:618, 1987a.

Gershenson DM, Kavanagh JJ, Copeland LJ, et al: High-dose doxorubicin infusion therapy for disseminated mixed mesodermal sarcoma of the uterus. Cancer 59:1264, 1987b.

Goldie J, Coldman A: A mathematical model for relating the drug sensitivity of tumors to the spontaneous mutation rate. Cancer Treat Rep 63:1727, 1979.

Gordon A, Bookman M, Malmstrom H, et al: Efficacy of topotecan in advanced epithelial ovarian cancer after failure of platinum and paclitaxel: International Topotecan Study Group trial. Proc Am Soc Clin Oncol 15:282, 1996.

Gore M, Mainwaring P, Macfarlane V, et al: A randomized study of high versus standard dose carboplatin in patients with advanced epithelial ovarian cancer. Proc Am Soc Clin Oncol 15:284, 1996.

Green MR: Gemcitabine safety overview. Semin Oncol 23: 32, 1996.

Grem JL, Tusch KD, Simon KJ, et al: Phase I study of taxol administered as a short I.V. infusion for five days. Cancer Treat Rep 71:1179, 1987.

Griffin TW, Bogden AE, Reich SD, et al: Initial clinical trials of the subrenal capsule assay as a predictor of tumor response to chemotherapy. Cancer 52:2185, 1983.

Gruppo Interegionale Cooperativo Oncologico Ginecologia: Randomized comparison of cisplatin with cyclophosphamide/cisplatin and with cyclophosphamide/doxorubicin/cisplatin in advanced ovarian cancer. Lancet 2:353, 1987.

Hacker N, Berek J, Pretorius R, et al: Intraperitoneal cisplatinum as salvage therapy for refractory epithelial ovarian cancer. Obstet Gynecol 70:759, 1987.

Hainsworth JD, Jones HW III, Burnett LS, et al: The role of hexamethylmelamine in the combination chemotherapy of advanced ovarian cancer: a comparison of hexamethylmelamine, cyclophosphamide, doxorubicin, and cisplatin (H-CAP) versus cyclophosphamide, doxorubicin, and cisplatin (CAP). Am J Clin Oncol 13:410, 1990.

Harker WG, Slade DL, Dalton WS, et al: Multidrug resistance in mitoxantrone-selected HL-60 leukemia cells in the absence of P-glycoprotein overexpression. Cancer Res 49: 4542, 1989.

Havsteen H, Bertelsen K, Gadeberg CC, et al: A phase 2 study with epirubicin as second-line treatment of patients with advanced epithelial ovarian cancer. Gynecol Oncol 63:210, 1996.

Hoskins WJ, Bundy BN, Thigpen JT, Omura GA: The influence of initial surgery on progression-free interval and survival in optimal stage III epithelial ovarian cancer. Gynecol Oncol 42:159, 1992.

Hreshchyshyn MM, Aron BS, Boronow RC, et al: Hydroxyurea or placebo combined with radiation to treat stage IIIB and IV cervical cancer confined to the pelvis. Int J Radiat Oncol Biol Phys 5:317, 1979.

Jakobsen A, Bertelsen K, Andersen JE, et al: Dose-effect study of carboplatin in ovarian cancer: a Danish Ovarian Cancer Group study. J Clin Oncol 15:193, 1997.

Kaldor JM, Day NE, Pettersson F, et al: Leukemia following chemotherapy for ovarian cancer. New Engl J Med 322:1, 1990.

Kaplan R, Markman M, Lucas W, et al: Infectious peritonitis in patients receiving intraperitoneal chemotherapy. Am J Med 78:49, 1985.

Kaye SB, Lewis CR, Paul J, et al: Randomised study of two doses of cisplatin with cyclophosphamide in epithelial ovarian cancer. Lancet 340:329, 1992.

Kaye S, Paul J, Cassidy J, et al: Mature results of a randomized trial of two doses of cisplatin for the treatment of ovarian cancer. J Clin Oncol 14:2113, 1996.

Kern DH, Wisenthal LM: Highly specific prediction of antineoplastic drug resistance with an in vitro assay using suprapharmacologic drug exposure. J Nat Cancer Inst 82:582, 1990.

Kochli OR, Sevin BU, Averette HE, et al: Overview of currently used chemosensitivity test systems in gynecologic malignancies and breast cancer. Contrib Gynecol Obstet 19:12, 1994.

Kotz K, Schilder R: High-dose chemotherapy and hematopoietic progenitor cell support for patients with epithelial ovarian cancer. Semin Oncol 22:250, 1995.

Kuhnle H, Meerpohl HG, Eiermann W, et al: Phase II study of carboplatin/ifosfamide in untreated advanced cervical cancer. Cancer Chemother Pharmacol 26(suppl):S33, 1990.

Lara PC, Garcia-Puche JL, Pedraza V: Cisplatin-ifosfamide as neoadjuvant chemotherapy in stage IIIB cervical uterine squamous cell carcinoma. Cancer Chemother Pharmacol 26(suppl):S36, 1990.

Levin L, Hryniuk W: Dose intensity analysis of chemotherapy regimens in ovarian carcinoma. J Clin Oncol 5:756, 1987.

Levin L, Simon R, Hryniuk W: Importance of multiagent chemotherapy regimens in ovarian carcinoma: dose intensity analysis. J Natl Cancer Inst 85:1732, 1993.

Lin JT, Bertino JR: Update on trimetrexate, a folate antagonist with antineoplastic and antiprotozoal properties. Cancer Invest 9:159, 1991.

Lira-Puerto V, Piccart M, Wiernik P: A comparison of U.S. and Mexican experience with single drug therapy in advanced cervical cancer. (NCI-PAHO and ECOG study). Proc Am Soc Clin Oncol 4:117, 1985.

Lum BL, Svec JM, Torti FM: Doxorubicin: alteration of dose scheduling as a means of reducing cardiotoxicity. Drug Intell Clin Pharmacol 19:259, 1985.

Maenpeaa JU, Heinonen E, Hinkka SM, et al: The subrenal capsule assay in selecting chemotherapy for ovarian cancer: a prospective randomized trial. Gynecol Oncol 57:294, 1995.

Manetta A, MacNeill C, Lyter JA, et al: Hexamethylmelamine as a single second-line agent in ovarian cancer. Gynecol Oncol 36:93, 1990.

Markman M: Intraperitoneal chemotherapy. Semin Oncol 18:248, 1991.

Markman M: Intraperitoneal chemotherapy. In Markman M, Hoskins W (eds): Cancer of the Ovary. New York, Raven Press, 1993, p 317.

Markman M, Cleary S, Lucas WE, Howell SB: Intraperitoneal chemotherapy with high-dose cisplatin and cytosine arabinoside for refractory ovarian carcinoma and other malignancies principally involving the peritoneal cavity. J Clin Oncol 3:925, 1985.

Markman M, Connelly B, Kennedy A, et al: Cisplatin (75 mg/m²) plus 3-hour infusional taxol (135 or 175 mg/m²): unexpected high incidence of peripheral neuropathy. Gynecol Oncol 60:9899, 1996a.

Markman M, Hakes T, Reichman B, et al: Intraperitoneal cisplatin and cytarabine in the treatment of refractory or recurrent ovarian carcinoma. J Clin Oncol 9:204, 1991a.

Markman M, Hakes T, Reichman B, et al: Ifosfamide and mesna in previously treated advanced epithelial ovarian cancer: activity in platinum-resistant disease. J Clin Oncol 10:243, 1992.

Markman M, Iseminger K, Hatch K, et al: Tamoxifen in platinum-refractory ovarian cancer: a Gynecologic Oncology Group ancillary report. Gynecol Oncol 62:4, 1996b.

Markman M, Muggia F: Intracavitary chemotherapy. CRC Crit Rev Oncol/Hematol 3:205, 1985.

Markman M, Reichman B, Hakes T, et al: Responses to second-line cisplatin-based intraperitoneal therapy in ovarian cancer: influence of a prior response to intravenous cisplatin. J Clin Oncol 9:1801, 1991b.

Markman M, Rothman R, Hakes T, et al: Second-line platinum therapy in patients with ovarian cancer previously treated with cisplatin. J Clin Oncol 9:389, 1991c.

Markman M, George M, Hakes T, et al: Phase II trial of intraperitoneal mitoxantrone in the management of refractory ovarian cancer. J Clin Oncol 8:146, 1990.

Martin PM, Rolland PH, Gammerre M, et al: Estradiol and progesterone receptors in normal and neoplastic endometrium: correlation between receptors, histopathologic examination, and clinical responses under progestin therapy. Int J Cancer 23:321, 1979.

Mather FJ, Simon RM, Clark GM, Von Hoff DD: Cardiotoxicity in patients treated with mitoxantrone: Southwest Oncology Group phase II studies. Cancer Treat Rep 71:609, 1987.

McCarty KS Jr, Barton TK, Fetter BF, et al: Correlation of estrogen and progesterone receptors with histologic differentiation in endometrial adenocarcinoma. Am J Pathol 96:171, 1979.

McGuire WP, Arseneau J, Blessing JA, et al: A randomized comparative trial of carboplatin and iproplatin in advanced squamous carcinoma of the uterine cervix: a Gynecologic Oncology Group study. J Clin Oncol 7:1462, 1989a.

McGuire WP, Hoskins WJ, Brady MF, et al: A phase III trial of dose intense versus standard dose cisplatin and cytoxan in advanced ovarian cancer. Proc Am Soc Clin Oncol 11:226, 1992.

McGuire WP, Hoskins W, Brady M, et al: Assessment of dose-intensive therapy in suboptimally debulked ovarian cancer: a Gynecologic Oncology Group study. J Clin Oncol 13:1589, 1995.

McGuire WP, Hoskins WJ, Brady NW, et al: Cyclophosphamide and cisplatin compared with paclitaxel and cisplatin in patients with stage III and stage IV ovarian cancer. N Engl J Med 334:1, 1996.

McGuire WP, Rowinsky EK, Rosenshein NB, et al: Taxol: a unique antineoplastic agent with significant activity in advanced ovarian epithelial neoplasms. Ann Intern Med 111:273, 1989b.

Minow R, Benjamin R, Gottlieb J: Adriamycin (NSC 123127) cardiomyopathy: an overview with determination of risk factors. Cancer Chemother Rep 6:195, 1975.

Moore DH, Fowler WC Jr, Jones CP, et al: Hexamethylmelamine chemotherapy for persistent or recurrent epithelial ovarian cancer. Am J Obstet Gynecol 165:573, 1991.

Muggia FM, Liu PY, Alberts DS, et al: Intraperitoneal mitoxantrone and floxuridine: effects on time-to-failure and survival in patients with minimal residual ovarian cancer after second-look laparotomy—a randomized phase II study by the Southwest Oncology Group. Gynecol Oncol 61:395, 1996.

Muggia FM, Braly PS, Brady MF, et al: Phase III trial of cisplatin or paclitaxel versus their combination in suboptimal stage III and IV epithelial ovarian cancer: Gynecologic Oncology Group study #132. Proc Am Soc Clin Oncol 16:352a, 1997a.

Muggia FM, Hainsworth J, Jeffers S, et al: Phase II study of liposomal doxorubicin in refractory ovarian cancer: antitumor activity and toxicity modification by liposomal encapsulation. J Clin Oncol 15:987, 1997b.

Muggia FM, McGuire W, Rozencweig M: Rationale, design and methodology of phase II clinical trials. In DeVita V Jr, Busch H (eds): Methods in Cancer Research, Vol. XVII. Cancer Drug Development, Part B. New York, Academic Press, 1979, p 199.

Muss HB, Bundy BN, DiSaia PJ, et al: Treatment of recurrent or advanced uterine sarcoma: a randomized trial of doxorubicin versus doxorubicin and cyclophosphamide (a phase III trial of the Gynecologic Oncology Group). Cancer 55:1648, 1985.

Myers C: The use of intraperitoneal chemotherapy in the treatment of ovarian cancer. Semin Oncol 11:275, 1984.

Neijt J, ten-Bokkel Huinink WW, van der Burg M, Dymant P: Randomized trial comparing two combination chemotherapy regimes (Hexa-CAF vs. CHAP-5) in advanced ovarian carcinoma. Lancet 2:594, 1984.

Neijt J, ten Bokkel Huinink W, van der Burg M, et al: Randomized trial comparing two combination chemotherapy regimens (CHAP-5 vs CP) in advanced ovarian carcinoma. J Clin Oncol 5:1157, 1987.

Neijt JP, ten Bokkel Huinink WW, van der Burg ME, et al: Long-term survival in ovarian cancer: mature data from The Netherlands Joint Study Group for Ovarian Cancer. Eur J Cancer 27:1367, 1991.

Ngan H, Choo Y, Cheung M, et al: A randomized study of high-dose versus low-dose cisplatinum combined with cyclophosphamide in the treatment of advanced ovarian cancer. Chemotherapy 35:221, 1989.

Nishida T, Nagasue N, Arimatsu T, et al: Ifosfamide, Adriamycin and cisplatin (IAP) plus bleomycin (B) combination chemotherapy in patients with recurrent cancer of the uterine cervix. Acta Obstet Gynaecol Jpn 41:590, 1989.

Ohnuma T, Zimet AS, Coffey VA, et al: Phase I study of taxol in a 24-hour infusion schedule. Proc Am Assoc Cancer Res 26:167, 1985.

Omura GA, Blessing JA, Ehrlich CE, et al: A randomized trial of cyclophosphamide and Adriamycin with or without cisplatin in advanced ovarian carcinoma: a Gynecologic Oncology Group study. Cancer 57:1725, 1986a.

Omura GA, Blessing JA, Major F, et al: A randomized clinical trial of adjuvant Adriamycin in uterine sarcomas: a Gynecologic Oncology Group study. J Clin Oncol 3:1240, 1986b.

Omura G, Blessing J, Vacarello L, et al: Randomized trial of cisplatin versus cisplatin plus mitolactol versus cisplatin plus ifosfamide in advanced squamous cell carcinoma of the cervix: a Gynecologic Oncology Group study. J Clin Oncol 15:165, 1997.

Omura G, Brady M, Delmore J, et al: A randomized trial of paclitaxel at 2 dose levels and filgastrim at 2 doses in platinum pretreated epithelial ovarian cancer: a Gynecologic Oncology Group, SWOG, NCCTG and ECOG study. Proc Am Soc Clin Oncol 15:280, 1996.

Omura GA, Brady MF, Homesley HD, et al: Long-term follow-up and prognostic factor analysis in advanced ovarian carcinoma: the Gynecologic Oncology Group experience. J Clin Oncol 9:1138, 1991.

Omura G, Bundy B, Berek J, et al: Randomized trial of cyclophosphamide plus cisplatin with or without doxorubicin in ovarian carcinoma: a Gynecologic Oncology Group study. J Clin Oncol 7:457, 1989.

Omura GA, Major F, Blessing JA: A randomized study of Adriamycin with and without dimethyl-triazenoimidazole carboxamide in advanced uterine sarcomas. Cancer 52:626, 1983a.

Omura GA, Morrow CP, Blessing JA, et al: A randomized comparison of melphalan versus melphalan plus hexamethylmelamine versus Adriamycin plus cyclophosphamide in ovarian carcinoma. Cancer 51:783, 1983b.

Ovarian Cancer Meta-Analysis Project: Cyclophosphamide plus cisplatin versus cyclophosphamide, doxorubicin, and cisplatin chemotherapy of ovarian carcinoma: a meta-analysis. J Clin Oncol 9:1668, 1991.

Ozols RF, Ostchega Y, Curt G, Young RC: High-dose carboplatin in refractory ovarian cancer patients. J Clin Oncol 5:197, 1987.

Ozols RF, Ostchega Y, Curt G, et al: High dose (HD) cisplatin (P) (40 mg/m^2) and HD carboplatinum (CBDCA) (400 mg/m^2 qd $\times$ 2) in refractory ovarian cancer: active salvage drugs with different toxicities. Proc Am Soc Clin Oncol 4:119, 1985.

Pecorelli S, Bolis G, Vassena L, et al: Randomized comparison of cisplatin and carboplatin in advanced ovarian cancer. Proc Am Soc Clin Oncol 7:136, 1988.

Perry MC (ed): The Chemotherapy Source Book, 2nd ed. Baltimore, Williams & Wilkins, 1996.

Piccart MJ, Bertelsen K, Stuart G, et al: Is cisplatin-paclitaxel the standard in first-line treatment of advanced ovarian cancer? The EORTC-GCCG, NOCOVA, NCI-C and Scottish Intergroup experience. Proc Am Soc Clin Oncol 16:352a, 1997.

Piotti P, Genitoni V, Comazzi R, et al: Relationship between pulmonary function tests and morphologic changes in the lung in bleomycin-treated patients. Tumori 70:439, 1984.

Piver MS, Lele S, Marchetti D, et al: Surgically documented response to intraperitoneal cisplatin, cytarabine, and bleomycin after intravenous cisplatin-based chemotherapy in advanced ovarian carcinoma. J Clin Oncol 6:1679, 1988.

Piver S: Hydroxyurea and radiation therapy in the treatment of carcinoma of the cervix. In Surwit E, Alberts D (eds): Cervix Cancer. Boston, Martinus Nijhoff, 1987, p 107.

Plosker GF, Faulds D: Epirubicin: a review of its pharmacodynamic and pharmacokinetic properties and therapeutic use in cancer chemotherapy. Drugs 45:788, 1993.

Plunkett W, Huang P, Searcy CE, et al: Gemcitabine: preclinical pharmacology and mechanism of action. Semin Oncol 23:3, 1996.

Potier P: The synthesis of Navelbine, prototype of a new series of vinblastine derivatives. Semin Oncol 16:2, 1989.

Reichman B, Markman M, Hakes T, et al: Intraperitoneal cisplatin and etoposide in the treatment of refractory/recurrent ovarian carcinoma. J Clin Oncol 7:1327, 1989.

Roila F, Tonato M, Cognetti F, et al: Prevention of cisplatin-induced emesis: a double-blind multicenter randomized crossover study comparing ondansetron and ondansetron plus dexamethasone. J Clin Oncol 9:675, 1991.

Rose PG, Blessing JA, Mayer AR, et al: Prolonged oral etoposide as second line therapy for platinum resistant and platinum sensitive ovarian carcinoma: a Gynecologic Oncology Group study. Proc Am Soc Clin Oncol 15:282, 1996.

Rosen GF, Lurain JR, Newton M: Hexamethylmelamine in ovarian cancer after failure of cisplatin-based multiple-agent chemotherapy. Gynecol Oncol 27:173, 1987.

Rowinsky EK, Donehower RC: Paclitaxel (taxol). N Engl J Med 332:1004, 1995.

Rowinsky EK, Donehower RC, Jones RJ, Tucker RW: Microtubule changes and cytotoxicity in leukemic cell lines treated with taxol. Cancer Res 48:4093, 1988.

Rowinsky ED, Gilbert MR, McGuire WP, et al: Sequences of taxol and cisplatin: a phase I and pharmacologic study. J Clin Oncol 9:1691, 1991a.

Rowinsky E, Mackey M, Goodman S: Meta-analysis of paclitaxel dose-response and dose-intensity in recurrent or refractory ovarian cancer. Proc Am Soc Clin Oncol 15:284, 1996.

Rowinsky EK, McGuire WP, Guarnieri T, et al: Cardiac disturbances during the administration of taxol. J Clin Oncol 9:1704, 1991b.

Rozencweig M, Martin A, Beltangady M, et al: Randomized trials of carboplatin versus cisplatin in advanced ovarian cancer. In Bunn P, Canetta R, Ozols R, Rozencweig M (eds): Carboplatin (JM-8): Current Perspectives and Future Directions. Philadelphia, WB Saunders, 1990, p 175.

Runowicz C, Dottino P, Shafir M, et al: Catheter complications associated with intraperitoneal chemotherapy. Gynecol Oncol 24:41, 1986.

Salmon SE, Hamburger AW, Soehnlen B, et al: Quantitation of differential sensitivity of human tumor stem cells to anticancer drugs. N Engl J Med 298:1321, 1978.

Shapiro J, Millward M, Rischin D, et al: Activity of gemcitabine in patients with advanced ovarian cancer: responses seen following platinum and paclitaxel. Gynecol Oncol 63:89, 1996.

Simon R: Designs for efficient clinical trials. Oncology 3:43, 1989.

Skipper H, Schabel F Jr, Wilcox W: Experimental evaluation of potential anticancer agents. XII. On the criteria and kinetics associated with "curability" of experimental leukemia. Cancer Chemother Rep 35:1, 1964.

Slayton RE, Park RC, Silverberg SG, et al: Vincristine, dactinomycin, and cyclophosphamide in the treatment of malignant germ cell tumors of the ovary. Cancer 56:243, 1985.

Sostman H, Matthay R, Putnam C: Cytotoxic-induced lung disease. Am J Med 62:608, 1977.

Speyer JL, Green MD, Dramer E, et al: Protective effect of the bis-piperazinedione (ICRF 187) against doxorubicin-induced cardiac toxicity in women with advanced breast cancer. New Engl J Med 319:745, 1988.

Stehman FB, Blessing JA, McGehee R, Barrett RJ: A phase II evaluation of mitolactol in patients with advanced squamous cell carcinoma of the cervix: a Gynecologic Oncology Group study. J Clin Oncol 7:1892, 1989.

Stehman F, Bundy B, Keys H, et al: A randomized trial of hydroxyurea versus misonidazole adjunct to radiation therapy in carcinoma of the cervix. Am J Obstet Gynecol 159:87, 1988.

Sutton GP, Blessing JA, Adcock L, et al: Phase II study of ifosfamide and mesna in patients with previously-treated carcinoma of the cervix: a Gynecologic Oncology Group study. Invest New Drug 7:341, 1989a.

Sutton GP, Blessing JA, Photopoulos G, et al: Phase II experience with ifosfamide/mesna in gynecologic malignancies: preliminary report of Gynecologic Oncology Group studies. Semin Oncol 16(suppl 3):68, 1989b.

Sutton GP, Blessing JA, Rosenshein N, et al: Phase II trial of ifosfamide and mesna in mixed mesodermal tumors of the uterus: a Gynecologic Oncology Group study. Am J Obstet Gynecol 161:309, 1989c.

Swenerton K, Jeffrey J, Stuart G, et al: Cisplatin-cyclophosphamide versus carboplatin-cyclophosphamide in advanced ovarian cancer: a randomized phase II study of the National Cancer Institute of Canada Clinical Trials Group. J Clin Oncol 10:718, 1992.

ten Bokkel Huinink WW, van der Burg MEL, van Oosterom AT, et al: Carboplatin in combination therapy for ovarian cancer. Cancer Treat Rev 15(suppl B):9, 1988.

Thigpen JT: Chemotherapy of gynecologic cancer. In Perry MC (ed): The Chemotherapy Source Book, 2nd ed. Baltimore, Williams & Wilkins, 1996, p 1253.

Thigpen JT, Blessing JA, Ball H, et al: A phase II trial of taxol in patients with ovarian carcinoma progressive after prior chemotherapy: a Gynecologic Oncology Group study. J Clin Oncol 12:1748, 1994.

Thigpen JT, Blessing JA, Beecham J, et al: Phase II trial of cisplatin as first-line chemotherapy in patients with advanced or recurrent uterine sarcomas: a Gynecologic Oncology Group study. J Clin Oncol 9:962, 1991a.

Thigpen JT, Blessing JA, DiSaia PJ, Ehrlich CE: A randomized comparison of Adriamycin with or without cyclophosphamide in the treatment of advanced or recurrent endometrial carcinoma. Proc Am Soc Clin Oncol 4:115, 1985.

Thigpen T, Blessing J, DiSaia P, Ehrlich C: Oral medroxyprogesterone acetate in advanced or recurrent endometrial carcinoma: results of therapy and correlation with estrogen and progesterone receptor levels. The Gynecologic Oncology Group experience. In Baulier E, Iacobelli S, McGuire W (eds): Endocrinology and Malignancy. Park Ridge, NJ, Parthenon, 1986a, p 446.

Thigpen JT, Blessing J, Hatch KD, et al: A randomized trial of oral medroxyprogesterone acetate 200 μg versus 1000 μg daily in advanced and recurrent endometreal carcinoma. Proc Am Soc Clin Oncol 10:185, 1991b.

Thigpen JT, Blessing JA, Homesley HD, Lewis G Jr: Phase II trials of cisplatin and piperazinedione in advanced or recurrent squamous cell carcinoma of the vulva: a Gynecologic Oncology Group study. Gynecol Oncol 23:358, 1986b.

Thigpen JT, Blessing JA, Homesley HD, et al: Phase II trial of cisplatin in advanced or recurrent cancer of the vagina: a Gynecologic Oncology Group study. Gynecol Oncol 23:101, 1986c.

Thigpen T, Blessing J, Homesley H, et al: Phase III trial of doxorubicin ± cisplatin in advanced or recurrent endometrial carcinoma: a Gynecologic Oncology Group study. Proc Am Soc Clin Oncol 12:261, 1993.

Thigpen JT, Blessing JA, Orr JW Jr, DiSaia PJ: Phase II trial of cisplatin in the treatment of patients with advanced or recurrent mixed mesodermal sarcomas of the uterus: a phase II trial of the Gynecologic Oncology Group. Cancer Treat Rep 70:271, 1986d.

Thigpen JT, Buchsbaum HJ, Mangan C, Blessing JA: Phase II trial of Adriamycin in the treatment of advanced or recurrent endometrial carcinoma: a Gynecologic Oncology Group study. Cancer Treat Rep 63:21, 1979.

Thigpen T, Lambuth B, Vance R: Ifosfamide in the management of gynecologic cancers. Semin Oncol 17:11, 1990.

Thigpen T, Lambuth BW, Vance RB: The role of ifosfamide in gynecologic cancer. Semin Oncol 19:30, 1992b.

Thigpen T, Vance R, Khansur T: The platinum compounds and paclitaxel in the management of carcinomas of the endometrium and uterine cervix. Semin Oncol 22:67, 1995.

Thigpen T, Vance R, Lambuth B, et al: Chemotherapy for advanced or recurrent gynecologic cancer. Cancer 60:2104, 1987.

Uziely B, Jeffers S, Isacson R, et al: Liposomal doxorubicin: antitumor activity and unique toxicities during two complementary phase I studies. J Clin Oncol 13:1777, 1995.

Vaage J, Mayhew E, Lasic D, et al: Therapy of primary and metastatic mouse mammary carcinomas with doxorubicin encapsulated in long circulating liposomes. Int J Cancer 51:942, 1992.

van der Burg ME, Hoff AM, van Lent M, et al: Carboplatin and cyclophosphamide salvage therapy for ovarian cancer patients relapsing after cisplatin combination chemotherapy. Eur J Cancer 27:248, 1991.

van der Burg ME, van Lent M, Buyse M, et al: The effects of debulking surgery after induction chemotherapy on the prognosis in advanced epithelial ovarian cancer: Gynecologic Cancer Cooperative Group of the European Organization for Research and Treatment of Cancer. N Engl J Med 332:675, 1995.

Vermorken JB, Kobierska A, van der Burg ME, et al: High dose epirubicin in platinum pretreated patients with ovarian carcinoma: the EORTC-GCCG experience. Eur J Gynecol Oncol 16:433, 1995.

Von Hoff DD: He's not going to talk about in vitro predictive assays again, is he? J Nat Cancer Inst 82:96, 1990.

Weisenthal LM, Marsden JA, Dill PL, Macaluso CK: A novel dye exclusion method for testing in vitro chemosensitivity of human tumors. Cancer Res 43:749, 1983.

Weiss G, Green S, Alberts DS, et al: Second-line treatment of advanced measurable ovarian cancer with iproplatin: a Southwest Oncology Group Study. Eur J Cancer 27:135, 1991.

Wiernik PH, Schwartz EL, Einzig A, et al: Phase I trial of taxol given as a 24-hour infusion every 21 days: responses observed in metastatic melanoma. J Clin Oncol 5:1232, 1987.

Williams SD, Blessing JA, Moore DH, et al: Cisplatin, vinblastine, and bleomycin in recurrent ovarian germ cell tumors: a trial of the Gynecologic Oncology Group. Ann Intern Med 111:22, 1989a.

Williams S, Blessing J, Slayton R, et al: Ovarian germ cell tumors: adjuvant trials of the Gynecologic Oncology Group (GOG). Proc Am Soc Clin Oncol 8:150, 1989b.

Wiltshaw E: Ovarian trials at the Royal Marsden. Cancer Treat Rev 12(suppl A):67, 1985.

Wiltshaw E, Evans B, Rustin G, et al: A prospective randomized trial comparing high-dose cisplatin with low-dose cisplatin and chlorambucil in advanced ovarian carcinoma. J Clin Oncol 4:722, 1986.

Yordan E, Bonomi P, Wilbanks G: Chemotherapy of vulvar and vaginal neoplasms. In Deppe G (ed): Chemotherapy of Gynecologic Cancer. New York, Alan R. Liss, 1984, p 85.

Zanaboni F, Scarfone G, Presti M, et al: Salvage chemotherapy for ovarian cancer recurrence: weekly cisplatin in combination with epirubicin or etoposide. Gynecol Oncol 43:24, 1991.

17

Principles of Radiation Therapy

John E. Byfield
Conley G. Lacey

Gynecologic oncology is almost unique in the level of integration that now exists between its surgical and radiation components. This integration, acquired over the past five decades, has resulted from the extensive experience of many medical centers. While areas of controversy still exist, the general principles of combined therapy are now reasonably well understood. To understand and to apply these principles, general comprehension of both the physics and the biology of radiation is required. With the growing administration of chemotherapy to many gynecologic cancer patients, the biology of the various organs within and surrounding the abdomen takes on added significance. It is the purpose of this chapter to give the reader a working knowledge of these principles and to illustrate their applications in gynecologic cancers. Specific topics and applications are discussed under the various disease categories elsewhere in this book.

INTRODUCTION TO RADIATION ONCOLOGY

Conventional clinical radiation sources can be divided into two basic types: (1) radiation sources used in the external regionalized treatment of cancer, of which cobalt units and linear accelerators are the most common representatives; and (2) internal radiation sources that are inserted into organ cavities or tissues, usually temporarily, to deliver localized therapy. For practical purposes, the gynecologist need be familiar only with external beam treatment methods and those intracavitary and interstitial treatments common to gynecologic oncology. External beam elec-

trical units (mainly linear accelerators) deliver high-energy photons, almost always with energies exceeding 1 MV. The electromagnetic radiation that emerges from some decaying isotopes (e.g., ^{60}Co) also consists of photons; these historically were termed *gamma rays*, but are identical to the radiation generated by electrical sources called *x-rays*. Most radiotherapy installations in the United States also have electron beam capacity. Electron beams are the primary particles produced by linear accelerators and can be used clinically if their energy is sufficiently high. Internal radiation emitters deliver either medium-energy photons (e.g., radioactive gold) or relatively high-energy electrons called *beta particles* (e.g., chromic phosphate [^{32}P]). Photons generate high-energy electrons within tissue water. Electrons are biologically equivalent to photon therapy in all respects save dosimetry. The use of one or more of these modalities to suppress the growth of cancer constitutes the medical practice of radiation oncology.

FUNDAMENTALS OF RADIATION PHYSICS

Structure of Matter

All matter consists of elemental particles, the most important of which make up the nuclei. The nucleus of every atom consists of positively charged particles (protons) and electrically neutral particles (neutrons); the simplest form is hydrogen, which consists of a single proton. The symbol for an atom (e.g., $^{60}_{27}$Co) includes two parts: (1) the subscript, which indicates the number of protons in the nucleus (the atomic number; e.g., $_{27}$Co), and (2) the superscript, which indicates the total number of protons plus neutrons (the mass number: e.g., ^{60}Co). The larger these numbers, the heavier the atomic nucleus. Surrounding the dense, heavy nucleus are the negatively charged orbital electrons, which, under electrochemically neutral conditions equal the number of protons. The weight of an electron is about 1/1,900th that of either nuclear particle, but electrons occupy a much larger volume of space. They may be conceptualized as a "cloud" around the nucleus and are responsible for the size of the atom. A neutron can be conceived as containing one proton and one electron (hence its neutrality). Atoms possessing identical numbers of protons but different numbers of neutrons are called *isotopes*. It is now known that the nucleus contains many other forms of particles, some of which appear to function as "glue" to hold it together. Other particles (e.g., pi mesons) are under study for potential therapeutic applications.

Origins of Natural Radioactivity: Radioactive Decay

When an imbalance exists between the number of protons and the number of neutrons in an atom, the atom may disintegrate by expelling a portion of the nucleus as either a particle or a gamma ray; this process will continue until a stable isotope is reached. This is termed *radioactive decay* and occurs in nature (e.g., radium). The useful radioactive isotopes are more commonly man made, the unstable atoms being generated by bombarding stable atoms with nuclear particles, creating new, heavier, unstable nuclei. As the number of protons in an atom increases, the potential number of both stable and unstable isotopes increases. From the standpoint of radiation therapy, the most important form of nuclear decay is one in which a portion of the imbalance within the nucleus is released as a packet of energy called a *photon* or gamma ray. A photon can be thought of as a package of energy traveling at the speed of light. Although photons are a form of electromagnetic energy, they have some properties similar to those of particles, especially in their interaction with other matter. Photons are commonly represented by the formula $h\nu$, where ν is the frequency and h is Planck's constant. As with all forms of electromagnetic energy, photons carry energy, the amount of which is proportional to their frequency ν and inversely related to their wavelength (λ). For all such ra-

diation $\nu = c$ (where $c = 3.0 \times 10^8$ m/sec, the speed of light in a vacuum). Thus the energy (E) carried by a photon is equal to $h\nu$. Photons used in radiation therapy vary from a few hundred thousand volts (kV) up to 50 million volts (MV).* While the basic principle of radioactive decay can be intuitively grasped without difficulty, the exact nature of this process is still only partially understood.

Three examples of clinically useful radioactive decay phenomena are shown in Figure 17–1. In cases such as ^{32}P, the radioactive decay phenomena are shown in Figure 17–1. In cases such as ^{32}P, the radioactive nucleus releases a pure beta particle (β^-, the atomic physicist's symbol for an electron). In this case, the negative particle (electron) can be envisioned as being ejected from a neutron in the nucleus, creating a new proton that converts the nucleus to a stable isotope of sulfur. A more complex process occurs when radioactive ^{60}Co decays. First a beta particle is released, and then the unstable intermediate nucleus immediately releases two photons, both of whose energies slightly exceed 1 MV. These two gamma rays are the source of the useful ^{60}Co treatment beam. The product is a stable isotope of nickel. An even more complex sequence of decay is shown in the third example, the decay of radiogold (^{108}Au). In this case, two significant alternative pathways exist, both of which are initiated by release of a beta particle. The beta particles can be distinguished by their different energies, but, more importantly, one pathway (release of the 0.959-MeV β^- particle) occurs 99 times as commonly as the other (release of the 0.282-MeV particle). The "extra" energy left behind by the low-energy β^- ejection is immediately released in the form of a 0.677-MV gamma ray. In both cases, the nucleus then either releases 0.412-MV gamma rays (95.6 percent of the time) or, in a small percentage of decays, is converted into an orbital electron. Once per 5,000 times, a third β^-, gamma ray release occurs. The complexity of such reactions is beyond the scope of this chapter; interested readers are referred to Johns and Cunningham (1983) for a more fundamental description. For the interested reader, the difference between maximum and average beta particle

---

*The reader will encounter the terms *MV* and *MeV* throughout the radiation oncology literature. Technically, MV should be used to denote the energy of photons per se, while MeV relates to the energy of electrons (*million* electron volts). However, the terms are frequently interchanged and are equivalent in their general meaning.

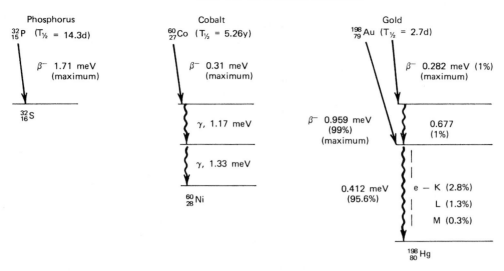

FIGURE 17-1. Three representative types of decay are illustrated for unstable isotopes used in gynecologic cancer therapy. See text for details.

energy is discussed by Rosenshein et al (1979).

In addition to the production of beta particles and gamma rays of different energies, each form of nuclear decay also has an intrinsic time constant termed the *half-life* ($T_{1/2}$). The $T_{1/2}$ of an unstable isotope is the length of time it would take for one half of the initial particles to undergo radioactive decay. The fact that a decay $T_{1/2}$ is a constant for each decay reaction is strong evidence for the randomness of the event for any given nucleus. The $T_{1/2}$ is important in therapy and indicates that, as time passes, the amount of radiation released decreases exponentially. Thus, in the first half-life, 50 percent of all the radiation remains, whereas after the fourth half-life only 1/16th remains (1/2 × 1/2 × 1/2 × 1/2). For example, 1 month after receiving an intraperitoneal injection of ^{198}Au ($T_{1/2}$ = 2.7 days), the maximum residual radiation in a patient's abdomen is very small, whereas after a dose of ^{32}P ($T_{1/2}$ = 14.3 days), about 25 percent can still remain. Note that the maximum amounts potentially present are precisely calculable. Similarly, a ^{60}Co source installed 5.26 years ago will have an output one-half that when new, and the treatment time must be twice as long. Half-lives vary from small fractions of a second to years—in the examples given, from 2.7 days (^{198}Au) to 5.26 years (^{60}Co). Isotopes used in interstitial or intraperitoneal treatments (Table 17–1) usually have a $T_{1/2}$ measured in days. Radioisotopes used for external beam therapy or as removable intracavitary sources (radium and cesium) have a $T_{1/2}$ measured in years. The reason for this is that far smaller amounts of radioactivity are usually used in interstitial therapy, so that the dose rate and total deposited useful energy need to be released faster, that is, within the time frame (days) that tumor cell damage occurs.

It is becoming increasingly common in the United States and Europe to replace intracavitary brachytherapy treatments (usually cesium) with high-dose-rate (HDR) outpatient intracavitary regimens. This approach eliminates the need for expensive hospitalization and for the general anesthesia that is usually employed for the conventional radium or cesium implants. While this approach is new, there already is sufficient information to justify its use in many forms of uterine cancer therapy. The most commonly available unit is called a *micro-Selectron*, which uses highly radioactive iridium-192. Special applicators are used for the tandem and colpostats. The variety of available applicators is increasing rapidly. Typically, a single, low-dose-rate cesium implant extending over approximately 48 hours is replaced by four to six or more HDR applications in which the radiation exposure is approximately 10 to 20 minutes. Examples of this are indicated later in this chapter.

TABLE **17–1**

Radioisotopes Used in Gynecologic Oncology

Name	Symbol	Decay Product	Half-Life	Energy (MV/MeV)	Usefulness
Cobalt	$^{60}_{27}$Co	Gamma ray	5.26 years	1.17	External beam radiotherapy
		Gamma ray	5.26 years	1.33	
		Beta particle	5.26 years	0.31	None
Cesium	$^{137}_{55}$Cs	Gamma ray	30 years	0.662	Common source of intracavitary radiation in place of radium
		Beta particle		0.51, 1.17	None
Radium, radon, and decay products	$^{226}_{86}$Ra	Gamma ray	1,620 years	0.18–2.2	Intracavitary treatments; major useful product is radon gas ($^{222}_{86}$Ra), which is troublesome because of leakage potential
		Alpha particle			
		Beta particle			
Iridium	$^{192}_{77}$Ir	Gamma ray	74.5 days	0.136–0.613	Interstitial therapy; effective gamma energy is about 0.340 MeV
		Beta particle	74.5 days	Maximum at 0.67	
Gold	$^{198}_{79}$Au	Gamma ray	2.7 days	0.071–1.09	Significant gamma rays are 0.677 (1.3%) and 0.412 (98.6%) MeV; colloidal preparation used for serosal radiation; seeds used occasionally as permanent interstitial sources
		Beta particle	2.7 days	0.959	
Phosphorus	$^{32}_{15}$P	Beta particle	14.3 days	0.698 (average)	Serosal radiation in ovarian cancer
Iodine	$^{125}_{53}$I	Gamma ray	60.2 days	0.035	Seeds, used occasionally; largely replaced by iridium

Physical Absorption of Ionizing Radiation

The generation of lethal damage in tumor and normal cells by x- or gamma rays depends on the conversion in tissues of photon energy into kinetic energy of electrons and subsequent chemical changes within target molecules. This represents the absorption of energy by tissue and is measured in *rad*. It has been agreed that the term *rad* will be replaced by the term *Gray* (Gy), where 1 Gy = 100 rad and 1 centiGray (cGy) = 1 rad. The unit cGy will be used throughout this chapter, but the vast majority of the existing literature uses the rad measurement system. However, cGy is now the correct technical term and is used in all current publications. To add further to the confusion, it may be noted that the correct plural form for rad is also rad, but frequently the more conventional term *rads* is used.

The mechanisms by which the first step in energy deposition takes place depend on the energy of the photon and the composition of the atoms in the target cells. Three distinct physical mechanisms exist: (1) photoelectric absorption, (2) Compton absorption, and (3) pair production. *Photoelectric absorption* occurs only with photons of relatively low en-

ergy (from about 0.5 to 100 kV) and can be envisioned as a transmission of photon energy into kinetic energy of inner shell electrons (K, L, and M shells). The variation in energy required to remove an inner electron is due to the higher forces required for removal of electrons closely "bound" by nuclei with more protons. Photoelectric absorption is proportional to the cube of the atomic number (Z). Thus calcium in bone ($Z = 20$) will absorb many more low-energy photons than the elements of soft tissue (the Z values for H, C, and O are 1, 6, and 8, respectively). The photoelectric effect is the basis for diagnostic x-ray pictures, which basically distinguish bones or high-Z contrast media from soft tissues.

The second mechanism for photon energy absorption is termed *Compton absorption* (named after its discoverer). Compton absorption predominates for photon energies in the therapeutic range (100 kV to 10 to 20 MV). It involves the transfer of some energy of the incoming photon to electrons of the outer shells whose binding energy is relatively small and much more easily set in motion. Thus the atomic number (number of protons) does not significantly influence Compton absorption, and all tissues, gram for gram, absorb about the same amount of energy. As the energy of the photon increases in this range, the energy of the "recoiling" Compton electron increases, and its destructive power becomes much greater. Compton absorption, which leads to highly energetic electrons, is responsible for most of the therapeutic effects of radiation treatments.

The third process, *pair production*, occurs only when the energy of the photon exceeds 1.02 MV. It results from the absorption of the photon by a nucleus with the emission of a positive and a negative electron pair (i.e., a positron and an electron). Since the "rest" energy of an electron (or positron) is 0.511 MeV, twice that amount of energy is needed for each pair production. For photon beams exceeding 1.02 MV some extra energy exists, and the process can involve an electron (rather than a nucleus), the extra energy then being taken up as kinetic energy of the affected electron (hence it is termed *triplet production*). For photon beams above 1.02 MV, pair production becomes increasingly important and Compton absorption declines; this change has no known biologic implications. The positron emitted by pair production interacts with (is "annihilated" by) a free electron, resulting in the emission of two photons of 0.511 MV, which then interact further in the cell (largely by Compton absorption). Since the field of a nucleus is a function of its size (atomic number), atoms with higher Z values will absorb more energy by pair production (Z^2).

A visual contrast between energy absorption by photoelectric absorption (which is Z dependent) and Compton absorption (Z independent) can be seen by comparing Figure 17–13 with Figure 17–14. The high concentration of calcium in bone results in the absorption of incident x-rays in the diagnostic (100-kV) x-ray picture (Fig. 17–13), whereas a port film (Fig. 17–14) taken with photons of a 6-MV linear accelerator shows only air-tissue interfaces, since at this energy Z-independent Compton absorption takes place. The relatively high incidence of bone necrosis in the early days of x-ray therapy has now been greatly reduced by the development of high-energy treatment beams in which undesirable photoelectric absorption by normal bone is greatly reduced.

Inverse Square Law

Of fundamental importance in understanding the clinical use of high-energy radiation is the inverse square law. This law, which applies to all electromagnetic radiation, including visible light, states that the amount of energy present at a point distant from a radiation source varies with the inverse square of the distance from the source. Thus the amount of light visible to a square unit of receptor on the human retina from a light source 1 cm away is four times that available if the same source were placed 2 cm away and nine times that from a 3-cm distance. This can be readily envisioned if one considers photons emanating from a point source of radiation as small packages of energy. As they fan out in space, the packages of energy become increasingly less "concentrated" in any square unit of the sphere as the sphere is drawn farther and farther away from the energy point source. Thus energy is diluted in a spherical configuration as it travels away from the source, and its concentration in space is inversely related to the square of the distance traveled.

The inverse square law is important in many aspects of radiation treatment. Its therapeutic importance becomes progressively less profound, however, as measurements are taken farther and farther from the energy source. The drop in energy over the distance of 1 cm is small if that 1 cm is added at 100 cm away from the radiation source (a typical treatment distance for modern linear accelerators). However, if the radiation source is a radium or cesium needle lying within the cervical canal, the rate of dose falloff with the addition of 1 cm is great. Thus in the previous illustration, the radiation dose at 3 cm from the source is one-ninth that at 1 cm from the source, whereas the dose at 101 cm is about 98 percent that at 100 cm.

The inverse square law is especially relevant in gynecologic cancer, where intracavitary and interstitial treatments are common. High-energy sources such as cesium placed in the uterus or vagina, or iridium needles in the lower parametrial tissues, deliver a much higher radiation dose to tissues immediately adjacent than to tissues just a short distance away. The efficacy of radiation treatment in the cure of cancer of the cervix lies primarily in the ability to deliver such high-energy radiation locally, sparing normal pelvic organs, a feature that is directly dependent on the inverse square law.

The inverse square law also has important implications for minimizing vaginal complications in radiation therapy. This can be seen in Figure 17–2, in which the radiation at point A (defined as 2 cm above the lateral vaginal fornix and 2 cm lateral to the endocervical canal) is contrasted for two colpostat applications for cervical cancer. In one case (right fornix, the mucosal contact line of the surface of the colpostats being shown by the dotted lines), the colpostat is placed in an extremely narrow vaginal vault with no plastic spacer cap. The surface dose rate to the vaginal mucosal tissues is 100 cGy/hr, whereas that at point A is 55 cGy/hr. When a spacer is used (left fornix) to increase the distance from the source to the surface of the ovoid (e.g., in a more capacious vaginal fornix), the dose rate to the mucosa is reduced to 60 to 70 cGy/hr, but the dose rate to point A remains 55 cGy/

hr. It can be seen that the ratio of the two is significantly more favorable when the spacer has been used. This is due to the energy dilution according to the inverse square law, which effectively reduces the vaginal mucosal dose rate and consequently leads to better dosimetry and a reduced likelihood of vault necrosis.

The inverse square law is also the single most important factor in maximizing radioprotection. Thus personnel involved in the handling of radioactive isotopes and caring for patients with radioactive implants should keep a maximum distance between all parts of their body and the radioactive material (sources). One additional foot of distance from the sources during bedside conversations dramatically reduces the radiation dose. A clear understanding of the inverse square law is important in all aspects of radiation oncology.

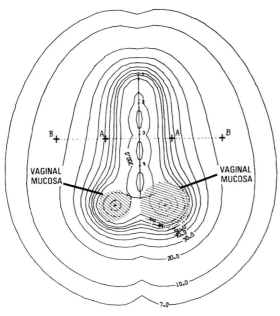

FIGURE 17–2. Isodose curve for a typical cesium insertion in cancer of the cervix. The numbers indicate the dose in centiGrays per hour at various sites around the colpostat (colpostat centers indicated by the cross). The location of points A and B is as indicated. On the left side of the figure a colpostat without plastic spacer (dotted lines in the outside circle) is shown, while on the right side the volume of the spacer has been increased by adding a large plastic cap. It can be seen that the larger spacer pushes the mucosa away from the radioactive source without significantly affecting the dose at point A or B. This improves the therapeutic ratio by significantly reducing the dose to the vaginal mucosa. The applicators themselves are shown in Figure 17–17.

RADIATION TREATMENT INSTRUMENTATION

Machinery currently used in the treatment of patients with gynecologic cancer can conveniently be divided into four types: (1) cobalt, (2) electrical x-ray sources, (3) high-dose-rate implant devices, and (4) experimental particle sources. Cobalt treatment units were first introduced in Canada in 1951 and almost immediately replaced the occasional teleradium units then in existence. Similarly, linear accelerators (linacs) began to replace cobalt units after 1960. In principle, it seems unlikely that further major evolutionary steps will occur, since the most desirable photon energies have now been obtained and current machinery is relatively inexpensive and acceptably reliable. However, there are theoretical advantages to some forms of particle therapy, as described later.

Cobalt Treatment Units

^{60}Co was for years the most common radiation treatment source worldwide because of its relatively low cost and its mechanical reliability. In most Western countries, it has been replaced by higher energy linear accelerators. ^{60}Co is generated in a radioactive pile by bombarding ^{59}Co with neutrons that originate from ^{235}U according to the reaction

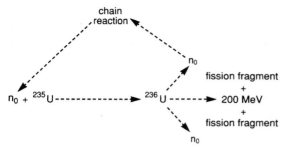

The neutrons released when ^{236}U decays are then used in part for the activation of several useful isotopes, such as

$$^{59}\text{Co} + n_0 \rightarrow {}^{60}\text{Co}$$

$$^{31}\text{P} + n_0 \rightarrow {}^{32}\text{P}$$

$$^{197}\text{Au} + n_0 \rightarrow {}^{198}\text{Au}.$$

Equivalent reactions can produce radioactive tracers such as radiopotassium, sodium, and iron.

^{60}Co instruments radiate gamma rays of 1.17 and 1.33 MV. The depth dose of ^{60}Co is quite satisfactory for most treatment situations except for deep-seated tumors in obese patients. In such cases, a more penetrating beam is highly desirable. Since many gynecology patients fit into this category, in general linac beams (4 to 20 MV or greater) are preferable. The other major difference between modern linacs and ^{60}Co is the *penumbra*, or shadow, at the edge of the treatment beam. This is a physical phenomenon that stems from the significantly larger size of the ^{60}Co source than is available from a linac source. It is represented as the convex "spreading" of the isodose lines shown in Figure 17–3. In practice one must choose some portion of this shadow to determine the defined treatment dose. Any area irradiated outside of this volume is extraneous and therefore can only add to complications. In gynecologic cancers, this is not particularly

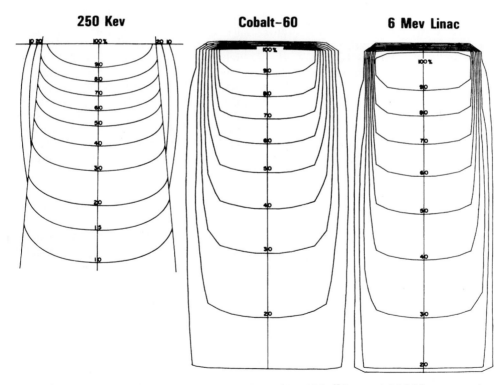

FIGURE 17–3. Typical isodose curves for orthovoltage (250-kV), ^{60}Co, and 6-MV linear accelerator. The most important difference between the megavoltage (^{60}Co and linac) beams in comparison with the 250-kV unit is the movement of the 100 percent isodose line several millimeters beneath the skin surface. This results in elimination of the severe skin reactions characteristic of earlier radiation sources. In addition, it can be seen that the higher energy leads to deeper penetration as the energy of the beam increases. The lateral spreading of the beam (penumbra or shadow) is less with ^{60}Co than with the 250-kV unit and is further reduced in the accelerator beam. The reduction of the penumbra with the accelerator beam is due to its possessing a source with smaller physical dimensions.

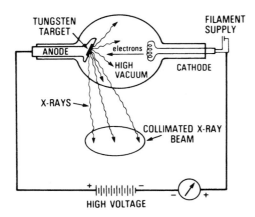

FIGURE 17–4. Diagram of the mechanism of x-ray production by a conventional x-ray (cathode ray) tube. These types of tubes are used in diagnostic machines and in therapy units in the treatment of superficial cancers.

important (at least its importance cannot be quantified). In areas where beam precision is vital, such as over the central nervous system or the lens of the eye, the use of a linac is preferred. The crisp edge of the accelerator treatment portal shown in Figure 17–14 demonstrates visually the sharp, box-like edge of the linac isodose lines shown in Figure 17–3.

Electrical Treatment Units

During the first half of this century, electrical treatment units using an x-ray tube predominated. The principle of this approach (Fig. 17–4) remained the same throughout this period. In an x-ray tube, a cathode filament is heated to very high temperatures and electrons are emitted from the heated surface. These are then accelerated by a voltage placed across the high-vacuum space between the cathode and the anode. The high-speed electrons strike a target (usually tungsten), and photons (x-rays) are emitted. The reaction therefore resembles a reversal of the phenomenon that occurs when photons strike tissue.

Throughout the period of development of electrical treatment units, the major challenge has been to increase the speed or energy of the electrons involved in generating the photons, since the photon energy is dependent on the energy of the generating electrons. Four different approaches were used: (1) development of improved cathode ray tubes, which are still useful in the treatment of superficial tumors and are called *orthovoltage* units; (2) Van de Graaff generators, which used mechanical transport of electrons followed by acceleration up to 10 MeV through a series of step electrodes; (3) betatrons, which employ a magnetic field to accelerate electrons up to 300 MeV; and (4) linacs, which employ a radiofrequency wave to accelerate the electrons (Fig. 17–5). As linacs have improved, they have essentially replaced all other forms of high-voltage therapy units. When linacs achieved energies of 12 MV or greater, clinically useful electron

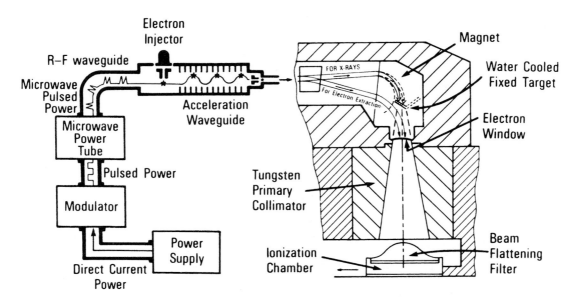

FIGURE 17–5. Diagram of a modern linac.

beams could be routinely obtained by removal of the target from the beam path, and the final advantage of other considerably more cumbersome generators, such as betatrons, disappeared. Today, clinically useful linacs are available with energies ranging from 4 to over 25 MV. In practice, a machine with variable energy output between 4 and 20 MV is ideal, with the higher energies having an advantage in only the most corpulent patients. In an era of cost-effective medical constraints, the volume and type of patient load must be considered in the choice of an instrument.

The other major advantage of high-energy linacs was the development of useful electron beams. As noted earlier, it is the release of electrons in tissue that is ultimately responsible for the biologic effects of ionizing radiation. In general, electron beams with mean energies below 6 MeV are not useful, since the capacity for penetration is insufficient. For example, the dose at 2.5 cm from an average (field)-size 6-MeV electron beam is only about 20 percent of the maximum dose, which occurs close to the surface. For 18-MeV electrons, the maximum dose also occurs near the surface, but the dose at even 7.0 cm is still 50 percent of the maximum dose. Electrons of intermediate energies correspondingly have different penetration curves; the lower the energy, the greater the rate of dose reduction (and energy deposition) with tissue penetration. Electron beams are therefore more useful in the treatment of relatively superficial tumors, such as inguinal lymph node lesions or localized skin recurrences. Because the energy of such electron beams is high, some of the advantages in terms of reduced bone absorption are retained.

High-Dose-Rate Implant Apparatus

One of the most useful advances in radiation oncology has been the introduction of HDR implant machines. The development of these machines began with the Brachytron and its analogs, which utilized radiocobalt as the radiation source. These units pushed a cobalt source through a long tube into applicators previously placed inside the patient. The cobalt units have now been replaced by markedly more sophisticated units that employ ^{192}Ir. The unit employed most commonly in the United States is called a micro-Selectron device.

These new units have been made doubly useful by the concomitant development of sophisticated computer-based planning units that can calculate the radiation dosimetry in about 15 minutes based on the appropriately made x-ray pictures. Fundamental to their use is the capacity of the derived dosimetric information to control the dwell time of the single ^{192}Ir source at any point along each portion of the relevant length of each applicator tube. Up to 18 channels (and 18 indwelling tubes) can be programmed for a single application. By controlling the dwell time at various positions, the computer plan can dictate the "shape" of the deposited radiation at any given point in and around the applicators during each application.

The introduction of these devices has eliminated the necessity for hospitalization and anesthesia in most gynecologic cancer applications. Although they are expensive, it is thought that these instruments will, over time, prove more cost-effective than were radium/cesium applications. Their use in the treatment of the common female pelvic cancers is discussed briefly in the sections on each type of malignancy later in this chapter. It must be acknowledged that with the introduction of HDR implant devices has come many new problems to solve at all levels of analysis. In only one area is their use an unqualified success: the personnel radiation protection problems associated with in-hospital radiation implants has been almost totally removed.

Experimental Instruments

A variety of experimental units are being tested for greater efficacy against human cancers. One approach is the reduction of the "oxygen effect." In contrast to photons, hypoxic cells are almost as sensitive to heavy particle bombardment as are oxygenated cells. To this end, medical cyclotrons have been used to accelerate positively charged particles such as protons, deuterons (^{2}H), and alpha particles (^{4}He), which are then used either directly or to bombard a target such as beryllium to produce neutron beams. Other particles such as pi mesons also appear to have a similarly useful potential. To date there is no convincing evidence that particle therapy will have any role in the treatment of gynecologic cancer. Much less expensive approaches to elimination of hypoxic cells are also being tested (see the discussion of radiosensitizers in the sections "Radiation Chemistry of X-Ray Damage," "Oxygen Effect," and "Chemotherapeutic Radiosensitizers" later in this chapter). The ultimate utility of these very expensive instruments is therefore still under study.

COMMON TERMS IN THERAPEUTIC RADIOLOGY

Figure 17–3 illustrates the shape of what are termed *depth dose curves* for three representative fields from orthovoltage, cobalt, and linac beams. Each line indicates the level at which a constant percentage of the maximum dose can be found. These are termed *isodose* lines. In each case, the line finds a maximum depth at the center of the field. This is called the *central axis depth dose* and is commonly used for calculations. For the linac curve, there is no greater deviation over the rest of the field at that depth (i.e., the depth dose curve is relatively flat). It may be noted that, as each of the beams penetrates, it is attenuated because energy has been absorbed. In the area at the edge of the beam, the dose falls from the maximum central axis dose (at that depth) to zero; this area is termed the *penumbra.*

In the application of megavoltage therapy, more than one beam is almost always used. The effect of the superimposition of these beams on the development of an appropriate treatment plan is discussed later in the chapter. Fundamentally, different beams (coming from different directions) are added together to get the desired pattern. This can be further influenced by *weighting* (giving more dose from one direction than from another), using blocks to remove part of one or more beams totally or using filters (e.g., wedges) to remove fixed components of the beam. Wedges of specific sizes are quite useful when beams must be directed at right angles to one another.

Finally, many therapists prefer to use beams that rotate around a fixed point in the center of a given field. Such treatments are termed *isocentric*, and calculations are made around the isocenter, which is measured as the source-to-(patient) axis distance (SAD) rather than the distance from the radiation source to the patient's surface (source-surface distance [SSD] calculation).

SPARING OF SKIN AND BONE

Of extreme importance in the delivery of radiation deep to the human body is the requirement for sparing both skin and bone. As the energy of the photon beam approaches and exceeds 1 MV, the high-energy photons penetrate the superficial tissues of the skin in excess of several millimeters before reaching their energy peak. This is illustrated in Figure 17–3, where the 100 percent isodose lines for both a ^{60}Co and a 6-MV linac are below the skin surface (5 and 15 mm, respectively), the actual surface doses being up to 38 percent for ^{60}Co and up to 30 percent for 6-MV linacs, depending on the field size. It can be readily understood that this phenomenon reduces the dose to the epidermal tissues, thereby introducing the phenomenon of skin sparing. This was highly important in order to reduce or eliminate the severe, acute skin reactions characteristic of kilovoltage radiation. As can be seen from Figure 17–3, the older x-ray units such as 250-kV units delivered the maximum (100 percent) dose to the skin, with a relatively rapid falloff of absorbed dose as the beam dissipated through absorption by the body tissues. It should be remembered, however, that even a megavoltage beam, which passes tangentially through skin (e.g., the perineum or gluteal folds), may cause skin reactions when the maximum build-up dose is delivered to portions of the skin surface perpendicular to the treatment beam. Thus skin sparing is not possible in all aspects of gynecologic cancer treatment, and it can be a significant clinical problem whenever the treatment field includes the curving surface of the skin in the regions of the umbilicus, perineum, and gluteal folds.

Less important in gynecologic oncology, but still significant, has been the reduction of bony complications characteristic of the initial low-energy radiotherapeutic treatment beams where photoelectric absorption predominated. The absorption of energy in tissue depends on both the primary energy of the beam and the types of elements concentrated in tissue. With megavoltage beams Compton absorption predominates, and the dose to bone becomes almost identical to that to soft tissue. This is clearly illustrated if one examines an x-ray picture taken with a linac beam, in which the bones of the pelvis (see Fig. 17–16) can barely be delineated because of the uniform nature of absorption of megavoltage energy photon beams. Clinically, the use of megavoltage beams has almost eliminated the bony and articular hip complications resulting from osteoradionecrosis that occurred after cervical cancer treatment with some degree of regularity earlier in the century. Thus the development of megavoltage treatment beams has led to a distinct reduction in the side effects characteristic of earlier radiation treatment machines.

TREATMENT PLANNING

The development and implementation of a radiation treatment plan involves a variety of people, including the radiation oncologist, radiation physicist, dosimetrist, and other support personnel, such as the technicians who will administer each treatment. Each of these individuals is specially trained and licensed for his or her task. The first step is for the radiation oncologist to identify the problem and develop an overall treatment approach. This should be done in close conjunction with the gynecologist. In many cases, the coordination of a planned surgical/radiation treatment program is involved. Once the overall program is projected, the radiation physicist becomes involved and the anatomic extent of known tumor is determined, frequently using computed tomography (CT) scans. Magnetic resonance imaging (MRI) and modern ultrasonography also can be useful in certain types of cases. Next, a three-dimensional, anatomically accurate treatment program is planned, using a modern computer dedicated to radiation treatment planning. Given the versatility of most modern radiation units, it is usually possible to develop a plan in which the dose can be varied almost exactly as needed in the pelvis and abdomen. Large clinics usually employ a dosimetrist to assist the physicist in treatment planning. Once completed, the plan is checked again with the radiation oncologist and treatment is initiated. Computerized computation of intracavitary and interstitial doses is also the modern standard, and it is now possible to monitor the dose of radiation to various accessible internal cavities, using special techniques. Radiation therapy has for many years been one of the most quantitatively accurate methods of administering medical therapy. The developments in both diagnostic radiology and radiation therapy itself have further enhanced its accuracy, but this has also re-emphasized the need for further knowledge about the biology of gynecologic malignancies.

Before completing this section we must mention *conformal radiation therapy.* This term is used to describe the most current attempt by radiation oncologists to tailor radiation treatments. The newest linear accelerators have been equipped with precise mechanisms both for shaping the treatment beams (beam shaping and collimation) and for the use of compensators (tools used to modify the beam to accommodate sloping skin surfaces). These additions to the available equipage are being studied with a view to reducing normal tissue damage and perhaps enhancing the therapeutic ratio. No conformal applications have achieved established usefulness in gynecologic oncology, whose proprietary tumors are notorious for their reluctance to candidly reveal their edges or, for that matter, where they have decided to conceal their progeny!

FUNDAMENTALS OF RADIATION BIOLOGY

DNA Damage

The great majority of useful radiation treatments employ high-energy photons. These photons penetrate tissue, interacting with all molecular species, until their energy is dissipated. Since the most common molecule by far in living tissue is water, most of the initial energy is dissipated through its absorption by water atoms. However, a wide variety of other products are formed by other molecules, many of which are free radicals containing a reactive electron. Virtually every component of the living cell can be affected by any form of radiation to some degree. Thus studies in which the dose of radiation inflicted on the cell greatly exceeds that known to be tolerable during clinical therapy have clearly illustrated that proteins, lipids, RNA, and so forth can be affected by irradiation. At intermediate levels of radiation, it would appear that cell membrane damage may be important.

Despite the complexity of the physicochemical reactions involved, it is well established that the lethal injury inflicted on all cells with clinical doses of x-rays stems from damage to DNA. At therapeutic doses, the overwhelming cause of cell proliferative death is a disruption of the cell's genetic apparatus so that it is impossible for the cell to deliver successfully a fully operative set of genes to either daughter cell. Early in the study of the biologic effects of radiation, it was shown that chromosome aberrations were a common effect of low-dose radiation exposure. When radiation is administered in significant doses to a fetus, the result is either developmental abnormalities or fetal death, indicating disruption of the ordered expression of genetic information. In the case of tumors, if either daughter cell contains genetic information sufficient to initiate sustained cell division, the damage to the mother tumor cell is nonlethal and ineffective. Thus, as far as we know at this stage of analysis, the most fundamental effect of useful x-rays is the damage to cellular DNA such that the cell is ultimately incapable of forming clonogenic daughter cells.

Radiation Chemistry of X-Ray Damage

As indicated in Figure 17–6, the first effect of an x-ray photon in tissue is usually the induction of a hydroxyl radical ($\cdot OH^-$). A multitude of other reactions can occur, but statis-

tically this is the most frequent, because water molecules are the most common single component of tissue. Such free radicals may then transfer the reaction to a DNA base such as the thymine base. In this particular case, the double bond in the thymine molecule is altered and a thymidyl radical is produced. In the cell, several possible secondary reactions can occur. In the presence of a sulfhydryl agent, the reaction may be reversed and the normal thymine base structure restored.

This reaction is the basis for the radioprotective potential of many reducing agents. However, if molecular oxygen is present, it may add to the intermediate, producing a peroxythymidyl radical. This is thought to be a common second-step reaction that results in the fixation of the damage, since this reaction is essentially irreversible. The only mechanism by which such damage can then be removed and the cellular DNA returned to the normal structure is through enzymatic repair.

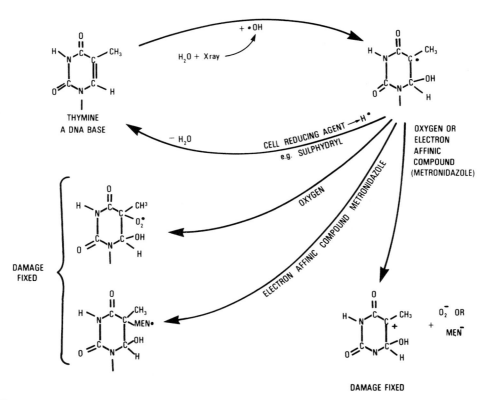

FIGURE 17–6. Radiochemistry of ionizing radiation. Photons penetrating tissue produce free radicals in water (·OH) that then react with a wide variety of other materials, including the bases of DNA. This interaction results in a complex series of events that may either reverse the reaction (as, for example, sulfhydryls) or lead to its fixation either by molecular oxygen or by other electron-affinic compounds such as mitronidazole (MEN). Once the damage is fixed, the cell must either repair it enzymatically or face mutation or a lethal event. (Courtesy of John F. Ward, Ph.D., University of California–San Diego.)

If oxygen is not present, the reaction is more likely to be reversed; hence hypoxic cells are radioresistant. Many other electron-affinic compounds, such as metronidazole (Flagyl), misonidazole, and related compounds, can react in a fashion similar to that of molecular oxygen. Several such compounds have been studied in an effort to determine whether or not the *oxygen effect* (i.e., the radioresistance resulting from hypoxia) can be eliminated. The development of thymidyl radicals with the addition of either the electron-affinic compound or oxygen are further intermediate steps. Ultimately, these additional compounds are lost, creating a thymine cation that will then react with free hydroxyl groups in the cell, which can in turn lead to permanent genetic damage if not repaired.

This sequence illustrates the critical role of oxygen in the process of fixing radiation damage. Without sufficient oxygen, cells can be up to three times as resistant to radiation as when oxygen is present. Oxygen can be regarded as in competition with reducing agents, largely sulfhydryls. Oxygen fixes the radiation damage, thereby killing the cell, whereas reducing agents remove the extra electron from the DNA component and spare the cell (Fig. 17–6). While the same chemistry applies to both normal and malignant cells, only the malignant cell can become hypoxic. Although the electron-affinic agents such as misonidazole and its congeners are seldom as active as oxygen in permitting damage fixation, unlike oxygen, they are not consumed by cellular metabolism and can thereby penetrate and persist in hypoxic tumor masses. This feature of tumor biology (the oxygen effect) is the basis of a great deal of current radiation research in sensitizer development, in the use of heavy particles (e.g., neutrons) with which the oxygen effect is minimized, and in the development of drug and x-ray regimens that result in rapid killing of oxygenated tumor cells and thereby facilitate the reoxygenation of tumors. All are aimed at eliminating the oxygen effect. To date no chemical oxygen replacer has been approved for use with radiation.

These radiochemical reactions should be considered only diagrammatic steps, but they indicate clearly the importance of oxygen in the development of permanent radiation damage. Interested readers are referred to reviews by Brown (1987) and Wasserman et al (1994) for a more sophisticated discussion of these topics.

Relative Biologic Effectiveness

There is one additional concept with which the reader should be familiar prior to discussing the cellular basis for radiation therapy: the relative biologic effectiveness (RBE). Not all radiation beams have an equivalent capacity for killing cells (or producing other biologic endpoints), even if the calculated or measured doses are identical. Differences in such effects are termed *RBE effects*. The standard is 250-kV x-rays. If a given dose of a certain radiation (e.g., pi mesons) doubles a specific effect produced by an identical dose of 250-kV x-rays, then the pi mesons' RBE is 2.0. If cobalt gamma rays require 125 cGy to produce the same effect as 100 cGy of 250-kV x-rays, then the cobalt RBE for that effect is 0.8. The RBE for most clinically relevant megavoltage effects (cobalt and linacs) is slightly less than that for 250-kV x-rays. Thus a slightly higher cobalt or linac dose is required to produce the same reaction (e.g., ovarian sterilization) than would be required with 250-kV x-rays. The RBE for many particles (e.g., neutrons) is significantly greater than megavoltage x-rays. RBEs are very dependent on a variety of factors (e.g., dose rate, size of the dose per fraction) and in principle must be measured for each radiation beam and phenomenon of interest (Hall, 1988).

Postradiation Repair and Cell Survival

Background Radiation

All living creatures are subjected to ionizing radiation exposure, both intracellular (e.g., radioactive potassium) and external (e.g., cosmic rays). The annual average dose from these sources approaches 0.13 cGy/year. To cope with this level of damage, living organisms have developed enzymatic mechanisms for cellular repair. These cellular repair mechanisms are moderately effective and work best at the biologic (background) dose levels, which deliver about 0.15×10^{-4} cGy/hr. The enzymology of x-ray damage repair is poorly understood, but it is known that all living cells can remove some forms of x-ray–damaged DNA bases and replace them with new nucleotides, restoring the DNA's integrity. By way of comparison, intracavitary radiation output approaches 100 cGy/hr, whereas megavoltage external treatment typically delivers about 100 cGy/min. These therapeutic sources cause, respectively, about 6,500 and 400,000 times the amount of damage that the mammalian cell is prepared to face. Therefore, it is not surprising that the cellular repair mechanisms become rapidly overwhelmed and that lethal events occur. Were this not so, ionizing radiation would not be effective in cancer treatment. However, cellular repair mechanisms do contribute to the recovery of cells from acute radiation exposure, and this recovery, in the acute sense, is termed *sublethal damage repair.* The contribution of these repair processes to cell recovery is thought to be responsible for the shape of the radiation survival curve and for the increase in the number of cells surviving a radiation dose when it is divided into two parts.

Repair of Sublethal Damage

A typical mammalian cell radiation survival curve is shown in Figure 17–7 (left curve, radiation in air). In this type of analysis, the cells' capacity to grow into a colony (clonogenicity) after a radiation exposure is measured (Puck and Marcus, 1955). Individual cells are plated out in a tissue culture dish and exposed to varying doses of radiation. The number of cells that survive and multiply (determined by subsequent colony formation) dictates the shape of the survival curve. In the case of almost all mammalian cells, both normal and malignant, the curve is characterized by an initial shoulder, followed by an exponential decrease in recovery as the radiation dose is increased. The efficiency of the radiation steadily increases as the survivorship passes through the shoulder of the curve and then becomes apparently log linear for all regions of the curve beyond the shoulder of threshold. An important aspect of the logarithmic portion of the survival curve (i.e., the region beyond the shoulder) is the observation that, for any constant incremental increase in dose, a constant proportion or fraction of the cells are killed. Thus, if 100 cGy kills 50 percent of the remaining viable cells, an additional 100 cGy will kill the same fraction of the cells surviving the previous dose. In a sense, therefore, the radiation becomes less and less efficient in terms of absolute numbers of cells killed. Almost all chemotherapeutic agents show survival curves whose initial components resemble the x-ray curve. Some chemotherapeutic drug curves have a resistant "tail" such that adding more

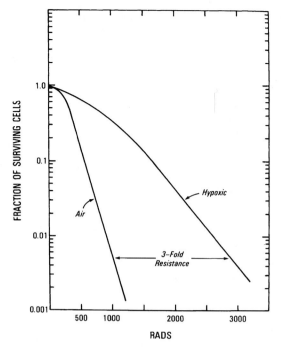

FIGURE 17–7. Typical radiation survival curve for mammalian cells. These cells have been irradiated and then plated out in culture, and the number of survivors has been determined by measuring the colonies (clones) of cells that survive. The curve is characterized by an initial shoulder followed by a log-linear region. Cells irradiated in air are considerably more sensitive than those irradiated in nitrogen (hypoxic), and the difference between the levels of killing is frequently about threefold. It is believed that most clinically demonstrable tumors have areas of hypoxia that lead to radioresistance.

drug does not lead to further killing. This phenomenon is not found with x-rays.

It is thought that the shoulder on the survival curve relates to the ability of the cell to accumulate and repair *sublethal* damage. Such damage becomes lethal as additional damage is inflicted. The extent of the shoulder of the curve is also presumed to reflect the capacity of the cell to repair the sublethal damage. One can also look at the situation in the opposite fashion and propose that the repair of damage is more efficient at lower radiation doses but is saturated above a certain dose level. Therefore, x-ray and drug repair processes are maximally efficient at the level of biologic radiation or drug damage.

A more conclusive way of demonstrating the cells' capacity to repair radiation damage is to divide a given radiation dose into two parts and to determine the effect of adding a period of rest between the two radiation fractions. When one measures the capacity of cells to survive such a split radiation dose, one encounters the type of curve shown in Figure 17–8. It can be seen that, as the interval between the two radiation exposures increases, the number of cells surviving increases. This is evidence that the cell has repaired some sublethal damage resulting from the first dose before the infliction of the second dose such that the second dose is relatively less damaging. This split-dose increase in cell survival in termed *Elkind-Sutton repair* after the scientists who first demonstrated it. If one constructs a second radiation survival time curve 4 hours or more after a radiation exposure that has initially reduced cell survival to the exponential part of an x-ray survival curve, one finds that the shoulder on the curve has been restored. This is additional evidence of a link between the increase in survivors after the split-dose repair and the shoulder on the x-ray survival curve. All of these phenomena are believed to reflect the same cellular mechanisms, namely, the capacity of the cells to recover from moderate doses of x-rays (Elkind and Whitmore, 1967).

It is important to note that the commonly used clinical radiation doses are those in the region of the terminal portion of the shoulder of the survival curve or slightly on the exponential part. Most radiation fractionation schemes operate at the limits of cell repair mechanisms, and modest increases in the radiation dose lead to significantly greater cell killing than equivalent amounts of radiation on the shoulder of the survival curve. Thus, clinically, the addition of 100 cGy to a 200-cGy fraction (total exposure dose, 300 cGy) is quantitatively quite different in terms of cell survival from the increase in radiation from 100 to 200 cGy. Both side effects and long-term complications can be significantly increased by only modest increases in individual dose fractions.

Also of great importance is the time to full recovery during a split-dose experiment, as illustrated in Figure 17–8. It can be seen that maximal recovery has been achieved at about 3 to 4 hours. It is therefore believed by some

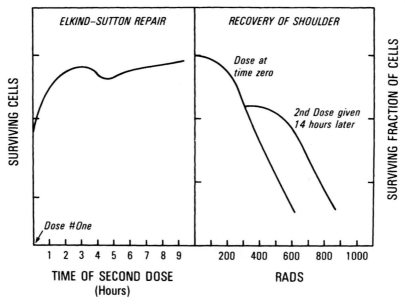

FIGURE 17–8. Experimental demonstration of the repair of sublethal x-ray damage. One means of demonstrating the cell's capacity to repair x-ray damage and to survive is to split the x-ray dose into two parts. The first part is administered at time 0 (arrow, left figure), and the second dose is administered at various times after the first dose. When this is done, the number of surviving cells increases and is consistent with the cellular repair of sublethal x-ray damage. This is termed *Elkind-Sutton repair.* Another means of demonstrating cell recovery is to irradiate cells down to some point on the exponential portion of the survival curve and then to administer the remainder of the dose at a subsequent time. In this case, the shoulder on the curve is restored. Both of these types of experiments are believed to demonstrate the repair of x-ray damage to cellular structures, most likely cellular DNA.

radiotherapists that multiple daily radiation fractions can probably be given without any substantial difference in toxicity if each successive dose of radiation is given 3 or more hours after the preceding dose. This proposal, however, is significantly limited by the phenomenon of repopulation, described later.

Survival curve analyses of human tumor cells in tissue culture have suggested that there may be significant differences in the absolute sensitivity of different cell types to ionizing radiation (Fertil and Malaise, 1985). It has been observed that seminoma cells, which are know to be quite sensitive to ionizing radiation, have radiation survival curves with much smaller shoulders than typical epithelial cells (Wells et al, 1977). Some melanoma cells (thought to be clinically radioresistant) have radiation survival curves with larger shoulders and less steep slopes than typical epithelial lines (Barranco et al, 1971; Dewey, 1971). The cells of radiosensitive granulosa cell tumors and dysgerminomas are probably similar to seminoma cells, although this has not as yet been studied in vitro. These observations suggest some correlation between the efficiency of cellular repair mechanisms and the capacity of the tumor to survive x-ray treatments. From the standpoint of gynecologic oncology, however, most of the tumors encountered are epithelial in origin and probably are not intrinsically different from their normal counterparts in their capacity to accumulate and repair sublethal x-ray damage and therefore in their net sensitivity to x-ray killing. The importance of the repair of sublethal x-ray damage in the development of improved radiation treatment protocols is considered in the discussion of fractionation later in this chapter.

Oxic Radiosensitizers

In addition to the use of hypoxic radiosensitizers (the electron-affinic compounds discussed previously), it is also possible to modify the sensitivity of mammalian cells to radiation by oxic radiosensitizers. These compounds are almost all halogenated pyrimidines, but they affect sensitization in two different ways. The first group includes bromouracil and iodouracil, both of which are analogs of thymine. These compounds in their nucleoside form can substitute for thymidine and are incorporated into cellular DNA (Szybalski, 1974). As such, they render the DNA up to three times more sensitive to radiation than it is in its nonsubstituted form.

Preliminary studies have shown that these compounds can be tolerable in humans, and their utility is under active investigation (Kinsella, 1991).

Potentially Lethal Damage

The second form of cellular repair that appears to assist the cell in recovering from toxic agents has been termed the *repair of potentially lethal damage*. This process is described as an increase in cell number if cells are allowed to rest after exposure to the agent (Phillips and Tolmach, 1966). Thus, if a cell continues through the cell cycle and attempts to divide after an x-ray exposure, it will die, whereas if the cell cycle is arrested, an increase in the number of surviving cells takes place, similar to Elkind-Sutton repair. In normal tissues in vivo, a similar increase in surviving cells can be demonstrated that is sometimes called *in situ repair*. This recovery in cell viability is probably an important feature in dictating the overall sensitivity of some of the major organs to radiation. In situ repair has been studied in organs such as the liver (Jirtle et al, 1984) and the thyroid gland (Clifton et al, 1978). These organs' cells show much greater survival after clinical-level radiation exposures if the assay for survival is delayed by about a day. In such organs, cell division after radiation is almost nonexistent; thus in situ repair is probably a major factor in such organ recovery.

The reader will appreciate the fact that the common denominator between in situ repair and the recovery from potentially lethal damage is a delay between the time of radiation exposure and the next cell division. In vivo, this is studied by varying the timing of removal of the glandular cells for clonogenic assay after x-ray exposure. In tissue culture, this can be demonstrated by the addition of various antimetabolites or by nutritional deprivation. In this case, damage that is potentially lethal becomes nonlethal, and it is assumed that the cell has repaired the damage during the rest period.

There is now evidence that the repair of potentially lethal damage in tumor cells and in situ repair of normal cells are important factors in both normal tissue tolerance and the response of tumors to therapy. The killing of cells by both x-rays and drugs appears to be influenced by these phenomena. For example, Weichselbaum (1984) has developed evidence suggesting that tumors that are resistant to radiation cure in humans are comprised of cells having a greater than usual capacity to repair potentially lethal x-ray damage. In a similar vein, it has been suggested that tumor cells that have an inadequate nutritional supply (and are therefore cycling slowly or not at all) can better recover from alkylating agent damage than normal cycling (growing) cells. Thus Fravel and Roberts (1979) showed that the recovery of cells from cis-platinum administration was a time-dependent phenomenon involving the slow removal of platinated sites from DNA. Each of these types of evidence suggests that cells that can repair damage before starting a new cell division cycle will have a preferential chance for survival. Therefore, manipulation of tumor cell kinetics and/or inhibition of tumor cell potential for damage repair are important current research topics.

Cell Cycle Stages and Their Radiosensitivity

Once a cell has received the stimulus to grow and multiply, it passes through the classic phases of the cell cycle. With autoradiography, whereby permanent incorporation of the tritiated thymidine into cellular DNA was first demonstrated, it was found that each cell underwent a discrete phase of DNA synthesis (S phase) before mitosis (M phase). S phase was always preceded by a phase in which the cell grew larger without incorporating any thymidine (growth phase I or G_1). S phase was also always followed by a second period lacking any thymidine incorporation (growth phase II or G_2). Subsequent to this, the quiescent period of G_0 was discovered, during which no growth occurs. The radiosensitivity of these various periods has been studied in vitro with synchronized cell populations. Almost always, some portion of S phase, usually late S, is considerably more resistant to x-rays than either G period. The short time when the mitotic apparatus is demonstrable is invariably the most sensitive portion of the cell cycle to x-rays. Numerous efforts have been made to utilize these latter observations in the clinic (e.g., by attempting to synchronize tumor cells with antimetabolites, followed by timed radiation), all without success.

Repopulation as a Form of Repair — Stem Cells

Both split-dose repair and potentially lethal damage/in situ repair reflect events that a cell undergoes prior to initiating the first cell division after x-ray (or drug) exposure. However, the major source of recovery in some normal tissues and their derivative tumors is simple cell multiplication after radiation. In tissues such as bone marrow, where there is essentially no shoulder on the radiation survival curve, cell multiplication is the sole source of tissue recovery. Therefore, while the increase in the number of both normal and tumor cells through multiplication or repopulation is not, in and of itself, a form of cellular repair, it is of great importance in the recovery from acute radiation injury. Because of this, it is important to understand some aspects of cellular kinetics in the context of x-ray damage. To do so, it is necessary to appreciate the role that stem cells play in many tissue recovery processes.

Normal tissues characterized by rapid cell turnover (best exemplified by bone marrow), contain stem cells that will form clones of normal cells that then undergo differentiation. Bone marrow stem cells are capable of forming red blood cell clones, neutrophil clones, megakaryocyte clones, and so forth. The growth of all cells along their various pathways of multiplication and differentiation can be traced to a small population of cells called *stem cells* (Potten, 1983). Intrinsic to the definition of a stem cell is its capacity to form two different daughter cells after some, but not all, divisions. From these differential divisions arise two types of cells: another stem cell and a cell from which the differentiated clone will derive (Fig. 17–9). When the cell population of a cell renewal tissue is drastically reduced, differentiation is suppressed and the stem cell population expands to ensure its preservation as a population (Fig. 17–9). These developmental switches are fundamental to the integrity of all multicellular organisms. They are beginning to be manipulated clinically. For example, the demonstration and use of bone marrow stem cells is the basis for bone marrow transplantation in cancer patients. Unfortunately, a disturbance of the control of this binary option appears to be intrinsic to the development of all malignancies in cell renewal systems, and therefore in the development of most gynecologic cancers.

Under normal circumstances, a portion of tissue stem cells are cycling at any one time, while others are resting. Resting cells are termed G_0, since they are not growing. When the normal population of cells has been re-

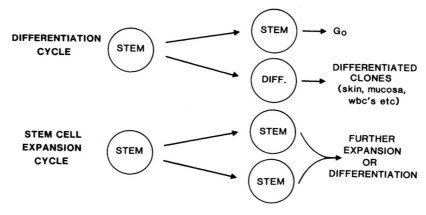

FIGURE 17–9. Alternative pathways for stem cell division cycles. In the upper example, the tissue stem cell initially produces two different daughter cells. One is another stem cell that returns to quiescence, while the other daughter cell goes on to form a differentiated clone. In the lower example, no differentiation occurs, with the result that the stem cell population doubles.

duced, for example, by exposure to x-rays or alkylating agents, the stem cells are stimulated to divide and the overall population is brought back to normal. It is now thought that tumors contain a variable number of stem cells (Salmon et al, 1978) and that such stem cells may also repopulate.

At this time, it is not clear whether all tumors actually contain true stem cells. We believe that only those tumors derived from true cell renewal systems (marrow, mucosa, skin, and so forth) contain real stem cells. Many cancers (e.g., melanoma and adult sarcomas) probably derive from transformed normal cells that were not themselves stem cells. Fibroblasts, endothelial cells, hepatocytes, and so on, while capable of cell division, simply reproduce two versions of themselves on multiplication. If this interpretation is correct, the reader will realize that any form of cytoreductive therapy will be less effective against the latter tumor types, as opposed to those derived from transformed stem cells. This is because a tumor derived from a transformed stem cell will contain many cells whose formal progeny are postmitotic, while all cells in non–stem cell tumors are potentially clonogenic. The current results of both x-ray therapy and chemotherapy suggest that this interpretation may be correct.

The great majority of gynecologic cancers are epithelial in origin and as such should contain true stem cells. The pathologic corollary of this is the evidence of differentiation seen in such tumors. Tumors such as epidermoid malignancies contain many cells (e.g., keratinized squamous cells) that are clearly postmitotic. Although many of these partially differentiated cells may still be capable of one or more further divisions, their entire progeny are destined to differentiate and are incapable of clonogenesis.

Thus the absolute number of clonogenic cells within 1 gm of well-differentiated squamous cell carcinoma may be significantly less than in an undifferentiated specimen, where many more cells may be capable of sustained repopulation. This concept of tumor stem cells is important in understanding differences in the sensitivity of tumors to radiation and in the capacity of the tumor cell mass to recover. Clearly, the more tumor stem cells capable of clonogenesis that exist within any given volume of tumor, the greater the chance that an x-ray treatment will fail. This is exemplified by an increase in the rate of repopulation of the tumor cell box within the normal tissue box (as shown in Fig. 17–10 later), which is explained more fully in the section "Tumor Versus Normal Cell Repopulation Kinetics" later in this chapter.

The repair of radiation damage and the repopulation of both normal and tumor tissues are extremely complex. We are just beginning to understand the mechanisms by which treatments succeed or fail. In any given tumor mass, there may be great variation in the physiologic milieu; treatment may be very successful in one part of the patient and fail in another for quite local, physiologic reasons. A clearer understanding of these various phenomena may well lead to improved treatment regimens.

Apoptosis

Apoptosis is the scientific term used to describe the process by which effete cells are removed from the body. It originally referred to phagocytosis. With a greater understanding of the cell cycle and differentiation, it became apparent that programmed cell death was fundamental to cell renewal systems and, indeed, to differentiation. Apoptosis is therefore clearly different from *necrosis*, the term used for nonscheduled cell death (Kerr et al, 1972). Radiation may lead to necrosis *or* apoptosis or both. In a tumor either effect is beneficial, but in a normal cell renewal system this can be a source of acute or chronic radiation toxicity (Kerr et al, 1994). It has been suggested that gynecologic cancers may vary in their sensitivity to apoptotic induction by radiation and that this may have clinical implications (Ling et al, 1994; Levine et al, 1995). Since cells capable of apoptosis exist in many tumor systems, they must contribute to hypoxia because pre-apoptotic cells are still consuming oxygen. This is another area in which preclinical research has the potential of further major advances in clinical radiotherapy.

Oxygen Effect

In the preceding sections, we described the phenomena associated with the development of molecular x-ray damage after exposure of mammalian tissues to ionizing radiation. Of fundamental importance to the infliction of lethal damage is the presence of molecular oxygen. This phenomenon, termed the *oxygen effect*, may provide an explanation for many radiation treatment failures. At the cellular level, it can be shown that, if a radiation survival curve is developed in the absence of oxygen, the cells show a two- to threefold increase in their capacity to survive radiation exposure (Fig. 17–7). Cells exposed to 100 percent oxygen are more sensitive to radiation than are cells exposed to air. Essentially all normal tissues are fully oxygenated, with the exception of skin and spermatogenic cells, which are very slightly hypoxic. The slightly reduced oxygen tension in these latter tissues has no clinical implications.

Tumor cells can rapidly outgrow their blood supply and become hypoxic, and therefore resistant to x-ray killing. Since the dose of x-rays administered to a patient usually approaches normal tissue tolerance, it is apparent that, if significant numbers of hypoxic cells exist, it is unlikely that x-ray therapy will be capable of sterilizing the tumor. The importance of the oxygen effect was first recognized by Gray et al (1953). Subsequently Thomlinson and Gray (1955) showed that tumor cells at a distance of more than 100 μm from a blood vessel are invariably hypoxic and will necrose. Intermediate regions must therefore contain relatively hypoxic (radioresistant), but potentially clonogenic, cells. In a certain sense, severe hypoxia may be beneficial and slow down the rate of tumor growth, since hypoxic cells are incapable of dividing. However, as the tumor grows, it develops its own blood supply, which tends to be created at the periphery of the tumor. In bulky tumor masses, which occur in many gynecologic malignancies, multiple microscopic areas of hypoxia must exist; thus the microanatomy of a tumor is extremely important.

The shape of the radiation survival curve under both oxygenated and hypoxic conditions is instructive. The full expression of hypoxic resistance is greatest when the curves have reached their exponential portion. Hypoxia is less important at lower radiation doses. In fact, it has been suggested that hypoxic tumors may be more readily treated by multiple low-dose fractions where the survival differential between oxic and hypoxic cells is minimal. This is an interesting area for further clinical investigation.

Clinically, the precapillary oxygen tension within normal tissues shows relatively little variation with changes in red blood cell mass, although the absolute amount of oxygen transported is a function of the hemoglobin concentration. When normal tissues are bathed in anemic blood, they extract relatively more oxygen, so that the venous O_2 tension is significantly less than it is in a nonanemic patient. Hypoxic tumors usually have areas of severe hypoxia, and oxygen is maximally removed from the perfusing blood. If a patient is severely anemic, tumor hypoxia may be exaggerated by the low oxygen-carrying capacity of anemic blood, in turn increasing the tumor's resistance to radiation. For this reason, it is important to transfuse the severely anemic patient before radiation therapy to raise the hemoglobin level to 12 gm/dl or more (Bush et al, 1978; Thomas, 1994).

The first efforts to reverse the potentially deleterious effects of low oxygen levels employed hyperbaric oxygen. In these clinical experiments, patients received their radiation treatments in chambers containing oxygen under several atmospheres of pressure. Unfortunately, in these early experiments the radiation fractionation schemes were altered such that the total radiation dose was delivered in fewer fractions. Nevertheless, some suggestion of benefit was obtained in randomized trials, including carcinoma of the cervix (Watson et al, 1978).

These initially promising studies using hyperbaric oxygen led to the ingenious hypothesis that certain chemicals, the electron-affinic radiosensitizers, might replace molecular oxygen (Adams, 1973). Compounds such as misonidazole are not consumed, as oxygen is, and therefore can accumulate in deeply hypoxic tumor areas. When such tumors are irradiated, the sensitizer then acts like molecular oxygen and "fixes" the x-ray damage, even in the hypoxic cells. Since oxygen is present in the irradiated surrounding normal cells, they cannot be further affected by the electron-affinic agents. Unfortunately, the compounds studied thus far have proven to be too neurotoxic for clinical use, but newer compounds might be capable of application in humans (Wasserman et al, 1994). Studies of these newer compounds are underway in many centers (Brown, 1987; Overgaard and Horsman, 1996).

Early Adverse Effects: Cellular Basis

During the clinical radiation treatment of a patient with radiotherapy, the patient will usually experience what are termed *acute side effects.* These will include local effects such as diarrhea or a perineal skin reaction and, less commonly, systemic side effects such as nausea. After cessation of the treatment, these complaints will dissipate. However, considerably more troublesome late effects may appear, including scar formation (fibrosis) and ischemic areas, which can lead to serious complications (discussed later in the chapter). It is important for the clinician to distinguish between these two phenomena because of their distinct prognostic implications.

Apart from nausea, almost all acute side effects of radiation therapy are caused by the depletion of cells from tissues characterized by renewing cell populations. In the pelvic area, these tissues include the skin and all major epithelial areas (vaginal, bladder and bowel mucosa, and so forth), together with the bone marrow. Radiation is capable of killing large numbers of normal stem cells in all tissues. For example, when mucosal stem cells have been reduced sufficiently, the mucosa will become thin and eventually the patient will experience painful symptoms as toxic substances penetrate to the nerve endings. If the skin is involved, a sunburn-like reaction appears. Other organs undergo similar cytoreductive phenomena as differentiated cells are lost and the stem cell population is depressed below the point where it can immediately replace the lost differentiated cells. Because of the built-in delay caused by the natural cell turnover time, the appearance of symptoms is typically delayed for about 2 weeks with conventional radiation fractionation. Provided that the cell depletion effect is not excessive (e.g., the epithelial barrier has not broken down sufficiently to permit a secondary infectious process), the mucosa will heal and the symptoms will pass.

In the case of bone marrow, some special features are apparent. While a portion of the pelvic bone marrow is included during standard radiation therapy for a typical gynecologic cancer, the volume treated is less than one might anticipate (see Fig. 17–13). However, the patient will experience a pronounced depression in the total white blood cell count. This occurs because a large amount of the total blood volume will flow through the treatment field in the 1 to 3 minutes occupied by each treatment. The mature lymphocytes contained in the irradiated blood are extremely sensitive to radiation, and all patients undergoing radiation to the body core, regardless of the specific treatment volume, will experience a significant, selective lymphocytopenia (Byfield, 1984). To this must be added the considerably more modest effect of the true hematosuppressive effects of the pelvic radiation. The most important aspect of this phenomenon is the combination of drug-containing regimens with radiation. If radiation-induced lymphopenia is not recognized and the total white blood cell count is employed in drug dosing, serious undertreatment may occur. The simplest way to avoid this pitfall is to adjust chemotherapeutic drug doses on the basis of the total granulocyte and platelet counts, which reflect real marrow activity, rather than using the total white blood cell count. This simple measure will prevent underdosing those patients who have received recent (within 1 year) radiotherapy.

Late Adverse Effects (Complications)

In addition to the acute effects of radiation, the physician must be aware of what are termed *late effects*. Some late effects are not of major consequence to the patient and may consist of no more than a slight increase in fibrosis in a small subcutaneous region. Others may produce major complications that can be life threatening (Fajardo, 1982). All are caused by the same biologic processes, which are only partially understood at this time.

When living tissue is irradiated, all forms of cells receive similar radiation damage. When the cell population involved turns over rapidly, cell depletion becomes clinically apparent after a brief delay. However, there are many tissues in the body in which cell turnover is slow, and a significant degree of cell depletion may take several months to years to produce symptoms.

The cell populations involved in late effects can be divided into two components. The first type are the cells of the connective tissues and their supportive elements (blood vessels, nerves), whose function is to ensure structural integrity and to provide neurologic and physiologic support to all of the body. Damage to these tissues leads to atrophy and fibrosis, which may appear months to years following the radiation. The loss of these components may then lead to serious secondary sequelae in the organ or area involved. For example, abdominal radiation may result in severe atrophic changes in the bowel itself, with obstruction and/or infarction of the bowel, as discussed later. If excessive acute cell loss from the primary cell renewal system(s) also occurs, then the degenerative processes may be accelerated (e.g., by superimposed infections). Cell loss from the capillary bed is thought to be the major contributor to the late effects of radiation in all parts of the body (see Fig. 17–10).

A second type of cell loss can occur in many of the major organs in the body that have slow turnover of their primary cells as part of the normal wear-and-tear processes. Such organs (the kidney, liver, thyroid gland, salivary glands) are not cell renewal systems in the ordinary sense, but all have a significant capacity to replace their cells, albeit slowly. Some, such as the liver, can grow very rapidly under select circumstances (e.g., partial hepatectomy), but ordinarily all of these organs have a very slow rate of replacement of parenchymal cells. These organs are not usually subject to variations in cell loss, as are the skin, mucosa, and marrow, and therefore have no real need for regular, substantial cell replacement. Radiation does not induce rapid cell death in these organs (at conventional therapeutic doses), and their cells remain viable and functioning for a considerable period of time after radiation, even when their clonogenic potential is lost. Thus x-ray exposure does not induce liver cell multiplication, as partial hepatectomy does, and the net liver cell mass remains unchanged for a prolonged period. Such organs are sensitive to radiation, but the deleterious effects do not become manifest until the normal slow loss of their cells has led to a significant net cell depletion. The result is a progressive loss of organ function. In the case of vital organs, such as the kidney or liver, the clinical effect may seem to be one of sudden organ failure. However, the process started the first day of radiation. These kinds of damage are frequently aggravated by concomitant vascular damage. In some cases, the clinical effects are not dramatic, but they may be very troublesome. The desiccating effect of radiation on the mucosal glands is an example of such an effect in the gynecologic population, especially when it is aggravated by the withdrawal of estrogen, as is frequently the case in most gynecologic cancers because of ovarian excision or radiation.

The absolute level of radiation tolerance varies from organ to organ and from tissue to tissue. Table 17–2 shows the 5 and 50 percent lethal doses for the common organs. These generally fall into three groups: (1) the very sensitive organs or organ functions, such as ovarian hormone production, the kidney, and the liver, in which sensitivity limits the tolerable dose (using fractions of 200 cGy/day or less) to 2,500 cGy or even much less; (2) the intermediate organs, such as bowel, heart, and spinal cord, where doses of between 4,000 and 5,000 cGy can be tolerated; and (3) the radioresistant organs, such as the cervix, brain, and skeletal muscle, where doses of between 5,000 and 7,000 cGy can be

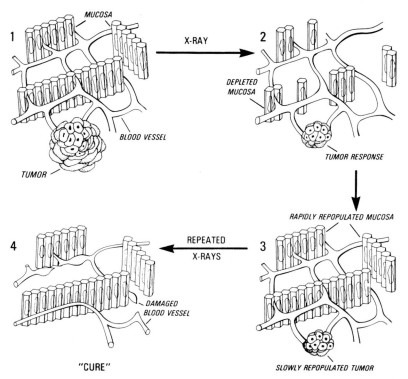

FIGURE 17–10. Biologic basis of radiation therapy. Human malignancies exist in an environment containing both acutely repopulating cells, such as intestinal or vaginal mucosa, bone marrow, and skin, and supportive structures, including blood vessels and peripheral nerves. Therapeutic x-ray doses kill both normal repopulating cells and tumor cells. This is indicated by a reduction in the number of both cell types. Most normal cells repopulate rapidly and regain normal epithelial integrity within hours to days. Excessive reduction in these cell layers leads to most of the acute effects of radiation therapy, including diarrhea, gastrointestinal bleeding, and mucosal blistering. Epithelial tumors tend to repopulate very slowly; therefore the ratio of tumor cells to normal tissue cells declines, and the tumor becomes smaller until it is eventually eliminated. Under ideal circumstances, normal tissue repopulation would not be damaged to the extent that full epithelial covering cannot be regained. All radiation exposures lead to damage in the mesenchymal structures, including blood vessels, some of which may be obliterated, as illustrated in the lower left corner. If blood vessel damage is excessive, areas are rendered avascular and may necrose, leading to radiation complications. (Drawing by Katharyne Jacobus.)

administered to limited volumes. The biologic basis of tissue and organ radioresistance is discussed later (see "The Linear Quadratic Survival Curve"). First, it is of interest to compare these rough tolerance doses to the known relationship between tumor volume and tumor sterilization. It has been clearly shown in a wide variety of clinical situations in most areas of the body that radiation doses of 4,000 to 5,000 cGy in 5 weeks can eliminate subclinical cancers in 80 to 90 percent of the cases (Fletcher, 1974). A gram of solid tumor tissue can contain a packed cell mass of approximately 10^9 cells; subclinical tumor masses therefore contain significantly less, perhaps having a variable level of 10^6 to 10^8

cells. Two things should be apparent: (1) any successful (tumoricidal) treatment usually requires doses above 5,000 cGy in 5 weeks when the tumor is palpable; and (2) to reduce or eliminate treatment complications, the treatment volume must be minimized throughout the period of therapy, since the tumoricidal dose ($\geq$7,000 cGy) for palpable epithelial tumors approximates maximum tissue tolerance. One might take these considerations further and ask: how do radiation treatments ever cure clinically apparent cancers if the cells constituting the tumor are not intrinsically more sensitive to x-rays than are their normal counterparts? What can be done to improve this situation?

TABLE 17-2

Radiation Tolerance Doses (cGy) and α/β Ratios for Various Organs*

Organ	TD$_5$[†]	TD$_{50}$[†]	α/β[‡]
Bone marrow	25	500	—
Ovary	250	1,000	—
Kidney	1,500	2,500	1.5–2.4
Lung	2,500	3,000	2.0–6.3
Liver	2,500	5,000	—
Heart	4,000	6,000	—
Intestine	4,250	6,250	—
Spinal cord	4,500	6,000	1.0–2.7
Brain	5,000	6,500	—
Bladder	5,750	6,500	3.0–7.0

*TD$_5$ = the radiation dose in cGy at which approximately 5 percent of all patients will develop a significant complication in that organ by 5 years; TD$_{50}$ = the same value for a 50 percent complication rate; α/β, see text for discussion.
[†]Values from Fajardo (1982).
[‡]Values from Fowler (1984).

CLINICAL IMPLICATIONS OF RADIATION BIOLOGY

Mechanisms of Tumor Destruction

The mechanisms by which x-rays kill tumors vary considerably with both the size and the location of the tumor. Small tumors, such as early carcinoma of the cervix, are essentially cauterized by the high radiation dose that can be locally administered because of the relative radioresistance of the uterine cervix and paravaginal tissues. The cancer is eliminated by bringing the resistant tissues to their radiation tolerance level. The cervical musculofibrous tissue can tolerate local doses in excess of 10,000 cGy. This tissue is readily replaced be dense scar tissue, usually without the development of necrosis. Such doses are possible only because the cervix is dispensable in a patient undergoing curative therapy. Tumor size is also important. For example, early carcinoma of the larynx commonly presents with a few milligrams of tumor manifested by a change in voice. Successful radiation therapy is possible, because the tumor stem cell population can be reduced to zero by a radiation dose tolerable to the surrounding normal tissues.

When tumors of even moderate volume occur in normal structures that are moderately radiosensitive, the mechanism of cure is rather more complicated. In most soft tissues where an intact (external or internal) epithelial covering must be retained, there seems to be an average tolerance of the normal struc-

tures that approximates 5,000 cGy delivered with conventional fractionation, about 200 cGy per treatment fraction, with five treatment fractions per week for 5 weeks.

Modern biologic studies suggest that the mechanism by which radiation sterilizes the larger human cancers focuses on the interplay of two disparate factors: (1) different rates of multiplication (repopulation) of tumor versus normal tissues, such that treatment may favor the more rapid growth of the normal, acutely dose-limiting cells; and (2) a slight relative radioresistance at low doses of those normal cells that limits the total administerable dose. These concepts, and their clinical implications, are discussed in the next two sections.

Tumor Versus Normal Cell Repopulation Kinetics

Most normal tissues, such as the gastrointestinal mucosa, skin, or bone marrow, have a phenomenal capacity to recover by simple cell division of the appropriate stem cells. Epithelial tumors, including both squamous cell carcinomas and adenocarcinoma, grow relatively slowly (Charbit et al, 1971) and are therefore depopulated by x-rays (Tubiana and Malaise, 1976) at a rate that can significantly exceed that of the surrounding normal tissues. If a tumor repopulates very slowly, then there is a much greater chance that the fractionated radiation treatment will successfully eliminate all tumor cells. If a tumor repopulates very rapidly, then it is probably not possible to cure a patient with conventional radiation treatments. In this context, it is convenient to envision a malignancy as a population of cells that exists as a volume within a larger volume of normal tissue (Fig. 17–10). The radiation oncologist must deliver a certain amount of energy to these tissues that includes both volumes, with the goal of reducing the volume of the tumor to zero at a dose rate (fractionation) that will not reduce the volume in the normal tissues to a level intolerable to the patient. Each radiation treatment reduces the cell population of both the tumor and the normal tissue (the latter shown in Fig. 17–10 as a reduced number of mucosal cells), and both tissues re-expand in the intertreatment time. If the rate of regrowth of the tumor is slow, then the tumor will eventually be eliminated, and only the normal tissue will remain. If one realizes that each treatment also weakens the mesenchymal structures that hold the normal tissues together, primarily the vascular tree supplying the normal tissues, and that they can only be stressed so much by a finite amount of radiation before they collapse (vascular obliteration leading to radionecrosis), it can readily be seen that the essence of successful radiation therapy is to bring the efficiency of each radiation fraction to a maximum. The developing study of cell kinetics, both normal and malignant, offers one approach to improving treatment results through the manipulation of radiation fractionation and cell kinetics in the future, especially through the coincident addition of chemotherapeutic agents that do not affect the supporting structures (blood vessels, nerves, and so forth) and through radiosensitizing compounds that eliminate tumor cell (hypoxic) radioresistance.

An alternative method of improving an initially unpromising situation is to reduce the number of tumor cells before embarking on the radiation treatments. This is the basis for surgical debulking of ovarian or other pelvic tumors before either x-ray therapy or chemotherapy. Pretreatment (frequently called *neoadjuvant*) chemotherapy offers another means of potentially improving treatment results. It will be readily understood that the development of optimum curative regimens in gynecologic cancers is complicated and likely to remain in flux for a considerable period of time. However, if one keeps in mind the biologic principles described earlier, it seems likely that improved therapeutic regimens will be forthcoming.

In this context, the reader will appreciate the critical importance of understanding normal stem cells and their repopulation kinetics, discussed previously.

The Linear Quadratic Survival Curve

The description of the radiation survival curve and its implications has been revised based on new data. It has been proposed that the typical radiation survival curve follows a linear quadratic formula rather than the straightforward semilogarithmic radiation survival curve described previously. This concept means that the curve can be regarded as having two major components analogous to the shoulder and straight portions of the semilogarithmic curve, but that both portions of the curve are curving downward. The curve then has the general formula

$$\text{Surviving fraction} = \alpha D + \beta D$$

where α and β are mathematical coefficients that can be derived from experimental data and D is the radiation dose. To study these topics, the experimental radiobiologist picks a specific endpoint (e.g., a given level of skin reaction or an adverse effect on the spinal cord) and then examines that endpoint over a wide variety of time-dose relationships. In the previous formula, the resulting curve will initially bend more rapidly if α (which dictates the shoulder) is larger than β (which dictates the rest of the curve), that is, if the α/β ratio is large. There is now evidence that the survival curves for the cells dictating acute reactions (primarily mucosa and skin reactions) have a larger α/β ratio than those dictating late reactions (e.g., spinal myelitis, pulmonary fibrosis, and radiation nephritis). The origins of the α/β ratio are shown in Figure 17–11.

These observations lend a theoretical basis for the well-confirmed clinical observation that fraction size (i.e., the dose per fraction) is very important in the clinical tolerance to radiation. Such observations were the basis of the earliest formulas developed by radiation oncologists (e.g., the Ellis formula, presented

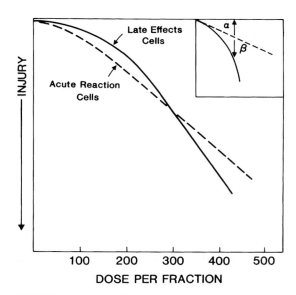

FIGURE 17–11. Diagrammatic example of the linear quadratic radiation survival curve, which is constantly bending (cf. Fig. 17–7). The rates of curvature of the initial and second components of the curve, termed α and β, differ. Cells believed to be responsible for late effects (complications) are initially somewhat more resistant to x-ray damage but eventually become more sensitive (where the curves cross). This difference is believed to dictate the clinical dose size and therefore the fractionation limits (see text).

later) to compare various treatment regimens. Radiobiologic studies have now shown that the α/β ratio is much greater for early radiation reactions (cell depletion reactions) than for late effects. Typical α/β values for early effects (bone marrow death, skin desquamation, mucosal denudation) are in the 5 to 25 range, while those for late effects, which include virtually all radiation complications, are less than 5 (Table 17–2). This indicates that the initial part of the radiation survival curve for the cells involved in early effects bends faster (the cells are more sensitive) at low doses of radiation than the curve for the cells involved in complications (late effects). At high radiation doses, the curves cross and late-effect cells are relatively more sensitive to higher doses. Because of these differences, high-dose-per-fraction regimens are more likely to lead to late reactions (complications).

It seems likely to the authors that the high α/β ratios of early-reactive cells (skin, mucosa, marrow) are retained in their derivative tumors, and these differences from late-reactive (normal) connective tissue cells are the basis for the usefulness of radiation therapy in the treatment of most cancers. This is further discussed later. Table 17–2 gives the approximate tolerance doses of the various important organs, as described by Fajardo (1982). The values given basically indicate the lowest radiation dose (using the conventional 200-cGy/day fractionation) at which a complication rate can be estimated (5 percent of all patients) and the dose at which 50 percent of all patients will develop the complication listed within 5 years. Also given are representative α/β ratios, as listed by Fowler (1984), from a wide variety of sources. It can be seen that all late effects (complications) have low α/β ratios.

Time-Dose Fractionation

It will be apparent to the reader that many different radiation regimens can lead to the same quantitative result measured in terms of tumor-cell killing. The principal variables include the individual dose (or dose per fraction), the total number of fractions, the total dose, and the overall treatment time. In clinical radiobiology these are considered the time-dose relationships for a given treatment regimen. While individual exposure might well vary between 1 and 1,000 cGy, acute radiation reactions tend to be dose limiting in clinical practice. Thus radiation-induced nausea, diarrhea, and skin de-epithelialization (moist desquamation or epitheliitis) tend to limit both individual daily exposure doses and overall weekly doses. Over the past five decades, a conventional dose for external beam treatment of 180 to 200 cGy/day has become customary.

Whether this daily fraction size is optimum has never really been established (Montague, 1968; Thames, 1992). Moreover, it is not the acute toxic reactions, but rather the damage inflicted on the supporting tissue components (vascular fine structures and possibly nerves), that basically limits the overall dose. While there is some correlation between the acute reaction level and long-term complications in gynecologic oncology (skin, bowel, and bone necrosis), this correlation is difficult to apply in any given patient, since other parameters such as treatment volume, bowel fixation, co-incident diseases, age, and infection all influence healing. Therefore the "science" of radiation fractionation remains empiric, and it is difficult to find many clinics that deviate significantly from the 180 to 200 cGy/day, 5 days/week, 5,000-cGy total dose that constrains the treatment of subclinical cancers.

A related problem that the gynecologic oncologist should be acquainted with is that of comparing different clinical regimens with respect to either results or complications. The pioneering efforts of Ellis (1968) were directed toward solving this problem. Ellis examined the time-dose relationships for skin complications from orthovoltage therapy and devised a formula designed to allow a comparison between various fractionation regimens. According to the Ellis formula

$$D = (NSD)T^{0.11}N^{0.24}$$

where D is the total dose, T is time in days, N is the number of treatment fractions, and NSD is the nominal standard dose. The NSD is measured in *rets*, which stands for *rad-equivalent therapy*. Representative NSDs might be as follows (assuming 200 cGy or rad per fraction delivered 5 days a week, commencing on Monday and subtracting Saturday and Sunday after the last treatment):

4,000 rad in 4 weeks, NSD = 1,362 rets

5,000 rad in 5 weeks, NSD = 1,572 rets

6,000 rad in 6 weeks, NSD = 1,768 rets

7,000 rad in 7 weeks, NSD = 1,987 rets

8,000 rad in 8 weeks, NSD = 2,128 rets

A NSD exceeding 1,800 rets will be required to sterilize a typical epithelial tumor. The most common application of the NSD concept is in comparing treatment results (and complications) of various regimens, especially when the dose per fraction and the number of fractions differ significantly from the 200-cGy/day convention. Note that the NSD concept is independent of field size and that it should be anticipated that tumor control and complications can be expected to increase as field size expands, independent of the NSD.

Orton and Ellis (1973) expanded the utility of the NSD concept of *partial tolerance* and tabulated the relationships between the time, dose, and fractionation (TDF) elements of the radiation prescription. NSDs for components of a treatment regimen, calculated from the basic Ellis equation, cannot be added, whereas partial tolerances (TDFs) can be added using the Orton-Ellis tables. This is possible because "decay factors" have also been calculated and can be used to estimate the recovery of normal tissues that occurs with time (as measured clinically by Ellis in the development of the NSD formula). This is especially useful in split-course regimens (Ellis, 1985). For example, if a patient with carcinoma of the cervix has 2 weeks of therapy and then requires a significant break in therapy (either planned or because of medical or social problems), it is possible, by using the Orton-Ellis tables of TDFs, to calculate the number of additional treatments required to deliver a similar biologic result. It is also possible to determine the fraction size (daily dose) required to give equivalent results if the treatment is given in one to five fractions per week. TDFs equivalent to the NSDs listed previously are 66, 82, 99, 115, and 132, going from 1,362 to 2,128 rets. Thus a TDF in excess of 100 is required to cure most common epithelial cancers.

It is important to emphasize that the NSD concept and its derivative, the TDF, are based ultimately on the tolerance of normal human connective tissue and have no intrinsic relationship to tumor control. However, they are widely used to compare different treatment regimens because they offer a convenient way of estimating to what degree a regimen approaches tolerance and of solving common clinical problems such as split-course treatments.

More recent studies have shown that the NSD formula (and its derivative, the TDF) are not applicable to tolerance comparisons for all human organs and structures (Thames et al, 1982). This stems from the significant variation in the slope of the isodose effect curve for different tissues. The Ellis formula is in essence a single-slope curve. The net effect of the differences demonstrated for different dose-limiting organs is to make the likelihood of the development of either a side effect or a complication somewhat different for the various organs involved when studied as a function of dose per fraction. Thus the likelihood of a complication developing increases much more rapidly with the size of the dose per fraction for some organs compared with others. This is under intense study at this time, especially because the evidence just discussed suggests that it may be possible to improve the results of radiation therapy through rational manipulations of the dose-per-fraction and fraction-per-day treatment scheduling. The interested reader is referred to reviews on this topic for further elaboration (Thames et al, 1982; Fowler, 1984; Withers and Horiot, 1988).

CHEMOTHERAPEUTIC RADIOSENSITIZERS

To the purist radiation biologist, only substances replacing oxygen or metabolites rendering DNA more subject to radiation damage are true radiosensitizers. However, a variety of chemotherapy drugs have been used as "radiosensitizers" (Hill and Bellamy, 1990). The literature on both the preclinical and clinical studies on these agents is immense (and confusing). It is only possible to present a brief summary of these agents with references that can lead the interested reader further if so inclined. Despite this meager introduction, the authors believe that this area has a bright future. We must remember that, while the combination of toxic cancer drugs and radiation is a potential minefield of acute and late complications, the Nobel prizes are funded each year by moneys derived from explosives!

1. *Hydroxyurea:* Hydroxyurea is an inhibitor of DNA synthesis long used by hematologists in the treatment of chronic myelogenous leukemia and now used for some applications in sickle cell anemia. Hydroxyurea is postulated to be a radi-

osensitizer with utility in cervical cancer (Hreschchyshyn et al, 1979).

2. *5-Fluorouracil (5-FU)*: 5-FU is an antimetabolite with well established uses in the treatment of several cancers. It is a known radiosensitizer, but its ability in this regard is schedule dependent. 5-FU must be presented to the tumor cell almost continuously following each radiation exposure for radiosensitivity to be demonstrated (Byfield et al, 1982). 5-FU is "active" against most epithelial cancers (Byfield, 1991), and randomized controlled trials of radiation and 5-FU in head-and-neck and esophageal cancers have shown statistically improved results (Lokich and Byfield, 1991; Herskovic et al, 1992).

3. *Cis-platinum*: *Cis*-platinum is thought to sensitize hypoxic cells to radiation (Douple, 1990) and has approximately the same objective single-agent activity in squamous cancers as 5-FU (about a 20 percent response rate). *Cis*-platinum is frequently combined with infused 5-FU. There are many trials of *cis*-platinum alone or with other drugs in gynecologic cancers with and without radiation. It is sometimes given as an intra-arterial infusion (Sueyama et al, 1995). To date there are no randomized trials that demonstrate improved survival when *cis*-platinum is combined with radiation.

4. *Mitomycin C*: Mitomycin C exerts its toxicity by preferentially killing hypoxic cells. Therefore, it is not a radiosensitizer but is a likely candidate for combination with radiation (Rockwell, 1982) because of the putative role of hypoxia in radiation treatment failure (Brown and Siim, 1996). Mitomycin C may cause severe and frequently unpredictable toxicity in many organ systems, a trait that has hampered its usefulness. A Gynecologic Oncology Group (GOG) phase II study demonstrated that this drug has a low level of activity in squamous cell carcinoma of the cervix (Thigpen et al, 1995).

5. *Paclitaxel*: Paclitaxel (Taxol) was reported by Steren et al (1993) and also Liebmann et al (1994) to radiosensitize ovarian cancer cells. These observations have been extended to human cervical cancer cells (Minarik and Hall, 1994; Rodriquez et al, 1995), and also refuted (Erlich et al, 1996). Paclitaxel has also been reported to enhance the oncogenicity of radiation (Hei et al, 1994)! Paclitaxel appears to act by binding to microtubules, thereby preventing successful mitosis. It has been questioned as to the semantic purity of its claim to be a radiosensitizer (van Rijn et al, 1995). Paclitaxel has also been reported to possibly sensitize the central nervous system to radiation (JM Liu et al, 1996). Under these contentious circumstances, it is undoubted that vigorous research on paclitaxel as a radiosensitizer will continue.

To date only hydroxyurea and 5-FU have survived randomized clinical trials with demonstrated clinical benefit as a radiosensitizer in any human tumor, and the study results with hydroxyurea are ambiguous. The relevant clinical studies on the use of these drugs as clinical radiosentizing agents and applications of interest are mentioned in subsequent sections on individual cancers.

RADIATION THERAPY FOR CERVICAL CARCINOMA

Choice of Modality

Elsewhere in this chapter, it is stated that the treatment for all but early stage I and some IIa cervical cancers lies primarily with radiation therapy. Even in the group of early cancers (including microinvasive), the results of surgery and radiation are equivalent in terms of 5-year survival, and consequently ancillary factors determine the best therapy. Thus we believe that vaginal changes, especially those leading to dyspareunia and preservation of the ovaries, make surgery a better option in most younger patients. Conversely, age or serious medical problems would favor x-ray therapy as the treatment of choice in older patients. As tumor volume increases in stage I and more of the cervix is involved, the likelihood of occult parametrial and lymphatic spread increases. Under these circumstances, it becomes necessary to treat the entire pelvis, and radiation therapy becomes the treatment of choice; surgery is held in reserve as an adjuvant (e.g., in the case of large, barrel-shaped lesions) or for radiation treatment failure salvage.

Having said this, it is incumbent on the radiation community to acknowledge that the decision to use surgery as the primary modality for a significant number of stage I cervical cancer patients is appropriate. Certainly, this number is larger now than it was a decade ago, because studies showing excellent surgical results can be obtained with tumors larger than the classical "early" stage I patients (e.g., Polednak, 1995). While the International Federation of Gynecology and Obstetrics (FIGO) staging system is *not* intended to dictate or suggest any specific therapeutic modality, it is the medical community's responsibility now to evaluate in an objective, multi-institutional study the appropriate role of surgery and radiation in FIGO stage IB2 lesions (tumors >4 cm in diameter) and possibly stage IB1 patients. Currently this decision remains arbitrary for many patients. Practicing clinicians need more objective guidance on this important topic (Curtin, 1996).

Until such studies are complete, it is the author's (JEB) practice to ask the gynecologic oncologist to re-examine those patients receiving radiation following the first intracavitary cesium insertion (or third HDR application) to get an opinion about the quality of each patient's response. In some cases the gynecologist will feel that surgical intervention is useful. By having this discussion at the appropriate watershed dose between preoperative radiation and a full course of radiation, we are sure that some patients have been spared central tumor recurrences. Two heads (and four hands) are better than one!

Treatment Dose and Dosimetry

External Beam Treatment

With modern instrumentation (either cobalt or linear accelerators), it is possible to individualize the configuration of the treatment beam isodose curves. The simplest illustration of this phenomenon is shown in Figure 17–12. Most patients with gynecologic cancers will undergo radiotherapy using parallel opposed portals (half of the treatment dose being administered in the anteroposterior [AP] direction and half in the posteroanterior [PA] direction). This produces a box-like series of isodose curves centered on the middle of the pelvis. By "loading" such treatment beams (i.e., giving more of the dose either AP or PA), it is possible to bring the maximum (100 percent isodose line) level forward or backward in the pelvis. Similarly, by the addition of one

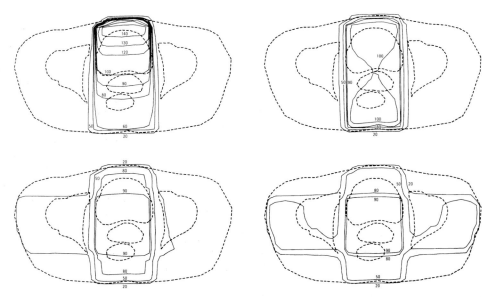

FIGURE 17–12. Isodose curves for single and multiple linac pelvic treatments. The construction of a typical patient's pelvis is indicated by the outer dotted lines. The rectum (lower inner circle), bladder (upper circle), and uterus (middle circle) are shown within the pelvic contours. In the upper left corner is a typical treatment beam for a single AP field. The isodose curves derived from the linac (Fig. 17–3) are superimposed on the anterior abdominal curvature. In the upper right corner a dose distribution for bilateral opposed fields (AP, PA) is shown, which yields a 100 percent isodose line in the shape of an hourglass. Through the introduction of a left lateral portal (lower left) and subsequently a right lateral portal (lower right), it can be seen that the isodose curves are pulled laterally into the pelvis. Asymmetrical tumors can be treated by the use of multiple treatment portals and parametrial boosts. By varying the beam angle and percentage contribution of individual beams, virtually any isodose distribution may be achieved.

or more lateral treatment portals, the maximum dose is pulled toward the side of the pelvis through which the beam is directed. In patients of more than medium thickness, multiple beams are required to reduce the entrance doses and achieve an optimum isodose configuration. This is done by altering the direction of the beam such that the dose distribution throughout the pelvis is manipulated to produce an ideal configuration. With the development of rotational units, which are now common, there is very little limitation to the potential ways by which the isodose distribution can be manipulated. For patients with localized disease, such as parametrial involvement in cervical carcinoma, smaller treatment volumes can be "boosted." It will be apparent to the reader, therefore, that there is great latitude in the dose distribution within the pelvis and in the volume of radiation. The treatment volume also can be altered on a daily basis such that great flexibility in following tumor responsiveness and altering treatment portals is available.

The most commonly accepted treatment dose recommendations for cervical cancer used in the United States today are those developed at the M.D. Anderson Hospital (MDAH) by Fletcher and his colleagues (Fletcher, 1980); these are listed in Table 17–3. In all cases, it is assumed that the best possible applicator position will be used, since less than ideal positioning must inevitably alter the overall treatment prescription. The MDAH approach, integrating external beam and intracavitary radiation with improved applicators, has clearly improved treatment results, especially in stage I and II lesions (Boronow and Hickman, 1977; Thomson and Spratt, 1978; Fletcher, 1980).

Several observations can be made regarding the recommended doses:

1. A wide variety of studies in both gynecologic and nongynecologic cancers have shown that occult metastatic tumor deposits from epithelial cancers require between 4,000 and 5,000 cGy for 90 to 100 percent sterilization (Fletcher, 1974). This is the minimum dose required to sterilize nodes involved with occult metastatic cervical cancer and must be administered to the area at risk in virtually all patients with easily visible ($\geq$1.0-cm) lesions (see Figs. 17–13 and 17–14).

2. Clinically apparent (palpable) tumor will require in excess of 6,000 cGy for sterilization, and in practice 7,000 to 8,000 cGy or more must usually be delivered. The dose dependence for tumor control is well illustrated by the Patterns of Care Study (Komaki et al, 1995), a radiation oncology comprehensive national survey currently being conducted under the supervision of the National Cancer Institute and the American College of Radiology. As part of this study, Montana et al (1991) showed that the central recurrence rate of stages I through III patients (on average, mainly of stage III patients) was reduced from 34 percent when the dose was less than 6,500 cGy to 14 percent for a dose of 7,500 cGy or higher. Doses above 8,500 cGy did not improve control and led to higher complication rates. Higher doses are best administered in at least two intracavitary sessions (when using cesium), which leads to better tolerance (Marcial et al, 1991). Doses of over 7,000 cGy exceed the tolerance of all but the most resistant normal tissues. Fortunately, the uterus itself is extremely radioresistant and can tolerate higher tumoricidal doses. However, parametrial tissues are considerably less resistant, and treatment of such tissues with a similarly high dose will inevitably produce complications in some patients, especially bowel necrosis and vesicovaginal fistulas (Strockbine et al, 1970; Pourquier et al, 1987).

3. When doses in excess of 5,000 cGy in 5 weeks must be prescribed, the complication rate will be a direct function of the required treatment volume; the smaller the tissue volume receiving the higher x-ray doses, the lower the complication rate.

4. To minimize giving a high radiation dose to a large volume, great reliance on the intracavity component is needed in order to deliver the medial parametrial dose, since the falloff resulting from the inverse square law allows maximum control over the parametrial dose.

5. For asymmetrical parametrial involvement, external beam boost to the involved side can be very useful, especially where optimum applicator placement cannot be achieved.

6. As tumor volume in the parametria increases, the possibility of delivering a tumoricidal dose to all clinical tumor decreases because large-volume external beam therapy is required (Table 17–3) and bowel tolerance is exceeded. Survival rates inevitably fall as a result of this problem.

T A B L E **17–3**

Summary of the M.D. Anderson Hospital Combination of External and Intracavitary Radiation for Carcinoma of the Cervix With an Intact Uterus*

Tumor Size	Whole Pelvis (cGy)	Radium† hr/interval/hr‡	Radium† mg × hr	Parametrial	Comment
≤1 cm	None	72/2 weeks/48	10,000	None	If anatomy is not good, radium is reduced and additional treatment is given with external radiation
1- to 3 cm lesions of exocervix with little or no extension to parametria or fornices	None 2,000 4,000	72/2 weeks/72 48/2 weeks/72 48/2 weeks/48	≤9,000 ≤8,000 ≤5,500	≤4,000 cGy‖ ≤2,000 cGy None	The amount of whole pelvis and parametrial irradiation depends on extent of disease, patient anatomy, and geometry and location in pelvis of radium system; if >7,500 mg × hr, ≤1,500 rad parametrial dose
Endocervical tumor or disease of moderate bulk, >3 to ≤6 cm, with or without extension to medial parametrium	4,000	48/2 weeks/48	5,500–6,500	None	If regression is poor and there is no parametrial involvement, one single radium insertion (72 hr or 5,000 mg × hr, whichever comes first) followed by an extrafascial hysterectomy
Bulky central disease, >6 cm "barrel-shaped" endo-cervical tumor	4,000	72§	5,000	None	Extrafascial hysterectomy performed 6 weeks after irradiation
Bulky central disease, >6 cm, extending near or to pelvic wall(s) and/or lower vagina	4,000 5,000 6,000	48/2 weeks/48 72 or 48/2 weeks/24–48 72 or 48/2 weeks/24	5,500–6,600 4,000–5,000 3,000–4,000	May add 1,000 cGy to side of major involvement	When major involvement is restricted to only one side, whole-pelvis radiation may be stopped at 4,000 cGy and the involved side may be boosted through the parametrial field After 5,000 rad, reduce fields to ≤12 × ≤12 cm
Massive disease or bladder or rectal involvement	Up to 7,000	None	None	None	After 5,000 rad, reduce fields to ≤12 × ≤12 cm; after 6,000 rad, reduce fields to ≤10 × ≤10 cm

*Courtesy of G.H. Fletcher, M.D.

†Use whichever maximum comes first, either the time or mg × hr. The longer time may be used first if vault size does not permit colpostats at second insertion. The larger figures for radium are used if lesions have not disappeared clinically at the time of the second insertion; the smaller figures are used if there has been excellent regression of disease.

‡Fractionated therapy: number of hours of first fraction/interval between fractions/number of hours of second fraction.

§Single-fraction therapy.

‖Midline block, both sides treated.

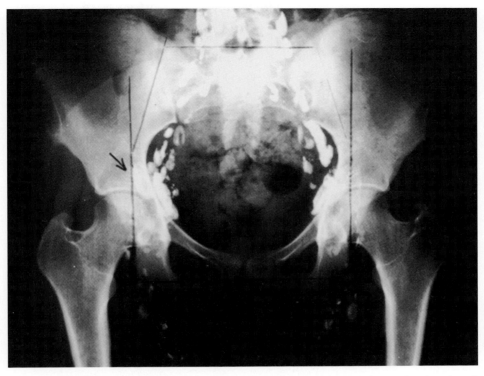

FIGURE 17–13. Treatment planning for cervical carcinoma. A lymphangiogram showing the distribution of lymph nodes within the pelvis is shown together with the treatment volume used by the authors. Note that lymph nodes are frequently found outside the shadow created by the true pelvis; therefore, the lateral treatment margins (arrow) in our clinic is 1 cm beyond the widest point in the pelvis. This by definition is more lateral than the classic point B. From this most lateral point, a line is drawn diagonally to the upper end of the sacroiliac joint. The lower treatment margins for early carcinoma of the cervix are the lower part of the symphysis pubis (which usually includes all of the obturator nodes) and the upper margin of the L5-S1 border. Note that the bone marrow treatment volume is quite small, while all draining lymph nodes up to the para-aortic chain are included. Many radiotherapists also block out the lower lateral ramus of the pubic bone.

7. The total treatment duration must not be extended by rest "breaks." Rests should be kept to a *minimum*. The data base on this topic is large and unequivocal (e.g., Petereit et al, 1994; Fyles et al, 1992). In a large MDAH series, the major complication rate with timely treatment was 14.4 percent at 20 years' follow-up (Eifel et al, 1995). With our current state of knowledge, we must accept this as part of the price for treating a potentially curable population with radiation.

Treatment Volume

Because lymphatic metastases occur early, the entire pelvis must be treated to the tolerance level by external beam radiation in most patients with cervical cancer (Lanciano et al, 1991). The recommended treatment volume (Figs. 17–13 and 17–14) is directly dictated by the distribution of the pelvic lymphatics. Two additional points can be made: (1) asymmetrical cancers may profitably be boosted through smaller external parametrial fields, especially if one side is clinically free of disease; and (2) a decision must be made whether to treat the para-aortic nodes (Boronow, 1991; Cunningham et al, 1991). Few patients die as a result of para-aortic recurrence alone. Almost all such patients die with coincident pelvic recurrence (Chism et al, 1975; Kademian and Bosch, 1977). Nevertheless, a controlled trial conducted by Rotman et al (1990) indicated a small but significant improvement in survivorship when para-aortic node radiation was carried out (Rotman et al, 1994). In our own clinics, the lower para-aortic nodes (to the lower L2 border; Figs. 17–15 and 17–16) are treated to 4,500

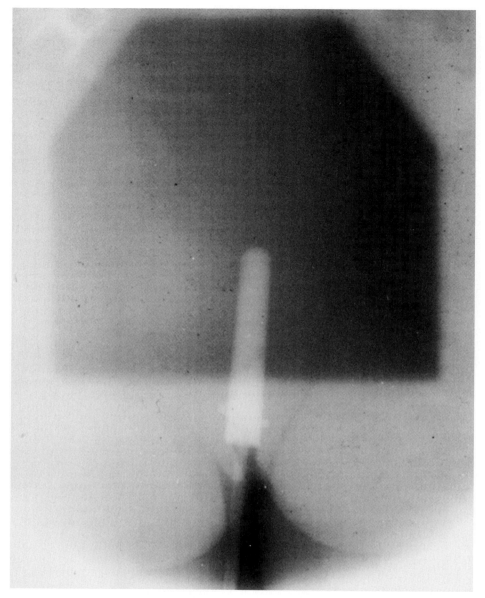

FIGURE 17–14. Linac treatment portal for early cervical carcinoma. An "ad-lux" x-ray film photograph of a typical treatment portal for stage I and II cervical carcinoma is shown. A lead vaginal marker is included indicating the vaginal volume. Toward the bottom part of the radiopaque vaginal marker is a loop of metal indicating the location of the urethral orifice. Patients with overt vaginal involvement or more extensive disease require a treatment portal extending to the level of the urethra to avoid occasional low periurethral recurrence. Note the relatively clean edge of the treatment portal, consistent with the small penumbra of a high-energy 6-MV linac beam.

cGy in all stage III, IV, and large stage IIb cases. We include para-aortic node radiation even in patients undergoing the concomitant chemoradiation described later. To date, bowel problems have not been excessively troublesome, but more time will be required to ensure this is the case. The reader must remember that this is limited to the 5-FU/cisplatin regimens. Other chemotherapeutic agents, particularly the intercalating agents such as doxorubicin, can be very troublesome when combined with radiation (Ransom et al, 1978). Most combined chemoradiation programs are carried out at a significantly

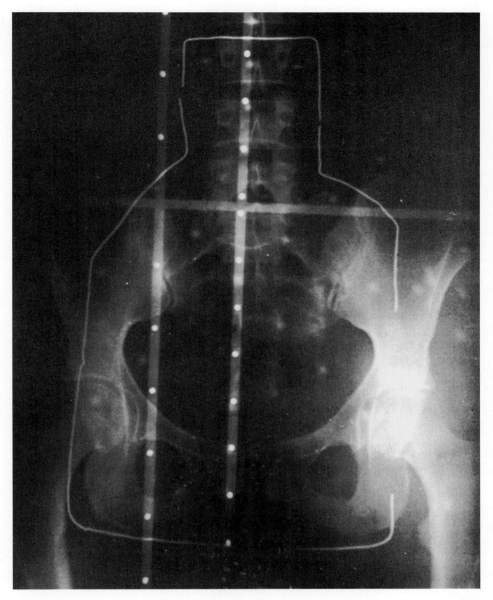

FIGURE 17–15. Confirmatory wire film of extended field cervical radiation. In the author's clinic, patients with stages IIIb and IVa tumors receive treatment to the lower para-aortic nodes (to the L2-3 border). In obese patients linac ad-lux beam films are frequently difficult to interpret, and confirmatory films taken with the treatment portal on the skin marked with flexible solder wires are useful. Note the considerably lower level of the treatment portal in patients who are highly at risk for lower vaginal recurrences.

reduced pace (we use 180 cGy/day), which may lend itself to improved bowel tolerance. This approach is reasonably well tolerated, provided no surgery is included (El Senoussi et al, 1979). The reader is referred to excellent articles in the literature for a fuller discussion of this still-controversial subject (Rotman et al, 1979, 1990; Brookland et al, 1984).

Intracavitary Treatment Applicators

All applicators now in use should be *afterloaded*, that is, the radioactive cesium should be inserted into the applicators after the patient has returned to her room following surgical placement of the applicators under anesthesia. In the United States, the most

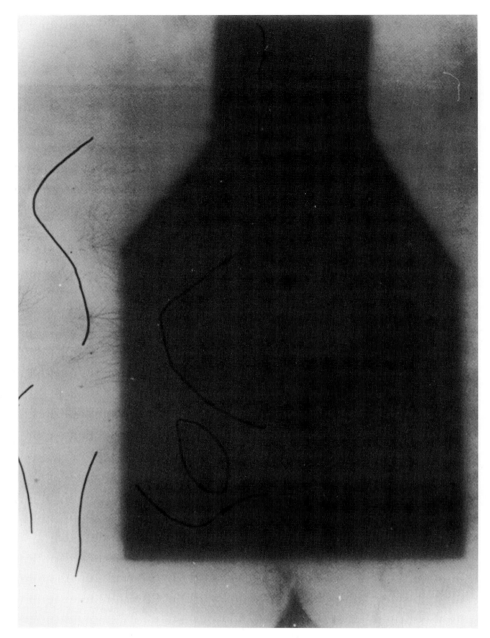

FIGURE 17–16. Extended field therapy port film. A confirmatory port film taken in an asthenic patient is shown. While difficult to reproduce, the bony structures of the pelvis can be seen on these films in most patients. These structures have been drawn on this film with a pen. Also shown are the edges of the vertebral bodies. In the author's opinion, full aortic node therapy (T12) for advanced cervical cancer is warranted only in an investigational setting.

commonly used applicator is the Fletcher-Suit afterloading apparatus (Fig. 17–17). Like all applicators, it consists of an intrauterine tandem and two vaginal colpostats. The colpostats have built-in tungsten shielding to reduce the bladder and rectal doses (Fig. 17–18). Various curvatures for the intrauterine com-

ponent are available, and, most importantly, the length of the intrauterine tandem and its loading can be varied. (This was not the case with many early applicators.) In the patient with a capacious, symmetrical, and supple vagina, the tandem and colpostats can be combined into a single unit by a built-in clamp.

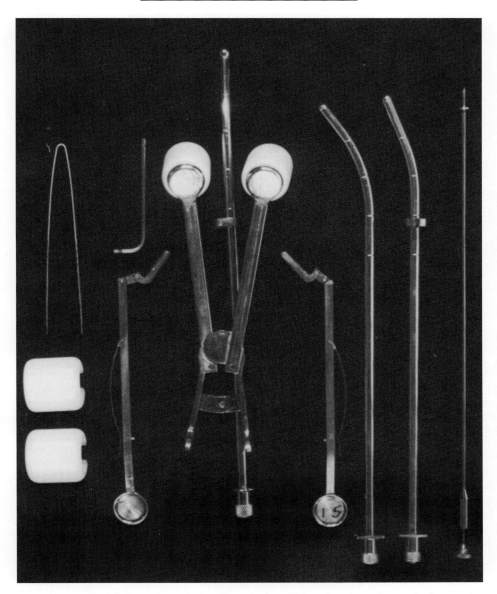

FIGURE 17–17. Fletcher-Suit uterine afterloading device. This type of applicator is the most commonly used in the United States today. It includes a uterine tandem, which is available in several contours and can be fixed in place under ideal circumstances to the two vaginal colpostats as shown. These instruments are afterloaded with radium or cesium, using the small tubes shown on either side of the applicator. Note the white spacers or caps placed over the colpostat to push the vaginal mucosa away from the radiation source. Also shown is a stylet for introducing inactive metallic seeds into the cervix for dosimetric determinations. The seeds should be placed at 90-degree angles to allow three-dimensional analysis.

With proper packing, such a combination produces ideal, stable geometry (Fig. 17–19). The vaginal colpostats are 2.0 cm in diameter and can be increased in size by adding plastic spacer caps. These spacers assist in placement and effectively increase the depth dose by moving the vaginal mucosa away from the sources (Fig. 17–2). Spacers should be used

whenever possible. In the older literature, the vaginal colpostats were called *ovoids* because of their shape.

There are many patients who have a naturally small vaginal vault or an upper vagina that is distorted by cancer or healing scar tissue from previous external beam treatment. It is sometimes difficult to place a conven-

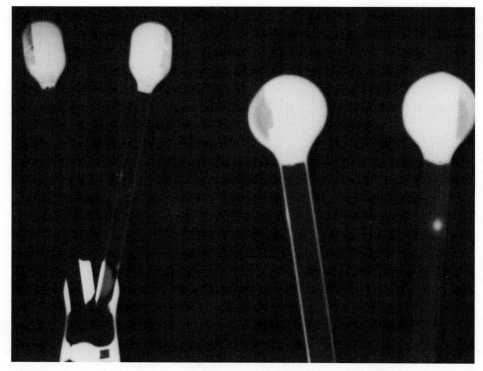

FIGURE 17–18. X-ray photographs of a Fletcher-Suit applicator. The more opaque (white) regions indicated on the AP and lateral views of the applicator show the lead shielding components. These are important in reducing the bladder and rectal doses. All applicators purchased should be checked to ensure the existence of these blocks, which are not visible from the surface of the applicator.

tional Fletcher-Suit applicator in these patients properly. For this reason, a smaller applicator, such as a reduced Fletcher-Suit or a Henschke (Fig. 17–20) applicator, may be useful. The newer version of the latter applicator also has bladder and rectum blocks (arrow, Fig. 17–20). The treatment of patients who cannot accept either type of applicator is discussed in the section "Interstitial Template Therapy" later in this chapter.

Sequence of External and Intracavitary Therapy

The innovative technique of using external beam radiation to shrink cervical cancer and to permit more efficient intracavitary treatment was developed by Fletcher and colleagues, and a detailed review of their approach is strongly recommended (Fletcher, 1980). Since it is the intracavitary component that is basically responsible for the cure of most patients, the patient should undergo intracavitary therapy as soon as reasonable anatomy has been achieved. The first intracavitary session should be given as soon after

2,000 cGy of external pelvic radiation as possible, provided that the applicator will deliver a tumoricidal dose (25 cGy/hr or more) to all palpable tumor. If physical examination suggests that this is not possible, then external beam therapy should be continued weekly with the clear understanding that each treatment will reduce the amount of intracavitary therapy that can be delivered.

Patients vary considerably in the rate of tumor regression, and radiotherapists similarly vary in their timing. The most important points to be made are that the external beam component is less likely to cure without the intracavitary component, but the latter is greatly limited in effective treatment volume by the inverse square law. Weekly examinations by the radiotherapist are necessary in decision making.

Initially, radium was used as the intracavitary radiation source for the treatment of cervical cancer, but in all United States hospitals it now has been replaced by cesium. At the same time, in-house cesium applications are rapidly being replaced by outpatient (HDR) treatments. The photon energy, and therefore

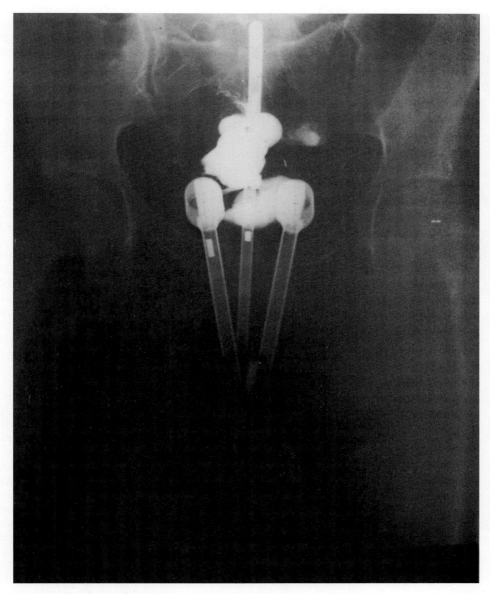

FIGURE 17–19. Fletcher-Suit applicator in place. Note that the implant is relatively symmetrical and that the colpostats are high in the pelvis at the upper level of the acetabulum. Radiopaque dye in the Foley catheter bulb and in the rectum allows calculation of rectal and bladder doses from lateral films. Although not easily seen, small, inert gold seeds placed at the 12 and 3 o'clock positions in the cervix aid in placement confirmation and physics calculations.

the depth dose of cesium, is slightly less than that of radium (Table 17–1), but cesium is quite adequate as an internal source provided that the small adjustment of depth dose is made in the calculations. By the same token, ^{192}Ir has a less penetrating gamma ray than cesium (Table 17–1), which further simplifies the mechanical aspects of radiation protection and facilitates outpatient treatment. However, its half-life is significantly briefer (Table

17–1) and ^{192}Ir sources must be replaced approximately every 3 months. The relatively rapid decay of ^{192}Ir also necessitates recalculation of its dosimetry essentially daily. Modern HDR computers fortunately do this easily, but the treatment duration for each treatment fraction varies significantly, and the patient must understand this aspect insofar as possible. Patients are sometimes amazingly perceptive about treatment duration changes!

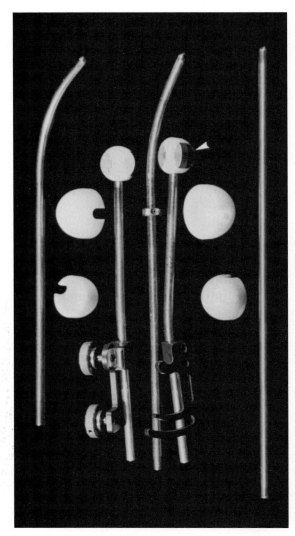

FIGURE 17–20. Henschke cervical applicator. This applicator is small and can be quite useful for patients with very narrow vaginal fornices. The newer applicators contain bladder and rectal blocks, as indicated by the arrow in the picture. Several sizes of vaginal colpostats are available. Since we use this applicator primarily in early cases, the tandem and colpostats are fixed with the clamps shown in the figure.

Special Situations in Radiation Therapy of Cervical Carcinoma

While many clinics report good survival rates for patients with early-stage cervical cancer, the results in patients with more advanced disease remain poor. Because cervical cancer staging is clinical in nature, comparison of the results between different clinics and regimens is difficult. Most importantly, unless all pa-

tients at risk are included, it becomes almost impossible to prove that one method is better than another. Examples of contemporary approaches to four problematic situations are presented in the following paragraphs.

ADJUVANT HYSTERECTOMY

Extensive tumor involvement of the entire cervix and its lymphatics can lead to dramatic enlargement of the lower uterine segment, resulting in what has been termed the *barrel-shaped cervix* (Durrance et al, 1969). A tumor fits into this category if the diameter of the midcervix exceeds 5.0 cm. Such patients have a poor prognosis for local control, and a sequence of modified radiotherapy (4,000 to 4,400 cGy of whole-pelvis radiation and one intracavitary insertion) followed by conservative extrafascial hysterectomy has become standard practice in many clinics (Mendenhall et al, 1994). Patients who show clinically persistent disease 2 to 3 weeks after the full insertion may benefit from one or two additional tandem-only insertions before hysterectomy. This sequence appears to improve the survival of this patient group (Nelson et al, 1975), although the absolute extent of improvement is more difficult to ascertain. This is because some patients who fail to respond do not go to surgery. Thus the impact on overall survival cannot be absolutely determined. Nevertheless, there seems little doubt that surgical removal of the uterus removes the source of treatment failure in many such patients without excessive complications, and the overall approach is eminently reasonable. It is clear, however, that including larger treatment portals or performing more radical surgery is deleterious (Rutledge et al, 1976). The reader is referred to Chapter 5 for further discussion of this clinical problem.

RADIATION AFTER RADICAL HYSTERECTOMY

The role of pelvic radiation in patients (usually stage Ib) with cervical cancer undergoing radical hysterectomy and pelvic lymph node dissection remains somewhat controversial. Given the known radiosensitivity of most forms of cervix cancer, it seemed natural to add pelvic radiation to treatment of patients who had undergone successful surgery but showed histologic involvement of lymph nodes. However, preradiation surgery—even for staging—may be associated with increasing morbidity (Potish et al, 1990). It should be noted that, while postoperative radiation in node-positive patients quite frequently is recommended and is done, it has not yet been possible to show survival benefit. For example, Morrow et al (1980) showed that no improvement in survival was encountered, although there was a suggestion of benefit in patients who had three or more involved nodes. Others have confirmed these findings (Baltzer and Zander, 1985; Remy et al, 1990). Most series have indicated that postoperative radiation in this context substantially reduces pelvic recurrence. With the growing application of chemotherapy in cervix cancer, control of pelvic disease with radiation may prove useful, provided better systemic therapy becomes available.

There is also a suggestion that high-risk patients may benefit from vaginal brachytherapy if not whole-pelvic radiation. For example, Photopulos et al (1990) found that postoperative treatment to the vagina and vaginal cuff using Fletcher-Suit colpostats reduced the local recurrence rate to zero. The indication for treatment was replacement of one half of the cervix with cancer. Their patients who refused this therapy recurred. In our clinic, postoperative patients with positive lymph nodes, especially those in whom a true lymph node dissection has not been done, are offered postoperative radiation, while those thought at risk for cuff recurrence (narrow or questionable margins) are also offered vaginal boost treatment.

Adenocarcinoma of the Cervix. It is commonly stated in otherwise exemplary textbooks that the prognosis of patients with adenocarcinoma of the cervix (any stage) is the same as squamous histology independent of treatment modality (e.g., Perez and Brady, 1992). Despite this confident statement, there remains the cold hand of doubt on the radiotherapist's shoulder when stage IB adenocarcinomas appear in the clinic. For example, Berek (1995) noted that "smaller lesions" (2 to 3 cm) respond well to either surgery or radiation but the local control rate was only 71 percent, and recurrences were seen even in very small lesions. Accordingly, he recommends adjunctive surgery (hysterectomy) for "bulky" stage I adenocarcinomas. In a large series from Toronto (Fyles et al, 1995), the survivorship of patients with adenocarcinoma seemed clearly less than with squamous cancers; an adenocarcinoma histology was described by the authors (diplomatically) as "a less powerful predictive factor" in terms of survival. Eifel et al (1995) reported the

same phenomenon when reporting on 1,767 radiation-treated patients from MDAH. Until this issue is clearly resolved, we will continue to recommend surgical removal of the uterus with appropriate modification of the radiation dose in patients with stage I adenocarcinoma in all but those patients for whom surgery could be unwise.

CHEMORADIATION (CERVIX AND VULVA)

The prognosis of patients with stage III and IV cervical cancer remains poor. Even in the most experienced hands, the 5-year survival of nonselected groups of such patients is significantly below one in three. Since the acceptable radiation dose (tolerance dose) already has been established, higher dose radiation per se cannot be employed. For this reason, researchers have begun to examine the potential for combining chemotherapy and radiation such that more than additive effects might be achieved (Patton et al, 1991; Christie et al, 1995).

Chemoradiation is the term now used for the more awkward phrase "concomitant chemotherapy and radiation therapy." There are myriad studies of chemotherapy before and after radiation in both gynecologic and non-gynecologic cancers. To date, there is no clear evidence that such neoadjuvant (before radiation) or adjuvant (following radiation) chemotherapy is of benefit (Grigsby, 1994). However, there is growing evidence that concomitant therapy (chemoradiation) may be useful. Two randomized studies have been reported that suggest the combination of hydroxyurea and x-rays gives better results than x-rays alone (Piver et al, 1977; Hreschchyshyn et al, 1979). However, in the larger GOG study, the large number of nonevaluable patients was troublesome, and this approach has never been established firmly.

The most promising studies have involved the use of slowly infused 5-FU, with or without additional drugs, based on the observation that 5-FU is a radiosensitizer (Bagshaw, 1961) but only when given as a continuous infusion (Byfield et al, 1982). The use of infused 5-FU has been shown to produce dramatic regression in squamous and squamous-like cancers in a variety of anatomic locations (Lokich and Byfield, 1991). Its application in gynecologic cancers has been reviewed by Maitra and Byfield (1991). The first application of 5-FU chemoradiation in cervix cancer was reported by Thomas et al (1984, 1990). They found a 3-year pelvic control rate of 85 percent and a survival rate of 71 percent in stage Ib/II, and rates of 50 and 42 percent, respectively, in stage III patients. They thought this was better than the results achieved with radiation alone at the Princess Margaret Hospital. Other studies reporting similar apparent improvements in control and survival rates have appeared (John et al, 1987; Ludgate et al, 1988; Kersh et al, 1990; Roberts et al, 1991a), but as yet no randomized trial has been completed.

These studies have been complemented by similar investigations in vulvar cancer. The tendency to attempt to reduce the extent of surgery in vulvar cancer and thereby reduce surgical morbidity has led to growing use of combined radiation therapy and surgery in that disease (Boronow, 1982; Hacker et al, 1984). These studies are described in Chapter 3. This led naturally to the use of chemoradiation involving infused 5-FU, since histologically vulvar cancers should be responsive to this regimen. Again, the first studies were reported by Thomas et al (1989) from the Princess Margaret Hospital. Confirmation of the utility of this approach was reported by Berek et al (1991). Complete response rates of about 70 percent or greater are reported, with many patients not requiring any surgery. These results are quite promising, since the treatment program is reasonably well tolerated and is not associated with any increase in complication rate (Thomas et al, 1990). This approach also can be carried out successfully and with good results when combined with hyperfractionated radiation (Heaton et al, 1990). Similarly, HDR afterloading brachytherapy can be employed in this context (Malviya et al, 1991). In vulvar cancer, it seems likely that some version of this approach ultimately may eliminate the need for use of radical vulvectomy and groin dissection, which has remained standard treatment for many years (Thomas et al, 1991).

Because cisplatin and mitomycin C are active against squamous cancers, it was natural to combine them with 5-FU and/or radiation. Both of these drugs are logical additions to a basic radiation regimen (Chang et al, 1992). Mitomycin C has been shown to be active specifically against hypoxic cells (Rockwell, 1982), while cisplatin has been proposed as a putative hypoxic cell radiosensitizer (Douple, 1990). Other drugs, such as vincristine and hydroxyurea, also have been employed occasionally. About the only thing certain thus far is that 5-FU is best given as an infu-

sion. Bolus 5-FU is quite toxic hematologically, and its combination with radiation to the pelvis subjects patients to severe hematologic and gastrointestinal complications. Infused 5-FU has minimal hematologic toxicity, and its mucosal toxicity is concentrated in the oropharynx. Both the daily dose and the *duration* of the infusion are critical. *The importance of schedules when using 5-FU as a radiosensitizer cannot be overemphasized.* Unfortunately the literature is not "user friendly." For example, the phrase "5-day infusion" is frequently used to describe either a Monday-through-Friday infusion (circa 96 hours) or a Monday-through-Saturday infusion (circa 120 hours). When given as a 4-day infusion, 5-FU has a response rate of 15 to 20 percent in typical squamous cancers (Jacobs et al, 1992), while 5-day infusions have reported objective response rates of as high as 100 percent (Tapazoglou et al, 1986). The duration of the infusion, the frequency of infusion, and the optimum scheduling with radiation have not been established; however, it is clear that they *must* be given concomitantly to achieve the desired increase in response rate. Many more studies will be required to establish the optimum use of 5-FU. One randomized study in esophageal cancer confirmed improved survival rates compared with radiation alone (Herskovic et al, 1992). The interested reader is referred to surveys of various tumor sites for more detailed information on these topics (Lokich and Byfield, 1991).

There are many small studies in which chemotherapy with putative radiosensitizing drugs has been evaluated. One representative study illustrates the difficulties that are encountered in such investigations. In this example, the "final results" of the RTOG phase 2 study of radiation in "advanced cervical cancer" became available (John et al, 1996). This study looked at three drugs (5-FU, mitomycin C, and cisplatin) administered concomitantly with radiation. The studied patients included 60 cases of stages IIB through IVA cervical cancer. A single injection of mitomycin C was given during the second week of radiation, along with a 96-hour infusion of 5-FU. The same dose of 5-FU was given with a single dose of cisplatin during one implant. Each patient received one or two brachytherapy implants if possible following external beam radiation. The radiation doses were indicated to be "in the lower range of acceptance." The drug doses given were (in terms of their accepted single dose): mitomycin C, 38 percent of recommended dose; 5-FU 80 percent; and cisplatin, 75 percent. Because a single (or at best double) injection of each drug was administered, the potential total dose of each agent in a 2-month treatment period was effectively further reduced as follows: mitomycin C was reduced to 19 percent of a standard dose, 5-FU (which can be given either continuously at 250 mg/m^2/d or every other week for 120 hours at 1 gm/m^2/d for 5 days) was reduced by a further fourfold to 20 percent of the optimal dose, and cisplatin was reduced by a further 50 percent to 38 percent of a standard dose. From the radiobiologic portions of this chapter, readers will understand the implications of *any* such reduction in dose of *either* radiation or chemotherapeutic agents. Such incrementally equivalent reductions will usually result in *logarithmic* reduction in tumor cell kill and thereby drug efficacy. John et al also reported incidences of 63 percent for nausea/vomiting, (less than expected for cisplatin alone) and 7 percent for severe leukopenia, and no lethal toxicity. Overall toxicity of the program was less than reported in the community for radiation alone (Patterns of Care Study). Not unexpectedly, survivorship was "not significantly" different from conventional results.

There are many such studies looking at polychemotherapy and radiation. Unfortunately, we do not have *any* studies looking at the tolerance of cervical cancer patients to any single agent when combined with radiation given at midrange to maximum radiation doses. In the construction of such clinical trials, it is essential to determine the goal of the study at the outset. The most immediate goal must be to learn how to use each chemotherapeutic agent to its maximum advantage as a single agent when used with radiation. We need then to fully understand the effects of dose reduction and schedule changes. The authors hope earnestly that some young gynecologists will achieve these rather straightforward goals, which have thus far eluded us!

Interstitial Template Therapy

There are a significant number of patients with advanced cervical carcinoma who never achieve sufficient regression with external radiotherapy to attain a satisfactory pelvic configuration for the intracavitary component. Included in this group of patients are some in whom the intracavitary tandem and colpos-

tats cannot be placed because of tumor distortion or replacement of the cervix by tumor. Significant advances in the treatment of these patients have been achieved by several investigative groups through the development of templates for interstitial therapy (Feder et al, 1978; Martinez et al, 1984). These applicators use interstitial needles that are held in place by a template, which is sewn into the perineal skin (Fig. 17–21). The applicator contains a variety of vaginal centermolds, some of which contain central apertures for the simultaneous placement of a conventional intrauterine tandem, which can be included as indicated. Both the depth and the number of needles used in the treatment can be controlled so that a butterfly distribution of radiation is achievable in the pelvis (Fig. 17–22). Once the applicator is in place, the patient is returned to her room and ^{192}Ir tubes are inserted into the various needles. The isodose distribution within the pelvis is then determined and can be manipulated by altering the number of loaded needles or the loading within individual needles. This system offers great flexibility in the distribution of radiation within the pelvis. A major feature of this type of applicator is its ability to increase the dose selectively to the parametrial regions.

For example, if one compares the isodose distributions through the level of point A in Figure 17–22 with that in Figure 17–2, it can be seen that the parametrial radiation is significantly increased with this interstitial applicator. Thus the ratio of doses to points A/B with the Syed-Neblett applicator is 100/60, whereas for a conventional application (Fig. 17–2) it is about 50/15. This indicates the enhanced capacity to irradiate the middle parametrial tissues with this approach. In addition, the entire uterine volume can be irradiated with needles if it is not feasible to insert a uterine tandem.

This system is quite useful also in the treatment of recurrences at the vaginal apex, lower parametrium, or periurethral regions. Since parametrial recurrences are a major problem, especially in the lower ureteral region, this technique has the potential to improve cure rates because of improved dosimetry. Although esthetically unpleasing in appearance, the applicators are surprisingly well tolerated by the patient. A minimum of analgesia is required, and the tissues heal rapidly after removal. The long-term results are not yet available, but the system has shown

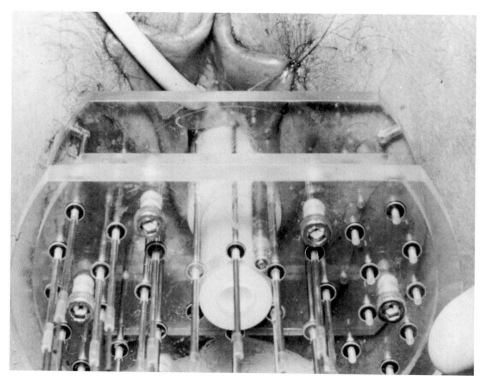

FIGURE 17–21. Syed-Neblett applicator. This patient with carcinoma of the cervix recurrent in the lower vagina and perirectal region is shown with the applicator in place. A Foley catheter has also been inserted.

great utility in the treatment of some subsets of patients with carcinoma of the cervix, vagina, and urethra, for whom conventional therapy presents difficult, and sometimes impossible, dosimetric challenges.

High-Dose-Rate Outpatient Brachytherapy

As mentioned previously, there is an increasing trend toward replacing in-hospital low-dose-rate cesium/radium implants with outpatient procedures. One of the original motivating forces behind this trend was an attempt to reduce the costs of hospitalization associated with conventional therapy. Another was to allow the intracavitary programs shown to be so successful using the classic low-dose-rate applicators to be used in high-volume clinics, particularly in developing countries. Thus these programs tended to evolve outside of the United States. The earliest instruments, such as the Cathetron, were first studied by Joslin and his group in England in the 1970s (Joslin et al, 1972). This was followed by the similar Brachytron studies in Canada and the United States (e.g.,

Utley et al, 1984). Both machines employed ^{60}Co. These units have now been largely replaced by units such as the micro-Selectron (Nucletron), which uses the more manageable isotope ^{192}Ir.

Results equivalent to those with conventional radium/cesium low-dose-rate brachytherapy have been obtained with all of these instruments (Brenner et al, 1991; Chen et al, 1991; Ito et al, 1991; Malviya et al, 1991; Orton et al, 1991; Roman et al, 1991; Kataoka et al, 1992). A study by Orton et al (1991) analyzed over 17,000 cervical cancer patients from 56 institutions who were treated with HDR remote afterloading therapy. They noted that the average fractionation for a typical carcinoma of the cervix was five fractions of 7.5 Gy (750 cGy) administered to point A, regardless of the stage of the disease. This dose was added to preimplant external beam treatment given in the same fashion as with low-dose-rate implants. These studies suggested that disease control was at least equivalent to, and perhaps slightly better than, that achieved with HDR therapy for stage III patients in particular, while (somewhat remarkably) morbidity and complications were less

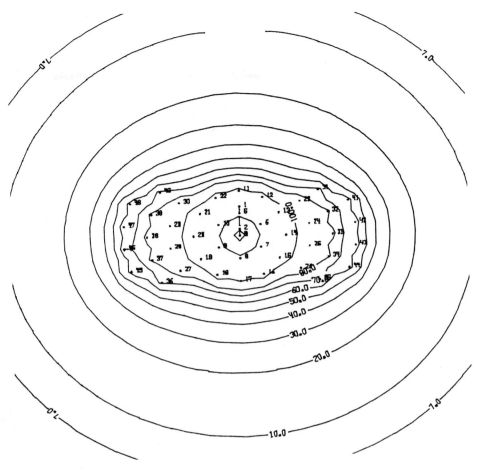

FIGURE 17–22. Isodose distribution around a Syed-Neblett applicator. The relatively regular isodose distribution in a butterfly configuration is shown. In this case, no central radium is in place. It can be seen that the dose distribution within the parametrium is somewhat better than that with a conventional applicator (see Fig. 17–2). However, virtually any dose distribution can be achieved with this type of interstitial treatment applicator.

with the HDR therapy. Orton et al suggested that this latter result was due to a "geometric" advantage for the newer approach. Others have suggested that, provided early effects are equivalent (mucosal reactions), then the "late effects," which fundamentally control total dose, will be equivalent for the classical and the new approach (Brenner et al, 1991). This suggests that early randomized trials with only modest numbers of patients (e.g., Joslin et al, 1972; Shigematsa et al, 1983; Utley et al, 1984) correctly indicated that the HDR approach is feasible and useful.

Patients with early cancers and reasonable anatomy typically can be treated with minimal anesthesia, frequently only intramuscular narcotic and numbing of the cervical mucosa with topical anesthetic. However, patients

with suboptimal anatomy, particularly common in advanced disease, typically present rather more difficult clinical problems. Such patients may require considerably more medication before they are sufficiently comfortable to tolerate the procedure. Some European clinics employ general anesthesia for some or all of their patients. In the United States, where many outpatient facilities are not hospital based, these difficulties can be substantial. For this reason, the American College of Radiology has begun to set forth standards that will be applied in the clinical application of HDR outpatient brachytherapy. In our clinic we typically employ a combination of midazolam and meperidine.

The rapidly expanding use of HDR therapy has generated many new technical questions that are as yet unanswered. There is no regimen determined to be ideal or even standard for the use of HDR therapy in the treatment of any gynecologic cancer. The authors employ a five-fraction (700-cGy) schedule in the treatment of most cervical cancers. These doses are given at weekly intervals. In some patients with advanced cancers, the tandem insertions become progressively more difficult because of progressive scarring. This is particularly true in patients who have undergone previous chemoradiation, in which the acceleration of the tumor response rate induces scarring and fibrosis very early in the treatment course. Orton (1995) noted in a review of the world data that the reported variation of HDR fraction size was 300 to 1,676 cGy, with a mean of 745 cGy, that is, from −40 to +225 percent! He also found that the reported variation of conventional (radium/cesium) dose *rates* had a similar distribution. The reader will therefore understand that much needs to be done to establish optimal regimens. Nevertheless, it is quite clear that HDR therapy is as effective in the cure of gynecologic cancers as low-dose-rate cesium therapy, and is therefore likely to replace cesium soon (Orton, 1993; Ito et al, 1994; Liu WS et al, 1996).

RADIATION THERAPY FOR ENDOMETRIAL CARCINOMA

The radiation component of endometrial carcinoma (EC) therapy is dictated explicitly by the clinical stage of the patient's disease at the time of diagnosis. In the past, many patients with EC received more radiation therapy than was required to achieve a maximum cure rate. Because of this, there has been a revision in the role of radiation therapy in EC treatment, especially for stage I lesions. The staging of EC, together with the known prognostic parameters, is reviewed in Chapter 6. Because other factors, especially the degree of differentiation and depth of myometrial invasion, strongly affect the likelihood of having disease outside the uterus, many patients without clinical involvement of the cervix will probably not require radiotherapy. To individualize patient therapy, the official staging of EC now is based on surgicopathologic information. For this reason, routine preoperative radiotherapy in all patients with EC cannot be recommended.

Stages I and IIa: Adjuvant Radiation

Patients with cancer apparently confined to the corpus or with only microscopic cervical involvement usually undergo laparotomy, simple extrafascial hysterectomy, and appropriate surgical staging. Postoperative radiation therapy is utilized for patients with significant muscle invasion, poorly differentiated tumor, lymph–vascular space invasion (LVSI), and other risk factors (see Chapter 6). Suitable candidates for radiation therapy who have risk factors usually receive a full course of pelvic radiotherapy (5,000 cGy in 5–6 weeks). Lower doses are not likely to be effective (Cox et al, 1980). Radiotherapy to the entire pelvis, including the vaginal cuff, is recommended (Wharam et al, 1976), since recurrences are frequent at the cuff and probably indicate lymphatic invasion. Whole-pelvis radiation considerably reduces the incidence of vaginal recurrence. Some therapists prefer to boost the vaginal cuff dose with a cesium application or HDR equivalent. Although it seems likely that this approach will enhance the cure rate of patients with EC (Joslin et al, 1977), an improved cure rate has not been proven in clinical trials. An individualized approach to EC will reduce to a minimum the number of patients requiring radiotherapy, since it permits a direct evaluation of the risk for extrauterine disease.

A Canadian study (Carey et al, 1995) of 384 patients showed that, when postoperative radiation was recommended for high-risk patients only, 59 percent of patients (low-risk group) were not irradiated, yet had a 95 percent 5-year relapse-free survival. The other 41 percent of patients (high risk) were irradiated and enjoyed an 81 percent 5-year relapse-free survival. The study also showed that 5 percent of the irradiated patients had a severe or live-threatening radiation reaction or complication. Such studies indicate that proper triage can minimize the number of patients treated and maximize the benefit of radiation. It also reminds us that there is always a price to be paid by the irradiated population. According to Lanciano and Greven (1995), remaining problems are (1) do grade 3 tumors with minimal muscle invasion (less than one third of the myometrium) or grade 1 tumors with "maximal" muscle invasion (more than two thirds of the myometrium) need any postoperative radiation? and (2) what level of cervical invasion or LVSI makes vaginal cuff radiation mandatory? In this vein, it is of interest to note that preoperative radiation of

170 patients achieved similar results, with 83 percent 5-year survival in grade 3 patients (Maingon et al, 1996). Only further studies will tell us what if any refinements are feasible in improving on these results, which already cure 86 percent of the stage I EC population.

Occasionally, postsurgical cuff radiation alone is given, using either vaginal ovoids or a specially designed vaginal applicator (Delclos et al, 1970). The recommended vaginal apical dose using the Delclos vaginal applicator is 4,000 cGy given in two separate sittings (2,000 cGy each at about 50 cGy/hr to a point 1 cm above the vaginal apex). However, for most patients, whole-pelvis radiation is preferable, the vaginal applicator approach being reserved for boost treatment of clinically apparent vaginal disease.

Clinical Stages I and II (Occult) Primary Radiation

Since many patients with stage I EC may have a variety of medical problems (obesity, heart disease, diabetes) that make surgery difficult or very risky, there are a significant number of patients who may require an attempt at cure by radiation alone. The principles of radiotherapy, outlined earlier in the chapter, apply explicitly to this patient group. Thus to adequately treat these patients, many of whom have bulky disease, a tumoricidal dose of at least 8,000 cGy to the primary cancer and 5,000 cGy to occult disease must be delivered. In the past, this has usually been done using Heyman's capsules, which are small, bullet-like metal containers, each of which contains a 5- to 10-mg radium or cesium source (Heyman et al, 1941). Heyman's capsules were packed, one by one, into the uterus, until the uterus was fully loaded. This approach, while quite effective, is seldom used anymore.

Following external beam radiation, almost all patients will have a modest-sized uterus, and a more conventional cervical cancer applicator can frequently be used. The dosimetry of an enlarged uterus is now most conveniently analyzed using either sonographic studies or CT. In this fashion, the exact size of the uterus can be determined, and a minimum calculated radiation dose of 7,500 to 8,000 cGy can be delivered to the serosal surface of the uterus. Studies show that this approach is successful with either conventional cesium applications (Chao et al, 1995) or

HDR therapy (e.g., Nguyen et al, 1995). In almost all cases the external beam treatment reduces the tumor volume and subsequent uterine contraction produces suitable conditions for intracavitary therapy with a conventional applicator. Since the endocervical canal is not often distorted by stage I endometrial cancer, HDR treatments can usually proceed in a timely fashion and with minimal patient discomfort. The authors prefer to approach these medically inoperable patients with 5,000 cGy whole-pelvis radiation, followed by intracavitary radiation using a micro-Selectron.

Kucera et al (1990) demonstrated the interaction between surgery and radiation in stage I EC, in this case combining conventional external beam pelvic radiation with HDR ^{192}Ir vaginal irradiation. They showed that irradiating only patients with poor prognostic factors (grade 2 or 3 tumor or invasion of the middle to external third of the myometrium) led to equivalent survivorship compared to good-prognosis patients. Intravaginal therapy was reserved for patients with grade 2 or 3 histology. External pelvic radiation was omitted when the level of infiltration of the myometrium was confined to the inner third regardless of histologic grade and when well-differentiated tumors invaded the middle third of the myometrium. These observations indicate that there is a clear-cut benefit when adding appropriate radiation measures for patients with the more aggressive stage I EC.

Clinical Stage II (Overt)

Patients with grossly demonstrable disease in the cervix are at higher risk for lymph node metastases, vaginal metastases, and distant recurrences than are stage I and IIa patients. Traditionally, such patients are treated in a fashion analogous to that of patients with bulky stage Ib cervical cancer. Thus they receive a total of 4,000 cGy of whole-pelvis radiotherapy, followed by one intracavitary treatment lasting for 48 to 72 hours administered with a typical cervical cancer treatment applicator (tandem and colpostats). This delivers a total radiation dose of between 6,500 and 7,500 cGy to the paracervical tissues (point A). Within 6 weeks after the radium application, the patient undergoes a total abdominal hysterectomy. For patients without bulky cervical involvement that would require initial external radiation, intracavitary therapy may be administered first, followed by immediate simple extrafascial hysterectomy and surgical staging. This approach provides critical surgicopathologic information that allows the radiation oncologist to plan external therapy more accurately. Stage II patients are a diverse group requiring individualization (Anderson, 1990). The prognosis of patients with stage II disease is discussed in Chapter 6.

Clinical Stages III and IV and Recurrent Carcinomas

In patients who are found to have stage III carcinomas (which local treatment is unlikely to cure), individualized therapy is warranted. The disease in a majority of these patients is classified as stage III by clinical evaluation that suggests parametrial, adnexal, or vaginal spread. The general principles of whole-pelvis radiation, as outlined earlier, should prevail in the treatment of these patients. In the case of an adnexal mass, laparotomy should be undertaken first to determine its nature. Patients with metastases to the submucosal regions of the vagina represent a specific treatment problem. They usually benefit from localized intensive radiation delivered through a specialized applicator for the upper vagina (Delclos et al, 1970) or from transvaginal orthovoltage treatment, if available; localized residual or recurrent metastases to the lower vagina in previously irradiated patients can be treated by either interstitial iridium or a vaginal mold applicator. These latter treatments may also be offered to patients who have received prior whole-pelvis radiotherapy and who subsequently suffered a recurrence in the vaginal region, provided they do not have widespread disease. HDR brachytherapy frequently is ideal in this clinical situation.

RADIATION THERAPY FOR OVARIAN CARCINOMA

The role of external radiation treatment in ovarian carcinoma is in continuous decline because of improvements in the results of systemic chemotherapy. The fundamental problem associated with irradiating ovarian carcinoma for cure lies in the need to deliver a tumoricidal dose to the whole abdomen, including the pelvis. There is no way to avoid full pelvic marrow irradiation in this context, and such irradiation has been shown to compromise seriously the capacity of a patient to

receive subsequent chemotherapy (Arian-Schad et al, 1990). The great majority of patients with ovarian carcinoma have disease disseminated at the visible or occult level throughout the abdomen, necessitating whole-abdomen radiation if cure is the goal of therapy. Since it is not possible to deliver, simultaneously or in sequence, full-dose whole-abdomen radiotherapy and full-dose systemic chemotherapy, the treatment today for most patients lies primarily with chemotherapy. However, it is important to remember that most ovarian cancers are relatively radiosensitive (subject only to the radioresistance inherent in all large tumor masses), and that radiotherapy can be very useful in the local reduction of tumor masses resistant to chemotherapy. There are many discrete factors that dictate the prognosis of ovarian cancers, and some patients can be cured with radiotherapy alone (Thomas, 1994). Selection of such patients is a major current clinical challenge (Dembo and Bush, 1982). Moreover, in patients with very limited macroscopic disease who are reluctant to embark on a chemotherapeutic regimen, abdominal radiotherapy can help to reduce or eliminate postsurgical residual tumor. Finally, because in early ovarian cancer the entire peritoneal cavity (including the diaphragm) is at risk for micrometastases, whereas systemic dissemination is rare, abdominal radiotherapy can be useful to treat most or all of this volume at risk with intraperitoneal radiocolloids. Three distinct types of radiotherapeutic maneuvers can be used to treat patients with ovarian cancer:

1. Palliative radiotherapy of locally obstructive tumor masses or local radiotherapeutic treatment of palpable but localized postchemotherapeutic residual disease
2. Treatment, frequently postoperative, of the entire abdomen, using an open-field (Dembo et al, 1992), a "moving strip" (Delclos and Murphy, 1966) or shrinking field technique (Martinez et al, 1988)
3. Postsurgical infusion of radiocolloids into the peritoneal cavity in patients whose tumor is microscopic or extremely limited in individual tumor volume

External Beam Therapy

Pelvic Field Irradiation

Selected patients may receive either definitive or palliative localized radiation treatments to the pelvis. This is most frequently offered to patients who are reluctant to receive systemic chemotherapy or to patients who are chemotherapeutic failures and have locally obstructive pelvic tumor masses. External beam treatment can then be given in the customary fashion, and frequently symptoms of intestinal obstruction and pain are significantly or completely relieved. To patients who have residual disease in the pelvis after undergoing debulking surgery and who are reluctant to consider chemotherapy, similar treatments may be offered.

Whole-Abdomen Radiation

In patients who have, or who are highly at risk for, peritoneal micrometastases, whole-abdomen radiotherapy can be offered as an alternative to systemic chemotherapy. There is evidence that, properly administered, it will achieve in the microscopic disease group as good a result overall as single-agent chemotherapy. Indeed, the end results of whole-abdomen radiation may be equivalent to the current best results obtained with systemic chemotherapy (Martinez et al, 1988; Dembo, 1992).

If whole-abdomen radiation is administered through a treatment beam covering the entire abdominal cavity, radiation enteritis and nausea are frequently problematic, and treatment can be quite protracted (typically 6 to 8 weeks). Alternatives to open-field whole-abdomen radiation are the moving strip and shrinking field procedures.

Because radiation is known to be effective in some patients with stage III ovarian carcinoma, it also has been studied in patients who have residual disease or who are thought to be at high risk for recurrence after an initial response to systemic chemotherapy. Typically, only approximately 25 to 30 percent of patients have no evidence of tumor at the time of second-look laparotomy (see Chapter 10). Even in the face of this good response, almost half of them will relapse and die within 5 years (Dembo, 1992). Thus the initial high response rate to platinum-based chemotherapy unfortunately has not markedly altered long-term survivorship. Quite naturally, whole-abdomen radiotherapy was added to this type of treatment program. However, a small randomized trial offered no promise when this was done (Bruzzone et al, 1990). In general, the results of this approach have been poor, and most authors recommend against it (Whelan et al, 1992). Toxicity, both hematologic and intestinal, is substantial, while survival benefit probably is not greater than an alternative form of chemotherapy (Bolis et al, 1990; Frachin et al, 1991; Whelan et al, 1992).

Intraperitoneal Radioactive Colloids

Radioactive colloids have been used intermittently for the treatment of ovarian and endometrial cancers since colloidal gold (^{198}Au) therapy was first introduced by Müller in 1950 (Table 17–4). In the United States, the colloidal suspension of chromic phosphate (^{32}P) replaced ^{198}Au as the preferred agent for intracavitary therapy of malignant effusions and microscopic residual disease, but the newer chemotherapeutic agents are more effective and safer for the treatment of ovarian cancer. For these reasons radioactive colloids have fallen into disfavor. For a review of the dosimetry, distribution, and physical properties of these two agents readers are referred to the reports by Rosenshein et al (1979), Currie et al (1981), Leichner et al (1981), Kaplan et al (1981), and Ott et al (1985). While ^{32}P intraperitoneal therapy is in general very well tolerated, some patients do experience a chemical peritonitis of various degrees, and there is approximately a 5 percent incidence of serious small bowel complications (Walton et al, 1991). Small bowel injury, either alone or associated with large bowel injury, commonly results from treatment plans combining radioactive isotopes and external beam therapy. Current data suggest that combining these modalities can be attended by a serious complication rate approaching 50 percent (Health, 1988; Klaasen et al, 1985, 1988).

ADVERSE EFFECTS OF RADIATION THERAPY

In gynecologic oncology, the majority of radiation injuries result from treatment of cervical and uterine carcinoma and usually involve epithelial-lined structures within the pelvis, where the dose-limiting normal tissues are the rectosigmoid, bladder, and small bowel, particularly the terminal ileum. Extension of the treatment field to the aortic region for cervical or endometrial cancer and to the whole abdomen in the management of ovarian cancer requires an even more restrictive

TABLE **17–4**

Properties of ^{32}P and ^{198}Au*

	^{32}P	^{198}Au
Color	Blue-green	Cherry red
Particle size	0.5–15 μm	0.003–0.007 μm
Half-life	14.3 days	2.69 days
Emission	Beta	Beta and gamma
Mean energy		
Beta	0.698 MeV	0.316 MeV
Gamma		0.411 MeV
Tissue penetration (maximum)		
Beta	8 mm	3.8 mm
Gamma		Infinity
Advantages	Minimal shielding required; outpatient administration; longer $T_{1/2}$; more penetrating beta; no radiation sickness	
Usual dose†	10–15 mCi	100–150 mCi

*Adapted from Rosenshein NB, Leichner PK, Vogelsang G; Radiocolloids in the treatment of ovarian cancer. Obstet Gynecol Surv 34:708, 1979, with permission.
†Intraperitoneal.

dose to protect the liver, kidneys, and small intestine, which tolerate radiation poorly (Table 17–2). Additional restraint is required when combining external radiation and radioactive nuclides, radiation and chemotherapy, or radiation after surgery(ies) resulting in extensive adhesions.

Pathology

Acute reaction to radiation consists of a rapid cessation of mitotic activity followed by cellular swelling and, if the injury is lethal, dissolution. Small-vessel edema appears with endothelial swelling and thrombosis. The connective tissue becomes edematous and congested with dilated lymphatics and small vessels. If the injury is severe enough, focal necrosis may be seen. Subsequent changes include intimal thickening with obliteration of the small vessels, fibrosis and hyalinization of vessel walls and connective tissue, and permanent reduction of the epithelial and parenchymal cell population. The extent to which these changes occur is dependent on the degree of injury.

Significant pathophysiologic effects of these changes are a reduction in the microcirculation (both vascular and lymphatic), loss of parenchymal tissue, and proliferation of fibrous tissue. These changes are progressive and may continue for many years. Consequently, irradiated tissue loses, in varying degrees, the specific function of its parenchymal component. For reasons that are not entirely clear, irradiated tissue is more susceptible to any type of injury, has a reduced capacity to repair itself, and is more vulnerable to bacterial infection. In these tissues, any injury may result in a self-sustaining cycle of necrosis and infection. Bacterial proliferation in the necrotic tissue leads to invasion of the viable tissue at the perimeter, producing additional metabolic stress that results in further necrosis and infection.

Acute Radiation Reactions

A number of side effects from radiation are commonly seen during the course of treatment, but these are usually transient and do not lead to permanent injury (Bourne et al, 1983). Individuals who show the most severe reactions during radiation have an increased probability of delayed radiation complications (Buchler et al, 1971). The skin reactions so important during the orthovoltage era are no longer a dose-limiting factor because modern high-energy machines can deliver the maximum dosage to a depth well below the skin surface. In some circumstances, as on the vulva or in the natal crease, folliculitis and moist desquamation can occur because the beam strikes the surface tangentially, producing forward scatter and intensification of the skin dose. The symptoms of radiation cystitis occur late in the treatment course and are usually well controlled with urinary analgesics, antispasmodics, and increased fluid intake. Superimposed bacterial infection requires antibiotic treatment. Radiation proctosigmoiditis, manifested by tenesmus, diarrhea, and cramps, usually responds well to a low-residue diet, antispasmodics, and steroid suppositories.

Enteritis is a frequent problem, particularly during whole-abdomen and extended field radiation for ovarian or cervical cancer. Dietary manipulation (Klimberg et al, 1990; Klimberg, 1991), antiemetics, and antispasmodics generally produce satisfactory control of the accompanying nausea, cramps, and diarrhea, but, since the diarrhea is at least partly due to bile salt malabsorption, cholestyramine therapy may be indicated (Stryker and Demers, 1979; Arlow et al, 1987). Occasionally, the severity of symptoms necessitates the interruption of treatment, at least temporarily. Rarely, acute radiation enteritis can produce a prolonged ileus simulating mechanical bowel obstruction. These patients require hospitalization, complete bowel rest, and nasogastric suction until the symptoms subside and bowel function is restored. Some evidence suggests that these severe symptoms can be prevented by utilizing glutamine-enriched elemental diets (Klimberg et al, 1990; Klimberg, 1991). Bone marrow suppression can be an important problem when irradiating both the abdomen and the pelvis. This is especially likely to occur in the patient who has previously received myelosuppressive chemotherapy. The interaction of radiation therapy and chemotherapy as they relate to chemotherapy dose adjustments was discussed earlier in this chapter.

Delayed Radiation Reactions

Proctitis

The majority of serious injuries from pelvic and abdominal irradiation are not manifest until 6 to 24 months after completion of therapy. Proctitis is usually seen in combination with sigmoiditis as part of a pelvic field injury. The close spatial relationship of the rectum to the upper vagina and cervix makes it especially vulnerable to cesium injuries or to a combination of cesium and external therapy injury. The symptoms of proctitis, with or without ulceration, include pain, tenesmus, intermittent diarrhea, constipation, and rectal bleeding. The symptoms may be mild, with ulceration persisting for years, or they may be severe and require vigorous therapy. Management includes low-residue diet, psyllium (Metamucil), antispasmodics, and mild analgesics. Steroid enemas and belladonna and opium suppositories may be especially useful. If medical management fails to relieve the symptoms or excessive bleeding is a problem, a diverting colostomy and/or resection is indicated.

When rectal bleeding occurs, proctosigmoidoscopy and contrast enema should be performed to confirm the source of bleeding and rule out a superimposed primary bowel carcinoma. However, a radiographic contrast study must always be undertaken with the utmost caution, because the injured rectosigmoid is vulnerable to perforation and barium-fecal peritonitis is usually fatal. Radiation-induced rectal ulcers are invariably located on the anterior rectal wall at the level of the cervix and have a punched-out appearance, with a dirty gray membrane covering the crater. Biopsies should be carried out cautiously, since the trauma may result in fistula formation.

Rectovaginal fistula is one of the most common complications of pelvic radiation requiring surgical intervention. If it is associated with vault necrosis, a proximal diverting colostomy should be performed as soon as possible. Even what seems to be an obvious rectovaginal fistula may represent multiple fistulas from other sections of the large or small bowel, so contrast studies should be performed before diversion is attempted. Occasionally, a very small fistula may heal spontaneously after fecal diversion, but usually a temporary colostomy and delayed surgical repair utilizing unirradiated new tissue (omentum, bulbocavernosus, gracilis muscle, or colon) to cover the defect is required (Aartsen and Sindram, 1988). The margins of the fistula should be clean and free of necrosis, and the colostomy is not taken down for 3 to 6 months to permit adequate healing. Successful repair is more likely to occur when the injury has been produced by radium or cesium, since the injury is more localized than the field injury resulting from large-volume external beam radiation therapy. Progressive fibrosis causing stricture is a more indolent radiation injury that sometimes requires a diverting colostomy.

The introduction of stainless steel surgical staples has greatly improved the outlook for patients with distal bowel injuries secondary to pelvic radiation. Anastomosis at or within a few centimeters of the anus is now being accomplished routinely with excellent results (Ravitch, 1984). Thus, for the irradiated patient with intractable proctitis, a stricture, or rectovaginal fistula, a permanent colostomy is not always necessary.

Sigmoiditis

Clinically significant radiation sigmoiditis increases in severity and frequency as the dose of external whole-pelvis radiation is raised. It is an infrequent problem when the external therapy is limited to 4,000 cGy in 4 weeks. However, the sigmoid is still subject to cesium injury because of its relatively fixed position in the hollow of the sacrum and its close association with the uterine fundus. Factors contributing to sigmoiditis, other than a high dose of external therapy and prior or concomitant chemotherapy, include age, inflammatory disease, and a posterior location of the radium system in the hollow of the sacrum (Strockbine et al, 1970). As with isolated proctitis, the symptoms of sigmoiditis include crampy pelvic pain, alternating diarrhea and constipation, and rectal bleeding. If the injury is severe, the pain may be disabling, and associated malaise, anorexia, and chronic weight loss are evident. This combination of severe, intractable pain and weight loss may be tragically misinterpreted as recurrent or persistent, unresectable carcinoma.

Milder forms of sigmoiditis may be managed medically, using a low-residue diet, Miller's bran or psyllium, mineral oil, and antispasmodics. Laxatives and enemas should be avoided. When there are severe symptoms or moderate symptoms unresponsive to medical management, or when evidence of obstruction or serious bleeding occurs, a proximal diverting colostomy is necessary. Undue delay must be avoided because of the constant threat of necrosis and perforation. Preoperative evaluation with a colon contrast radiographic study carries the risk of perforation, and this risk may be increased by the use of enemas and laxatives.

Flexible sigmoidoscopy is a safer method to use in evaluating the lesion and allows a more accurate assessment of the extent of damage. In the case of a segmental injury to the sigmoid, resection and anastomosis may be feasible at the time the diverting colostomy is performed. As with rectal injuries, anastomosis with stainless steel staples has often avoided permanent colostomy. A temporary colostomy should be done outside the field of radiation, preferably in the left transverse colon, to protect the anastomosis for 3 to 6 months. The colon is completely divided to ensure total diversion of the fecal stream. Whether or not reanastomosis is possible, resection of the injured sigmoid colon is recommended to prevent continued pain or bleeding. A distal descending or left transverse colostomy is selected in this situation, because sigmoid colostomy is more likely to result in stenosis or infarction (DeCosse et al, 1969).

Small Bowel Injury

Radiation small bowel injury, either alone or associated with large bowel injury, is commonly the result of treatment plans combining radioactive isotopes and external beam therapy. Isotopes alone usually will not result in small bowel obstruction or perforation (Proctor et al, 1990; Walton et al, 1991). Current data suggest that combining these modalities can be extremely toxic, with serious complication rates approaching 50 percent (Pezner et al, 1978; Bakri and Given, 1984; Klaassen et al, 1985, 1988; Heath et al, 1988; Potter et al, 1989).

The terminal ileum is the most common site of radiation small bowel injury because it is immobilized within the pelvic radiation portal just proximal to the cecum, has a relatively poor blood supply, and is the narrowest portion of the small bowel. Furthermore, it is the portion of the small bowel most likely to be adherent in the pelvis as a result of previous surgery (staging laparotomy, hysterectomy, cesarean section, adnexal surgery) or inflammatory disease such as chronic salpingitis, appendicitis, endometriosis, granulomatous inflammations of the bowel, and diverticulitis. When whole-pelvis external irradiation has been less than 4,000 to 5,000 cGy in 4 to 5 weeks, a clinically significant injury to the small bowel is more likely the result of brachytherapy from a uterine tandem perforation or bowel directly adherent to the uterus. Injury from the brachytherapy is focal, producing progressive obstruction or necrosis and perforation. Multiple sites or types of injury significantly reduce survival (Covens et al, 1991).

The symptoms of small bowel injury are usually those of an incomplete obstruction, with delayed postprandial cramping, nausea, and vomiting that relieves the pain and bloating. Diarrhea and progressive weight loss are often prominent symptoms. The clinical picture often suggests recurrent, advanced carcinoma and hence may result in nonintervention for a surgically curable problem. Radiation reduces the inflammatory response of the peritoneum and bowel wall to ischemia, necrosis, and infection (Fig. 17–23), thus masking the occurrence of these events. The patient may have a florid peritonitis without the anticipated signs of abdominal rigidity or rebound tenderness. There may be no elevation of the temperature or white blood cell count. Generalized peritonitis after radiation is almost always fatal, because the tissues are unable to heal. For this reason, conservative management is especially hazardous (O'Brien et al, 1987; Sher and Bauer, 1990). An upper gastrointestinal radiographic series or CT scan may demonstrate the injury but should not be relied on if negative.

The management of radiation-caused small bowel injury is complex and requires fine surgical judgment. In the presence of generalized peritonitis, exteriorization of the fistulous loops is required, and the patient should be maintained on hyperalimentation and antibiotics until the infection resolves. When necrosis and perforation with a localized infection are present, resection and anastomosis (ileoileostomy or ileocolostomy) are carried out, provided relatively normal proximal and distal bowel is available. Resection with anasto-

mosis, rather than bypass, is the procedure of choice for long- or short-segment injuries, provided there is adequate mobility (Smith et al, 1985; Fenner et al, 1989; Fisher et al, 1989). When there is obstruction related to extensive interloop adhesions and fixation to pelvic structures, an end-to-side or side-to-side bypass anastomosis to the ascending or transverse colon with the exclusion of the involved segment is preferable (Smith et al, 1984; O'Brien et al, 1987). Resection of small bowel, requiring extensive dissection of adhesions from the pelvis, frequently results in numerous enterotomies in adjacent small or large bowel. The remaining small bowel readheres to the pelvis, where it is subject to recurrent obstruction. Thus such complex adhesions should be left undisturbed.

When the terminal ileum and the sigmoid colon have been injured, the symptoms of one injury may mask the presence of the other. This possibility should always be kept in mind and both areas should be assessed preoperatively as well as at surgery. Radiation enteropathy and related intestinal complications can be prevented to some extent by careful patient selection, individualization of treatment volume and dose, and appropriate nutritional support. The risk of bowel injury can be further reduced by employing continuous course, rather than split-course, pelvic radiation (Sigmon et al, 1994) and by utilizing

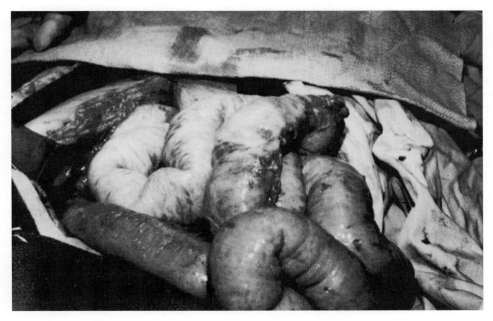

FIGURE 17–23. Radiation injury to the small bowel. Note the thickened, blanched, edematous wall compared with the dilated but more normal adjacent loops (foreground).

the extraperitoneal approach for staging laparotomy (Potish and Dusenbery, 1990; Whelan et al, 1992; Hindley and Cole, 1993; Fine et al, 1995).

Displacement of the small bowel out of the pelvis during therapy is a desirable goal because it would decrease the incidence of small bowel injury and might allow for the administration of higher and potentially more curable doses of radiation. A variety of methods have been tried. The omental hammock and mesh sling (Trimbos et al, 1991; van Kasteren et al, 1993; Choi and Lee, 1995) are sometimes successful but require considerable surgical skill and can result in serious complications. Peritoneal insufflation (Hindley and Cole, 1993) has very limited experience. The volumetric tissue expander has not received much attention, but the concept is attractive because it is simple and temporary and seems to be associated with fewer serious complications than the surgical methods (Herbert et al, 1993).

Vulvar and Vaginal Injuries

The vagina and vulva are not immune to the ischemic effects of microcirculatory injury from irradiation. It is estimated that more than 80 percent of women have at least partial vaginal stenosis and occlusion following pelvic irradiation (Poma, 1980). The resultant dyspareunia and loss of sexual function from these complications can be avoided to some degree by frequent intercourse or the use of dilators and estrogen cream (Pitkin and van Voorhis, 1971). Patients should be encouraged to use these measures, even during therapy, once reasonably normal anatomy has been restored and there is no danger of serious bleeding from local trauma. Sexual dysfunction is often an unavoidable consequence of vaginal irradiation. A willingness to discuss this problem with the patient and, if necessary, to institute more intensive counseling is an important aspect of her treatment.

Vault necrosis results from severe vascular compromise. The process may respond to local measures, such as antiseptic douches and estrogen cream, or it may progress relentlessly, resulting in severe pain that is unresponsive to narcotic analgesics. Extreme malaise, anorexia, progressive weight loss, and psychological withdrawal usually accompany such severe pain. These patients often are so exquisitely tender that examination is impossible without anesthesia. Bowel or urinary tract fistulas or life-threatening hemorrhage may ensue. This clinical syndrome must not be mistaken for advanced, terminal carcinoma.

In the presence of a urinary or fecal fistula, the necrosis, pain, and infection cannot be controlled without diversion (Looser et al, 1979). Conservative management of radiation ulcers is rarely successful. Modern management includes wide debridement of the necrotic bed and transposition of unirradiated tissue into the defect, usually utilizing a full-thickness or myocutaneous flap (Wang et al, 1987; Roberts et al, 1991b). Biopsies are indicated to rule out persistent or recurrent cancer, but they must be performed cautiously in the irradiated vaginal apex, bladder, or rectum to avoid inducing a fistula. This complication is less likely with needle biopsy or fine-needle aspiration. Isolated rectovaginal fistulas sometimes can be closed effectively utilizing the bulbocavernosus muscle (Martius procedure), but the gracilis muscle usually yields a better flap, since it provides more tissue and a better blood supply. When unresectable, recurrent cancer is present, the most conservative diverting procedure should be selected. For patients with urinary fistulas and a limited life expectancy, bilateral percutaneous nephrostomy, with occlusion of the distal ureters utilizing cyanoacrylate, can provide temporary continence. Selected patients with a longer life expectancy may be considered for ureterostomy or ileal conduit diversion. In the absence of recurrence, the procedure of choice will be determined by the site and extent of injury and by the long-term goals of the procedure, consistent with optimal quality of life. In some instances, total pelvic exenteration with musculocutaneous flap vaginal replacement is the only safe and effective method to deal with the multifarious problems of severe radiation vault necrosis and multiple fistulas. Untreated, these patients may die from inanition or sepsis, despite the fact that the process is reversible and there may be no persistent cancer.

The association between *vaginal dysplasia* and previous pelvic radiation for cervical cancer is well known (Choo and Anderson, 1982). The patient is usually asymptomatic, and the dysplasia can appear more than 20 years following radiation exposure, underscoring the need for lifetime cytologic follow-up of these patients. These dysplastic lesions are sometimes mistakenly interpreted as harmless radiation-induced changes, but they can progress to invasive cancer (Geelhoed et al, 1976). Colposcopy, Lugol's staining, and biopsy are used to identify high-grade dysplasias, which always require aggressive treatment. Mild dysplasia may respond to topical estrogen cream (see Chapter 1). Laser therapy and topical 5-FU tend to produce further vaginal shrinkage and are not highly effective.

Urinary Tract Injury

Urinary tract infection is common during radiation therapy for locally advanced cervical cancer (Prasad et al, 1995). Hemorrhagic cystitis is an uncommon complication of pelvic radiation that tends to appear later (10 to 20 years after therapy) than bowel complications. It is usually mild and associated with a superimposed bacterial cystitis, but deaths have been reported when the cystitis results from a combination of cyclophosphamide or ifosfamide and radiation (Price and Keldahl, 1990). Uncomplicated cases respond to appropriate antibiotics and continuous bladder irrigation with saline. If bleeding persists, cytoscopic removal of the clots and electrocautery of the bleeding vessels may be helpful. Cystoscopy is performed in all cases, but biopsy should be avoided unless a highly suspicious lesion is present. With contemporary radiotherapy, the need for urinary conduit diversion for intractable cases of radiation hemorrhagic cystitis has all but disappeared. Cyclophosphamide should be used with caution in patients who have received previous pelvic radiation.

Ureteral obstruction from radiation fibrosis is a rare complication (0.8 to 1.6 percent), but it comprises about 35 percent of all cases of postradiation ureteral blockage (Kaplan, 1977; Muram et al, 1981). Predisposing factors include chronic urinary tract infection, antecedent surgery, and high-dose parametrial radiation from external beam or brachytherapy. It is usually unilateral and most frequently occurs more than 24 months following treatment for early-stage disease. When recurrent cancer is the cause, usually the obstruction is bilateral and the patient has been irradiated for late-stage disease less than 24 months previously. Laparotomy is indicated in all patients if directed needle biopsies do not establish the presence of recurrence as the cause of the obstruction. For patients without recurrence, ureteral stents inserted retrograde or anterograde may relieve the obstruction.

The stents need to be changed on a regular schedule because they tend to harden or become plugged. Because surgical attempts to release the ureteral obstruction usually fail, ureteroneocystostomy is the treatment of choice for long-term management.

In selected cases, vesicovaginal fistulas caused by brachytherapy injury may be successfully repaired if a new source of blood supply is available to nourish the repair. Fistulas associated with high-dose, external beam therapy are best managed by conduit diversion (Boronow and Rutledge, 1971). Symptomatic colovesical fistulas always require resection of the disease segment of bowel and primary anastomosis of adequately prepared bowel. The fistulous tract should be resected, and a new source of blood supply applied to the bladder repair to ensure complete healing.

Miscellaneous Injuries

Bilateral femoral artery occlusion from radiation fibrosis has been reported after high-dose pelvic radiation. Skin atrophy and telangiectasia may occasionally be observed in patients who were treated with orthovoltage units. Dense subcutaneous fibrosis, even simulating a pelvic mass, is common following irradiation with low-megavoltage machines, especially ^{60}Co units. Aseptic necrosis of the femoral head also occasionally follows pelvic radiation therapy.

Radiation-induced *second cancers* are a justifiable concern for gynecologic oncology patients. A comprehensive study of patients treated with radiation therapy for cervical cancer identified significantly increased relative risks 10 or more years after treatment for bladder (relative risk = 2.8), rectal (1.7), and genital cancers other than those of the uterine corpus and ovary (3.1) (Boice et al, 1985). These risks increase with age. At 30 or more years after treatment, the cancer relative risk is 8.5, 4.1, and 4.8, for the respective organs. The risk of uterine corpus cancer and ovarian cancer after pelvic irradiation also tends to increase with age, although the trend is less clear, probably as a result of confounding variables such as hysterectomy and oophorectomy.

Radiation and Surgery

There are few challenges in gynecologic oncology to compare with operating in a previously irradiated field; at no time are surgical

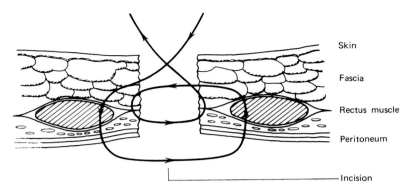

FIGURE 17–24. The internal retention suture of Smead-Jones. Instead of wire, we use No. 1 monofilament nylon. The security of this closure is comparable to that of through-and-through abdominal wall retention sutures. (From Morrow CP, Hernandez WL, Townsend DE, DiSaia PJ: Pelvic celiotomy in the obese patient. Am J Obstet Gynecol 127:335, 1977, with permission.)

experience, judgment, and skill called more into play (O'Brien et al, 1987; Fenner et al, 1989). The subliminal effects of ionizing radiation on tissue are usually clinically inapparent or unrecognized until an additional insult occurs within the irradiated area. The surgical risks for these patients, which rise rapidly with the dose of previous radiation, may be greatly underestimated.

As with all gynecology patients at risk for wound disruption, the recommended method for closing the abdominal incision is the running or interrupted internal retention closure of Smead-Jones (Jones et al, 1941; Fig. 17–24), utilizing monofilament nylon or polypropylene. In thin women, one of the new monofilament, absorbable sutures may provide sufficient tensile strength for a sufficient period of time and avoid the problems associated with leaving permanent knots just below the skin surface. Management of wound infection and wound disruption does not differ significantly from that of unirradiated wounds. Local debridement, and irrigation with dilute Dakin's or povidone iodine solution until the wound is clean, followed by moist saline packs, will promote new granulations. Dry packs impede surface fibroblasts by removing the surface layer each time the pack is changed.

CONCLUSIONS

Optimizing the integration of radiation therapy and surgery into the treatment of patients with gynecologic cancers remains a continuing challenge. From the foregoing discussion, the reader will understand that exposure of

human patients to ionizing radiation sets in motion a complex series of events, some of which will clearly lead to patient cure, some to palliation, and some to complications. The dialogue between the gynecologic surgeon and the radiation therapist is necessarily a continuing one. A clear understanding of the basic biologic principles involved makes this dialogue more useful to all concerned—patient, surgeon, and radiation oncologist.

REFERENCES

Aartsen EJ, Sindram IS: Repair of the radiation induced rectovaginal fistulas without or with interposition of the bulbocavernosus muscle (Martius procedure). Eur J Surg Oncol 14:171, 1988.

Adams GE: Chemical radiosensitization of hypoxic cells. Br Med Bull 29:48, 1973.

Anderson ES: Stage II endometrial carcinoma: prognostic factors and the results of treatment. Gynecol Oncol 38:220, 1990.

Arian-Schad KS, Kapp DS, Hackl A, et al: Radiation therapy in stage III ovarian cancer following surgery and chemotherapy: prognostic factors, patterns of relapse, and toxicity: a preliminary report. Gynecol Oncol 39:47, 1990.

Arlow FL, DeKovich AA, Priest RJ, Beher WT: Bile acids in radiation-induced diarrhea. South Med J 80:259, 1987.

Bagshaw MA: Possible role of potentiation in radiation therapy. Am J Roentgenol 85:822, 1961.

Bakri YN, Given FT Jr: Radioactivity in blood and urine following intraperitoneal instillation of chromic phosphate in patients with and without ascites. Am J Obstet Gynecol 150:184, 1984.

Baltzer J, Zander J: Adjuvant radiotherapy in the surgical treatment of carcinoma of the cervix. Biomed Pharmacol Ther 39:422, 1985.

Barranco SC, Romsdahl MM, Humphrey R: The radiation response of human malignant melanoma cells grown in vitro. Cancer Res 31:830, 1971.

Berek JS: Radiation therapy for adenocarcinoma of the uterine cervix: does the histology matter? Int J Radiat Oncol Biol Phys 32:1543, 1995.

Berek JS, Heaps JM, Fu YS, et al: Concurrent cisplatin and 5-fluorouracil chemotherapy and radiation therapy for advanced-stage squamous carcinoma of the vulva. Gynecol Oncol 42:197, 1991.

Boice JD Jr, Day NE, Andersen A, et al: Second cancers following radiation treatment for cervical cancer: an international collaboration among cancer registries. J Natl Cancer Inst 74:955, 1985.

Bolis G, Zanaboni F, Vanoli P, et al: The impact of whole-abdomen radiotherapy on survival in advanced ovarian cancer patients with minimal residual disease after chemotherapy. Gynecol Oncol 39:150, 1990.

Boronow RC: Combined therapy as an alternative to exenteration for locally advanced vulvovaginal cancer: rationale and results. Cancer 49:1085, 1982.

Boronow RC: Should whole pelvic radiation therapy become past history? A case for the routine use of extended field therapy and multimodality therapy. Gynecol Oncol 43:71, 1991.

Boronow RC, Hickman BT: A comparison of two radiation therapy treatment plans for carcinoma of the cervix. II. Complications and survival rates. Am J Obstet Gynecol 128:99, 1977.

Boronow RC, Rutledge F: Vesicovaginal fistula, radiation, and gynecologic cancer. Am J Obstet Gynecol 111:85, 1971.

Bourne RG, Kearsley JH, Grove WD, Roberts SJ: The relationship between early and late gastrointestinal complications of radiation therapy for carcinoma of the cervix. Int J Radiat Oncol Biol Phys 9:1445, 1983.

Brenner DJ, Huang Y, Hall EJ: Fractionated high dose-rate versus low dose-rate regimens for intracavitary brachytherapy of the cervix: equivalent regimens for combined brachytherapy and external irradiation. Int J Radiat Oncol Biol Phys 21:1415, 1991.

Brookland RK, Rubin S, Danoff BF: Extended field irradiation in the treatment of patients with cervical carcinoma involving biopsy-proven para-aortic nodes. Int J Radiat Oncol Biol Phys 10:1875, 1984.

Brown JM, Siim BG: Hypoxia-specific cytotoxins in cancer therapy. Semin Radiat Oncol 6:22, 1996.

Brown JM: Sensitizers in radiotherapy. In Withers HR, Peters LJ (eds): Innovations in Radiation Oncology. New York, Springer-Verlag, 1987, p 247.

Bruzzone M, Repetto L, Chiara S, et al: Chemotherapy versus radiotherapy in the management of ovarian cancer patients with pathological complete response or minimal residual disease at second look. Gynecol Oncol 38:392, 1990.

Buchler DA, Kline JC, Peckham BM: Radiation reactions in cervical cancer therapy. Am J Obstet Gynecol 111:745, 1971.

Bush RS, Jenkin RDT, Allt WE, et al: Definitive evidence for hypoxic cells influencing cure in cancer therapy. Br J Cancer 37:302, 1978.

Byfield JE: Hematologic parameters in the adjustment of chemotherapy doses in combined modality treatment using radiation. Am J Clin Oncol 7:319, 1984.

Byfield JE: Radiosensitizing effect of 5-fluorouracil by continuous infusion of gastrointestinal cancer. In Rotman M, Rosenthal J (eds): Concomitant Continuous Infusion Chemotherapy and Radiation: Theoretical Basis and Clinical Application of 5-Fluorouracil as a Radiosensitizer—an Overview. New York, Springer-Verlag, 1991, p 115.

Byfield JE, Calabro-Jones P, Klisak I, Kulhanian F: Pharmacologic requirements for obtaining sensitization of human tumor cells in vitro to combined 5-fluorouracil or ftorafur and x-rays. Int J Radiat Oncol Biol Phys 8:1923, 1982.

Carey MS, O'Connell GJ, Johanson CR, et al: Good outcome associated with a standardized treatment protocol using selective postoperative radiation in patients with clinical stage I adenocarcinoma of the endometrium. Gynecol Oncol 57:138, 1995.

Chang H-C, Lai C-H, Chen M-S, et al: Preliminary results of concurrent radiotherapy and chemotherapy with cis-platinum, vincristine, and bleomycin in bulky, advanced cervical carcinoma: a pilot study. Gynecol Oncol 44:182, 1992.

Chao CK, Grigsby PW, Perez CA, et al: Brachytherapy-related complications for medically inoperable stage I endometrial carcinoma. Int J Radiat Oncol Biol Phys 31:37, 1995.

Charbit A, Malaise EP, Tubiana M: Relation between the pathological nature and growth rate of human tumors. Eur J Cancer 7:307, 1971.

Chen M-S, Lin F-J, Hong C-H, et al: High-dose-rate afterloading technique in the radiation treatment of uterine cervical cancer: 399 cases and 9 years experience in Taiwan. Int J Radiat Oncol Biol Phys 20:915, 1991.

Chism SE, Park RE, Keys HM: Prospects for para-aortic irradiation in treatment of cancer of the cervix. Cancer 35:1505, 1975.

Choi JH, Lee HS: Effect of omental pedicle hammock in protection against radiation-induced enteropathy in patients with rectal cancer. Dis Colon Rectum 38:276, 1995.

Choo YC, Anderson DG: Neoplasms of the vagina following cervical carcinoma. Gynecol Oncol 14:125, 1982.

Christie DRH, Bull CA, Gebski V, et al: Concurrent 5-fluorouracil, mitomycin C and irradiation in locally advanced cervix cancer. Radiother Oncol 37:181, 1995.

Clifton KH, DeMott RK, Mulcahy RT, Gould MN: Thyroid gland formation from inocula of monodispersed cells: early results on quantitation, function, neoplasia and radiation effects. Int J Radiat Oncol Biol Phys 4:987, 1978.

Covens A, Thomas G, DePetrillo A, et al: The prognostic importance of site and type of radiation-induced bowel injury in patients requiring surgical management. Gynecol Oncol 43:270, 1991.

Cox JD, Komaki R, Wilson JF, Greenberg M: Locally advanced adenocarcinoma of the endometrium: results of irradiation with and without subsequent hysterectomy. Cancer 45:715, 1980.

Cunningham MJ, Dunton CJ, Corn B, et al: Extended-field radiation therapy in early-stage cervical carcinoma: survival and complications. Gynecol Oncol 43:51, 1991.

Currie JL, Bagne F, Harris C, et al: Radioactive chromic phosphate suspension: studies on the distribution, dose absorption and effect of therapeutic radiation in phantoms, dogs, and patients. Gynecol Oncol 12:193, 1981.

Curtin JP: Radical hysterectomy—the treatment of choice for early-stage cervical carcinoma. Gynecol Oncol 62:137, 1996.

DeCosse JJ, Rhodes RS, Wentz WB, et al: The natural history and management of radiation induced injury of the gastrointestinal tract. Ann Surg 170:369, 1969.

Delclos L, Fletcher GH, Suit HD, et al: Afterloading vaginal applicators. Radiology 96:666, 1970.

Dembo AJ: Epithelial ovarian cancer: the role of radiotherapy. Int J Radiat Oncol Biol Phys 22:835, 1992.

Dembo AJ, Bush RS: Current concepts in cancer. Ovary: treatment of stages III and IV. Choice of postoperative therapy based on prognostic factors. Int J Radiat Oncol Biol Phys 8:893, 1982.

Dewey DL: The radiosensitivity of melanoma cells in culture. Br J Radiol 44:816, 1971.

Double EG: Interactions between platinum coordination complexes and radiation. In Hill BT, Bellamy AS (eds): Antitumor Drug-Radiation Interactions. Boca Raton, FL, CRC Press, 1990, p 171.

Durrance FY, Fletcher GH, Rutledge FN: Analysis of central recurrent disease in stage I and II squamous cell carcinomas of cervix on intact uterus. Am J Roentgenol 106:831, 1969.

Eifel PJ, Burke TW, Morris M, et al: Adenocarcinoma as an independent risk factor for disease recurrence in patients with stage IB cervical carcinoma. Gynecol Oncol 59:38, 1995.

Elkind MM, Whitmore GF: The Radiobiology of Cultured Mammalian Cells. New York, Gordon and Breach, 1967.

Ellis F: The relationship of biological effect to time-dose-fractionation factors in radiotherapy. Curr Top Radiat Res 4:359, 1968.

Ellis F: Is NSD-TDF useful to radiotherapy? Int J Radiat Oncol Biol Phys 11:1685, 1985.

El Senoussi MA, Fletcher GH, Burlase BC: Correlation of radiation and surgical parameters in complications in the extended technique for carcinoma of the cervix. Int J Radiat Oncol Biol Phys 5:927, 1979.

Erlich E, McCall AR, Potkul RK, et al: Paclitaxel is only a weak radiosensitizer of human cervical carcinoma cell lines. Gynecol Oncol 60:251, 1996.

Fajardo L: Pathology of Radiation Injury. New York, Masson, 1982.

Feder BH, Syed AMN, Neblett D: Treatment of extensive carcinoma of the cervix with the transperineal parametrial butterfly: a preliminary report on the revival of Waterman's approach. Int J Radiat Oncol Biol Phys 4:735, 1978.

Fenner MN, Sheehan P, Nanavati PJ, Ross DS: Chronic radiation enteritis: a community hospital experience. J Surg Oncol 41:246, 1989.

Fertil B, Malaise EP: Intrinsic radiosensitivity of human cell lines is correlated with radioresponse of human tumors: analysis of 101 published survival curves. Int J Radiat Oncol Biol Phys 11:1699, 1985.

Fine BA, Hempling RE, Piver MS, et al: Severe radiation morbidity in carcinoma of the cervix: impact of pretherapy surgical staging and previous surgery. Int J Radiat Oncol Biol Phys 31:717, 1995.

Fisher L, Kimose HH, Spjeldnaes N, Wara P: Late radiation injuries of the small intestine—management and outcome. Acta Chir Scand 155:47, 1989.

Fletcher GH: Radiation therapy and subclinical disease. In Neoplasia of the Head and Neck. Chicago, Year Book Medical Publishers, 1974, p 19.

Fletcher GH: Textbook of Radiotherapy, 3rd ed. Philadelphia, Febiger, 1980.

Fowler JF: What next in fractionation radiotherapy? Br J Cancer 49(suppl VI):285, 1984.

Franchin G, Tumolo S, Scarabelli C, et al: Whole abdomen radiation therapy after a short chemotherapy course and second-look laparotomy in advanced ovarian cancer. Gynecol Oncol 41:206, 1991.

Fravel HNA, Roberts JJ: Excision repair of cis-diamminedichloroplatinum (II)-induced damage to DNA in Chinese hamster cells. Cancer Res 39:1793, 1979.

Fyles AW, Keane TJ, Barton M, Simms J: The effect of treatment duration in the local control of cervix cancer. Radiother Oncol 25:273, 1992.

Fyles AW, Pintilie M, Kirkbride P, et al: Prognostic factors in patients with cervix cancer treated by radiation therapy: results of a multiple regression analysis. Radiother Oncol 35:107, 1995.

Geelhoed GW, Henson DE, Taylor PT, Ketcham AS: Carcinoma in situ of the vagina following treatment for carcinoma of the cervix: a distinctive clinical entity. Am J Obstet Gynecol 124:510, 1976.

Gray LH, Conger AD, Ebert M: The concentration of oxygen dissolved in tissues at the time of irradiation as a factor in radiotherapy. Br J Radiol 26:638, 1953.

Grigsby PW: Lack of proven efficacy of chemotherapy for patients with carcinoma of the uterine cervix. Semin Radiat Oncol 4:30, 1994.

Hacker NF, Berek JS, Julliard GJF, Lagasse LD: Preoperative radiation therapy for locally advanced vulvar cancer. Cancer 54:2056, 1984.

Hall EJ: Radiobiology for the Radiologist, 4th ed. New York, Harper & Row, 1988.

Heath R, Rosenman J, Varia M, Walton L: Peritoneal fluid cytology in endometrial cancer: its significance and the role of chromic phosphate (32P) therapy. Int J Radiat Oncol Biol Phy 15:815, 1988.

Heaton D, Yordan E, Reddy S, et al: Treatment of 29 patients with bulky squamous cell carcinoma of the cervix with simultaneous cisplatin, 5-fluorouracil, and split-course hyperfractionated radiation therapy. Gynecol Oncol 38:323, 1990.

Hei TK, Piao CQ, Geard CR, et al: Taxol and ionizing radiation: interaction and mechanisms. Int J Radiat Oncol Biol Phys 29:267, 1994.

Herbert SH, Solin LJ, Hoffman JP, et al: Volumetric analysis of small bowel displacement from radiation portals with the use of a pelvic tissue expander. Int J Radiat Oncol Biol Phys 25:885, 1993.

Herskovic A, Martz K, Al-Sarraf M, et al: Combined chemotherapy and radiotherapy compared with radiotherapy alone in patients with cancer of the esophagus. N Engl J Med 326:1593, 1992.

Heyman J, Reuterwall O, Benner S: The Radiumhemmet experience with radiotherapy in cancer of the corpus of the uterus: classification, method of treatment and results. Acta Radiol 22:11, 1941.

Hill BT, Bellamy AS: Antitumor Drug Interactions. Boca Raton, FL, CRC Press, 1990.

Hindley A, Cole H: Use of peritoneal insufflation to displace the small bowel during pelvic and abdominal radiotherapy in carcinoma of the cervix. Br J Radiol 66:67, 1993.

Hreschchyshyn MM, Aron BS, Boronow RC, et al: Hydroxyurea or placebo combined with radiation in stages IIIB and IV cervical cancer confined to the pelvis. Int J Radiat Oncol Biol Phys 5:17, 1979.

Ito H, Kumaga H, Shigmatsu N, et al: High dose rate intracavitary brachytherapy for recurrent cervical cancer of the vaginal stump following hysterectomy. Int J Radiat Oncol Biol Phys 20:927, 1991.

Ito H, Kutuki S, Nishiguchi I, et al: Radiotherapy for cervical cancer with high-dose rate brachytherapy: correlation between tumor size, dose and failure. Radiother Oncol 31:240, 1994.

Jacobs C, Lyman G, Velez-Garcia E, et al: A phase III randomized study comparing cisplatin and fluorouracil as single agents and in combination for advanced squamous cell carcinoma of the head and neck. J Clin Oncol 10:257, 1992.

Jirtle RL, Michalopoulos SC, Strom PM, et al: The survival of parenchymal hepatocytes irradiated with high and low LET radiation. Br J Cancer 49:197, 1984.

John M, Cooke KJ, Flam M, et al: Preliminary results of concomitant radiotherapy and chemotherapy in advanced cervical carcinoma. Gynecol Oncol 28:101, 1987.

John M, Flam M, Caplan R, et al: Final results of a phase II chemoradiation protocol for locally advanced cervical cancer: RTOG 85-15. Gynecol Oncol 61:221, 1996.

Johns HE, Cunningham JR: The Physics of Radiology, 4th ed. Springfield, IL, Charles C Thomas, 1983.

Jones TE, Newell ET Jr, Brubaker RE: The use of alloy steel wire in the closure of abdominal wounds. Surg Gynecol Obstet 72:1056, 1941.

Joslin CA, Smith CW, Mallik A: The treatment of cervix cancer using high activity Co-60 sources. Br J Radiol 45:275, 1972.

Joslin CA, Vaishampayan GV, Mallik A: The treatment of early cancer of the corpus uteri. Br J Radiol 50:38, 1977.

Kademian MT, Bosch A: Staging laparotomy and survival in carcinoma of the uterine cervix. Acta Radiol Ther Phys Biol 16:314, 1977.

Kaplan AL: Postradiation ureteral obstruction. Obstet Gynecol Surv 32:1, 1977.

Kaplan WD, Zimmerman RE, Bloomer WD, et al: Therapeutic intraperitoneal ^{32}P: a clinical assessment of the dynamics of distribution. Radiology 138:683, 1981.

Kataoka M, Kawamura M, Nishiyama Y, et al: Results of the combination of external-beam and high-dose-rate intracavitary irradiation for patients with cervical carcinoma. Gynecol Oncol 44:48, 1992.

Kerr JFR, Winterford CM, Harmon BV: Apoptosis: its significance in cancer and cancer therapy. Cancer 73:2013, 1994.

Kerr JFR, Wyllie AH, Currie AR: Apoptosis: a basic biological phenomenon with wide-ranging implications in tissue kinetics. Br J Cancer 26:239, 1972.

Kersh CR, Constable WC, Spalding CA, et al: A phase I-II trial of multimodality management of bulky gynecologic malignancy. Cancer 66:30, 1990.

Kinsella TJ: Radiosensitization of nonhypoxic cells by halogenated pyrimidines. In Rotman M, Rosenthal CJ (eds): Concomitant Continuous Infusion Chemotherapy and Radiation. New York, Springer-Verlag, 1991, p 91.

Klaassen D, Shelley W, Starreveld A, et al: Early stage ovarian cancer: a randomized clinical trial comparing whole abdominal radiotherapy, melphalan and intraperitoneal chromic phosphate. A National Cancer Institute of Canada Clinical Trials Group report. J Clin Oncol 6:1254, 1988.

Klaassen D, Starreveld A, Shelly W, et al: External beam pelvis radiotherapy plus intraperitoneal radioactive chromic phosphate in early stage ovarian cancer: a toxic combination. A National Cancer Institute of Canada Clinical Trials Group report. J Radiat Oncol Biol Phys 11:1801, 1985.

Klimberg VS: Prevention of radiogenic side effects using glutamine-enriched elemental diets. Recent Results Cancer Res 121:283, 1991.

Klimberg VS, Salloum RM, Kasper M, et al: Oral glutamine accelerates healing of the small intestine and improves outcome after whole abdominal radiation. Arch Surg 125:1040, 1990.

Komaki R, Brickner TJ, Hanlon AL, et al: Long-term results of treatment of cervical carcinoma in the United States in 1973, 1978 and 1983: Patterns of Care Study (PCS). Int J Radiat Oncol Biol Phys 31:973, 1995.

Kucera H, Vavra N, Weghaupt K: Benefit of external irradiation in pathologic stage I endometrial carcinoma: a prospective clinical trial of 605 patients who received postoperative vaginal irradiation and additional pelvic irradiation in the presence of unfavorable prognostic factors. Gynecol Oncol 38:99, 1990.

Lanciano RM, Greven KM: Adjuvant treatment of endometrial cancer: who needs it? Gynecol Oncol 57:135, 1995.

Lanciano RM, Martz K, Coia LR, Hanks GE: Tumor and treatment factors improving outcome in stage III-B cervix cancer. Int J Radiat Oncol Biol Phys 20:95, 1991.

Leichner PK, Cash SA, Backx C, Durand RE: Effects of injection volume on the tissue dose, dose rate, and therapeutic potential of intraperitoneal ^{32}P. Radiology 141:193, 1981.

Leichner PK, Rosenshein NB, Leibel SA, Order SE: Distribution of tissue dose of intraperitoneally administered radioactive chromic phosphate ^{32}P in New Zealand white rabbits. Radiology 134:729, 1980.

Levine EL, Renehan A, Gossiel R, et al: Apoptosis, intrinsic radiosensitivity and prediction of radiotherapy response in cervical carcinoma. Radiother Oncol 37:1, 1995.

Liebmann J, Cook JA, Fisher J, et al: Changes in radiation survival curve parameters in human tumor and rodent cells exposed to paclitaxel (Taxol). Int J Radiat Oncol Biol Phys 29:559, 1994.

Ling CC, Chen CH, Li WX: Apoptosis induced at different dose rates: implication for the shoulder region of cell survival curves. Radiother Oncol 32:129, 1994.

Liu JM, Chen YM, Chao Y, et al: Paclitaxel-induced severe neuropathy in patients with previous radiotherapy to the head and neck region. J Natl Cancer Inst 88:1000, 1996.

Liu WS, Yen SH, Chan CH, et al: Determination of the appropriate fraction number and size of the HDR brachytherapy for cervical cancer. Gynecol Oncol 60:295, 1996.

Lokich JJ, Byfield JE (eds): Combined Modality Cancer Therapy—Radiation and Infusional Chemotherapy. Chicago, Precept Press, 1991.

Looser KG, Quan SHQ, Clark DGC: Colo-urinary-tract fistula in the cancer patient. Dis Colon Rectum 22:143, 1979.

Ludgate SM, Crandon AJ, Hudson CJ, et al: Synchronous 5-fluorouracil, mitomycin C and radiation therapy in the treatment of locally advanced carcinoma of the cervix. Int J Radiat Oncol Biol Phys 15:893, 1988.

Maingon P, Horiot JC, Fraisse J, et al: Preoperative radiotherapy in stage I/II endometrial adenocarcinoma. Radiother Oncol 39:201, 1996.

Maitra AJ, Byfield JE: Gynecologic cancer. In Lokich JJ, Byfield JE (eds): Combined Modality Cancer Therapy—Radiation and Infusional Chemotherapy. Chicago, Precept Press, 1991, p 209.

Malviya VK, Han I, Deppe G, et al: High-dose-rate afterloading brachytherapy, external radiation therapy, and combination chemotherapy in poor-prognosis cancer of the cervix. Gynecol Oncol 42:233, 1991.

Marcial LV, Marcial VA, Krall JM, et al: Comparison of 1 vs 2 or more intracavitary brachytherapy applications in the management of carcinoma of the cervix, with irradiation alone. Int J Radiat Oncol Biol Phys 20:81, 1991.

Martinez A, Cox RS, Edmundson GK: A multiple-site perineal applicator (MUPIT) for treatment of prostatic, anorectal and gynecologic malignancies. Int J Radiat Oncol Biol Phys 10:297, 1984.

Martinez A, Schray M, Hoes AE, Bagshaw MA: Postoperative radiation therapy for epithelial ovarian cancer: the curative role based on a 24-year experience. J Clin Oncol 3:901, 1988.

Mendenhall WM, Sombeck MD, Freeman DE, et al: Stage IB and IIA-B carcinoma of the intact uterine cervix: impact of tumor volume and the role of adjuvant hysterectomy. Semin Radiat Oncol 4:16, 1994.

Minarik L, Hall EJ: Taxol in combination with acute and low dose rate irradiation. Radiother Oncol 32:124, 1994.

Montague ED: Experience with altered fractionation on radiation therapy of breast cancer. Radiology 90:962, 1968.

Montana GS, Martz KL, Hanks GE: Patterns and sites of failure in cervix cancer treated in the U.S.A. in 1978. Int J Radiat Oncol Biol Phys 20:87, 1991.

Morrow CP, Shingleton HM, Averette HE, et al: Is pelvic radiation beneficial in the postoperative management of stage IB squamous cell carcinoma of the cervix with pelvic node metastasis treated by radical hysterectomy and pelvic lymphadenectomy? A report from the Presidential Panel at the 1979 Annual Meeting of the Society of Gynecologic Oncologists. Gynecol Oncol 10:105, 1980.

Morrow CP, Hernandez WL, Townsend DE, DiSaia PJ: Pelvic celiotomy in the obese patient. Am J Obstet Gynecol 127:335, 1977.

Müller JH: Weiter entwicklungen der therapic von peritoneal carcinomen beit ovarial carcinoma mit kunstlicher radioaktivitat ^{198}Au. Gynecologia 129:289, 1950.

Muram D, Oxorn H, Curry RH, et al: Postradiation ureteral obstruction: a reappraisal. Am J Obstet Gynecol 139:289, 1981.

Nelson AJ III, Fletcher GH, Wharton JT: Indications for adjunctive conservative extrafascial hysterectomy in selected cases of carcinoma of the uterine cervix. Am J Roentgenol 123:91, 1975.

Nguyen C, Souhami L, Roman TN, et al: High-dose-rate brachytherapy as the primary treatment of medically inoperable stage I-II endometrial carcinoma. Gynecol Oncol 59:370, 1995.

O'Brien PH, Jenrette JM III, Garvin AJ: Radiation enteritis. Am Surg 53:501, 1987.

Orton CG: High dose rate versus low dose rate brachytherapy for gynecologic cancer. Semin Radiat Oncol 3: 232, 1993.

Orton CG: Width of the therapeutic window: what is the optimal dose-per-fraction for high dose rate cervix cancer brachytherapy? Int J Radiat Oncol Biol Phys 31:1011, 1995.

Orton CG, Ellis F: A simplification in the use of the NSD concept in practical radiotherapy. Br J Radiol 46:529, 1973.

Orton CG, Seyedsadr M, Somnay A: Comparison of high and low dose rate remote afterloading for cervix cancer and the importance of fractionation. Int J Radiat Oncol Biol Phys 21:1425, 1991.

Ott RJ, Flower MA, Jones A, McCready VR: The measurement of radiation doses from ^{32}P chromic phosphate therapy of the peritoneum using SPECT. Eur J Nucl Med 11: 305, 1985.

Overgaard J, Horsman MR: Modification of hypoxia-induced radioresistance in tumors by the use of oxygen and sensitizers. Semin Radiat Oncol 6:10, 1996.

Patton TJ, Kavanagh JJ, Delclos L, et al: Five-year survival in patients given intra-arterial chemotherapy prior to radiotherapy for advanced squamous carcinoma of the cervix and vagina. Gynecol Oncol 42:54, 1991.

Perez CA, Brady LW: Principles and Practice of Radiation Oncology. Philadelphia, JB Lippincott, 2nd ed, 1992.

Petereit DG, Fowler JF, Kinsella TJ: Optimizing the dose rate and technique in cervical carcinoma—balancing cases versus complications. Int J Radiat Oncol Biol Phys 29: 1195, 1994.

Pezner RD, Stevens KR Jr, Tong D, Allen CV: Limited epithelial carcinoma of the ovary treated with curative intent by the intraperitoneal installation of radiocolloids. Cancer 42:2563, 1978.

Phillips RA, Tolmach LF: Repair of potentially lethal damage in x-irradiated HeLa cells. Radiat Res 29:413, 1966.

Photopulos GJ, Vander Zwaag R, Miller B, et al: Vaginal radiation brachytherapy to reduce central recurrence after radical hysterectomy for cervical carcinoma. Gynecol Oncol 38:187, 1990.

Pitkin RM, van Voorhis LW: Postirradiation vaginitis: an evaluation of prophylaxis with topical estrogen. Radiology 99: 417, 1971.

Piver MS, Barlow JJ, Vongtama V, Blumenson L: Hydroxyurea as a radiation sensitizer in women with carcinoma of the uterine cervix. Am J Obstet Gynecol 129:379, 1977.

Polednak AP: Declining use of radiotherapy for invasive cervical cancer in Connecticut: 1983–1990. Gynecol Oncol 58:226, 1995.

Poma PA: Postirradiation vaginal occlusion: nonoperative management. Int J Gynaecol Obstet 18:90, 1980.

Potish RA, Dusenbery KE: Enteric morbidity of postoperative pelvic external beam and brachytherapy for uterine cancer. Int J Radiat Oncol Biol Phys 18:1005, 1990.

Potish RA, Twiggs LB, Prem KA, et al: Surgical intervention following multimodality therapy for advanced cervical cancer. Gynecol Oncol 38:175, 1990.

Potten CS: Stem Cells: Their Identification and Characterization. Edinburgh, Churchill Livingstone, 1983.

Potter ME, Partridge EE, Singleton HM, et al: Intraperitoneal chromic phosphate in ovarian cancer: risks and benefits. Gynecol Oncol 32:314, 1989.

Pourquier H, Delard R, Achille E, et al: A quantified approach to the analysis and prevention of urinary complications in radiotherapeutic treatment of cancer of the cervix. Int J Radiat Oncol Biol Phys 13:1025, 1987.

Prasad KN, Pradhan S, Datta NR: Urinary tract infection in patients of gynecological malignancies undergoing external pelvic radiotherapy. Gynecol Oncol 57:380, 1995.

Price WE, Keldahl LR: Fatal hemorrhagic cystitis induced by pelvic irradiation and cyclophosphamide therapy. Minn Med 73(5):39, 1990.

Proctor J, Doering D, Barnhill D, Park R: Bowel perforation associated with intraperitoneal chromic phosphate instillation. Gynecol Oncol 36:125, 1990.

Puck TT, Marcus PI: A rapid method for viable cell titration and clone production with HeLa cells in tissue culture: the use of x-irradiated cells to supply conditioning factors. Proc Natl Acad Sci USA 41:432, 1955.

Ransom JL, Novak RW, Kumer AP, et al: Delayed gastrointestinal complications after combined modality therapy of childhood rhabdomyosarcoma. Int J Radiat Oncol Biol Phys 5:1275, 1978.

Ravitch MM: Varieties of stapled anastomoses in rectal resection. Surg Clin North Am 64:543, 1984.

Remy JC, Di Maio T, Fruchter RG, et al: Adjunctive radiation after radical hysterectomy in stage Ib squamous cell carcinoma of the cervix. Gynecol Oncol 38:161, 1990.

Roberts WS, Hoffman MS, Kavanagh JJ, et al: Further experience with radiation therapy and concomitant intravenous chemotherapy in advanced carcinoma of the lower female genital tract. Gynecol Oncol 43:233, 1991a.

Roberts WS, Hoffman MS, LaPolla JP, et al: Management of radionecrosis of the vulva and distal vagina. Am J Obstet Gynecol 164:1235, 1991b.

Rockwell S: Cytotoxicities of mitomycin C and x-rays to aerobic and hypoxic cells in vitro. Int J Radiat Oncol Biol Phys 8:1035, 1982.

Rodriguez M, Sevin BU, Perras J, et al: Paclitaxel: a radiation sensitizer of human cervical cancer cells. Gynecol Oncol 57:165, 1995.

Roman TN, Souhami L, Freeman CR, et al: High dose rate afterloading intracavitary therapy in carcinoma of the cervix. Int J Radiat Oncol Biol Phys 20:921, 1991.

Rosenshein NB, Leichner PK, Vogelsang G: Radiocolloids in the treatment of ovarian cancer. Obstet Gynecol Surv 34: 708, 1979.

Rotman M, Aziz H, Eifel PJ: Irradiation of pelvic and para-aortic nodes in carcinoma of the cervix. Semin Radiat Oncol 4:23, 1994.

Rotman M, Choi K, Goze C, et al: Prophylactic irradiation of the para-aortic lymph node chain in stage IIB and bulky IB carcinoma of the cervix: initial treatment results of RTOG 7920. Int J Radiat Oncol Biol Phys 19:513, 1990.

Rotman M, John MJ, Moon SH, et al: Limitations of adjunctive surgery in carcinoma of the cervix. Int J Radiat Oncol Biol Phys 5:327, 1979.

Rutledge FN, Wharton JT, Fletcher GH: Clinical studies with adjunctive surgery and irradiation therapy in the treatment of carcinoma of the cervix. Cancer 38:596, 1976.

Salmon SE, Hamburger AW, Soehnlen B, et al: Quantitation of differential sensitivity of human-tumor stem cells to anticancer drugs. N Engl J Med 298:1321, 1978.

Sher ME, Bauer J: Radiation-induced enteropathy. Am J Gastroenterol 85:121, 1990.

Shigematsa Y, Nishigama K, Masaki N, et al: Treatment of carcinoma of the uterine cervix by remotely controlled afterloading intracavitary radiotherapy with high-dose rate: a comparative study with a low-dose rate system. Int J Radiat Oncol Biol Phys 9:351, 1983.

Sigmon WR, Randall ME, Olds WW, et al: Increased chronic bowel complications with split-course pelvic irradiation. Int J Radiat Oncol Biol Phys 28:349, 1994.

Smith DH, Pierce VK, Lewis JL Jr: Enteric fistulas encountered on a gynecologic oncology service from 1969 through 1980. Surg Gynecol Obstet 158:71, 1984.

Smith ST, Seski JC, Copeland LJ, et al: Surgical management of irradiation-induced small bowel damage. Obstet Gynecol 65:563, 1985.

Steren AJ, Sevin BU, Perras JP, et al: Taxol sensitizes human ovarian cancer cells to radiation. Gynecol Oncol 48:252, 1993.

Strockbine MF, Hancock JE, Fletcher GH: Complications in 831 patients with squamous cell carcinoma of the intact uterine cervix treated with 3,000 rads or more whole pelvis irradiation. Am J Roentgenol 108:293, 1970.

Stryker JA, Demers LM: The effect of pelvic irradiation on the absorption of bile acids. Int J Radiat Oncol Biol Phys 5:935, 1979.

Sueyama H, Nakano M, Sakumoto K, et al: Intra-arterial chemotherapy with cisplatin followed by radical radiotherapy for locally advanced cervical cancer. Gynecol Oncol 59:327, 1995.

Szybalski W: X-ray sensitization by halopyrimidines. Cancer Chemother Rep 58:539, 1974.

Tapazoglou E, Kish J, Ensley J, Al-Sarrat M: The activity of a single agent 5-fluouracil infusion in advanced and recurrent head and neck cancer. Cancer 57:1105, 1986.

Thames HD: On the origin of dose fractionation regimens in radiotherapy. Semin Radiat Oncol 2:3, 1992.

Thames HD, Withers HR, Peters LJ, Fletcher GH: Changes in early and late radiation response with altered dose-fractionation: implications for dose-survival relationships. Int J Radiat Oncol Biol Phys 8:219, 1982.

Thigpen JT, Blessing JA, Gallup DG, et al: Phase II trial of mitomycin-C in squamous cell carcinoma of the uterine cervix: a Gynecologic Oncology Group study. Gynecol Oncol 57:376, 1995.

Thomas GM: Hypoxia and carcinoma of the cervix. Semin Radiat Oncol 4:9, 1994.

Thomas GM, Dembo AJ, Beale E, et al: Concurrent radiation, mitomycin-C and 5-fluorouracil in poor prognosis cancer of cervix: preliminary results of a phase I-II trial. Int J Radiat Oncol Biol Phys 10:1785, 1984.

Thomas GM, Dembo AJ, Bryson SCP, et al: Changing concepts in the management of vulvar cancer. Gynecol Oncol 42:9, 1991.

Thomas GM, Dembo AJ, DePetrillo A, et al: Concurrent radiation and chemotherapy in vulvar carcinoma. Gynecol Oncol 34, 263, 1989.

Thomas GM, Dembo AJ, Fyles A, et al: Concurrent chemoradiation in advanced cervical cancer. Gynecol Oncol 38:446, 1990.

Thomlinson RH, Gray LH: The histological structure of some human lung cancers and the possible implications for radiotherapy. Br J Cancer 9:539, 1955.

Thomson JM, Spratt JS Jr: Treatment policies affecting survival in patients with carcinoma of the cervix. Radiology 127:771, 1978.

Trimbos JB, Snijders-Keilhotz T, Peters AA: Feasibility of the application of a reasorbable polyglycolic-acid mesh (Dexon mesh) to prevent complications of radiotherapy following gynaecological surgery. Eur J Surg 157:281, 1991.

Tubiana M, Malaise E: Comparison of cell proliferation kinetics in human and experimental tumors: response to irradiation. Cancer Treat Rep 60:1887, 1976.

Utley JF, von Essen CF, Horn RA, Moeller JH: High-dose-rate afterloading brachytherapy in carcinoma of the uterine cervix. Int J Radiat Oncol Biol Phys 10:2259, 1984.

Van Kasteren YM, Burger CW, Meijer OW, et al: Efficacy of a synthetic mesh sling in keeping the small bowel in the upper abdomen to prevent radiation enteropathy in gynecologic malignancies. Eur J Obstet Gynecol Reprod Biol 50:211, 1993.

van Rijn J, van den Berg J, Meijer OWM: Proliferation and clonal survival of human lung cancer cells treated with fractionated irradiation in combination with paclitaxel. Int J Radiat Oncol Biol Phys 33:635, 1995.

Walton LA, Yadusky A, Rubinstein L: Intraperitoneal radioactive phosphate in early ovarian carcinoma: an analysis of complications. Int J Radiat Oncol Biol Phys 20:939, 1991.

Wang TN, Whetzel T, Mathes SJ, Vasconez LO: A fasciocutaneous flap for vaginal and perineal reconstruction. J Plast Reconst Surg 80:95, 1987.

Wasserman T, Siemann D, Suguhara T: The 8th International Conference on Chemical Modifiers of Cancer Treatment. Int J Radiat Oncol Biol Phys 29:419, 1994.

Watson ER, Halnan KE, Dische E, et al: Hyperbaric oxygen and radiotherapy: a Medical Council Research Trial in cancer of the cervix. Br J Radiol 51:879, 1978.

Weichselbaum RR: The role of DNA repair processes in the response of human tumors to fractionated radiation. Int J Radiat Oncol Biol Phys 10:1127, 1984.

Wells J, Berry RJ, Laing AH: Reproductive survival of explanted human tumor cells after exposure to nitrogen mustard or x-irradiation: differences in response with subsequent subcultures in vitro. Radiat Res 69:90, 1977.

Wharam MD, Phillips TL, Bagshaw MA: The role of radiation therapy in clinical stage I carcinoma of the endometrium. Int J Radiat Oncol Biol Phys 1:1081, 1976.

Whelan TJ, Dembo AJ, Bush RS, et al: Complications of whole abdominal and pelvic radiotherapy following chemotherapy for advanced ovarian cancer. Int J Radiat Oncol Biol Phys 22:853, 1992.

Withers HR, Horiot JC: Hyperfractionation. In Withers HR, Peters LJ (eds): Innovations in Radiation Oncology. New York, Springer-Verlag, 1988, p 223.

18

Principles of Immunology and Immunotherapy

Malcolm S. Mitchell
Revised by Cheryl C. Gurin

An understanding of the biologic mechanisms a tumor-bearing individual, the "host," possesses for rejecting the tumor is fundamental to any therapeutic approach to cancer biology. Even when immunotherapy is not specifically considered as an option in a particular patient, it is nonetheless important for the clinician to be aware of the ways in which standard methods of treatment affect the patient's natural defenses against the cancer. This alone could justify the study of tumor immunology, but there is also increasing evidence that appropriately designed modifications of the immune response can be useful as treatment for several types of cancer. Gynecologic cancers are no exception to these general remarks. In this chapter the general principles of tumor immunology are presented, followed by an outline of the categories of immunotherapy that are currently being investigated, with special reference to their application to gynecologic oncology.

BASIC PRINCIPLES OF IMMUNOLOGY

The Immune System

The primary function of the immune system is to recognize "self" or host substance as different from "nonself" or foreign substance, and to eliminate foreign substances. The components central to the function of the immune system are (1) circulating cells, the most important of which are lymphocytes; (2) protein products of immune cells, such as antibodies and cytokines; and (3) the complement system.

Lymphocytes and Macrophages

The three major classes of lymphocytes—T cells, B cells, and large granular lymphocytes—originate from a common stem cell. T-cell (thymus-derived) lymphocytes originate in the bone marrow. Late in fetal development the T cells migrate to the thymus for further differentiation. T cells are the primary effectors of cell-mediated immunity. They also exert a regulatory function over other cells in the immune system. Based on expression of cluster designation (CD) molecules, there are two major subsets of T cells: CD4 and CD8. The CD4 cells induce B-cell and cytotoxic T-cell (CD8) proliferation, function as cytotoxic effector cells, and recognize antigens associated with major histocompatibility (MHC) class II molecules on antigen-presenting cells. CD8 cells suppress antibody synthesis, function as cytotoxic T cells, and recognize antigens associated with MHC class I molecules. B cells are also derived from the bone marrow. In the presence of specified antigen, B cells can both produce and secrete antibody; they are also capable of maturing into plasma cells. B-cell function can be regulated by lymphokines produced by T cells and macrophages. The large granular lymphocyte class of cells includes null cells, natural killer (NK) cells, and lymphokine-activated killer (LAK) cells. These cells mediate antibody-dependent cellular cytotoxicity (ADCC) and natural killer activity.

Another group of cells within the immune system are the monocytes and macrophages. They possess a wide variety of functions, including the production and secretion of lymphokines, prostaglandins, interferons, and tumor necrosis factor (TNF); antigen presentation; and phagocytosis. Other cells that function within the immune system, but with less direct application to tumor immunology, are neutrophils, eosinophils, basophils, dendritic cells, and the cells of the reticuloendothelial system.

Antibodies and Cytokines

The two major protein products of the immune system are antibodies and cytokines. Antibodies, which are produced and secreted by B cells, consist of one to several units each containing two heavy and two light chains. The heavy chain region (Fc) is constant and is bound to the surface membrane of the immune cell. The light chain region (Fab) is hypervariable and is responsible for binding to an antigenic determinant. Antibodies function to mediate cell destruction either by acting as an opsonin, leading to phagocytosis and cell lysis, or through activation of the complement system. Cytokines are soluble protein products involved in the regulation, proliferation, and differentiation of cells of the immune system. They are named according to a function they perform (e.g., TNF, colony-stimulating factor) or by their cell of origin (e.g., lymphokines are derived from lymphocytes, monokines from macrophages).

The Complement System

The complement system consists of at least 12 different plasma proteins that interact in a complex manner with the cells of the immune system. The fragments of the complement system are potent mediators of the immune response. There are two pathways in the complement system, the classic and the alternative. Both pathways eventually lead to cleavage of the C3 fragment, which opsonizes the target antigen, leading to phagocytosis and cell lysis.

Tumor Antigens

Fundamental to this entire discussion of tumor immunology is the concept that tumors have substances on their surfaces (combinations of proteins, lipids, and carbohydrates) that are different qualitatively or quantitatively from those on normal tissues in the host. These substances, called tumor-associated antigens (TAAs), can be detected by the immune system, allowing it to differentiate between the tumor cells and normal cells. In general "spontaneous" tumors, those that arise without purposeful induction by chemicals or viruses, are weakly immunogenic, a feature that obscures their differences from normal tissues and makes tumor recognition by the immune system more problematic.

Since the discovery of blood group antigens by Landsteiner in 1900, antigens specific for the surface of a tumor have been actively sought, mainly through transplantation experiments. It was only with the development of inbred strains of mice that these experiments could be properly performed. Before then, experiments investigating the ability of an animal to accept a tumor transplant were far more a measure of histocompatibility differences than of TAAs, and, of course, gave entirely erroneous conclusions about the immunogenic strength of tumor antigens. Carcinogen-induced tumors were the subject of the first conclusive investigations on the existence of tumor antigens in the 1950s. Prehn and Main (1957) demonstrated that inbred mice could be made specifically resistant to a methylcholanthrene-induced sarcoma by allowing the tumor to grow briefly and then amputating it. Thus true immunity to the tumor developed in the autologous host. Since then, a number of chemically and virally induced tumors have been studied in rodents, always with the finding that TAAs are present on the tumor cells.

It is important to distinguish TAAs from *tumor-specific antigens*, because the former term implies only that the tumor has antigens that are preferentially expressed on it, and not that those antigens are necessarily unique. Thus such things as differentiation antigens and embryonic (fetal) antigens are tumor associated but not unique in the ontogeny of the host. It should be stressed that tumor-specific antigens (i.e., antigens found on tumors and nowhere else in nature) have not been conclusively demonstrated either in animals or in humans. Nevertheless, testing for TAAs may be very useful in detecting the tumor amid normal tissues, or detecting tumor antigens shed into the circulation, provided that there are no cells or soluble materials that are antigenically similar in that environment. Because TAAs appear to be relatively weak immunogens in the autologous host, they may be difficult to demonstrate with the patient's own serum or lymphoid cells as the reactants. However, if antigens are present in higher quantity on tumor cells than on normal tissue, they can be considered functionally "tumor specific" in their distribution (Kan-Mitchell and Mitchell, 1988).

Ethical constraints and genetic heterogeneity prevent transplantation of the tumors among humans to generate a stronger immunologic reaction. The alternative of injecting animals with human tissues to obtain antisera is more feasible, but this approach is subject to several limitations. So many strong antigens on human cells are preferentially recognized by an animal's lymphoid cells that only a small minority of the lymphocytes might detect the weaker tumor antigens. Also, some TAAs might resemble antigens present on normal cells in the animal, which could prevent them from being recognized as immunogens.

Monoclonal antibodies (mAbs), derived mainly from mice, and, more recently, cloned helper or cytotoxic T lymphocytes derived from patients bearing a specific type of cancer, have been the means by which human TAAs have been most conclusively demonstrated. mAbs are prepared by in vitro fusion of lymphoid cells from immunized mice (or more rarely spleen cells from donors immunized with TAAs) with immortalized mouse myeloma cells. These mAbs react to a single antigenic determinant (epitope) and are thus an exquisitely specific and sensitive way of detecting differences between a tumor cell and a normal cell of the same histologic background. In this manner, one can seek the proverbial "needle in the haystack"—that is, the TAAs amid the many other antigens on the tumor cell. Widespread availability of mAbs has revolutionized the histologic diagnosis of malignancies of all kinds, but the therapeutic application of mAbs has been limited by the development of human antimouse antibodies (HAMAs). It is not uncommon for a patient's natural defense system to generate antibodies against the murine markers of epithelial differentiation found on the mAbs, precluding the mAbs from functioning in vivo. Strategies being investigated to reduce the development of HAMAs include immunosuppression of the host, use of smaller murine antibody fragments, recombinant antibodies with substitution of human sequences for murine sequences, and direct cloning of human hypervariable regions with desired binding specificity (Shaw et al, 1988).

Carcinogen-induced tumors in rodents appear to have unique antigens. They are even different from other tumors induced by the same carcinogen in inbred littermates. In direct contrast, virus-induced tumor antigens are characteristic of the inducing virus (Klein, 1968). Specifically, a methylcholanthrene-induced tumor in one DBA/2 mouse is different from a methylcholanthrene-induced tumor in another DBA/2 mouse, whereas a polyoma virus–induced tumor in a C57BL/6 mouse (or even a rat, for that matter) has antigens that indicate that polyoma virus was the inducing agent. This major difference has made it difficult to develop a unitary theory of the cause of cancer, because if, as some suggest, carcinogens simply release latent tumor viruses in the cell, why are not more common antigens found? It is very possible that the individual modifications of fundamentally similar proteins, perhaps belonging to a 96-kDa glycoprotein family (gp96) represented on the tumor cell surface, lead to the apparent uniqueness of carcinogen-induced antigens on each tumor (Srivastava and Old, 1989).

The Immune Response to Tumor Antigens

Many clinical anecdotes suggest that antitumor immunity exists in humans and, in fact, influences the course of malignant disease. The possible involvement of tumor immunity is suggested by the following findings:

1. Spontaneous regression of tumors (rare)
2. Prolonged survival or cure of patients after incomplete removal of malignant lesions
3. Sudden appearance of metastases many years after successful therapy, the tumor having been ostensibly "dormant" in the interim
4. Regression of metastases after removal of the primary lesion (rare)

More direct evidence exists documenting that humans as well as animals can mount an antibody or cell-mediated immune response against tumor cells. Reactivity to autologous tumors, and often to histologically similar tumors, but not to different histotypes of tumors or to normal tissues, has provided the most compelling evidence for specificity. In fact, the reactivity of cloned T cells, derived from single lymphocytes, as well as blocking experiments with the specific histotype of the tumor, have largely resolved earlier controversies surrounding whether the reactivity of peripheral blood lymphocytes, shown in the 1970s, was really tumor specific.

There are two principal components of immunity to tumors, as there are to any antigenic material: (1) humoral immunity (antibodies) and (2) cell-mediated immunity. The latter appears to be more universally important in the rejection of tumors, although some cells (NK cells, LAK cells, and macrophages) require the cooperative participation of antibodies to achieve their maximal effectiveness.

T-cell lymphocytes, including CD4 helper/inducer cells and CD8 cytotoxic cells, are probably the most important type of cell involved in tumor rejection. That distinction is far from absolute, however, because macrophages are the predominant cells found in tumor rejection in animals, and they can also be directly responsible for cytotoxicity in human cancers. Macrophages appear to be influenced by helper T cells in their migration into, and their activation at the site of, the tumor. NK cells, and perhaps polymorphonuclear leukocytes, appear to be more involved in surveillance against tumors rather than rejection of overt masses. Functional classification of lymphocytes (helper, suppressor, cytotoxic) is no longer usefully assigned to specific cluster designations because cells from both clusters have been shown to perform the same functions.

In vitro, sensitized CD8 T cells can lyse tumor cells within 4 to 6 hours after exposure. CD4 T cells also have in vitro cytolytic properties, demonstrating tumor cell death in 16- to 20-hour assays. Nevertheless, it is likely that their major role in vivo is to recruit other effector cells, particularly macrophages, through the production of lymphokines. Interleukin-2 (IL-2), interferon-alpha (INF-α), and interferon-gamma (INF-γ) are lymphokines of interest in tumor immunology in general, and in gynecologic oncology in particular. LAK cells and tumor-infiltrating lymphocytes (TILs), most of which are derived from NK cells, can be stimulated in vitro with high doses of IL-2 to kill transformed cells but not normal cells. The cytolytic activity of NK cells does not depend upon the presence of antibody or the induction of specific immunity (i.e., MHC independent). NK cell activity is most pronounced against established tumor cell lines; in fact there is little histologic evidence that such cells are operative in tumor rejection in vivo. CD4 and CD8 T cells, and especially macrophages, are present at the site of active experimental tumor rejection. Macrophages, after activation by various means, can eliminate tumor cells nonspecifi-

cally (i.e., with or without antibody). The monokines produced by macrophages affect the function of B cells, T cells, and macrophages, thus demonstrating the endocrine and autocrine pathways of these hormones. TNF and IL-1 are examples of monokines. Macrophages also process and present antigens to T cells for antibody production.

Cell-mediated immunity and antibody synthesis are regulated by helper and suppressor cells, which are subpopulations of T cells and macrophages. T cells and macrophages are thus not simply effector cells that kill tumor cells; they also interact considerably with each other as well as the other cells of the immune system. Regulatory cytokines with both stimulatory and inhibitory functions have been isolated from each type of cell.

Antibody synthesis in response to cancer cells occurs in all animals, including humans. Cytotoxic antibodies, which kill tumor cells through the activation of the complement system, may not be as important in vivo as cytophilic antibodies, which arm macrophages and other cells that have receptors for the Fc portion of an antibody. Cytophilic (arming) antibodies enable immunologically neutral macrophages, NK, and active LAK cells to seek out and destroy tumor cells. Together with nonspecific activators of macrophages, such as lymphokines and monokines, the cytophilic antibodies help to create a very potent, directed antitumor cellular response.

The detection of tumor antigens with a patient's serum was a seminal influence of reaffirming the existence of TAAs in humans (Old, 1981). Based on this serologic analysis, three "classes" of antigens were defined. Class 1 antigens are those found uniquely on a patient's own tumor and not on any other, even of the same histologic type of tumor; class 2 antigens are found on all tumors of a certain histologic class (histotype) and on a few other related tumors; and class 3 antigens are found on a wide variety of tumor cells and normal cells. Old and colleagues found that antibody response was most frequent to class 3 antigens, less frequent to class 2 antigens, and rare to class 1 antigens.

Although the T cells are often restricted in their activity by the need to recognize the entire self-MHC complex in addition to the TAAs, in many cases recognition of only one shared allele is sufficient. This recognition process is discussed in more detail here because it has important ramifications for immunotherapy. If one retains Old's terminology, anti-class 2 reactivity is clearly dominant in the cell-mediated response, while anti-class 1 reactivity is rare.

Immunologic Surveillance

If cancer cells are antigenic, why are they not detected when they are present in small numbers and rejected before they can become a frank malignancy? This question has not been completely answered, but it must not be taken as a criticism fatal to the idea that endogenous tumor immunity exists and is important. In fact, to the contrary, it may well be that only when immunity is defective do we develop a malignant tumor. The immunosurveillance theory, first postulated by Thomas and popularized by Burnet (1970), states in its simplest form that cancer cells arise frequently by somatic mutation in every individual, but they are recognized as foreign and destroyed by immunologic mechanisms before a tumor develops.

In patients with an established tumor, there is no question that an antitumor response exists, but it is logistically impossible to determine whether there is antitumor immunity at the time the tumor first develops from a single cell. Thus the evidence for immunologic surveillance against cancer necessarily comes mainly from examples in which its predictions seem to have been borne out clinically. Patients with an immunodeficiency disorder, such as those with T-cell deprivation, would be expected to have a greater than normal frequency of cancers. In fact, this is true. Patients with ataxia-telangiectasia, variable immunodeficiency, or Wiskott-Aldrich syndrome have at least a 200-fold excess risk of cancer over age- and sex-matched controls. Most of these cancers are lymphomas or Hodgkin's disease, and are particularly aggressive forms of these diseases. Similarly, among renal transplant patients, all of whom receive long-term immunosuppressive therapy, there is at least a 300-fold increased incidence of malignancies. Virally induced tumors are more common in animals given antilymphocyte serum chronically, or exposed to thymectomy. Finally, individuals with the acquired immunodeficiency syndrome, whose total lymphocyte count (and particularly CD4 T cell count) is decreased, have a high incidence of Kaposi's sarcoma, Burkitt's lymphoma, carcinoma of the tongue, cloacogenic carcinoma of the rectum, and perhaps other tumors as well (Levine, 1982).

It is not necessary to postulate a complete loss of immunocompetence to explain the loss of surveillance. The extreme examples of profound immunodeficiency states described previously are simply more dramatic evidence supporting the immunosurveillance hypothesis. It is, in fact, more likely that the immunodeficiency that allows for the development of a malignancy is highly selective for the cancer cell (or its etiologic agent) and of short duration. Evidence for the complex nature of immunosurveillance can be found in the immune system alterations in response to certain gynecologic cancers. For example, ovarian cancer patients have been shown to have a decrease in the absolute number of both T and B cells. The T-cell function, however, appears to remain intact in these patients, while B-cell function is defective (Nalick et al, 1974; Mandell et al, 1979). In patients with cervical cancer, defects have been demonstrated in T-cell function, NK cell activity, and the number of effector cells available for antibody-dependent cytotoxicity (Satam et al, 1986). Surveillance is most likely an integrated process performed by many different components of the immune system. Fundamentally, however, the immunosurveillance theory remains a useful hypothesis with which to assess observations on the occurrence of cancer under various circumstances.

Recognition of Tumor-Associated Antigen Peptides by T Cells: Major Histocompatibility Complex Restriction

It was originally thought that only surface antigens were recognized by the immune system. However, T cells can recognize peptides derived from internal (cytoplasmic and inner membrane) antigens, including TAAs, when presented at the surface of a cell bound to a MHC molecule. The peptide becomes associated with a MHC class I molecule in the endoplasmic reticulum and the two make their way to the surface. MHC class I molecules can be found on the cells of most normal tissues as well as on tumor cells. MHC class II molecules are found on lymphocytes, macrophages, endothelial cells, some epithelial cells, and less often cancer cells. Eighty percent of ovarian cancer cell lines express MHC class I molecules, but only 40 percent express MHC class II molecules. Cytotoxic T cells have receptors that recognize the antigenic peptide and the MHC class I molecule together. Inducer T cells recognize peptides presented by MHC class II molecules, and then stimulate the function of other T cells, B cells, and monocytes. If MHC molecules are downregulated in the tumor cells, tumor-associated peptides cannot be presented on the surface and the tumor is functionally non-immunogenic. However, if the tumor cells continue to produce TAA epitopes, the afferent portion of immune stimulation will continue. This immediately suggests a strategy for immunotherapy: upregulation of MHC class I molecules (and at the same time TAAs) on the surface of the tumor cell. The interferons and TNF-α have this ability.

The Escape of Established Tumors from Immunologic Rejection

Regardless of whether immunity plays a role in preventing the occurrence of a cancer, once a frank malignancy is established, there is little doubt that the host can mount an immune response against it. The response may, however, be relatively deficient, failing to reject the cancer. It seems that the mechanisms originally intended to regulate immune responses are in general exaggerated by the presence of the tumor, and may paradoxically foster the tumor's growth. Tumors shed antigens into the circulation, which, by themselves or admixed with host antibody, can stimulate T cells and initiate the secretion of regulatory cytokines (Hellstrom and Hellstrom, 1978; Mitchell, 1976). The secreted cytokines interact through multiple feedback loops and can effect a net increase in immunocompetence or a relative immunosuppression. For example, INF-γ and IL-2, both produced by CD4 cells, increase NK effector cells and cytotoxic T cell–mediated immunity, whereas IL-10, produced by another subtype of CD4 cell, downregulates IFN production and MHC class I expression (Fiorentino et al, 1991; Taga and Tosato, 1992). Other humoral factors, such as alpha$_1$ acid glycoprotein, that are elicited by tumors and can inhibit cell-mediated immunity also may be involved in tumor escape from immunity. It is known that macrophages can produce IL-12, which stimulates production of IFN-γ and IL-2, which in turn feed back positively on macrophages and other cytotoxic cells (Gately, 1993). IL-10, as described earlier, can inhibit IL-12 production.

The role of macrophage suppressor cells in the perpetuation of a cancer is beginning to be delineated. IL-1, IL-6, and TNF-α, which are cytokines produced by activated macrophages, have all been shown to have immunosuppressive properties and to inhibit the growth and function of T and B cells. Macrophage suppressor functions may also be related to epiphenomena associated with cancers, such as the impaired hypersensitivity seen in skin test anergy and the deficient cell-mediated reactivity to microorganisms in Hodgkin's disease.

Tumor cells, usually only weekly immunogenic to begin with, further lose immunogenicity through prolonged residency in the host and immunoselection, a phenomenon called "antigenic modulation." Not only are TAAs lost, but MHC molecules are also lost, most critically MHC class I molecules. This makes it difficult or impossible for the T-cell receptor of killer T cells to recognize the peptide epitopes of the TAAs, because they cannot be brought to the cell surface in the proper context.

Types of Immunotherapy

There are five categories by which to classify most existing forms of immunotherapy. However, it should be noted that the field is rapidly expanding and new strategies that affect the growth and regulation of tumor cells are constantly being investigated. In practice, immunotherapy may actually consist of a combination of two or three treatment categories. The divisions described here are used mainly by convention.

Active Immunotherapy

Active immunotherapy attempts to stimulate the tumor-bearing host to respond more vigorously against the tumor, through augmentation of either specific (T) cells or nonspecific (macrophage, NK) cells. Most of the agents used during the 1970s were nonspecific stimulants of active immunity, such as bacillus Calmette-Guérin and *Propionibacterium acnes* (formerly, *Corynebacterium parvum*). Many of the agents in current use are cytokines produced through molecular engineering. They are best used in humans in combination with specific immunizing substances, such as killed tumor cells or antigenic extracts, rather than by themselves, because they are principally stimulants of macrophages and can affect immunity better, longer, and more specifically when used as true adjuvants.

Adoptive Immunotherapy

Adoptive immunotherapy transfers immunologically active histocompatible (often autologous) lymphoid cells that will be accepted by the host. Adoptive immunotherapy, particularly with transferred T lymphocytes, has been very effective for treatment of rodent leukemias and lymphomas (Greenberg et al, 1982). With the present ability to immunize and clone T cells in vitro, and then expand the number of highly specific cytolytic and helper T cells for adoptive transfer, the capacity to attack tumors by this means is now greater than ever. Bone marrow transplantation, in addition to being a means of replacing hematopoietic stem cells, is also a form of adoptive immunotherapy through its transfer of immunocompetent cells and their precursors.

Restorative Immunotherapy

Restorative immunotherapy attempts to boost the immune response of a host to normal levels before an attempt is made to augment it above those levels. Restorative immunotherapy entails the replenishment of competent effector cells by the administration of thymic hormones or agents such as levamisole that have a similar effect. These materials stimulate precursor cells to differentiate into mature T cells. Antagonism of suppressor T cells by the administration of low-dose cyclophosphamide, and antagonism of suppressor macrophages by the administration of prostaglandin inhibitors (by which suppressor macrophages produce their effect), are other forms of restorative immunotherapy.

Passive Immunotherapy

Passive immunotherapy attempts to supplement the host's existing antibody response by the transferrance of antibodies, particularly mAbs, to attack cancer cells dispersed in the circulation or in ascites, an environment where they are most easily accessible to direct coating by antibodies. Passive immunotherapy was the form of immunotherapy that seemed in the past to have the least likelihood of profound usefulness, since it is by definition a short-lived therapy. Antibodies transferred as part of sera have been of some use in treating rodent leukemias, primarily by "arming" effector cells, but raising the antisera posed a significant problem, as did the transfusion of large amounts of foreign proteins (albumin and globulin) into humans. The advent of mAbs, with their great inherent specificity and potency, has made it possible to give relatively small amounts of protein from foreign species (usually a mouse), reducing the risk of an anaphylactic reaction. Recombinant human mAbs are now being developed and produced in bacteria with a further reduction in cross-reactivity, and cell selection is being used to improve the binding affinity of the antibodies. Conjugates of mAbs with toxins, drugs, and radionuclides are most commonly used.

Cytomodulatory Immunotherapy

Cytomodulatory immunotherapy refers to the upregulation of TAAs, MHC molecules, and accessory molecules on the tumor cell surface to promote recognition of the tumor cell by the immune system. The interferons and certain cytokines, particularly IFN-γ, and IL-2 are cytomodulatory in this way. Lymphokines are also included in this category because they are often injected as growth factors and further stimulants of host-derived cells. The administration of interferons and TNF-α adjunctively with cytotoxic T cells for more efficient and less toxic targeted treatments, may prove to be their major use. The interferons can also have biochemical effects on the cell through upregulation of growth factor receptors and subsequent alterations in the sensitivity of the cell to various chemotherapies (Boente et al, 1992). This activity is cytomodulatory in the larger context of biologic response modification. In fact, the interferons, with their antiviral, antitumor, and immunostimulatory effects, do not fit into any single category of immunotherapy. Similarly the retinoids, which are vitamin A derivatives, have anticarcinogenic and immunostimulatory effects and are another good example of biomodulators that transcend the older category of "immunotherapy."

IMMUNOLOGY OF GYNECOLOGIC CANCER

Although the foregoing principles of tumor immunology and immunotherapy probably apply to all gynecologic cancers, and indeed all malignant diseases, by far the most information regarding the immunology of gynecologic cancer has been accrued from studies on carcinoma of the ovary and carcinoma of the cervix. This is partly attributable to the facts that tumors at both sites are accessible and that ovarian carcinomas in particular grow readily in culture, making in vitro tests of immunologically active cells most feasible. In addition, the growth of ovarian carcinoma in ascites is conducive to immunotherapeutic investigations in which imunnologically active materials are injected directly into the peritoneal cavity in the vicinity of the dispersed tumor cells. Thus, although most examples of the application of immunologic principles in gynecologic cancers are drawn from these two malignancies, the same approaches should be valid for all gynecologic tumors.

Tumor Antigens

Most of the ample evidence that there are TAAs in ovarian cancer is derived from studies with mAbs. It should be noted, however, that none of the antigens thus far identified is tumor specific; rather, all are found in several other tumors, such as gastrointestinal adenocarcinomas, and usually in normal tissues as well (Steplewski et al, 1985).

Bast and his colleagues (1984) developed a monoclonal antibody, OC-125, that detects an antigen known as CA-125 in ovarian carcinomas. CA-125 is released into the blood in quantities that crudely reflect the tumor volume in the patient. Like carcinoembryonic antigen and the antigens detected by mAbs CA-19-9 and CA-15-3, CA-125 is not a tumor-specific antigen. CA-125 is found in many other gynecologic and nongynecologic malignancies, especially adenocarcinomas. However, its near-ubiquitousness in the common epithelial ovarian carcinomas and its absence from most normal tissues, notably normal mesothelial cells, has made CA-125 a useful marker of ovarian cancer. Approximately 85 percent of all ovarian carcinomas have measurable serum levels of the antigen, permitting the course of the disease to be monitored by radiomimetric determinations. The value of serum CA-125 measurements for the early diagnosis of ovarian cancer is limited, particularly in premenopausal women, because serum levels are often elevated by chronic inflammatory conditions such as endometriosis, uterine leiomyomas, and salpingitis.

A number of other mAbs have been developed, some of which detect different antigenic determinants (epitopes) on the same molecule as CA-125, but none has been shown to be superior to CA-125 in monitoring the course of ovarian or any other gynecologic cancer in which CA-125 is expressed. Several researchers have examined the use of multiple tumor markers to distinguish preoperatively benign from malignant ovarian tumors. In general, it can be said that the sensitivity increases as the number of tumor markers in the panel increases. This approach has not proven to be practical, however, because there is a decline in diagnostic specificity with the addition of each tumor marker (Woolas et al, 1995).

A mouse mAb has identified a squamous cell carcinoma antigen (SCA) of cervical origin. The antigen has been employed to monitor the course of that disease. Although the specificity of the SCA radioimmunoassay has been high (approximately 95 percent), its sensitivity is reported to be only 50 to 68 percent. However, when it is present, it has been useful for monitoring the effectiveness of treatment and for post-therapy surveillance (Yazigi et al, 1991).

A valuable study on MHC class I antigen expression in squamous cell carcinoma of the cervix, reported in the Japanese literature by Honma et al (1989), has noted that 21 of 23 cases had a monomorphic (public) determinant of that antigen. However, the full expression of the class I molecule was absent in 9 of 14 cases in which the patient's normal cells had that haplotype. As the authors themselves point out, this may have important implications for the effectiveness of immunotherapy in cervical cancer, emphasizing the possible need for upregulating MHC class I molecules in addition to applying other modes of specific targeted antitumor immunotherapy.

Antibody-Mediated Immunity

As described earlier, patients with ovarian carcinoma have impaired B-cell function and a decrease in the absolute number of circulating B cells. Nonetheless, antibodies that react with ovarian cancer cells, indicating that they are either anti-tumor or autoimmune, have been recovered from the sera and ascites of ovarian cancer patients. The antigens to which these antibodies were bound, however, have not been characterized (Old, 1981; Dawson et al, 1983).

Mitchell and Kohorn (1976) had earlier found "blocking factors" in the serum of patients with ovarian cancer, in a study to be discussed in more detail later. It was not proved that the blocking factors were immune complexes, but studies of similar serum factors in other laboratories have noted many of the same characteristics in their inhibitory activities upon cell-mediated immunity as are seen in (tumor) antigen–(antitumor) antibody complexes purposely produced in vitro (Hellstrom and Hellstrom, 1974). Dawson et al (1983) found that natural killing of ovarian carcinoma cells in vitro is also inhibitable by immune complexes from the serum or ascites of ovarian cancer patients, but they too did not fully demonstrate the element of specificity. Studies with mAbs have re-emphasized that the cytophilic ("arming") property of mAbs is most responsible for their in vivo activity against tumors; this arming effect is more important than the in vitro tumor cell cytotoxicity of the antibodies (Herlyn and Koprowski, 1982).

Cell-Mediated Immunity

DiSaia and colleagues (1971) were among the first to demonstrate the cytotoxicity of partially purified peripheral blood lymphocytes against ovarian carcinoma cells. At approximately the same time, Hellstrom and Hellstrom (1974) showed that cell-mediated immunity to ovarian and several other cancers often coexisted with serum "blocking factors," complexes of tumor antigens and antitumor antibodies that were able to block cell-mediated cytotoxicity in vitro. Later, Mitchell and Kohorn (1976) found lymphocyte-mediated cytotoxicity to short-term cultures of tumor cells obtained from 37 ovarian carcinoma patients. Very little cross-reactivity against nonovarian target cells was noted, and there was likewise little reactivity against ovarian carcinoma cells by lymphocytes from normal subjects or patients with a different type of tumor. The most notable exceptions were the endometrial and cervical cancer patients, who had reactivity in the same range as the ovarian cancer patients. There was no correlation between the clinical stage of the tumor and the level of cell-mediated immunity, and in the 16 patients with serial follow-up, there was no correlation between the level of cell-mediated cytotoxicity and the status of the disease or response to therapy. However, serum blocking factors, which profoundly inhibit the cell-mediated immune response in vitro, were found in the serum preceding or accompanying relapse in 14 of 16 patients, and were lost in two patients during remission. Therapy with alkylating agents such as L-phenylalanine mustard (melphalan) and cyclophosphamide failed to influence cellular immune response.

Some of the strongest support for an in vivo role of NK cells in surveillance against spontaneously occurring human cancer resulted from laboratory studies employing human ovarian cancer cell lines. Shau et al (1983) found that the large granular lymphocytes enriched for NK cells from normal individuals could kill primary and established ovarian carcinoma cell cultures. A common NK recognition determinant was demonstrated on the ovarian cells that was shared by the K562 cell line (a standard myeloid leukemia cell line) through specific inhibition of killing by unlabeled ("cold") target cells. Monocytes did not appear to be involved in this reaction.

More recently, Ioannides and his colleagues (1990, 1991a,b; Ioannides and Freedman, 1991) have provided conclusive evidence of T-cell–mediated specific reactivity against ovarian cancers. Both proliferative and cytotoxic responses to ovarian carcinoma lysates have been noted with peripheral blood lymphocytes, tumor-infiltrating (tumor-associated) lymphocytes, T-cell lines, and several T-cell clones. These lymphocytes reacted against autologous tumors for the most part, but in some instances allogeneic cancers were also killed. As in parallel studies conducted by other investigators in melanoma, each T-cell clone from ovarian cancer appears to recognize one of a rather small number of different epitopes. The presence of a limited number of important antigenic determinants is a favorable sign for success of targeted immunotherapy, with either antibodies or effector lymphocytes, in ovarian carcinoma.

IMMUNOTHERAPY OF GYNECOLOGIC CANCER

The field of tumor immunology is rapidly evolving, and advances in immunotherapy of gynecologic malignancies in particular will certainly continue for many years to come. As outlined previously, studies reported thus far have been conducted principally with ovarian and cervical cancers. For the most part, immunotherapeutic approaches to gynecologic cancer have focused on four areas: (1) the targeting of tumor growth and regulation, including studies on cytokines, interferons, and tumor angiogenesis; (2) cellular immunotherapy; (3) antibody therapy, including the conjugation of antibodies with radionuclides, immunotoxins, and cytotoxic drugs; and (4) tumor vaccines.

Immunotherapy of Tumor Growth and Regulation (Cytomodulatory Immunotherapy)

Most of the work on growth factors and growth factor receptors has focused on the transmembrane tyrosine kinase growth factor receptors. Epidermal growth factor (EGF) receptor (*erb*-B1) and HER-2/*neu* receptor (*erb*-B2) can both be overexpressed in ovarian carcinoma. EGF receptor is thought to be a negative prognostic indicator in ovarian cancer, and overexpression of HER-2/*neu* is associated with a worse prognosis in ovarian, endometrial, and cervical cancer (Khalifa et al, 1994; Kihana et al, 1994). In vitro treatment of normal ovarian epithelial cells with exogenous EGF stimulates growth, whereas growth in ovarian cancer cell lines is often inhibited. Similarly, activation of HER-2/*neu* in ovarian cancer cells can result in growth inhibition. Anti–*erb*-B2 antibodies have a direct antitumor effect both in cell culture and in animal studies (Drebin et al, 1988). In addition, repair of chemotherapy-induced DNA damage is inhibited when anti–*erb*-B2 antibodies are given concomitantly with the chemotherapy. Overexpression of *erb*-B2 has also been shown to increase tumor cell recognition and susceptibility to cytotoxic T cells (Yoshino et al, 1994). This suggests that an antigenic determinant exists on *erb*-B2 that is easily recognized by cytotoxic T cells and could possibly serve as a TAA. Several clinical trials are currently underway targeting *erb*-B2 with anti–*erb*-B2 antibodies and antitumor vaccines.

The cytokines are a group of soluble proteins produced by cells of the immune system whose functions are numerous and diverse, many of them having opposing effects. One of the approaches to immunotherapy has been to increase the effect of the cytokines that inhibit tumor cell growth and/or decrease the activity of those cytokines that suppress the immune system or stimulate tu-

mor growth. As detailed in an earlier section, IFN-γ is produced by cells that mediate delayed hypersensitivity reactions and eliminate chronic infections. IFN-γ, along with other stimulatory cytokines, is involved in the activation of cytotoxic effector cells. In contrast, IL-10 and the class of CD4 cells that produce IL-10 accentuate atopic reactions and perpetuate chronic infections. IL-10 has also been shown to inhibit the production of stimulatory cytokines and to prevent upregulation of MHC molecules on cell surface membranes (Malefyt et al, 1991). It is this negative feedback loop of IL-10 on stimulatory cytokines that is thought to contribute, at least in part, to the relative state of immunosuppression found in the peritoneal cavity. This hypothesis is further supported by the presence of high concentrations of IL-10 in the ascites of ovarian cancer patients (Gotlieb et al, 1992). Interestingly, lymphocytes obtained from the ascites of ovarian cancer patients show an increase in cytotoxic effector cell activity when treated with exogenous IL-2 and IL-12, both of which are stimulatory cytokines (DeCesare et al, 1995).

Intraperitoneal therapy, designed to alter the endogenous immunoregulatory balance, has met with varied success in clinical trials. Edwards et al (1995) reported on the use of intraperitoneal IL-2 in patients with chemorefractory ovarian cancer. They reported an overall response rate of 26 percent, with seven complete responses and two partial responses confirmed at laparotomy. Six of the 34 evaluable patients in the study were alive and free of disease at 5-year follow-up. Studies using intraperitoneal recombinant IFN-α have consistently yielded a response rate of 30 to 45 percent in patients with advanced or recurrent ovarian carcinoma (Berek et al, 1985; Willemse et al, 1990). Responses were limited to patients whose residual tumor was not greater than 5 mm in maximum diameter, a rather surprising finding because manipulation of the "immune environment" would not seem to be dependent upon absorption of the cytokine into the solid tumor. Intraperitoneal IFN-γ has been shown to increase the tumoricidal activity of cytotoxic effector cells and to increase the expression of MCH class II molecules on cancer cells. In a study of 108 ovarian cancer patients with residual disease confirmed at second-look laparotomy, Pujade-Lauraine et al (1996) reported a 32 percent response rate with twice-weekly administration of intraperitoneal IFN-γ for 3 to 4 months. The complete response rate improved to 41 percent for patients younger than 60 years with residual tumor less than 2 cm in maximum diameter. The median duration of response was 20 months, and the 3-year survival of responders was 62 percent. These results indicate that adjuvant intraperitoneal cytokine therapy may be effective in ovarian cancer.

Clinical trials employing systemic IFN therapy have been less successful. Overall response rates in advanced ovarian cancer trials have been in the range of 10 to 18 percent. Dose escalation has been limited by the high frequency of severe cytokine toxicity. Improved response rates have been reported in patients with advanced cervical cancer. In one study, IFN-α was given in combination with *cis*-retinoic acid. An overall response rate of 58 percent was reported, but the responses were of short duration and no responses were seen in previously treated patients (Hallum et al, 1995).

TNF-α is a regulatory cytokine that has been isolated from monocytes and macrophages as well as from tumor cells. Because TNF-α is a potent agent against certain murine tumors in vitro, it was thought that it could be used for direct cytotoxic therapy. Human studies, however, have failed to show any antitumor effect, although the dose tolerable in humans is far less than that in mice. Further research has demonstrated that most ovarian cancer cell lines are resistant to TNF-α (although this resistance can be overcome with the use of buthionine sulfoximine, which depletes cellular glutathione), and growth is actually stimulated in some cell lines. In animal studies, exogenous TNF-α has been shown to increase the metastatic behavior of human ovarian cancer cells, leading to an increase in tumor cell growth and implantation. The significance of this finding is unclear because proteins that block the activity of TNF-α receptors have been found in high concentration in the ascites of patients with ovarian cancer. These endogenous blocking factors may therefore limit the biologic effect of TNF-α in vivo. Research efforts have also been directed toward the TNF-α receptor. Clarification of the biologic function(s) of TNF-α will aid in defining its potential as an immunotherapeutic agent.

Other agents involved in tumor growth and regulation that are currently being investigated include tumor angiogenesis factors. Vascular endothelial growth factor (VEGF) and its receptor have been found in high concentrations in the ascites of ovarian cancer patients (Yeo et al, 1993). VEGF is a vascular endothelial mitogen and may contribute to the increased vascular permeability frequently found in ovarian cancer patients. In addition, VEGF is thought to promote tumor angiogenesis. Animal studies have demonstrated a decrease in tumor cell proliferation using antibodies directed against the VEGF receptor (Kim et al, 1993). Phase I and II clinical trials are currently underway using other molecules that selectively inhibit tumor angiogenesis.

Cellular Immunotherapy (Adoptive Immunotherapy)

Cellular immunotherapy transfers cytotoxic effector cells into the host. Non—MHC-restricted cells, such as LAK cells, NK cells, and macrophages, are able to kill tumor cells after systemic adoptive transfer, but they localize to tumor sites poorly. Concomitant use of IL-2 has been successful in improving antitumor activity of these cells; however, despite the improved efficacy, frequent cytokine toxicity continues to limit the systemic use of these cytotoxic effector cells. Given the pattern of spread of ovarian carcinoma, there has been enthusiasm for direct intraperitoneal transfer of activated effector cells with IL-2 as a way of reducing systemic toxicity and improving the localization of the immune response. Unfortunately, intraperitoneal administration has not resulted in improved tumor regression, and, in fact, such treatment has been further complicated by the development of abdominal pain, ascites, and peritoneal fibrosis (Stewart et al, 1990).

Efforts to improve tumor targeting have included the use of autologous antigen-specific cells such as TILs and lymphocytes retargeted with bispecific mAbs. Activation of TILs into CD8 cytotoxic effector cells has been demonstrated in several ovarian carcinoma lines (Wang et al, 1989). The preliminary results from clinical studies using TILs to treat patients with advanced ovarian cancer have been difficult to interpret because the TILs have been used in combination with several different chemotherapeutic agents (Aoki et al, 1991). A phase II trial in women with advanced ovarian cancer employing serial intraperitoneal infusions of IL-2 and autologous lymphocytes retargeted with a mAb to the folate receptor on ovarian cancer cells showed an overall intraperitoneal response rate of 27 percent (Canevari et al, 1995). Of the 28 patients who entered the trial, 3 showed a complete response (11 percent) and 4 had a partial response, although one of these had complete clearing of the intraperitoneal disease. Twelve patients had progression of disease documented at the conclusion of the treatment. Side effects were reported to be mild to moderate. Nonetheless, because of the severity of the toxicity in previous studies and the overall limited therapeutic benefit, clinical trials utilizing cellular immunotherapy for gynecologic malignancies have been relatively few.

Antibody Therapy (Passive Immunotherapy)

mAbs have been investigated in a large number of immunotherapeutic studies on gynecologic malignancies. In these studies the mAbs are typically of murine origin and directed against ovarian cancer TAAs. Murine mAbs are not commonly known to have directed antitumor activity, so their therapeutic application often depends upon conjugation to a radionuclide, drug, or other agent that is toxic to the tumor cell. One exception to this general statement is the group of mAbs directed against growth factors and their receptors. As previously discussed, antibodies directed against *erb*-B2 have been shown to have direct antitumor effects.

Conjugates composed of mAbs and radionuclides have been used both for imaging and for therapy. The dose of radiation delivered is dependent upon the type of isotope employed, the specificity of the tumor binding, the depth of tumor penetration, and the systemic clearance. Approaches designed to improve the specificity of binding and delivery of the radionuclide to the tumor cell hold the most promise. Intraperitoneal administration of mAbs conjugated with radionuclides represents a potentially effective form of therapy for ovarian cancer. This route of delivery increases tumor localization and minimizes the potential for systemic side effects. Most clinical studies have used conjugates of ^{131}I. This isotope is readily available, and because it emits both gamma and beta particles, it has both imaging and therapeutic applications. One conjugate of interest is ^{131}I-labeled OC-125. However, although theoretically useful, Finkler et al (1989) reported only 3 responses, all partial, among 20 ovarian cancer patients

treated intraperitoneally with this conjugate. The failure of this therapy may be related to circulating CA-125 antigen, which is thought to interfere with the ability of the mAb to bind preferentially to the tumor. Other factors may also determine the efficacy of this form of therapy. For example Epenetos et al (1987) treated 24 women with drug-resistant ovarian cancer using intraperitoneal ^{131}I-conjugated mAbs directed against four different TAAs. The outcome was directly related to the size of the residual tumor. Three of six patients with microscopic disease had a complete tumor response, whereas there were no responses among the eight patients with residual disease treater than 2 cm.

Other isotopes that have been used in clinical trials are ^{99m}Tc and ^{90}Y. The former is ideal for imaging studies because of its single-photon decay and 6-hour half-life. ^{90}Y, which has a decay path of several millimeters, is capable of delivering a therapeutic dose of radiation to adjacent tumor cells not bound to the mAb.

Immunotoxins and cytotoxic drugs have also been conjugated to mAbs in an attempt to improve tumor localization and to decrease systemic toxicity. Included among the numerous agents that have been conjugated to mAbs are plant and bacterial toxins, in addition to conventional cytotoxic drugs. mAbs to CA-125 conjugated with daunorubicin can lead to the selective killing of ovarian cancer cells in vitro (Sweet et al, 1989). Conjugated daunorubicin enters the cell in higher concentrations than does the free drug or the drug conjugated to nonspecific protein carriers, a phenomenon that was noted previously in studies on melanoma patients by Young and Riesfeld (1988). Most of the clinical trials in this field of immunotherapy have been limited by the development of severe, unexpected toxicity. For the conjugated agent to have its cytotoxic effect, the cell must internalize the antigen-antibody-toxin complex. Many antigens have been found in normal human tissues that cross-react with mAbs directed against tumor cells. This cross-reactivity, which may not be detected prior to the clinical trial, need not be very strong for a toxic level of the cytotoxic agent to accumulate within normal cells. Antibodies must be developed that are directed less against shared epitopes and more specifically against TAAs. Animal studies may aid in predicting toxic side effects, but they too are quite limited in their usefulness because human tissues do not share many antigens in common with nonprimates.

Tumor Vaccines (Specific Active Immunotherapy)

Freedman and colleagues have described the use of tumor cells infected with harmless viruses, usually influenza virus, as a vaccine to treat or prevent the recurrence of ovarian, vulvar, and cervical carcinomas (Freedman et al, 1988, 1989; Ioannides and Freedman, 1989; Ioannides et al, 1989). Preparations of crude tumor cell membranes from virus-infected cultures elicited stronger delayed-type hypersensitivity skin reactions in patients with these tumors than did unmodified tumor cell membrane preparations. There was a tendency to cross-reactivity, such that patients with cervical cancer often reacted to the virus-augmented ovarian carcinoma skin test material.

Forty patients with advanced ovarian cancer, 31 of whom had ascites and 5 with pleural effusions, were treated with intraperitoneal injections of viral oncolysates of two cultured ovarian cell lines (Freedman et al, 1988). Ascites disappeared in seven patients, five of whom had a decrease in malignant cells in the ascites. Two of these five patients, and two others without ascites, had masses that shrank after treatment. Pleural effusions were successfully treated with a single intrapleural injection of the oncolysates in two of the nine patients who responded to intraperitoneal injections.

Responses lasted from 3 to 19 months, with survivals ranging from 4 to 42 months. The long survivals in some of he patients are very promising and may represent a feature of biologic treatment that is at once more difficult to prove and yet more pronounced than any other. Suggestions of the same effect (i.e., longer overall survival) have been found in many other studies with tumor vaccines, even where patients have not experienced a major clinical regression of tumor masses (Mitchell, 1992). The toxicity of the regimen, characterized by fever, nausea, anorexia, malaise, abdominal pain, and arthralgias, was generally tolerable. Only two of the patients in the study were forced to discontinue treatment because of toxicity.

It was somewhat disappointing that a randomized trial of adjunctive viral oncolysate added to radiation therapy in the treatment of cervical cancer failed to show an advantage for the combination regimen (Freedman et al, 1989). Of the 75 patients in this study, 51 relapsed by the time of the report, with a median survival time of 29 months and a median progression-free interval of 18 months, with no differences between the two arms. Clinical trials are continuing in ovarian and cervical cancer patients, as well as in nongynecologic malignancies such as melanoma, with analogous materials.

Nonspecific Active Immunotherapy

Scarification with bacillus Calmette-Guérin has been reported to improve the rate of remission, its duration, and the survival of patients receiving chemotherapy for ovarian cancer (Alberts et al, 1989). Intraperitoneal administration of *P. acnes* has been used to nonspecifically enhance the antitumor activity of leukocytes in the ascitic fluid of ovarian carcinoma patients. NK activity and antibody-dependent cellular cytotoxicity in the peritoneal cavity were both augmented (Bast et al, 1983). These studies have not been substantiated and represent rare examples of apparent therapeutic benefit conferred by nonspecific active immunotherapy in any type of tumor. However, with the advent of better forms of immunotherapy, it is unlikely that this type of therapy will be addressed in the foreseeable future.

SUMMARY AND CONCLUSIONS

Although development of the field of cancer immunology as applied to gynecologic malignancies is only in its early stages, it is already clear that these tumors are governed by the same immunologic principles as other tumors. Fundamental observations remain to be made about the nature of the antigens in these tumors, which should be facilitated by the advent of several important new mAbs. The application of newer immunologically active agents, such as IL-2, mAbs with killer molecules attached to them, and immunogenic tumor vaccines, promises interesting results judging from experience with other types of tumors. Although surgery, radiation therapy, and chemotherapy are often useful in the standard treatment of gynecologic cancers, and are not likely to be supplanted, immunologically based therapy (biomodulation) has a vast potential to improve the outlook with these difficult tumors.

REFERENCES

Alberts DS, Mason-Liddil N, O'Toole RV, Abbott TM: Randomized phase III trial of chemoimmunotherapy in patients with previously untreated stages III and IV suboptimal disease ovarian cancer: a Southwest Oncology Group Study. Gynecol Oncol 32:8, 1989.

Aoki Y, Takakuwa K, Kodama S, et al: Use of adoptive transfer of tumor-infiltrating lymphocytes alone or in combination with cisplatin-containing chemotherapy in patients with epithelial ovarian cancer. Cancer Res 51:1934, 1991.

Bast JS, Berek J, Obrist R, et al: Intraperitoneal immunotherapy of human ovarian carcinoma with Corynebacterium parvum. Cancer Res 43:1395, 1983.

Bast RC, Klug TL, Schaetzl E, et al: Monitoring human ovarian carcinoma with a combination of CA 125, CA 19-9 and carcinoembryonic antigen. Am J Obstet Gynecol 149:553, 1984.

Berek JS, Hacker NF, Lichtenstein A, et al: Intraperitoneal recombinant alpha-interferon for "salvage" immunotherapy in stage III epithelial ovarian cancer: a Gynecologic Oncology Group study. Cancer Res 45:4447, 1985.

Boente MP, Berchuck A, Rodriguez GC, et al: The effect of interferon-gamma on epidermal growth factor receptor expression in normal and malignant ovarian epithelium. Am J Obstet Gynecol 167:1877, 1992.

Burnet FM: The concept of immunologic surveillance. Prog Exp Tumor Res 13:1, 1970.

Canevari S, Stoter G, Arienti F, et al: Regression of advanced ovarian carcinoma by intraperitoneal treatment with autologous T lymphocytes retargeted by a bispecific monoclonal antibody. J Natl Cancer Inst 87:1463, 1995.

Dawson JR, Lutz PM, Shau H: The humoral response to gynecologic malignancies and its role in the regulation of tumor growth: a review. Am J Reprod Immunol 3:12, 1983.

DeCesare SL, Michelini-Norris B, Blanchard DK, et al: Interleukin-12-mediated tumoricidal activity of patient lymphocytes in an autologous in vitro ovarian cancer assay system. Gynecol Oncol 57:86, 1995.

DiSaia PJ, Rutledge FW, Smith JP, et al: Cell mediated immunologic response in two gynecologic tumors. Cancer 28:1129, 1971.

Drebin JA, Link VC, Greene MI: Monoclonal antibodies specific for the *neu* oncogene product directly mediate antitumor effects in vivo. Oncogene 2:387, 1988.

Edwards RP, Lembersky BC, Kunschner AJ, et al: Intraperitoneal interleukin-2 (IL-2) produces durable responses for refractory ovarian cancer. Proc Am Soc Clin Oncol 14:333, 1995.

Epenetos AA, Munro AJ, Stewart S, et al: Antibody-guided irradiation of advanced ovarian cancer with intraperitoneally administered radiolabeled monoclonal antibodies. J Clin Oncol 5:1890, 1987.

Finkler NJ, Muto MG, Kassis AI, et al: Intraperitoneal radiolabeled OC 125 in patients with advanced ovarian cancer. Gynecol Oncol 34:339, 1989.

Fiorentino DF, Zlotnick A, Vieira P, et al: IL-10 acts on the antigen-presenting cell to inhibit cytokine production by Th1 cells. J Immunol 146:3444, 1991.

Freedman RS, Bowen JM, Atkinson EN, et al: Randomized comparison of viral oncolysates plus radiation and radiation alone in uterine cervix carcinoma. Am J Clin Oncol 12:244, 1989.

Freedman RS, Edwards CL, Bowen JM, et al: Viral oncolysates in patients with advanced ovarian cancer. Gynecol Oncol 29:337, 1988.

Gately MK: Interleukin-12: a recently discovered cytokine with potential for enhancing cell-mediated immune responses to tumors. Cancer Invest 11:500, 1993.

Gotlieb WH, Abrams JS, Watson JM, et al: Presence of interleukin-10 (IL-10) in the ascites of patients with ovarian and other intra-abdominal cancers. Cytokine 4:385, 1992.

Greenberg PD, Cheever MA, Fefer A: Prerequisite for successful adoptive immunotherapy: nature of effector cells and role of H-2 restriction. In Fefer A, Goldstein AL (eds): The Potential Role of T Cells in Cancer Therapy. New York, Raven Press, 1982, p 31.

Hallum AV III, Alberts DS, Lippman SM, et al: Phase II study of 13-cis-retinoic acid plus interferon-alpha 2a in heavily pretreated squamous carcinoma of the cervix. Gynecol Oncol 56:382, 1995.

Hellstrom KE, Hellstrom I: Evidence that tumor antigens enhance tumor growth *in vivo* interacting with a radiosensitive (suppressor?) cell population. Proc Natl Acad Sci USA 75:436, 1978.

Hellstrom KE, Hellstrom I: Lymphocyte-mediated cytotoxicity and blocking serum activity to tumor antigens. Adv Immunol 18:209, 1974.

Herlyn D, Koprowski H: IgG$_{2a}$ monoclonal antibodies inhibit human tumor growth through interaction with effector cells. Proc Natl Acad Sci USA 49:4761, 1982.

Honma S, Nakamura M, Maruhashi T, et al: Immunohistochemical study on the MHC class I antigen expression on squamous cell carcinoma of the uterine cervix. Nippon Sanka Fujinka Gakkai Zasshi 41:813, 1989.

Ioannides CG, Freedman RS: T cell responses to ovarian tumor vaccines: identification and significance for future immunotherapy. Int Rev Immunol 7:349, 1989.

Ioannides CG, Freedman RS: Selective usage of TCR V beta in tumor-specific CTL lines isolated from ovarian tumor-associated lymphocytes. Anticancer Res 11:1919, 1991.

Ioannides CG, Platsoucas CD, Freedman RS: Immunologic effects of tumor vaccines: II. T cell responses directed against cellular antigens in the viral oncolysates. In Vivo 4:17, 1990.

Ioannides CG, Platsoucas CD, O'Brian CA, et al: Viral oncolysates in cancer treatment: immunological mechanisms of action. Anticancer Res 9:535, 1989.

Ioannides CG, Platsoucas CD, Rashed S, Kim YP: Cytotoxic T cell clones isolated from ovarian tumor-infiltrating lymphocytes recognize multiple antigenic epitopes on autologous tumor cells. J Immunol 146:1700, 1991a.

Ionnides CG, Platsoucas CD, Rashed S, et al: Tumor cytolysis by lymphocytes infiltrating ovarian malignant ascites. Cancer Res 51:4257, 1991b.

Kan-Mitchell J, Mitchell MS: Human monoclonal antibodies for the diagnosis of tumors. In Kupchik HZ (ed): In Vitro Diagnosis of Human Tumors Using Mono-clonal Antibodies. New York, Marcel Dekker, 1988, p 289.

Khalifa MA, Mannel RS, Haraway SD, et al: Expression of EGFR, HER-2/neu, P53, and PCNA in endometrioid, serous papillary, and clear cell endometrial adenocarcinomas. Gynecol Oncol 53:84, 1994.

Kihana T, Tsuda H, Teshima S, et al: Prognostic significance of the overexpression of c-*erb*B-2 protein in adenocarcinoma of the uterine cervix. Cancer 73:148, 1994.

Kim KJ, Li B, Winer J, et al: Inhibition of vascular endothelial growth factor-induced angiogenesis suppresses tumor growth in vivo. Nature 362:841, 1993.

Klein G: Tumor specific transplantation antigens: GHA Clowes Memorial Lecture. Cancer Res 28:625, 1968.

Levine AS: The epidemic of acquired immune dysfunction in homosexual men and its sequelae—opportunistic infections, Kaposi's sarcoma, and other malignancies: an update and interpretation. Cancer Treat Rep 1391, 1982.

Malefyt RW, Abrams J, Bennett B, et al: Interleukin 10 (IL-10) inhibits cytokine synthesis by human monocytes: an autoregulatory role of IL-10 produced by monocytes. J Exp Med 174:1209, 1991.

Mandell GL, Fisher FI, Bostick F, Young RC: Ovarian cancer: a solid tumor with evidence of normal cellular immune function but abnormal B-cell function. Am J Med 66:621, 1979.

Mitchell MS: Role of "suppressor" T-lymphocytes in antibody-induced inhibition of cytophilic antibody receptors. Ann N Y Acad Sci 276:229, 1976.

Mitchell MS (ed): The Biological Approach to Cancer Treatment: Biomodulation. New York, McGraw-Hill, 1992.

Mitchell MS: Principles of tumor immunology and their application to the biomodulation of cancer. In Calabresi P, Schein PS (eds): Medical Oncology, 2nd ed. New York, McGraw-Hill, 1993, p 323.

Mitchell MS, Kohorn EI: Cell-mediated immunity and blocking factor in ovarian carcinoma. Obstet Gynecol 48:590, 1976.

Nalick RH, DiSaia PJ, Rea TH, Morrow CP: Immunocompetence and prognosis in patients with gynecologic cancer. Gynecol Oncol 2:81, 1974.

Old LJ: Cancer immunology: the search for specificity. GHA Clowes Memorial Lecture. Cancer Res 41:361, 1981.

Prehn RT, Main JM: Immunity to methylcholanthrene-induced sarcoma. J Natl Cancer Inst 18:769, 1957.

Pujade-Lauraine E, Guastalla J-P, Columbo N, et al: Intraperitoneal recombinant interferon gamma in ovarian cancer patients with residual disease at second-look laparotomy. J Clin Oncol 14:343, 1996.

Satam MN, Suraiya JN, Nadkarm JJ: Natural killer and antibody-dependent cellular cytotoxicity in cervical carcinoma patients. Cancer Immunol Immunother 23:56, 1986.

Shau H, Koren HS, Dawson JR: Human natural killing against ovarian carcinoma. Br J Cancer 47:687, 1983.

Shaw DR, Khazaeli MB, LoBuglio AF: Mouse/human chimeric antibodies to a tumor-associated antigen: biologic activity of the four human IgG subclasses. J Natl Cancer Inst 80:1553, 1988.

Srivastava PK, Old LJ: Gp96 molecules: recognition elements in tumor immunity. In Metzgar RS, Mitchell MS (eds): Human Tumor Antigens and Specific Tumor Immunity. New York, Alan R. Liss, 1989, p 63.

Steplewski Z, Sears HF, Koprowski H: Monoclonal antibodies against gastrointestinal tumor associated antigens. In Reif AE, Mitchell MS (eds): Immunity to Cancer. Orlando, FL, Academic Press, 1985, p 97.

Stewart JA, Belinson JL, Moore AL, et al: Phase I trial of intraperitoneal recombinant interleukin-2/lymphokine-activated killer cells in patients with ovarian cancer. Cancer Res 50:6302, 1990.

Sweet F, Roski LO, Sommers GM, Collins JL: Daunorubicin conjugated to a monoclonal anti-CA125 antibody selectivity kills human ovarian cancer cells. Gynecol Oncol 34:305, 1989.

Taga K, Tosato G: IL-10 inhibits T cell proliferation and IL-2 production. J Immunol 148:1143, 1992.

Wang YL, Si LS, Kanbour A, et al: Lymphocytes infiltrating human ovarian tumors: synergy between TNF alpha and IL-2 in the generation of CD8+ effectors from TILS. Cancer Res 49:5979, 1989.

Willemse PHB, DeViries EGE, Mulder NH, et al: Interperitoneal human recombinant interferon-alpha-2b in minimal residual ovarian cancer. Eur J Cancer 26:353, 1990.

Woolas RP, Conaway MR, Xu FJ, et al: Combinations of multiple serum markers are superior to individual assays for discriminating malignant from benign pelvic masses. Gynecol Oncol 59:111, 1995.

Yazigi R, Munoz AK, Richardson B, Risser R: Correlation of squamous cell carcinoma antigen levels and treatment response in cervical cancer. Gynecol Oncol 41:135, 1991.

Yeo K-T, Wang HH, Nagy JA, et al: Vascular permeability factor (vascular endothelial growth factor) in guinea pig and human tumor and inflammatory effusions. Cancer Res 52:2912, 1993.

Yoshino I, Peoples GE, Goedegebuure PS, et al: Association of Her-2/*neu* expression with sensitivity to tumor-specific CTL in human ovarian cancer. J Immunol 152:2393, 1994.

Young HM, Reisfeld RA: Doxorubicin conjugated with a monoclonal antibody directed to a human melanoma-associated proteoglycan suppresses the growth of established xenografts in nude mice. Proc Natl Acad Sci USA 85:1189, 1988.

19

Molecular Genetics of Gynecologic Cancers

Jeff Boyd

PRINCIPLES OF CANCER MOLECULAR GENETICS

All cancers are genetic in origin, in the sense that the driving force of tumor development is genetic mutation. A given tumor may arise through the accumulation of mutations that are exclusively somatic in origin, or through the inheritance of a mutation(s) through the germline, followed by the acquisition of additional somatic mutations. These two genetic scenarios distinguish what are colloquially referred to as "sporadic" and "hereditary" cancers, respectively (Fig. 19–1). Although the neoplastic phenotype is partially derived from epigenetic alterations in gene expression, the sequential mutation of cancer-related genes, with their subsequent selection and accumulation in a clonal population of cells, are the determinant factors as to whether a tumor develops and the time required for its development and progression. The data to support this multistep, multigenic paradigm are extensive (Bishop, 1991; Boyd and Barrett, 1990; Vogelstein and Kinzler, 1993; Weinberg, 1989), but perhaps the most compelling evidence is that the age-specific incidence rates for most human epithelial tumors increase at roughly the fourth to eighth power of elapsed time, suggesting that a series of four to eight genetic alterations are rate limiting for cancer development (Renan, 1993).

Genetic alterations in cancer cells have been described thus far in two major families of genes: oncogenes (Hunter, 1991) and tumor suppressor genes (Weinberg, 1991). Proteins encoded by oncogenes may generally be viewed as stimulatory and those encoded by tumor suppressor genes as inhibitory to the neoplastic phenotype; mutational activation of proto-oncogenes to oncogenes and mutational inactivation of tumor suppressor genes must both occur for cancer development to take place. Proto-oncogene mutations are nearly always somatic; two known exceptions involve the *RET* and *MET* proto-oncogenes, mutations of which may be inherited through the germline, predisposing to multiple endocrine neoplasia type 2 (Hofstra et al, 1994), and papillary renal carcinoma (Schmidt et al, 1997), respectively. Tumor suppressor gene mutations may be inherited or acquired somatically. Other than the previously noted exceptions, all hereditary cancer syndromes for which predisposing genes have been identified are linked to tumor suppressor genes.

Oncogenes

Oncogenes result from gain-of-function mutations in their normal cellular counterpart proto-oncogenes, the normal function of which is to drive cell proliferation in the appropriate contexts. Activated oncogenes behave in a dominant fashion at the cellular level; that is, cell proliferation or development of the neoplastic phenotype is stimulated following the mutation of only one allele. This class of genes was originally discovered through studies of the mechanism of retroviral tumorigenesis (Bishop, 1983), which involves viral transduction of the vertebrate proto-oncogene and re-integration into the host genome under the transcriptional control of viral promoters, such that expression is constitutive and thus oncogenic. The most common mechanisms for muta-

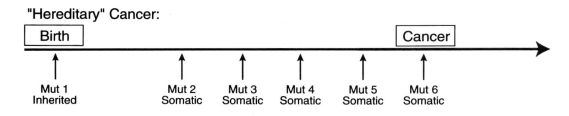

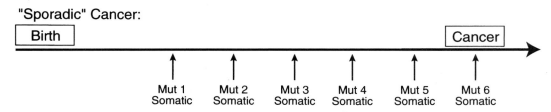

FIGURE 19–1. All cancers are genetic. "Hereditary" cancers differ from "sporadic" cancers by virtue of association with a predisposing mutation inherited through the germline. In contrast, all of the mutations associated with sporadic tumorigenesis are acquired somatically.

tional activation of human proto-oncogenes are gene amplification, typically resulting in overexpression of an otherwise normal protein product; point mutation, generally leading to constitutive activation of a mutant form of the protein product; and chromosomal translocation, which usually results in juxtaposition of the oncogene with the promoter region of a constitutively expressed gene, thus resulting in overexpression of the oncogene-encoded protein. This latter mechanism is most common in hematopoietic malignancies, while the first two are more common in solid cancers. The oncogenes most relevant to human solid malignancies, their mechanism of activation and biochemical function, and the tumor types most often affected by each are summarized in Table 19–1.

Tumor Suppressor Genes

The protein products of tumor suppressor genes normally function to inhibit cell proliferation and are inactivated through loss-of-function mutations. Knudson's two-hit model established the paradigm for tumor suppressor gene recessivity at the cellular level, wherein both alleles must be inactivated in order to exert a phenotypic effect on tumor-

igenesis (Knudson, 1985). The most common mutations observed in tumor suppressor genes are point mutations, either missense or nonsense, microdeletions or insertions of one or several nucleotides causing frameshifts, large deletions, and, rarely, translocations. A mutation in one allele, whether germline or somatic, is then revealed following somatic inactivation of the homologous wild-type allele. In theory, the same spectrum of mutational events could contribute to inactivation of the second allele, but what is typically observed in tumors is homozygosity or hemizygosity for the first mutation, indicating loss of the wild-type allele. As originally demonstrated for the retinoblastoma susceptibility gene (Cavenee et al, 1983), loss of the second allele may occur through mitotic nondisjunction or recombination mechanisms, or large deletions. This so-called loss of heterozygosity (LOH) has become recognized as the hallmark of tumor suppressor gene inactivation at a particular genomic locus. Laboratory methods for detection of LOH are discussed later in this chapter. Table 19–2 summarizes the known tumor suppressor genes, their chromosomal locations and suspected biochemical functions, and the hereditary and sporadic tumors with which they are most commonly associated.

TABLE **19–1**

Summary of Representative Oncogenes Mutated in Human Solid Cancers

Gene	Chromosomal Location	Function	Mutation	Tumor*
RAS (K-, H-, N-)	12p12, 11p15, 1p13	Membrane-associated GTPase; signal transduction	Point mutation (codons 12, 13, or 16)	Many
ERBB-2[†]	17q12-q21	Transmembrane tyrosine kinase receptor	Gene amplification	Breast, ovary, endometrium
MYC (C-, N-, L-)	8q24, 1p34, 2p24	Transcription factor	Gene amplification	C: many N: neuroblastoma L: lung
MDM2	12q14-q15	p53-binding protein	Gene amplification	Sarcomas
RET	10q11	Transmembrane tyrosine kinase receptor	Point mutation	Endocrine
MET	7q31	Transmembrane tyrosine kinase receptor	Point mutation	Renal
CCND2 (cyclin D1)	11q13	Cell cycle regulator	Gene amplification	Many

*Carcinoma, unless otherwise specified.
[†]ERBB-2 same as HER-2/neu.

TABLE **19–2**

Summary of Representative Tumor Suppressor Genes Mutated in Human Solid Cancers

Gene	Chromosomal Location	Function	Tumors* Hereditary	Sporadic
RB1	13q14	Cell cycle regulator	Retinoblastoma, osteosarcoma	Retinoblastoma, sarcomas, bladder, breast, lung
WT1	11p13	Transcription factor	Wilms' tumor	Wilms' tumor
P53	17p13	Transcription factor; regulator of cell cycle, apoptosis	Li-Fraumeni syndrome	Many
APC	5q21-q22	Signal transduction	Familial adenomatous polyposis	Colorectal, gastric
VHL	3p26-p25	Transcriptional elongation	von Hippel-Lindau syndrome	Renal
hMSH2, hMLH1, hPMS2	2p16, 3p21, 7p22	DNA mismatch repair	Hereditary nonpolyposis colorectal cancer syndrome	Colorectal, endometrial
BRCA1	17q12-21	Transcription factor; DNA repair	Breast, ovary, prostate	Ovary (rare)
BRCA2	13q12	DNA repair	Breast, ovary, others	Ovary (rare)
NF1	17q11	Negative regulator of Ras	Neurofibromatosis	None
DPC4	18q21	TGF-β signaling pathway	None	Pancreatic
CDKN2A (p16)	9p21	Negative regulator of cyclin D	Melanoma	Many
PTEN (MMAC1)	10q24	Phosphatase	Cowden disease	Many

*Carcinoma, unless otherwise specified.

Molecular Tumorigenesis

A human cancer represents the endpoint of a long and complex process involving multiple changes in genotype and phenotype. Human solid tumors are monoclonal in nature; every cell in a given malignancy may be shown to have arisen from a single progenitor cell. As proposed by Nowell (1976), the process through which a cell and its offspring sustain and accumulate multiple mutations, with the stepwise selection of variant sublines, is known as clonal evolution or clonal expansion (Fig. 19–2). A long-term goal in studying the molecular genetics of a particular tumor type is to catalog the specific genes that are affected by mutations and the relative order in which they are affected, and, ultimately, to use this molecular blueprint to improve methods of diagnosis, prognostication, and treatment. This task will undoubtedly prove difficult, however, because a defining characteristic of cancer is genetic instability (Loeb, 1991). There are multiple types of such instability, operative at both the chromosomal and molecular levels. Distinguishing the genetic mutations that are simply the by-product of genetic instability from those that are critical to the neoplastic phenotype or, indeed, responsible for increasing genetic instability of one form or another is among the greatest challenges to be faced in cancer research.

The greatest progress in this context has clearly been achieved for colorectal cancer, and a model has been proposed that applies molecular detail for this particular cancer type to the general paradigm of multistep tumorigenesis and clonal evolution. In addition to the demonstration that most colon cancer cell lines are affected by one of two types of genetic instability (Lengauer et al, 1997), specific molecular genetic alterations have been shown to occur at discrete stages of neoplastic progression in the colon: for example, mutation of the *APC* tumor suppressor gene at a very early stage of hyperproliferation, mutation of the *K-RAS* oncogene in the progression of early to intermediate adenoma, and mutation of the *P53* tumor suppressor gene in the progression of late adenoma to carci-

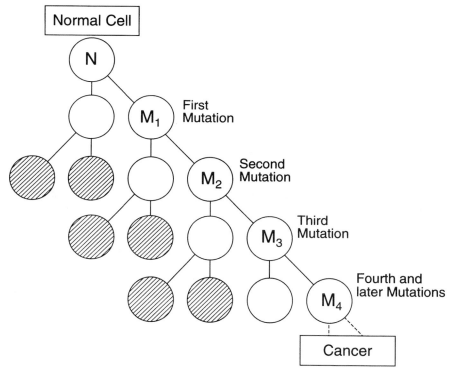

FIGURE 19–2. Model of clonal evolution in neoplasia. Following the initiating mutation in a normal cell, stepwise genetic mutations and selective pressures result in a cancer consisting of a clonal population of cells all derived from the original progenitor cell. Each critical mutation in the evolving tumor may be viewed as having provided a selective advantage leading to clonal expansion.

noma (Fearon and Vogelstein, 1990). Several features of colorectal cancer facilitate this type of characterization, including the well-defined histopathologic progression of normal colonic epithelium to cancer and the accessibility of the various premalignant lesions for molecular analyses, as well as the occurrence of some of these genetic mutations in unusually large fractions of all colorectal tumors. The model is limited in applicability to other cancer types, however, because nonmalignant precursor lesions for many solid tumor types (e.g., ovarian cancer) are not readily detectable, and few molecular genetic changes have been described that occur in major fractions of other cancer types.

HEREDITARY GYNECOLOGIC CANCERS

It has long been recognized that a family history of cancer confers one of the greatest risks of all known factors, and endometrial carcinoma and epithelial ovarian carcinoma both occur as components of cancer predisposition syndromes. As defined earlier, hereditary cancers are those associated with the inheritance of a mutant genetic allele through the germline, conferring predisposition to the development of one or more cancer types. Extraordinary progress has been made in identifying the molecular basis for essentially all of the autosomal dominant, highly penetrant manifestations of endometrial and ovarian carcinoma. It should be stressed that there are likely many other gene variants that confer predisposition to one or another cancer type with lower penetrance, in a recessive fashion, or through interactions with other susceptibility loci, but much less is currently known regarding these types of genes. Thus it is likely that a much larger fraction of all cancers eventually will be regarded as "hereditary" in nature; for the purposes of this discussion, however, "hereditary cancer" will refer to those cancers associated with dominant, highly penetrant loci.

Virtually all hereditary endometrial cancers, probably less than 5 percent of all cases, occur within the context of the hereditary nonpolyposis colorectal cancer (HNPCC) syndrome. The existence of a "site-specific" endometrial cancer syndrome has been postulated (Boltenberg et al, 1990; Lynch et al, 1994; Sandles et al, 1992), but no genetic data exist to support the occurrence of such a phe-

nomenon, which likely represents a rare manifestation of HNPCC. Hereditary ovarian cancers, about 10 percent of all cases, occur primarily within the context of the breast and ovarian cancer syndrome and to a lesser extent as part of the HNPCC syndrome. A "site-specific" form of hereditary ovarian cancer has also been described (Lynch et al, 1991; Narod et al, 1994; Steichen-Gersdorf et al, 1994) but, similarly, this phenomenon appears to represent a variant of the breast and ovarian cancer syndrome, because the same genetic locus (*BRCA1*) is responsible for both.

Hereditary Nonpolyposis Colorectal Cancer Syndrome

Known previously as the cancer family syndrome and Lynch syndromes I and II (depending upon the absence or presence of extracolonic malignancies, respectively), HNPCC is an autosomal dominant genetic syndrome characterized by three or more first-degree relatives with colon or endometrial cancer, at least two of whom were diagnosed with colon cancer at age 50 or younger (Lynch et al, 1993). In addition to cancers of the colon and endometrium, HNPCC family members are at an increased risk for malignancies of other gastrointestinal sites, the upper urologic tract, and the ovary (Watson and Lynch, 1993). Limited data on the risk of ovarian cancer in these families indicate a 3.5-fold increase in the number of cases observed over that expected in the general population (Watson and Lynch, 1993); HNPCC accounts for approximately 10 to 15 percent of all familial ovarian cancer cases (Bewtra et al, 1992). Significant heterogeneity in ovarian cancer frequency is seen among HNPCC families (Watson and Lynch, 1993), suggestive of genetic heterogeneity. Consistent with this observation are linkage data indicative of at least three genetic loci that contribute to the HNPCC phenotype (Lindblom et al, 1993; Nicolaides et al, 1994; Nystrom-Lahti et al, 1994; Peltromäki et al, 1993). The cloning and characterization of the genes responsible for HNPCC have provided significant insights into the etiology of HNPCC-associated tumors and the potential for genetic screening for this disorder.

The HNPCC syndrome arises from an inherited defect in any one of three known genes, *hMSH2* (chromosome 2p), *hMLH1* (chromosome 3p), or *hPMS2* (chromosome

7p) (Fishel and Kolodner, 1995; Marra and Boland, 1995). Although mutations have been described in all three genes, the great majority of HNPCC kindreds appear to be linked to either *hMSH2* or *hMLH1*, and more than 90 percent of all reported mutations affect one of these two genes. The proteins encoded by these genes participate in the same DNA mismatch repair (MMR) pathway, and loss-of-function mutations are associated with genetic instability in the tumors of affected family members (Fishel and Kolodner, 1995; Kolodner, 1995). The MMR genes appear to function as classical tumor suppressors, insofar as the wild-type allele inherited from the unaffected parent is lost or mutated somatically in HNPCC-linked tumors (Hemminki et al, 1994; Leach et al, 1993; Liu et al, 1995).

The genetic instability phenotype associated with defective MMR genes is most readily observed through somatic length alterations in simple repeat sequences [e.g., $(CA)_n$], located throughout the genome and known as "microsatellites." Replication errors in these repeat sequences are probably common, and their inefficient repair results in the "microsatellite instability" phenotype. Since the discovery of mutant MMR genes and the corresponding microsatellite instability, a large number of studies have documented microsatellite instability in many sporadic tumor types, including those not associated with the HNPCC syndrome (Loeb, 1994; Modrich, 1994). Whereas mutations of the MMR genes have been readily identified in many HNPCC kindreds, somatic MMR gene mutations in sporadic tumors with the microsatellite instability phenotype are not commonly detected (Katabuchi et al, 1995; Liu et al, 1995). Thus it is possible that this type of genetic instability arises in sporadic tumors through a different mechanism than in HNPCC-associated cancers. Hypermethylation of the *hMLH1* promoter, resulting in downregulation of its expression, is one such potential mechanism (Kane et al, 1997).

It is not clear how microsatellite instability per se contributes to tumorigenesis in the ovary or in other organs affected by the HNPCC syndrome. Microsatellites exist throughout the genome in predominantly noncoding regions of DNA. Simple repeat sequences are known to occur in the coding regions of genes, however, and their somatic mutation may result in loss of function for genes critical to the regulation of proliferation, invasion, or metastasis. Examples include genes encoding the transforming growth factor (TGF)-beta receptor type II (Markowitz et al, 1995; Parsons et al, 1995), the regulator of apoptosis, Bax protein (Rampino et al, 1997), and the insulin-like growth factor II receptor (Ouyang et al, 1997), all of which contain homopolymeric microsatellite repeats that are mutated in one or another tumor type with microsatellite instability.

Breast and Ovarian Cancer Syndrome

The breast and ovarian cancer syndrome accounts for 85 to 90 percent of all familial ovarian cancer cases (Bewtra et al, 1992; Narod et al, 1994). The probable genetic relationship of these two malignancies in a hereditary context has been demonstrated in population-based, case-control epidemiologic studies (Go et al, 1983; Lynch et al, 1978; Schildkraut et al, 1989). Families with a total of five or more breast or ovarian cancers in first- or second-degree relatives have been suggested to qualify as having the breast and ovarian cancer syndrome (Easton et al, 1993); alternatively, families that contain at least three cases of early-onset (before age 60 years) breast or ovarian cancer have been similarly classified (Narod et al, 1995a). Following the original report of genetic linkage of early-onset breast cancer families to the *BRCA1* locus (Hall et al, 1990), some breast and ovarian cancer families were shown to demonstrate linkage to *BRCA1* as well (Narod et al, 1991). This finding has been extended such that it is now clear that most breast and ovarian cancer families (76 to 92 percent) are linked to *BRCA1* (Easton et al, 1993; Narod et al, 1995a,b). The variable estimates of linkage are the probable result of genetic heterogeneity. Lower estimates are obtained if all families, including those with cases of male breast cancer, are considered, whereas higher estimates (approaching 100 percent) are obtained if families with cases of male breast cancer or less than two cases of ovarian cancer are excluded (Narod et al, 1995a,b). Most of the breast and ovarian cancer families not linked to *BRCA1* are linked to the *BRCA2* locus on chromosome 13q12-13, especially those with cases of male breast cancer (Narod et al, 1995a,b; Wooster et al, 1994). The incidence of ovarian cancer compared to breast cancer appears to be much lower in *BRCA2*-linked families, however, raising questions pertaining to the penetrance of this gene for ovarian cancer.

BRCA1

Genetic linkage analyses confirmed the existence of a gene on chromosome 17q12-21, named *BRCA1*, that is responsible for approximately 45 percent of early-onset hereditary breast cancers and most cases (>80 percent) of hereditary ovarian cancers occurring within the context of site-specific ovarian cancer, and breast and ovarian cancer syndrome (Easton et al, 1993; Hall et al, 1990; Narod et al, 1991; Steichen-Gersdorf et al, 1994). The discovery of a candidate *BRCA1* gene (Miki et al, 1994) was confirmed by several subsequent studies describing the segregation of inactivating mutations in this gene with disease phenotype in numerous breast and ovarian cancer families (Castilla et al, 1994; Friedman et al, 1994; Simard et al, 1994). Germline mutations in *BRCA1* are commonly seen in ovarian cancer patients with remarkable medical or family histories, such as early age at diagnosis, dual primary cancers of the breast and ovary, and relatives affected by breast or ovarian cancer (Futreal et al, 1994; Shattuck-Eidens et al, 1995; Takahashi et al, 1995), consonant with the linkage data implicating *BRCA1* in most of these cancers.

The *BRCA1* gene consists of 22 coding exons distributed over approximately 100 kb of genomic DNA on chromosome 17q21 (Miki et al, 1994). The 7.8-kb mRNA transcript is expressed most abundantly in the testis and thymus, and at lower levels in the breast and ovary, and encodes a 1,863-residue protein (Miki et al, 1994). Multiple *BRCA1*-specific antibodies detect a 220-kDA protein in the nucleus of cultured cells and normal tissues (Chapman and Verma, 1996; Chen et al, 1995, 1996; Scully et al, 1996). Several domains of potential functional significance include an N-terminal RING-finger domain, a negatively charged region in the C-terminus, and C-terminal sequences partially homologous to yeast RAD9 and a cloned p53-binding protein (Koonin et al, 1996; Miki et al, 1994), consistent with the ability of *BRCA1* to activate gene transcription in vitro (Chapman and Verma, 1996; Monteiro et al, 1996). Evidence that *BRCA1* is a component of the RNA polymerase II transcription complex strongly supports its probable function as a transcription factor (Scully et al, 1997a). Thus mutational

inactivation of *BRCA1* might be expected to affect the expression of other genes, involved presumably in the regulation of growth or differentiation in breast and ovarian epithelium. The expression pattern of *BRCA1* during mouse development, and the cell cycle− and hormone-regulated expression of *BRCA1*, suggest a relationship with differentiation and cell proliferation (Gudas et al, 1995, 1996; Lane et al, 1995; Marquis et al, 1995; Vaughn et al, 1996). A role for *BRCA1* in conjunction with the hRAD51 protein has been implicated in the repair of double-strand DNA breaks, suggesting that an additional function may lie in the maintenance of genomic stability (Scully et al, 1997b). Finally, functional studies on tumorigenesis support the classification of *BRCA1* as a tumor suppressor protein (Holt et al, 1996; Rao et al, 1996; Shao et al, 1996).

Known mutations of *BRCA1* are located throughout the gene with little evidence of clustering; about 80 percent of the mutations are loss-of-function nonsense or frameshift alterations, consistent with the classification of *BRCA1* as a tumor suppressor gene (Couch and Weber, 1996; Shattuck-Eidens et al, 1995). Other studies have shown that allelic deletions (as detected by loss of heterozygosity) affecting the 17q21 region in *BRCA1*-linked breast or ovarian cancers invariably involve the wild-type chromosome (Merajver et al, 1995a; Smith et al, 1992), as would be expected if *BRCA1* were behaving as a typical tumor suppressor gene. Two specific mutations, 185delAG and 5382insC, are present in approximately 1.0 and 0.25 percent of the Ashkenazi Jewish population, respectively (Roa et al, 1996; Struewing et al, 1995). An important research priority is to understand how specific mutations of *BRCA1* may preferentially contribute to breast or ovarian cancer, and how other genetic and/or environmental factors may affect penetrance and tissue specificity. Several possible clues relating to these phenomena have emerged in two studies. A study of 32 breast and ovarian cancer families revealed a significant correlation between the location of the mutation in the gene and the ratio of breast to ovarian cancer incidence within each family; specifically, mutations within the 3′ third of the gene are associated with a lower proportion of ovarian cancer (Gayther et al, 1995). Ovarian cancer risk is increased in women with germline mutations of *BRCA1* when one or two rare alleles of the *HRAS1* variable number of tandem repeats polymorphism are present, compared to carriers with only common alleles (Phelan et al, 1996b). The mechanism of this effect remains obscure, but the data are consistent with the concept that modifying genetic loci may affect penetrance of hereditary ovarian cancer.

The data linking BRCA1 to most hereditary ovarian cancers are now unequivocal. It has been thought that this gene would be found to play a major role in sporadic ovarian carcinomas as well. This speculation centered around the observation that LOH, the genetic hallmark of tumor suppressor gene inactivation, is observed on chromosome 17q in up to 80 percent of sporadic ovarian carcinomas (Cliby et al, 1993; Eccles et al, 1992; Foulkes et al, 1991; Russell et al, 1990; Sato et al, 1991; Yang-Feng et al, 1993). Analyses of unselected ovarian carcinomas, most of which would be sporadic, suggest that somatic mutations of BRCA1 are very rare, however (Futreal et al, 1994; Hosking et al, 1995; Matsuhima et al, 1995; Merajver et al, 1995b; Stratton et al, 1997; Takahashi et al, 1995). This finding is supported by fine deletion mapping studies, which implicate one and perhaps two regions distal to BRCA1 as harboring an additional tumor suppressor gene(s) (Godwin et al, 1994; Jacobs et al, 1993; Saito et al, 1993). These data suggest that mutational inactivation of BRCA1 is necessary at a relatively early stage of development in order to contribute to ovarian tumorigenesis. Under this hypothesis, somatic mutation of BRCA1 in the adult ovarian epithelium does not provide a significant selective advantage in a developing malignancy, and thus rarely leads to clonal selection and manifestation as a somatic mutation in the ovarian cancer. Finally, the analysis of unselected ovarian cancers (Matsushima et al, 1995; Stratton et al, 1997; Takahashi et al, 1995) indicates that germline mutations in BRCA1 are associated with approximately 5 percent of all ovarian cancers.

BRCA2

Similar approaches were used to localize and clone the BRCA2 cancer susceptibility gene. Genetic linkage analysis of high-risk breast cancer families that were unlinked to BRCA1 revealed a locus at chromosome 13q12-13 to which some of these families were linked (Wooster et al, 1994). A candidate gene from this region of chromosome 13 was determined to represent BRCA2 based on the presence of germline-inactivating mutations that segregated with disease in linked families (Wooster et al, 1995). Confirmation of this finding was provided by additional studies in which inactivating mutations were identified in breast cancer families, especially those with male breast cancer (Couch et al, 1996; Phelan et al, 1996a; Tavtigian et al, 1996; Thorlacius et al, 1996). Unlike BRCA1, inherited mutations in BRCA2 appear to confer a substantially lower risk of ovarian cancer compared to breast cancer, as inferred from tumor incidence rates in linked families (Couch et al, 1996; Gudmundsson et al, 1996; Narod et al, 1995a,b; Phelan et al, 1996a; Tavtigian et al, 1996; Thorlacius et al, 1996; Wooster et al, 1994, 1995). Furthermore, an analysis of unselected ovarian cancer cases suggests that germline-inactivating mutations of BRCA2 may be found in patients with late-onset disease and no remarkable medical or family histories in regard to breast or ovarian cancer (Foster et al, 1996; Takahashi et al, 1996). Taken together, these findings are consistent with the hypothesis that inherited mutations in BRCA2 contribute to ovarian cancer with a lower penetrance than BRCA1, and that the fraction of all ovarian cancers resulting from hereditary predisposition may be higher than previously suspected based on estimates derived from highly penetrant genetic loci.

The BRCA2 gene consists of 26 coding exons distributed over approximately 70 kb of genomic DNA, encoding a transcript of 11 to 12 kb (Tavtigian et al, 1996). As for BRCA1, the BRCA2 mRNA is most highly expressed in testis and thymus, with lower levels in breast and ovary (Tavtigian et al, 1996). In addition to tissue-specific expression profiles, BRCA1 and BRCA2 share a number of additional structural and functional similarities. Both are unusually large genes in terms of the number of exons and size of the encoded message, both have a large exon 11 that contains approximately half of the entire coding region, both contain translation start sites in exon 2, and both are relatively A/T-rich. Expression of both genes appears to be coordinately regulated during cell cycle progression (Wang et al, 1997) and in response to estrogen (Spillman and Bowcock, 1996) in human cells and in embryonic and adult mouse tissues (Conner et al, 1997; Rajan et al, 1997). Studies on the role of Brca2 in mouse development indicate that loss of the protein confers radiation hypersensitivity, consistent with its interaction with the Rad51 protein involved in repair of double-strand DNA breaks (Sharan et al, 1997). Remarkably, *BRCA1* and *BRCA2* proteins are thus likely to be involved in the same biochemical pathway, mediated by hRAD51, regulating genomic integrity (Scully et al, 1997b; Sharan et al, 1997). Preliminary findings suggest that *BRCA2* may also function as a transcription factor, because a small portion of the protein shares homology with the known transcription factor c-Jun and is capable of activating transcription in vitro (Milner et al, 1997).

Mutations of *BRCA2* reported to date are, as for *BRCA1*, dispersed throughout the gene with little evidence for hotspots or clustering (Couch et al, 1996; Phelan et al, 1996a; Takahashi et al, 1996; Tavtigian et al, 1996; Thorlacius et al, 1996; Wooster et al, 1995). The great majority of mutations are frameshift in nature, with microdeletions being most common; microinsertions, nonsense, and missense mutations occur rarely. Loss of heterozygosity at the *BRCA2* locus in tumors from linked individuals invariably involves the wild-type allele, consistent with the classification of *BRCA2* as a tumor suppressor gene (Collins et al, 1995; Gudmundsson et al, 1995). Some mutations have been observed in multiple unrelated families, suggesting that a subset of *BRCA2* mutations may also occur relatively frequently. A single mutation in *BRCA2*, 6174delT, is found in approximately 1.4 percent of the Ashkenazi Jewish population (Neuhausen et al, 1996; Oddoux et al, 1996; Roa et al, 1996); this mutation together with those in *BRCA1* are thus present in approximately 1 in 40 Ashkenazi Jewish individuals. These findings have profound implications for genetic screening in this population. As might be expected, a relatively large fraction of all ovarian cancer cases in Ashkenazi Jews may be associated with germline mutations in *BRCA1* or *BRCA2*; one study suggests that as many as 62 percent of ovarian cancers in this population are attributable to one of these three founder mutations (Abeliovich et al, 1997).

As was the case for *BRCA1*, it was believed that somatic mutations of *BRCA2* might be involved in a significant fraction of sporadic ovarian cancers, based on the high frequency of allelic loss observed on chromosome 13q in these tumors (Cliby et al, 1993; Gallion et al, 1992; Yang-Feng et al, 1993). Analysis of a large sample of unselected ovarian cancers indicates that, although LOH that includes the *BRCA2* locus is seen in over half of the tumors, somatic mutations of the gene are rare (Foster et al, 1996; Takahashi et al, 1996) but probably more common than for *BRCA1*. These studies further indicate that approximately 3 percent of all ovarian cancers are associated with germline mutations in *BRCA2*.

MOLECULAR GENETICS OF COMMON GYNECOLOGIC CANCERS

The greatest progress in defining critical molecular genetic alterations in gynecologic cancers has been achieved for the most commonly occurring malignancies, epithelial ovarian carcinoma and carcinomas of the uterine endometrium and cervix (Table 19–3). The degree to which the *RAS* and *ERBB*-2 oncogenes, the p53 tumor suppressor gene, and microsatellite instability affect the sporadic manifestations of these cancers has been reasonably well established. In addition, allelotype analyses have pointed to the involvement of additional tumor suppressor genes for each tumor type. Research into the molecular biology and genetics of gynecologic cancers has provided important insights pertaining to the clinical distinction of two types of endometrial carcinoma, the biologic behavior of various types of ovarian tumors, and the mechanism through which human papillomaviruses initiate tumorigenesis in the cervix.

Endometrial Carcinoma

Epidemiologic observations support the existence of two forms of endometrial carcinoma, one of which is related to estrogen and is most common in North America and Western Europe and the other of which is unrelated to estrogen and occurs similarly throughout the world (Parazzini et al, 1991). Additional lines of clinical and pathologic evidence have led to the development of two classifications for endometrial carcinoma, type I (estrogen related) and type II (non-estrogen related) (Boyd, 1996; Deligdisch and Holinka, 1987; Kurman et al, 1994). Type I tumors, in addition to their relationship to estrogen, occur in relatively younger, perimenopausal women, are frequently associated with endometrial hyperplasia, are of low grade and minimal myometrial invasion, exhibit a

TABLE **19–3**

Summary of Known Molecular Alterations in Common Gynecologic Cancers

Cancer	RAS	ERBB-2[§]	C-MYC	P53	Microsatellite Instability	LOH*
Endometrial	10–30% (type I)	10–15% (type II)	Rare[†]	10–30% (type II)	20% (type I)	3p, 6p, 8p, 9q, 10q, 14q, 16q, 17q, 18q
Ovarian	30–50% (mucinous) 10–30% (serous)	20–30%	Rare	10–15% (stage I/II) 40–50% (stage III/IV)	Rare	6q, 11p, 13q, 14q, 17p, 17q, 18q, 22q, Xp
Cervical	Rare	Rare	30–50%	Rare	Rare	3p, 4q, 5p, 6p, 11q, 18q
Sarcomas	ND[‡]	ND	ND	30–50%	Rare	ND

*Chromosome arms affected relatively frequently by LOH.
[†]Involved in less than 5 percent of all cases reported.
[‡]Few or no data reported.
[§]ERBB-2 same as HER-2/neu.

stable clinical course, and are associated with a good prognosis. In contrast, type II tumors occur in relatively older, postmenopausal women with an absence of estrogen-related risk history, are not preceded or accompanied by hyperplasia, are of high grade and deep myometrial invasion, exhibit a progressive clinical course, and are associated with a poorer prognosis. Histologically, the type I tumors are typically well-differentiated endometrioid adenocarcinomas; less commonly, secretory, ciliated, villoglandular, and squamous variants occur. The type II tumors include adenosquamous, papillary serous, and clear cell carcinomas (Kurman et al, 1994). Presumably, there is a molecular genetic basis for the existence of these two categories of tumor, and any attempt to address the molecular etiology of endometrial carcinoma must be founded in the recognition of this distinction (Table 19–4).

Although endometrial carcinoma is the most common gynecologic malignancy encountered, the molecular characterization of this cancer remains very limited in comparison to other common solid tumor types. Among published studies examining abnormalities in oncogene structure or expression, several of the genes most commonly altered in human solid tumors have also been implicated in carcinomas of the endometrium, including RAS and ERBB-2, although it should be emphasized that no single oncogene has been found to be altered in greater than approximately 20 percent of the endometrial cancers studied. Activating point mutation of a member of the RAS gene family is, in general, the most commonly found oncogene aberration in human cancers. Several studies have confirmed that a RAS mutation, predominantly in codon 12 of the K-RAS gene, is present in 10 to 30 percent of endometrial cancers (Duggan et al, 1994a; Enomoto et al, 1993; Mizuuchi et al, 1992; Sasaki et al, 1993). In those tumors that contain RAS mutations, this event appears to occur early in the neoplastic process, because the incidence of mutant RAS is the same in endometrial hyperplasia as that found in carcinoma. Attempts to correlate RAS mutation with clinical outcome have produced conflicting data (Mizuuchi et al, 1992; Sasaki et al, 1993), possibly reflecting an age dependency of this phenomenon (Ito et al, 1996).

TABLE **19–4**

Two Types of Endometrial Carcinoma

Type I	Type II
Clinicopathologic Features	
Hyperestrogenism	No estrogen risk factors
Younger age	Older age
Endometrioid histology	Nonendometrioid histology
Associated with hyperplasia	No hyperplasia
Low grade	High grade
Good prognosis	Poor prognosis
Genetic Features	
Diploid	Aneuploid
Low LOH	High LOH
K-RAS	K-RAS
Microsatellite instability	p53
PTEN	ERBB-2

Involvement of the *ERBB-2* (also known as HER-2/*neu*) oncogene in tumorigenesis is through overexpression, with or without gene amplification. It is clear that 10 to 15 percent of endometrial cancers display overexpression of ERBB-2 protein compared to normal endometrial epithelium, as quantitated by immunohistochemistry (Berchuck et al, 1991; Hetzel et al, 1992). Some studies have also documented *ERBB-2* gene amplification in endometrial cancers, although in only a subset of those tumors showing overexpression (Czerwenka et al, 1995; Esteller et al, 1995; Saffari et al, 1995). Overexpression of *ERBB-2* appears to be confined to a subset of high-grade and/or advanced-stage tumors. Correlation of expression with clinical outcome has been less conclusive, although the trend has been toward a positive correlation between overexpression and worsening of prognosis.

Mutation of the p53 tumor suppressor gene is the single most common genetic abnormality currently recognized in human cancers. Relative overexpression of the p53 protein is frequently observed in conjunction with many of the common missense mutations that the gene is subject to; thus immunohistochemical analysis of p53 expression is frequently used as an endpoint in many human tumor studies. Through the analysis of overexpression, mutation, or both, the presence of p53 mutations in endometrial carcinomas has now been well established, although the incidence is clearly limited to a subset (10 to 30 percent) of all tumors studied (Enomoto et al, 1993; Honda et al, 1993; Kohler et al, 1992; Okamoto et al, 1991a; Risinger et al, 1992). Overexpression and/or mutation are associated with poor prognostic features, such as high grade, advanced stage, nonendometrioid histology, and disease recurrence (Inoue et al, 1994; Ito et al, 1994; Kohler et al, 1992; Soong et al, 1996). Several studies have also focused on papillary serous endometrial carcinomas, a majority of which display p53 mutations or overexpression (Khalifa et al, 1994; King et al, 1995; Prat et al, 1994; Tashiro et al, 1997a; Zheng et al, 1996). In a study of over 100 premalignant endometrial hyperplasia specimens, p53 mutations are uniformly absent (Kohler et al, 1993b).

As discussed earlier, all cancers associated with germline mutations in a mismatch repair gene, occurring within the context of the HNPCC syndrome, display somatic genetic instability of microsatellite repeat sequences. Endometrial carcinoma is one of several tumor types in which a fraction of sporadic, nonhereditary forms of the cancer also display microsatellite instability. This phenomenon is evident in approximately 20 percent of all endometrial carcinomas (Burks et al, 1994; Duggan et al, 1994b; Peiffer et al, 1995; Risinger et al, 1993). Although it was assumed that these cases probably result from somatic mutations in the same mismatch repair genes that cause HNPCC, it appears that only a fraction of sporadic endometrial cancers with microsatellite instability have acquired mutations in *hMSH2*, *hMLH1*, or *hPMS2* (Katabuchi et al, 1995). Microsatellite instability in endometrial carcinoma may result from somatic mutations in other genes encoding proteins involved in mismatch repair or, alternatively, from epigenetic alterations of the known mismatch repair genes, such as that which occurs in some sporadic colorectal carcinomas (Kane et al, 1997). Preliminary data suggest that microsatellite instability occurs in diploid tumors of endometrioid histology with good prognosis (Risinger et al, 1993) and may be present in atypical hyperplasia lesions associated with adenocarcinoma (Jovanovic et al, 1996). Conversely, microsatellite instability is not seen in papillary serous carcinomas of the endometrium (Tashiro et al, 1997b).

Most recently, a novel tumor-suppressor gene responsible for the hereditary cancer syndrome, Cowden's disease, was cloned and characterized (Li et al, 1997; Steck et al, 1997 Liaw et al, 1997). Named *PTEN* or *MMAC1*, this gene appears to encode a tyrosine phosphatase with additional significant homology to the cytoskeletal proteins tensin and auxilin. Although endometrial cancer is not recognized as a component of the Cowden's syndrome, sporadic endometrial carcinomas frequently exhibit LOH in a region of chromosome 10q with reasonably close proximity to the *PTEN* gene (Peiffer et al, 1995; Nagase et al, 1997). Mutation analyses of *PTEN* in endometrial carcinomas indicate that this gene is somatically inactivated in 30–50% of all such tumors (Tashiro et al, 1997c; Kong et al, 1997; Risinger et al, 1997), representing the most frequent molecular genetic alteration in endometrial cancers yet defined. Interestingly, there is a strong correlation between the presence of microsatellite instability and *PTEN* mutation (Tashiro et al, 1997c; Kong et al, 1997).

Clues to the involvement of additional tumor suppressor genes in endometrial carcinogenesis have emerged from "allelotyping" studies, in which LOH is quantitated throughout the genome. The principle of this type of analysis is discussed in the section "Tumor Suppressor Genes" earlier in this chapter. At least five studies have published partial or complete allelotyping data for endometrial cancers, allowing for several conclusions (Fujino et al, 1994; Imamura et al, 1992; Jones et al, 1994; Okamoto et al, 1991b; Peiffer et al, 1995). In a general sense, LOH occurs at a relatively low frequency in endometrial carcinoma compared to other common solid tumor types. Sites at which frequent LOH has been observed include chromosomes 3p, 6p, 8p, 9q, 10q, 14q, 16q, 17p, and 18q. Chromosome arms for which the underlying tumor suppressor gene defects have been established with reasonable certainty are 17p and 10q, LOH at which generally correlates with mutation of p53 and PTEN, respectively. The only chromosomal region for which a clinical correlation has been noted is 14q, LOH at which is correlated with a poor prognosis (Fujino et al, 1994).

In conclusion, a relatively limited body of data on the molecular genetics of endometrial carcinoma suggests that mutations of K-RAS codon 12, microsatellite instability, and PTEN mutations may be associated with Type I tumors, whereas amplification or overexpression of ERBB-2, mutation of p53, and LOH at chromosome 14q are features of some type II cancers (Table 19–4). Further studies are clearly warranted to define the molecular bases of these two subtypes of endometrial cancer.

Epithelial Ovarian Carcinoma

As the most lethal of all gynecologic cancers, epithelial carcinoma of the ovary has been the focus of intense research. Several features of this cancer type, however, present problems relating to its study. Foremost are the tendency for clinical presentation at an advanced stage and the absence of a well-defined premalignant lesion associated with progression to invasive cancer. It is now well accepted that benign and borderline (or low-malignant-potential) ovarian tumors are generally not precursor lesions for invasive ovarian carcinomas, but rather represent distinct biologic entities (see later). The available molecular genetic characterization of borderline and invasive cancers supports this distinction. Another common feature of ovarian cancers is the diffuse nature of intrapelvic disease evident at diagnosis, causing confusion as to the primary site of tumor origin or even the clonal nature of the cancer. Molecular studies have supported the clinicopathologic impression that papillary serous tumors of the peritoneum may be multifocal in origin, while serous tumors arising in the ovary are monofocal in origin (Muto et al, 1995; Tsao et al, 1993).

As in the case of endometrial carcinoma, a significant literature exists pertaining to the status of RAS, ERBB-2, and p53 genes in ovarian carcinoma. Activating point mutations of K-RAS, primarily at codon 12, are found in 30 to 50 percent of both borderline and invasive cancers of mucinous histology, and at a lower frequency in serous tumors (Ichikawa et al, 1994; Mok et al, 1993; Teneriello et al, 1993). Gene amplification and overexpression of the ERBB-2 gene are observed in 20 to 30 percent of invasive cancers and have been associated with a poorer prognosis in some but not all studies (Berchuck et al, 1990; Felip et al, 1995; Rubin et al, 1993, 1994; Slamon et al, 1989). Mutations of the p53 gene accompanied by allelic deletions on chromosome 17p are found in 10 to 15 percent of early-stage and 40 to 50 percent of advanced-stage ovarian cancers (Jacobs et al, 1992; Kohler et al, 1993a; Marks et al, 1991; Okamoto et al, 1991b; Teneriello et al, 1993) but not in benign or borderline tumors (Berchuck et al, 1994; Wertheim et al, 1994). Overexpression of the p53 protein correlates with shorter survival time in advanced-stage disease (Henriksen et al, 1994; Herod et al, 1996; Levesque et al, 1995). In contrast to endometrial cancer, microsatellite instability is very rare in sporadic ovarian carcinomas and is not likely to play a significant role in this tumor type (Iwabuchi et al, 1995; Osborne and Leech, 1994; Phillips et al, 1996).

Chromosomal instability and allelic deletions are common in ovarian carcinoma, and allelotyping data implicate many, if not most, chromosome arms as sites of potential tumor suppressor gene mutations (Cliby et al, 1993; Osborne and Leech, 1994; Sato et al, 1991; Yang-Feng et al, 1993). Chromosome 17 is subject to LOH in 50 to 80 percent of all ovarian cancers. High-frequency deletion on the short arm is often associated with p53 mutation, but there is likely an additional 17p tumor suppressor locus as well (Phillips et al,

1996). The common LOH observed on 17q is not associated with somatic mutation of the *BRCA1* gene (Takahashi et al, 1995), and there are likely to be one or more novel tumor suppressor genes distal to this locus (Godwin et al, 1994; Jacobs et al, 1993). Other frequently affected chromosomal sites include 6q (Cliby et al, 1993; Ehlen and Dubeau, 1990; Lee et al, 1990); 11p (Ehlen and Dubeau, 1990; Lee et al, 1990; Lu et al, 1997; Vandamme et al, 1992); 13q (Cliby et al, 1993; Dodson et al, 1994; Kim et al, 1994; Takahashi et al, 1996; Yang-Feng et al, 1993); 14q (Bandera et al, 1997); 18q (Chenevix-Trench et al, 1992; Cliby et al, 1993); 22q (Bryan et al, 1996; Cliby et al, 1993); and Xp (Osborne and Leech, 1994; Yang-Feng et al, 1993). The technique of comparative genomic hybridization also allows for the detection of increases in copy number, which may reflect the location of amplified oncogenes. Increases in copy number on chromosomes 3q, 8q, and 20q appear to be common in ovarian cancers (Iwabuchi et al, 1995).

Cervical Carcinoma

Squamous cell carcinomas constitute the majority of invasive cervical cancers, with much of the remaining fraction attributable to adenocarcinomas of various types, and there is now considerable evidence that all of these tumors arise from cervical intraepithelial neoplasia and that human papillomavirus (HPV) is critically involved in their initiation (Wright et al, 1994). Consequently, a large body of research has elucidated in great detail the molecular biology of HPV function in tumorigenesis. It should be emphasized, however, that cervical cancers undoubtedly conform to the paradigm of multistep, multigenic carcinogenesis, and that additional oncogenes and tumor suppressor genes are certain to be involved in their etiology.

The more than 60 known types of HPV may generally be categorized into one of two groups: low-risk types associated with benign lesions and oncogenic, high-risk types associated with invasive cancers. In cervical cancers and derived cell lines, the HPV DNA is usually integrated into the host genome and there appears to be selection for the integrity of the region encoding two proteins, E6 and E7, that are regularly expressed in cancers (Howley, 1993). The mechanism through which E6 and E7 contribute to cellular transformation involves physical interaction with two tumor suppressor proteins that play critical roles in mammalian cell cycle regulation, p53 and Rb. The E6 protein of high-risk HPV types binds to p53 with a higher affinity than E6 of low-risk types and promotes p53 degradation (Scheffner et al, 1990; Werness et al, 1990). Similarly, E7 binds and inactivates the Rb protein (Dyson et al, 1989; Munger et al, 1989). The combined effects of p53 and Rb inactivation in infected cells are likely to provide a proliferative advantage that is conducive to further genetic alterations leading to cancer. That only a small fraction of those infected by HPV eventually develop cervical cancer is further evidence that HPV alone is insufficient for malignant transformation.

The prevalence of *RAS* oncogene mutations in cervical cancers has been inadequately surveyed. The absence of published data, however, suggests that such mutations are probably rare. Activating point mutations of codon 12 of the *H-RAS* gene were found in 24 percent of advanced-stage squamous carcinomas (Riou et al, 1988), and *K-RAS* codon 12 mutations were identified in 13 percent of invasive endocervical adenocarcinomas (Koulos et al, 1993). Amplification and overexpression of the *ERBB*-2 oncogene are present in only small fractions of squamous carcinomas and adenocarcinomas of the cervix (Kihana et al, 1994; Mandai et al, 1995; Mitra et al, 1994b), and a correlation with poor prognosis exists for adenocarcinomas (Kihana et al, 1994; Mandai et al, 1995). A thorough analysis of cervical cancers for p53 status indicates that mutations are rare, and that there is no correlation with HPV status (Benjamin et al, 1996; Busby-Earle et al, 1994; Fujita et al, 1992; Kurvinen et al, 1994; Paquette et al, 1993; Park et al, 1994). In contrast to other gynecologic cancers, the *C-MYC* oncogene may play a significant role in cervical carcinogenesis, with amplification and/or rearrangement of *C-MYC* observed in 30 to 50 percent of cervical carcinomas (Baker et al, 1988; Ocadiz et al, 1987). Microsatellite instability appears to be very rare in cervical carcinoma (Larson et al, 1996). Allelotyping analyses implicate potential tumor suppressor genes for cervical carcinoma on chromosomes 3p, 4q, 5p, 6p, 11q, and 18q (Kohno et al, 1993; Misra and Srivatsan, 1989; Mitra et al, 1994a; Mullokandov et al, 1996; Srivatsan et al, 1991), and deletions on chromosome 3p appear to represent a frequent and early event in cervical tumorigenesis (Wistuba et al, 1997).

Sarcomas

Gynecologic sarcomas account for only about 3 percent of all female reproductive tract cancers, and, perhaps because of their rarity, they have not been studied at the molecular level in great detail. By far the most well-characterized genetic alteration in these cancers is mutation of the p53 tumor suppressor gene (Randall and Boyd, 1998). In a study of 46 uterine and ovarian sarcomas, 27 (59 percent) were found to harbor p53 mutations (Liu et al, 1994), including 26 of 41 mixed mesodermal tumors and one of four leiomyosarcomas. Mutations were identified in both early- and late-stage disease, suggesting that, unlike many epithelial tumor types, p53 inactivation is a critical early event in sarcoma development. Other studies substantiate the role of p53 in about a third of leiomyosarcomas but never in benign leiomyomas of the uterus (de Vos et al, 1994; Jeffers et al, 1995). Microsatellite instability is also present in a minority of sarcomas of the uterus and ovary, primarily in high-grade, anaplastic lesions (Risinger et al, 1995).

LABORATORY TECHNIQUES IN MOLECULAR GENETICS

The mutations in cancer-related genes described in this chapter all may be characterized using a small number of standard laboratory techniques that are now in widespread use in molecular genetics laboratories. A brief overview of the most commonly employed techniques, along with their original citations and a visual presentation of representative data, is presented in this section.

The Polymerase Chain Reaction

Many procedures are based on the polymerase chain reaction (PCR), which has revolutionized the practice of molecular genetics. The procedure employs a thermostable DNA polymerase (e.g., *Taq* polymerase) and oligodeoxynucleotide primers to exponentially amplify a small target DNA sequence (Mullis and Faloona, 1986). Template DNA is combined with primers, polymerase, and the appropriate buffer and, using a thermal cycler, subjected to multiple cycles each consisting of three steps: DNA template denaturation, primer annealing, and enzymatic elongation of the target sequence. The amplified target sequence may then be cloned, screened for mutations, sequenced, or otherwise subjected to the analysis of DNA structure and expression. Genomic DNA obtained from any number of sources, including fresh-frozen or fixed and embedded tissues, is amenable to PCR analysis, and a single-copy DNA sequence present in several picograms of genomic DNA template may be routinely amplified to large (several billion-fold) quantities. The ability to amplify tumor tissue DNA obtained from archival paraffin blocks has greatly facilitated the molecular genetic analysis of human cancers.

Mutation Screening Procedures

Several screening procedures have been developed that allow rapid analysis of a large number of DNA samples for the presence of potential mutations that may be confirmed subsequently by direct sequence analysis. A representative screening procedure that is also the most commonly used is single-strand conformation polymorphism (SSCP) analysis (Orita et al, 1989). Radiolabeled PCR products are denatured, and the single-strand DNA molecules are electrophoresed in nondenaturing polyacrylamide gels under certain conditions. The procedure is based on the principle that any sequence change usually will cause an altered three-dimensional conformation and thus altered mobility of the PCR product through the gel. Variant bands may then be sequenced directly to determine the sequence change (Fig. 19–3A). Disadvantages of the SSCP analysis are that complete sequence information of the target gene is necessary in order to design PCR primers, conformation variants can be detected reliably only in relatively small PCR products (100 to 300 bp), and that the procedure is generally only 75 to 100 percent sensitive in variant detection, depending on the target sequence. Other indirect screening procedures for the detection of small (one or several base pairs) mutations include denaturing gradient gel electrophoresis, heteroduplex analysis, RNase A cleavage, and chemical mismatch cleavage (Grompe, 1993).

Another screening procedure has been developed to detect mutations resulting in truncated protein products such as occur with frameshift, nonsense, and splice-site alterations affecting tumor suppressor genes. Known as the in vitro synthesized protein assay or protein truncation test, this procedure first was described in the analysis of truncat-

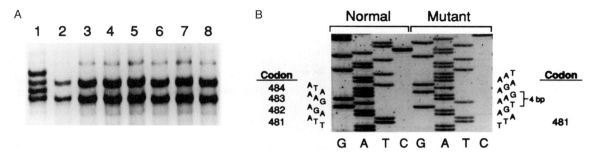

FIGURE 19–3. Detection of an *hMSH2* gene mutation by SSCP and sequencing analyses. *A*, Following the PCR amplification of exon 9 of the *hMSH2* gene, an autoradiogram of the SSCP gel reveals a wild-type pattern of DNA single-strand mobility in patients 2 through 8; DNA from patient 1 shows an additional set of bands migrating with slower (larger) mobility than the wild-type bands. *B*, Dideoxy sequence analysis comparing one of the altered bands (mutant) to the product from a normal individual (normal) reveals a 4-bp insertion beginning at codon 482 resulting in a frameshift mutation.

ing mutations in the *APC* gene (Powell et al, 1993). RNA from blood or tumor is used to synthesize first-strand cDNA, which is then used as template for the PCR amplification of overlapping products spanning the coding region of interest. PCR primers are constructed such that the necessary sequences for translation initiation are included and the amplified product remains in the correct reading frame for protein translation. The PCR product is added to a reaction mixture containing the necessary enzymes and reagents for in vitro mRNA transcription and protein translation that includes a radiolabeled amino acid. Analysis of the in vitro synthesized protein fragments by gel electrophoresis reveals the presence of smaller protein fragments in cases where truncating mutations are present in the original template. The original PCR products may then be sequenced to identify the relevant mutations. This procedure has been employed successfully to screen for mutations in most tumor suppressor genes, including *BRCA1* (Hogervorst et al, 1995) and the mismatch repair genes involved in HNPCC (Liu et al, 1995). The major advantage of this procedure is that relatively large PCR products may be screened, but the disadvantage is that RNA, rather than the generally more readily available DNA, is required from the tissue to be screened.

Gene amplification may be detected with quantitative PCR procedures, but the more sensitive and still preferred technique is that of Southern blotting. This relatively old procedure (Southern, 1975) may also be used to detect mutations in which substantial (several hundred base pairs or more) portions of

genes are deleted, duplicated, or translocated. Genomic DNA is digested with one or more restriction enzymes, and the resulting fragments are separated by size on a horizontal agarose gel, transferred to a solid nylon support, and subjected to hybridization with a radiolabeled probe from within (or near) the gene of interest. Advantages of this technique are that relatively large regions (several kilobase pairs) of DNA may be examined for alterations and that no knowledge of the target gene sequence is necessary for the analysis. The major disadvantage is that relatively large amounts of high-quality genomic DNA, generally from fresh-frozen tissues, are required.

DNA sequencing is generally accomplished using one or another modification of the dideoxy termination protocol originally described by Sanger et al (1977). Genomic DNA fragments or PCR products may be subcloned and sequenced with a DNA polymerase, or small quantities of PCR products may be "cycle-sequenced" using a modified PCR (Innis et al, 1988). The procedure is performed manually using one radiolabeled nucleotide substrate, polyacrylamide gel electrophoresis, and autoradiography (Fig. 19–3B), or in an automated format that employs fluorescently labeled dye terminators. Although the direct sequencing of DNA is the most straightforward and reliable method for mutation detection, it is technically and economically prohibitive for most routine research applications. More typically, variant DNA samples identified by an indirect screening procedure such as SSCP analysis are then characterized by sequencing.

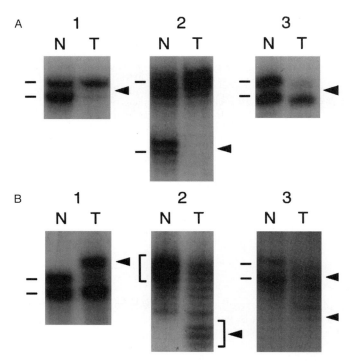

FIGURE 19–4. Use of polymorphic microsatellite repeats to identify LOH and microsatellite instability. *A*, Examples of LOH at three different microsatellite loci in tumor DNA (T) compared to normal DNA (N) from the same individual. Clonal absence of one or the other allele in tumor DNA from an informative (heterozygous) individual indicates LOH. Bars on the left side of each autoradiogram indicate two alleles, and arrowheads on the right side indicate position of allele lost in the tumor. *B*, Examples of microsatellite instability at three different loci in tumor DNA (T) compared to normal DNA (N) from the same individual. Presence of an additional allele or alleles (larger or smaller) in tumor DNA, rather than loss, indicates microsatellite instability. Bars on the left side of each autoradiogram indicate normal alleles, and arrowheads on the right side indicate new (additional) alleles.

Analysis of Polymorphic Alleles

As explained earlier, LOH at a particular genomic locus is taken to indicate the presence of a mutant tumor suppressor gene on the remaining allele. LOH may be characterized by comparing any polymorphic locus in tumor and normal tissue DNA from a person heterozygous (informative) at that locus; clonal loss of one or the other allele in the tumor DNA is defined as LOH. Originally performed using Southern blotting to detect restriction fragment length polymorphisms near the gene of interest (Cavenee et al, 1983), the procedure is now based almost exclusively on the use of the PCR to amplify highly polymorphic microsatellite repeats, many thousands of which have been mapped throughout the human genome (Dib et al, 1996). The PCR/microsatellite-based technique is used to perform allelotype analyses for particular tumor types as a means to identify potential novel tumor suppressor loci, or as a means to define the boundaries of a relatively small subchromosomal region such that positional cloning strategies may be employed (Fig. 19–4A). This is also the technique used to perform genetic linkage analyses, utilized when hunting for novel hereditary disease loci. The same procedure is used to quantitate microsatellite instability. Instead of loss of one allele, this phenomenon manifests as one or more additional alleles in tumor compared to normal DNA samples from an individual (Fig. 19–4B).

REFERENCES

Abeliovich D, Kaduri L, Lerer I, et al: The founder mutations 185delAG and 5382insC in BRCA1 and 6174delT in BRCA2 appear in 60% of ovarian cancer and 30% of early-onset breast cancer patients among Askenazi women. Am J Hum Genet 60:505, 1997.
Baker VV, Hatch KD, Shingleton HM: Amplification of the c-myc proto-oncogene in cervical carcinoma. J Surg Oncol 39:225, 1988.

Bandera CA, Takahashi H, Behbakht K, et al: Deletion mapping of two potential chromosome 14 tumor suppressor gene loci in ovarian carcinoma. Cancer Res 57:513, 1997.

Benjamin I, Saigo P, Finstad C, et al: Expression and mutational analysis of *P53* in stage IB and IIA cervical cancers. Am J Obstet Gynecol 175:1266, 1996.

Berchuck A, Kamel A, Whitaker R, et al: Overexpression of *HER-2/neu* is associated with poor survival in advanced epithelial ovarian cancer. Cancer Res 50:4087, 1990.

Berchuck A, Kohler MF, Hopkins MP, et al: Overexpression of p53 is not a feature of benign and early-stage borderline epithelial ovarian tumors. Gynecol Oncol 52:232, 1994.

Berchuck A, Rodriguez G, Kinney RB, et al: Overexpression of HER-2/*neu* in endometrial cancer is associated with advanced disease stage. Am J Obstet Gynecol 164:15, 1991.

Bewtra C, Watson P, Conway T, et al: Hereditary ovarian cancer: a clinicopathological study. Int J Gynecol Pathol 11:180, 1992.

Bishop JM: Cellular oncogenes and retroviruses. Annu Rev Biochem 52:301, 1983.

Bishop JM: Molecular themes in oncogenesis. Cell 64:235, 1991.

Boltenberg A, Furgyik S, Kullander S: Familial cancer aggregation in cases of adenocarcinoma corporis uteri. Acta Obstet Gynecol Scand 69:249, 1990.

Boyd J: Estrogen as a carcinogen: the genetics and molecular biology of human endometrial carcinoma. In Huff JE, Boyd J, Barrett JC (eds): Cellular and Molecular Mechanisms of Hormonal Carcinogenesis: Environmental Influences. New York, John Wiley & Sons, 1996, p 151.

Boyd J, Barrett JC: Genetic and cellular basis of multistep carcinogenesis. Pharmacol Ther 46:469, 1990.

Bryan EJ, Watson RH, Davis M, et al: Localization of an ovarian cancer tumor suppressor gene to a 0.5-cM region between *D22S284* and *CYP2D*, on chromosome 22q. Cancer Res 56:719, 1996.

Burks RT, Kessis TD, Cho KR, et al: Microsatellite instability in endometrial carcinoma. Oncogene 9:1163, 1994.

Busby-Earle RM, Steel CM, Williams AR, et al: p53 mutations in cervical carcinogenesis—low frequency and lack of correlation with human papillomavirus status. Br J Cancer 69:732, 1994.

Castilla LH, Couch FJ, Erdos MR, et al: Mutations in the *BRCA1* gene in families with early-onset breast and ovarian cancer. Nature Genet 8:387, 1994.

Cavenee WK, Dryja TP, Phillips RA, et al: Expression of recessive alleles by chromosomal mechanisms in retinoblastoma. Nature 305:779, 1983.

Chapman MS, Verma IM: Transcriptional activation by BRCA1. Nature 382:678, 1996.

Chen Y, Chen C-F, Riley DJ, et al: Aberrant subcellular localization of BRCA1 in breast cancer. Science 270:789, 1995.

Chen Y, Farmer AA, Chen C-F, et al: BRCA1 is a 220-kDa nuclear phosphoprotein that is expressed and phosphorylated in a cell cycle-dependent manner. Cancer Res 56:3168, 1996.

Chenevix-Trench G, Leary J, Kerr J, et al: Frequent loss of heterozygosity on chromosome 18 in ovarian adenocarcinoma which does not always include the DCC locus. Oncogene 7:1059, 1992.

Cliby W, Ritland S, Hartmann L, et al: Human epithelial ovarian cancer allelotype. Cancer Res 53:2393, 1993.

Collins N, McManus R, Wooster R, et al: Consistent loss of the wild-type allele in breast cancers from a family linked to the *BRCA2* gene on chromosome 13q12-13. Oncogene 10:1673, 1995.

Conner F, Smith A, Wooster R, et al: Cloning, chromosomal mapping and expression pattern of the mouse Brca2 gene. Hum Mol Genet 6:291, 1997.

Couch FJ, Farid LM, DeShano ML, et al: *BRCA2* germline mutations in male breast cancer cases and breast cancer families. Nature Genet 13:123, 1996.

Couch FJ, Weber BL: Mutations and polymorphisms in the familial early-onset breast cancer (BRCA1) gene. Breast Cancer Information Core. Hum Mutat 8:8, 1996.

Czerwenka K, Lu Y, Heuss F: Amplification and expression of the c-erbB-2 oncogene in normal, hyperplastic, and malignant endometria. Int J Gynecol Pathol 14:98, 1995.

De Vos S, Wilczynski SP, Fleischhacker M, et al: p53 alterations in uterine leiomyosarcomas versus leiomyomas. Gynecol Oncol 54:205, 1994.

Deligdisch L, Holinka CF: Endometrial carcinoma: two diseases? Cancer Detect Prev 10:237, 1987.

Dib C, Faure S, Fizames C, et al: A comprehensive genetic map of the human genome based on 5,264 microsatellites. Nature 380:152, 1996.

Dodson MK, Cliby WA, Xu H-J, et al: Evidence of functional RB protein in epithelial ovarian carcinomas despite loss of heterozygosity at the *RB* locus. Cancer Res 54:610, 1994.

Duggan BD, Felix JC, Muderspach LI, et al: Early mutational activation of the c-Ki-*ras* oncogene in endometrial carcinoma. Cancer Res 54:1604, 1994a.

Duggan BD, Felix JC, Muderspach LI, et al: Microsatellite instability in sporadic endometrial carcinoma. J Natl Cancer Inst 86:1216, 1994b.

Dyson N, Howley P, Munger K, et al: The human papillomavirus-16 E7 oncoprotein is able to bind to the retinoblastoma gene product. Science 243:934, 1989.

Easton DF, Bishop DT, Ford D, et al: Genetic linkage analysis in familial breast and ovarian cancer: results from 214 families. The Breast Cancer Linkage Consortium. Am J Hum Genet 52:678, 1993.

Eccles DM, Russell SEH, Haites NE, et al: Early loss of heterozygosity on 17q in ovarian cancer. Oncogene 7:2069, 1992.

Ehlen T, Dubeau L: Loss of heterozygosity on chromosomal segments 3p, 6q and 11p in human ovarian carcinomas. Oncogene 5:219, 1990.

Enomoto T, Fujita M, Inoue M, et al: Alterations of the *p53* tumor suppressor gene and its association with activation of the c-K-*ras*-2 protooncogene in premalignant and malignant lesions of the human uterine endometrium. Cancer Res 53:1883, 1993.

Esteller M, Garcia A, Martinez i Palones JM, et al: Detection of c-erbB-2/neu and fibroblast growth factor-3/INT-2 but not epidermal growth factor gene amplification in endometrial cancer by differential polymerase chain reaction. Cancer 75:2139, 1995.

Fearon ER, Vogelstein B: A genetic model for colorectal tumorigenesis. Cell 61:759, 1990.

Felip E, Del Campo JM, Rubio D, et al: Overexpression of c-*erb*B-2 in epithelial ovarian cancer: prognostic value and relationship with response to therapy. Cancer 75: 2147, 1995.

Fishel R, Kolodner R: Identification of mismatch repair genes and their role in the development of cancer. Curr Opin Genet Dev 5:382, 1995.

Foster KA, Harrington P, Kerr J, et al: Somatic and germline mutations of the *BRCA2* gene in sporadic ovarian cancer. Cancer Res 56:3622, 1996.

Foulkes W, Black D, Solomon E, et al: Allele loss on chromosome 17q in sporadic ovarian cancer. Lancet 338:444, 1991.

Friedman LS, Ostermyer EA, Szabo CI, et al: Confirmation of *BRCA1* by analysis of germline mutations linked to breast and ovarian cancer in ten families. Nature Genet 8:399, 1994.

Fujino T, Risinger JI, Collins NK, et al: Allelotype of endometrial carcinoma. Cancer Res 54:4294, 1994.

Fujita M, Inoue M, Tanizawa O, et al: Alterations of the p53 gene in human primary cervical carcinoma with and without human papillomavirus infection. Cancer Res 52:5323, 1992.

Futreal PA, Liu Q, Shattuck-Eidens D, et al: BRCA1 mutations in primary breast and ovarian cancers. Science 266: 120, 1994.

Gallion HH, Powell DE, Morrow JK, et al: Molecular genetic changes in human epithelial ovarian malignancies. Gynecol Oncol 47:137, 1992.

Gayther SA, Warren W, Mazoyer S, et al: Germline mutations of the BRCA1 gene in breast and ovarian cancer families provide evidence for a genotype-phenotype correlation. Nature Genet 11:428, 1995.

Go RCP, King M-C, Bailey-Wilson J, et al: Genetic epidemiology of breast cancer and associated cancers in high risk families. I. Segregation analysis. J Natl Cancer Inst 71: 455, 1983.

Godwin AK, Vanderveer L, Schultz DC, et al: A common region of deletion on chromosome 17q in both sporadic and familial epithelial ovarian tumors distal to BRCA1. Am J Hum Genet 55:666, 1994.

Grompe M: The rapid detection of unknown mutations in nucleic acids. Nature Genet 5:111, 1993.

Gudas JM, Li T, Nguyen H, et al: Cell cycle regulation of BRCA1 messenger RNA in human breast epithelial cells. Cell Growth Diff 7:717, 1996.

Gudas JM, Nguyen H, Li T, et al: Hormone-dependent regulation of BRCA1 in human breast cancer cells. Cancer Res 55:4561, 1995.

Gudmundsson J, Johannesdottir G, Arason A, et al: Frequent occurrence of BRCA2 linkage in Icelandic breast cancer families and segregation of a common BRCA2 haplotype. Am J Hum Genet 58:749, 1996.

Gudmundsson J, Johannesdottir G, Bergthorsson JT, et al: Different tumor types from BRCA2 mutation carriers show wild-type chromosome deletions on 13q12-q13. Cancer Res 55:4830, 1995.

Hall JM, Lee NK, Newman B, et al: Linkage of early-onset familial breast cancer to chromosome 17q21. Science 250: 1684, 1990.

Hemminki A, Peltomaki P, Mecklin J-P, et al: Loss of the wild-type MLH1 gene is a feature of hereditary non-polyposis colorectal cancer. Nature Genet 8:405, 1994.

Henriksen R, Strang P, Wilander E, et al: p53 expression in epithelial ovarian neoplasms: relationship to clinical and pathological parameters, Ki-67 expression and flow cytometry. Gynecol Oncol 53:301, 1994.

Herod JJO, Eliopoulos AG, Warwick J, et al: The prognostic significance of Bcl-2 and p53 expression in ovarian carcinoma. Cancer Res 56:2178, 1996.

Hetzel DJ, Wilson TO, Keeney GL, et al: HER-2/neu expression: a major prognostic factor in endometrial carcinoma. Gynecol Oncol 47:179, 1992.

Hofstra RMW, Landsvater RM, Ceccherini I, et al: A mutation in the RET proto-oncogene associated with multiple endocrine neoplasia type 2B and sporadic medullary thyroid carcinoma. Nature 367:375, 1994.

Hogervorst FBL, Cornelis RS, Bout M, et al: Rapid detection of BRCA1 mutations by the protein truncation test. Nature Genet 10:208, 1995.

Holt JT, Thompson ME, Szabo C, et al: Growth retardation and tumour inhibition by BRCA1. Nature Genet 12:298, 1996.

Honda T, Kato H, Imamura T, et al: Involvement of p53 gene mutations in human endometrial carcinomas. Int J Cancer 53:963, 1993.

Hosking L, Trowsdale J, Nicolai H, et al: A somatic BRCA1 mutation in an ovarian tumor. Nature Genet 9:343, 1995.

Howley PM: Principles of carcinogenesis: viral. In DeVita VT, Hellman S, Rosenberg SA (eds): Cancer: Principles and Practice of Oncology. Philadelphia, JB Lippincott, 1993, p 182.

Hunter T: Cooperation between oncogenes. Cell 64:249, 1991.

Ichikawa Y, Nishida M, Suzuki H, et al: Mutation of K-ras protooncogene is associated with histological subtypes in human mucinous ovarian tumors. Cancer Res 54:33, 1994.

Imamura T, Arima T, Kato H, et al: Chromosomal deletions and K-ras gene mutations in human endometrial carcinomas. Int J Cancer 51:47, 1992.

Innis MA, Myambo KB, Gelfand DH, et al: DNA sequencing with Thermus aquaticus DNA polymerase chain reaction amplified DNA. Proc Natl Acad Sci USA 85:9436, 1988.

Inoue M, Okayama A, Fujita M, et al: Clinicopathological characteristics of p53 overexpression in endometrial cancers. Int J Cancer 58:14, 1994.

Ito K, Watanabe K, Nasim S, et al: Prognostic significance of p53 overexpression in endometrial cancer. Cancer Res 54:4667, 1994.

Ito K, Watanabe K, Nasim S, et al: K-ras point mutations in endometrial carcinoma: effect on outcome is dependent on age of patient. Gynecol Oncol 63:238, 1996.

Iwabuchi H, Sakamoto M, Sakunaga H, et al: Genetic analysis of benign, low-grade, and high-grade ovarian tumors. Cancer Res 55:6172, 1995.

Jacobs IJ, Kohler MF, Wiseman RW, et al: Clonal origin of epithelial ovarian carcinoma: analysis by loss of heterozygosity, p53 mutation, and X-chromosome inactivation. J Natl Cancer Inst 84:1793, 1992.

Jacobs IJ, Smith SA, Wiseman RW, et al: A deletion unit on chromosome 17q in epithelial ovarian tumors distal to the familial breast/ovarian cancer locus. Cancer Res 53:1218, 1993.

Jeffers MD, Farquharson MA, Richmond JA, et al: p53 immunoreactivity and mutation of the p53 gene in smooth muscle tumors of the uterine corpus. J Pathol 177:65, 1995.

Jones MH, Koi S, Fujimoto I, et al: Allelotype of uterine cancer by analysis of RFLP and microsatellite polymorphisms: frequent loss of heterozygosity on chromosome arms 3p, 9q, 10q, and 17p. Genes Chromosom Cancer 9: 119, 1994.

Jovanovic AS, Boynton KA, Mutter GL: Uteri of women with endometrial carcinoma contain a histopathological spectrum of monoclonal putative precancers, some with microsatellite instability. Cancer Res 56:1917, 1996.

Kane MF, Loda M, Gaida GM, et al: Methylation of the hMLH1 promoter correlates with lack of expression of hMLH1 in sporadic colon tumors and mismatch repair-defective human tumor cell lines. Cancer Res 57:808, 1997.

Katabuchi H, van Rees B, Lambers AR, et al: Mutations in DNA mismatch repair genes are not responsible for microsatellite instability in most sporadic endometrial carcinomas. Cancer Res 55:5556, 1995.

Khalifa MA, Mannel RS, Haraway SD, et al: Expression of EGFR, HER-2/neu, P53, and PCNA in endometrioid, serous papillary, and clear cell endometrial adenocarcinomas. Gynecol Oncol 53:84, 1994.

Kihana T, Tsuda H, Teshima S, et al: Prognostic significance of the overexpression of c-erbB-2 protein in adenocarcinoma of the uterine cervix. Cancer 73:148, 1994.

Kim TM, Benedict WF, Xu H-J, et al: Loss of heterozygosity on chromosome 13 is common only in the biologically more aggressive subtypes of ovarian epithelial tumors and is associated with normal retinoblastoma gene expression. Cancer Res 54:605, 1994.

King SA, Adas AA, LiVolsi VA, et al: Expression and mutation analysis of the p53 gene in uterine papillary serous carcinoma. Cancer 75:2700, 1995.

Knudson AG: Hereditary cancer, oncogenes, and antioncogenes. Cancer Res 45:1437, 1985.

Kohler MF, Berchuck A, Davidoff AM, et al: Overexpression and mutation of *p53* in endometrial carcinoma. Cancer Res 52:1622, 1992.

Kohler MF, Marks JR, Wiseman RW, et al: Spectrum of mutation and frequency of allelic deletion of the p53 gene in ovarian cancer. J Natl Cancer Inst 85:1513, 1993a.

Kohler MF, Nishii H, Humphrey PA, et al: Mutation of the p53 tumor-suppressor gene is not a feature of endometrial hyperplasias. Am J Obstet Gynecol 169:690, 1993b.

Kohno T, Takayama H, Hamaguchi M, et al: Deletion mapping of chromosome 3p in human uterine cervical cancer. Oncogene 8:1825, 1993.

Kolodner RD: Mismatch repair: mechanisms and relationship to cancer susceptibility. Trends Biochem Sci 20:397, 1995.

Kong D, Suzuki A, Zou T-T, et al: *PTEN* is frequently mutated in primary endometrial carcinomas. Nature Genet 17:143, 1997.

Koonin EV, Altschul S, Bork P: BRCA1 protein products: functional motifs. Nature Genet 13:266, 1996.

Koulos JP, Wright TC, Mitchell MF, et al: Relationships between c-Ki-ras mutations, HPV types, and prognostic indicators in invasive endocervical adenocarcinomas. Gynecol Oncol 48:364, 1993.

Kurman RJ, Zaino RJ, Norris HJ: Endometrial carcinoma. In Kurman RJ (ed): Blaustein's Pathology of the Female Genital Tract. New York, Springer-Verlag, 1994, p 439.

Kurvinen K, Tervahaut A, Syrjanen S, et al: The state of the p53 gene in human papillomavirus (HPV)-positive and HPV-negative genital precursor lesions and carcinomas as determined by single-strand conformation polymorphism analysis and sequencing. Anticancer Res 14:177, 1994.

Lane TF, Deng C, Elson A, et al: Expression of BRCA1 is associated with terminal differentiation of ectodermally and mesodermally-derived tissues in mice. Genes Dev 9:2712, 1995.

Larson AA, Kern S, Sommers RL, et al: Analysis of replication error (RER+) phenotypes in cervical carcinoma. Cancer Res 56:1426, 1996.

Leach FS, Nicolaides NC, Papadopoulos N, et al: Mutations of a *mutS* homolog in hereditary nonpolyposis colorectal cancer. Cell 75:1215, 1993.

Lee JH, Kavanagh JJ, Wildrick DM, et al: Frequent loss of heterozygosity on chromosomes 6q, 11, and 17 in human ovarian carcinomas. Cancer Res 50:2724, 1990.

Lengauer C, Kinzler KW, Vogelstein B: Genetic instability in colorectal cancers. Nature 386:623, 1997.

Levesque MA, Katsaros D, Yu H, et al: Mutant p53 protein overexpresion is associated with poor outcome in patients with well or moderately differentiated ovarian carcinoma. Cancer 75:1327, 1995.

Li J, Yen C, Liaw D, et al: *PTEN*, a putative protein tyrosine phosphatase gene mutated in human brain, breast, and prostate cancer. Science 275:1943, 1997.

Liaw D, Marsh DJ, Li J, et al: Germline mutations of the *PTEN* gene in Cowden disease, an inherited breast and thyroid cancer syndrome. Nature Genet 16:64, 1997.

Lindblom A, Tannergård P, Werelius B, et al: Genetic mapping of a second locus predisposing to hereditary nonpolyposis colon cancer. Nature Genet 5:279, 1993.

Liu B, Nicolaides NC, Markowitz S, et al: Mismatch repair gene defects in sporadic colorectal cancers with microsatellite instability. Nature Genet 9:48, 1995.

Liu F-S, Kohler MF, Marks JR, et al: Mutation and overexpression of the P53 tumor suppressor gene frequently occurs in uterine and ovarian sarcomas. Obstet Gynecol 83:118, 1994.

Loeb LA: Mutator phenotype may be required for multistage carcinogenesis. Cancer Res 51:3075, 1991.

Loeb LA: Microsatellite instability: marker of a mutator phenotype in cancer. Cancer Res 54:5059, 1994.

Lu KH, Weitzel JN, Kodali S, et al: A novel 4-cM minimally deleted region on chromosome 11p15.1 associated with high grade nonmucinous epithelial ovarian carcinomas. Cancer Res 57:387, 1997.

Lynch HT, Conway T, Lynch J: Hereditary ovarian cancer: pedigree studies, part II. Cancer Genet Cytogenet 52:161, 1991.

Lynch HT, Harris RE, Guirgis HA, et al: Familial association of breast/ovarian carcinoma. Cancer 41:1543, 1978.

Lynch HT, Lynch J, Conway T, et al: Familial aggregation of carcinoma of the endometrium. Am J Obstet Gynecol 171:24, 1994.

Lynch HT, Smyrk TC, Watson P, et al: Genetics, natural history, tumor spectrum, and pathology of hereditary nonpolyposis colorectal cancer. Gastroenterology 104:1535, 1993.

Mandai M, Konishi I, Koshiyama M, et al: Altered expression of *nm23-H1* and c-*erb*B-2 proteins have prognostic significance in adenocarcinoma but not in squamous cell carcinoma of the uterine cervix. Cancer 75:2523, 1995.

Markowitz S, Wang J, Myeroff L, et al: Inactivation of the type II TGF-β receptor in colon cancer cells with microsatellite instability. Science 268:1336, 1995.

Marks JR, Davidoff AM, Kerns BJ, et al: Overexpression and mutation of p53 in epithelial ovarian cancer. Cancer Res 51:2979, 1991.

Marquis ST, Rajan JV, Wynshaw-Boris A, et al: The developmental pattern of *BRCA1* expression implies a role in differentiation of breast and other tissues. Nature Genet 11:17, 1995.

Marra G, Boland CR: Hereditary nonpolyposis colorectal cancer: the syndrome, the genes, and historical perspectives. J Natl Cancer Inst 87:1114, 1995.

Matsushima M, Kobayashi K, Emi M, et al: Mutation analysis of the *BRCA1* gene in 76 Japanese ovarian cancer patients: four germline mutations, but no evidence of somatic mutation. Hum Mol Genet 4:1953, 1995.

Merajver SD, Frank TS, Xu J, et al: Germline *BRCA1* mutations and loss of the wild-type allele in tumors from families with early-onset breast and ovarian cancer. Clin Cancer Res 1:539, 1995a.

Merajver SD, Pham TM, Caduff RF, et al: Somatic mutations in the *BRCA1* gene in sporadic ovarian tumours. Nature Genet 9:439, 1995b.

Miki Y, Swensen J, Shattuck-Edens D, et al: A strong candidate for the breast and ovarian cancer susceptibility gene *BRCA1*. Science 266:66, 1994.

Milner J, Ponder B, Hughes-Davies L, et al: Transcriptional activation functions in BRCA2. Nature 386:772, 1997.

Misra BC, Srivatsan ES: Localization of HeLa cell tumor-suppressor gene to the long arm of chromosome 11. Am J Hum Genet 45:565, 1989.

Mitra AB, Murty VVVS, Li RG, et al: Allelotype analysis of cervical carcinoma. Cancer Res 54:4481, 1994a.

Mitra AB, Murty VVVS, Pratap M, et al: *ERBB2* (*HER2/neu*) oncogene is frequently amplified in squamous cell carcinoma of the uterine cervix. Cancer Res 54:637, 1994b.

Mizuuchi H, Nasim S, Kudo R, et al: Clinical implications of K-*ras* mutations in malignant epithelial tumors of the endometrium. Cancer Res 52:2777, 1992.

Modrich P: Mismatch repair, genetic stability, and cancer. Science 266:1959, 1994.

Mok SC, Bell DA, Knapp RC, et al: Mutation of K-ras protooncogene in human ovarian epithelial tumors of borderline malignancy. Cancer Res 53:1489, 1993.

Monteiro ANA, August A, Hanafusa H: Evidence for a transcriptional activation function for BRCA1 C-terminal region. Proc Natl Acad Sci USA 93:13595, 1996.

Mullis K, Faloona F: Specific synthesis of DNA in vitro via a polymerase-catalyzed chain reaction. Meth Enzymol 155:335, 1986.

Mullokandov MR, Kholodilov NG, Atkin NB, et al: Genomic alterations in cervical carcinoma: losses of chromosome heterozygosity and human papilloma virus tumor status. Cancer Res 56:197, 1996.

Munger K, Werness BA, Dyson N, et al: Complex formation of human papillomavirus E7 proteins with the retinoblastoma tumor suppressor gene product. EMBO J 8:4099, 1989.

Muto MG, Welch WR, Mok SC-H, et al: Evidence for a multifocal origin of papillary serous carcinoma of the peritoneum. Cancer Res 55:490, 1995.

Nagase S, Yamakawa H, Sato S, Yajima A, Horii A: Identification of a 790-kilobase region of common allelic loss in chromosome 10q25-q26 in human endometrial cancer. Cancer Res 57:1630, 1997.

Narod SA, Feunteun J, Lynch HT, et al: Familial breast-ovarian cancer locus on chromosome 17q12-q23. Lancet 338:82, 1991.

Narod SA, Ford D, Devilee P, et al: An evaluation of genetic heterogeneity in 145 breast-ovarian cancer families. Am J Hum Genet 56:254, 1995a.

Narod SA, Ford D, Devilee P, et al: Genetic heterogeneity of breast-ovarian cancer revisited. Am J Hum Genet 57:957, 1995b.

Narod SA, Madlensky L, Bradley L, et al: Hereditary and familial ovarian cancer in Southern Ontario. Cancer 74:2341, 1994.

Neuhausen S, Gilewski T, Norton L, et al: Recurrent BRCA2 6174delT mutations in Ashkenazi Jewish women affected by breast cancer. Nature Genet 13:126, 1996.

Nicolaides NC, Papadopoulos N, Liu B, et al: Mutations of two PMS homologues in hereditary nonpolyposis colon cancer. Nature 371:75, 1994.

Nowell P: The clonal evolution of tumor cell populations. Science 194:23, 1976.

Nystrom-Lahti M, Parsons R, Sistonen P, et al: Mismatch repair genes on chromosomes 2p and 3p account for a major share of hereditary nonpolyposis colorectal cancer families evaluable by linkage. Am J Hum Genet 55:659, 1994.

Ocadiz R, Sauceda R, Cruz M, et al: High correlation between molecular alterations of the c-myc oncogene and carcinoma of the uterine cervix. Cancer Res 47:4173, 1987.

Oddoux C, Struewing JP, Clayton CM, et al: The carrier frequency of the BRCA2 6174delT mutation among Askenazi Jewish individuals is approximately 1%. Nature Genet 14:188, 1996.

Okamoto A, Sameshima Y, Yamada Y, et al: Allelic loss on chromosome 17p and p53 mutations in human endometrial carcinoma of the uterus. Cancer Res 51:5632, 1991a.

Okamoto A, Sameshima Y, Yokoyama S, et al: Frequent allelic losses and mutations of the p53 gene in human ovarian cancer. Cancer Res 51:5171, 1991b.

Orita M, Iwahana H, Kanazawa H, et al: Detection of polymorphisms of human DNA by gel electrophoresis as single-strand conformation polymorphisms. Proc Natl Acad Sci USA 86:2766, 1989.

Osborne RJ, Leech V: Polymerase chain reaction allelotyping of human ovarian cancer. Br J Cancer 69:429, 1994.

Ouyang H, Shiwaku HO, Hagiwara H, et al: The insulin-like growth factor II receptor gene is mutated in genetically unstable cancers of the endometrium, stomach, and colorectum. Cancer Res 57:1851, 1997.

Paquette RL, Lee YY, Wilczynski SP, et al: Mutations of p53 and human papillomavirus infection in cervical carcinoma. Cancer 72:1272, 1993.

Parazzini F, La Vecchia C, Bocciolone L, et al: The epidemiology of endometrial cancer. Gynecol Oncol 41:1, 1991.

Park DJ, Wilczynski SP, Paquette RL, et al: p53 mutations in HPV-negative cervical carcinoma. Oncogene 9:205, 1994.

Parsons R, Myeroff L, Liu B, et al: Microsatellite instability and mutations of the transforming growth factor β type II receptor gene in colorectal cancer. Cancer Res 55:5548, 1995.

Peiffer SL, Herzog TJ, Tribune DJ, et al: Allelic loss of sequences from the long arm of chromosome 10 and replication errors in endometrial cancers. Cancer Res 55:1922, 1995.

Peltomäki P, Aaltonen LA, Sistonen P, et al: Genetic mapping of a locus predisposing to human colorectal cancer. Science 260:810, 1993.

Phelan CM, Lancaster JM, Tonin P, et al: Mutation analysis of the BRCA2 gene in 49 site-specific breast cancer families. Nature Genet 13:120, 1996a.

Phelan CM, Rebbeck TR, Weber BL, et al: Ovarian cancer risk in BRCA1 carriers is modified by the HRAS1 variable number of tandem repeat (VNTR) locus. Nature Genet 12:309, 1996b.

Phillips NJ, Ziegler MR, Radford DM, et al: Allelic deletion on chromosome 17p13.3 in early ovarian cancer. Cancer Res 56:606, 1996.

Powell SM, Petersen GM, Krush AJ, et al: Molecular diagnosis of familial adenomatous polyposis. N Engl J Med 329:1982, 1993.

Prat J, Oliva E, Lerma E, et al: Uterine papillary serous adenocarcinoma: a 10-case study of p53 and c-erbB-2 expression and DNA content. Cancer 74:1778, 1994.

Rajan JV, Marquis ST, Gardner HP, et al: Developmental expression of Brca2 co-localizes with Brca1 and is associated with proliferation and differentiation in multiple tissues. Dev Biol 184:385, 1997.

Rampino N, Yamamoto H, Ionov Y, et al: Somatic frameshift mutations in the BAX gene in colon cancers of the microsatellite mutator phenotype. Science 275:967, 1997.

Randall TC, Boyd J: Genetics of gynecologic sarcomas. CME J Gynecol Oncol 2:182, 1998.

Rao VN, Shao N, Ahmad M, et al: Antisense RNA to the putative tumor suppressor gene BRCA1 transforms mouse fibroblasts. Oncogene 12:523, 1996.

Renan MJ: How many mutations are required for tumorigenesis? Implications from human cancer data. Mol Carcinog 7:139, 1993.

Riou G, Barrois M, Sheng Z-M, et al: Somatic deletions and mutations of c-Ha-ras gene in human cervical cancers. Oncogene 3:329, 1988.

Risinger JI, Berchuck A, Kohler MF, et al: Genetic instability of microsatellites in endometrial carcinoma. Cancer Res 53:5100, 1993.

Risinger JI, Dent GA, Ignar-Trowbridge D, et al: p53 gene mutations in human endometrial carcinoma. Mol Carcinog 5:250, 1992.

Risinger JI, Hayes AK, Berchuck A, Barrett JC: PTEN/MMAC1 mutations in endometrial cancers. Cancer Res 57:4736, 1997.

Risinger JI, Umar A, Boyer JC, et al: Microsatellite instability in gynecological cancers and in hMSH2 mutant uterine sarcoma cell lines defective in mismatch repair activity. Cancer Res 55:5664, 1995.

Roa BB, Boyd AA, Volcik K, et al: Ashkenazi Jewish population frequencies for common mutations in BRCA1 and BRCA2. Nature Genet 14:185, 1996.

Rubin SC, Finstad CL, Federici MG, et al: Prevalence and significance of HER-2/neu expression in early epithelial ovarian cancer. Cancer 73:1456, 1994.

Rubin SC, Finstad CL, Wong GY, et al: Prognostic significance of HER-2/neu expression in advanced epithelial ovarian cancer: a multivariate analysis. Am J Obstet Gynecol 168:162, 1993.

Russell SEH, Hickey GL, Lowry WS, et al: Allele loss from chromosome 17 in ovarian cancer. Oncogene 5:1581, 1990.

Saffari B, Jones LA, el-Naggar A, et al: Amplification and overexpression of the HER-2/neu (c-erbB2) in endometrial cancers: correlation with overall survival. Cancer Res 55:5693, 1995.

Saito H, Inazawa J, Saito S, et al: Detailed deletion mapping of chromosome 17q in ovarian and breast cancers: 2-cM region on 17q21.3 often and commonly deleted in tumors. Cancer Res 53:3382, 1993.

Sandles LG, Shulman LP, Elias S, et al: Endometrial adenocarcinoma: genetic analysis suggesting heritable site-specific uterine cancer. Gynecol Oncol 47:167, 1992.

Sanger F, Nicklen S, Coulson AR: DNA sequencing with chain-terminating inhibitors. Proc Natl Acad Sci USA 74:5463, 1977.

Sasaki H, Nishii H, Takahashi H, et al: Mutation of the Ki-ras protooncogene in human endometrial hyperplasia and carcinoma. Cancer Res 53:1906, 1993.

Sato T, Saito H, Morita R, et al: Allelotype of human ovarian cancer. Cancer Res 51:5118, 1991.

Scheffner M, Werness BA, Huibregtse JM, et al: The E6 oncoprotein encoded by human papillomavirus types 16 and 18 promotes the degradation of p53. Cell 63:1129, 1990.

Schildkraut JM, Risch N, Thompson WD: Evaluating genetic association among ovarian, breast, and endometrial cancer: evidence for a breast/ovarian cancer relationship. Am J Hum Genet 45:521, 1989.

Schmidt L, Duh F-M, Chen F, et al: Germline and somatic mutations in the tyrosine kinase domain of the MET proto-oncogene in papillary renal carcinomas. Nature Genet 16:68, 1997.

Scully R, Anderson SF, Chao DM, et al: BRCA1 is a component of the RNA polymerase II holoenzyme. Proc Natl Acad Sci USA 94:5605, 1997a.

Scully R, Chen J, Plug A, et al: Association of BRCA1 with Rad51 in mitotic and meiotic cells. Cell 88:265, 1997b.

Scully R, Ganesan S, Brown M, et al: Location of BRCA1 in human breast and ovarian cancer cells. Science 272:123, 1996.

Shao N, Chai YL, Shyam E, et al: Induction of apoptosis by the tumor suppressor protein BRCA1. Oncogene 13:1, 1996.

Sharan SK, Morimatsu M, Albrecht U, et al: Embryonic lethality and radiation hypersensitivity mediated by Rad51 in mice lacking Brca2. Nature 386:804, 1997.

Shattuck-Eidens D, McClure M, Simard J, et al: A collaborative survey of 80 mutations in the BRCA1 breast and ovarian cancer susceptibility gene. JAMA 273:535, 1995.

Simard J, Tonin P, Durocher F, et al: Common origins of BRCA1 mutations in Canadian breast and ovarian cancer families. Nature Genet 8:392, 1994.

Slamon DJ, Godolphin W, Jones LA, et al: Studies of the HER-2/neu proto-oncogene in human breast and ovarian cancer. Science 244:707, 1989.

Smith SA, Easton DF, Evans DG, et al: Allele losses in the region 17q12-21 in familial breast and ovarian cancer involve the wild-type chromosome. Nature Genet 2:128, 1992.

Soong R, Knowles S, Williams KE, et al: Overexpression of p53 protein is an independent prognostic indicator in human endometrial carcinoma. Br J Cancer 74:562, 1996.

Southern EM: Detection of specific sequences among DNA fragments separated by gel electrophoresis. J Mol Biol 98:503, 1975.

Spillman MA, Bowcock AM: BRCA1 and BRCA2 mRNA levels are coordinately elevated in human breast cancer cells in response to estrogen. Oncogene 13:1639, 1996.

Srivatsan ES, Misra BC, Venugopalan M, et al: Loss of heterozygosity for alleles on chromosome 11 in cervical carcinoma. Am J Hum Genet 49:868, 1991.

Steck PA, Pershouse MA, Jasser SA, et al: Identification of a candidate tumour suppressor gene, MMAC1, at chromosome 10q23.3 that is mutated in multiple advanced cancers. Nature Genet 15:356, 1997.

Steichen-Gersdorf E, Gallion HH, Ford D, et al: Familial site-specific ovarian cancer is linked to BRCA1 on 17q12-21. Am J Hum Genet 55:870, 1994.

Stratton JF, Gayther SA, Russell P, et al: Contribution of BRCA1 mutations to ovarian cancer. N Engl J Med 336:1125, 1997.

Struewing JP, Abeliovich D, Peretz T, et al: The carrier frequency of the BRCA1 185delAG mutation is approximately 1% in Ashkenazi Jewish individuals. Nature Genet 11:198, 1995.

Takahashi H, Behbakht K, McGovern PE, et al: Mutation analysis of the BRCA1 gene in ovarian cancers. Cancer Res 55:2998, 1995.

Takahashi H, Chiu H-C, Bandera CA, et al: Mutations of the BRCA2 gene in ovarian carcinomas. Cancer Res 56:2738, 1996.

Tashiro H, Blazes MS, Wu R, et al: Mutations in PTEN are frequent in endometrial carcinoma but rare in other common gynecological malignancies. Cancer Res 57:3935, 1997c.

Tashiro H, Isacson C, Levine R, et al: p53 gene mutations are common in uterine serous carcinoma and occur early in their pathogenesis. Am J Pathol 150:177, 1997a.

Tashiro H, Lax SF, Gaudin PB, et al: Microsatellite instability is uncommon in uterine serous carcinoma. Am J Pathol 150:75, 1997b.

Tavtigian SV, Simard J, Rommens J, et al: The complete BRCA2 gene and mutations in chromosome 13q-linked kindreds. Nature Genet 12:333, 1996.

Teneriello MG, Ebina M, Linnoila RI, et al: p53 and Ki-ras gene mutations in epithelial ovarian neoplasms. Cancer Res 53:3103, 1993.

Thorlacius S, Olafsdottir G, Tryggvadottir L, et al: A single BRCA2 mutation in male and female breast cancer families from Iceland with varied cancer phenotypes. Nature Genet 13:117, 1996.

Tsao SW, Mok SCH, Knapp RC, et al: Molecular genetic evidence for a unifocal origin for human serous ovarian carcinomas. Gynecol Oncol 48:5, 1993.

Vandamme B, Lissens W, Amfo K, et al: Deletion of chromosome 11p13-11p15.5 sequences in invasive human ovarian cancer is a subclonal progression factor. Cancer Res 52:6646, 1992.

Vaughn JP, Davis PL, Jarboe MD, et al: BRCA1 expression is induced before DNA synthesis in both normal and tumor-derived breast cells. Cell Growth Differ 7:711, 1996.

Vogelstein B, Kinzler KW: The multistep nature of cancer. Trends Genet 9:138, 1993.

Wang SC, Lin SH, Su LK, et al: Changes in BRCA2 expression during progression of the cell cycle. Biochem Biophys Res Commun 234:247, 1997.

Watson P, Lynch HT: Extracolonic cancer in hereditary nonpolyposis colorectal cancer. Cancer 71:677, 1993.

Weinberg RA: Oncogenes, antioncogenes, and the molecular basis of multistep carcinogenesis. Cancer Res 49:3713, 1989.

Weinberg RA: Tumor suppressor genes. Science 254:1138, 1991.

Werness BA, Levine AJ, Howley PM: Association of human papillomavirus types 16 and 18 E6 proteins with p53. Science 248:76, 1990.

Wertheim I, Muto MG, Welch WR, et al: p53 gene mutation in human borderline epithelial ovarian tumors. J Natl Cancer Inst 86:1549, 1994.

Wistuba II, Montellano FD, Milchgrub S, et al: Deletions of chromosome 3p are frequent and early events in the pathogenesis of uterine cervical carcinoma. Cancer Res 57:3154, 1997.

Wooster R, Bignell G, Lancaster J, et al: Identification of the breast cancer susceptibility gene BRCA2. Nature 378:789, 1995.

Wooster R, Neuhausen SL, Mangion J, et al: Localization of a breast cancer susceptibility gene, BRCA2, to chromosome 13q12-13. Science 265:2088, 1994.

Wright TC, Ferenczy A, Kurman RJ: Carcinoma and other tumors of the cervix. In Kurman RJ (ed): Blaustein's Pathology of the Female Genital Tract. New York, Springer-Verlag, 1994, p 279.

Yang-Feng TL, Han H, Chan KC, et al: Allelic loss in ovarian cancer. Int J Cancer 54:546, 1993.

Zheng W, Cao P, Zheng M, et al: p53 overexpression and bcl-2 persistence in endometrial carcinoma: comparison of papillary serous and endometrioid subtypes. Gynecol Oncol 61:164, 1996.

20

Principles of Statistics

John A. Blessing

Statistics can be viewed as a language that enables scientists to discuss their hypotheses, results, and conclusions in comparable terms. As with any language, idiomatic phrases, slang jargon, proper terminology, and improper application of limited knowledge are but a few contingencies. The objective of this chapter is not to impart "statistical fluency" but rather to enable one to develop the ability to understand and partake in casual "conversational statistics."

Just as a limited vocabulary must be developed before a sentence is constructed, a minimal understanding of probability is requisite to any examination of statistics. Following a discussion of two basic probability distributions and their characteristics, statistical techniques of sampling, confidence intervals, and hypothesis formulation and testing are addressed. Additionally, application of these topics in a clinical trial setting are developed. Finally, often-encountered terminology is discussed with regard to interpretation and limitation.

PROBABILITY

When a scientific investigator conducts an experiment, the outcome generally cannot be predicted with certainty. That is, if the same experiment were conducted repeatedly under identical conditions, the result would not necessarily be the same. Since the results are earmarked by variability and affected by chance, we use the term *random variable* to denote the outcome of interest. The set of all possible outcomes of a random variable and the associated probability of occurrence of each outcome constitutes the *probability distribution* of the random variable.

If the possible number of outcomes is finite, then the random variable is called *discrete*. Examples of experiments described by discrete random variables include

1. A coin is tossed three times and the number of heads is noted.
2. A patient suffering from advanced measurable ovarian cancer is treated with a chemotherapeutic agent, and her response is determined.

If the possible outcomes of an experiment are not countable, the random variable is called *continuous*. One of the most commonly encountered continuous random variables is survival time. Others include disease-free survival and response duration.

Our purposes do not require that we become familiar with all probability distributions; it is sufficient to understand that there are many distinct distributions and that proper analysis and interpretation are contingent upon selection of the appropriate one for each set of circumstances. A brief examination of those most relevant to clinical investigation follows.

Binomial Distribution

A *Bernoulli trial* is one that has only two possible outcomes (called *binary* outcomes), which can be labeled as success or failure. It is common practice to denote the probability of success by p. If n independent Bernoulli trials are conducted and if the probability of success is p for all trials, then the discrete random variable representing the total number of successes observed has a *binomial* probability distribution. The values n and p are called *parameters*; they are constants for the individual experiment, but can and will vary from setting to setting. The true value of p is generally unknown. However, it is possible to make statistical inferences about p from the outcomes of experiments. This is discussed in later sections.

Probabilities for the binominal distribution have been tabulated and are widely available for values of p between 0.05 and 0.95 and for values of n from 1 to 20 (Freund, 1971). If p is very small and n is very large, the binomial distribution is well approximated by the *Poisson distribution*; additionally, if n is large, say, greater than 20, the *normal distribution* may be employed to approximate the binomial distribution. This is pointed out not to muddy the water at this point, but to reiterate that use of the appropriate distribution for the specific problem at hand must be considered.

As an example, suppose that 14 patients suffering from the same disease have all been treated independently with the same agent. Also assume that the outcome will be quantified as a response or a nonresponse and that the probability of a response for all patients is approximately 0.40. The binomial distribution would seem to apply. The probability distribution for $n = 14$ and $p = 0.40$ is presented in Table 20–1 and depicted in Figure 20–1. The probability of observing exactly five responses is approximately 0.20; the probability of observing five or fewer responses is found by adding the individual probabilities and is approximately 0.48.

TABLE 20–1

The Binomial Probability Distribution
($n = 14, p = 0.40$)

No. of Successes	Probability of Occurrence
0	.0008
1	.0073
2	.0317
3	.0845
4	.1549
5	.2066
6	.2066
7	.1574
8	.0918
9	.0408
10	.0136
11	.0083
12	.0005
13	.0001
14	.0000

Normal Distribution

Many distributions that are encountered in the real world can be well approximated by a specific probability distribution called the *normal* (or *Gaussian*) *distribution*. This is a smooth, symmetrical, bell-shaped curve that depends on two parameters, μ, the population *mean*, and σ, the population *standard deviation*. The former is the arithmetic average of all items in the population under consideration, and the latter may be thought of

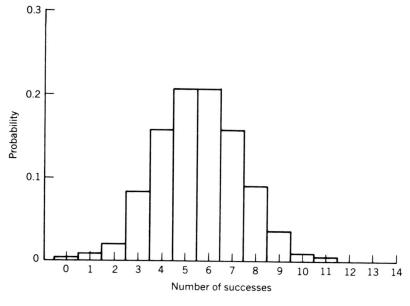

FIGURE 20–1. Binomial distribution.

as an approximate average deviation of the individual items from the population mean. Although μ may take on any value and σ may take on any positive value, for the probability distribution it is only necessary for $\mu = 0$ and $\sigma = 1$ to be tabulated. This is true since, if we denote a random variable having a normal probability distribution with a population mean μ and a population standard deviation σ by X, the new random variable defined as

$$Z = \frac{X - \mu}{\sigma}$$

has a normal probability distribution with mean 0 and standard deviation 1. Z is called a *standard normal random variable* defined by the so-called *Z transformation*.

Again, it is not necessary (or practical) to understand the mathematics of the normal distribution; rather, an appreciation of its properties is of value to the nonstatistician

1. The interval within 1 standard deviation (σ) from the mean contains 68 percent of the total area under the curve (i.e., 68 percent of the total probability of the distribution).
2. The interval within 2 standard deviations (2σ) contains 95.4 percent of the total area under the curve.
3. Virtually all of the area under the curve is contained within 3σ of the mean.

The normal curve is shown in Figure 20–2, and the standard normal distribution is tabulated in Table 20–2. Since the total area under the curve (total probability) is 1.00 and since the curve is symmetrical about its mean ($\mu = 0$ for the standardized normal), it is only necessary to tabulate the area under the curve for the right half.

As an example, denote the average daily high temperature in a certain city during the month of May by X. Assume that the probability distribution for this random variable is normal, with $\mu = 71$ and $\sigma = 3$, and consider the following:

1. What is the probability that the average temperature will be less than 76°F?

$$\text{Prob}(X < 76) = \text{Prob}\left(\frac{X - 71}{3} < \frac{76 - 71}{3}\right)$$

$$= \text{Prob}(Z < 1.67)$$

$$= 0.5 + 0.4525$$

$$= 0.9525$$

2. What is the probability that the average temperature will be greater than 68°F?

$$\text{Prob}(X > 68) = \text{Prob}\left(\frac{X - 71}{3} > \frac{68 - 71}{3}\right)$$

$$= \text{Prob}(Z > -1.00)$$

$$= \text{Prob}(Z < 1.00) \text{ (by symmetry)}$$

$$= 0.5 + 0.3413$$

$$= 0.8413$$

3. What is the probability that the average temperature will fall between 74° and 75° F?

$$\text{Prob}(72 < X < 75)$$

$$= \text{Prob}\left(\frac{72 - 71}{3} < \frac{X - 71}{3} < \frac{75 - 71}{3}\right)$$

$$= \text{Prob}(0.33 < Z < 1.33)$$

$$= \text{Prob}(Z < 1.33) - \text{Prob}(Z < 0.33)$$

$$= (0.5 + 0.4082) - (0.5 + 0.1293)$$

$$= 0.2789$$

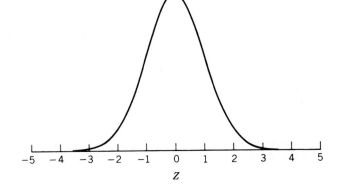

FIGURE 20–2. Standardized normal probability distribution.

T A B L E **20–2**

The Standard Normal Probability Distribution

Z	.00	.01	.02	.03	.04	.05	.06	.07	.08	.09
0.0	.0000	.0040	.0080	.0120	.0160	.0199	.0239	.0279	.0139	.0359
0.1	.0398	.0438	.0478	.0517	.0557	.0596	.0636	.0675	.0714	.0753
0.2	.0793	.0832	.0871	.0910	.0948	.0987	.1026	.1064	.1103	.1141
0.3	.1179	.1217	.1255	.1293	.1331	.1368	.1406	.1443	.1480	.1517
0.4	.1554	.1991	.1628	.1664	.1700	.1736	.1772	.1808	.1844	.1879
0.5	.1915	.1950	.1985	.2019	.2054	.2088	.2123	.2157	.2190	.2224
0.6	.2257	.2291	.2324	.2357	.2389	.2422	.2454	.2486	.2517	.2549
0.7	.2580	.2611	.2642	.2673	.2704	.2734	.2764	.2794	.2823	.2852
0.8	.2881	.2910	.2939	.2967	.2995	.3023	.3051	.3078	.3106	.3133
0.9	.3159	.3186	.3212	.3238	.3264	.3289	.3315	.3340	.3365	.3389
1.0	.3413	.3438	.3461	.3485	.3508	.3531	.3554	.3577	.3599	.3261
1.1	.3643	.3665	.3686	.3708	.3729	.3749	.3770	.3790	.3810	.3830
1.2	.3849	.3869	.3888	.3907	.3925	.3944	.3962	.3980	.3997	.4015
1.3	.4032	.4049	.4066	.4082	.4099	.4115	.4131	.4147	.4162	.4177
1.4	.4192	.4207	.4222	.4236	.4251	.4265	.4279	.4292	.4306	.4319
1.5	.4332	.4345	.4357	.4370	.4382	.4394	.4406	.4418	.4429	.4441
1.6	.4452	.4463	.4474	.4484	.4495	.4505	.4515	.4525	.4535	.4545
1.7	.4554	.4564	.4573	.4582	.4591	.4599	.4608	.4616	.4625	.4633
1.8	.4641	.4649	.4656	.4664	.4671	.4678	.4686	.4693	.4699	.4706
1.9	.4713	.4719	.4726	.4732	.4738	.4744	.4750	.4756	.4761	.4767
2.0	.4772	.4778	.4783	.4788	.4793	.4798	.4803	.4808	.4812	.4817
2.1	.4821	.4826	.4830	.4834	.4838	.4842	.4846	.4850	.4854	.4857
2.2	.4861	.4864	.4868	.4871	.4875	.4878	.4881	.4884	.4887	.4890
2.3	.4893	.4896	.4898	.4901	.4904	.4906	.4909	.4911	.4913	.4916
2.4	.4918	.4920	.4922	.4925	.4927	.4929	.4931	.4932	.4934	.4936
2.5	.4938	.4940	.4941	.4943	.4945	.4946	.4948	.4949	.4951	.4952
2.6	.4953	.4955	.4956	.4957	.4959	.4960	.4961	.4962	.4963	.4964
2.7	.4965	.4966	.4967	.4968	.4969	.4970	.4971	.4972	.4973	.4974
2.8	.4974	.4975	.4976	.4977	.4977	.4978	.4979	.4979	.4980	.4981
2.9	.4981	.4982	.4982	.4983	.4984	.4984	.4985	.4985	.4986	.4986
3.0	.4987	.4987	.4987	.4988	.4988	.4989	.4989	.4989	.4990	.4990

The binomial and normal distributions are by no means the only distributions encountered in scientific investigations, but they will serve as a convenient springboard to a discussion of topics in statistical inference.

STATISTICAL TOPICS

Sampling Theory

In any scientific investigation, it is possible to identify a *population*, which is the entire collection of individuals or items under consideration. However, in most instances, it is neither practical nor possible to investigate or test all elements of the population. Therefore, it is customary to obtain a *sample*, which is a subset of the population employed to examine the properties of the parent population. Statistical techniques are based on the assumption that there is an element of randomness in the sample. For each object sampled, a measurement (or measurements) will be obtained. All information obtained will be used to provide some insight regarding the population. Recall that the true values of population parameters are not known; the information obtained in the sample will be used to draw inferences regarding the total population and its parameters.

A function of the observations that does not depend on any unknown parameters is called a *statistic*. The most frequently encountered statistic is the *sample mean* $(\bar{X})$. If a sample of size n is taken from a population and $X_1, X_2, \ldots X_n$ denotes the individual measurements taken of some characteristic (random variable) of interest, then the sample mean is denoted by

$$\bar{X} = \frac{X_1 + X_2 + \ldots + X_n}{n}$$

Note that the sample mean is a function of random variables and is therefore a random variable itself with its own probability distribution. If μ and σ denote the population mean and standard deviation, respectively, of the individual observations and if $\mu_{\bar{x}}$ and $\sigma_{\bar{x}}$, respectively, denote the mean and standard deviation of the sample mean (commonly called the *standard error of the mean*), then

$$\mu_{\bar{x}} = \mu$$

and

$$\sigma_{\bar{x}} = \frac{\sigma}{\sqrt{n}}$$

There are three important implications of these facts:

1. The sample mean appears to be a good candidate for estimating the unknown population mean.
2. The standard deviation of the mean depends on the variation from item to item in the parent population and upon n, the sample size.
3. The larger the sample size, the smaller the standard deviation of the mean.

One last characteristic of the sample mean is extremely important; it has been shown that if a random sample is taken from some population with mean μ and standard deviation σ, then the sample mean $\bar{X}$ has a distribution that is approximately normal, with mean μ and standard deviation $\sigma\sqrt{n}$. As the sample size increases, the approximation becomes more accurate. This is called the *Central Limit Theorem*, and it enhances the usefulness of the normal distribution. It is noteworthy that this theorem holds true regardless of the probability distribution of the population.

A corollary of this result will show that, if one samples observations from a Bernoulli distribution, then the total number of successes (a binomial random variable), denoted by X, may also be approximated by the normal distribution with $\mu = np$ and $\sigma = \sqrt{np(1 - p)}$.

As an example, suppose that 16 patients are treated independently with the same agent. Additionally, the outcome will be quantified as either a response or a nonresponse, and the probability of a response is 0.50 for all patients. Using the binomial tables to find the exact probability of between 6 and 10 responses, we find

$$\text{Prob}(6 \leq X \leq 10) = 0.7900$$

We will now approximate this probability using the normal distribution, with $\mu = np = 8$ and $\sigma = \sqrt{np(1 - p)} = 2$.

$$\text{Prob}(6 \leq X \leq 10) = \text{Prob}\left(\frac{6 - 8}{2} \leq Z \leq \frac{10 - 8}{2}\right)$$

$$= \text{Prob}(-1 \leq Z \leq 1)$$

$$= 0.6826$$

This approximation is not particularly good; could it be that n is not large enough to obtain accuracy? Recall that the binomial distribution is discrete, whereas the normal distribution is continuous. It has been shown that in this type of situation the accuracy can be greatly improved if a *continuity correction* is employed. This consists of adding 0.5 of a unit to each end of the range of the original probability statement (only to one end if the original statement is one-sided, such as Prob[$X \leq 7$]). In the present example,

$$\text{Prob}(6 \leq Z \leq 10) = \text{Prob}(5.5 \leq X \leq 10.5)$$

(continuity correction)

$$= \text{Prob}\left(\frac{5.5 - 8}{2} \leq Z \leq \frac{10.5 - 8}{2}\right)$$

$$= \text{Prob}(-1.25 \leq Z \leq 1.25)$$

$$= 0.7888$$

This approximation is quite good and reinforces the fact that the binomial probability distribution need only be tabulated for values of n up to 20. For values of n greater than 20, the normal approximation is appropriate.

Confidence Intervals

As previously noted, we generally do not know the true values of all population parameters; rather, we seek to draw some inference from our sample regarding the unknown parameter(s). We have also seen that the sample mean $\bar{X}$ is a logical choice for an estimate of μ.

If we are sampling from a normal distribution and if we denote by $Z_{\alpha/2}$ the tabulated value of 2 such that the area under the normal curve from $Z_{\alpha/2}$ to ∞ is then

$$\text{Prob}\left(-Z_{\alpha/2} \leq \frac{X - \mu}{\sigma/\sqrt{n}} \leq Z_{\alpha/2}\right) = 1 - \alpha$$

Equivalently,

$$\text{Prob}\left(\bar{X} - Z_{\alpha/2} \cdot \frac{\alpha}{\sqrt{n}} \leq \mu \leq \bar{X} + Z_{\alpha/2} \cdot \frac{\sigma}{\sqrt{n}}\right) = 1 - \alpha$$

Although μ is not a random variable, intuitively we have a degree of confidence equal to $1 - \alpha$ that μ will fall somewhere in the interval defined by $\bar{X} \pm Z_{\alpha/2} \cdot \sigma/\sqrt{n}$. We refer to this as a *two-sided confidence interval* for μ and to $(1 - \alpha)$ percent as the *degree of confidence*.

For example, suppose we have 49 observations from a normal population with $\sigma = 14$ and desire a 95 percent confidence interval for μ. Here $\alpha/2 = 0.025$ and $Z_{\alpha/2} = 1.96$. If the sample mean is 53.6, then the 95 percent confidence interval is given by

$$53.6 \pm 1.96 \cdot \frac{14}{\sqrt{49}}$$

or

$$53.6 \pm 3.92$$

This confidence interval was designed for use in circumstances in which the population being sampled has a normal distribution. However, due to the Central Limit Theorem, it can also be used to estimate the means of other populations with known variances if n is sufficiently large (in practice, if n is 30 or more).

Note that the endpoints of the confidence interval depend on the sample mean, a value from the normal table, and the standard error of the mean, $\sigma/\sqrt{n}$. In practice, it is not likely that σ will be known. The standard deviation of a sample, denoted by s, is defined as

$$s = \sqrt{\frac{1}{n} \sum_{i=1}^{n} X_i^2 - \bar{X}^2}$$

where

$$\sum_{i=1}^{n} X_i^2$$

denotes the sum of the squares of the n observations.

It would appear logical to substitute the sample standard deviation, s, for the unknown population standard deviation, σ. For the moment, we will again restrict our attention to situations in which the population has a normal probability distribution. In such instances,

$$\frac{\bar{X} - \mu}{s/\sqrt{n}}$$

has a Student's t distribution with $n - 1$ degrees of freedom. The *Student's t distribution* comprises a family of distinct curves, one for each positive integer, n. The probability distribution is tabulated for degrees of freedom up to 29. For larger values the distribution is virtually identical to the normal distribution. If we denote by $t_{\alpha/2, n-1}$ the tabulated value such that the area under the curve for $n - 1$ degrees of freedom from $t_{\alpha/2, n-1}$ to ∞ is $\alpha/2$, then

$$\text{Prob}\left(-t_{\alpha/2, n-1} \leq \frac{\bar{X} - \mu}{s/\sqrt{n}} \leq t_{\alpha/2, n-1}\right) = 1 - \alpha$$

In an analogous fashion to the previous discussions, we find that the interval defined by

$$\bar{X} \pm t_{\alpha/2, n-1} \cdot \frac{s}{\sqrt{n}}$$

provides a $(1 - \alpha)$ percent confidence interval for μ when σ is unknown. Moreover, if the population is not known to be normal, this methodology will provide an approximate large-sample confidence interval.

The construction of one-sided confidence intervals proceeds in a similar fashion. However, in selecting tabulated values, care must be taken to employ α rather than $\alpha/2$. For example, suppose that 25 patients received the same dose and schedule of chemotherapy for the treatment of recurrent ovarian carcinoma. If the average white blood cell count nadir following course 1 is of interest and our testing reveals that

$$\bar{X} = 2{,}900 \text{ mm}^3$$

$$s = 532 \text{ mm}^3$$

then a 95 percent confidence interval for the true average white blood cell count following course 1 is given by

$$2{,}900 \pm 2.064 \cdot \frac{532}{5}$$

That is,

$$2{,}900 \pm 219.6 \ mm^3$$

If the underlying distribution is known to be normal, the confidence interval is exact; otherwise, it is approximate. Various other confidence intervals can be constructed, but those outlined in this chapter are apt to be of the most use in a clinical setting.

Estimation

It is helpful to be able to construct confidence intervals for unknown population parameters. However, it is frequently more desirable to obtain actual estimates of the values of the parameters. We have seen that the sample mean and the sample standard deviation are intuitive choices to use in estimating their population analogs. Sample proportions might also be considered in estimating unknown population proportions. The statistic employed is called an *estimator*, and the actual value realized is called an *estimate*. Fortuitously, the statistics considered do possess the desired statistical properties that make them judicious choices. These properties include lack of bias, minimum variance, consistency, relative efficiency, and sufficiency. A description of these topics is beyond the scope of this chapter. Likewise, the method of deriving estimators in situations in which intuition is of no value is not appropriate in this context. It is sufficient to note that a methodology exists for determining appropriate estimators and that they do not contradict our "gut feelings" in these elementary situations.

Hypothesis Testing

One of the fundamental elements of the scientific process is the formulation and testing of hypotheses. In designing the investigation, a *null hypothesis*, denoted by H_0, is postulated. As its name suggests, the null hypothesis often features no substantial positive result, consequently, the scientist often hopes to reject this statement. The null hypothesis must be stated precisely in statistical terms. Similarly, an alternative hypothesis, H_a, must

also be formulated and precisely stated. The ultimate result of experimentation will be either to accept or reject the null hypothesis on the basis of a test statistic. As shown in Table 20–3, two types of error are possible. If the sample data lead to a rejection of H_0 but in reality H_0 is true, the resulting error is termed a *type I error*. Conversely, if H_0 is accepted and in reality H_a is true, the resulting error is known as a *type II error*. Generally, the erroneous rejection of H_0 with its implied acceptance of H_a constitutes a false endorsement of a positive concept. Consequently, the type I error is often referred to as a *false-positive error*. Similarly, erroneous acceptance of H_0, the type II error, is referred to as a *false-negative error*.

It is mathematically impossible to minimize the probabilities of both errors simultaneously without increasing the sample size. In practice, the probability of committing a type I error is usually fixed at some tolerable level, denoted by α. It is called the *level of significance*. The probability of committing a type II error is denoted by β. The power of the test refers to the probability of rejecting H_0 when it is false. It is therefore seen to be equal to $1 - \beta$.

Having specified the level of significance, α, and the sample size, n, an appropriate test statistic is determined. The set of possible outcomes for the test statistic is then partitioned into a rejection region and an acceptance region. Upon collection of the data and calculation of the test statistic, a decision is made. If the calculated statistic falls into the rejection region, H_0 is rejected; if the statistic falls into the acceptance region, H_0 is accepted. The actual determination of the appropriate test statistic and the rejection region cannot be addressed in this context. The basic premise is that if the collected data are not consistent with H_0, it will be rejected, otherwise, H_0 will not be rejected.

Alternative hypotheses may be either one sided or two sided, depending on the logic

T A B L E 20–3
Possible Outcomes in a Test of Hypothesis

Reality	Decision	
	Accept Null	*Reject Null*
Null true	Correct decision	Type I error (false positive)
Null false	Type II error (false negative)	Correct decision

of the experiment. To illustrate, we will suppose that it is desired to compare the proportion of observed responses achieved with chemotherapy regimens I and II. We denote these by P_I and P_{II}, respectively. If the logistics of experimentation rule out the contingency that I would be superior to II (e.g., if regiment I consisted of drug A and regimen II consisted of a combination of drugs A and B, and the properties of each are well known), then the appropriate hypotheses might be

$$H_0 : P_I = P_{II}$$

$$H_a : P_{II} \geq P_I \text{ (one-sided alternative)}$$

Conversely, if either regimen could protentially prove superior to the other, the more appropriate hypotheses would be

$$H_0 : P_I = P_{II}$$

$$H_a : P_I \neq P_{II} \text{ (two-sided alternative)}$$

As an example of a test of a hypothesis, suppose that it is desired to examine the first-course platelet count nadirs of 36 patients receiving a chemotherapeutic agent under identical circumstances. The drug manufacturer states that the average nadir is $100,000/mm^3$. It is desired to compare this against the alternative that the average nadir is actually lower (a one-sided alternative), subject to $\alpha = 0.05$ and $n = 25$. Our hypotheses are

$$H_0 : \mu_0 = 100,000$$

$$H_a : \mu_a < 100,000$$

The appropriate test of H_0 is to reject H_0 if

$$\frac{\bar{X} - \mu_0}{s/\sqrt{n}} < -t_{.05, 24} = -1.711$$

This is the case since, if H_0 is true, then

$$\frac{\bar{X} - \mu_0}{s/\sqrt{n}}$$

has a t distribution with 24 degrees of freedom. Consequently,

$$\text{Prob} \left(\frac{\bar{X} - \mu_0}{s/\sqrt{n}} < -t_{.05, 24} \right) = .05$$

If, when the data are collected, $\bar{X} = 95,000$ and $s = 12,500$, then

$$\frac{\bar{X} - \mu_0}{s/\sqrt{n}} = \frac{95,000 - 100,000}{12,500/5}$$

$$= \frac{-5,000}{2,500}$$

$$= -2 < -1.711$$

Therefore, H_0 must be rejected.

The previous example is but one of various problems encountered. The difficulty lies not in calculating the test statistic but rather in knowing which distribution and associated test statistic to apply in a given situation. For example, if n is greater than 30, the Central Limit Theorem would allow the normal distribution to apply. It would be unwise to attempt most tests of hypotheses without consultation with a trained statistician. A very readable presentation of many frequently encountered hypothesis testing problems has been compiled by Brown and Hollander (1977).

CLINICAL TRIAL APPLICATIONS

The discussion is here limited to medical investigations designed to study the therapeutic efficacy of treatment agents. Zelen (1983) has defined a *clinical trial* as "a scientific experiment to generate clinical data for the purpose of evaluating one or more therapies on a population." The importance of determining a well-designed, feasible study prior to initiation of the investigation cannot be overemphasized. Medical journals are filled with anecdotal studies that are of little or no predictive value regarding the population. Such articles may do more harm than good, since the casual reader may become convinced of the existence of unproven efficacy. Moreover, the lack of a proven significant result in such studies in no way precludes the existence of such a result.

Several types of clinical trials are employed in clinical trials methodology. Once a new regimen is devised and tested in animal studies, a phase I study is conducted to determine the optimal dose and schedule. Next, a phase II study is planned to examine the response and the possible adverse effects. If warranted by the results, a phase III study is initiated to compare the new regimen with the standard therapy. This latter study, conducted in a prospective, randomized fashion, is the appropriate vehicle for carrying out the comparative clinical trial. More detailed discussions of the various types of clinical trials are found in Gehan and Schneiderman (1982) and Blessing (1985).

The results may either determine a new mode of therapy or rule out any further investigation. Therefore, careful planning is required to provide definitive, unambiguous results. In designing a study, the following guidelines are suggested:

1. Interaction between the medical investigator and the statistician at the outset will enhance the chance of achieving a sound study design and quality results.
2. The appropriateness and feasibility of applying a phase II or phase III study to the question being posed must be determined.
3. If a phase II study is desired, the precision of the confidence interval estimate of the response rate (or other binary variables) and the associated level of confidence should be determined. The sample size can then be considered. Serious consideration should be given to implementing a two-stage sampling design to minimize the expenditure of patient resources on inactive agents.
4. If a phase III study of the response rate is desired, it should be determined whether a one-sided or two-sided test of the hypothesis is appropriate, what values of α and β are desirable, what the baseline response rate is, and how large a difference is to be sought. The sample size can then be considered.
5. Similar considerations must be made regarding studies of survival and other time variables.

It is appropriate to consider phase II and phase III studies separately.

Phase II Studies

The key concept in conducing a phase II clinical trial is the required sample size. If we wish to estimate the true probability of getting a response (as opposed to a nonresponse), we recall that we are really trying to estimate the parameter, p, of a binomial distribution. Using methodology similar to, but more complicated than, that employed in obtaining confidence intervals, the appropriate sample size can be determined so that our estimate will be within a specified range of

the true value of p and we have a given degree of confidence that we are correct. For example, in order to have 90 percent confidence that an estimate is within ± 15 percent of the true value of p, we would require 30 patients. To tighten the 15 percent restraint to 10 percent would require 68 cases, while increasing the confidence level to 95 percent would necessitate 43 observations.

One must balance the extremes of anecdotal cases and extremely precise estimates in designing the phase II study. If estimates are required to be ultraprecise, the ability to test each new agent will be restricted. It is advisable to settle for being 90 percent confident of being within ± 15 percent unless the patient resources are abundant. The investigation of 30 patients provides a reasonable idea of therapeutic efficacy while enabling the evaluation process to proceed.

Agents may be found to be ineffective at an earlier stage. Consequently, it is now customary to build early stopping rules into study designs. One such stopping rule was developed by Gehan (1961). However, it has been frequently misinterpreted and incorrectly applied. In his paper, Gehan gave an example of a study designed to investigate the existence of a 20 percent response rate. If 14 consecutive nonresponses were observed at the outset, using the binomial distribution with $n = 14$, $p = 0.20$, and X denoting the number of responses, then

$$\text{Prob}(X = 0) = 0.044$$

Therefore Gehan stated that if an agent "were 20% effective or more, there would be more than a 95% chance that one or more successes would be obtained in 14 consecutive cases." His paper gave corresponding values for various true values of p; the 20 percent figure was but one example to clarify the tabulated values. It is decidedly false that consecutive failures among the first 14 cases are always an indication for early stopping. This is the case only if the investigation hinges on a hypothesized value of $p = 0.20$. For example, if the true value of p is 0.05, the probability of zero successes in the first 14 trials is 0.4877; thus the occurrence of 14 failures is not at all unlikely and is not an indication for early stopping. Likewise, if the true value of p were 0.50, the probability of consecutive failures in the first five trials is 0.0312. This would indicate that stopping should be considered at this early stage. If stopping rules are employed, a thorough understanding of their use and consequences is required.

Flemming (1982) has proposed a multiple testing procedure that accrues patients in several stages. Following the completion of each stage of patient accession, either early terminal or initiation of the next stage of accrual can occur, based on the observed results. If the initial response rate is very low (or in some instances very high), it may be unnecessary to continue the second phase, thereby maintaining ethical standards and conserving patient resources.

For example, suppose that the current response rate observed with standard salvage therapy for a specific disease process is 20 percent. In testing a new agent in a phase II setting, we will denote the true response rate of the new agent by P. We might then be interested in testing the hypothesis

$$H_0 : P \leq 10$$

versus the alternative

$$H_0 : P \geq 30$$

If we set the level of significance at 0.05 and desire power of at least 0.80, then our required sample size would be 25.

However, if we employ a two-stage sampling plan, we might consider entering 15 patients in the first phase of accrual. If less than two responses are noted, we conclude that H_0 is true, while we reject H_0 if five or more responses are seen. Only if two to four responses are observed, we will resume patient entry and accession an additional 10 patients. In this instance, upon final analysis of the 25 cases, we will accept H_0 if five or fewer responses are noted, while we reject H_0 if six or more responses occur. The resulting power is 0.807. If the agent does not possess the desired efficacy, there is a very good chance that the study will determine this after only 15 patients.

The above example is one possibility. Another would feature three accession stages of 10, 10, and 5 patients. However, the preceding example suffices to exhibit the preservation of size and power while allowing early termination if indicated.

Phase III Studies

As is the case with phase II studies, required sample size is a central concept of phase III studies. Here we are concerned not only with the precision of estimation but also with the feasibility of the study itself. The number of patients required to conduct an appropriate phase III study varies with the type of outcome variable required to address the study objectives. We will examine here the two objectives most commonly encountered: tumor response and survival.

Tumor Response

Although objective tumor response is usually defined in four categories (complete response, partial response, stable disease, and increasing disease), it is preferable in gynecologic investigations to examine the complete response (versus the other three categories combined). Nonetheless, this discussion is readily generalized into responders versus nonresponders. Without loss of generality, we assume response to be a binary random variable. Thus, once again, the binomial distribution is the underlying model.

In determining sample size, four factors are to be considered:

1. *The magnitude of the difference thought to be clinically significant.* Detection of smaller differences requires a greater number of observations than detection of larger differences. Conversely, there must be valid clinical evidence to suggest that a large difference might exist. Detection of 15 or 20 percent differences is most commonly sought. Looking for a 10 percent difference generally requires a prohibitive number of cases, while the medical setting seldom justifies studies to look for 25 percent or greater differences.

2. *The baseline response rate of the standard group, if applicable.* While not intuitively obvious, detection of the same magnitude of difference requires more patients if the baseline is closer to 50 percent than if it is one of the extremes.

3. *The probabilities of type I and type II errors.* As previously noted, the only way to minimize both simultaneously is to increase the sample size. Common choices for α and β are 0.05 and 0.20, respectively (a 95 percent probability that an observed difference is not due to chance and an 80 percent probability that, if a difference exists, it will be detected). In certain circumstances, α may be relaxed to 0.10 or β decreased to 0.10. Actual choice is dependent on the specific investigation and on

the possible consequences of each error. A detailed discussion of this aspect is found in Blessing (1985).

4. *The type of alternative hypothesis.* Two-sided tests require a greater sample size than do their one-sided counterparts. In general, if one of the regimens constitutes (or may be viewed as) a standard or control regimen, then a one-sided test may be indicated. For example, consider Figure 20–3, which depicts the schema of Gynecologic Oncology Group (GOG) Protocol 48. The two treatment regimens differ by the presence of cyclophosphamide in one regimen. There was little reason to believe that the addition of cyclophosphamide would lessen the activity of Adriamycin (doxorubicin), so only a one-sided test was envisioned.

Conversely, if the composition of the regimens is such that either might prove superior, then a two-sided alternative is appropriate. Figure 20–4 depicts the schema for GOG Protocol 77, a phase III randomized study of carboplatin and CHIP (iproplatin) in patients with advanced or recurrent cervical carcinoma. In designing this study, the superiority of either drug was considered a possibility, and thus a two-sided alternative was required.

To visualize how these four factors interact, Table 20–4 presents the number of patients required in each regimen to demonstrate a 15 percent treatment difference for various combinations of baseline response, α and β, and type of alternative based on methodology presented by Cochran and Cox (1957). Casagrande et al (1980) have revised the figures for one-sided tests, resulting in a slight increase in sample size. The figures of Cochran and Cox are nonetheless employed here to facilitate presentation of the interaction of the four factors noted previously. While the number of patients required to investigate the existence of a 15 percent difference varies considerably, one fact is clear: the credibility of comparative studies featuring multiple regimens composed of only 25 patients must be severely questioned. Such studies are trivial and constitute a substantial waste of resources.

O'Brian and Flemming (1979) have proposed a multiple testing procedure applicable to this situation that enables early testing if one regimen has markedly better efficacy than the other. In this instance, the number of tests and the number of patients between each test is fixed in advance. The mathematical details are beyond the scope of this chapter. It is sufficient to state that ethical consid-

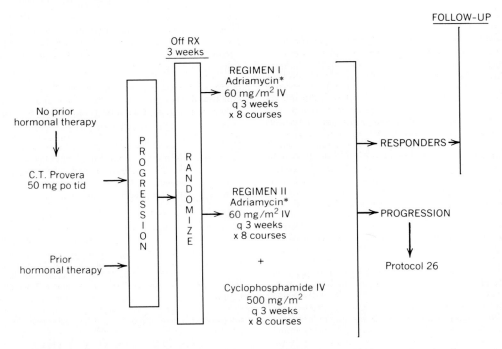

FIGURE 20–3. Algorithm of Gynecologic Oncology Group Protocol 48. A randomized comparison of Adriamycin (doxorubicin) versus Adriamycin plus cyclophosphamide in patients with advanced endometrial carcinoma after hormonal failure. *Maximum cumulative dose 480 mg/m^2.

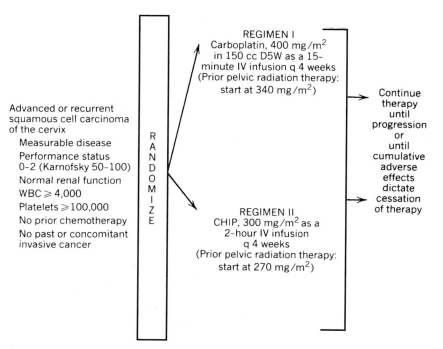

FIGURE 20–4. Algorithm of Gynecologic Oncology Group Protocol 77. A randomized study of carboplatin versus CHIP (iproplatin) in advanced carcinoma of the cervix.

erations can be accommodated in phase III trials.

Survival

We have interpreted *response* as a discrete random variable with two possible outcomes. Survival (or response duration, progression-free interval, and so forth) is a continuous random variable measured in time and may be visualized as having an infinite number of possible outcomes. Moreover, at any given point, many observations may be censored by time (i.e., still alive, in response, disease free). It is not surprising, then, that studies whose main objective is a comparison of sur-

vival require a different methodology than do studies whose main objective is a comparison of response rates. Once again, consideration must be given to the values of α and β, the type of alternative hypothesis, and the magnitude of the difference sought. However, the latter aspect is not particularly intuitive. Statistical methodology is sophisticated, and even resulting sample size tables require interpretation by someone trained in this area.

George and Desu (1974) have presented the number of observed *failures* (not entries) required in each regimen to determine a significant difference in two survival distributions. Table 20–5 depicts sample size requirements based on this methodology. This information is difficult to employ appropriately, but it does underscore the need for a substantial number of failures (and a large number of entries) for a meaningful study. Publications making sweeping generalizations based on a small number of patients must be viewed with considerable skepticism.

CONTINGENCY TABLES

Suppose that a phase III study has been designed to compare the complete response

TABLE **20–4**

Number of Patients Required in Each Regimen to Detect a 15% Treatment Difference (α = 0.05)

Response Rates of Each Regimen	β	No. of Patients	
		One-Sided	Two-Sided
5–20%	0.20	55	69
	0.10	76	93
25–40%	0.20	120	150
	0.10	165	200
45–60%	0.20	135	175
	0.10	190	230

TABLE 20-5

Number of Patients (d^*) Required to Detect a Significant Difference in Two Survival Distributions

$1 - \beta^\dagger$	$\Delta^\ddagger$													
	1.1	1.2	1.3	1.4	1.5	1.6	1.7	1.8	1.9	2.0	2.5	3.0	3.5	4.0
0.95	3,479	951	460	280	193	144	113	92	77	66	38	27	21	17
	2,384	652	315	192	132	98	77	63	53	46	26	18	14	12
0.90	2,870	785	379	231	159	118	93	76	64	55	32	22	17	14
	1,884	515	249	152	105	78	61	50	42	36	21	15	11	9
0.80	2,213	605	292	178	123	91	72	59	49	42	24	17	13	11
	1,360	372	180	110	76	56	44	36	30	26	15	11	8	7

*The number of patients required for each treatment group, all followed until failure.
†The probability of detecting a significant difference at the 0.01 level (upper figure) or the 0.05 level (lower figure) when the true ratio is Δ.
‡The ratio of the median survival for the experimental treatment group to the median survival for the control treatment group (the ratio of means could be substituted for the ratio of medians).

rates of two chemotherapeutic agents. We denote the true response rate for each agent by P_1 and P_2, respectively. Furthermore, the number of observations will be denoted by n_1 and n_2, respectively. We are essentially comparing the proportions of two binomial populations. If we assume that a two-sided test is warranted, then the hypothesis of interest is $H_0 : P_1 \neq P_2$. If we cross-classify the results, as shown in Table 20-6, we have what is called a *contingency table*. Since the patients have been dichotomized in two different ways (treatment agent and response), this is called a *2 × 2 contingency table*. The general form, called an *r × c contingency table*, classifies all observations with respect to two qualitative variables, one having *r* categories and the other having *c* categories.

How does one test this hypothesis? We will define a test statistic as

$$\chi^2 = \frac{(n_1 + n_2)(ad - bc)^2}{n_1 n_2 (a + c)(b + d)}$$

When H_0 is true, then χ^2 has an approximate chi-square distribution with 1 degree of freedom. Like Student's *t* distribution, there is a family of continuous probability distributions, one for each positive integer (degree of freedom). If we denote by $\chi^2_{\alpha\nu}$ the tabulated value

such that the area under the curve for ν degrees of freedom from $\chi^2_{\alpha\nu}$ to ∞ is α, then

$$\text{Prob}(\chi^2 \geq \chi^2_{\alpha,\nu}) = \alpha$$

Thus our test criterion is to reject H_0 if $\chi^2 \geq \chi^2_{\alpha,1}$. For example, if a $\alpha = 0.05$ and if the results of the trial are as shown in Table 20-7, then

$$\chi^2 = 5.128 > \chi^2_{0.05,1} = 3.84$$

Thus H_0 is rejected.

Once again, we have used a continuous distribution to address a problem arising out of a discrete distribution. *Yates' continuity correction* has been suggested as an alternative approach that modifies the calculation of χ^2 as follows:

$$\chi^2 = \frac{[(n_1 + n_2)(|ad - bc| - 0.05(n_1 + n_2)]^2}{n_1 n_2 (a + c)(b + d)}$$

where the term $|ad - bc|$ denotes the absolute value of $(ad - bc)$. If the sample size is suitably large, the correction will have little effect on the value of χ^2. In the example, the resultant value of χ^2 would be 4.467 and H_0 would still be rejected.

Finally, we note that when H_0 is true, χ^2 has an approximately chi-square distribution.

TABLE 20-6

Format of a Contingency Table

Treatment Agent	Complete Response	Others	Total
I	a	$b(= n_1 - a)$	n_1
II	c	$d(= n_2 - c)$	n_2
Total	$a + c$	$b + d$	$n_1 + n_2$

TABLE 20-7

Example of a Contingency Table

Regimen	Complete Response	Others	Total
I	40	60	100
II	25	75	100
Total	65	135	200

Are there situations in which the approximation should not be used? If the individual entries in the table are small, usually five or fewer, an alternative is *Fisher's exact test*. Its actual use is not described here, but we note its existence for completeness.

The chi-square distribution is applicable to many practical problems, not just the 2×2 contingency tables. Other more complex problems include $r \times c$ contingency tables, tests for both homogeneity and independence, and tests for trends in proportions. Although the calculation of the test statistic may become more complex and the degrees of freedom may increase, the methodology consists of calculating the test statistic, comparing it to the appropriate entry in the chi-square probability distribution table, and deciding to accept or reject H_0.

Life Tables

We have seen in the preceding section that discrete random variables such as response are conveniently presented in contingency tables and analyzed employing the chi-square statistic. How to we proceed when dealing with time variables such as survival? Data are most conveniently presented in a life table.

For each treatment regimen, a separate table depicts the following for each interval of time:

1. The number of patients alive at the beginning of the interval.
2. The number of patients dying during the interval.
3. The number of censored observations during the interval.
4. An estimate of the cumulative probability of surviving the interval.

Table 20–8 presents a hypothetical life table for one sample of 25 patients. These data are presented in a *survival curve* in Figure 20–5. In comparing two therapies, a separate life table is constructed for each, and both are displayed on one graph. The actual calculation of probabilities is best accomplished via appropriate computer programs for all but the simplest problems.

Various statistics have been proposed to test for differences between two (or more) survival curves. Our purpose is not to develop or distinguish among them, but rather to be familiar with the general concept. All of the suggested tests involve the calculation (usually by computer) of a test statistic and

TABLE **20–8**

Example of a Life Table

Interval (in Months)	Alive at Start	Failed	Censored*	Cumulative Probability of Survival
0–1	25	1	0	96.0
1–2	24	1	0	92.0
2–3	23	1	0	88.0
3–4	22	1	0	84.0
4–5	21	1	0	80.0
5–6	20	0	1	80.0
6–7	19	0	1	80.0
7–8	18	1	0	75.6
8–9	17	2	0	66.7
9–10	15	1	1	62.1
10–11	13	1	0	57.3
11–12	12	1	0	52.5
12–13	11	0	1	52.5
13–14	10	0	1	52.5
14–15	9	1	0	46.7
15–16	8	0	1	46.7
16–17	7	1	0	40.0
17–18	6	0	1	40.0
18–19	5	0	1	40.0
19–20	4	0	1	40.0
20–21	3	0	1	40.0
21–22	2	0	1	40.0
22–23	1	0	1	40.0

*The number of patients whose observed survival at the time of analysis falls within the given interval but whose actual survival is censored by time (unknown), since they are alive.

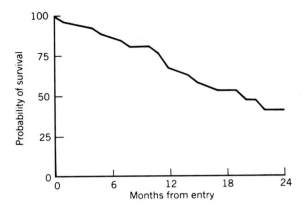

FIGURE 20–5. Example of survival curve.

the comparison of the value to an appropriate tabulated entry that separates the region of acceptance from the region of rejection. By now it should not be surprising that the probability distributions most often employed are the chi-square and normal distributions.

P VALUES

As anyone who has ever read the medical literature knows, analyses proclaiming "significant differences" between two treatments always give a so-called P value. Scientists have a particular affection for 0.05, accepting results with accompanying P values less than 0.05 as "significant." What is a P value, and how does it relate to the items previously discussed?

Recall that when we test a hypothesis, we generally define H_0 such that its rejection would constitute a positive finding. The P value gives the probability of observing data at least as inconsistent with the null hypothesis as the data observed if the null hypothesis is actually true. The more inconsistent our data are with the null hypothesis, the smaller the P value. Recall in our example on contingency tables we tested $H_0:P_1 \neq P_2$ versus $H_a:P_1 = P_2$ and rejected H_0 because of the calculated value of our test statistic,

$$\chi^2 = 5.128 > \chi^2_{0.05,1} = 3.84$$

How discrepant from H_0 were our observed data? If H_0 was true, then

$$\text{Prob}(\chi^2 \geq 5.128) = 0.0235$$

That is, for the significant result proclaimed,

$P = 0.0235$. Glancing at the chi-square table, it is apparent that, for a given problem, the larger the value of the calculated statistic, the smaller the P value.

In conclusion, the level of significance, α, gives the maximum probability of a type I error that we are willing to tolerate; this is determined before the data are collected. Assume that we have chosen $\alpha = 0.05$; after the data have been collected and the test statistic calculated, if H_0 is rejected, we can then state that the observed difference is significant at the 0.05 level (also noted as $P < 0.05$). If desired, one can also give the exact P value corresponding to the results. The 0.05 P value means that the probability of the observed differences resulting from chance is 5 percent, or 1 in 20.

OTHER TOPICS

Randomization

To allow an unbiased assessment of therapeutic efficacy, treatment assignment in phase III studies should be accomplished by randomization. This will minimize the possibility that positive findings are due to an advantageous distribution of good-prognosis patients. If there is an observed difference in efficacy, we must be certain that this is due to the therapy itself and not to the patient composition of the regimens. Randomization will not guarantee complete comparability of the regimens with respect to prognostic factors, but it enhances the chance of its occurring. The usual pattern of randomization provides equal allocation of patients to each therapeutic regimen. Randomization designs may feature stratification. Prognostic variables are categorized at specific "levels." Mutually exclusive subsets of patients are defined by the various combinations of these levels, and each stratum is then randomized separately. However, it is noted that excessive use of stratification is worse than no stratification at all.

Prognostic Factors

The previous discussions would not be complete without mentioning a few other topics that cannot be presented in detail in the present context. Analysis and interpretation of both response and survival data are often more complex than the preceding descriptions indicate. In practice, the investigator will have information about other variables that may have an impact on the outcome. Hopefully, the composition of all regimens will be such that they are comparable with regard to these *prognostic factors*. Employing randomization will enhance this likelihood. Nonetheless, this aspect must be considered. When there are prognostic factors that must be taken into account, there are statistical techniques to do so. In this regard, frequently encountered statistical terminology includes the following:

1. *Correlation*—enables a determination to be made of the interdependence of two variables. Neither variable is held fixed.
2. *Regression*—enables the examination of the distribution of one variable while another is held fixed at each of several levels.
3. *Linear regression*—employed when the relationship between variables is believed to be best described as fitting a straight line.
4. *Multiple regression* (analyses of covariance)—the most common method of statistical adjustment employed when the outcome is believed to be influenced by the treatment *and* by several prognostic factors.
5. *Multiple logistic model*—the equivalent of multiple regression for qualitative variables such as response.
6. *Log rank test*—used to adjust for prognostic factors when comparing survival.

This list is not exhaustive, nor are these topics readily understandable. They are presented merely to indicate that routine application of the elementary procedures discussed in this chapter is dangerous.

Interpretation of Negative Results

It cannot reasonably be expected that a statistician will be consulted to interpret every clinical paper one reads. Therefore, a few concepts should be considered.

In light of the sample size requirements for definitive clinical trials, one must question negative studies. That is, if no significant treatment difference is proclaimed, is this conclusion warranted? It may well be that an insufficient number of patients were entered into a well-designed study and the difference sought in the initial design was not detected. The results must be interpreted within this context. It is not appropriate to state that there is "no difference"; rather, a difference of the predetermined magnitude or greater does not exist. The study was not designed to investigate the existence of smaller magnitudes.

CONCLUSION

This chapter was begun with the goal of developing the ability to partake in conversational statistics. Derivations and mathematical concepts have been deliberately minimized or eliminated in an attempt to make the language palatable and to encourage its use. Topics covered in this chapter may prove useful in understanding articles and interacting on analyses, but they do not prepare the clinician to analyze his or her own data.

REFERENCES

Blessing JA: Design, analysis and interpretation of chemotherapy trials in gynecologic cancer. In Deppe G (ed): Chemotherapy of Gynecologic Cancer. New York, Alan R Liss, 1985, p 49.

Brown BW Jr, Hollander M: Statistics: A Biomedical introduction. New York, John Wiley & Son, 1977.

Casagrande JT, Pike MC, Smith PG: The power function of the "exact" test for comparing two binomial distributions. Appl Stat 27:176, 1980.

Cochran WG, Cox GM: Experimental Designs, 2nd ed. New York, John Wiley & Son, 1957.

Flemming TR: One-sample multiple testing procedure for phase II clinical trials. Biometrics 38:143, 1982.

Freund JE: Mathematical Statistics, 2nd ed. Englewood Cliffs, NJ, Prentice-Hall, 1971.

Gehan EA: The determination of the number of patients required in a preliminary and a follow-up trial of a new chemotherapeutic agent. J Chronic Dis 13:346, 1961.

Gehan EA, Schneiderman MA: Experimental design of clinical trials. In Holland JF, Frei E (eds): Cancer Medicine, 2nd ed. Philadelphia, Lea & Febiger, 1982, p 531.

George SL, Desu MM: Planning the size and duration of a clinical trial studying the time to some critical event. J Chronic Dis 27:15, 1974.

O'Brian PC, Flemming TR: A multiple testing procedure for clinical trials. Biometrics 35:549, 1979.

Zelen M: Guidelines for publishing papers on cancer clinical trials: responsibilities of editors and authors. J Clin Oncol 1:164, 1983.

Key to Abbreviations and Acronyms

5-FU: 5-fluorouracil

5-HIAA: 5-hydroxyindoleacetic acid

AA: adenoacanthoma

ACC: adenoid cystic carcinoma (cylindroma)

AcFuCy: actinomycin-D, 5-fluorouracil, Cytoxan

ACIS: adenocarcinoma in situ

ACOG: American College of Obstetricians and Gynecologists

ACT-D: actinomycin D; dactinomycin

ACTH: adrenocorticotrophic hormone

ADR: Adriamycin; doxorubicin

AFP: α-fetoprotein; alpha-fetoprotein

AIDS: acquired immunodeficiency syndrome

AN: acanthosis nigricans

AP: anteroposterior

APA: atypical polypoid adenomyoma

ASC: adenosquamous carcinoma

BEP: bleomycin, etoposide, cisplatin

BML: benign metastasizing leiomyoma

BSE: breast self-examination

BSO: bilateral salpingo-oophorectomy

BUN: blood urea nitrogen

CAF: Cytoxan, Adriamycin, 5-fluorouracil (also FAC)

CAP: Cytoxan, Adriamycin, cisplatin (also PAC)

CBE: clinical breast examination

CCC: clear cell carcinoma

CDDP: cis-diamminedichloroplatinum; cisplatin

CEA: carcinoembryonic antigen

cGy: centiGray

CHAMOCA: Cytoxan, hydroxyurea, actinomycin D, methotrexate, Oncovin, citrovorum factor, Adriamycin

CIN: cervical intraepithelial neoplasia

CMF: Cytoxan, methotrexate, 5-fluorouracil

CNS: central nervous system

CP: Cytoxan, cisplatin (also PC)

CR: complete response

CS: carcinosarcoma

CT: computed tomography

CTX: Cytoxan; cyclophosphamide

DCIS: ductal carcinoma in situ

DES: diethylstilbestrol

DESAD: DES Adenosis (Project)

DFP: dermatofibrosarcoma protuberans

DHEAS: dehydroepiandrosterone sulfate

DM: distant metastasis

DPL: disseminated peritoneal leiomyomatosis (leiomyomatosis peritonealis disseminata)

DTIC: dimethyl-triazenoimidazole carboxamide; dacarbazine

EC: endometrial carcinoma

ECC: endocervical curettage

EGF: epidermal growth factor

EH: endometrial hyperplasia

ELISA: enzyme-linked immunosorbent assay

EMA/CE: etoposide, methotrexate, actinomycin D, cisplatin, etoposide

EMA/CO: etoposide, methotrexate, actinomycin D, Cytoxan, Oncovin

EMB: endometrial biopsy

ER: estrogen (estradiol) receptor

ERT: estrogen replacement therapy

ESI: early stromal invasion

ESM: endolymphatic stromal myosis

ESS: endometrial stromal sarcoma

EST: endodermal sinus tumor

FA: folinic acid; citrovorum factor; Leukovorin

FAC:	5-fluorouracil, Adriamycin, Cytoxan (also CAF)	Laser:	light amplification by stimulated emission of radiation
FIA:	fluoro-immunoassay	LCIS:	lobular carcinoma in situ
FIGO:	International Federation of Gynecology and Obstetrics	LD_{10}:	lethal dose 10 percent
		LDH:	lactate dehydrogenase
FNA:	fine-needle aspiration	LEEP:	loop electrosurgical excision procedure
FNAC:	fine-needle aspiration cytology	LLETZ:	large loop excision of the transformation zone
FSH:	follicle-stimulating hormone	LGESS:	low-grade endometrial stromal sarcoma
G:	histologic grade	LH:	luteinizing hormone
GCM:	granular cell myoblastoma	LMM:	lentigo malignant melanoma
GI:	gastrointestinal	LMP:	low malignant potential
GOG:	Gynecologic Oncology Group	LMS:	leiomyosarcoma
		L-PAM:	L-phenylalanine mustard; Alkeran; melphalan
GTD:	gestational trophoblastic disease (also GTN)	LS:	lichen sclerosus
GTN:	gestational trophoblastic neoplasia (also GTD)	LSA:	lichen sclerosus et atrophicus
Gy:	Gray	LVSI:	lymph–vascular space invasion
hCG:	human chorionic gonadotropin	mAb:	monoclonal antibody
HGESS:	high-grade endometrial stromal sarcoma	MAC:	methotrexate, actinomycin D, Cytoxan (Chlorarubucil)
HIP:	health insurance plan	MAS:	müllerian adenosarcoma
HIV:	human immunodeficiency virus	Mesna:	mercaptoethane sulfonate sodium
HLA:	human leukocyte antigen	MFH:	malignant fibrous histiocytoma
HM:	hydatidiform (hydatid) mole	MHC:	major histocompatibility complex
HMM:	hexamethylmelamine		
HPC:	hemangiopericytoma	MM:	mucocutaneous melanoma
hpf:	high-power field	MMMT:	malignant mixed mesodermal tumor (mixed mesodermal sarcoma; carcinosarcoma)
hPL:	human placental lactogen		
HPV:	human papillomavirus		
HSV-2:	herpes simplex virus type 2		
HU:	hydroxyurea		
IM:	intramuscular	MPA:	medroxyprogesterone acetate
IP:	intraperitoneal	MR(I):	magnetic resonance (imaging)
IRMA:	immunoradiometric assay		
IRS:	Intergroup Rhabdomyosarcoma Study	MTD:	maximum tolerable dose
		MTX:	methotrexate
IT:	immature teratoma	MV:	million electron volts (also MeV)
IV:	intravenous		
IVL:	intravenous leiomyomatosis		
IVP:	intravenous pyelogram (urogram)	NCI:	National Cancer Institute
		NIH:	National Institutes of Health
		NM:	nodular melanoma
kV:	kilo (electron) volts	NSD:	nominal standard dose
		PA:	posteroanterior
LAK:	lymphokine-activated killer cell	PAC:	cisplatin, Adriamycin, Cytoxan (also CAP)
LAM:	lymphangioleiomyomatosis	Pap:	Papanicolaou
		PCO:	polycystic ovary syndrome

PE: cisplatin, etoposide
PEG: percutaneous endoscopic
            gastrostomy
PFI: progression-free interval
PO: by mouth
PR: partial response
PgR: progesterone receptor
PSC: papillary serous carcinoma
PSTT: placental site trophoblastic
            tumor

RBE: relative biologic
            effectiveness
RIA: radioimmunoassay
RS: rhabdomyosarcoma
RT: radiation therapy

SAD: source-to-axis (patient)
            distance
SCC: squamous cell carcinoma
SCJ: squamocolumnar junction
SCTAT: sex cord tumor with annular
            tubules

SEER: Surveillance, Epidemiology,
            and End-Result (a National
            Cancer Institute program)
SIL: squamous intraepithelial
            lesion
SLCT: Sertoli-Leydig cell tumor
SRTDC: Southeastern Regional Tro-
            phoblastic Disease Center

SSD: source to surface (skin)
            distance
SSM: superficial spreading
            melanoma

T: testosterone
TAA: tumor-associated antigen
TAH: total abdominal
            hysterectomy
TDF: time-dose-fractionation
TDLU: terminal duct lobular unit
TNF: tumor necrosis factor
TNM: tumor, nodes, metastasis
TRAM: transverse rectus abdominis
            myocutaneous flap
TSA: tumor-specific antigen
TSH: thyroid-stimulating hormone

USO: unilateral salpingo-
            oophorectomy
UTZ: ultrasound

VAC: vincristine, actinomycin D,
            Cytoxan
VAIN: vaginal intraepithelial
            neoplasia
VBP: Velban, bleomycin, cisplatin
VIN: vulvar intraepithelial
            neoplasia

WAR: whole-abdomen radiation
            therapy
WHO: World Health Organization

Staging and Classification of Malignant Tumors in the Female Pelvis[1]

The classification and staging of tumors in the female pelvis are considered not only by the Gynecologic Oncology Committee of the International Federation of Gynecology and Obstetrics (FIGO), but also by the Union Internationale Contre Cancer (UICC), especially its *Tumor, Nodes, Metastasis* (TNM) Committee, by the Cancer Unit of the World Health Organization (WHO), by the Reference Centers of WHO for histopathologic classification of ovarian tumors as well as tumors in the uterus and the vagina, by the American Joint Committee, and finally by the International Congress of Radiology, especially its ICPR committee. For several years opinions differed concerning the classification and staging of malignant tumors in the female pelvis. The Gynecologic Oncology Committee of FIGO has aimed at adjusting these opinions. It has been possible to reach international agreement on several main issues that are considered to be of great importance for research.

The TNM classification makes it possible to describe in detail the anatomic extent of the disease. However, if it is used as the only method of classification, it will divide a series of treated cases into so many small groups that statistical evaluation of the material is not possible. The Gynecologic Oncology Committee of FIGO stresses the importance of staging, and experience has shown that, from a statistical as well as a prognostic point of view, it is advisable to group every type of malignant tumor into four stages.

CARCINOMA OF THE VULVA

Cases should be classified as carcinoma of the vulva when the primary site of the growth is in the vulva. Tumors present in the vulva as secondary growths from either a genital or extragenital site should be excluded. A car-

cinoma of the vulva that has extended to the vagina should be considered as a carcinoma of the vulva.

FIGO Stages in Carcinoma of the Vulva (Surgical)

Stage	Definition
0 (Tis)	Carcinoma in situ, intraepithelial carcinoma
1* (T1N0M0)	Tumor ≤2 cm in size confined to the vulva or perineum; no nodal metastasis
Ia	Stromal invasion ≤1.0 mm[†]
Ib	Stromal invasion >1.0 mm
II (T2N0M0)	Tumor >2 cm in size confined to the vulva or perineum; no nodal metastasis
III (T3N0M0, T3N1M0, T1N1M0, T2N1M0)	Tumor of any size with (1) adjacent spread to the lower urethra or vagina or anus, or (2) unilateral regional lymph node metastasis
IV	
IVa (T1N2M0, T2N2M0, T3N2M0, T4M0)	Tumor invades the upper urethra, bladder mucosa, rectal mucosa, pelvic bone, or bilateral regional node metastases
IVb (any T, any N, M1)	Any distant metastasis, including pelvic lymph nodes

*Changed in 1995 (Creasman WT: New gynecologic cancer staging [editorial]. Gynecol Oncol 58:157, 1995).
†The depth of invasion is defined as the measurement of the tumor from the epithelial–stromal junction of the adjacent most superficial dermal papilla to the deepest point of invasion.

Definition of TNM

TNM classification of carcinoma of the vulva is based on the FIGO classification.

Primary Tumor (T)

T0   No evidence of primary tumor
Tis   Carcinoma in situ (preinvasive carcinoma)
T1   Tumor confined to the vulva or to the vulva and perineum, 2 cm or less in greatest dimension
T2   Tumor confined to the vulva or to the vulva and perineum, more than 2 cm in greatest dimension
T3   Tumor invades any of the following: lower urethra, vagina, or anus

[1]Adapted from Pettersson F: Annual report on the results of treatment in gynecological cancer. Int J Gynecol Obstet 36(suppl):1, 1991; and Pettersson F: Staging rules for gestational trophoblastic tumors and fallopian tube cancer. Acta Obstet Gynecol Scand 71:224, 1992, with permission.

T4   Tumor invades any of the following: bladder mucosa, upper urethral mucosa, or rectal mucosa, or is fixed to the bone

Regional Lymph Nodes (N)

Nx   Lymph nodes cannot be assessed
N0   No regional lymph node metastasis
N1   Unilateral regional lymph node metastasis
N2   Bilateral regional lymph node metastases

Distant Metastasis (M)

Mx   Presence of distant metastasis cannot be assessed
M0   No distant metastasis
M1   Distant metastasis (including pelvic lymph node metastasis)

Notes on Staging Carcinoma of the Vulva

Carcinoma of the vulva is staged by surgical and/or pathologic findings. Carcinoma of the vulva is the only gynecologic malignancy that routinely includes the TNM classification.

CARCINOMA OF THE VAGINA

Cases should be classified as carcinoma of the vagina when the primary site of the growth is in the vagina. Tumors present in the vagina as secondary growths from either genital or extragenital sites should be excluded from registration. A growth that has extended to the portio and reached the area of the exter-

FIGO Stages in Carcinoma of the Vagina (Clinical)

Stage	Definition
0	Carcinoma in situ, intraepithelial carcinoma
I	The carcinoma is limited to the vaginal wall
II	The carcinoma has involved the subvaginal tissue but has not extended onto the pelvic wall
III	The carcinoma has extended onto the pelvic wall
IV	The carcinoma has extended beyond the true pelvis or has clinically involved the mucosa of the bladder or rectum; bullous edema as such does not permit a case to be allotted to stage IV
IVa	Spread of the growth to adjacent organs and/or direct extension beyond the true pelvis
IVb	Spread to distant organs

nal or should always be allotted to carcinoma of the cervix. A growth that is limited to the urethra should be classified as carcinoma of the urethra.

Rules for Staging Carcinoma of the Vagina

The rules for staging carcinoma of the vagina are similar to those for carcinoma of the cervix.

CARCINOMA OF THE CERVIX

FIGO Stages in Carcinoma of the Cervix (Clinical)

Stage	Definition
0	Carcinoma in situ; intraepithelial carcinoma
I*	Carcinoma strictly confined to the cervix (extension to the corpus is disregarded)
Ia	Invasive cancer identified only microscopically; all gross lesions even with superficial invasion are stage Ib; invasion limited to measured stromal invasion with a maximum depth of 5.0 mm and no wider than 7.0 mm[†]
Ia1	Stromal invasion not >3.0 mm deep, not >7.0 mm wide
Ia2	Stromal invasion 3.0–5.0 mm deep, not >7.0 mm wide
Ib	Clinical lesions confined to the cervix or preclinical lesions greater than stage Ia
Ib1	Clinical lesions not >4 cm in size
Ib2	Clinical lesions >4 cm in size
II	Carcinoma extends beyond the cervix but has not extended onto the pelvic wall; carcinoma involves the vagina but not as far as the lower third
IIa	No obvious parametrial involvement
IIb	Obvious parametrial involvement
III	The carcinoma has extended onto the pelvic wall; on rectal examination there is no cancer-free space between the tumor and the pelvic wall; the tumor involves the lower third of the vagina; all cases with a hydroureter or nonfunctioning kidney should be included unless they are due to another cause
IIIa	No extension onto the pelvic wall but involvement of the lower third of the vagina
IIIb	Extension to the pelvic wall or hydronephrosis or nonfunctioning kidney
IV	Carcinoma has extended beyond the true pelvis or has clinically involved the mucosa of the bladder or rectum
IVa	Spread of the growth to adjacent organs
IVb	Spread to distant organs

*Changed in 1995 (Creasman WT: New gynecologic cancer staging [editorial]. Gynecol Oncol 58:157, 1995).
[†]The depth of invasion should not be more than 5 mm taken from the base of the epithelium, either surface or glandular, from which it originates. Vascular space involvement, either venous or lymphatic, should not alter the staging.

Rules for Staging Carcinoma of the Cervix

The staging should be based on careful clinical examination and should be performed before any definitive therapy. It is desirable that the examination be performed by an experienced examiner and under anesthesia. The clinical stage must under no circumstances be changed on the basis of subsequent findings. When it is doubtful to which stage a particular case should be allotted, the case must be referred to the earlier stage.

For staging purposes the following examination methods are permitted: palpation, inspection, colposcopy, endocervical curettage, hysteroscopy, cystoscopy, proctoscopy, intravenous urography, and radiographic examination of the lungs and skeleton. Suspected bladder or rectal involvement should be confirmed by biopsy and histologic evidence. Findings by examinations such as lymphangiography, arteriography, venography, and laparoscopy are of value for the planning of therapy but, because these are not yet generally available, and also because the interpretation of results varies, the findings of such studies should not be the basis for changing the clinical staging.

Infrequently, hysterectomy is carried out in the presence of unsuspected extensive invasive cervical carcinoma. Such cases cannot be clinically staged or included in therapeutic statistics, but it is desirable that they be reported separately.

Notes on Staging Carcinoma of the Cervix

Stage Ia

The diagnosis of both stage Ia1 and Ia2 should be based on microscopic examination of removed tissue, preferably a cone biopsy, which must include the entire lesion. The depth of invasion should be measured from the base of the epithelium, either surface or glandular, from which it originates. The second dimension, the horizontal spread, must not exceed 7 mm. Vascular space involvement, either venous or lymphatic, should not alter the staging but should be specifically recorded because it may affect treatment decisions in the future.

Stage Ib

The remaining stage I cases should be allotted to stage Ib. As a rule these cases can be diagnosed by routine clinical examination. It is not possible to estimate clinically whether a cancer of the cervix has extended to the corpus or not. Extension to the corpus should therefore be disregarded in staging.

Stages II and III

A patient with a growth fixed to the pelvic wall by a short and indurated but not nodular parametrium should be allotted to stage IIb. It is impossible at clinical examination to decide whether a smooth and indurated parametrium is truly cancerous or only inflammatory. Therefore, the case should be placed in stage III only if the parametrium is nodular out on the pelvic wall or if the growth itself extends out on the pelvic wall.

The presence of hydronephrosis or a nonfunctional kidney resulting from stenosis of the ureter by cancer permits a case to be allotted to stage III even if, according to the other findings, the case should be allotted to stage I or stage II.

Stage IV

The presence of bullous edema as such should not permit a case to be allotted to stage IV. Ridges and furrows into the bladder wall should be interpreted as signs of submucosal involvement of the bladder if they remain fixed to the growth at palposcopy (i.e., examination from the vagina or the rectum during cystoscopy). A finding of malignant cells in cytologic washing from the urinary bladder requires further examination and biopsy.

CARCINOMA OF THE CORPUS UTERI (ENDOMETRIUM)

Histopathology—Degree of Differentiation

Cases of carcinoma of the corpus should be graded according to the degree of histologic differentiation as follows:

G1 = 5 percent or less of a nonsquamous or nonmorular solid growth pattern

G2 = 6 to 50 percent of a nonsquamous or nonmorular solid growth pattern

G3 = more than 50 percent of a nonsquamous or nonmorular growth pattern

FIGO Stages in Carcinoma of the
Corpus Uteri (Surgical)

Stage*	Definition
I	The cancer is limited to the corpus uteri
Ia	Tumor limited to the endometrium
Ib	Invasion to <50% of the myometrium
Ic	Invasion to ≥50% of the myometrium
II	The cancer involves the cervix
IIa	Endocervical glandular involvement only
IIb	Cervical stromal invasion
III	The cancer extends outside the uterus to the pelvis or retroperitoneal lymph nodes
IIIa	Tumor invades serosa and/or adnexa, and/or positive peritoneal cytology
IIIb	Vaginal metastases
IIIc	Metastases to pelvic and/or aortic lymph nodes
IV	The cancer involves the bladder or bowel, or has distant metastases
IVa	Tumor invasion of bladder and/or bowel mucosa
IVb	Distant metastases including intra-abdominal and/or inguinal lymph nodes

*The stage is not affected by the tumor grade.

Notes on Histologic Grading

1. Nuclear atypia inappropriate for the architectural grade raises the grade of a grade 1 or grade 2 tumor by one.
2. In serous, clear cell, and squamous carcinomas, nuclear grading takes precedence.
3. Adenocarcinomas with squamous differentiation are graded according to the nuclear grade of the glandular component.

Rules Related to Surgical Staging of Carcinoma of the Corpus Uteri

1. Corpus cancer is now staged surgically. Procedures previously used for determination of stages are no longer applicable, such as the findings from fractional dilation and curettage (D&C) to differentiate between stages I and II.
2. There may be a small number of patients with corpus cancer who will be treated primarily with radiation therapy. If that is the case, the clinical staging adopted by FIGO in 1971 would still apply, but designation of that staging system would be noted.
3. Ideally, width of the myometrium should be measured along with the width of tumor invasion.

The previously accepted FIGO rules (1971) for clinical staging are still relevant and should be used for cases not primarily operated and cases treated with radiation only.

FIGO Stages in Carcinoma of
the Corpus Uteri (Clinical)

Stage	Definition
0	Atypical hyperplasia, carcinoma in situ
I	The carcinoma is confined to the corpus
Ia	The length of the uterine cavity is ≤8 cm
Ib	The length of the uterine cavity is >8 cm
II	The carcinoma has involved the corpus and the cervix but has not extended outside the uterus
III	The carcinoma has extended outside the uterus but not outside the true pelvis
IV	The carcinoma has extended outside the true pelvis or has obviously involved the mucosa of the bladder or rectum; bullous edema as such does not permit a case to be allotted to stage IV
IVa	Spread of the growth to adjacent organs such as urinary bladder, rectum, sigmoid, or small bowel
IVb	Spread to distant organs

Rules for Clinical Staging of Carcinoma of the Corpus Uteri

The staging should be based on careful clinical examination and should be performed before any definitive therapy. It is desirable that the examination is performed by an experienced examiner and under anesthesia. The clinical stage must under no circumstances be changed on the basis of subsequent findings. When it is doubtful to which stage a particular case should be allotted, the case must be referred to the earlier stage.

The following examinations are permitted for carcinoma of the corpus: palpation, inspection, endocervical curettage, hysteroscopy, cystoscopy, proctoscopy, and radiographic examination of the lungs and skeleton. Findings by examinations such as lymphangiography, arteriography, venography, and laparoscopy are of value for the planning of therapy but, because these are not yet generally available, and also because the interpretation of results is variable, the findings of such studies should not be the basis for changing the clinical staging.

Fractional curettage is essential with separation of endometrial and endocervical curettings. Extension of the carcinoma to the endocervix is confirmed by fractional curettage. Scraping the cervix should be the first step of the curettage, and the specimens from the cervix should be examined separately. Occasionally it may be difficult to decide whether the endocervix is involved by the cancer. In such cases, the simultaneous presence of normal cervical glands and cancer in the same section will give the final diagnosis. Extension of the carcinoma outside the uterus should refer a case to stage III or IV. The presence of metastases in the vagina or in the ovary permits allotment of a case to stage III.

CARCINOMA OF THE OVARY

FIGO Stages for Carcinoma of the Ovary (Surgical)

Stage	Definition
I	Growth limited to the ovaries
Ia	Growth limited to one ovary; no ascites; no tumor on the external surface; capsule intact
Ib	Growth limited to both ovaries; no ascites; no tumor on the external surfaces; capsules intact
Ic	Tumor either stage Ia or Ib but with tumor on surface of one or both ovaries; or with capsule ruptured; or with ascites present containing malignant cells or with positive peritoneal washings
II	Growth involving one or both ovaries with pelvic extension
IIa	Extension and/or metastases to the uterus and/or tubes
IIb	Extension to other pelvic tissues
IIc*	Tumor either stage IIa or IIb but with tumor on surface of one or both ovaries; or with capsule(s) ruptured; or with ascites present containing malignant cells or with positive peritoneal washings
III	Tumor involving one or both ovaries with peritoneal implants outside the pelvis and/or positive retroperitoneal or inguinal nodes; superficial liver metastasis equals stage III; tumor is limited to the true pelvis but with histologically proven malignant extension to small bowel or omentum
IIIa	Tumor grossly limited to the true pelvis with negative nodes but with histologically confirmed microscopic seeding of abdominal peritoneal surfaces
IIIb	Tumor involving one or both ovaries with histologically confirmed implants of abdominal peritoneal surfaces, none exceeding 2 cm in diameter; nodes are negative
IIIc	Abdominal implants greater than 2 cm in diameter and/or positive retroperitoneal or inguinal nodes
IV	Growth involving one or both ovaries with distant metastases; if pleural effusion is present there must be positive cytology to allot a case to stage IV; parenchymal liver metastasis equals stage IV

*In order to evaluate the impact on prognosis of the different criteria for allotting a case to stage Ic or IIc, it would be of value to know (1) if the source of malignant cells detected was (a) peritoneal washings or (b) ascites; and (2) if rupture of the capsule was (a) spontaneous or (b) caused by the surgeon.

Rules for Staging Carcinoma of the Ovary

Only rarely is it possible to come to a final diagnosis of ovarian carcinoma by inspection or palpation or by any of the other methods recommended for clinical staging of carcinoma of the uterus and vagina. Therefore, the Committee on Gynecologic Oncology of FIGO recommends that the staging of primary carcinoma of the ovary should be based on findings by laparoscopy or laparotomy as well as on the usual clinical examination and roentgen studies.

Thus, laparotomy and resection of ovarian masses, as well as hysterectomy, form the basis for staging. Biopsies of all suspicious sites, such as the omentum, mesentery, liver, diaphragm, and pelvic and para-aortic nodes, are required. The final histologic findings after surgery (and cytologic findings when available) are to be considered in the staging. Clinical studies, if carcinoma of the ovary is diagnosed, include routine radiography of the chest. Computed tomography (CT) may be helpful in both initial staging and follow-up of tumors.

Histologic Classification of the Common Primary Epithelial Tumors of the Ovary

1. Serous Cystomas

a. Serous benign cystadenomas
b. Serous cystadenomas with proliferating activity of the epithelial cells and nuclear abnormalities but with no infiltrative destructive growth (borderline cases; low potential malignancy)
c. Serous cystadenocarcinomas

2. Mucinous Cystomas

a. Mucinous benign cystadenomas
b. Mucinous cystadenomas with proliferating activity of the epithelial cells and nuclear abnormalities but with no infiltrative destructive growth (borderline cases; low potential malignancy)
c. Mucinous cystadenocarcinomas

3. Endometrioid Tumors

a. Endometrioid benign cysts
b. Endometrioid tumors with proliferating activity of the epithelial cells and nuclear abnormalities but with no infiltrative de-

structive growth (borderline cases; low potential malignancy)
c. Endometrioid adenocarcinomas

4. *Clear Cell Tumors*

a. Benign clear cell tumors
b. Clear cell tumors with proliferating activity of the epithelial cells and nuclear abnormalities but with no infiltrative destructive growth (borderline cases; low potential malignancy)
c. Clear cell cystadenocarcinomas

5. *Undifferentiated Tumors*

A malignant tumor of epithelial structure that is too poorly differentiated to be placed in any of the groups 1 through 4 or 6.

6. *Mixed Epithelial Tumors*

Tumors composed of a mixture of two or more of the malignant groups 1c through 4c described previously and where none of them is predominant. Thus a case should be listed as "mixed epithelial tumor" only if it is not possible to decide which is the predominant structure.

7. *No Histology or Unclassifiable*

Cases where explorative surgery has shown that obvious ovarian epithelial malignant tumor is present but where no biopsy has been taken, or where the specimen is unclassifiable because of, for instance, necrosis.

CARCINOMA OF THE FALLOPIAN TUBE

FIGO Stages in Carcinoma of the Fallopian Tube (Surgical)*

Stage	Definition
0	Carcinoma in situ (limited to tubal mucosa)
I	Growth limited to the fallopian tubes
Ia	Growth limited to one tube with extension into the submucosa and/or muscularis but not penetrating the serosal surface; no ascites
Ib	Same as Ia except growth limited to both tubes
Ic	Ia or Ib with tumor extension through or onto the tubal serosa, or with ascites containing malignant cells or with positive peritoneal washings
II	Growth involving one or both fallopian tubes with pelvic extension
IIa	Extension and/or metastasis to the uterus and/or ovaries
IIb	Extension to other pelvic tissues
IIc	IIa or IIb with ascites containing malignant cells or positive peritoneal washings
III	Tumor involves one or both fallopian tubes with peritoneal implants outside the pelvis and/or retroperitoneal or inguinal lymph node metastases; superficial liver metastasis equals stage III
IIIa	Tumor is grossly limited to the true pelvis with negative nodes but with histologically confirmed seeding of abdominal peritoneal surfaces
IIIb	Histologically confirmed gross implants of the abdominal peritoneal surfaces, ≤2 cm in diameter; lymph nodes negative
IIIc	Abdominal implants >2 cm in diameter and/or retroperitoneal or inguinal lymph node metastasis
IV	Distant metastases present; pleural effusion with malignant cells equals stage IV; parenchymal liver metastases equal stage IV

*Staging for fallopian tube cancer is by the surgicopathologic system. Operative findings designating stage are determined before tumor debulking.

GESTATIONAL TROPHOBLASTIC TUMORS

FIGO Stages for Trophoblastic Tumors (Clinical)

Stage	Definitions
I	Disease confined to the uterus
Ia	No risk factors
Ib	One risk factor
Ic	Two risk factors
II	Disease extends outside the uterus but is limited to the genital structures (adnexa, vagina, broad ligament)
IIa	No risk factors
IIb	One risk factor
IIc	Two risk factors
III	Disease extends to the lungs with or without known genital tract involvement
IIIa	No risk factors
IIIb	One risk factor
IIIc	Two risk factors
IV	All other metastatic sites
IVa	No risk factors
IVb	One risk factor
IVc	Two risk factors

Rules for Staging Gestational Trophoblastic Tumors

The staging should be based on actual clinical examination, chest radiograph, and other appropriate studies. It should be performed before any definitive therapy is begun. It is desirable that the evaluation be conducted by experienced physicians. The clinical stage must under no circumstances be changed on the basis of subsequent findings. Those cases that do not fulfill the criteria for any given stage should be listed separately as "unstaged."

Different opinions may be expressed as to which findings should serve as a basis for clinical staging of gestational trophoblastic tumors. The Committee on Gynecologic Oncology of FIGO considers it important that exclusively those examinations be used that can be carried out at any hospital by physicians and surgeons. The following examinations fulfill this requirement: palpation, inspection, cystoscopy, intravenous pyelography, electroencephalography, radiographic examinations of the lungs, pelvic examinations, CT scan of the brain, liver function tests, liver scan, and (uterine) curettage. Findings by examinations such as arteriography, laparoscopy, and hysteroscopy are of value for planning of therapy, but they should have no influence on the staging. They are not carried out as a routine and the interpretation of the results is not uniform.

The clinical staging of gestational trophoblastic tumors should be based on the examination methods mentioned previously. Hysterectomy and D&C should also be regarded as clinical examinations.

Notes on Staging Gestational Trophoblastic Tumors

The following factors should be considered and noted in reporting:

1. Prior chemotherapy
2. Placental site tumors should be reported separately
3. Histologic verification of disease is not required

Risk factors affecting staging include the following:

1. Human chorionic gonadotropin level greater than 100,000 mIU/ml
2. Duration of disease greater than 6 months from termination of the antecedent pregnancy

The Revised Bethesda System for Reporting Cervical/Vaginal Cytologic Diagnoses

Adequacy of the Specimen

Satisfactory for evaluation
Satisfactory for evaluation but limited by (specify reason)
Unsatisfactory for evaluation (specify reason)

General Categorization (Optional)

Within normal limits
Benign cellular changes: *see* Descriptive Diagnosis
Epithelial cell abnormality: *see* Descriptive Diagnosis

Descriptive Diagnosis

Benign cellular changes
　Infection
　Vaginalis
　Fungal organisms morphologically consistent with *Candida* spp.
　Predominance of coccobacilli consistent with shift in vaginal flora
　Bacteria morphologically consistent with *Actinomyces*
　Cellular changes associated with herpes simplex virus
　Other
Reactive Changes—Cellular Changes Associated with:
　Inflammation (includes typical repair)
　Atrophy with inflammation ("atrophic vaginitis")
　Radiation
　Intrauterine contraceptive device (IUD)
　Other
Epithelial Cell Abnormalities
　Squamous cells

Squamous cells of undetermined significance: Qualify*
Low-grade squamous intraepithelial lesion encompassing: HPV,[†] mild dysplasia/CIN 1
High-grade squamous intraepithelial lesion encompassing: Moderate and severe dysplasia, CIS/CIN 2 and CIN 3
Squamous cell carcinoma
Glandular Cell Abnormalities
　Endometrial cells, cytologically benign, in a postmenopausal woman
　Atypical glandular cells of undetermined significance: Qualify*
　Endocervical adenocarcinoma
　Endometrial adenocarcinoma
　Extrauterine adenocarcinoma
　Adenoarcinoma, NOS

Other Malignant Neoplasms (Specify)

Hormonal Evaluation (Applies to Vaginal Smears Only)

Hormonal pattern compatible with age and history
Hormonal pattern incompatible with age and history (specify reason)
Hormonal evaluation not possible due to (specify reason)

---

*Atypical squamous or glandular cells of undetermined significance should be further qualified as to whether a reactive or premalignant/malignant process is favored.
[†]Cellular changes of human papillomavirus (HPV)—previously termed koilocytosis, koilocytotic atypia, or condylomatous atypia—are included in the category of low-grade squamous intraepithelial lesion.
　From The Revised Bethesda System for reporting cervical/vaginal cytologic diagnoses: report of the 1991 Bethesda Workshop. Acta Cytologica 36:273, 1992, with permission.

Index

ISBN 0-443-07509-3

9 780443 075094

90038